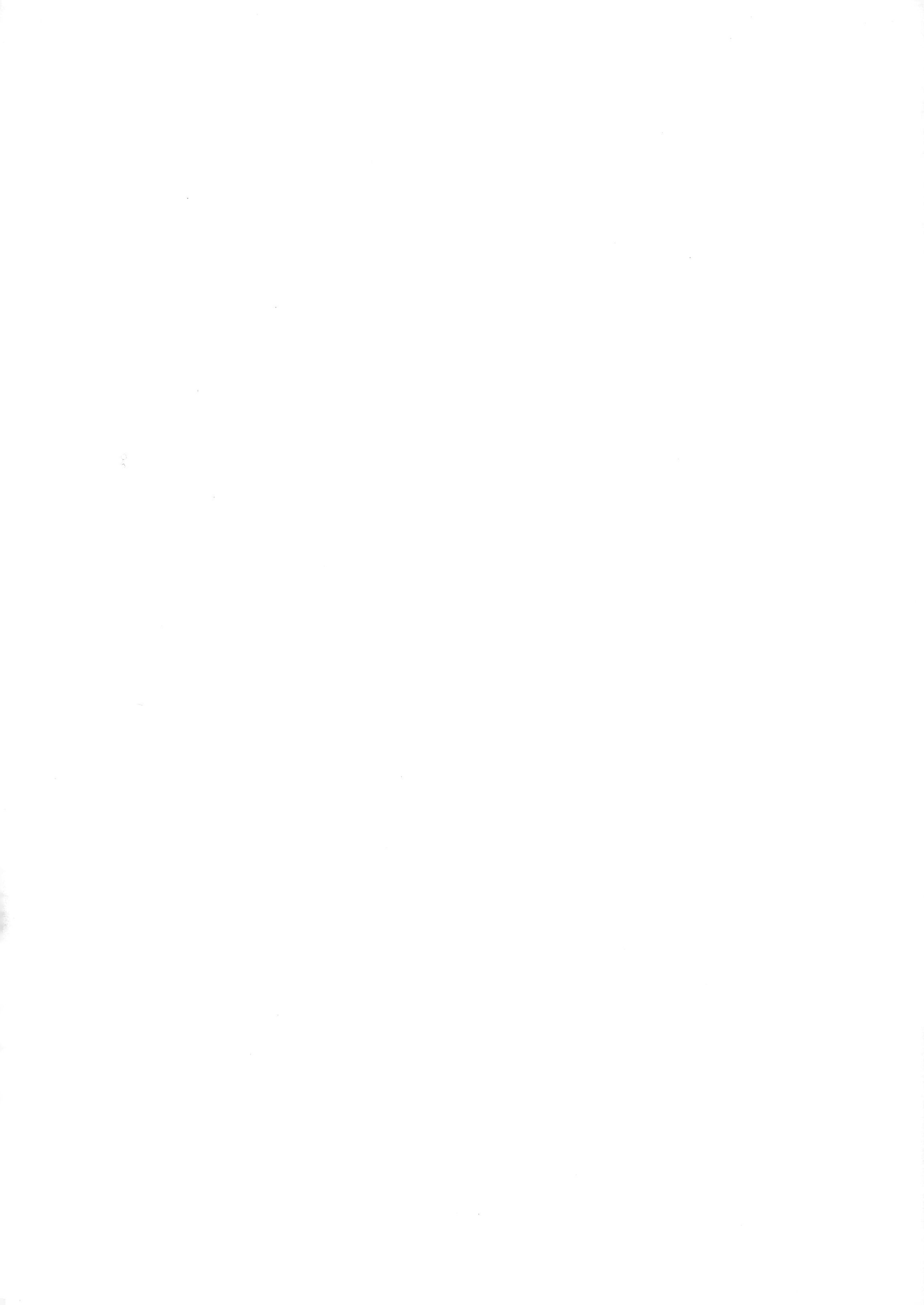

Gastrointestinal Oncology

A Critical Multidisciplinary Team Approach

Gastro-intestinal Oncology

A Critical Multidisciplinary Team Approach

EDITED BY

Janusz Jankowski **MD, PhD, FRCP, FACG**
Consultant Gastroenterologist, Digestive Diseases Centre UHL Trust, Leicester, UK
James Black Senior Fellow and Professor, University of Oxford, UK
Fellow and Professor, Cancer Research UK and Queen Mary University of London, UK

Richard Sampliner **MD**
Professor of Medicine, University of Arizona College of Medicine, USA
Chief of Gastroenterology, Southern Arizona VA Health Care System, USA

David Kerr **CBE, MA, MD, DSc, FRCP, FMedSci**
Rhodes Professor of Cancer Therapeutics and Clinical Pharmacology, University of Oxford, UK
Head of Department of Clinical Pharmacology, University of Oxford, UK

Yuman Fong **MD**
Murray F. Brennan Chair in Surgery, Memorial Sloan-Kettering Cancer Center, New York, USA
Professor of Surgery, Weill Cornell Medical Center, New York, USA

FOREWORD BY

Ernest Hawk **MD, MPH** & Jaye L. Viner **MD, MPH**
National Cancer Institute, Bethesda, USA

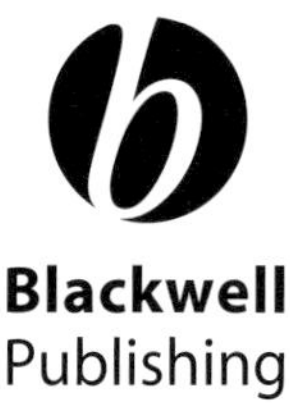

Blackwell
Publishing

Blackwell Publishing, Inc., 350 Main Street, Malden, Massachusetts 02148-5020, USA
Blackwell Publishing Ltd, 9600 Garsington Road, Oxford OX4 2DQ, UK
Blackwell Publishing Asia Pty Ltd, 550 Swanston Street, Carlton, Victoria 3053, Australia

First published 2008
1 2008

Library of Congress Cataloging-in-Publication Data

Gastrointestinal oncology : a critical multidisciplinary team approach / edited by Janusz Jankowski . . . [et al.].
p. ; cm.
Includes bibliographical references and index.
ISBN 978-1-4051-2783-7 (alk. paper)
1. Digestive organs–Cancer. 2. Health care teams. 3. Medical cooperation. I. Jankowski, Janusz
[DNLM: 1. Gastrointestinal Neoplasms–diagnosis. 2. Gastrointestinal Neoplasms–therapy. 3. Liver Neoplasms–diagnosis. 4. Liver Neoplasms–therapy. WI 149 G257442 2008]

RC280.D5G3783 2008
616.99′43–dc22

2007048809

A catalogue record for this title is available from the British Library

Set in 9.5/12 pt Minion by SNP Best-set Typesetter Ltd., Hong Kong
Printed and bound in Singapore by Markono Print Media Pte Ltd

Commissioning Editor: Alison Brown
Editorial Assistant: Cathryn Gates
Development Editor: Helen Harvey
Production Controller: Debbie Wyer

For further information on Blackwell Publishing, visit our website:
http://www.blackwellpublishing.com

The publisher's policy is to use permanent paper from mills that operate a sustainable forestry policy, and which has been manufactured from pulp processed using acid-free and elementary chlorine-free practices. Furthermore, the publisher ensures that the text paper and cover board used have met acceptable environmental accreditation standards.

The contents of this work are intended to further general scientific research, understanding, and discussion only and are not intended and should not be relied upon as recommending or promoting a specific method, diagnosis, or treatment by physicians for any particular patient. The publisher and the author make no representations or warranties with respect to the accuracy or completeness of the contents of this work and specifically disclaim all warranties, including without limitation any implied warranties of fitness for a particular purpose. In view of ongoing research, equipment modifications, changes in governmental regulations, and the constant flow of information relating to the use of medicines, equipment, and devices, the reader is urged to review and evaluate the information provided in the package insert or instructions for each medicine, equipment, or device for, among other things, any changes in the instructions or indication of usage and for added warnings and precautions. Readers should consult with a specialist where appropriate. The fact that an organization or Website is referred to in this work as a citation and/or a potential source of further information does not mean that the author or the publisher endorses the information the organization or Website may provide or recommendations it may make. Further, readers should be aware that Internet Websites listed in this work may have changed or disappeared between when this work was written and when it is read. No warranty may be created or extended by any promotional statements for this work. Neither the publisher nor the author shall be liable for any damages arising herefrom.

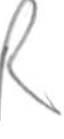

Contents

List of Contributors

Editors

Yuman Fong MD
Memorial Sloan-Kettering Cancer Center
New York, NY
USA

Janusz Jankowski MD, PhD, FRCP, FACG
Department of Clinical Pharmacology
University of Oxford
Oxford
UK

David Kerr CBE, MA, MD, DSc, FRCP, FMedSci
Department of Clinical Pharmacology
University of Oxford
Oxford
UK

Richard Sampliner MD
University of Arizona College of Medicine
Tuscon, AZ
USA

Contributors

Kerin Adelson MD
Mount Sinai School of Medicine
New York, NY
USA

Håkan Ahlman MD, PhD
Department of Clinical Sciences
Sahlgrenska Academy
University of Göteborg
Sweden

Jaffer Ajani MD
Department of Radiation Oncology
University of Texas MD Anderson Cancer Center
Houston, TX
USA

Goran Akerström PhD, MD
Department of Surgery
University Hospital
Uppsala
Sweden

Peter J. Allen MD
Department of Surgery
Memorial Sloan-Kettering Cancer Center
New York, NY
USA

Mitual B Amin MD
Department of Anatomic Pathology
William Beaumont Hospital
Royal Oak, MI
USA

Christopher D. Anderson MD
Section of Abdominal Transplant Surgery
Washington University in St. Louis
St Louis, MI
USA

Mark R. Anderson MBBChir, PhD, MRCP
City Hospital
Birmingham
UK

Salim M. Anjarwalla MD, MBChB, MRCPath
Department of Histopathology
Gloucestershire Royal Hospital
Gloucester
UK

Nadir Arber MD, MSc, MHA
Integrated Cancer Prevention Center
Tel Aviv Medical Center and Tel Aviv University
Israel

Rudolf Arnold MD, FRCP
Division of Gastroenterology and Endocrinology
Department of Internal Medicine Philipps
University
Marburg
Germany

Christoph J. Auernhammer MD
Medizinische Klinik II, Grosshadern
Klinikum der Ludwig-Maximilians-Universität
München
München
Germany

Nahida Banu MBBS, PhD
Department of Pathology
Bristol Royal Infirmary
Bristol
UK

Hugh Barr MD, ChM, FRCS, FRCS, FHEA
Cranfield Health
Gloucestershire Royal Hospital
Gloucester
UK

Shantanu Battacharyja MS, FRCSEd
BGS Global Hospital
Kengeri
Bangalore
India

Regina G.H. Beets-Tan MD
University Hospital Maastrict
Maastricht
The Netherlands

Jordan Berlin MD
Vanderbilt University
Vanderbilt-Ingram Medical Center
Nashville, TN
USA

Rossella Bettini MD
Chirurgia Generale B
Dipartimento di Scienze Chirurgiche e
Gastroenterologiche Policlinico 'GB Rossi'
Verona
Italy

Margaret Betts MBChB, MRCP, FRCR
John Radcliffe Hospital
Oxford
UK

Chetan Bhan MBBS
Department of Surgery
Eastbourne Hospital
Eastbourne
UK

Shailender Bhatia MBBS
Division of Hematology-Oncology
Fred Hutchinson Cancer Research Center
University of Washington
Seattle, WA
USA

Cesare Bordi MD
Universita Degli Studi di Parma
Parma
Italy

Jan Bornschein MD
Department of Gastroenterological Surgery
Yale University School of Medicine
New Haven, CT
USA

Yulia Bronstein MD
Diagnostic Radiology
Body Imaging
MD Anderson Cancer Center
Houston, TX
USA

Navtej S. Buttar MD
Miles and Shirley Fiterman Center for Digestive Diseases
Mayo Clinic
Rochester, MN
USA

Darren Carpizo MD, PhD
Memorial Sloan-Kettering Cancer Center
Department of Surgery
New York, NY
USA

Annemieke Cats MD, PhD
Netherlands Cancer Institute/Antoni van Leeuwenhoek Hospital
Amsterdam
The Netherlands

Amitabh Chak MD
Division of Gastroenterology
Case Western Reserve University School of Medicine
Cleveland, OH
USA

A. Bapsi Chakravarthy MD
Radiation Oncology
Vanderbilt University Medical Center
Nashville, TN
USA

Annie O.O. Chan MBBS, MRCP, FHKAM, MD, PhD, FRCP
Department of Medicine
Queen Mary Hospital
Pokfulam Road
Hong Kong

Ravi S. Chari MD, FRCSC, FACS
Division of Hepatobiliary
Surgery and Liver
Transplantation
Vanderbilt University Medical Center
Nashville, TN
USA

Yu Jo Chua MD, MBBS
Department of Medicine
Royal Marsden Hospital
Surrey
UK

Matthew Clark MBChB, MD, FRACS
University of Auckland
Auckland
New Zealand

Anne M. Covey MD
Memorial Sloan-Kettering Cancer Center
New York, NY
USA

Chris Cunningham MD, FRCSEd
Department of Colorectal Surgery
John Radcliffe Hospital
Oxford
UK

David Cunningham MD, FRCP
Royal Marsden Hospital
Surrey
UK

Brian G. Czito MD
Department of Radiation Oncology
Duke University Medical Center
Durham, NC
USA

Ananya Das MD, FACP, FASGE
Associate Professor
Mayo Clinic Arizona
Scottsdale, AZ
USA

Evan S. Dellon MD
Center for Esophageal Diseases and Swallowing
Division of Gastroenterology and Hepatology
University of North Carolina School of Medicine
Chapel Hill, NC
USA

Ronald P. DeMatteo MD, FACS
Department of Surgery
Memorial Sloan-Kettering Cancer Center
New York, NY
USA

M. Dicato MD, FRCP
Hematology-Oncology Service
Laboratory of Research on Cancer and Blood Disorders
Luxembourg Medical Center
Luxembourg

Tomislav Dragovich MD, PhD
Arizona Cancer Center /University Medical Center
Tucson, AZ
USA

Ronelle Dubrow MS, MD
MD Anderson Cancer Center
Houston TX
USA

T. Markley Earl MD
Department of Surgery
Vanderbilt University School of Medicine
Nashville, TN
USA

Rami Eliakim MD
Rambam Health Care Campus
Technion-Israe Institute of Technology
Haifa
Israel

Hashem B El-Serag MD, MPH
Michael E. DeBakey VA Medical Center and Baylor College of Medicine
Houston, TX
USA

William D. Ensminger MD
Upjohn Center SPC 5504
Ann Arbor, MI
USA

Barbro Eriksson MD, PhD
Department of Medical Sciences
Uppsala University Hospital'
Uppsala
Sweden

Carlos Escriu MD, MRCP
Clatterbridge Centre for Oncology
Liverpool
UK

Massimo Falconi MD
Chirurgia Generale B
Dipartimento di Scienze Chirurgiche e Gastroenterologiche
Policlinico 'GB Rossi'
Verona
Italy

Gianfranco Delle Fave MD
Università di Roma 'La Sapienza'
Rome
Italy

John Fetsch MD
Department of Soft Tissue Pathology
Armed Forces Institute of Pathology
Washington, DC
USA

Elliot K. Fishman MD
Johns Hopkins Hospital
Department of Radiology
Baltimore, MD
USA

Peter J. Friend MA, MB, FRCS, MD
Nuffield Department of Surgery
University of Oxford
UK

Helmut Friess MD
Department of Surgery
Klinikum rechts der Isar
Technical University of Munich
Munich
Germany

Paula Ghaneh MBChB, MD, FRCS
University of Liverpool
School of Cancer Studies
Liverpool
UK

Fergus Gleeson FRCP, FRCR
Department of Radiology
The Churchill Hospital
Oxford
UK

Ian M. Gralnek MD, MSHS, FASGE
Department of Gastroenterology
Rambam Health Care Campus
Haifa
Israel

Mark Greaves MD
Memorial Sloan-Kettering Cancer Center
New York, NY
USA

William Greenhalf BSc, PhD
University of Liverpool
School of Cancer Studies
Liverpool
UK

Nicole C.T. van Grieken MD, PhD
Department of Pathology
Vrije Universiteit Medical Center
Amsterdam
The Netherlands

Rebecca F. Harrison BSc, MBChB, FRCPath
Department of Pathology
Leicester General Hospital
Leicester
UK

Per Hellman PhD, MD
Department of Surgery
University Hospital
Uppsala
Sweden

Fernando Herbella MD
Fellow, Department of Surgery
University of Rochester
Rochester, NY
USA

Wouter W. de Herder MD PhD
Department of Internal Medicine
Sector of Endocrinology
Erasmus MC
Rotterdam
The Netherlands

Joseph Herman MD, MSc
Department of Radiation Oncology
Sidney Kimmel Cancer Center
The Johns Hopkins University
Baltimore, MD
USA

David Hewin BSc, MD, FRCS
Consultant Upper Gastrointestinal Surgeon
Gloucestershire Royal Hospital
Gloucester
UK

Manuel Hidalgo MD, PhD
The Johns Hopkins University School of Medicine
Baltimore, MD
USA

Karen M. Horton MD
Johns Hopkins Medical Institutions
Baltimore, MD
USA

Ralph H. Hruban MD
The Sol Goldman Pancreatic Cancer Research Center
The Johns Hopkins Medical Institutions
Baltimore, MD
USA

Hero K. Hussain MBChB, FRCR
Department of Radiology / MRI
University of Michigan Health System
Ann Arbor, MI
USA

Jeffrey Infante MD
Sarah Cannon Research Institute
Nashville, TN
USA

Lincoln Israel BHB, MBChB, FRACS
Middlemore Hospital
Otahuhu
Auckland
New Zealand

Christopher Jackson MBChB
Gastrointestinal Unit
Royal Marsden Hospital
Surrey
UK

Edwin P.M. Jansen MD
The Netherlands Cancer Institute/Antoni van Leeuwenhoek Hospital
Department of Radiotherapy
Amsterdam
The Netherlands

Aminah Jatoi MD
Department of Oncology
Mayo Clinic
Rochester, MN
USA

Jayamarx Jayaraman MBBS, MPH
Vanderbilt University Medical Center
Nashville, TN
USA

Heikki Joensuu MD
Department of Oncology
Helsinki University Central Hospital
Helsinki
Finland

Elizabeth I. Johnston MD
Department of Pathology
Vanderbilt University School of Medicine
Nashville, TN
USA

Robert Glynne Jones BA, MBBS, FRCR, FRCP
Mount Vernon Cancer Centre
UK

Gregory Kaltsas MD, FRCP
Department of Pathophysiology
National University of Athens
Athens
Greece

Boen L. Kam MD
Nuclear Medicine Physician
Dept of Nuclear Medicine
Erasmus MC, Rotterdam
the Netherlands

Malathy Kapali MD
University of Arizona
College of Medicine
Tucson, AZ
USA

Burnett S. Kelly MD
Department of Surgery
Vanderbilt University Medical Center
Nashville, TN
USA

Nancy Kemeny MD
Memorial Sloan-Kettering Cancer Center
Gastrointestinal Solid Tumor Service
Department of Medicine
New York, NY
USA

Knut Ketterer MD
Department of Surgery
Klinikam rechts der Isar
Technical University of Munich
Munich
Germany

Omar Khan BSc, MBBS, MRCP
Cancer Research UK
Department of Medical Oncology
Churchill Hospital
Oxford
UK

Mark Kidd PhD
Department of Gastroenterological Surgery
Yale University School of Medicine
New Haven, CT
USA

Joseph M. Klausner MD
Department of Surgery
The Tel Aviv Sourasky Medical Center
Sackler School of Medicine
Tel Aviv University
Tel Aviv
Israel

James A. Knol MD, FACS
Division of Gastrointestinal Surgery
University of Michigan Department of Surgery
Ann Arbor, MI
USA

Ritsuko Komaki MD, FACR
Anderson Cancer Center
Houston, TX
USA

Eric P. Krenning MD
Erasmus MC
Rotterdam
The Netherlands

Dik J. Kwekkeboom MD, PhD
Erasmus MC
University Hospital Rotterdam
Department of Nuclear Medicine
Rotterdam
The Netherlands

Daniel Laheru MD
Department of Medical Oncology
The Johns Hopkins University School of Medicine
The Sidney Kimmel Comprehensive Cancer Center
Baltimore, MD
USA

Jerzy Lasota MD, PhD
Department of Soft Tissue Pathology
Armed Forces Institute of Pathology
Washington, DC
USA

Theodore Lawrence MD, PhD
Department of Radiation Oncology
University of Michigan
USA

Angela D. Levy MD
Uniformed Services University of the Health Sciences
Bethesda, Maryland
USA

Zhongxing Liao MD
Department of Radiation Oncology
The University of Texas M. D. Anderson Cancer Center
Houston, TX
USA

Julia Liddi BSc
John Radcliffe Hospital
Oxford
UK

Matthew Lovell MBBS
Department of Clinical Pharmacology
St Bartholomew's and the London School of Medicine and Dentistry
London
UK

Frédérique Maire MD
Service de Gastroentérologie et Pancréatologie
Pôle des maladies de l'Appareil Digestif
Hôpital Beaujon
Clichy
France

Gary N. Mann MBBCh, FACS
Department of Surgery
Section of Surgical Oncology
University of Washington Medical Center
Seattle, WA
USA

John Mansour MD
Department of Surgery
Memorial Sloan-Kettering Cancer Center
New York, NY
USA

Jorge A. Marrero MD, MS
Multidisciplinary Liver Tumor Program
University of Michigan
Taubman Center
Ann Arbor, MI
USA

Colin McArdle FRCS
Department of Surgery
Royal Infirmary
Glasgow, UK

Stuart McDonald BSc, PhD
Department of Clinical Pharmacology
GI Oncology Group
University of Oxford
Oxford
UK

Angus H. McGregor MBChB, Bsc, MD
Department of Histopathology
Leicester Royal Infirmary
Leicester
UK

Robert A. Meguid MD
Department of Surgery
Johns Hopkins University School of Medicine
Baltimore, MD
USA

Gerrit A. Meijer MD, PhD
Vrije Universiteit Medical Center
Amsterdam
The Netherlands

Zsombor Melegh MD, MSc
Department of Cellular and Molecular Medicine
Histopathology Division
Bristol Royal Infirmary
Bristol
UK

Steven J. Meranze MD
Vanderbilt University Medical Center
Nashville, TN
USA

Wells Messersmith MD
Division of Medical Oncology
Department of Medicine
University of Colorado
Aurora, CO
USA

Mark Middleton MD
University of Oxford
Cancer Research UK
Department of Medical Oncology
Churchill Hospital
Oxford
UK

Rachel S. Midgley BSc, MB ChB, MRCP, PhD
Department of Clinical Pharmacology
University of Oxford
UK

Markku Miettinen MD, PhD
Department of Soft Tissue Pathology
Armed Forces Institute of Pathology
Washington, DC
USA

Luka Milas MD, PhD
Department of Experimental Radiation Oncology
The University of Texas M. D. Anderson Cancer Center
Houston, TX
USA

Paul Moayyedi BSc, MB ChB, PhD, MPH, FRCP, FRCPC, FACG, AGAF
Department of Medicine
McMaster University Medical Centre
Hamilton, ON
Canada

Irvin M. Modlin MD, PhD, DSC, FRCS
Yale University School of Medicine
New Haven, CT
USA

Vidu B. Mokkala MD
Miles and Shirley Fiterman Center for Digestive Diseases
Mayo Clinic
Rochester, MN
USA

Daniela Molena MD
Department of Surgery
University of Rochester Medical Center
Rochester, NY
USA

Ido Nachmany MD
Department of Surgery
Tel Aviv Sourasky Medical Center
Sackler School of Medicine
Tel Aviv University
Tel Aviv
Israel

John P. Neoptolemos MBChB, MD, FRCS, FMedSci
University of Liverpool
School of Cancer Studies
Liverpool
UK

Alfred I. Neugut MD, PhD
Columbia University Medical Center
New York, NY
USA

Zhannat Nurgalieva MD
Michael E. DeBakey VA Medical Center and Baylor College of Medicine
Houston, TX
USA

Michael Olausson MD
Division of Transplantation and Liver Surgery
University of Göteborg
Göteborg
Sweden

Dermot O'Toole MD, MRCPI
St James's Hospital and Trinity College Dublin
Dublin
Ireland

Charlie Pan MD
Department of Radiation Oncology
University of Michigan Medical School
Ann Arbor, MI
USA

Dimitrios Papadogias MD
General Hospital 'G. Gennimatas'
Athens
Greece

Marianne Pavel MD
Internistin, Endokrinologin
Medizinische Klinik I mit Poliklinik
Universitätsklinikum Ulmenweg
Erlangen
Germany

Timothy M. Pawlik MD, MPH, FACS
Division of Surgical Oncology
Department of Surgery
Johns Hopkins School of Medicine
Baltimore, MD
USA

Benjamin Paz MD
City of Hope National Medical Center
California, CA
USA

Pascal Peeters MD
Digestive Oncology Unit
University Hospital Gasthuisberg
Leuven
Belgium

Shawn J. Pelletier MD
General and Transplantation Surgery
Taubman Center
University of Michigan Health System
Ann Arbor, Michigan
USA

Daniel O. Persky MD
University of Arizona Health Sciences Center
Tucson, AZ
USA

Jeffrey H. Peters MD
Department of Surgery
University of Rochester
Rochester, NY
USA

Rachel R. Phillips FRCP, DCH, FRCR
University of Oxford
Department of Radiology
The Churchill Hospital
Oxford
UK

Massimo Pignatelli MD, PhD, FRCPath
Department of Cellular and Molecular Medicine
Histopathology Division
Bristol Royal Infirmary
Bristol
UK

Ursula Plöckinger MD
Interdisziplinäres Stoffechsel-Centrum
Charité-Universitätsmedizin Berlin
Campus-Virchow-Klinikum
Berlin
Germany

Anil R. Prasad MD, FASCP, FCAP
University of Arizona Health Sciences Center
Tucson, AZ
USA

Asif Rashid MD, PhD
Department of Pathology
MD Anderson Cancer Center
Houston, TX
USA

Ann MacArthur Rgn Enb
The Horton Hospital
Oxford Radcliffe Hospitals NHS Trust
Oxford
UK

Guido Rindi MD, PhD
Anatomic Pathology Section
Department of Pathology and Laboratory Medicine
University of Parma
Parma
Italy

Anja Rinke MD
Philipps Universität Marburg
Marburg
Germany

Matthias Rothmund MD
Philipps Universität Marburg
Marburg
Germany

Daniel Royston MBChB, BMSc
Department of Cellular Pathology
John Radcliffe Hospital
Oxford
UK

Philippe Ruszniewski MD, PhD
Beaujon Hospital
Clichy
Université Denis Diderot
Paris
France

Ami Sabharwal MD
Department of Clinical Pharmacology
University of Oxford
Oxford
UK

Eyal Sagiv PhD
Tel Aviv Medical Center
Tel Aviv
Israel

Sanjay Saluja MD
Department of Radiology
Yale University School of Medicine
New Haven, CT
USA

Alastair Sammon MD, FRCS
Department of General Surgery
Gloucestershire Hospitals NHS Foundation Trust
Gloucester
UK

Mark Schattner MD, FACP
Gastroenterology and Nutrition Service
Memorial Sloan-Kettering Cancer Center
New York, NY
USA

Lawrence Schwartz MD
Memorial Sloan-Kettering Cancer Center
New York, NY
USA

Nicholas J. Shaheen MD, MPH
University of North Carolina School of Medicine
Chapel Hill NC
USA

Neil A. Shepherd DM, FRCPath
Department of Histopathology
Gloucestershire Royal Hospital
Gloucester
UK

Cen Si MD
Department of Pathology
Vrije Universiteit Medical Center
Amsterdam
The Netherlands

Baljit Singh FRCS, DPhil
Nuffield Department of Surgery
John Radcliffe Hospital
Oxford
UK

Ferdinandos Skoulidis MD, MRCP
MRC/Hutchison Research Centre
University of Cambridge
UK

Thomas C. Smyrk MD
Department of Lab medicine and Pathology
Mayo Clinic
Rochester, MN
USA

Louis M. Wong Kee Song MD
Miles and Shirley Fiterman Center for Digestive Diseases
Mayo Clinic
Rochester, MN
USA

Ilfet Songun MD, PhD
Leiden University Medical Center
Department of Surgery
Leiden
The Netherlands

Zahir Soonawalla FRCS, MS, DNB
John Radcliffe Hospital
Oxford
UK

Naureen Starling MBBS, BSc, MRCP
Gastrointestinal Unit
Department of Medicine
Royal Marsden Hospital
Surrey
UK

Robert J. C. Steele MD, FRCS
Ninewells Hospital and Medical School
Dundee
UK

Paul H. Sugarbaker MD
Peritoneal Surface Malignancy Program
Washington Cancer Institute
Washington Hospital Center
Washington DC
USA

Anders Sundin MD, PhD
Department of Radiology
Karolinska University Hospital Solna
Stockholm
Sweden

Jaap J.M. Teunissen MD
Erasmus MC
University Hospital Rotterdam
Department of Nuclear Medicine
Rotterdam
The Netherlands

John L. Thompson MD
Fred Hutchinson Cancer Research Center
University of Washington
Seattle, WA
USA

Roelf Valkema MD, PhD
Department of Nuclear Medicine
Erasmus MC
Rotterdam
The Netherlands

Eric Van Cutsem MD, PhD
Digestive Oncology Unit
University Hospital Gasthuisberg
Leuven
Belgium

Cornelius J.H. van de Velde FRCS, FRCPS, MD, PhD
Leiden University Medical Center
Department of Surgery
Leiden
The Netherlands

Marcel Verheij MD, PhD
Department of Radiation Oncology
The Netherlands Cancer Institute/ Antoni van Leeuwenhoek Hospital
Amsterdam
The Netherlands

Mark Vipond MS, FRCS
Gloucestershire Royal NHS Foundation Trust
Gloucester
UK

Kenneth K. Wang MD
Mayo Clinic
Department of Gastroenterology and Hepatology
Rochester, MN
USA

Bryan F. Warren MBChB, FRCP, FRCPath
John Radcliffe Hospital
Oxford
UK

Mary Kay Washington MD, PhD
Vanderbilt University Medical Center
Nashville, TN
USA

Andrew Weaver MD, MRCP, FRCR
John Radcliffe Hospital
Oxford
UK

Donna White PhD
Baylor College of Medicine
Houston, TX
USA

Bertram Wiedenmann
University Medicine Berlin, Charite
Department of Internal Medicine
Division of Hepatology and Gastroenterology
Berlin
Germany

Jonathon Willatt MBChB, FRCR
Radiology Department
University of Michigan
Ann Arbor, MI
USA

Christopher Willett M.D.
Duke University Medical Center
Department of Radiation Oncology
Durham, NC
USA

Laura A. Williams MD
Vanderbilt University
Vanderbilt-Ingram Medical Center
Nashville, TN
USA

Christopher L. Wolfgang MD, PhD, FACS
Johns Hopkins Hospital
Baltimore, MD
USA

Herbert C. Wolfsen MD
Mayo Clinic College of Medicine
Rochester, MN
USA

Benjamin C.Y. Wong MD, PhD
Department of Medicine
University of Hong Kong
Hong Kong

Tristan D. Yan BSc, MBBS
Peritoneal Surface Malignancy Program
Washington Cancer Institute
Washington Hospital Center
Washington DC
USA

Preface

Gastrointestinal Oncology: A Critical Multidisciplinary Team Approach takes an entirely novel approach to the management of cancer. Since we accept that cancer medicine has changed over the last decade so must the approach to learning in this complex area, nowhere more so than the many multidisciplinary needs of the single patient. The rationale for the book is as the reference text for multidisciplinary meetings dealing with esophageal, gastric, intestinal, colonic, hepatobiliary, pancreatic and other GI tumors. It recapitulates the many expert opinions that are needed to weigh up the best management for a particular cancer sufferer. This text book will enable the expert not only to stay up to date with their speciality, but also make themselves experts in allied disciplines. This compendium is also aimed at those in training as we have used an evidence based approach to prioritise the themes of each chapter. Therefore, anyone who is a gastroenterologist, oncologist, radiologist, pathologist, GI surgeon or clinical scientist should refer to this book so their conceptual understanding is given breadth and depth.

The book is divided up into specific tumour areas for immediate and easy access and then subdivided into the specialities relating to an individual tumour. The unique advantage is that an expert in one area can refresh his knowledge in one area while quickly grasping the fundamentals in related clinical specialities. The task of getting the worlds' experts to write and submit their texts to such an exceptional standard is due in part to the excellent publishing team. We hope you enjoy this book and feel sure that your patients will benefit time and again from the tried and tested effective advice as well as help to manage recalcitrant disease. As doctors we are tasked on a daily basis to make a real difference to every one of our patients each day. This book will help make this privilege manageable for the individual doctor and will allow doctors to think and act as a team. If one expert is not available then the book will provide the expertise needed – the immortal cancer specialist.

Janusz Jankowski
Leicester, 2008

Foreword

As a group, gastrointestinal (GI) cancers are the most frequent cause of cancer-related mortality worldwide. Recent data suggest that annual deaths exceed an estimated 2.4 million, and incident cases number more than 3.2 million. Even though relatively preventable, mortality rates approach incidence rates because GI cancers typically come to attention only at advanced clinical stages when current therapies are of limited benefit.

GI cancers vary greatly in their pathogenesis and global occurrence. For example, cancers of the esophagus, stomach, and liver occur more commonly in men and in economically developing countries, whereas colorectal cancer typically occurs without preference to gender, but is more common in industrialized countries. Variations in GI cancer—and changing patterns observed in migrant populations that tend to assume the cancer risks of their host countries, often within one generation—suggest a prominent role for environmental influences at most sites. In some cases, significant environmental contributors have been identified, such as *Helicobacter pylori* infection (stomach cancer), chronic viral hepatitis B and C and alcohol abuse (liver cancer), and alcohol abuse and tobacco exposure (esophageal squamous cell carcinoma). Our understanding of etiologic associations for other GI cancers is less complete and/or the associations appear to be more complex. Colorectal cancer risk, for example, is influenced by a broad range of lifestyle and environmental factors, such as dietary nutrients, dietary fiber, physical activity, tobacco exposure, and diabetes mellitus.

Key cellular and molecular derangements underlying the development of GI cancer are becoming clearer, and this knowledge is informing advances in cancer risk assessment, screening, early detection, and diagnosis. Molecular data have already translated into more effective and less toxic approaches to prevent, treat, and palliate certain GI cancers. Now, in all but the earliest clinical settings, a multidimensional approach has proven most effective for clinical management. Multidisciplinary approaches draw upon the expertise of gastroenterologists, surgeons, radiologists, radiotherapists, medical oncologists, specialized nurses, and supportive health specialists and have paved the way for multi-specialty clinics that attend to the diverse needs of patients with GI cancer.

Despite these conceptual and practical advances, many patients suffer serious morbidity from their disease and/or its management, and advanced GI cancer remains highly lethal. This underscores the critical role that basic, translational, and clinical research play in improving patient care. Indeed, as genetic susceptibility, molecular characterization, and tailored interventions play an expanding role in clinical decision making, molecular biologists, cancer geneticists, and other translationally-oriented researchers are increasingly integrated into multidisciplinary teams.

Finally, our improved molecular understanding of GI cancers suggests that we might one day be able to reduce their incidence altogether. This possibility has already been realized in colorectal carcinoma, where screening, polypectomy, and most recently, chemoprevention have not only proven to be feasible, but more importantly, effective. Furthermore, colorectal cancer screening of average risk individuals has demonstrated that issues of long-term health risks/benefits and cost-effectiveness ultimately drive dissemination of medical approaches. This final hurdle may prove the most difficult to overcome, particularly if such advances are to be extended across all sectors of the population. Nevertheless, high-quality research offers the best opportunity to provide care for our patients, and to generate data that improve options for future generations.

This text, edited by Janusz Jankowski, Richard Sampliner, David Kerr and Yuman Fong, provides a timely and comprehensive summary of our knowledge of GI cancer from a multidisciplinary perspective—highlighting its pathogenesis, as well as its translation into clinical measures that can be applied by health care practitioners to benefit those at risk for, or living with, GI cancers. In addition, it provides insights into pressing discovery needs that may guide bench researchers, clinical researchers, and population scientists in the search for more effective, safe, and cost-effective interventions.

Ernest Hawk MD, MPH & Jaye L. Viner MD, MPH
National Cancer Institute, Bethesda, USA
2008

1 Gastroesophageal Cancer

Edited by Richard Sampliner

1 Epidemiology of Gastroesophageal Cancer

Evan S. Dellon & Nicholas J. Shaheen

Malignancies of the esophagus and stomach represent a diverse group of disease processes. The epidemiology of these conditions has changed substantially over the last half-century, likely due to interactions between genetic predisposition and environmental factors. The goal of this chapter is to provide a review of the epidemiology of the major forms of gastroesophageal cancer. The first part of the chapter will focus on the two major forms of esophageal neoplasm: adenocarcinoma and squamous cell carcinoma. In the second part of the chapter, gastric malignancies including adenocarcinoma, lymphoma, and stromal tumors will be discussed.

Epidemiology of esophageal cancer

Esophageal cancer is the eighth most common malignancy worldwide, responsible for an estimated 462,000 incident cases in 2002, and squamous cell carcinoma (SCC) is felt to be the most common subtype (Parkin *et al.* 2005). During the first part of the twentieth century, SCC was also the most prevalent form in the US, but over the past several decades the incidence of adenocarcinoma of the esophagus (ACE) has risen dramatically (Jemal *et al.* 2006). In fact, the rate of increase has been faster than that of any other type of cancer (see Fig. 1.1) and has been measured at between 4 and 10% per year, with an overall increase of 300–500% (Daly *et al.* 1996; Devesa *et al.* 1998). While the cause of this shift is not fully understood, it may be a combination of factors such increasing obesity, alteration in known risk factors including treatment of *Helicobacter pylori*, and changes in the US population from the standpoint of aging and immigration (Daly *et al.* 1996; Devesa *et al.* 1998). Misclassification bias from improved detection alone does not appear to explain this finding (Pohl & Welch 2005). Specific risk factors for each subtype of esophageal cancer will be discussed separately below.

Gastrointestinal Oncology: A Critical Multidisciplinary Team Approach. Edited by J. Jankowski, R. Sampliner, D. Kerr, and Y. Fong.

While there has been a substantial increase in the number of ACEs, there has been a relative decline in the incidence of SCC such that the overall burden of esophageal cancer has increased only slightly in the US. The 14,550 estimated cases of esophageal cancer in the US in 2006 were responsible for approximately 13,770 deaths, making esophageal cancer the 19th most common cancer, but the sixth leading cause of cancer death in men and the 16th cause in women (Jemal *et al.* 2006). Compared to 1970 when approximately 5% of new diagnoses of esophageal cancer were ACE, over half now are ACE with the remainder largely comprised of SCC (Devesa *et al.* 1998). The overall 5-year survival rate for esophageal cancer of 15% is poor and has not significantly improved over the past quarter-century (Eloubeidi *et al.* 2003; Jemal *et al.* 2006).

Risk factors for adenocarcinoma of the esophagus

Demographic

Multiple risk factors for ACE have been established (see Table 1.1), and these also pertain to adenocarcinoma of the gastric cardia (see below). The incidence of ACE increases with increasing age, with a mean onset in the seventh and eighth decade of life; males are two to four times more likely to be affected than females, and Caucasians are approximately 5 times more likely than African-Americans to develop ACE; an association with socioeconomic status has not yet been seen (Blot *et al.* 1991; Daly *et al.* 1996; Devesa *et al.* 1998). There is regional variation in both incidence and ethnicity (Kubo & Corley 2002) but it has yet to be determined whether this is related to geographical factors or to issues pertaining to detection and diagnosis. Finally, to date, a strong heritable component of ACE has yet to be described, though in limited familial studies it appears that host factors are important (Chak *et al.* 2002).

Obesity

With the ongoing obesity epidemic in the US, there has been interest in obesity as a risk factor for malignancy. Several studies have linked increasing body mass index (BMI) with a stepwise

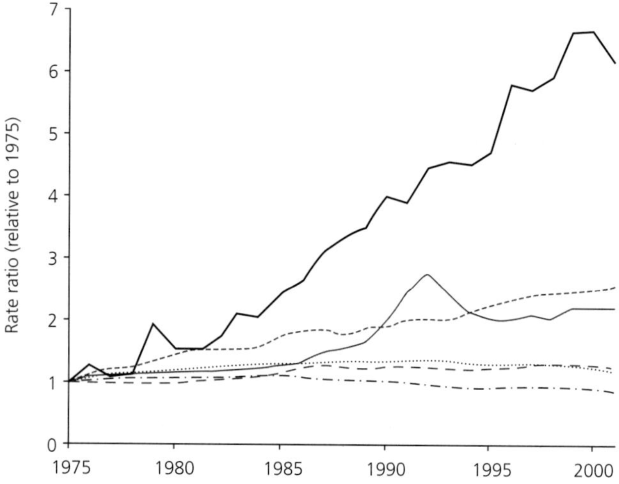

Fig. 1.1 Comparison of relative rates of increase of esophageal adenocarcinoma (solid black line) and other malignancies in the US (red short dashed line, melanoma; red thin solid line, prostate cancer; red dashed line, breast cancer; grey dotted line, lung cancer; black dashed and dotted line, colorectal cancer). From Pohl and Welch (2005).

increase in ACE risk (Chow *et al.* 1998b; Lagergren *et al.* 1999b). This finding is more prominent in men than women, and appears to be most directly related to central (visceral) adiposity. Additionally, a high-fat diet has been associated with increased risk of ACE (Mayne *et al.* 2001).

Acid exposure

Acid exposure is pertinent to the pathogenesis of ACE (direct injury) and is also a well-established risk factor. A number of investigations have linked gastroesophageal reflux disease (GERD) to ACE, demonstrating that the risk increases with increasing severity and duration of GERD symptoms (Lagergren *et al.* 1999a; Farrow *et al.* 2000; Ye *et al.* 2001). However, it should be noted that in these same studies, as many as 40–50% of patients eventually diagnosed with ACE did not have previous symptoms of GERD. In a similar vein, medications that reduce the pressure of the lower esophageal sphincter (LES) such as anticholinergics, nitrates, and others, have also been associated with ACE (Lagergren *et al.* 2000). The role of *Helicobacter pylori* will be discussed below.

Barrett's esophagus

Barrett's esophagus (BE), defined as metaplasia of the normal esophageal squamous mucosa to specialized (intestinalized)

Table 1.1 Risk factors for the major types of esophageal and gastric cancers.

Esophageal adenocarcinoma	Esophageal squamous cell carcinoma	Gastric adenocarcinoma
Geographic location*	Geographic location*	Geographic location*
Demographics Increasing age Male White	Demographics Increasing age Male Ethnic minorities Low socioeconomic status	Demographics Increasing age (except where *H. pylori* is endemic) Male Ethnic minorities Low socioeconomic status
Diet, nutrition, and habits Tobacco Obesity High fat diet	Diet, nutrition, and habits Tobacco Alcohol Few fruits and vegetables Low selenium or zinc Vitamin deficiency*	Diet, nutrition, and habits Tobacco Alcohol Few fruits and vegetables Vitamin deficiency*
Increased acid exposure		
Barrett's esophagus		*H. pylori* infection
Heritability possible	Heritability not established	Heritability established
Other Cholecystectomy	Other Achalasia Caustic injury Radiation Plummer–Vinson Zenker's diverticulum Tylosis palmaris Human papillomavirus	Other Partial gastrectomy Pernicious anemia Epstein–Barr virus Ménétrier's disease

* See text.

columnar epithelium with goblet cells present, is a widely studied risk factor for ACE (Sharma *et al.* 2004). There is significant interest in this condition because it appears that ACE frequently arises in an area of BE, and that BE can progress from metaplasia, to dysplasia, and finally to carcinoma (Hameeteman *et al.* 1989; Shaheen & Ransohoff 2002). As noted above, while GERD and obesity are risk factors for ACE, they have also been found to be risk factors for BE (Avidan *et al.* 2002; El-Serag *et al.* 2005). These relations, however, do not explain the entire association; other studies show that a significant proportion of subjects without GERD also have BE (Rex *et al.* 2003; Ronkainen *et al.* 2005). While an interaction between genetic predisposition and environmental exposures is implied, specific genes have not yet been identified.

A large number of studies provide estimates that BE increases the risk of ACE 30 to 400 times, but more accurate projections place the increased risk at between 30 and 60 times (Lagergren 2005). The current best estimate of the rate of progression from non-dysplastic BE to ACE is approximately 0.5% per year in the USA but 1% in the UK (Shaheen *et al.* 2000). In BE with high-grade dysplasia (HGD), however, the rate of progression is substantially higher at 10–30% per year (Miros *et al.* 1991; Buttar *et al.* 2001) and synchronous cancers are often found on esophagectomy specimens (Heitmiller *et al.* 1996; Cameron & Carpenter 1997).

The relation between BE, dysplasia, and ACE is not straightforward, and the dysplasia to carcinoma pathway is not inevitable. Observations of the natural history of BE and from structured treatment trials have repeatedly demonstrated cases of spontaneous regression from BE to normal squamous epithelium, HDG to low-grade dysplasia (LGD), and LGD to non-dysplastic Barrett's mucosa (Schnell *et al.* 2001; Overholt *et al.* 2005; Shaheen 2005). The presence of BE has not been shown to affect mortality or life expectancy, and even in cases of BE where ACE develops, because ACE is a disease of the elderly competing comorbidities are often the cause of death (van der Burgh *et al.* 1996; Eckardt *et al.* 2001; Anderson *et al.* 2003).

Other

Several other risk factors for ACE have also been studied. Cigarette smoking likely increases the risk of ACE, but the results of population-based studies have been mixed (Brown *et al.* 1994; Zhang *et al.* 1996). Similarly, alcohol consumption has not been shown to be a strong risk factor (Brown *et al.* 1994). One study, which has yet to be replicated, found that cholecystectomy was associated with ACE (Freedman *et al.* 2001).

Possible preventive factors

While a number of risk factors for ACE have been identified, there are also several factors that may be potentially protective, though these have not been rigorously tested in clinical trials. As summarized in a recent meta-analysis, multiple studies have reported that non-steroidal anti-inflammatory drugs (NSAIDs) reduce the risk of BE and ACE (Hur *et al.* 2004). The use of these medications specifically for BE, however, is not currently recommended outside of ongoing clinical trials which will define the relative merits of chemoprevention with aspirin alone or in combination with proton pump inhibitors (PPIs). Several studies have also found that PPIs were associated with regression of BE and reduction of incidence of dysplasia (Sharma *et al.* 1997; El-Serag *et al.* 2004). Though there are no direct data showing that PPIs prevent ACE, given their favorable risk–benefit profile many experts now recommend that all patients with BE should be treated with PPIs. The value of aspirin as a chemoprevention agent is being tested in the world's largest BE brial, ASPECT (Aspirin Chemoprevention Trial). Last, limited data suggest that the presence of *H. pylori* may decrease the development of dysplasia, so routine testing and treatment for this microorganism in reflux and BE may not be warranted (Chow *et al.* 1998a, Ye *et al.* 2004).

Risk factors for squamous cell carcinoma of the esophagus

Geographic

While some risk factors between the two major forms of esophageal cancer overlap, in general the risk factors for SCC are distinct (see Table 1.1). Incidence of SCC varies much more substantially by global geographic region that does ACE, with low rates (1–5 cases per 100,000) reported in the US and Western European countries and higher rates (50–200 cases per 100,000) in sections of Asia, India, and Africa (Parkin *et al.* 2005). While country of origin is a non-modifiable risk factor, this information may be useful in risk stratification.

Demographic

Similar to ACE and other gastrointestinal malignancies, SCC of the esophagus is most frequently diagnosed in the 7th and 8th decades of life (Engel *et al.* 2003). White males are 2–4 times more likely to be affected than white women, and African-Americans are at 4–5 times higher risk for SCC than Caucasians (Gammon *et al.* 1997). Low socioeconomic status has also been related to elevated risk of SCC (Gammon *et al.* 1997).

Tobacco and alcohol

Tobacco and alcohol have repeatedly been shown not only to increase the risk of SCC in a dose-dependent manner, but also to act synergistically. The majority of studies report an elevated risk of 2–10 times, but some find increases as high as 25 times (Brown *et al.* 1997; Thun *et al.* 1997). While there is a dose-dependent relationship between smoking and cancer risk, the total quantity of alcohol consumed, rather than the specific type, is likely the more important measure.

Diet and nutrition

The wide geographic variability in SCC of the esophagus may be explained, in part, by environmental factors such as diet and nutrition. Higher rates of SCC have been associated with consumption of foods rich in N-nitrosamines, which in turn can cause either direct esophageal toxicity, DNA damage, or both (Siddiqi *et al.* 1988). Similarly, local practices such as the Iranian custom of imbibing extremely hot tea (Ghadirian 1987) or betel nut chewing in Asia (Pickwell *et al.* 1994) have been associated with SCC. An increased risk of SCC has also been associated with deficiencies in a number of micronutrients, such as vitamins A, C, and E, folate, riboflavin, B12, selenium, and zinc (Santhi Swaroop *et al.* 1989; Blot *et al.* 1993; Mark *et al.* 2000).

Non-malignant esophageal disease

Non-malignant processes affecting the esophagus have also been associated with SCC. Though the mechanism is not fully understood, patients with achalasia are 15–30 times more likely to develop SCC of the esophagus compared with expected cancer registry rates (Sandler *et al.* 1995). Caustic ingestions (Appelqvist & Salmo 1980), radiation exposure (Ogino *et al.* 1992), Plummer–Vinson syndrome (Larsson *et al.* 1975), and Zenker's diverticula (Huang *et al.* 1984) have been linked to SCC as well.

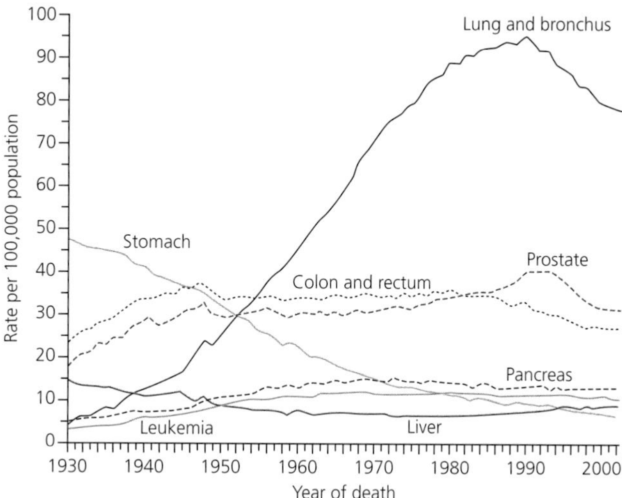

Fig. 1.2 Decline in the annual age-adjusted cancer death rate from gastric cancer (pink line) for males; a similar trend has been seen in females as well (graph not shown). From Jemal *et al.* (2006).

Other

A number of miscellaneous diseases are also thought to be associated with SCC. Infection with human papillomavirus (HPV) has been implicated in SCC, just as it has been in neoplastic transformation of squamous epithelium of the anus and cervix (Chang *et al.* 2000). There is also a very strong link between tylosis palmaris and SCC of the esophagus, with as many as 50% of patients affected by this autosomal dominant disorder developing a malignancy by age 45, and 95% doing so by age 65 (Iwaya *et al.* 1998). Because of this, screening with upper endoscopy is recommended for all patients with tylosis starting at age 30 (Brown & Shaheen 2004).

Epidemiology of gastric cancer

Gastric cancer is the fourth most common malignancy worldwide (behind lung, breast, and colorectal cancers) and the second most common cause of cancer death (behind only lung cancer), responsible for an estimated 934,000 new cases and 700,000 deaths in 2002 (Parkin *et al.* 2005). This burden of disease falls most heavily on developing countries, where two-thirds of incident cases occur, and on China, where 42% of all cases are diagnosed (Parkin *et al.* 2005). Over the past several decades, however, there has been a general decline in the age-adjusted incidence rate of gastric cancer (Parkin *et al.* 1988). As with the rapidly evolving epidemiology of ACE, this decline implies a changing environmental milieu interacting with host factors rather than primary changes in genetics. Potential causes of this decline including sanitation and refrigeration, diet, and *H. pylori* will be discussed below.

In the US the epidemiology of gastric cancer does not reflect the global picture. Incidence of gastric cancer has declined by more than 60–80% since 1930 (see Fig. 1.2). In 2006, 22,280 new cases were estimated to occur, accounting for 11,430 deaths and making gastric cancer the 14th most common cancer and the 15th cause of cancer death (Jemal *et al.* 2006). Additionally, the 5-year survival rate has increased from 15% for the period 1974–1976 to 23% for the period 1995–2001 (Jemal *et al.* 2006). It is important to note that these trends are representative of non-cardia (or distal) gastric cancer, and will be the focus of this section. Because adenocarcinoma of the gastric cardia is felt to be closely related to ACE, risk factors for this disease are similar to those for ACE.

Gastric adenocarcinoma (GAC) comprises 90% of all non-cardia gastric cancer pathologic subtypes, with lymphomas, stromal tumors, and rare malignancies accounting for the remainder (Fuchs & Mayer 1995; Crew & Neugut 2006). GAC has been further subdivided into two histologic classes: an intestinal type which tends to maintain a distinct glandular structure and develops in the setting of atrophic gastritis, and a diffuse type which is generally poorly differentiated, features signet-ring cells, and arises in non-atrophic gastritis (Lauren 1965; Crew & Neugut 2006). It appears that the incidence of intestinal-type tumors is falling noticeably, while that of diffuse-type tumors is stable or rising slowly (Lauren & Nevalainen 1993; Kaneko & Yoshimura 2001; Henson *et al.* 2004). The specific characteristics of these individual types of cancer will be discussed in further detail in Chapters 6 and 7. The general epidemiology of GAC is discussed below, and any significant differences between the intestinal and diffuse types are noted. The chapter concludes with a discussion of the epidemiology of gastric lymphomas and stromal tumors.

Risk factors for gastric adenocarcinoma

Geographic

A large number of studies have investigated risk factors for GAC, and while some of these overlap with esophageal cancer, many are unrelated (see Table 1.1). First, there is a substantial amount of geographic variability in the worldwide incidence of gastric cancer (see Fig. 1.3). In North America and selected regions of Africa and South Asia, rates are low (less than 10 per 100,000). By contrast, Japan has the highest rates in the world for both males and females (62 and 26 per 100,000, respectively), with comparatively high rates (approximately 20 per 100,000 or higher) also seen in China, Eastern Europe, and Central and South America (Parkin *et al.* 2005).

These wide differences in incidence almost certainly point to environmental factors placing inhabitants of certain regions at higher risk for GAC. Studies of migrants who emigrated from regions of high to low incidence help to confirm this theory in multiple population types (McMichael *et al.* 1980; Kamineni *et al.* 1999). Specifically, when subjects emigrate from areas of high GAC incidence to low GAC incidence, they initially retain their 'native' incident rate. However, over time and especially over subsequent generations, descendants acquire the GAC incidence rate of their adopted country.

Demographic

In the US and other areas with a low incidence of GAC, the diagnosis of gastric cancer is most commonly made between the ages of 50 and 70. In high-incidence areas such as East Asia and parts of Central America, however, diagnosis may be made at a much earlier age (Fuchs & Mayer 1995; Crew & Neugut 2006). In general, males are approximately 2 times more likely to be affected than females, as are certain ethnic minorities including African-Americans, Hispanic-Americans, and Native Americans (Fuchs & Mayer 1995). Low socioeconomic class has also been associated with an increased risk of GAC (Barker *et al.* 1990).

Helicobacter pylori and gastritis

Inflammation, especially when related to *H. pylori*, is likely central to GAC pathogenesis (see Chapters 2 and 3). There appears to be a progression from gastritis, to atrophic gastritis, to intestinal metaplasia, to gastric dysplasia, and finally to carcinoma (Correa 2005). Epidemiologic studies of the role of *H. pylori* support this association in several ways. First, prevalence rates of *H. pylori* correlate with GAC incidence rates (Dooley *et al.* 1989; Parkin 2006). In other words, areas of the world in which *H. pylori* prevalence is high and infection is acquired at an early age are the same geographic areas in which some of the highest incidence rates of GAC can be found.

While the overlap of these distributions is suggestive, further investigations have confirmed the association. A number of

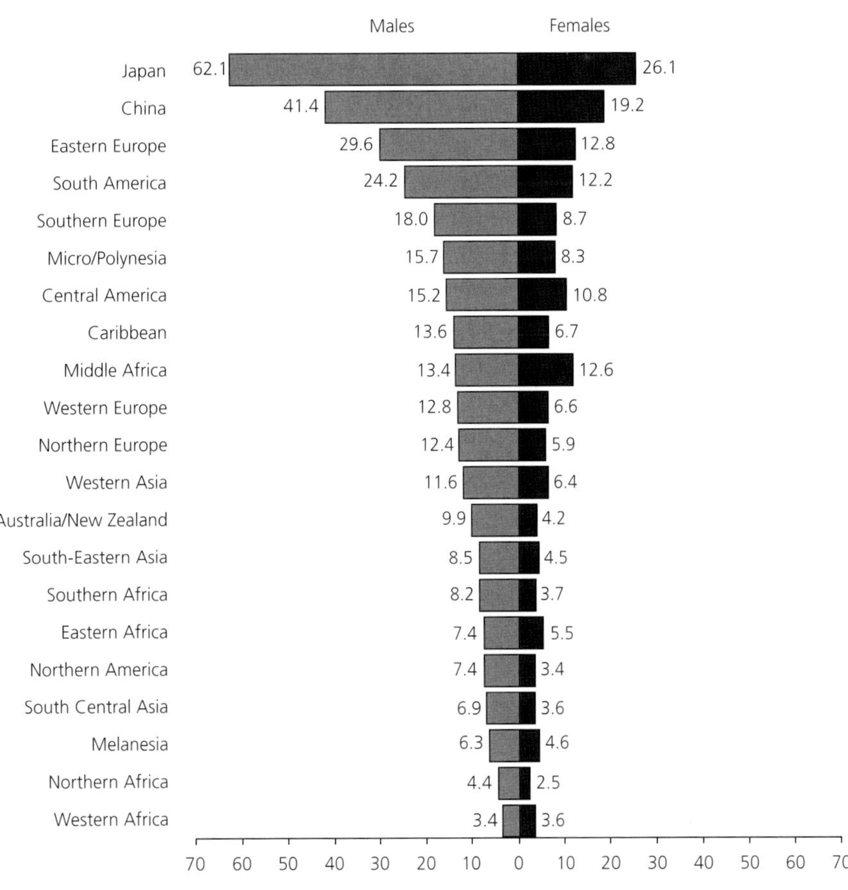

Fig. 1.3 Distribution of age-standardized incidence rates of gastric cancer by gender and location. From Parkin *et al.* (2005).

case–control studies report associations between *H. pylori* and non-cardia GAC of both intestinal and diffuse types with odds ratios (ORs) in the 2.5–4 range (Hansson *et al.* 1993; Hu *et al.* 1994; Kokkola *et al.* 1996). Nested case–control studies in both prospective and retrospective cohorts have been convincing as well. ORs in selected studies ranged from 2.7 to 6.0 and a meta-analysis found the pooled OR to be 2.5 (Danesh 1999). More recently, a prospective cohort of 1526 Japanese patients with either peptic ulcer disease, non-ulcer dyspepsia, or gastric hyperplasia were followed for a mean of 7.8 years to find 36 GACs (Uemura *et al.* 2001). All of the 36 malignancies occurred in the 2.9% of patients with prior *H. pylori;* none were detected in patients without *H. pylori.* Taken together, the preponderance of the evidence strongly associates *H. pylori* infection with non-cardia GAC.

While *H. pylori* is a strong risk factor, it is also very common; perhaps 50% of the population worldwide are infected, and the majority of patients with *H. pylori* infection do not develop GAC. Ostensibly, host factors interact with bacterial and environmental factors to make progression to malignancy more or less likely. While this topic will be discussed in more detail in Chapter 2, one example involves the *H. pylori* virulence factor cytotoxin-associated gene A (cagA) (Al-Marhoon *et al.* 2004). Multiple case–control studies have shown that the presence of this virulence factor increases the risk for GAC above the risk of *H. pylori* alone, and a recent meta-analysis reported an overall OR of approximately 2.0 (Huang *et al.* 2003). Further, new data suggest that the presence of the cagA virulence factor interacts with host factors such as severity of atrophic gastritis to further modulate risk of GAC (Sasazuki *et al.* 2006).

While there are strong data to support the role of *H. pylori* in the development of GAC, whether the presence of gastric ulcer in the absence of *H. pylori* infection is a risk factor for GAC remains controversial (Hansson *et al.* 1996).

Diet and nutrition

Because the role of environment is so important in understanding GAC epidemiology, dietary factors have been well studied. Early investigations found that the use of refrigeration was a protective factor, suggesting that either preservatives or breakdown products in spoiling food might be risk factors for GAC (Coggon *et al.* 1989; La Vecchia *et al.* 1990). Subsequent investigations focused on the role of salt. A multinational ecologic study linked increasing salt intake to countries with higher incidences of GAC (Joossens *et al.* 1996), and case–control studies as well as animal models suggest that high-salt diets are a risk factor (Kono & Hirohata 1996). A recent large prospective cohort study also supports this, with ORs in the 2–3 range (Shikata *et al.* 2006).

A different type of preservative, N-nitroso compounds in meat, has been shown to be a risk factor for GAC. The same ecologic study evaluating the role of salt also examined rates of nitrate intake (Joossens *et al.* 1996). It found that increasing nitrate consumption was associated with increased risk of GAC, and that the risk was additive to the risk of a high-salt diet. Case–control studies have also found an association between nitrates and GAC (Fraser *et al.* 1980; Kato *et al.* 1992). More recently, a multicenter prospective cohort demonstrated that both increased meat intake and increased processed meat intake were linked to an increased risk of GAC (Gonzalez *et al.* 2006). This study further showed that high levels of meat consumption acted synergistically with *H. pylori* to elevate risk.

A wide range of studies have looked at the role of fruit, vegetables, and micronutrients in GAC risk. While some of the results of these studies have been conflicting, consumption of fruit and vegetables is felt to be protective, and vitamin C, beta-carotene, vitamin A, and vitamin E have also been found to decrease risk; consistent findings have not been reported for other minerals (Kono & Hirohata 1996; Jenab *et al.* 2006a,b). While obesity has been linked to EAC and gastric cardia neoplasms, it has not been associated with non-cardia GAC (Lindblad *et al.* 2005).

Tobacco and alcohol

Use of tobacco has clearly been shown to be related to GAC in a dose-dependent fashion in a number of studies, with ORs in the 1.5–2.5 range (Nomura *et al.* 1990; Kneller *et al.* 1991; Kato *et al.* 1992; Tredaniel *et al.* 1997; Gonzalez *et al.* 2003; Koizumi *et al.* 2004). The relation of alcohol to GAC, however, has not been clearly established. Most studies support either a minimal association (Kato *et al.* 1992) or no association (Nomura *et al.* 1990; D'Avanzo *et al.* 1994), while one recent retrospective cohort suggested that wine intake could be protective (Barstad *et al.* 2005).

Genetics and heritability

The role of genetics and heritability in gastric malignancy will be fully addressed in Chapters 2 and 3. However, early epidemiologic work associating GAC with blood group A (Hoskins *et al.* 1965) and other heritable cancer syndromes such as hereditary non-polyposis colorectal cancer (HNPCC or Lynch syndrome), familial adenomatous polyposis (FAP), and Peutz–Jeghers (Fuchs & Mayer 1995) highlighted the importance of host factors and laid the groundwork for current genomic and molecular research. Epidemiologic studies have also demonstrated that GAC likely has a heritable component (Palli *et al.* 1994; Zhao *et al.* 1994) and that this risk is independent from a shared environmental factor such as *H. pylori* (Brenner *et al.* 2000; Yatsuya *et al.* 2004). A recently described syndrome of hereditary diffuse gastric cancer has been linked to a germline mutation of the E-cadherin gene and confers a lifetime risk of GAC of 67% in males and 83% in females by the age of 80 (Blair *et al.* 2006). Finally, ongoing studies are examining the effect of inherited polymorphisms in interleukin-1-beta (El-Omar *et al.* 2003) and the interferon gamma receptor (Thye *et al.* 2003) on the host response in gastric inflammation and *H. pylori* infection.

Other

In addition to the major risk factors for GAC discussed above, a number of other associations have been reported. Two meta-analyses found that approximately 15 years after partial gastrectomy for benign gastric conditions, the risk of subsequent GAC was elevated by 1.5–3 times (Stalnikowicz & Benbassat 1990; Tersmette *et al.* 1990). A retrospective cohort found that this risk continued to increase as time from surgery increased (Tersmette *et al.* 1991).

While pernicious anemia is more frequently associated with gastric carcinoid (see Chapter 10), it has also been associated with GAC, potentially through a common pathway of atrophic gastritis. Two studies have found that GAC was 2–3 times more likely to develop in the setting of pernicious anemia (Brinton *et al.* 1989; Hsing *et al.* 1993). Of note, long-term use of anti-secretory therapy has not been associated with GAC (Moller *et al.* 1992; Klinkenberg-Knol *et al.* 1994).

Other associations that have been reported include infection with Epstein–Barr virus (EBV) (Levine *et al.* 1995), and hypertrophic gastropathy conditions such as Ménétrier's disease (Fuchs & Mayer 1995).

Risk factors for other gastric neoplasias

Of the 10% of non-GAC gastric malignancies, the majority are comprised of gastric lymphomas and gastric stromal tumors. These are discussed in detail in Chapters 9 and 10. Because they are less common than GAC, their epidemiology is correspondingly less well studied.

Gastric lymphoma

Comprising a diverse group of malignancies, gastric lymphomas account for 3–5% of all gastric cancers and approximately 10% of all lymphomas, and the stomach is the most common site for extranodal lymphoma (Parsonnet *et al.* 1994; Al-Akwaa *et al.* 2004). In general, the peak incidence is between 50 and 65 years of age, and a small male predominance has been reported (Koch *et al.* 2001; Al-Akwaa *et al.* 2004).

As for GAC, the best-studied risk factor for gastric lymphoma is infection with *H. pylori*. In particular, a number of studies have reported a strong association between this bacterium and mucosa-associated lymphoid tissue (MALT) lymphoma, now termed extranodal marginal zone B-cell lymphoma (Parsonnet *et al.* 1994; Eck *et al.* 1997). In general, *H. pylori* is detected in nearly all patients with MALT lymphoma, and a large nested case–control study demonstrated an OR of greater than 6 (Parsonnet *et al.* 1994).

In addition to *H. pylori*, different types of gastric lymphoma have been associated with immunosuppression from medications used in the post-transplant setting (Aull *et al.* 2003) as well as immunosuppression from the human immunodeficiency virus (HIV) (Powitz *et al.* 1997; Srinivasan *et al.* 2004). Lastly, infection with EBV has been associated with gastric lymphoma (Thompson & Kurzrock 2004).

Gastric stromal tumors

Gastric stromal tumors account for up to 3% of all gastric neoplasias, but comprise approximately 60% of all gastrointestinal stromal tumors (GISTs) (Trent & Benjamin 2006). The peak incidence is between 50 and 70 years of age, and there may be a very slight male predominance (Miettinen *et al.* 2005; Nilsson *et al.* 2005; Trent & Benjamin 2006). While a substantial amount of research has focused on the pathogenesis of GISTs, and specifically on the role of an activating mutation in the Kit tyrosine kinase receptor, little to no epidemiologic research has yet been done to identify specific population-based risk factors (Trent & Benjamin 2006).

Conclusions

This chapter has reviewed the epidemiology of gastroesophageal cancers, a diverse group of conditions with a correspondingly varied epidemiology and set of risk factors. While esophageal malignancies are less common, gastric adenocarcinoma in particular exerts a large burden of disease worldwide. Additionally, the epidemiology of both types of tumors has changed substantially in recent decades. While the incidence of ACE has been rising quickly and the worldwide incidence of GAC continues a slow decline, the decline of GAC in the US has been particularly dramatic. Explanations for these changing epidemiologic patterns involve an interaction between environmental, host, and genetic factors that differ for each disease. In GAC and gastric lymphoma, infection with *H. pylori* is of particular importance, both for understanding pathogenesis and for providing a target for treatment and prevention. For ACE, obesity, GERD, and BE play a major role, but do not account for all cases. And for most of the conditions discussed in this chapter, modifiable risk factors such as diet, nutrition, and tobacco use remain significant. Ongoing research will likely clarify the role of genetics and heritability for all of these conditions, and help to further our knowledge of these processes.

Box 1.1 Level 1 evidence* for prevention of upper GI malignancies

Esophageal cancers

There is no level 1 evidence for prevention of either adenocarcinoma of the esophagus or squamous cell carcinoma of the esophagus but aspirin is being tested in a large RCT ASPECT.

Gastric cancers

There is no level 1 evidence for prevention of gastric adenocarcinoma.

*Level 1 evidence is defined as a significant effect either in one or more randomized controlled trials or in a meta-analysis of randomized controlled trials without heterogeneity.

References

al-Akwaa AM, Siddiqui N, Al-Mofleh IA. (2004) Primary gastric lymphoma. *World J Gastroenterol* 10: 5–11.

Al-Marhoon MS, Nunn S, Soames RW. (2004) The association between cagA+ H. pylori infection and distal gastric cancer: a proposed model. *Dig Dis Sci* 49: 1116–22.

Anderson LA, Murray LJ, Murphy SJ *et al.* (2003) Mortality in Barrett's oesophagus: results from a population based study. *Gut* 52: 1081–4.

Appelqvist P, Salmo M. (1980) Lye corrosion carcinoma of the esophagus: a review of 63 cases. *Cancer* 45: 2655–8.

Aull MJ, Buell JF, Peddi VR *et al.* (2003) MALToma: a *Helicobacter pylori*-associated malignancy in transplant patients: a report from the Israel Penn International Transplant Tumor Registry with a review of published literature. *Transplantation* 75: 225–8.

Avidan B, Sonnenberg A, Schnell TG, Chejfec G, Metz A, Sontag SJ. (2002) Hiatal hernia size, Barrett's length, and severity of acid reflux are all risk factors for esophageal adenocarcinoma. *Am J Gastroenterol* 97: 1930–6.

Barker DJ, Coggon D, Osmond C, Wickham C. (1990) Poor housing in childhood and high rates of stomach cancer in England and Wales. *Br J Cancer* 61: 575–8.

Barstad B, Sorensen TI, Tjonneland A *et al.* (2005) Intake of wine, beer and spirits and risk of gastric cancer. *Eur J Cancer Prev* 14: 239–43.

Blair V, Martin I, Shaw D *et al.* (2006) Hereditary diffuse gastric cancer: diagnosis and management. *Clin Gastroenterol Hepatol* 4: 262–75.

Blot WJ, Devesa SS, Kneller RW, Fraumeni JF Jr. (1991) Rising incidence of adenocarcinoma of the esophagus and gastric cardia. *JAMA* 265: 1287–9.

Blot WJ, Li JY, Taylor PR *et al.* (1993) Nutrition intervention trials in Linxian, China: supplementation with specific vitamin/mineral combinations, cancer incidence, and disease-specific mortality in the general population. *J Natl Cancer Inst* 85: 1483–92.

Brenner H, Arndt V, Sturmer T, Stegmaier C, Ziegler H, Dhom G. (2000) Individual and joint contribution of family history and *Helicobacter pylori* infection to the risk of gastric carcinoma. *Cancer* 88: 274–9.

Brinton LA, Gridley G, Hrubec Z, Hoover R, Fraumeni JF Jr. (1989) Cancer risk following pernicious anaemia. *Br J Cancer* 59: 810–3.

Brown A, Shaheen NJ. (2004) Screening for upper gastrointestinal tract malignancies. *Semin Oncol* 31: 487–97.

Brown LM, Silverman DT, Pottern LM *et al.* (1994) Adenocarcinoma of the esophagus and esophagogastric junction in white men in the United States: alcohol, tobacco, and socioeconomic factors. *Cancer Causes Control* 5: 333–40.

Brown LM, Hoover R, Gridley G *et al.* (1997) Drinking practices and risk of squamous-cell esophageal cancer among Black and White men in the United States. *Cancer Causes Control* 8: 605–9.

van der Burgh A, Dees J, Hop WC, Van Blankenstein M. (1996) Oesophageal cancer is an uncommon cause of death in patients with Barrett's oesophagus. *Gut* 39: 5–8.

Buttar NS, Wang KK, Sebo TJ *et al.* (2001) Extent of high-grade dysplasia in Barrett's esophagus correlates with risk of adenocarcinoma. *Gastroenterology* 120: 1630–9.

Cameron AJ, Carpenter HA. (1997) Barrett's esophagus, high-grade dysplasia, and early adenocarcinoma: a pathological study. *Am J Gastroenterol* 92: 586–91.

Chak A, Lee T, Kinnard MF *et al.* (2002) Familial aggregation of Barrett's oesophagus, oesophageal adenocarcinoma, and oesophagogastric junctional adenocarcinoma in Caucasian adults. *Gut* 51: 323–8.

Chang F, Syrjanen S, Shen Q, Cintorino M, Santopietro R, Tosi P, Syrjanen K. (2000) Human papillomavirus involvement in esophageal carcinogenesis in the high-incidence area of China. A study of 700 cases by screening and type-specific in situ hybridization. *Scand J Gastroenterol* 35: 123–30.

Chow WH, Blaser MJ, Blot WJ *et al.* (1998a) An inverse relation between cagA+ strains of *Helicobacter pylori* infection and risk of esophageal and gastric cardia adenocarcinoma. *Cancer Res* 58: 588–90.

Chow WH, Blot WJ, Vaughan TL *et al.* (1998b) Body mass index and risk of adenocarcinomas of the esophagus and gastric cardia. *J Natl Cancer Inst* 90: 150–5.

Coggon D, Barker DJ, Cole RB, Nelson M. (1989) Stomach cancer and food storage. *J Natl Cancer Inst* 81: 1178–82.

Correa P. (2005) New strategies for the prevention of gastric cancer: *Helicobacter pylori* and genetic susceptibility. *J Surg Oncol* 90: 134–8; discussion 138.

Crew KD, Neugut AI. (2006) Epidemiology of gastric cancer. *World J Gastroenterol* 12: 354–62.

D'Avanzo B, La Vecchia C, Franceschi S. (1994) Alcohol consumption and the risk of gastric cancer. *Nutr Cancer* 22: 57–64.

Daly JM, Karnell LH, Menck HR. (1996) National Cancer Data Base report on esophageal carcinoma. *Cancer* 78: 1820–8.

Danesh J. (1999) *Helicobacter pylori* infection and gastric cancer: systematic review of the epidemiological studies. *Aliment Pharmacol Ther* 13: 851–6.

Devesa SS, Blot WJ, Fraumeni JF Jr. (1998) Changing patterns in the incidence of esophageal and gastric carcinoma in the United States. *Cancer* 83: 2049–53.

Dooley CP, Cohen H, Fitzgibbons PL, Bauer M, Appleman MD, Perez-Perez GI, Blaser MJ. (1989) Prevalence of *Helicobacter pylori* infection and histologic gastritis in asymptomatic persons. *N Engl J Med* 321: 1562–6.

Eck M, Schmausser B, Haas R, Greiner A, Czub S, Muller-Hermelink HK. (1997) MALT-type lymphoma of the stomach is associated with *Helicobacter pylori* strains expressing the CagA protein. *Gastroenterology* 112: 1482–6.

Eckardt VF, Kanzler G, Bernhard G. (2001) Life expectancy and cancer risk in patients with Barrett's esophagus: a prospective controlled investigation. *Am J Med* 111: 33–7.

El-Omar EM, Rabkin CS, Gammon MD *et al.* (2003) Increased risk of noncardia gastric cancer associated with proinflammatory cytokine gene polymorphisms. *Gastroenterology* 124: 1193–201.

El-Serag HB, Aguirre TV, Davis S, Kuebeler M, Bhattacharyya A, Sampliner RE. (2004) Proton pump inhibitors are associated with reduced incidence of dysplasia in Barrett's esophagus. *Am J Gastroenterol* 99: 1877–83.

El-Serag HB, Kvapil P, Hacken-Bitar J, Kramer JR. (2005) Abdominal obesity and the risk of Barrett's esophagus. *Am J Gastroenterol* 100: 2151–6.

Eloubeidi MA, Mason AC, Desmond RA, El-Serag HB. (2003) Temporal trends (1973–1997) in survival of patients with esophageal adenocarcinoma in the United States: a glimmer of hope? *Am J Gastroenterol* 98: 1627–33.

Engel LS, Chow WH, Vaughan TL *et al.* (2003) Population attributable risks of esophageal and gastric cancers. *J Natl Cancer Inst* 95: 1404–13.

Farrow DC, Vaughan TL, Sweeney C *et al.* (2000) Gastroesophageal reflux disease, use of H2 receptor antagonists, and risk of esophageal and gastric cancer. *Cancer Causes Control* 11: 231–8.

Fraser P, Chilvers C, Beral V, Hill MJ. (1980) Nitrate and human cancer: a review of the evidence. *Int J Epidemiol* 9: 3–11.

Freedman J, Ye W, Naslund E, Lagergren J. (2001) Association between cholecystectomy and adenocarcinoma of the esophagus. *Gastroenterology* 121: 548–53.

Fuchs CS, Mayer RJ. (1995) Gastric carcinoma. *N Engl J Med* 333: 32–41.

Gammon MD, Schoenberg JB, Ahsan H *et al.* (1997) Tobacco, alcohol, and socioeconomic status and adenocarcinomas of the esophagus and gastric cardia. *J Natl Cancer Inst* 89: 1277–84.

Ghadirian P. (1987) Thermal irritation and esophageal cancer in northern Iran. *Cancer* 60: 1909–14.

Gonzalez CA, Pera G, Agudo A *et al.* (2003) Smoking and the risk of gastric cancer in the European Prospective Investigation Into Cancer and Nutrition (EPIC). *Int J Cancer* 107: 629–34.

Gonzalez CA, Jakszyn P, Pera G *et al.* (2006) Meat intake and risk of stomach and esophageal adenocarcinoma within the European Prospective Investigation Into Cancer and Nutrition (EPIC). *J Natl Cancer Inst* 98: 345–54.

Hameeteman W, Tytgat GN, Houthoff HJ, Van Den Tweel JG. (1989) Barrett's esophagus: development of dysplasia and adenocarcinoma. *Gastroenterology* 96: 1249–56.

Hansson LE, Engstrand L, Nyren O *et al.* (1993) *Helicobacter pylori* infection: independent risk indicator of gastric adenocarcinoma. *Gastroenterology* 105: 1098–103.

Hansson LE, Nyren O, Hsing AW *et al.* (1996) The risk of stomach cancer in patients with gastric or duodenal ulcer disease. *N Engl J Med* 335: 242–9.

Heitmiller RF, Redmond M, Hamilton SR. (1996) Barrett's esophagus with high-grade dysplasia. An indication for prophylactic esophagectomy. *Ann Surg* 224: 66–71.

Henson DE, Dittus C, Younes M, Nguyen H, Albores-Saavedra J. (2004) Differential trends in the intestinal and diffuse types of gastric carcinoma in the United States, 1973–2000: increase in the signet ring cell type. *Arch Pathol Lab Med* 128: 765–70.

Hoskins LC, Loux HA, Britten A, Zamcheck N. (1965) Distribution of ABO blood groups in patients with pernicious anemia, gastric carcinoma and gastric carcinoma associated with pernicious anemia. *N Engl J Med* 273: 633-7.

Hsing AW, Hansson LE, Mclaughlin JK *et al.* (1993) Pernicious anemia and subsequent cancer. A population-based cohort study. *Cancer* 71: 745–50.

Hu PJ, Mitchell HM, Li YY, Zhou MH, Hazell SL. (1994) Association of *Helicobacter pylori* with gastric cancer and observations on the detection of this bacterium in gastric cancer cases. *Am J Gastroenterol* 89: 1806–10.

Huang BS, Unni KK, Payne WS. (1984) Long-term survival following diverticulectomy for cancer in pharyngoesophageal (Zenker's) diverticulum. *Ann Thorac Surg* 38: 207–10.

Huang JQ, Zheng GF, Sumanac K, Irvine EJ, Hunt RH. (2003) Meta-analysis of the relationship between cagA seropositivity and gastric cancer. *Gastroenterology* 125: 1636–44.

Hur C, Nishioka NS, Gazelle GS. (2004) Cost-effectiveness of aspirin chemoprevention for Barrett's esophagus. *J Natl Cancer Inst* 96: 316–25.

Iwaya T, Maesawa C, Ogasawara S, Tamura G. (1998) Tylosis esophageal cancer locus on chromosome 17q25.1 is commonly deleted in sporadic human esophageal cancer. *Gastroenterology* 114: 1206–10.

Jemal A, Siegel R, Ward E *et al.* (2006) Cancer statistics 2006. *CA Cancer J Clin* 56: 106–30.

Jenab M, Riboli E, Ferrari P *et al.* (2006a) Plasma and dietary carotenoid, retinol and tocopherol levels and the risk of gastric adenocarcinomas in the European prospective investigation into cancer and nutrition. *Br J Cancer* 95: 406–15.

Jenab M, Riboli E, Ferrari P *et al.* (2006b) Plasma and dietary vitamin C levels and risk of gastric cancer in the European Prospective Investigation into Cancer and Nutrition (EPIC-EURGAST). *Carcinogenesis* 27: 2250–7.

Joossens JV, Hill MJ, Elliott P *et al.* (1996) Dietary salt, nitrate and stomach cancer mortality in 24 countries. European Cancer Prevention (ECP) and the INTERSALT Cooperative Research Group. *Int J Epidemiol* 25: 494–504.

Kamineni A, Williams MA, Schwartz SM, Cook LS, Weiss NS. (1999) The incidence of gastric carcinoma in Asian migrants to the United States and their descendants. *Cancer Causes Control* 10: 77–83.

Kaneko S, Yoshimura T. (2001) Time trend analysis of gastric cancer incidence in Japan by histological types, 1975–1989. *Br J Cancer* 84: 400–5.

Kato I, Tominaga S, Matsumoto K. (1992) A prospective study of stomach cancer among a rural Japanese population: a 6-year survey. *Jpn J Cancer Res* 83: 568–75.

Klinkenberg-Knol EC, Festen HP, Jansen JB *et al.* (1994) Long-term treatment with omeprazole for refractory reflux esophagitis: efficacy and safety. *Ann Intern Med* 121: 161–7.

Kneller RW, Mclaughlin JK, Bjelke E *et al.* (1991) A cohort study of stomach cancer in a high-risk American population. *Cancer* 68: 672–8.

Koch P, Del Valle F, Berdel WE *et al.* (2001) Primary gastrointestinal non-Hodgkin's lymphoma: I. Anatomic and histologic distribution, clinical features, and survival data of 371 patients registered in the German Multicenter Study GIT NHL 01/92. *J Clin Oncol* 19: 3861–73.

Koizumi Y, Tsubono Y, Nakaya N *et al.* (2004) Cigarette smoking and the risk of gastric cancer: a pooled analysis of two prospective studies in Japan. *Int J Cancer* 112: 1049–55.

Kokkola A, Valle J, Haapiainen R, Sipponen P, Kivilaakso E, Puolakkainen P. (1996) *Helicobacter pylori* infection in young patients with gastric carcinoma. *Scand J Gastroenterol* 31: 643–7.

Kono S, Hirohata T. (1996) Nutrition and stomach cancer. *Cancer Causes Control* 7: 41–55.

Kubo A, Corley DA. (2002) Marked regional variation in adenocarcinomas of the esophagus and the gastric cardia in the United States. *Cancer* 95: 2096–102.

La Vecchia C, Negri E, D'Avanzo B, Franceschi S. (1990) Electric refrigerator use and gastric cancer risk. *Br J Cancer* 62: 136–7.

Lagergren J. (2005) Adenocarcinoma of oesophagus: what exactly is the size of the problem and who is at risk? *Gut* 54 Suppl 1: i1–5.

Lagergren J, Bergstrom R, Lindgren A, Nyren O. (1999a) Symptomatic gastroesophageal reflux as a risk factor for esophageal adenocarcinoma. *N Engl J Med* 340: 825–31.

Lagergren J, Bergstrom R, Nyren O. (1999b) Association between body mass and adenocarcinoma of the esophagus and gastric cardia. *Ann Intern Med* 130: 883–90.

Lagergren J, Bergstrom R, Adami HO, Nyren O. (2000) Association between medications that relax the lower esophageal sphincter and risk for esophageal adenocarcinoma. *Ann Intern Med* 133: 165–75.

Larsson LG, Sandstrom A, Westling P. (1975) Relationship of Plummer–Vinson disease to cancer of the upper alimentary tract in Sweden. *Cancer Res* 35: 3308–16.

Lauren P. (1965) The two histological main types of gastric carcinoma: diffuse and so-called intestinal-type carcinoma. an attempt at a histo-clinical classification. *Acta Pathol Microbiol Scand* 64: 31–49.

Lauren PA, Nevalainen TJ. (1993) Epidemiology of intestinal and diffuse types of gastric carcinoma. A time-trend study in Finland with comparison between studies from high- and low-risk areas. *Cancer* 71: 2926–33.

Levine PH, Stemmermann G, Lennette ET, Hildesheim A, Shibata D, Nomura A. (1995) Elevated antibody titers to Epstein–Barr virus prior to the diagnosis of Epstein–Barr-virus-associated gastric adenocarcinoma. *Int J Cancer* 60: 642–4.

Lindblad M, Rodriguez LA, Lagergren J. (2005) Body mass, tobacco and alcohol and risk of esophageal, gastric cardia, and gastric non-cardia adenocarcinoma among men and women in a nested case–control study. *Cancer Causes Control* 16: 285–94.

McMichael AJ, McCall MG, Hartshorne JM, Woodings TL. (1980) Patterns of gastro-intestinal cancer in European migrants to Australia: the role of dietary change. *Int J Cancer* 25: 431–7.

Mark SD, Qiao YL, Dawsey SM *et al.* (2000) Prospective study of serum selenium levels and incident esophageal and gastric cancers. *J Natl Cancer Inst* 92: 1753–63.

Mayne ST, Risch HA, Dubrow R *et al.* (2001) Nutrient intake and risk of subtypes of esophageal and gastric cancer. *Cancer Epidemiol Biomarkers Prev* 10: 1055–62.

Miettinen M, Sobin LH, Lasota J. (2005) Gastrointestinal stromal tumors of the stomach: a clinicopathologic, immunohistochemical, and molecular genetic study of 1765 cases with long-term follow-up. *Am J Surg Pathol* 29: 52–68.

Miros M, Kerlin P, Walker N. (1991) Only patients with dysplasia progress to adenocarcinoma in Barrett's oesophagus. *Gut* 32: 1441–6.

Moller H, Nissen A, Mosbech J. (1992) Use of cimetidine and other peptic ulcer drugs in Denmark 1977–1990 with analysis of the risk of gastric cancer among cimetidine users. *Gut* 33: 1166–9.

Nilsson B, Bumming P, Meis-Kindblom JM *et al.* (2005) Gastrointestinal stromal tumors: the incidence, prevalence, clinical course, and prognostication in the preimatinib mesylate era—a population-based study in western Sweden. *Cancer* 103: 821–9.

Nomura A, Grove JS, Stemmermann GN, Severson RK. (1990) A prospective study of stomach cancer and its relation to diet, cigarettes, and alcohol consumption. *Cancer Res* 50: 627–31.

Ogino T, Kato H, Tsukiyama I *et al.* (1992) Radiation-induced carcinoma of the esophagus. *Acta Oncol* 31: 475–7.

Overholt BF, Lightdale CJ, Wang KK *et al.* (2005) Photodynamic therapy with porfimer sodium for ablation of high-grade dysplasia in Barrett's esophagus: international, partially blinded, randomized phase III trial. *Gastrointest Endosc* 62: 488–98.

Palli D, Galli M, Caporaso NE *et al.* (1994) Family history and risk of stomach cancer in Italy. *Cancer Epidemiol Biomarkers Prev* 3: 15–8.

Parkin DM. (2006) The global health burden of infection-associated cancers in the year 2002. *Int J Cancer* 118: 3030–44.

Parkin DM, Laara E, Muir CS. (1988) Estimates of the worldwide frequency of sixteen major cancers in 1980. *Int J Cancer* 41: 184–97.

Parkin DM, Bray F, Ferlay J, Pisani P. (2005) Global cancer statistics, 2002. *CA Cancer J Clin* 55: 74–108.

Parsonnet J, Hansen S, Rodriguez L *et al.* (1994) *Helicobacter pylori* infection and gastric lymphoma. *N Engl J Med* 330: 1267–71.

Pickwell SM, Schimelpfening S, Palinkas LA. (1994) 'Betelmania'. Betel quid chewing by Cambodian women in the United States and its potential health effects. *West J Med* 160: 326–30.

Pohl H, Welch HG. (2005) The role of overdiagnosis and reclassification in the marked increase of esophageal adenocarcinoma incidence. *J Natl Cancer Inst* 97: 142–6.

Powitz F, Bogner JR, Sandor P, Zietz C, Goebel FD, Zoller WG. (1997) Gastrointestinal lymphomas in patients with AIDS. *Z Gastroenterol* 35: 179–85.

Rex DK, Cummings OW, Shaw M *et al.* (2003) Screening for Barrett's esophagus in colonoscopy patients with and without heartburn. *Gastroenterology* 125: 1670–7.

Ronkainen J, Aro P, Storskrubb T *et al.* (2005) Prevalence of Barrett's esophagus in the general population: an endoscopic study. *Gastroenterology* 129: 1825–31.

Sandler RS, Nyren O, Ekbom A, Eisen GM, Yuen J, Josefsson S. (1995) The risk of esophageal cancer in patients with achalasia. A population-based study. *JAMA* 274: 1359–62.

Santhi Swaroop V, Damle SR, Advani SH, Desai PB. (1989) Nutrition and esophageal cancer. *Semin Surg Oncol* 5: 370–2.

Sasazuki S, Inoue M, Iwasaki M *et al.* (2006) Effect of *Helicobacter pylori* infection combined with CagA and pepsinogen status on gastric cancer development among Japanese men and women: a nested case–control study. *Cancer Epidemiol Biomarkers Prev* 15: 1341–7.

Schnell TG, Sontag SJ, Chejfec G *et al.* (2001) Long-term nonsurgical management of Barrett's esophagus with high-grade dysplasia. *Gastroenterology* 120: 1607–19.

Shaheen NJ. (2005) Advances in Barrett's esophagus and esophageal adenocarcinoma. *Gastroenterology* 128: 1554–66.

Shaheen N, Ransohoff DF. (2002) Gastroesophageal reflux, Barrett esophagus, and esophageal cancer: scientific review. *JAMA* 287: 1972–81.

Shaheen NJ, Crosby MA, Bozymski EM, Sandler RS. (2000) Is there publication bias in the reporting of cancer risk in Barrett's esophagus? *Gastroenterology* 119: 333–8.

Sharma P, Sampliner RE, Camargo E. (1997) Normalization of esophageal pH with high-dose proton pump inhibitor therapy does not result in regression of Barrett's esophagus. *Am J Gastroenterol* 92: 582–5.

Sharma P, McQuaid K, Dent J *et al.* (2004) A critical review of the diagnosis and management of Barrett's esophagus: the AGA Chicago Workshop. *Gastroenterology* 127: 310–30.

Shikata K, Kiyohara Y, Kubo M *et al.* (2006) A prospective study of dietary salt intake and gastric cancer incidence in a defined Japanese population: the Hisayama study. *Int J Cancer* 119: 196–201.

Siddiqi M, Tricker AR, Preussmann R. (1988) The occurrence of preformed N-nitroso compounds in food samples from a high risk area of esophageal cancer in Kashmir, India. *Cancer Lett* 39: 37–43.

Srinivasan S, Takeshita K, Holkova B *et al.* (2004) Clinical characteristics of gastrointestinal lymphomas associated with AIDS (GI-ARL) and the impact of HAART. *HIV Clin Trials* 5: 140–5.

Stalnikowicz R, Benbassat J. (1990) Risk of gastric cancer after gastric surgery for benign disorders. *Arch Intern Med* 150: 2022–6.

Tersmette AC, Offerhaus GJ, Tersmette KW *et al.* (1990) Meta-analysis of the risk of gastric stump cancer: detection of high risk patient subsets for stomach cancer after remote partial gastrectomy for benign conditions. *Cancer Res* 50: 6486–9.

Tersmette AC, Goodman SN, Offerhaus GJ *et al.* (1991) Multivariate analysis of the risk of stomach cancer after ulcer surgery in an Amsterdam cohort of postgastrectomy patients. *Am J Epidemiol* 134: 14–21.

Thompson MP, Kurzrock R. (2004) Epstein–Barr virus and cancer. *Clin Cancer Res* 10: 803–21.

Thun MJ, Peto R, Lopez AD *et al.* (1997) Alcohol consumption and mortality among middle-aged and elderly US adults. *N Engl J Med* 337: 1705–14.

Thye T, Burchard GD, Nilius M, Muller-Myhsok B, Horstmann RD. (2003) Genomewide linkage analysis identifies polymorphism in the human interferon-gamma receptor affecting *Helicobacter pylori* infection. *Am J Hum Genet* 72: 448–53.

Tredaniel J, Boffetta P, Buiatti E, Saracci R, Hirsch A. (1997) Tobacco smoking and gastric cancer: review and meta-analysis. *Int J Cancer* 72: 565–73.

Trent JC, Benjamin RS. (2006) New developments in gastrointestinal stromal tumor. *Curr Opin Oncol* 18: 386–95.

Uemura N, Okamoto S, Yamamoto S *et al.* (2001) *Helicobacter pylori* infection and the development of gastric cancer. *N Engl J Med* 345: 784–9.

Yatsuya H, Toyoshima H, Tamakoshi A *et al.* (2004) Individual and joint impact of family history and *Helicobacter pylori* infection on the risk of stomach cancer: a nested case–control study. *Br J Cancer* 91: 929–34.

Ye W, Chow WH, Lagergren J, Yin L, Nyren O. (2001) Risk of adenocarcinomas of the esophagus and gastric cardia in patients with gastroesophageal reflux diseases and after antireflux surgery. *Gastroenterology* 121: 1286–93.

Ye W, Held M, Lagergren J *et al.* (2004) *Helicobacter pylori* infection and gastric atrophy: risk of adenocarcinoma and squamous-cell carcinoma of the esophagus and adenocarcinoma of the gastric cardia. *J Natl Cancer Inst* 96: 388–96.

Zhang ZF, Kurtz RC, Sun M *et al.* (1996) Adenocarcinomas of the esophagus and gastric cardia: medical conditions, tobacco, alcohol, and socioeconomic factors. *Cancer Epidemiol Biomarkers Prev* 5: 761–8.

Zhao L, Blot WJ, Liu WD *et al.* (1994) Familial predisposition to precancerous gastric lesions in a high-risk area of China. *Cancer Epidemiol Biomarkers Prev* 3: 461–4.

2 Factors involved in Carcinogenesis and Prevention

Mark R. Anderson & Janusz Jankowski

Introduction

The incidence of esophageal adenocarcinoma is increasing rapidly, at a rate of 4–10% annually in some Western countries. Despite continuing advances in neoadjuvant therapy and surgery, the 5-year survival rate remains less than 20%.

Gastric cancer has shown a declining incidence, but is still one of the leading causes of cancer-related death worldwide. The prognosis is closely related to the stage of disease at presentation, but the disease is often relatively asymptomatic in the early stages.

These grim statistics surrounding curative approaches have fuelled interest in the possibilities of risk reduction, screening and chemoprevention. In this chapter we discuss the lifestyle factors that may influence an individual's risk of developing upper gastrointestinal (GI) cancer, the role of screening and surveillance programs, and the potential effects of chemoprevention.

Modifiable lifestyle and dietary factors

Many of the identifiable risk factors for gastric and esophageal cancer cannot be altered by an individual. The sex and race of a person exert a large influence on cancer risk. Being Caucasian and male increases the risk of esophageal adenocarcinoma, and the incidence rates in US white males are over four times higher than in US black people. Gastric cancer shows a marked preponderance for high-risk ethnic groups (e.g. Japanese, Korean) and first-generation migrants bring their native risk rate with them.

Smoking and alcohol are most commonly quoted as modifiable risk factors. However, the role of these potential carcinogens is not clear cut. Smokers have a two-fold increased risk of squamous esophageal carcinoma and proximal gastric cancer, but the association with esophageal adenocarcinoma is weaker. The percentage of adults who smoke has steadily fallen since 1975 in the UK, but the annual rise in incidence of esophageal adenocarcinoma has continued unabated. Alcohol is also linked to squamous esophageal carcinoma but large case–control studies have failed to show a strong association between alcohol intake and either gastric cancer or esophageal adenocarcinoma (Lindblad *et al.* 2005).

Obesity is arguably a risk factor that is modifiable by the individual. The prevalence of obesity in most populations has risen alongside the rising incidence of esophageal adenocarcinoma. Obesity has been established as an independent risk factor for gastric cardia and esophageal adenocarcinoma in several studies, with up to a 16-fold increase in risk being defined in patients with the highest body mass index quartile (Chow *et al.* 1998a; Lagergren *et al.* 1999).

Dietary factors are thought to play a significant role in the development of esophageal and gastric cancer and much work has centered on elucidating the relevant dietary components. Diets high in total fat, saturated fat and cholesterol have been

Table 2.1 Factors that are postulated to increase the risk of upper gastrointestinal malignancy.

Esophageal	Gastric
Male sex	Chronic gastritis
Chronic gastroesophageal reflux disease	*Helicobacter pylori*
Barrett's metaplasia	High-salt diet
Bile acid exposure	Nitrates
Chronic inflammation	Obesity
Smoking (squamous cell)	Hypergastrinemia
Obesity	Low socioeconomic status
Alcohol	Genetic predisposition
High-fat diet	Smoking (proximal gastric)
Micronutrient deficiencies	Red meat intake
Hypergastrinemia	
Caucasian	
N-nitroso compounds	

Gastrointestinal Oncology: A Critical Multidisciplinary Team Approach.
Edited by J. Jankowski, R. Sampliner, D. Kerr, and Y. Fong.

associated with esophageal adenocarcinoma (Mayne *et al.* 2001). Diets containing high levels of fruit and vegetables have long been associated with reduced risk of several GI cancers. Fruit and vegetables have been thought to protect against esophageal cancer (Steinmetz & Potter 1996) and attempts have been made to isolate the specific dietary micronutrients that are beneficial. It is suggested that vitamin and mineral supplementation may reduce esophageal cancer risk (Blot *et al.* 1993). Oxidative damage to DNA is recognized as playing an important role in the pathogenesis of many cancers. Reflux disease in the esophagus and chronic gastritis in the stomach are both causes of chronic inflammation associated with the production of reactive oxygen species that cause DNA damage. It has been suggested therefore that dietary supplementation with antioxidant vitamins (e.g. vitamins C and E) may inhibit development of these cancers, although evidence is limited to animal models and case–control studies that use food intake as a surrogate marker for antioxidant potential. Certainly the available epidemiological data suggest a weakly protective effect of diets that are rich in fruit, green vegetables and fish, and that are low in red meat. This is different from showing that a specific dietary supplement will reduce cancer risk. There have even been concerns raised that some high-dose multivitamin preparations may actually promote carcinogenesis.

Until recently most supporting evidence for diet-associated risk modification was from meta-analyses and case–control studies only. The recent European Prospective Investigation into Cancer and Nutrition (EPIC) study reported findings from a large cohort study that included over half a million participants. Despite the size of the study, only weak non-significant associations were found between vegetable or citrus intake and reduced risk of gastric cancer and esophageal adenocarcinoma. An association between total meat intake and increased gastric non-cardia cancer was shown, but not cancers of the gastric cardia (Gonzalez *et al.* 2006a,b).

A cancer-promoting effect has been ascribed to nitrates and N-nitroso compounds following data from case–control studies (Hansson *et al.* 1994). Most dietary nitrate comes from fertilizer use. Absorbed dietary nitrates are secreted in saliva where buccal bacteria then convert them into nitrite. When this mixes with gastric acid the nitrite is converted into nitrous acid and other potentially carcinogenic N-nitroso compounds (McColl 2005). The production of reactive nitrogen species is thought to be maximal at the esophagogastric junction and it has been postulated that this nitrite chemistry contributes to the incidence of esophageal adenocarcinoma. Certainly the mixing of saliva and gastric acid would occur in different anatomical sites in patients with reflux disease than in normal individuals, and reflux episodes have been shown to cause marked rises in nitric oxide levels. However, there is no evidence that changes in agricultural techniques have ever influenced national cancer incidence rates, and a large cohort study concluded that exposure to N-nitroso compounds may be associated with an increased risk of colorectal but not upper GI malignancies (Knekt *et al.* 1999).

High dietary salt intake has also been proposed as a promoter of gastric carcinogenesis. However, the consumption of highly salted food tends to occur in diets also low in fresh fruit and vegetables, so it is hard to assess this as an independent variable.

What is clear from the above is that there is a need for evidence from large randomized controlled studies before we can assess with certainty the long-term effects of specific dietary modifications.

Table 2.2 Factors suggested to be protective in upper gastrointestinal malignancy.

Esophageal	Gastric
Proton pump inhibitors	Low-salt diet
Aspirin	*H. pylori* eradication
NSAIDs	NSAIDs
H. pylori	Prophylactic gastrectomy (if E-cadherin gene mutation)
Micronutrient supplementation	
Fiber	
Fruit and vegetables	

NSAIDs, non-steroidal anti-inflammatory drugs.

Helicobacter pylori

No definite association has been established between *Helicobacter pylori* and esophageal adenocarcinoma. In fact, a possible protective role has been suggested. Chronic gastritis caused by the infection can result in gastric atrophy and reduced gastric acidity (Chow *et al.* 1998b). It has even been postulated that the rising incidence of esophageal adenocarcinoma may be related to a declining incidence of *H. pylori* colonization in the Western world.

However, when it comes to gastric cancer, *H. pylori* colonization of the gastric mucosa is probably the most prevalent and least debatable carcinogen considered to increase gastric carcinogenesis. In 1994 *H. pylori* was classified as a type 1 carcinogen by the World Health Organization International Agency for Research on Cancer. The exact pathogenetic mechanisms are still being debated but certainly there is interplay between environmental, bacterial, host and genetic factors, with interleukin-1 and tumor necrosis factor-alpha playing key roles in the chronic inflammation. Epidemiological studies suggest that the presence of *H. pylori* infection with Cag-A antigen causes a 20-fold increase in gastric cancer risk.

However, what is less clear is whether *H. pylori* eradication will prevent or reduce gastric cancer. Nearly 50% of the world's population is colonized by *H. pylori*, but no more than 1% will ever develop gastric neoplasia.

The best proof of a reduction in cancer risk by *H. pylori* eradication would come from a prospective randomized clinical trial. However, attempts at such trials are fraught with difficulties, not least concerning ethical approval, recruitment and the large sample size needed. It is hard to convince a patient to have their type-1 carcinogen treated only with placebo. Consequently smaller trials have been performed and surrogate endpoints have been studied such as intestinal metaplasia or cancer recurrence to serve as possible markers of reduced cancer risk. A non-randomized study of 132 Japanese patients who had undergone endoscopic resection of gastric cancer showed that 9% had recurrence at 2 years if *H. pylori* had not been eradicated, compared to none of those who had been treated (Uemura *et al.* 1997). In China a placebo-controlled randomized study to assess the effect of eradication ran for 7 years and showed a reduced incidence of gastric cancer, but only in the subgroup of patients without atrophy or intestinal metaplasia at baseline (Wong & Lam 2004). Furthermore, these studies are from high-risk ethnic groups and it is not known whether these results can be extrapolated to Western populations. It seems feasible that widespread eradication of *helicobacter pylori* may lead to a measurable risk reduction only in groups with a high incidence of gastric cancer. A recent international panel reported their conclusions from an evidence-based workshop (Malfertheiner *et al.* 2005). They suggested that a screen-and-treat strategy should only be focused on first-degree relatives of gastric cancer patients and recognized high-risk populations.

Endoscopic screening and surveillance

Whilst the presence of Barrett's metaplasia is a recognized risk factor for the development of esophageal adenocarcinoma, much debate has continued around the benefit of regular surveillance endoscopy and biopsy sampling for high-grade dysplasia or neoplasia in those patients. It has been shown in case series of individuals under surveillance that esophageal cancers detected as part of a screening program are found at an earlier stage than in non-surveyed patients. However, there is less evidence that surveillance programs significantly reduce mortality. The cost-effective interval for surveillance endoscopy varies according to incidence in the population. In the UK, where the cancer risk in Barrett's patients is approximately 1% every 2 years, current guidelines suggest that 2-yearly surveillance will cost over £19,000 per life saved, although this is based on a Markov model with many assumptions made (BSG 2005). The evidence from cohort data is liable to bias, in particular lead-time bias (cancers merely detected earlier but time of death unchanged) and length-time bias (slower-growing lesions more likely to be found at the next surveillance procedure). In any case it should not be forgotten that surveillance is only of relevance in those patients who have their Barrett's metaplasia diagnosed, and over 90% of cases go undetected. Currently less than 4% of esophageal adenocarcinomas are detected from a surveillance program. Given this scenario, it is unlikely that surveillance endoscopy for Barrett's metaplasia can ever influence national mortality rates overall.

The survival from gastric cancer is also closely linked to the stage of disease at diagnosis. Early gastric cancer (EGC), where the disease is confined to the mucosa or submucosa, has a 5-year survival rate of over 90% in some series. This has prompted the development of mass-screening programs in high-incidence populations. Japan has one such population, where over 100,000 cases of gastric cancer are diagnosed every year. In 1960, the Japanese government funded a screening program of endoscopy for asymptomatic individuals over the age of 40. Since then reports of the proportion of gastric cancer that is found as EGC have shown an increase from 8% before screening to over 50% since. The 5-year survival rate for gastric cancer in Japan has doubled since the 1960s. By comparison, in Western countries the proportion of gastric cancers diagnosed at an early stage remains less than 20%. However, the incidence of gastric cancer is much lower in the US and Western Europe, and so mass screening with endoscopy would have a low yield, making it not cost effective. In these areas, endoscopic screening needs to be targeted at high-risk groups, and those groups are hard to define (Tan & Fielding 2006). Certainly dyspepsia is common in the majority of EGC cases, and the development of open-access endoscopy for individuals with new dyspeptic symptoms could be viewed as a screening approach to detecting gastric cancer early. Of course dyspepsia itself is common, and leads to many primary care contacts. Whilst it may seem pragmatic for general practitioners to try treatment with acid suppression first, before referral for endoscopy, this should probably be avoided in the over-45s. Early gastric cancer may temporarily heal and epithelialize over following acid suppression, rendering it invisible at endoscopy. Several case studies have reported the temporary healing of a malignant ulcer with proton pump inhibitors (PPIs). Therefore the injudicious use of PPIs prior to investigation may reduce the benefit of screening dyspeptic patients and lead to false-negative endoscopy reports.

Other high-risk groups have been suggested, including those with chronic gastritis and post-gastrectomy patients. *Helicobacter pylori*-associated atrophic gastritis is linked to a sixfold increased risk of gastric cancer. Intestinal metaplasia may occur with patches of altered gastric mucosa that appear histologically similar to small bowel mucosa. In the presence of altered glandular architecture, this metaplasia is associated with an estimated 10-fold increased lifetime risk of gastric cancer. Screening of these patients has also been suggested, although no hard data exist to confirm benefit. Similarly, although a history of gastric surgery is associated with an increased risk, an endoscopic screening program of post-gastrectomy patients failed to show a significant detection rate (Schafer *et al.* 1983). Patients with hereditary non-polyposis colorectal cancer are known to be at increased of gastric cancer but surveillance of this group was also shown to carry no significant benefit.

One rare group are those families with hereditary diffuse gastric cancer, a syndrome described by the International Gastric Cancer Linkage Consortium (IGCLC) (Caldas *et al.* 1999). It presents early in families carrying a germline-inactivating mutation of the E-cadherin gene. Penetrance for gastric cancer in these families is thought to be around 70%. Germline and somatic mutations in the E-cadherin gene (which encodes a cell adhesion protein) seem solely associated with the diffuse type of gastric cancer and the IGCLC have stressed the need to ensure familial cases are of diffuse type before undergoing mutation analysis. Currently they define the syndrome as i) two or more cases of diffuse-type gastric cancer in first/second-degree relatives with one diagnosed before the age of 50, or ii) three or more cases of diffuse-type gastric cancer in first/second-degree relatives regardless of age. In families that fit these criteria, the E-cadherin gene mutation is found in nearly 30% of cases. However, it has been suggested that an individual found to be carrying this mutation should be considered for more than just screening endoscopy and should be offered prophylactic gastrectomy.

It seems therefore that endoscopic screening programs are of benefit in populations with high incidence rates, such as in the far East. In Western countries we are still left trying to target our screening approaches at high-risk groups, and these remain hard to identify.

Chemoprevention

The term 'chemoprevention' has been in use since the late 1970s, and is defined as the prevention or retardation of cancer by using agents or drugs to suppress or reverse the carcinogenic processes. In recent years, two theoretical approaches to chemoprevention have arisen with regard to gastric and esophageal cancer. Those are acid suppression and inflammatory modulation, in the form of aspirin or cyclo-oxygenase inhibition.

Chemoprevention by acid suppression

Acid suppression is already the cornerstone of management in reflux disease and Barrett's metaplasia. Patients with metaplasia are known to have more frequent and prolonged periods of esophageal acid exposure, and at first it seems theoretically possible that acid suppression may impede the progress of carcinogenesis. Certainly, *in vitro* studies have shown that biopsy specimens of Barrett's epithelium have been shown to exhibit hyperproliferation and increased expression of cyclo-oxygenase 2 (COX-2) when exposed to acid (Fitzgerald *et al.* 1996). Acid exposure has also been shown to activate the mitogen-activated protein kinase (MAPK) pathways that have a role in increasing cell proliferation and survival and in decreasing apoptosis (Souza *et al.* 2002).

However, there is an absence of clear clinical data to show that acid suppression alters long-term consequences of this disease. Clinical studies showing slight regressions in the surface area of Barrett's metaplasia following PPI therapy have not been widely replicated, and even then it is not known whether a less than 10% regression of the surface area of metaplastic epithelium makes any difference to long-term cancer risk. It is an inescapable fact that the incidence of esophageal adenocarcinoma has continued to rise throughout the era of PPIs. The doses of PPI needed to abolish reflux symptoms are lower than those needed to achieve full acid suppression, a fact that further hampers attempts to find consistent clinical data regarding effects on cancer incidence. One prospective study that focused on the progression to dysplasia in a cohort of over 200 patients has provided evidence suggesting that PPIs are linked to a reduced risk of dysplasia (El-Serag *et al.* 2004), but larger prospective trials are needed.

One opposing line of thought is that PPIs may actually increase the risk of adenocarcinoma, with the suggested mechanisms including hypoacidity, hypergastrinemia and subsequent enterochromaffin-like cell hyperplasia. Gastrin can give a pro-proliferation signal to cells *in vitro*. This theory would fit with the epidemiological observations of rising incidence rates alongside the use of more potent acid suppression medication. However, the incidence of esophageal adenocarcinoma was

Table 2.3 Factors affecting the strength of proposed cancer prevention strategies.

Cancer prevention strategy	Cost per person	Evidence from RCT or case–control studies	Applicable to whole population	Advice likely followed by public, or tests acceptable to public	Risks
Reduce alcohol/smoking	Low	Weak	Yes	Yes	Nil
Reduce fat intake/obesity	Low	Weak	Yes	No? Obesity increasing.	Nil
Dietary supplements (e.g. vitamins)	Low	No	Yes	Yes	Low
Endoscopic surveillance	High	Weak	No, high-risk groups only	Yes	High
Endoscopic screening	High	Yes	No, high-risk groups only	Unknown	High
H. pylori eradication	Moderate	No	Yes, test and treat	Yes	Low
Chemoprevention	Moderate/high (depends on drug used)	Yes	Yes, but may be targeted at symptomatic groups	Yes	Moderate (depends on drug used)

already rising before the introduction of the first PPI, and a recent study of 18,000 patients treated with omeprazole found no increased incidence of gastric or esophageal cancer (Bateman *et al.* 2003).

Long-term studies show that PPIs have a very low side-effect profile overall and still merit further research into their potential for modulating the carcinogenesis sequence. At the very least they may have an important role in reducing the risk of the second approach to chemoprevention, by combining them with the inhibitors of the inflammatory pathway.

Chemoprevention by aspirin/COX inhibition

Chronic inflammation appears intricately linked to the process of carcinogenesis in the upper GI tract, whether as a consequence of acid reflux in the esophagus or of chronic gastritis in the stomach. In addition, population-based studies have shown associations between long-term use of non-steroidal anti-inflammatory drugs (NSAIDs) and reduced incidence of several cancers. These two facts have led to a focus on anti-inflammatory agents as potential chemopreventive drugs.

The principal target of NSAIDs is cyclo-oxygenase (COX), which converts arachidonic acid to prostaglandins. COX exists in two distinct isoforms. COX-1 is expressed constitutively in many tissues where it may be viewed as maintaining physiologic housekeeping functions. COX-2, however, is only present in very low levels in normal tissues, but is upregulated pathologically by pro-inflammatory cytokines, growth factors and tumor promoters, and as such is viewed as a harbinger of inflammation. It has been linked to inhibition of apoptosis, an increase in cell growth and survival, and also neoangiogenesis, and has come to be seen as important in carcinogenesis. Prostaglandin-E2, a product of COX-2, has procarcinogenic effects. It stimulates the antiapoptotic protein bcl-2 and induces IL-6, an interleukin associated with tumor metastasis, invasion, implantation, and angiogenesis. The overexpression of COX-2 has been well described in patients with Barrett's metaplasia, esophageal adenocarcinoma, *H. pylori*-induced gastritis and gastric adenocarcinoma, and tumors with a high COX-2 content may have a more aggressive course (Buskens *et al.* 2002). COX-2 inhibition may limit the disease in animal models with esophageal adenocarcinoma (Buttar *et al.* 2002).

Aspirin has multiple effects on the inflammatory process, whilst NSAIDs and the newer COX-2 inhibitors show more selectivity. In light of this, several large population studies have assessed whether chronic users of aspirin or NSAIDs have an associated reduced risk of esophageal or gastric cancers.

One of the largest studies by Thun *et al.* (1993) observed a cohort of around 650,000 individuals for up to 10 years. They showed a risk reduction for both esophageal and gastric cancer in recurrent users of aspirin or NSAIDs. In particular, the risk of gastric cancer was halved in those people reporting regular use of aspirin more than 16 times a month, and the risk of esophageal adenocarcinoma was reduced by 40%. Similarly other cohort and case–control studies have reported risk reductions of between 40% and 90%, varying with the level of drug use, the duration of follow-up, and the cancer concerned. The risk reductions seen in case–control studies have been greater for non-cardia gastric adenocarcinoma than for cancers of the cardia. A meta-analysis of these studies has estimated a 43% risk reduction for esophageal adenocarcinoma in individuals on aspirin or NSAIDs (Corley *et al.* 2003). From this meta-analysis, the potential for chemopreventive efficacy of aspirin appears greater than that of NSAIDs. The overall protective effect of aspirin is suggested as 50% compared to 25% for NSAIDs. Also, the use of these drugs has to be frequent to achieve this associated effect.

Obviously such epidemiological data are prone to confounding factors. The regular use of aspirin may be associated with additional lifestyle factors that have not been excluded, for instance vitamin supplementation or health-seeking behavior. Conversely those individuals with chronic dyspeptic symptoms may have been less likely to be prescribed aspirin or NSAIDs, all of which may lead to false associations.

A recent prospective study that followed a cohort of 350 people with Barrett's metaplasia for 21,000 person-months, calculated hazard ratios for esophageal adenocarcinoma according to use of NSAIDs. The ratio for current NSAID users was 0.32 compared to never-users (Vaughan *et al.* 2005). However, evidence from prospective studies is limited and randomized clinical trials are needed. Furthermore, the enthusiasm for the widespread use of NSAIDs in healthy individuals is hampered by concerns over toxicity. At one time it was expected that the risk of GI hemorrhage would be overcome by the use of selective COX-2 inhibitors, which cause less injury to GI mucosa. However, considerable attention has been recently focused on the cardiovascular side-effects of these agents, with some high-profile cases against the makers of Rofecoxib appearing in the media. Concerns have also arisen over the side-effect profile of other COX-2 inhibitors, and it seems unlikely these will ever be used as chemopreventive agents in healthy populations. Most commentators have excluded them as viable candidates for use in low-risk groups. If non-selective NSAIDs were to be used, the fundamental questions around safety, efficacy, choice of agent, dosing, and duration of use would all need to be answered. In any case, if the epidemiological data are proven correct, it may be that aspirin is the most potent chemopreventive agent of all. There are certainly several biochemical reasons why aspirin may be more effective. Multiple inflammatory pathways are active in Barrett's metaplasia and chronic gastritis, and it seems logical that agents designed to be inhibitory against a single pathway (e.g. COX activity) may be rendered less suitable by the very selectivity they were designed to have. Aspirin, on the other hand, has been associated with multiple anti-inflammatory mechanisms *in vitro*, including the suppression of MAPK pathways, inhibition of cytokine signaling via NFkappaB, proapoptotic effects, and reduced beta-catenin signaling. Additionally, aspirin has more long-term safety data than any of the other suggested agents. Concerns about GI bleeding may be circumvented by the coadministration of a PPI. Whilst aspirin alone increases the GI bleed risk by two- to fourfold, this is dramatically cut when it is given in conjunction with a PPI.

When it comes to chemoprevention by anti-inflammatory agents, or by acid suppression for that matter, it is data from a randomized clinical trial that are really needed. In the UK, the AspECT trial (Aspirin and Esomeprazole Chemoprevention Trial) is attempting to address this need. This is a national multicenter phase III randomized clinical trial aiming to recruit 2000 male patients and 1000 female patients with Barrett's metaplasia to one of four treatment arms, consisting of low- or high-dose acid suppression, and aspirin or no aspirin long term. The trial then plans to survey these patients for up to 10 years and will report on the incidence rates of high-grade dysplasia and esophageal adenocarcinoma as clinical endpoints. Recruitment, which began in 2005, is well under way with 2000 already recruited. The potential to prevent the progression of Barrett's metaplasia to cancer by the use of PPIs and aspirin certainly holds clinical appeal. The results of such trials will be eagerly awaited.

Conclusions

Gastric and esophageal cancers remain a major health concern globally and despite advances in surgery and neoadjuvant therapies, prevention remains the only convincing approach to reducing morbidity and mortality on a wide scale. Endoscopic screening programs may have a role in certain high-risk populations, but in most parts of the world the high-risk groups are not readily identifiable and surveillance will not significantly reduce the national burden of disease. Similarly, the widespread eradication of *H. pylori* may be of benefit in some groups, but overall there is still a lack of evidence to show this will significantly reduce national incidence rates of gastric cancer.

Interest surrounds dietary factors and lifestyle modification, but the actual key elements of the diet that are of importance have proven elusive to identify. Evidence as it stands amounts to general advice to eat 'healthily', a suggestion that has been made many times in the past regarding cardiovascular disease but which has been met with rising obesity rates.

Therefore it may transpire that the real chance of significant risk reduction lies with chemoprevention using simple and safe agents that are acceptable to the healthy population. Large clinical trials are needed, but these will be rare and costly, and will take several years until they bear fruit. It may one day be the case that an aspirin–PPI combi-pill a day keeps the cancer away, but until then we can expect to see a significant disease burden for many years to come.

References

Bateman DN, Colin-Jones D, Hartz S *et al.* (2003) Mortality study of 18,000 patients treated with omeprazole. *Gut* 52: 942–6.

Blot WJ, Li JY, Taylor PR *et al.* (1993) Nutrition intervention trials in Linxian, China: supplementation with specific vitamin/mineral combinations, cancer incidence, and disease-specific mortality in the general population. *J Natl Cancer Inst* 85(18): 1483–92.

British Society of Gastroenterology (BSG). (2005) *Guidelines for the Diagnosis and Management of Barrett's Columnar-Lined Oesophagus. A Report of the Working Party of the British Society of Gastroenterology.* www.bsg.org.uk [accessed 2005]

Buskens CJ, Van Rees BP, Sivula A *et al.* (2002) Prognostic significance of elevated cyclooxygenase-2 expression in patients with adenocarcinoma of the oesophagus. *Gastroenterology* 122: 1800–07.

Buttar NS, Wang KK, Leontovich O *et al.* (2002) Chemoprevention of esophageal adenocarcinoma by COX-2 inhibitors in an animal model of Barrett's esophagus. *Gastroenterology* 112: 1101–12.

Caldas C, Carneiro F, Lynch H *et al.* (1999) Familial gastric cancer: overview and guidelines for management. *J Med Genet* 36: 873–80.

Chow WH, Blot WJ, Vaughan TL. (1998a) Body mass index and risk of adenocarcinomas of the esophagus and gastric cardia. *J Natl Cancer Inst* 90: 150–55.

Chow WH, Blaser MJ, Blot WJ, Gammon MD, Vaughan TL, Risch HA *et al.* (1998b) An inverse relation between cagA+ strains of *Helicobacter pylori* infection and risk of esophageal and gastric cardia adenocarcinoma. *Cancer Research* 58: 588–90.

Corley DA, Kerlikowske K, Verma R, Buffler P. (2003) Protective association of aspirin/NSAIDs and oesophageal cancer: a systematic review and meta-analysis. *Gastroenterology* 124: 47–56.

El-Serag HB, Aguirre TV, Davis S, Kuebeler M, Bhattacharyya A, Sampliner RE. (2004) Proton pump inhibitors are associated with reduced incidence of dysplasia in Barrett's esophagus. *Am J Gastroenterol* 99: 1877–83.

Fitzgerald RC, Omary MB, Triadafilopoulos G. (1996) Dynamic effects of acid on Barrett's esophagus. An ex vivo proliferation and differentiation model. *J Clin Invest* 98: 2120–28.

Gonzalez CA, Jakszyn P, Pera G *et al.* (2006a) Meat intake and risk of stomach and esophageal adenocarcinoma within the European Prospective Investigation into Cancer and Nutrition (EPIC). *J Natl Cancer Inst* 98: 345–54.

Gonzalez CA, Pera G, Agudo A *et al.* (2006b) Fruit and vegetable intake and the risk of stomach and oesophagus adenocarcinoma in the European Prospective Investigation into Cancer and Nutrition (EPIC-EURGAST). *Int J Cancer* 118: 2559–66.

Hansson LE, Nyren O, Bergstrom R. (1994) Nutrients and gastric cancer risk: a population-based case–control study in Sweden. *Int J Cancer* 57: 638–44.

Knekt P, Jarvinen R, Dich J, Hakulinen T. (1999) Risk of colorectal and other gastrointestinal cancers after exposure to nitrates, nitrites and N-nitroso compounds: a follow-up study. *Int J Cancer* 80(6): 852–56.

Lagergren J, Bergstrom R, Nyren O. (1999) Association between body mass and adenocarcinoma of the esophagus and gastric cardia. *Ann Intern Med* 130(11): 883–90.

Lindblad M, Rodriguez LA, Lagergren J. (2005) Body mass, tobacco and alcohol and risk of esophageal, gastric cardia, and gastric non-cardia adenocarcinoma among men and women in a nested case–control study. *Cancer Causes Control* 16: 285–94.

McColl KE. (2005) When saliva meets acid: chemical warfare at the oeosphagogastric junction. *Gut* 54(1): 1–3.

Malfertheiner P, Sipponen P, Naumann M *et al.* (2005) *Helicobacter* eradication has the potential to prevent gastric cancer: A state of the art critique. *Am J Gastroenterol* 100: 2100–115.

Mayne ST, Risch HA, Dubrow R *et al.* (2001) Nutrient intake and risk of subtypes of esophageal and gastric cancer. *Cancer Epidemiol Biomarkers Prev* 10(10): 1055–62.

Schafer LW, Larson DE, Melton LJ III, Higgins JA, Ilstrup DM. (1983) The risk of gastric carcinoma after surgical treatment for benign disease. *N Engl J Med* 309: 1210–13.

Souza RF, Shewmake K, Terada LS, Spechler S. (2002) Acid exposure activates the mitogen activated protein kinase pathways in Barrett's oesophagus. *Gastroenterology* 122: 299–307.

Steinmetz KA, Potter JD. (1996) Vegetables, fruit and cancer prevention: a review. *J Am Diet Assoc* 96(10): 1027–39.

Tan YK, Fielding JW. (2006) Early diagnosis of early gastric cancer. *Eur J Gastroenterol Hepatol* 18: 821–9.

Thun MJ, Namboodiri MM, Calle EE, Flanders WD, Heath CW. (1993) Aspirin use and risk of fatal cancer. *Cancer Research* 53: 1322–7.

Uemura N, Mukai T, Okamoto S *et al.* (1997) Effect of *Helicobacter pylori* eradication on subsequent development of cancer after endoscopic resection of early gastric cancer. *Cancer Epidemiol Biomarkers Prev* 6: 639–42.

Vaughan TL, Dong LM, Blount PL *et al.* (2005) Non-steroidal anti-inflammatory drugs and risk of neoplastic progression in Barrett's oesophagus: a prospective study. *Lancet Oncol* 6: 945–52.

Wong BC, Lam SK. (2004) *Helicobacter pylori* eradication to prevent gastric cancer in a high-risk region of China: A randomized controlled trial. *JAMA* 291: 187–94.

3 Molecular Biology of Gastroesophageal Cancers: the Role of Mutational Analysis in Prognosis

Matthew Lovell, Chetan Bhan, Janusz Jankowski & Stuart McDonald

Upper gastrointestinal tract malignancies are some of the most commonly diagnosed cancers worldwide. They are complex diseases and consequently the biological pathways involved in their development are similarly complex. It is beyond the scope of this chapter to give a detailed description of each of the pathways involved. Instead, we have endeavored to provide an insight into the role of the molecular biology involved and its clinical relevance in terms of prognosis of gastric and esophageal cancer.

Molecular biology of esophageal cancer

Unfortunately, a diagnosis of esophageal cancer is usually a preterminal event. Mortality statistics back this view up—it has one of the highest mortality rates of any cancer (Holmes & Vaughan 2007). There are two major forms of this disease, esophageal squamous cell carcinoma (ESSC) and adenocarcinoma. Although ESSC remains the most common form worldwide, its incidence has been declining consistently over the last 20 years (Williams *et al.* 1971). During the same period the incidence of esophageal adenocarcinoma has risen remarkably (Holmes & Vaughan 2007).

ESSC is thought to originate as an epithelial dysplasia, which initially develops as a mild to severe dysplasia and eventually becomes invasive carcinoma. Smoking and substantial alcohol intake are the risk factors for the vast majority of ESSC cases, with only a small proportion being familial (Lagergren *et al.* 2000). Adenocarcinoma, on the other hand, is linked not to smoking (Wu *et al.* 2001) but to chronic gastroesophageal reflux disease (GERD) which can lead to the development of metaplasia (Barrett's esophagus; 5–8% of GERD population). Progression occurs from metaplasia to dysplasia and ultimately to adenocarcinoma in 0.5% per year (Shaheen & Ransohoff 2002). Here we discuss the molecular biology of these diseases and concentrate on the major implicated mechanisms that lead to cancer development in the esophagus.

Gastrointestinal Oncology: A Critical Multidisciplinary Team Approach.
Edited by J. Jankowski, R. Sampliner, D. Kerr, and Y. Fong.

Esophageal squamous cell carcinoma

Growth factors

The epidermal growth factor receptor (EGFR) family consists of four members: erbB1 and erbB2–4, all of which possess an extracellular domain and signal through tyrosine kinase pathways upon binding with their ligands. Activation of the receptor initiates other signaling molecules such as mitogen-activated protein kinase (MAPK) and phosphatidylinositol-3-kinase (PI_3K). EGFR-mediated gene transcription has been implicated in cell growth, survival and chemotaxis (Burgess *et al.* 2003). It has long been recognized that EGFRs are overexpressed in stratified squamous carcinomas (SSCs) and there is a relationship between high EGFR expression and poor prognosis of ESSC, possibly due to a reduced efficacy of chemoradiotherapy (Hirai *et al.* 1998). As a prognostic marker EGFRs could be useful, but as yet there have been no specific genetic defects associated with this family. The targeting of EGFRs may, however, provide potential novel therapies, especially when targeted towards the prevention of EGFR signaling.

Transforming growth factor beta (TGFβ) is a pleiotropic cytokine, which appears to play a central role in epithelial homeostasis. It binds to two receptors, type I and type II (Fig. 3.1). TGFβ-mediated gene transcription, through activation of these receptors, involves Smad proteins (Massague & Wotton 2000). Of these, a reduction in Smad4 expression leads to a dysfunction in TGFβ signaling and this has been implicated in the development of epithelial cancers (Akhurst & Derynck 2001). This results in a decrease in *c-myc* expression (Chen *et al.* 2001; Feng *et al.* 2002), and a subsequent G1 arrest of the cell cycle due to inhibition of promoters of the cell cycle such as *p21*. Mutations in the TGFβ type II receptor gene have been reported in hereditary non-polyposis colon cancer but are extremely rare in ESSC. Similarly, mutations in the *SMAD4* gene have been reported in pancreatic and colonic cancer but mutation in *SMAD* genes is

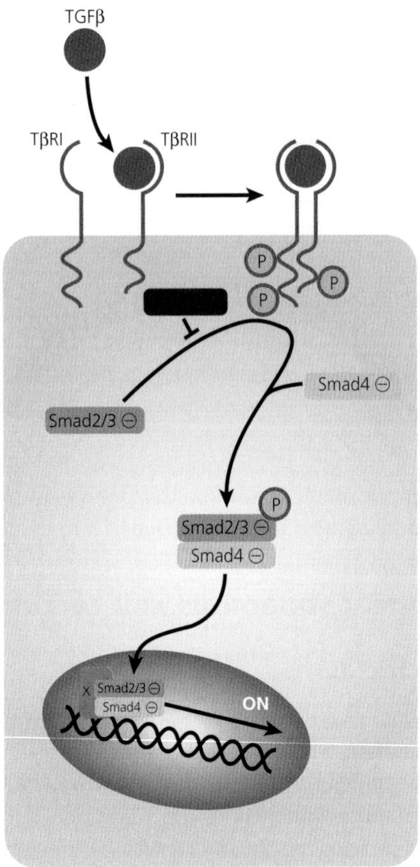

Fig. 3.1 The TGFβ signaling pathway. TGFβ binds to TGFβRII which sequesters TGFβR1 and the intracellular tail of this complex is phosphorylated, allowing binding of Smad2/3 with Smad4. This transcription complex can then bind to specific TGFβ-dependent gene promoters. This pathway is effectively blocked by Smad7 interacting with Smad2/3.

rare in ESSC (Osawa *et al.* 2000). As for use as prognostic markers, a reduction in Smad4 expression has correlated well with poor outcome (Fukuchi *et al.* 2002).

Cell-cycle proteins

As with all cancers, changes in expression of factors that regulate the control of the cell cycle (cell division) have been heavily implicated, in particular p53 and p21. Fig. 3.2 illustrates a summary of the major p53/p21 pathways.

p53

Dysfunction of p53 protein is a characteristic of the majority of human cancers. It serves as a tumor suppressor protein and is produced in response to events such as DNA damage, inflammation and hypoxia. One of its major functions is to downregulate *bcl-2* while upregulating *bax,* with the consequence that apoptosis is induced. As well as DNA damage, p53 may be induced by oncogenes such as *myc, E1A* and *E2F* (Fridman & Lowe 2003). If p53 is absent, cells are unable to undergo DNA damage induced- or oncogene-mediated apoptosis and therefore these cells sustain a growth advantage and can continue to expand. p53 knockout mice are resistant to radiation-induced apoptosis (Clarke *et al.* 1993), and p53 deficiency has been shown to correlate with tumor progression (Symonds *et al.* 1994; Parant & Lozano 2003) and is in itself strong evidence that defects in p53 are important in development and progression of tumors (Van Dyke 2007). *p53* is the most commonly mutated gene in human cancers and has been described as the 'guardian of the genome' (Lane 1992; Kuwano *et al.* 2005). Analysis of ESCCs within the IARC *TP53* database reveals that numerous *p53* mutations have been detected. They centre around a cluster region between exons 5–8 and the vast majority are point mutations with hot spots at Arg175, Cys176, Arg248, Arg273 and Arg282 (Kuwano *et al.* 2005). As a marker of prognosis of ESCC, however, p53 has not been conclusively shown to be useful. Some studies have found correlations with survival times (Ikeda *et al.* 1999) and some have found no correlation (Lam *et al.* 1999), so the jury is still out regarding using loss of *p53* as a prognostic tool.

p21

$p21^{waf/CIP1}$ activation occurs downstream of p53 signaling. $p21^{waf/CIP1}$ belongs to the CIP/KIP family of CDK inhibitors (Gartel *et al.* 1996). As its family name suggests, it inhibits cyclin/CDK2 and suppresses cell-cycle progression (Brugarolas *et al.* 1999). It can bind to proliferating cell nuclear antigen (PCNA) and this inhibits DNA synthesis. $p21^{waf/CIP1}$ is a transcriptional target of p53. Arrest of the cell cycle in response to irradiation-mediated DNA damage requires expression of both to be effective in maintaining cells at the G2 checkpoint (el-Deiry *et al.* 1994), as $p21^{waf/CIP1}$ –/– cells fail to undergo p53-mediated cell arrest in response to such stimuli and develop tumors (Martin-Caballero *et al.* 2001).

Unlike *p53*, mutations and deletions in the $p21^{waf/CIP1}$ gene in human tumors are very rare (Shiohara *et al.* 1996), although polymorphisms have been identified at codon 31 and 49 on exon 2 in ESCCs (Bahl *et al.* 2000). As a marker of ESCC prognosis, expression of $p21^{waf/CIP1}$ has been shown to correlate with disease progression, with some reports suggesting that downregulation (Natsugoe *et al.* 1999, Nita *et al.* 1999) indicates poor prognosis, and others overexpression (Sarbia *et al.* 1998). Additionally, there have been reports that have suggested that there is no significant correlation so the issue remains unclear. However, Michel *et al.* (2002) and Shimoyama *et al.* (1998) have demonstrated that p53 and p21 expression are markers of a good response to chemoradiation therapy for ESCC.

$p16^{INK4a}$

The INK4 family of cell-cycle inhibitors (which includes $p15^{INK4b}$, $p16^{INK4a}$, $p18^{INK4c}$ and $p19^{INK4d}$) are homologous inhibitors of the

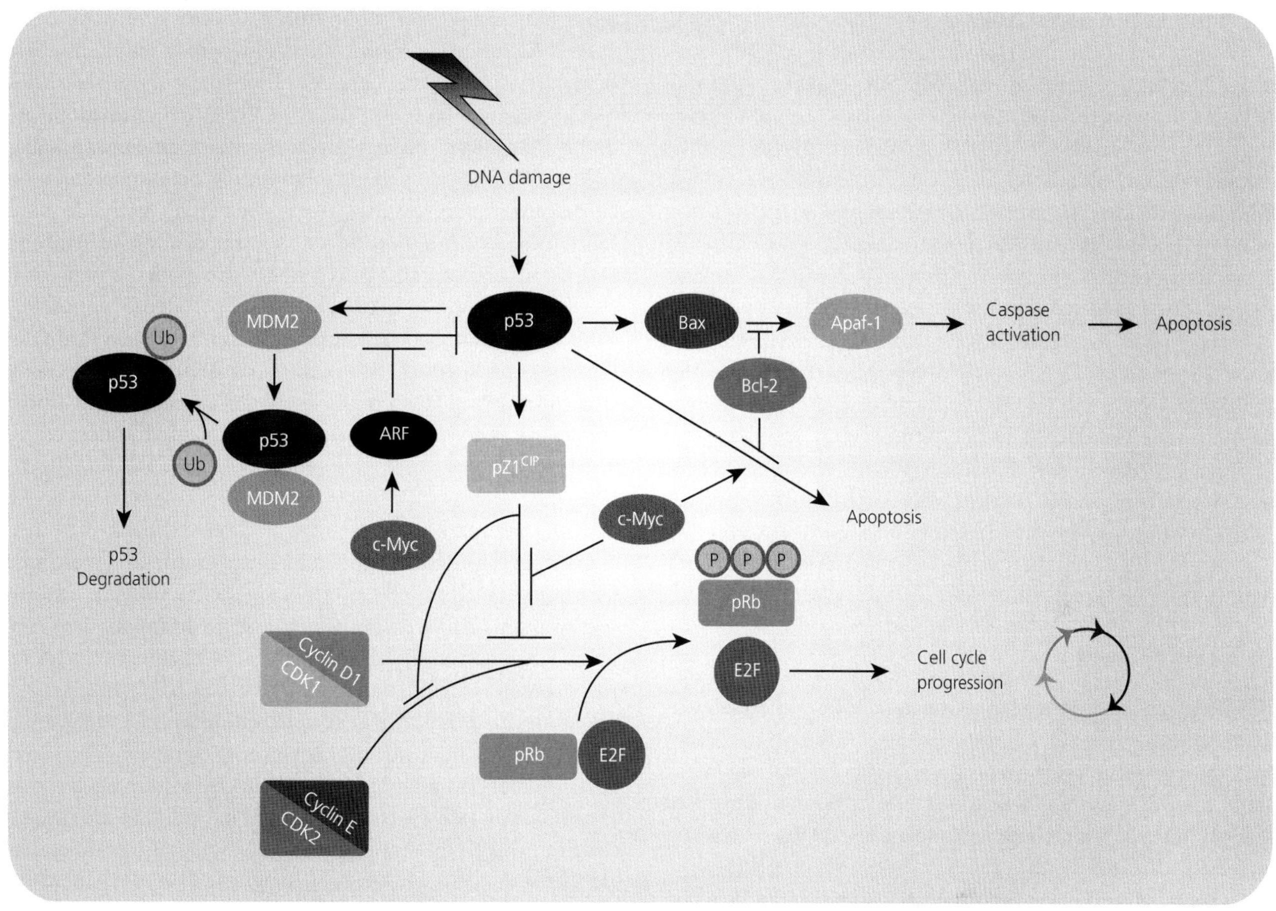

Fig. 3.2 The complexities of the p53/p21 signaling pathways in response to DNA damage. This illustrates how p53 induces the caspase cascade that leads to apoptosis via Bax. Bcl-2 can prevent this process. A reduction in p53 expression in this system prevents expression of p21, an important negative regulator of cell proliferation. Mutations that result in a loss of p53 or p21 are invariably present in human gastroesophageal cancers.

cyclin-dependent kinases (CDKs) CDK4 and CDK6. The binding of p16^{INK4a} to CDKs prevents CDKs binding to D-type cyclins, inhibiting the phosphorylation of retinoblastoma (Rb) family members (Sharpless 2005); this hypophosphorylation results in G1 cell-cycle arrest. Mutations in the *p16^{INK4a}* gene are common in human cancers and are generally associated with deletions in *p15* and *ARF* genes as they are all located at the same locus (CDKN2B) on chromosome 9p21 (Kim & Sharpless 2006). There has been debate as to which gene of this locus is the primary tumor suppressor gene. Knockout studies have shown that absence of all three genes in mice results in the spontaneous development of tumors. But *p16^{INK4a}/ARF* double knockouts appear to be the most susceptible to tumor growth (Latres *et al.* 2000; Sharpless *et al.* 2004), and conversely, animals who overexpress these proteins are resistant to spontaneous tumor formation (Matheu *et al.* 2004).

In human tumors, p16^{INK4a} appears to be frequently mutated with a myriad of deletions, transitions or aberrant DNA methylation (Nobori *et al.* 1994; Okamoto *et al.* 1994; Herman *et al.* 1995). Many ESCC cell lines have high incidences of homozygous deletions (Igaki *et al.* 1994) and are greatly variable in type (Tanaka *et al.* 1997). Loss of p16^{INK4a} appears to be an early event in ESCC development and takes the form of loss of heterozygosity (LOH) or silencing of the p16^{INK4a} promoter by aberrant methylation (Xing *et al.* 1999; Fong *et al.* 2000; Tokugawa *et al.* 2002). As a prognostic tool, expression of p16^{INK4a} has been shown to correlate with poor outcome, especially when taken with expression of cyclin D1 (Takeuchi *et al.* 1997), but as p16^{INK4a} loss appears to be an early event in ESCC it may also be a useful screening tool (Hibi *et al.* 2001; Nie *et al.* 2002).

Esophageal adenocarcinoma

Esophageal adenocarcinoma (EA) is the most predominant form of esophageal cancer in Europe (Powell *et al.* 2002). This is thought to be primarily due to the incidence of Barrett's esophagus (BE) which is seen as a premalignant disease with a risk of progression into adenocarcinoma. BE is characterized by a metaplastic change in the esophageal epithelium with squamous epithelial cells being replaced with columnar epithelial cells and subsequent formation of crypts or glands resembling gastric/colonic mucosa. Current dogma is that BE is caused by chronic reflux of bile and acid; a familial element is also involved. BE lesions are also associated with inflammation and this may promote a field of genetic instability within the epithelium and promote progression from metaplasia to dysplasia to adenocarcinoma. The factors and events that lead to the development of BE are poorly understood. As stated above, BE is hypothesized to be a consequence of prolonged exposure of the squamous epithelium to bile and stomach acid (reflux). However, there is no conclusive evidence demonstrating how BE develops, nor are there any reliable models. Hence, all research has been based on tissue obtained from patients with BE that only allows one 'snapshot' in time or serial 'snapshots' in follow-up. Here we discuss the major molecular events and changes in BE and their significance in adenocarcinoma.

Growth factors

EGFR expression appears to be increased along the metaplasia–dysplasia–adenocarcinoma pathway (Gibson *et al.* 2003). This may be related to one of the original observations made about the *EGFR* gene. Al-Kasspooles *et al.* (1993) demonstrated that in human esophageal adenocarcinomas there was an increase in the number of copies of the *EGFR* gene in 30% of the tumors studied. They also reported a similar finding in a case of BE. Latterly, it has been shown that EGFR can predict poor survival only in cases of adenocarcinoma (Gibson *et al.* 2003). Functional studies have revealed that there are mutations in the EGFR kinase domain (Kwak *et al.* 2006) and the fact that these are activating mutations helps to explain the increase in EGFR expression in esophageal adenocarcinoma. C-met expression has recently been shown to be a poor prognostic factor in esophageal adenocarcinoma (Anderson *et al.* 2006).

A characteristic of BE is the presence of a strong T helper-2 inflammatory response, and a reduction in the ability to signal through TGFβ primarily due to loss of downstream signaling components such as members of the Smad family (Onwuegbusi *et al.* 2006) which can inhibit cell-cycle arrest (Onwuegbusi *et al.* 2007). The authors, however, were unsure if this was a consequence of BE or a fundamental of BE and hopefully future work will enlighten us. Despite a lack of signaling potential TGFβ is overexpressed in BE and adenocarcinoma, and is associated with a poor prognosis (von Rahden *et al.* 2006).

Cell-cycle proteins

p53

Mutations or loss of expression of p53 are found frequently in esophageal adenocarcinomas arising from BE. LOH for *p53* is an early event in the progression from BE to adenocarcinoma because it develops in diploid cells before aneuploidy and before other LOH events that occur (Blount *et al.* 1993, 1994). *p53* LOH is found in 14% of BE, 42% of low-grade dysplasias, 79% of high-grade dysplasias (HGDs) and 75–80% of adenocarcinomas (Morgan *et al.* 1998; Wu *et al.* 2001). *p53* mutations are found in 40–88% of high-grade dysplasias/adenocarcinomas and in 29–66% of low-grade dysplasias/BE. *p53* mutations can be detected before the development of HGD, and may have some value as a prognostic tool due to their high incidence in HGD and adenocarcinoma. Furthermore, patients with both *p53* mutations and/or overexpression of p53 in the tumor after surgical resection had significantly poorer 5-year survival than those that had neither (Schneider *et al.* 2000). Although there is a consensus that *p53* mutations are an early event, more studies are needed to elucidate their role as biomarkers.

p16

The tumor suppressor protein p16^{ink4a} can be inactivated by a two-hit mechanism that occurs by one or more of a multitude of processes such as LOH, homozygous deletion, or CpG island methylation (a process by which a gene promoter becomes methylated preventing the binding of transcription factors). p16 promoter methylation (with or without *p16* LOH) is a frequent mechanism of *p16* gene inactivation in BE and becomes even more frequent during neoplastic progression. However, allelic loss of *p16* at 9p21 has been described in many reports (Tarmin *et al.* 1994; Barrett *et al.* 1996) but point mutations are relatively rare when compared with squamous carcinomas (Esteve *et al.* 1996). It has been suggested that *p16* mutations are the earliest molecular event in cases of BE. The Reid group has provided evidence to suggest that *p16* mutations rapidly and clonally expand throughout the Barrett's lesion (known as a 'selective sweep'), providing a 'primed' epithelium that can accumulate further mutations (Wong *et al.* 2001). Due to the relative frequency of *p16* loss at an early stage of the metaplasia–adenocarcinoma pathway, the presence of *p16* mutations probably has little prognostic value.

Mismatch repair genes

The mismatch repair (MMR) system is a vital mechanism by which DNA damage is repaired. Essentially, this system removes mismatched DNA base pairs made by DNA polymerases and insertion/deletion loops resulting from slippage during DNA replication or recombination. Mitochondrial DNA is notable for its absence of such repair mechanisms, making it particularly susceptible to DNA mutations (Greaves *et al.* 2006), which increase with age. Failure of MMR results in the accumulation of single-base DNA insertions and alterations of length of simple, repetitive microsatellite regions throughout the genome, known as microsatellite instability (MSI) (Koppert *et al.* 2005). Mutations in MMR genes such as *MLH1* and *MSH2* are found in diseases such as hereditary non-polyposis coli colorectal cancer. Such cancers can be categorized as MSI-high (2–5/5 markers) or MSI-low (1/5 marker; can be called MSI-stable).

Various studies on MSI have been performed attempting to rank gastric cancers according to MSI ranking. Evans *et al.* (2004) investigated the presence of 15 markers in 80 cases of adenocarcinoma arising from BE and showed that 65% of the carcinomas investigated had between 1 and 5/15 markers present. Although not conclusive, this does indicate that such MSI regions are present in the BE–adenocarcinoma pathway. It must be stated that overall the results from all studies currently published on MMR genes in BE adenocarcinoma are highly variable, with the majority showing a low incidence of MSI markers. It is estimated that there is typically 5–10% MSI within BE adenocarcinomas. Consequently, MSI is currently not a suitable biomarker of prognosis, and far more work is required before it can be used as such (Koppert *et al.* 2005).

Wnt signaling pathway

The Wnt glycoproteins comprise a family of extracellular signaling ligands that play an important role in cell differentiation, cell proliferation and motility. There are at least 19 members of the Wnt family, and at least 10 members of their receptor, frizzled (FZ). The Wnt receptor complex is made up of FZ and LRP5/6 (homologues of the LDL receptor) (McDonald *et al.* 2006). In the absence of Wnt, cytosolic β-catenin (which is normally bound to membranous E-cadherin) interacts with a destruction complex of adenomatous polyposis coli (APC), glycogen synthase kinase 3(GSK3) and axin, and becomes phosphorylated and degraded by the ubiquitin pathway. However, if Wnt binds to FZ, the kinase activity of the destruction complex is blocked, and β-catenin remains unphosphorylated and builds up in the cytosol. Beta-catenin is then able to bind to a transcription factor TCF-4, the targets of which include genes such as *c-myc* which promote the cell into the S phase of the cell cycle (Bailey *et al.* 1998; reviewed in McDonald *et al.* 2006) (Fig. 3.3).

A large number of Wnt genes including *WNT2*, *WNT5A*, and *WNT7* have been implicated in a wide variety of human cancers (Bui *et al.* 1997; Holcombe *et al.* 2002). Furthermore, there are widespread mutations of downstream molecules such APC and β-catenin. One of the most well known mutations of *APC* results in familial adenomatous polyposis (FAP), where one allele of the *APC* gene is mutated in the germline. Over a number of years a second hit occurs, resulting in a loss of APC and an increase in nuclear β-catenin, an increase in cell proliferation, and subsequent development of large numbers of polyps. Patients normally undergo a prophylactic colectomy before the development of cancer.

Unlike colon cancer, EA and the preceding Barrett's does not have a strong association with mutations of *APC* or β-catenin. LOH at the APC locus has been identified in patients with high-grade dysplasia and adenocarcinoma but is often preceded by 17p LOH and is not considered to be an early event; furthermore, mutations in APC and β-catenin are rare (Powell *et al.* 1994) and are therefore unlikely to play a major role in the pathogenesis of EA. Indeed, in models of EA, APC is redundant in mice, and tumors still develop in its absence (Fein *et al.* 1999). Methylation of the APC promoter is a common event in BE and persists through to the development of EA (Clement *et al.* 2006), and Kawakami *et al.* (2000) have demonstrated that there is an increase in plasma APC methylation in the progression towards EA and this associates with poor prognosis. Overall, it is becoming clear that mutations in the Wnt–APC pathway are rare, if not absent, but other epigenetic alterations such as hypermethylation have some potential in revealing poor prognosis.

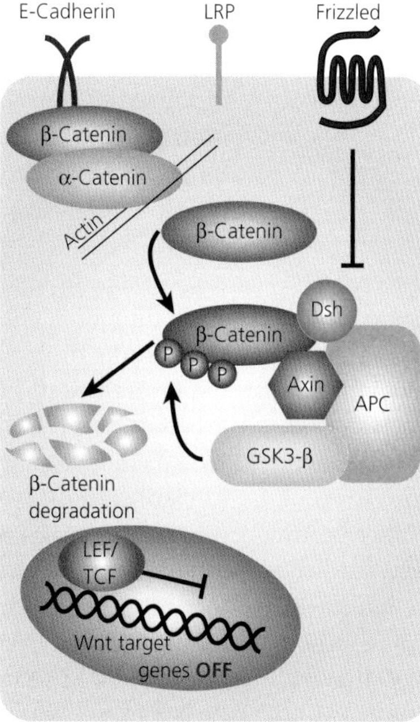

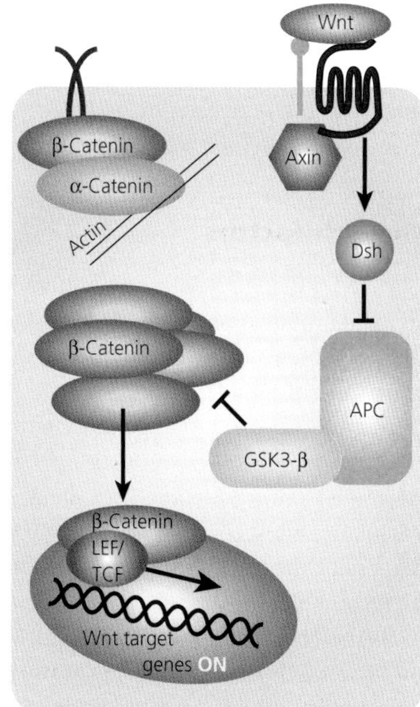

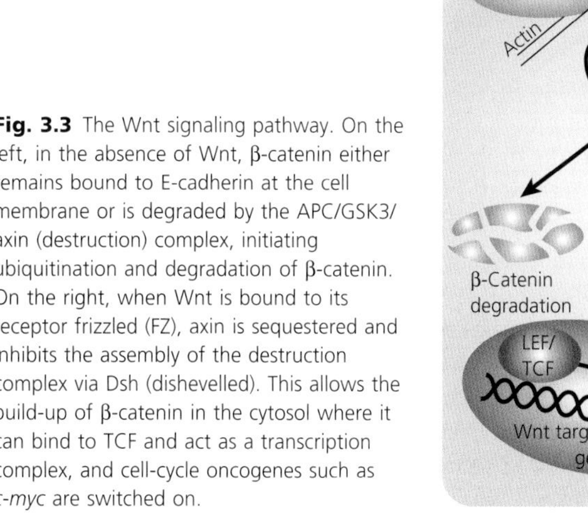

Fig. 3.3 The Wnt signaling pathway. On the left, in the absence of Wnt, β-catenin either remains bound to E-cadherin at the cell membrane or is degraded by the APC/GSK3/axin (destruction) complex, initiating ubiquitination and degradation of β-catenin. On the right, when Wnt is bound to its receptor frizzled (FZ), axin is sequestered and inhibits the assembly of the destruction complex via Dsh (dishevelled). This allows the build-up of β-catenin in the cytosol where it can bind to TCF and act as a transcription complex, and cell-cycle oncogenes such as *c-myc* are switched on.

Molecular biology of gastric cancer

Introduction

Gastric cancer is still one of the commonest malignancies in the world. Until the mid-eighties it was the most common malignancy and has now been surpassed only by lung cancer worldwide. Approximately 876,000 new cases are diagnosed globally, and 649,000 people die from it each year (Parkin *et al.* 2001). Unfortunately, it is still most commonly diagnosed after invasion of the muscularis propria has occurred, and as a result the 5-year survival of these patients is less than 20%. The majority of cases are sporadic, only 1–3% being familial. Infection with *Helicobacter pylori* is the most important risk factor for development. In 1994 the World Health Organization (WHO) classified *H. pylori* as a class 1 carcinogen.

The best-known classification of gastric cancer differentiates between poorly differentiated diffuse and well-differentiated intestinal types (Lauren 1965). There have been more recent attempts at classification, but this is the most widely used method today. The diffuse-type adenocarcinoma tends to have a stronger genetic preponderance and presents at an earlier age. The intestinal type affects an older age group, tends to be acquired, and is characterized by the formation of gland-like structures. Increasingly it is thought that the two are completely different diseases.

In colorectal cancer a clear multistep process with accumulation of genetic defects has been characterized as the adenoma carcinoma sequence. With respect to gastric cancer our knowledge is fragmentary. Although no clear multistep process has been identified in diffuse gastric cancer an attempt has been made to delineate the intestinal type. This consists of three possible pathways: the intestinal metaplasia–adenoma–carcinoma sequence, the intestinal metaplasia–carcinoma sequence, and *de novo* formation (Tahara 2004).

This section concentrates on the various molecular pathways involved in the development of gastric cancer and evaluates their use as potential biomarkers.

Growth factors

The TGFβ signaling pathway is altered in gastric cancer. TGFβ signaling induces phosphorylation of cytoplasmic signal transducing proteins (Smads). Translocation of this Smad complex, consisting of Smad2, 3 and 4, to the nucleus results in transcription of various target genes (Heldin *et al.* 1997). Han *et al.* recently demonstrated reduction of Smad3 in gastric cancer cells. The reintroduction of Smad3 decreased expression of vascular endothelial growth factor (VEGF), consequently decreasing the cells' ability to go through the angiogenic switch. They also demonstrated the ability of Smad3 to induce E-cadherin (Han *et al.* 2004). In addition, Smad7 is a negative regulator of Smad-dependent signaling, is present in one-third of gastric cancer cells, and infers a poor prognosis (Kim *et al.* 2004).

The function of TGFβ signaling itself in cancer appears to be biphasic. In the early stages it has a tumor suppressor function. However, in the later stages it appears to enhance carcinogenesis by suppressing the immune system, producing extracellular matrix and promoting angiogenesis. TGFβ signaling can be affected by mutation of its receptors or epigenetic silencing via hypermethylation of CpG islands in the region of its receptor genes (Pinto *et al.* 2003).

Upregulation of the EGFR has been implicated in gastric cancer. It is a possible point of attack for targeted therapy by monoclonal antibodies. Cetuximab has been licensed for use in metastatic colorectal cancer and is an anti-EGFR antibody. Clinical trials in gastric carcinoma have provided minimal evidence of the efficacy of anti-EGFR antibodies as therapeutic agents. In a multicenter phase II Japanese trial only 13/75 (18.3%) of patients with metastatic gastric cancer receiving 250 or 500 mg/day anti-EGFR (gefitinib) showed any clinical improvement, and grade III and IV toxicities were observed (Rojo *et al.* 2006). Subsequent studies have revealed that the kinase domain of EGFR in gastric cancers is highly conserved and that this would predict poor outcome of such therapies (Mimori *et al.* 2006).

Cell-cycle proteins

p53

There has been extensive analysis of the role of p53 in the development of gastric cancer. In non-neoplastic gastric lesions there is an increase in frequency of p53 abnormalities, particularly in metaplastic lesions (Yamada *et al.* 1991), with up to 50% of areas of intestinal metaplasia having DNA substitutions (Shiao *et al.* 1994). They are rarely detected in gastritis and in normal glands (Blok *et al.* 1998). p53 is readily detectable in gastric dysplasia (Joypaul *et al.* 1993) and mutations occur within a broad range of cases (0–67%) (Tohdo *et al.* 1993; Strickler *et al.* 1994; Wang *et al.* 1994). These studies also included adenomas, which had a high incidence of missense mutations (Sakurai *et al.* 1995) which could be a useful indicator of progression to neoplasia. LOH of the *p53* 3′ untranslated region is found in 0–22% of gastric adenomas (Tahara *et al.* 1996).

p53 expression has been shown to be reduced in non-metastatic tumors as compared with invasive ones, and mutations seen in p53 from patients with metastatic gastric cancer that result in a loss of p53-mediated apoptosis may prove a useful prognostic tool (Uchino *et al.* 1993; Scartozzi *et al.* 2004). There are a plethora of *p53* mutation analysis studies in gastric adenocarcinoma, most concentrating on the exon 5–8 region of the gene. In summary, the majority are base substitutions (Renault *et al.* 1993; Hongyo *et al.* 1995; Fenoglio-Preiser *et al.* 2003) but there does not appear to be any significant relationship between the presence of *p53* mutations and tumor stage. A detailed summary of all *p53* mutation studies can be found in Fengolio-Preiser *et al.* (2003).

Wnt signaling pathway

As previously discussed, the Wnt signaling pathway is important for the control of cellular proliferation and differentiation within the gastrointestinal tract. Nearly 60% of intestinal-type gastric cancers contain mutations for LOH of the *APC* gene (Horii *et al.* 1992; Tahara 1995). These are uncommon in diffuse-type gastric cancer, but there may be some correlation with signet ring carcinomas (Nakatsuru *et al.* 1992). A consequence of *APC* mutation is increased levels of cytosolic β-catenin, and subsequent binding to TCF leads to increased gene transcription of cell-cycle promoters such as *c-myc*. Beta-catenin mutations have been discovered in intestinal-type but not diffuse-type gastric cancer (Candidus *et al.* 1996). Besides playing a role in the Wnt signaling pathway β-catenin also binds to E-cadherin, an adhesion molecule important in epithelial–epithelial cell adhesion. Overexpression of E-cadherin can suppress the levels of cytoplasmic β-catenin and downstream cell-cycle promoter genes (Gottardi *et al.* 2001). Studies have shown that there is reduced membranous β-catenin in 83% of diffuse gastric cancers and 29% of intestinal-type gastric cancers, but in both cases nuclear β-catenin expression appeared to be low (Ramesh *et al.* 1999). There is therefore some ambiguity as to the role of mutations in the Wnt signaling pathway and consequently their use as prognostic tools or biomarkers is limited.

E-Cadherin

E-cadherin is one of the most extensively studied proteins in gastric cancer. It is a 120-kDa adhesion molecule that binds to cytoplasmic β-catenin below the cellular membrane, and extracellularly is part of the tight junction complex. It is expressed on all epithelial cells and appears to be one of the most commonly mutated or silenced genes in gastric cancer. The protein has been routinely shown to have reduced expression in all gastric cancers, ranging from 17 to 92% (Shimoyama & Hirohashi 1991; Mayer *et al.* 1993) although loss of expression is skewed more towards diffuse gastric cancer. There is a clear correlation between expression of E-cadherin and the grade of tumor differentiation. Patients with E-cadherin-positive tumors have a higher 3- and 5-year survival rates as compared with E-cadherin-negative tumors (Gabbert *et al.* 1996).

It is primarily in diffuse gastric cancers that mutations account for the reduction in E-cadherin expression (Becker *et al.* 1994). However, it is the methylation status of the E-cadherin promoter that has generated the most interest. Grady *et al.* (2000) have shown that hypermethylation of the CDH1 promoter (of the E-cadherin gene) is the 'second hit' in familial diffuse gastric cancer. Furthermore, it has been shown that *H. pylori* (which has been associated with a downregulation of E-cadherin (Terres *et al.* 1998a,b) can induce hypermethylation of CDH1 and that eradication of *H. pylori* may have the potential to reverse this (Chan *et al.* 2003). Whether or not *H. pylori* eradication reduces gastric cancer risk by means of restoring E-cadherin expression remains to be seen.

Conclusion

It is obvious that mutational analysis of gastroesophageal cancers has progressed exponentially over the last decade and our understanding of the pathways that govern the development of such tumors has risen similarly. However, as yet there appears to be no ideal molecular signature that can predict prognosis. The clinician must comprehend the limitations of the current biomarkers of prognosis when evaluating patients, while at the same time remaining aware that they may be useful indicators in the future. The basic research, which has identified the major genes involved in cancer development, is complex, and future therapeutic strategies will be similarly complicated. Infection by *H. pylori* is considered to be oncogenic according to the WHO. The understanding of how this fits into the development of gastric cancer has advanced tremendously over recent years and is covered in another chapter.

Box 3.1 'Take-home' messages

1 As yet no mutation or genetic defect has been conclusively shown, on its own, to be an effective prognostic marker.
2 There is promise! Potentially, screening of a range of genetic or epigenetic events may prove useful in future and therefore the gastroenterologist must keep abreast of this field.
3 Different upper gastrointestinal cancers display different molecular biology.

References

Akhurst RJ, Derynck R. (2001) TGF-beta signaling in cancer—a double-edged sword. *Trends Cell Biol* 11: S44–51.

Al-Kasspooles M, Moore JH, Orringer MB, Beer DG. (1993) Amplification and over-expression of the EGFR and erbB-2 genes in human esophageal adenocarcinomas. *Int J Cancer* 54: 213–9.

Anderson MR, Harrison R, Atherfold PA, *et al.* (2006) Metreceptor signalling: a key effector in esophageal adenocarcinoma. *Clin Can Res* 12: 5936–43.

Bahl R, Arora S, Nath N, Mathur M, Shukla NK, Ralhan R. (2000) Novel polymorphism in p21(waf1/cip1) cyclin dependent kinase inhibitor gene: association with human esophageal cancer. *Oncogene* 19: 323–8.

Bailey T, Biddlestone L, Shepherd N, *et al.* (1998) Altered cadherin and catenin complexes in Barrett's esophagus. *Am J Pathol* 152: 135–44.

Barrett MT, Sanchez CA, Galipeau PC, Neshat K, Emond M, Reid BJ. (1996) Allelic loss of 9p21 and mutation of the CDKN2/p16 gene develop as early lesions during neoplastic progression in Barrett's esophagus. *Oncogene* 13: 1867–73.

Becker KF, Atkinson MJ, Reich U *et al.* (1994) E-cadherin gene mutations provide clues to diffuse type gastric carcinomas. *Cancer Res* 54: 3845–52.

Blok P, Craanen ME, Dekker W, Offerhaus GJ, Tytgat GN. (1998) No evidence for functional inactivation of wild-type p53 protein by MDM2 overexpression in gastric carcinogenesis. *J Pathol* 186: 36–40.

Blount PL, Meltzer SJ, Yin J, Huang Y, Krasna MJ, Reid BJ. (1993) Clonal ordering of 17p and 5q allelic losses in Barrett dysplasia and adenocarcinoma. *Proc Natl Acad Sci U S A* 90: 3221–5.

Blount PL, Galipeau PC, Sanchez CA *et al.* (1994) 17p allelic losses in diploid cells of patients with Barrett's esophagus who develop aneuploidy. *Cancer Res* 54: 2292–5.

Brugarolas J, Moberg K, Boyd SD, Taya Y, Jacks T, Lees JA. (1999) Inhibition of cyclin-dependent kinase 2 by p21 is necessary for retinoblastoma protein-mediated G1 arrest after gamma-irradiation. *Proc Natl Acad Sci U S A* 96: 1002–7.

Bui TD, Zhang L, Rees MC, Bicknell R, Harris AL. (1997) Expression and hormone regulation of Wnt2, 3, 4, 5a, 7a, 7b and 10b in normal human endometrium and endometrial carcinoma. *Br J Cancer* 75: 1131–6.

Burgess AW, Cho HS, Eigenbrot C *et al.* (2003) An open-and-shut case? Recent insights into the activation of EGF/ErbB receptors. *Mol Cell* 12: 541–52.

Candidus S, Bischoff P, Becker KF, Hofler H. (1996) No evidence for mutations in the alpha- and beta-catenin genes in human gastric and breast carcinomas. *Cancer Res* 56: 49–52.

Chan AO, Lam SK, Wong BC, Kwong YL, Rashid A. (2003) Gene methylation in non-neoplastic mucosa of gastric cancer: age or *Helicobacter pylori* related? *Am J Pathol* 163: 370–1; author reply 371–3.

Chen CR, Kang Y, Massague J. (2001) Defective repression of c-myc in breast cancer cells: A loss at the core of the transforming growth factor beta growth arrest program. *Proc Natl Acad Sci U S A* 98: 992–9.

Clarke AR, Purdie CA, Harrison DJ *et al.* (1993) Thymocyte apoptosis induced by p53-dependent and independent pathways. *Nature* 362: 849–52.

Clement G, Braunschweig R, Pasquier N, Bosman FT, Benhattar J. (2006) Alterations of the Wnt signaling pathway during the neoplastic progression of Barrett's esophagus. *Oncogene* 25: 3084–92.

el-Deiry WS, Harper JW, O'Connor PM *et al.* (1994) WAF1/CIP1 is induced in p53-mediated G1 arrest and apoptosis. *Cancer Res* 54: 1169–74.

Esteve A, Martel-Planche G, Sylla BS, Hollstein M, Hainaut P, Montesano R. (1996) Low frequency of p16/CDKN2 gene mutations in esophageal carcinomas. *Int J Cancer* 66: 301–4.

Evans SC, Gillis A, Geldenhuys L *et al.* (2004) Microsatellite instability in esophageal adenocarcinoma. *Cancer Lett* 212: 241–51.

Fein M, Peters JH, Baril N *et al.* (1999) Loss of function of Trp53, but not Apc, leads to the development of esophageal adenocarcinoma in mice with jejunoesophageal reflux. *J Surg Res* 83: 48–55.

Feng XH, Liang YY, Liang M, Zhai W, Lin X. (2002) Direct interaction of c-Myc with Smad2 and Smad3 to inhibit TGF-beta-mediated induction of the CDK inhibitor p15(Ink4B). *Mol Cell* 9: 133–43.

Fenoglio-Preiser CM, Wang J, Stemmermann GN, Noffsinger A. (2003) TP53 and gastric carcinoma: a review. *Hum Mutat* 21: 258–70.

Fong LY, Nguyen VT, Farber JL, Huebner K, Magee PN. (2000) Early deregulation of the p16ink4a-cyclin D1/cyclin-dependent kinase 4-retinoblastoma pathway in cell proliferation-driven esophageal tumorigenesis in zinc-deficient rats. *Cancer Res* 60: 4589–95.

Fridman JS, Lowe SW. (2003) Control of apoptosis by p53. *Oncogene* 22: 9030–40.

Fukuchi M, Fukai Y, Masuda N *et al.* (2002) High-level expression of the Smad ubiquitin ligase Smurf2 correlates with poor prognosis in patients with esophageal squamous cell carcinoma. *Cancer Res* 62: 7162–5.

Gabbert HE, Mueller W, Schneiders A *et al.* (1996) Prognostic value of E-cadherin expression in 413 gastric carcinomas. *Int J Cancer* 69: 184–9.

Gartel AL, Serfas MS, Tyner AL. (1996) p21—negative regulator of the cell cycle. *Proc Soc Exp Biol Med* 213: 138–49.

Gibson MK, Abraham SC, Wu TT *et al.* (2003) Epidermal growth factor receptor, p53 mutation, and pathological response predict survival in patients with locally advanced esophageal cancer treated with preoperative chemoradiotherapy. *Clin Cancer Res* 9: 6461–8.

Gottardi CJ, Wong E, Gumbiner BM. (2001) E-cadherin suppresses cellular transformation by inhibiting beta-catenin signaling in an adhesion-independent manner. *J Cell Biol* 153: 1049–60.

Grady WM, Willis J, Guilford PJ *et al.* (2000) Methylation of the CDH1 promoter as the second genetic hit in hereditary diffuse gastric cancer. *Nat Genet* 26: 16–7.

Greaves LC, Preston SL, Tadrous PJ *et al.* (2006) Mitochondrial DNA mutations are established in human colonic stem cells, and mutated clones expand by crypt fission. *Proc Natl Acad Sci U S A* 103: 714–9.

Han SU, Kim HT, Seong DH *et al.* (2004) Loss of the Smad3 expression increases susceptibility to tumorigenicity in human gastric cancer. *Oncogene* 23: 1333–41.

Heldin CH, Miyazono K, Ten Dijke P. (1997) TGF-beta signalling from cell membrane to nucleus through SMAD proteins. *Nature* 390: 465–71.

Herman JG, Merlo A, Mao L *et al.* (1995) Inactivation of the CDKN2/p16/MTS1 gene is frequently associated with aberrant DNA methylation in all common human cancers. *Cancer Res* 55: 4525–30.

Hibi K, Taguchi M, Nakayama H *et al.* (2001) Molecular detection of p16 promoter methylation in the serum of patients with esophageal squamous cell carcinoma. *Clin Cancer Res* 7: 3135–8.

Hirai T, Kuwahara M, Yoshida K *et al.* (1998) Clinical results of transhiatal esophagectomy for carcinoma of the lower thoracic esophagus according to biological markers. *Dis Esophagus* 11: 221–5.

Holcombe RF, Marsh JL, Waterman ML, Lin F, Milovanovic T, Truong T. (2002) Expression of Wnt ligands and Frizzled receptors in colonic mucosa and in colon carcinoma. *Mol Pathol* 55: 220–6.

Holmes RS, Vaughan TL. (2007) Epidemiology and pathogenesis of esophageal cancer. *Semin Radiat Oncol* 17: 2–9.

Hongyo T, Buzard GS, Palli D *et al.* (1995) Mutations of the K-ras and p53 genes in gastric adenocarcinomas from a high-incidence region around Florence, Italy. *Cancer Res* 55: 2665–72.

Horii A, Nakatsuru S, Miyoshi Y *et al.* (1992) The APC gene, responsible for familial adenomatous polyposis, is mutated in human gastric cancer. *Cancer Res* 52: 3231–3.

Igaki H, Sasaki H, Kishi T *et al.* (1994) Highly frequent homozygous deletion of the p16 gene in esophageal cancer cell lines. *Biochem Biophys Res Commun* 203: 1090–5.

Ikeda G, Isaji S, Chandra B, Watanabe M, Kawarada Y. (1999) Prognostic significance of biologic factors in squamous cell carcinoma of the esophagus. *Cancer* 86: 1396–405.

Joypaul BV, Newman EL, Hopwood D *et al.* (1993) Expression of p53 protein in normal, dysplastic, and malignant gastric mucosa: an immunohistochemical study. *J Pathol* 170: 279–83.

Kawakami K, Brabender J, Lord RV *et al.* (2000) Hypermethylated APC DNA in plasma and prognosis of patients with esophageal adenocarcinoma. *J Natl Cancer Inst* 92: 1805–11.

Kim WY, Sharpless NE. (2006) The regulation of INK4/ARF in cancer and aging. *Cell* 127: 265–75.

Kim YH, Lee HS, Lee HJ *et al.* (2004) Prognostic significance of the expression of Smad4 and Smad7 in human gastric carcinomas. *Ann Oncol* 15: 574–80.

Koppert LB, Wijnhoven BP, Van Dekken H, Tilanus HW, Dinjens WN. (2005) The molecular biology of esophageal adenocarcinoma. *J Surg Oncol* 92: 169–90.

Kuwano H, Kato H, Miyazaki T *et al.* (2005) Genetic alterations in esophageal cancer. *Surg Today* 35: 7–18.

Kwak EL, Jankowski J, Thayer SP *et al.* (2006) Epidermal growth factor receptor kinase domain mutations in esophageal and pancreatic adenocarcinomas. *Clin Cancer Res* 12: 4283–7.

Lagergren J, Ye W, Lindgren A, Nyren O. (2000) Heredity and risk of cancer of the esophagus and gastric cardia. *Cancer Epidemiol Biomarkers Prev* 9: 757–60.

Lam KY, Law S, Tin L, Tung PH, Wong J. (1999) The clinicopathological significance of p21 and p53 expression in esophageal squamous cell carcinoma: an analysis of 153 patients. *Am J Gastroenterol* 94: 2060–8.

Lane DP. (1992) Cancer. p53, guardian of the genome. *Nature* 358: 15–6.

Latres E, Malumbres M, Sotillo R *et al.* (2000) Limited overlapping roles of P15(INK4b) and P18(INK4c) cell cycle inhibitors in proliferation and tumorigenesis. *EMBO J* 19: 3496–506.

Lauren P. (1965) The two histological main types of gastric carcinoma: diffuse and so-called intestinal-type carcinoma. An attempt at a histo-clinical classification. *Acta Pathol Microbiol Scand* 64: 31–49.

Martin-Caballero J, Flores JM, Garcia-Palencia P, Serrano M. (2001) Tumor susceptibility of p21(Waf1/Cip1)-deficient mice. *Cancer Res* 61: 6234–8.

Massague J, Wotton D. (2000) Transcriptional control by the TGF-beta/Smad signaling system. *EMBO J* 19: 1745–54.

Matheu A, Pantoja C, Efeyan A *et al.* (2004) Increased gene dosage of Ink4a/Arf results in cancer resistance and normal aging. *Genes Dev* 18: 2736–46.

Mayer B, Johnson JP, Leitl F *et al.* (1993) E-cadherin expression in primary and metastatic gastric cancer: down-regulation correlates with cellular dedifferentiation and glandular disintegration. *Cancer Res* 53: 1690–5.

McDonald SA, Preston SL, Lovell MJ, Wright NA, Jankowski JA. (2006) Mechanisms of disease: from stem cells to colorectal cancer. *Nat Clin Pract Gastroenterol Hepatol* 3: 267–74.

Michel P, Magois K, Robert V *et al.* (2002) Prognostic value of TP53 transcriptional activity on p21 and bax in patients with esophageal squamous cell carcinomas treated by definitive chemoradiotherapy. *Int J Radiat Oncol Biol Phys* 54: 379–85.

Mimori K, Nagahara H, Sudo T *et al.* (2006) The epidermal growth factor receptor gene sequence is highly conserved in primary gastric cancers. *J Surg Oncol* 93: 44–6.

Morgan RJ, Newcomb PV, Bailey M, Hardwick RH, Alderson D. (1998) Loss of heterozygosity at microsatellite marker sites for tumour suppressor genes in oesophageal adenocarcinoma. *Eur J Surg Oncol* 24: 34–7.

Nakatsuru S, Yanagisawa A, Ichii S, Tahara *et al.* (1992) Somatic mutation of the APC gene in gastric cancer: frequent mutations in very well differentiated adenocarcinoma and signet-ring cell carcinoma. *Hum Mol Genet* 1: 559–63.

Natsugoe S, Nakashima S, Matsumoto M *et al.* (1999) Expression of p21WAF1/Cip1 in the p53-dependent pathway is related to prognosis in patients with advanced esophageal carcinoma. *Clin Cancer Res* 5: 2445–9.

Nie Y, Liao J, Zhao X *et al.* (2002) Detection of multiple gene hypermethylation in the development of esophageal squamous cell carcinoma. *Carcinogenesis* 23: 1713–20.

Nita ME, Nagawa H, Tominaga O *et al.* (1999) p21Waf1/Cip1 expression is a prognostic marker in curatively resected esophageal squamous cell carcinoma, but not p27Kip1, p53, or Rb. *Ann Surg Oncol* 6: 481–8.

Nobori T, Miura K, Wu DJ, Lois A, Takabayashi K, Carson DA. (1994) Deletions of the cyclin-dependent kinase-4 inhibitor gene in multiple human cancers. *Nature* 368: 753–6.

Okamoto A, Demetrick DJ, Spillare EA *et al.* (1994) Mutations and altered expression of p16INK4 in human cancer. *Proc Natl Acad Sci U S A* 91: 11045–9.

Onwuegbusi BA, Aitchison A, Chin SF *et al.* (2006) Impaired transforming growth factor beta signalling in Barrett's carcinogenesis due to frequent SMAD4 inactivation. *Gut* 55: 764–74.

Onwuegbusi BA, Rees JR, Lao-Sirieix P, Fitzgerald RC. (2007) Selective loss of TGFbeta Smad-dependent signalling prevents cell cycle arrest and promotes invasion in oesophageal adenocarcinoma cell lines. *PLoS ONE* 2: e177.

Osawa H, Shitara Y, Shoji H *et al.* (2000) Mutation analysis of transforming growth factor beta type II receptor, Smad2, Smad3 and Smad4 in esophageal squamous cell carcinoma. *Int J Oncol* 17: 723–8.

Parant JM, Lozano G. (2003) Disrupting TP53 in mouse models of human cancers. *Hum Mutat* 21: 321–6.

Parkin DM, Bray FI, Devesa SS. (2001) Cancer burden in the year 2000. The global picture. *Eur J Cancer* 37 Suppl 8: S4–66.

Pinto M, Oliveira C, Cirnes L *et al.* (2003) Promoter methylation of TGFbeta receptor I and mutation of TGFbeta receptor II are frequent events in MSI sporadic gastric carcinomas. *J Pathol* 200: 32–8.

Powell SM, Papadopoulos N, Kinzler KW, Smolinski KN, Meltzer SJ. (1994) APC gene mutations in the mutation cluster region are rare in esophageal cancers. *Gastroenterology* 107: 1759–63.

Powell J, McConkey CC, Gillison EW, Spychal RT. (2002) Continuing rising trend in oesophageal adenocarcinoma. *Int J Cancer* 102: 422–7.

von Rahden BH, Stein HJ, Feith M *et al.* (2006) Overexpression of TGF-beta1 in esophageal (Barrett's) adenocarcinoma is associated with advanced stage of disease and poor prognosis. *Mol Carcinog* 45: 786–94.

Ramesh S, Nash J, McCulloch PG. (1999) Reduction in membranous expression of beta-catenin and increased cytoplasmic E-cadherin expression predict poor survival in gastric cancer. *Br J Cancer* 81: 1392–7.

Renault B, Van Den Broek M, Fodde R *et al.* (1993) Base transitions are the most frequent genetic changes at P53 in gastric cancer. *Cancer Res* 53: 2614–7.

Rojo F, Tabernero J, Albanell J *et al.* (2006) Pharmacodynamic studies of gefitinib in tumor biopsy specimens from patients with advanced gastric carcinoma. *J Clin Oncol* 24: 4309–16.

Sakurai S, Sano T, Nakajima T. (1995) Clinicopathological and molecular biological studies of gastric adenomas with special reference to p53 abnormality. *Pathol Int* 45: 51–7.

Sarbia M, Stahl M, Zur Hausen A *et al.* (1998) Expression of p21WAF1 predicts outcome of esophageal cancer patients treated by surgery alone or by combined therapy modalities. *Clin Cancer Res* 4: 2615–23.

Scartozzi M, Galizia E, Freddari F, Berardi R, Cellerino R, Cascinu S. (2004) Molecular biology of sporadic gastric cancer: prognostic indicators and novel therapeutic approaches. *Cancer Treat Rev* 30: 451–9.

Schneider PM, Stoeltzing O, Roth JA *et al.* (2000) P53 mutational status improves estimation of prognosis in patients with curatively resected adenocarcinoma in Barrett's esophagus. *Clin Cancer Res* 6: 3153–8.

Shaheen N, Ransohoff DF. (2002) Gastroesophageal reflux, Barrett esophagus, and esophageal cancer: clinical applications. *JAMA* 287: 1982–6.

Sharpless NE. (2005) INK4a/ARF: a multifunctional tumor suppressor locus. *Mutat Res* 576: 22–38.

Sharpless NE, Ramsey MR, Balasubramanian P, Castrillon DH, Depinho RA. (2004) The differential impact of p16(INK4a) or p19(ARF) deficiency on cell growth and tumorigenesis. *Oncogene* 23: 379–85.

Shiao YH, Rugge M, Correa P, Lehmann HP, Scheer WD. (1994) p53 alteration in gastric precancerous lesions. *Am J Pathol* 144: 511–7.

Shimoyama Y, Hirohashi S. (1991) Expression of E- and P-cadherin in gastric carcinomas. *Cancer Res* 51: 2185–92.

Shimoyama S, Konishi T, Kawahara M *et al.* (1998) Expression and alteration of p53 and p21(waf1/cip1) influence the sensitivity of chemoradiation therapy for esophageal cancer. *Hepatogastroenterology* 45: 1497–504.

Shiohara M, Spirin K, Said JW *et al.* (1996) Alterations of the cyclin-dependent kinase inhibitor p19 (INK4D) is rare in hematopoietic malignancies. *Leukemia* 10: 1897–900.

Strickler JG, Zheng J, Shu Q, Burgart LJ, Alberts SR, Shibata D. (1994) p53 mutations and microsatellite instability in sporadic gastric cancer: when guardians fail. *Cancer Res* 54: 4750–5.

Symonds H, Krall L, Remington L *et al.* (1994) p53-dependent apoptosis suppresses tumor growth and progression in vivo. *Cell* 78: 703–11.

Tahara E. (1995) Genetic alterations in human gastrointestinal cancers. The application to molecular diagnosis. *Cancer* 75: 1410–7.

Tahara E. (2004) Genetic pathways of two types of gastric cancer. *IARC Sci Publ*: 327–49.

Tahara E, Semba S, Tahara H. (1996) Molecular biological observations in gastric cancer. *Semin Oncol* 23: 307–15.

Takeuchi H, Ozawa S, Ando N *et al.* (1997) Altered p16/MTS1/CDKN2 and cyclin D1/PRAD-1 gene expression is associated with the prognosis of squamous cell carcinoma of the esophagus. *Clin Cancer Res* 3: 2229–36.

Tanaka H, Shimada Y, Imamura M, Shibagaki I, Ishizaki K. (1997) Multiple types of aberrations in the p16 (INK4a) and the p15(INK4b) genes in 30 esophageal squamous-cell-carcinoma cell lines. *Int J Cancer* 70: 437–42.

Tarmin L, Yin J, Zhou X *et al.* (1994) Frequent loss of heterozygosity on chromosome 9 in adenocarcinoma and squamous cell carcinoma of the esophagus. *Cancer Res* 54: 6094–6.

Terres AM, Pajares JM, Hopkins AM *et al.* (1998a) *Helicobacter pylori* disrupts epithelial barrier function in a process inhibited by protein kinase C activators. *Infect Immun* 66: 2943–50.

Terres AM, Pajares JM, O'Toole D, Ahern S, Kelleher D. (1998b) *H. pylori* infection is associated with downregulation of E-cadherin, a molecule involved in epithelial cell adhesion and proliferation control. *J Clin Pathol* 51: 410–2.

Tohdo H, Yokozaki H, Haruma K, Kajiyama G, Tahara E. (1993) p53 gene mutations in gastric adenomas. *Virchows Arch B Cell Pathol* incl *Mol Pathol* 63: 191–5.

Tokugawa T, Sugihara H, Tani T, Hattori T. (2002) Modes of silencing of p16 in development of esophageal squamous cell carcinoma. *Cancer Res* 62: 4938–44.

Uchino S, Noguchi M, Ochiai A, Saito T, Kobayashi M, Hirohashi S. (1993) p53 mutation in gastric cancer: a genetic model for carcinogenesis is common to gastric and colorectal cancer. *Int J Cancer* 54: 759–64.

Van Dyke T. (2007) p53 and tumor suppression. *N Engl J Med* 356: 79–81.

Wang DY, Xiang YY, Tanaka M *et al.* (1994) High prevalence of p53 protein overexpression in patients with esophageal cancer in Linxian, China and its relationship to progression and prognosis. *Cancer* 74: 3089–96.

Williams G, Krajewski C, Dagher F, Ter Haar A, Roth J, Santos G. (1971) Host repopulation of endothelium. *Transplant Proc* III: 869–872.

Wong DJ, Paulson TG, Prevo LJ *et al.* (2001) p16(INK4a) lesions are common, early abnormalities that undergo clonal expansion in Barrett's metaplastic epithelium. *Cancer Res* 61: 8284–9.

Wu AH, Wan P, Bernstein L. (2001) A multiethnic population-based study of smoking, alcohol and body size and risk of adenocarcinomas of the stomach and esophagus (United States). *Cancer Causes Control* 12: 721–32.

Xing EP, Nie Y, Wang LD, Yang GY, Yang CS. (1999) Aberrant methylation of p16INK4a and deletion of p15INK4b are frequent events in human esophageal cancer in Linxian, China. *Carcinogenesis* 20: 77–84.

Yamada Y, Yoshida T, Hayashi K *et al.* (1991) p53 gene mutations in gastric cancer metastases and in gastric cancer cell lines derived from metastases. *Cancer Res* 51: 5800–5.

4 Esophageal Adenocarcinoma

Edited by Kenneth K. Wang

Diagnosis

Endoscopic diagnosis of Barrett's esophagus

Vidu B. Mokkala, Navtej S. Buttar & Louis M. Wong Kee Song

Barrett's esophagus (BE) results from the metaplastic transformation of normal squamous epithelium to a specialized columnar epithelium in the distal esophagus. This change to columnar epithelium is readily recognized at endoscopy by its salmon-colored appearance, and can be categorized as short-segment (<3 cm) or long-segment (≥3 cm) BE (Spechler 1994). Columnar-lined esophageal mucosa can contain three different histologic subtypes of epithelium including intestinal metaplasia (IM), and fundic and junctional-type epithelium. IM, with the presence of goblet cells, is a premalignant condition which can progress to dysplasia and eventually to adenocarcinoma of the esophagus. Although the detection of BE currently relies on the use of a conventional white-light endoscope and biopsy, diagnosis may be enhanced by several emerging techniques, including chromoendoscopy, magnification endoscopy, optical coherence tomography, narrow-band imaging, spectroscopy, miniprobe endosonography and autofluorescence endoscopy.

Standard white-light endoscopy

BE is suspected when the squamocolumnar junction appears proximal to the gastroesophageal junction (Figs 4.1a & 4.2a). Although it is relatively straightforward to recognize the squamocolumnar junction by the whitish squamous mucosa to salmon pink-colored columnar mucosa interface, the identification of the gastroesophageal junction is more problematic. The gastroesophageal junction coincides with the proximal-most extent of gastric longitudinal folds, but there is potential for error since excessive air insufflation in the esophagus may efface the longitudinal gastric folds. To confirm the diagnosis of BE, current guidelines recommend obtaining four-quadrant biopsy specimens at 2-cm intervals using standard biopsy forceps from the columnar-appearing mucosa (Sampliner 2002; Wang *et al.* 2005). Moreover, lesions that appear suspicious at white-light endoscopy, such as those with nodularity or ulceration, should be specifically biopsied and submitted separately.

Principles

White light from a Xenon lamp is passed through a rotary RGB filter that separates the white light into the colors red, green, and blue which are then sequentially illuminated on to the mucosa. The red, green, and blue reflected light is detected separately by a monochromatic charged-coupled device (CCD) located at the tip of the endoscope, and the three images are integrated into a single color image by the video processor that is synchronized with the rotation speed of the RGB filter (Sampliner 2002; Wang *et al.* 2005).

Standard biopsy forceps

Standard pinch biopsy forceps that fit through 2.8-mm biopsy channels are most commonly used. The aim is to get full-thickness mucosa in the biopsy.

Jumbo/large cup forceps

These forceps fit through a therapeutic endoscope with a 3.2-mm biopsy channel and have an open span of 9 mm. The large cup forceps is safe and provides a larger surface area of the Barrett's mucosa than standard forceps.

Limitations of standard endoscopy with biopsy

Four-quadrant biopsies of Barrett's esophagus with endoscopic monitoring are not ideal since they involve blind biopsy

Gastrointestinal Oncology: A Critical Multidisciplinary Team Approach. Edited by J. Jankowski, R. Sampliner, D. Kerr, and Y. Fong.

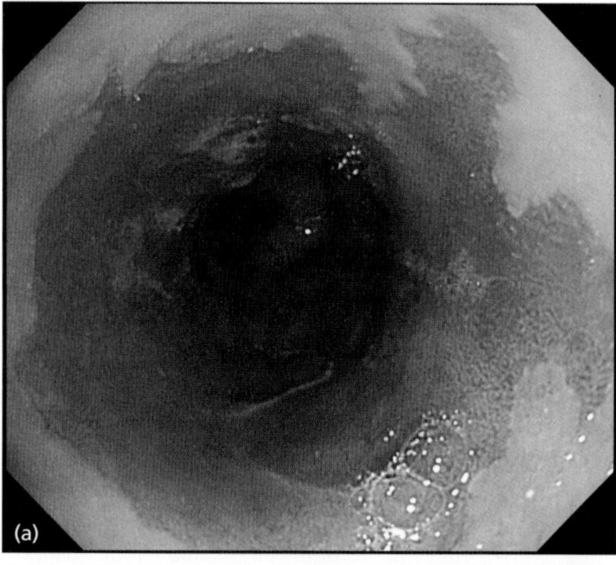

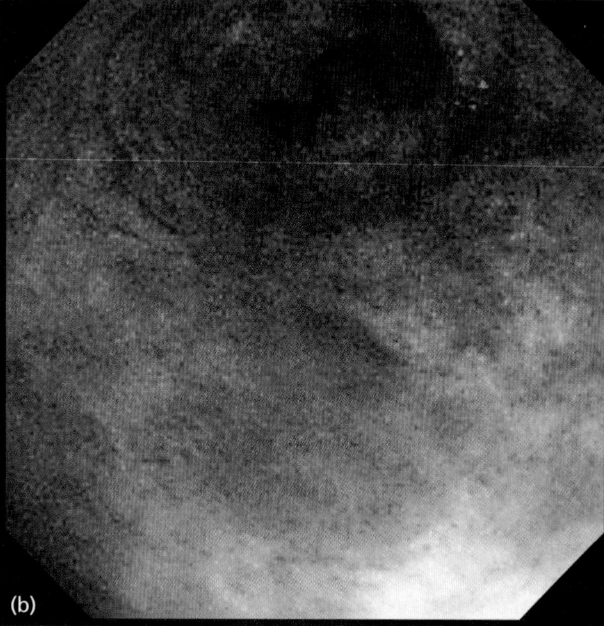

Fig. 4.1 (a) White-light imaging of BE; no suspicious lesions readily identified. (b) Autofluorescence imaging of BE; suspicious lesion (purplish color) identified at 6 o'clock amid surrounding normal-appearing green background.

sampling, taken randomly. Moreover, standard endoscopy provides only few details about the mucosal surface of the esophagus. It is difficult to distinguish specialized intestinal metaplasia (SIM) from gastric-type metaplasia or to detect dysplastic epithelium with standard white-light endoscopy, although this is changing with better-resolution endoscopes, processors and monitors. The use of jumbo biopsy forceps is not recommended for routine surveillance and has not proven to provide increased benefit in patients with high-grade dysplasia. There is evidence that routine biopsy forceps are acceptable providing at least 8 biopsies are taken (Harrison *et al.* 2007).

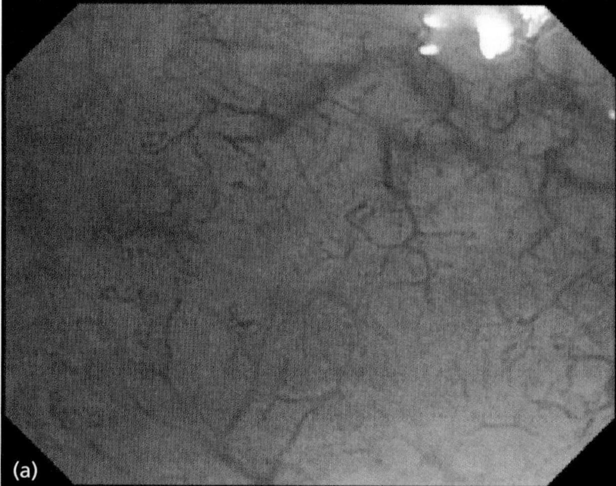

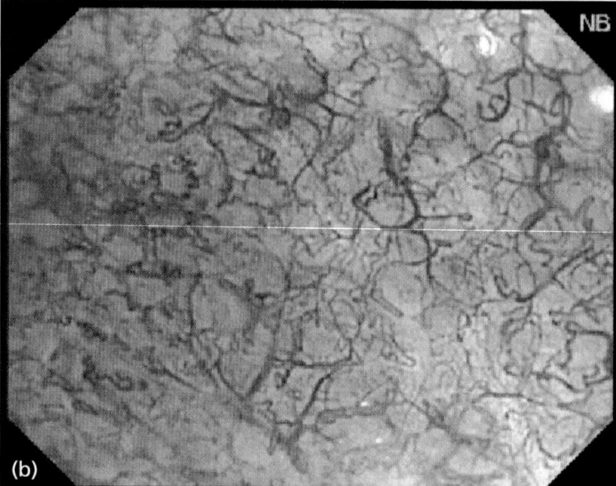

Fig. 4.2 (a) White-light imaging of Barrett's mucosa (b) NBI of Barrett's mucosa enhancing vasculature.

Side-effects

Complications of standard endoscopy include:

1 bleeding from the biopsy site or polyp removal site
2 tear or perforation in the gastrointestinal lining being examined
3 aspiration of fluid or food into the lungs
4 reactions to sedative medication used for the procedure
5 trouble swallowing or sore throat after the procedure
6 bloating of the abdomen from the air used during the procedure.

The first three complications are rare.

Chromoendoscopy

Chromoendoscopy refers to a technique in which stains or pigments are applied to the mucosa of the gastrointestinal tissues to improve characterization, to localize mucosal abnormalities and for diagnosis during endoscopy. Even though Barrett's esophagus is readily visible to the naked eye using ordinary endoscopy, staining helps to improve the diagnosis of Barrett's esophagus. The aim of staining in Barrett's esophagus is to provide more information about the dysplastic and cancerous areas within the Barrett's mucosa to target the biopsies. The various stains in chromoendoscopy are broadly classified as absorptive/vital stains, contrast stains, and reactive stains. When compared to novel diagnostic methods for the Barrett's esophagus, chromoendoscopy equipment is readily available, inexpensive, quick, and safe.

Absorptive/vital stains

These stains identify specific epithelial cells or cellular contents by preferential absorption or diffusion across the cell membrane. These help to identify cellular changes in the mucosa such as metaplasia, dysplasia, or neoplasia in patients with flat lesions which are difficult to detect by standard endoscopy.

Lugol's solution

Named after the 19th century French physician Jean Guilliaume Auguste Lugol. It contains potassium iodide and iodine which preferentially bind to the glycogen in the non-keratinized squamous epithelium.

Technique

Between 20 and 50 mL of 1.2% glycerin-free Lugol's solution which contains 24 g of potassium iodide and 12 g of iodine in 1000 mL of water is applied proximally from the gastroesophageal junction using a spray catheter. Squamous epithelium stains black, dark brown or green brown within seconds and this remains for 5 to 8 minutes.

Clinical uses

In Barrett's esophagus, the normal squamous epithelium which stains dark brown with Lugol's iodine solution is clearly demarcated from the metaplastic columnar epithelium by the absence of dye. After photodynamic therapy or multipolar electrocoagulation of Barrett's esophagus the regenerating squamous islands and normal squamous epithelium will appear dark brown and the residual areas of Barrett's esophagus will not stain.

Limitations

Application of Lugol's solution during endoscopy is not standardized, with no uniform concentrations (1–3%) or volumes (10–50 mL).

Side-effects

Bronchospasm and transient retrosternal discomfort occur. Patients allergic to iodine should not undergo Lugol's staining.

Toluidine blue

Also called tolonium chloride, this is a basic vital dye which has affinity for the cellular nuclei. It stains nuclei of columnar epithelium but cannot differentiate between subtypes of columnar epithelium (i.e. intestinal, fundic, and junctional). Malignant and inflammatory tissues which have an increased nuclear to cytoplasmic ratio due to increased mitotic activity stain blue.

Technique

A 1% mucolytic acetic acid rinse is followed by application of 1% aqueous solution of toluidine blue with a spray catheter. Another wash with 1% acetic acid is performed within 30 seconds to remove excess dye.

Clinical uses

Columnar mucosa (gastric and intestinal) stains blue, while squamous mucosa remains unstained with toluidine blue (TB). IM of BE stains blue with TB.

Chobanian *et al.* (1987) studied 58 patients with reflux symptoms. In these patients, standard endoscopy was performed first, followed by toluidine blue-aided visualization of the mucosa and targeted biopsies. IM was detected with 98% sensitivity and 80% specificity. Six patients were diagnosed with BE with TB chromoendoscopy which was missed by standard endoscopy.

Limitations

The technique cannot differentiate between gastric and intestinal metaplasia. False-positive results are seen in esophageal ulcers and erosive esophagitis.

Side-effects

No adverse side-effects have been reported.

Methylene blue (MB)

Also called methylthionine chloride, this is a vital stain which is taken up by actively absorbing tissues like small intestinal and colonic epithelium but not by non-absorptive tissues such as squamous and gastric epithelium.

Technique

As the surface mucus impairs the uptake of the dye into the epithelium, 10% N-acetyl cysteine, 16 mL for each 5 cm of circumferential Barrett's esophagus, or another mucolytic agent like pronase, is used to wash the superficial mucous layer using a spray catheter. The mucolytic action is related to the breakage of disulfide linkages in the mucus, thereby decreasing its viscosity. Two minutes later, 20 mL of 0.5–1% solution of MB is sprayed for every 5 cm of circumferential Barrett's esophagus and left for another 2 minutes, followed by a wash with 100–300 mL of tap water to remove excess MB.

Clinical uses

Intestinal metaplasia of Barrett's esophagus stains dark blue. Areas of dysplasia or neoplasia appear white or pink stained because of less uptake of the stain. Differential staining intensity and heterogenicity of dysplastic and neoplastic tissue when compared to metaplastic tissue is due to decreased cytoplasm, increase in the nuclear–cytoplasmic ratio and loss of goblet cells which are characteristic of the dysplastic and neoplastic tissues. Long-segment Barrett's mucosa stains diffusely with MB because of the diffuse nature of specialized columnar epithelium. Focal unstained areas may represent dysplastic foci within the background of heterogeneous MB staining or areas lacking IM. Methylene blue-directed biopsies (MBDBs) provide better yield than standard endoscopy. MB staining helps in differentiating dysplastic or malignant areas for endoscopic therapies like mucosal resection or photodynamic therapy. The histologic features of Barrett's esophagus can be detected when MB staining is combined with magnification endoscopy. Short-segment (less than 3 cm long) Barrett's esophagus can be easily detected by MB staining which is often missed with standard endoscopy.

Four randomized (2) controlled trials have been conducted to examine the utility of chromoendoscopy without magnification: two with positive results and two with negative results. A study conducted in the UK showed 7% improvement in the detection of intestinal metaplasia but none in the detection of dysplasia on MBDB compared with random biopsies. Another study by Canto (2001) found a significant improvement in the diagnosis of dysplasia or cancer with MB (12% vs 6%, $p = 0.004$). However, Wo *et al.* (2001) in a study of 47 patients in a prospective randomized crossover trial and Saporiti *et al.* (2003) in a study of 45 patients, comparing the MB-guided biopsy technique versus conventional biopsy technique found no significant difference in the relative frequencies for the detection of dysplasia or intestinal metaplasia between these techniques. MB chromoendoscopy is not clearly beneficial and should not be used in the routine assessment of Barrett's esophagus.

Limitations

Chromoendoscopy with MB requires pretreatment of the mucosa with the mucolytics, a dwell time for the dye to take effect, and the rinse phase to remove the excess dye. The MB staining pattern in Barrett's tissue in different studies is inconsistent. MB dye binds non-specifically to exudates or fails to stain denuded epithelial areas, thereby missing microscopic or macroscopic ulcerations. A uniform classification system for mucosal topographic patterns needs to be devised.

Side-effects

Concerns about oxidative damage to the DNA and potential for carcinogenesis in premalignant tissues in the presence of white light and methylene blue during endoscopy has been raised. Passage of green urine and stool within the next day is distressing to the patient.

Indigo carmine

Blue contrast stain is derived from indigo, a blue plant dye and carmine, a red coloring agent. The dye is not absorbed by the gastrointestinal mucosal epithelium like the vital stains are. Endoscopy with higher-resolution instruments like magnification endoscopy provides better mucosal architecture.

Clinical uses

Indigo carmine seeps into epithelial cell crevices providing mucosal topography. It identifies surface villiform pattern of the intestinal metaplasia and irregularities.

Sharma *et al.* (2003) studied 80 patients with suspected BE with a mean length of columnar-lined distal esophageal mucosa of 3.7 cm using high-magnification chromoendoscopy (MCE). Three types of mucosal pattern were noted within the columnar mucosa using 0.4–0.8% of indigo carmine and ×115 high-magnification endoscopy: ridge/villous, circular, and irregular/distorted patterns. Fifty-seven of 62 patients (97%) with rich or villous patterns showed IM. Two of 12 patients (17%) with a circular pattern had IM. Six out of 6 of patients with an irregular/distorted pattern had high-grade dysplasia (HGD). Low-grade dysplasia (LGD) was found in 18 patients at biopsy, all of whom had ridged/villous patterns. The drawback of this MCE is that it is unable to differentiate LGD from non-dysplastic epithelium.

Technique

Using a spray catheter 0.1–0.5% solution can be sprayed directly onto the mucosa.

Limitations

The dye disappears rapidly after mucosal application because of the gut motility and the effects of the mucosal secretions.

Magnification endoscopy

Magnification endoscopy or enhanced magnification endoscopy (EME) provides better visualization of mucosal details that are not provided by standard endoscopy. This can be achieved using fiberoptic, videoscopic or ultra-high magnification endoscopes. High-resolution endoscopes are capable of discriminating between two closely approximated objects 10–71 microns in diameter as compared with the naked eye which can discriminate objects 125–165 microns in diameter. Prototype ultra-high ME uses a moveable lens controlled by the operator to vary the degree of magnification, which generally ranges from ×8 to ×170. Additional time is needed compared to standard endoscopy. The resolving power of the standard endoscope is only 0.1 cm but the resolving power is up to 0.01 mm with ultra-high ME which can detect the nuclei and cellular contents more clearly. New electronic videoendoscopes are equipped with CCD chips of high pixel density of up to 400 K, enabling high-image resolution. Commercially available endoscopes with megapixel density as high as 850 K have been introduced, which better enhances the image.

Clinical use

Magnification endoscopy provides better visualization of epithelial patterns in patients with Barrett's dysplasia or early cancer. It can also provide information about the vascular architecture for early diagnosis of carcinoma in Barrett's mucosa.

Ferguson *et al.* (2006) conducted a prospective, randomized trial of 137 patients with gastroesophageal reflux disease to compare the effectiveness of EME-directed biopsies (×115) and random biopsies with standard endoscopy. Patterns classified with EME were reticular, villous and ridged, similar to the classification of Guelrud. They concluded that there is no difference in the ability of EME-directed biopsies to identify SIM in patients with or without the endoscopic appearance of BE compared with standard endoscopy with random biopsies.

Limitations of ME

At a magnified view, a smaller range of mucosa is observed and unless the magnifying lens is kept very close to the mucosa, the image obtained is out of focus. The technique requires more time and effort to learn than other techniques. For this reason the tip of the magnification endoscope has a 2-mm soft tissue distal attachment that stabilizes the tissue. This method needs standardization of the mucosal patterns.

Magnification chromoscopy or enhanced magnification endoscopy

This is a technique in which high-resolution and high-magnification endoscopes are used in conjunction with tissue stains or pigments to further enhance the image and reduce procedure length. The stains used in magnification chromoscopy are methylene blue, acetic acid and indigo carmine.

Methylene blue magnification chromoscopy

Technique

Endo *et al.* (2002) used magnification endoscopy with MB for better identification of SIM and dysplasia. MB dye staining was performed according to Canto's method (2001, 2005) and staining status of the selected regions was classified as either positive or negative. The biopsy specimens were taken from the selected regions with ×80 magnification endoscopy.

Thirty patients with BE with a total of 67 biopsy specimen regions were analyzed for five types of pit pattern:

1 small round (dot) type with relatively uniform size and shape

2 straight type with long straight lines

3 long oval and curved type with long extended pits larger than those of the dot type

4 tubular type with complicated and twisted patterns similar to a branch or gyrus-like structure

5 villous type with flat, finger-like projections.

The percentage of positive staining with MB was 0% for pits 1 and 2, 23% for pit 3, 60% for pit 4, and 50% for pit 5. The percentages of specialized columnar epithelium (SEC) for pit types 3, 4, and 5 were 40%, 100%, and 100% respectively. Pit types 1 and 2 contain scarcely any SCE. Pits 3, 4 and 5 had abundant SCE. Mucin phenotype analysis showed a predominance of gastric phenotype mucin in pit 1 and 2 patterns. Pit 4 and 5 patterns had a high proportion of cells with intestinal-type mucin. Pit 3 had mixed gastric and intestinal-type mucin.

Limitations

The frequency of SCE in pit 3 was not high enough to discriminate fundic or junctional-type mucosa from SCE by magnification endoscopy. More precise subclassification of the pit 3 pattern is awaited in the future.

Acetic acid magnification chromoscopy

The aceto white reaction is a procedure in which the red translucent epithelial surface is converted into white opaque epithelial surface with the application of acetic acid.

Technique

Between 5 and 10 ml of 1.5% acetic acid is sprayed over esophageal mucosa suspected of Barrett's using a spray catheter from the distal end of the esophagus and then moving proximally. Both the esophageal and gastric epithelium whitens initially, and within 2–3 minutes the gastric and metaplastic columnar epithelium of Barrett's mucosa turns reddish but the normal squamous epithelium of esophagus remains white.

Clinical uses

Helps to differentiate normal tissue from metaplastic tissue. Useful for metaplasia and dysplasia-directed biopsies for screening and surveillance of Barrett's esophagus and for monitoring response to ablative therapy.

Guelrud *et al.* (2001) used acetic acid application in the distal esophagus for better endoscopic visualization of BE and islands of specialized columnar epithelium not ablated by endoscopic therapy in 21 patients. In 11 of the 21 patients, acetic acid installation improved the detection of islands of columnar epithelium not visualized before acetic acid installation. The same authors used acetic acid in conjunction with ×35 magnification endoscopy to identify IM in 49 patients with suspected SSBE. In this study, four mucosal patterns were identified: round (round pits with regular and orderly arranged circular dots), reticular (pits were circular or oval and were regular in shape and arrangement), villous (no pits were present but there was a fine villiform appearance with regular shape and arrangement), and ridged (no pits were present but there was a thick villous convoluted shape with a cerebriform appearance with regular shape and arrangement). Mucosa exhibiting the villous and ridged pattern yielded IM in 87% and 100% of biopsy specimens, respectively. Enhanced magnification endoscopy enabled the detection of IM with a higher success rate compared with standard endoscopic methods.

Limitations

Helps to identify an increasing number of patients with very short segment Barrett's esophagus, the malignant risk of which is unclear. A high level of interobserver variability has been recognized.

Stevens *et al.* (1994) combined ×35 magnification endoscopy with chromoendoscopy (Lugol's iodine with indigo carmine) for the evaluation of BE in 13 of 46 patients with gastroesophageal reflux symptoms. The Lugol's solution was used to identify and highlight the squamocolumnar junction. The abnormal raised or depressed areas seen by magnification chromoscopy are selected for biopsy.

Discrimination of dysplasia from metaplasia is not possible.

Narrow-band imaging

NBI is a technique that reveals fine superficial mucosal pattern and vascular pattern without the use of dyes. RGB-based NBI systems are available with white light illumination along with a color CCD chip.

Principles

A xenon lamp provides white light which, when passed through a rotating RGB filter, separates into red, green, and blue colors to illuminate the mucosa sequentially. The depth of penetration of light depends on its wavelength. Blue light has a shorter wavelength than the red light which penetrates more superficially when compared to red light. The tip of the endoscope is fitted with a monochromatic CCD that detects the red, green, and blue reflected light, and the three images are integrated by the video processor into a single color image. The RGB filters used in NBI have a band-pass range which is narrowed, with highest contribution from the blue light that reveals optimal superficial imaging. During endoscopy, the NBI filter can be enabled or disabled making it easy to switch between NBI mode and standard mode. NBI provides visualization of the superficial mucosal pattern because of the optimal superficial imaging by the blue light and superficial vasculature because of the absorption of blue light by hemoglobin.

Advantages over chromoendoscopy

It is user friendly, staining agents are not required, and the whole endoscopic field is visualized in NBI. It also visualizes the superficial vascular pattern clearly.

Clinical uses

NBI is useful for differentiating high-grade intraepithelial neoplasia (HGIN) from non-dysplastic specialized intestinal metaplasia (SIM). In non-dysplastic SIM (Kara *et al.* 2006a) the mucosa pattern is regular with flat or villous/gyrus pattern (80%) and a regular vascular pattern: the blood vessels are located along or between the mucosal ridges and have regular honeycomb structures. In dysplastic tissue the mucosal pattern is irregular (disrupted pattern and destroyed villi) with an irregular vascular pattern (disorganized vessels that are irregular). Three important factors for differentiating HGIN from non-dysplastic tissue are irregular mucosal pattern, irregular vascular pattern, and abnormal blood vessels (Figs 4.2 & 4.3). In 85%

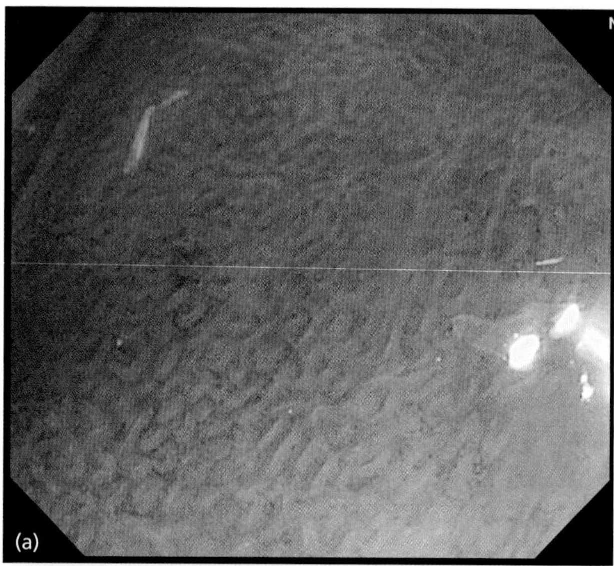

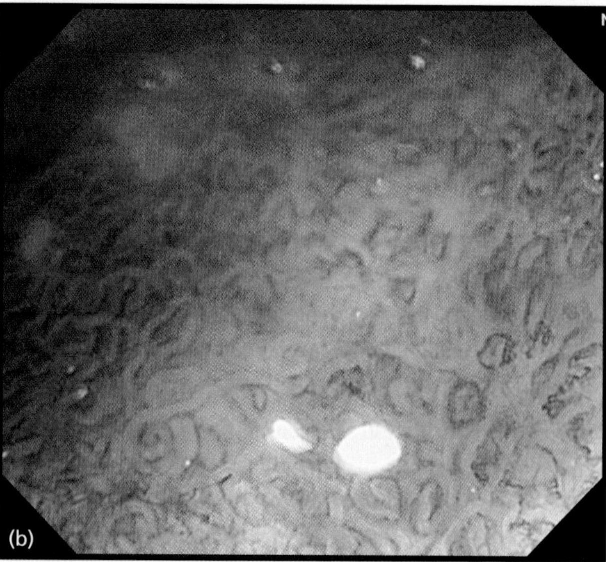

Fig. 4.3 (a) NBI or non-dysplastic BE with regular mucosal pattern. (b) NBI of BE with HGD with irregular mucosal pattern and abnormal vascular pattern (corkscrew vessels).

of cases two or more of the above factors are detected. When differentiating non-dysplastic SIM from low-grade and high-grade dysplasia, the above factors are also useful.

Kara *et al.* (2006a) reported magnified NBI imaging of 62 patients with non-dysplastic SIM characterized by either villous/gyrus patterns (80%), which were mostly regular and had regular vascular patterns, or a flat mucosa with normal-appearing long branching vessels (20%). All areas with HGIN had at least one abnormality and 85% had two or more abnormalities. The frequency of the abnormalities showed a significant rise with increasing grades of dysplasia. The magnified NBI images had a sensitivity of 94%, a specificity of 76%, a positive predictive value of 64%, and a negative predictive value of 94% for HGIN.

Sharma *et al.* (2005, 2006a) recently correlated the NBI pattern in 51 patients with known or suspected BE. Of 51 patients (mean BE length 3.5 cm), 28 had IM without dysplasia, 8 had LGD, 7 had HGD and 8 had cardiac-type mucosa. The sensitivity, specificity, and positive predictive value of the ridge/villous (regular) pattern for diagnosis of IM without HGD were 93.55, 86.7%, and 94.7% respectively. The sensitivity, specificity, and positive predictive value of an irregular/distorted pattern for HGD were 100%, 98.7%, and 95.3% respectively. This study is limited by the lack of a control group.

Limitations

Low-grade dysplasia cannot be distinguished from intestinal metaplasia by NBI. As yet, a randomized controlled trial (RCT) has not critically examined the usefulness of NBI in patients with BE.

Optical coherence tomography

Optical coherence tomography (OCT) (Chak *et al.* 2005a) is an interferometric, non-invasive optical tomographic imaging technique offering millimeter penetration with submicrometer axial and lateral resolution. OCT remains the imaging technology with the highest available endoscopic resolution of any available technology. OCT, first described in 1991, is an optical analog of B-mode ultrasonography. OCT is similar to B-scan ultrasonography, but uses light as opposed to sound, and the resolution is 10 times greater than high-frequency ultrasound. OCT (Chak *et al.* 2005a) is a novel emerging biomedical imaging technology which depends on the backscattering of light from subsurface tissue microstructures to obtain high-resolution (1–2-μm) cross-sectional images. This high resolution allows visualization of microscopic mucosal features like villi, glands, crypts, lymphatic aggregates and blood vessels. OCT measures the back-reflected signal of light to generate a two-dimensional map of the esophagus in a longitudinal and radial fashion.

Principles

Low coherence interferometry is the main principle of OCT. The incident light from super luminescent diode which is a source of low-coherence infrared light is split into two by a 50/50 optical beam splitter, with half directed to the tissue via an optical fiber and the other half directed to a moveable reference mirror, located at a controlled distance. The backscattered light from both the mirror and tissue is directed towards a detector which produces interference signal only when the reflected light travels the same distance from both the mirror and tissue. The interference signal provides information about the magnitude of the backscattered light intensity from the microstructures within the tissue at a particular depth.

Potential clinical uses

The current *in vivo* endoscopic optical coherence tomography (EOCT) (Isenberg *et al.* 2005) probes are 2–2.7 mm in diameter, providing end-on scanning, longitudinal scanning (along the length of the esophagus) or 360° radial scanning. OCT provides details up to the inner circular layer of the muscularis propria but cannot visualize the outer longitudinal layer of the muscularis propria in the normal esophagus because of the limitation of the sampling depth in the tissue (4–6 mm). In specialized intestinal metaplasia (Poneros *et al.* 2001) of Barrett's esophagus there is glandular morphology with presence of submucosal glands and lack of normal esophageal morphology because of loss of signal from light scattering within the metaplastic epithelium. In Barrett's adenocacinoma OCT provides pronounced morphologic distortion characterized by abnormal configuration of the neoplastic epithelium containing large pockets of mucin surrounded by a cellular stroma. OCT may help endoscopists in the surveillance of patients with Barrett's esophagus (Poneros 2005) by obtaining targeted biopsies from worrisome morphologic areas.

In a prospective double-blinded study Isenberg *et al.* (2005) used EOCT in the detection of dysplasia in BE in 33 patients with a total of 314 biopsies. By using histology as the standard, EOCT detected BE dysplasia with a sensitivity of 68%, specificity of 82, positive predictive value of 53%, negative predictive value of 89%, and diagnostic accuracy of 78%. Diagnostic accuracy for the four endoscopists ranged from 56% to 98%, the main limitation of the study.

Recently computer-aided diagnosis of dysplasia in BE was used with EOCT by Qi *et al.* (2006) in 13 patients with 106 images. Using histology as a reference standard it had a sensitivity of 82%, specificity of 74% and accuracy of 83%. With further refinements, computer-aided diagnosis could also improve the accuracy of EOCT identification of dysplasia in BE.

Limitations

OCT is an evolving technique requiring refinement for accurate diagnosis of preneoplastic lesions. Biopsy correlation of OCT-visualized areas is technically challenging. Variations in the esophageal peristalsis and cardiothoracic movements can result in the biopsy of a different area from that initially imaged by

OCT. The procedure is expensive and cumbersome and only a small volume of tissue is assessed. Compression artifacts can be seen with OCT probe–tissue interaction.

Point spectroscopy

Point spectroscopy is a technique in which light is passed into tissue in a non-destructive fashion providing structural, molecular composition and biochemical information by analyzing light–tissue interactions. Examples described below are elastic scattering spectroscopy, fluorescence spectroscopy, and Raman scattering. The point spectroscopic techniques provide histopathologic diagnosis in real time for the recognition of metaplasia and dysplasia. Such point spectroscopic techniques are useful both alone or as adjuncts to optical imaging devices that are capable of visualizing larger mucosal surfaces.

Elastic scattering spectroscopy (ESS)

ESS is a relatively simple spectroscopic technique that provides structural information about tissues in less than 1 second. The main advantages over fluorescence spectroscopy are the use of white light instead of laser and the use of a stronger signal.

Principles

ESS is based on white light reflectance. The incident white light on the tissue is scattered back by scatterers like cell nuclei and mitochondria without change in wavelength or energy. ESS measures the intensity of the backscattered light (reflectance spectra), providing details about the changes in the density and size of the tissue scatterers. Reflectance spectra contain both multiple scattered photons mostly from the stroma and singly backscattered photons. The reflectance spectrum in diffuse reflectance spectra provides information about the structural composition of connective tissues such as collagen. The reflectance spectrum in light-scattering spectroscopy (LSS) provides information about the nuclear size, density, enlargement and crowding which makes up 2–5% of the total reflectance spectrum. Because of limited penetration of white light only structural composition and morphologic information is obtained from the epithelial layers.

Clinical uses

ESS helps to detect the dysplastic changes in Barrett's esophagus by providing information regarding the nuclear size, number, enlargement and crowding through the backscattered light from the epithelial nuclei.

Georgakoudi and Van Dam (2003) used diffuse reflectance spectra in 16 patients (40 samples) for evaluating LGD and HGD in patients with BE. In reflectance spectroscopy, white light from a xenon flash lamp was coupled into a 6 collected fiber probe to detect biochemical and morphologic changes in mucosa progressing to dysplasia in less than 1 second. This procedure has specificity and sensitivity of 100% and 86%, respectively.

Lovat and Bown (2004) and Lovat *et al.* (2006) used ESS for detection of HGD and cancer in BE. The optical spectra from ESS measurement were compared with 181 matched histologic biopsy specimens taken from identical sites within BE from 81 patients. Three gastrointestinal pathologists classified the biopsies as either low risk (non-dysplastic or LGD) or high risk (HGD or cancer). ESS detected high-risk sites with a sensitivity of 92% and specificity of 60% and differentiated from low-risk sites with 79% sensitivity and specificity. This method requires validation in prospective studies for BE surveillance.

Wallace *et al.* (2000, 2006) conducted LSS for detecting dysplasia in 66 sites in 13 patients with BE compared with histologic findings from biopsy specimens. Each suspected mucosal site was sampled using a fiberoptic probe in LSS. The reflected white light was spectrally analyzed to obtain the distribution of cell nuclei for enlargement and crowding in the Barrett's mucosa. If 30% of cell nuclei exceeded 10 μm, then the mucosa was classified as dysplastic. Four different histologic grades: non-dysplastic Barrett's, indefinite for dysplasia, LGD, and HGD, were determined by four different pathologists, who were blinded to spectroscopic diagnosis and diagnosis of the other pathologists. The specificity and sensitivity of LSS for detecting LGD or HGD were 90% and 90% respectively.

Limitations

As for fluorescence spectroscopy below, the limited volume of tissue sampled is the main drawback when compared to conventional biopsy.

Fluorescence spectroscopy (FS)

Also called light/laser-induced fluorescence spectroscopy (LIFS) or autofluorescence spectroscopy (AFS). Tissue fluorescence is a phenomenon in which short wavelength light is absorbed and long wavelength light is emitted by the molecules within the tissue. Fluorescence diagnosis can be achieved by autofluorescence or drug-enhanced autofluorescence. Autofluorescence is a phenomenon in which numerous endogenous molecules in biologic tissue fluoresce when illuminated by short wavelength visible light or ultraviolet light. Multiple endogenous molecules (flurophores) in biologic tissue that produce autofluoresence are connective tissue elements (collagen, elastin), aromatic amino acids (tryptophan, tyrosine, phenylalanine), porphyrin, flavins, coenzymes (reduced NADH), and lipofuscin. Each flurophore has a characteristic fluorescence excitation spectrum (wavelength region at which light is absorbed) and characteristic fluorescence emission spectrum (wavelength region at which fluorescent light is emitted).

Principles

FS is usually passed through the working channel of an endoscope. FS contains a light source and a fiberoptic probe with fibers to carry the excitation light to the tissue and to transmit back the fluorescence signal to a spectrographic photon detector which is then optically analyzed by computer. The light source is usually short wavelength laser that emits light at 337-nm wavelength. The fluorescence signal usually has a long wavelength in the range of 350–700 nm. Fluorescence spectra from different tissue fluorophores is broad and line shaped and based on re-emission of incident light at longer wavelength by either endogenous or exogenous fluorophores. Drug-enhanced autofluoresence (Brand *et al.* 2002) is a phenomenon in which exogenous agents like aminolevulinic acid (ALA)-induced protoporphyrin IX (PpIX) fluorescence is administered which has selectivity for neoplasia. Generally drug-enhanced autofluoresence emits stronger fluorescence signals than autofluoresence.

Clinical uses

FS differentiates Barrett's esophagus with high-grade dysplasia and adenocarcinoma from low-grade and no dysplasia accurately.

Panjehpour *et al.* (1996) used 410-nm laser light to induce autofluoresence in 36 patients (308 samples) with BE. The fluorescence spectra were analyzed from all patients collectively using differential normalized fluorescence (DNF) indices individually at 480-nm and 660-nm intensity. Using the 480-nm index to classify the spectra, specificity was 96% for detecting benign tissue in non-dysplastic Barrett's mucosa (208 of 216), and specificity was 100% for detecting benign tissue in low-grade dysplasia samples (36 of 36). The sensitivity was 28% (13 of 46) and 90% (9 of 10) for detecting premalignant tissue for samples with low-grade with focal high-grade dysplasia and for samples with HGD. Using DNF 660-nm index to classify the spectra, the results were similar. This method is rapid, accurate and a less invasive technique for detecting HGD in patients with BE compared with standard methods but a false-positive rate of 30% is seen for inflammatory and reactive changes in the esophagus.

Bourg-Heckly *et al.* (2000) used ultraviolet autofluoresence spectroscopy. Ultraviolet light of 330-nm excitation was used in 24 patients (218 samples) to identify early malignant lesions in the esophagus. The fluorescence spectra were analyzed by three dimensionless indices using distinct fluorophores, R1 (ratio of intensities at 390 nm and 450 nm, collagen, and NADPH), R2 (ratio of intensities at 450 nm and 550 nm, NADPH, and flavins), R3 (ratio of intensities at 390 nm and 550 nm, collagen, and flavins). Comparison of spectral shapes of the autofluoresence spectra can be done by comparing the values of R1, R2, and R3 ratios. The method showed a sensitivity of 86% and specificity of 95% for distinguishing specialized columnar epithelium and neoplastic tissue from normal esophageal mucosa.

Georgakoudi *et al.* (2001) used fluorescence spectroscopy in 16 patients (40 samples) for evaluating LGD and HGD in patients with BE. In fluorescence spectroscopy, a 1-mm diameter optical fiber probe was used to deliver 11 different excitation wavelengths between 337 and 620 nm to detect intrinsic tissue fluorescence which provides tissue biochemistry in early detection of mucosa progressing to dysplasia. This procedure has a specificity and sensitivity of 97% and 100% respectively.

Pfefer *et al.* (2003) used temporal and spectral fluorescence spectroscopy for the detection of HGD in BE. Excitation wavelengths of 337 and 400 nm were used to obtain 148 fluorescence spectra and 108 transient delay profiles in 37 patients. The biopsy specimens from BE were classified as carcinoma, HGD or low-risk tissue (LGD, indefinite for dysplasia and non-dysplastic tissue). A linear discriminant analysis diagnostic algorithm was developed retrospectively to differentiate HGD from low-risk tissue. The sensitivity and specificity were 74% and 67–85%, respectively. Improved accuracy is necessary.

Brand *et al.* (2002) used 5-ALA in 20 patients for detecting HGD in BE by fluorescence spectroscopy. Three hours before endoscopy, patients were given 10 mg/kg of 5-ALA orally. Administration of 5-ALA leads to accumulation of PpIX, the precursor of heme in malignant and premalignant tissues. PpIX has florescence intensity at 635 nm wavelength. Nitrogen-pumped dye laser spectrography was used to measure quantitative fluorescence spectra from 97 spectra. This 5-ALA-PpIX spectrum was compared with histopathologic mucosal biopsy specimens taken immediately after fluorescence measurement. The PpIX fluorescence intensity was greater for HGD than for non-dysplastic Barrett's epithelium. HGD was distinguished from non-dysplastic tissue types with 77% sensitivity and 71% specificity. Nodular HGD had decreased fluorescence and could be differentiated from non-dysplastic tissue with 100% sensitivity and 100% specificity by using the fluorescence intensity ratio of 635 nm/480 nm.

Ortner *et al.* (2003) used 5-ALA time-gated PpIX fluorescence spectroscopy in 53 patients to differentiate LGD from non-dysplastic Barrett's mucosa. 5-ALA was sprayed 1–2 hours before biopsy. Biopsy specimens were interpreted by two different pathologists and 141 of 168 samples were further analyzed immunohistochemically for P53 protein expression. Significant fluorescence intensity (ratio of delayed PpIX fluorescence intensity to immediate fluorescence intensity) was seen between non-dysplastic SIM and LGD. There was a 2.8-fold increased rate of dysplasia detection compared to screening endoscopy. This method also helps to differentiate SIM from junctional or gastric fundic-type epithelium in short-segment Barrett's esophagus. The sensitivity and specificity of this method was 76% and 63% respectively. High interobserver variability of 40% is reported.

Limitations

False positives are seen in the esophagus with reactive and inflammatory change. Because of the small sample depth and volume of the mucosa FS is not used as a surveillance tool. Drug-enhanced autofluoresence has obstacles in current endoscopic practice because of adverse effects, cost, variable pharmacokinetics, and the need for prior regulatory approval before usage.

Raman spectroscopy

Raman spectroscopy (RS) or inelastic spectroscopy (IS) provides the biochemical details (Kendall *et al.* 2003) of the biologic molecules in tissues. RS has high molecular specificity providing more specific tissue diagnosis than ESS or FS. RS has a narrower and more detailed peak than FS.

Principles

When incident light is passed through tissue, the molecules comprising the tissue produce vibrational frequencies resulting in tiny shifts in the wavelength of inelastically scattered light. This shift in wavelength is called the Raman shift and the effect is called the Raman effect. Raman spectra can be obtained with good signal-to-noise ratio in 5 seconds (Fig. 4.4).

Clinical uses

Two different studies by Wong Kee Song *et al.* (Wong Kee Song & Marcon 2003; Wong Kee Song 2005) reported the diagnostic accuracy and potential of Raman spectroscopy. In one study of 65 patients assessed for non-dysplastic Barrett's, LGD and HGD/early AC, the diagnostic accuracy was 88%, 81% and 92% respectively. In another study of 192 samples from 65 patients, the Raman spectra collected from near-infrared Raman spectroscopy (NIRS) were compared with histologic biopsies. NIRS differentiates dysplastic from non-dysplastic Barrett's samples with 86% sensitivity, 88% specificity, and 87% accuracy. NIRS also identifies high-risk lesions (HGD/early AC) with 88% sensitivity, 89% specificity, and 89% accuracy. Although the volume size of tissue sample is small, RS provides detailed information from the spectra with good diagnostic accuracy.

Limitations

The Raman signal of tissues *in vivo* is weak due to interference from tissue fluorescence and spectral contamination of Raman and fluorescence signals produced by fiberoptic materials. RS requires sophisticated instruments, intensive signal processing and complex statistical technique for spectral analysis and classification.

Multimodal or trimodal spectroscopy

Georgakoudi and Feld (2004) and Georgakoudi *et al.* (2001) used three different spectroscopic techniques (fluorescence, reflectance, and light-scattering spectroscopy) in 16 patients (40 samples) to evaluate LGD and HGD in patients with BE. In fluorescence spectroscopy, a 1-mm diameter optical fiber probe was used to deliver 11 different excitation wavelengths between 337 and 620 nm to detect intrinsic tissue fluorescence which provides tissue biochemistry. In reflectance spectroscopy, white light from Xe flash lamp was coupled into a 6 collected fiber probe to get biochemical and morphologic changes in detection of dysplasia in less than 1 second. In light scattering spectroscopy, a small fraction of reflected light caused by photons are singly backscattered by the cell nuclei providing the number,

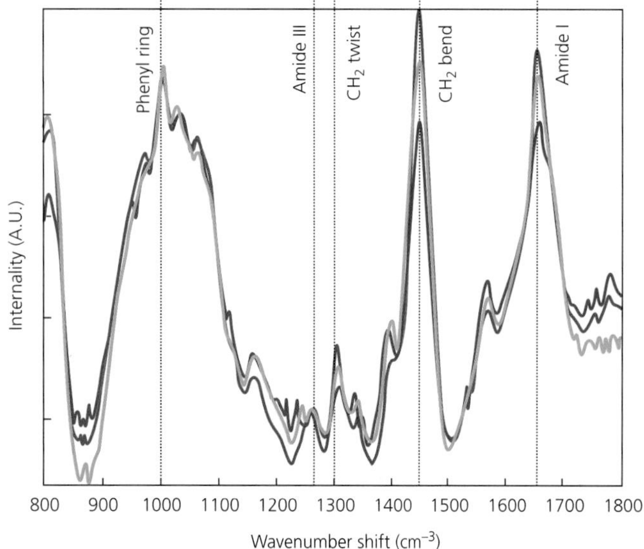

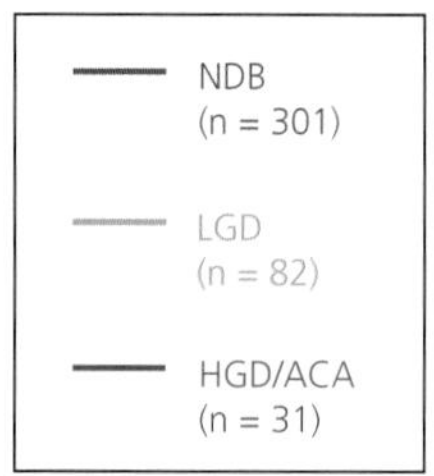

Fig. 4.4 Raman spectra of Barrett's epithelia. Spectral differences among tissue types can be exploited using multivariate statistical techniques for spectral algorithm development and tissue discrimination.

size, enlargement and crowding. This procedure has a very high specificity and sensitivity. In the future, software development will allow data analysis of three types of spectroscopic information in real time, providing a rapid guide for performing biopsies from desired areas.

Autofluorescence imaging (AFI)

Light-induced fluorescence endoscopy (LIFE) or endoscopic fluorescence imaging allows visualization of the entire endoscopic mucosal field at once when compared to spectroscopy. The prototype LIFE II device allows endoscopists to switch between white light imaging and fluorescence imaging mode in less than 4 seconds. LIFE uses a metal halide light source that delivers photons of desired wavelength, typically about 400–450 nm (blue light) and receives light at the desired fluorescence range by a sensitive intensified camera. In the LIFE II camera the emitted fluorescence in the green wavelength (490–560 nm) and red wavelength (630–750 nm) ranges are measured by two separate intensified CCDs.

Clinical uses

The fluorescence image from the dysplastic tissue is displayed as a brick red color against a green/cyan colored normal background on the video monitor. When AFI is used, non-dysplastic BE appears green and the dysplastic lesions appear blue or violet (see Fig. 4.1b).

Haringsma (2002) presented promising data on the capability of autofluoresence endoscopy to detect the presence of HGD and early adenocarcinoma (EAC) in BE.

Two RCTs have been conducted, both using fiberoptic AFI endoscopes with low-quality images and did not incorporate information from reflected light. The first multicenter RCT by Borovicka *et al.* (2006) reported that autofluoresence endoscopy alone was not suitable for replacing the standard four-quadrant biopsy protocol. Another prospective randomized crossover study of 50 patients with Barrett's esophagus showed no significant benefit over a standard surveillance biopsy for the detection of high-grade dysplasia and early adenocarcinoma. Both of the above studies had very high false-positive rates.

A recent feasibility trial by Kara and Bergman (2006) using video AFI in 21 patients suggested that it may improve the detection of HGD/EC in patients with BE compared to white light endoscopy (WLE). Introduction of a novel concept of multimodality imaging (AFI-NBI) by Kara *et al.* (2006b) increased the accuracy of detecting HGIN in BE. Twenty patients with BE with suspected HGIN were examined initially by AFI followed by NBI. AFI detected 47 suspicious lesions; 28 contained HGIN (60%) and 19 were false positive (40%). With NBI, 25 of the true positive lesions had definitely suspicious patterns (89%) and 3 had possibly suspicious patterns (11%). Of the 19 false positives, 14 were not suspicious on NBI (suggesting non-dysplastic tissue). Low-grade dysplasia was found in 4 of the remaining 5 false positives (10%). The false-positive rate was therefore reduced from 40% to 10%.

Limitations

This technique has limited diagnostic utility in Barrett's esophagus because of high false-positive results. There is no significant benefit of LIFE-guided biopsies over standard WLE surveillance biopsy protocol for the detection of high-grade dysplasia and early carcinoma. LIFE is an evolving technique not yet optimized for clinical use.

Miniprobe endosonography

While white light endoscopy can assess the extent of intraluminal spread of a tumor, endosonography can assess the depth of tumor invasion into surrounding areas including the status of lymph nodes.

Principles

Endoscopic ultrasound is a device with a 360° sector, a penetration depth of 10 cm, and frequency ranging from 7.5 to 12 MHz. Miniprobes with a frequency of 15–20 MHz are thin probes that can be introduced and used for detecting mucosal and submucosal areas.

Clinical uses

Endosonographic techniques have been used and adapted for staging TNM (Pech *et al.* 2006) classification. They have also been used for detection of paraesophageal lymph nodal invasion. Miniprobes are used for staging early esophageal carcinoma with submucosal assessment.

Limitations

The technique has an accuracy rate of 90% for T and of up to 80% for lymph node status for pretherapeutic tumor staging. Despite the good sensitivity of 80% for lymph node involvement, the specificity for lymph node metastasis is still 40%. Another limitation of miniprobe endosonography is detection of invasion of the submucosa.

Confocal endomicroscopy

Confocal endomicroscopy is a study which provides *in vivo* histology of the mucosa during ongoing endoscopy. Confocal laser endomicroscopy is set up with a miniature confocal microscope in the distal tip of a conventional video endoscope.

Principles

Confocal endomicroscopy uses focal laser illumination of the tissue with excitation wavelength of 488 nm by an optic fiber. The confocal cross-sectional images are detected at a rate of 0.8–1.6 frames per second through a pinhole, rejecting out-of-focus light to provide clear images of the mucosa. This technique provides <1-μm high-resolution histologic imaging of the mucosa. The imaging depth ranges from 100 to 300 μm, allowing subsurface mucosal analysis. Newer fluorescence-aided endomicroscopy uses contrast agents: topical (acriflavine) or intravenous (fluorescein sodium) (Wang *et al.* 2005) in combination with confocal endomicroscopy to provide clear details of the cellular architecture.

Clinical uses

Kiesslich *et al.* (2005, 2006) and Kiesslich and Neurath (2006) performed confocal laser endomicroscopy in 63 patients. The endomicroscopy distinguished between different types of epithelial cells and also detected changes in the cellular and vascular architecture in the BE. *In vivo* histology of BE and associated neoplasia were compared with histologic biopsy specimens. The sensitivity, specificity, and accuracy for BE were 98.1%, 92.9%, and 96.8%. The sensitivity, specificity, and accuracy for Barrett's-associated neoplasia were 94.1%, 98.4%, and 97.4% (Fig. 4.5).

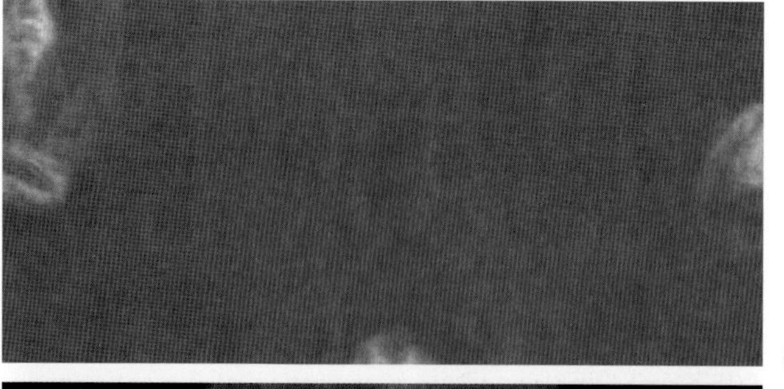
(a)

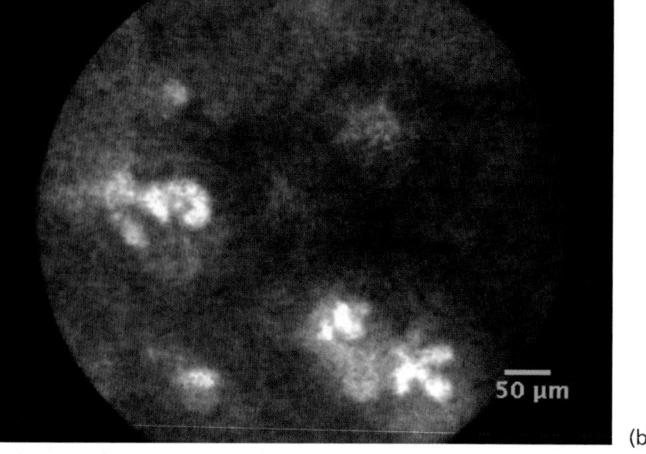

(b)

Fig. 4.5 Confocal endoscopic probe. Images of (a) squamous, non-dysplastic Barrett's and (b) Barrett's with high-grade dysplasia, represented by irregular cells and fluorescin leakage (white spots). A small area of non-dysplastic Barrett's is also present at the three o'clock position.

Limitations

Because of the small sampling size, the routine use of confocal endomicroscopy for screening and surveillance needs further assessment.

Endocytoscopy

The shift from histologic confirmation to imaging confirmation recently with the concept of optical biopsy has led to the development of endocytoscopy. This is another *in vivo* histologic technique which gives very high magnification of ×1100 through contact microscopy and simultaneous use of the vital staining dyes (MB) (Kumagai *et al.* 2004).

Principles

The prototype endocytoscopy systems are 3.2 mm in diameter and can pass through the working channel of therapeutic endoscopes.

Clinical uses

Kumagai *et al.* (2004) tested the feasibility of prototype endocytoscopy after MB staining in 20 patients with known epithelial cell characteristics in esophageal carcinoma. Endoscopic images obtained were compared across normal cells and esophageal cancers. In normal squamous cells, the arrangement was homogeneous and the nuclear cytoplasmic ratio was uniform and low. In esophageal carcinoma the cells were irregular and extremely heterogeneous, with the nuclei having different staining, size and shape. The nuclear cytoplasmic ratio was also very irregular, with high density.

Inoue *et al.* (2006) used prototype magnification endocytoscopy for *in vivo* evaluation of tissue atypia in 28 patients. The standard endoscope was supplemented with NBI and magnification endocytoscopy. 0.5% MB was also used for further enhancing the mucosa. The average time of examination was 9 minutes. The endoscopic images were classified into five grades of endocytoscopic atypia. Histologic assessment of the biopsies and resected specimens was based on the Vienna classification. The positive predictive value for malignancy was 94%. The overall accuracy was 82% in differentiating benign from malignant tissue.

Limitations

Histologic imaging methods are difficult to perform in organs like the esophagus because of constant peristalsis, saliva and reflux of gastric contents. There is a high rate of interobserver variability in interpreting the cellular and nuclear images.

String capsule endoscopy

Wireless esophageal capsule imaging has recently been introduced as an alternate modality to diagnose Barrett's esophagus.

Principles

This device contains miniaturized image sensors with low power consumption, based on complementary metal oxide semiconductor technology. Images are wirelessly transferred to a storage device.

Clinical uses

This is an innovative, effective and less invasive strategy than endoscopy for the diagnosis of Barrett's esophagus. Ramirez and colleagues (2005) evaluated the accuracy, safety, and patient tolerance of capsule endoscopy as a technique to identify patients with Barrett's esophagus. Using a wireless capsule device with attached strings, to allow controlled movement along the length of the esophagus, 50 patients with known Barrett's esophagus (28 had short segment and 22 long segment) were studied. The capsule was swallowed without sedation, and patient acceptance of the procedure was assessed by use of a questionnaire. In addition, a single endoscopist (blinded to the patient's previous diagnosis) reviewed the pictures and classified the patient's likelihood of having Barrett's esophagus on the basis of the wireless capsule pictures. All 50 patients who completed the study were correctly diagnosed. In addition, when asked which technique they would prefer if a study of the esophagus had to be repeated, 92% (46 patients) selected the capsule. Although capsule endoscopy appears to hold some promise as a screening technique, larger randomized studies and cost analysis for those requiring subsequent endoscopy for histologic confirmation will need to be conducted (Ramirez *et al.* 2005).

Limitations

There are several limitations in the use of the string-capsule endoscopy. These include the rather large size of the capsule, the frequent presence of bubbles that may interfere with the images, its inability to provide clear images at distances further than 30 mm, and its current inability to generate 'live' or 'real-time' pictures.

The histologic diagnosis of Barrett's esophagus

Thomas C. Smyrk & Navtej S. Buttar

Barrett's esophagus is defined as the replacement of normal squamous epithelium in the distal esophagus by a columnar epithelium, specifically intestinal metaplasia (IM) of the esophagus (Fig. 4.6). This metaplastic epithelium can develop dysplastic changes, which can lead to adenocarcinoma of the esophagus (Sampliner *et al.* 2002). The diagnostic feature of Barrett's esophagus is that the intestinal metaplasia is an incomplete form of IM, similar to type II and type III IM of the stomach. The metaplastic epithelium contains goblet cells interspersed between intermediate mucous cells; however, normal absorptive intestinal cells with a well-defined brush border are rare. A mosaic of cardiac-type and fundic-type mucosa is also present in this predominantly intestinal type of epithelium. Most definitions include incomplete IM as an absolute diagnostic criterion (Chandrasoma *et al.* 2000; Kilgore *et al.* 2000; Ormsby *et al.* 2000; Sandick *et al.* 2002), including the recent American Gastroenterological Association Chicago workshop statement that 'esophageal IM documented by histology is a prerequisite criterion for the diagnosis of Barrett's esophagus'(Sharma *et al.* 2004b). This definition has been challenged recently by the new British Society of Gastroenterology guidelines for the diagnosis and management of Barrett's esophagus, which consider that 'the presence of areas of IM, although often present, is not a requirement for diagnosis'. The rationale behind this change is that sampling errors at the initial endoscopy may miss an area of IM, leading to the exclusion of patients from the surveillance protocols purely due to inappropriate biopsy sampling. In the following paragraphs, we will attempt to clarify the key concepts that are relevant to the histologic diagnosis of Barrett's esophagus. At least 8 biopsies should be taken to identify IM in Barrett's esophagus (Harrison *et al.* 2007).

The gastroesophageal junction and gastric cardia

The gastroesophageal junction (GEJ) is the line at which the esophagus ends and the stomach begins. It can be defined manometrically as the lower border of the lower esophageal sphincter, endoscopically as the top of the gastric folds, and grossly as the point at which the tubular esophagus flares to become the stomach. In the normal setting, the squamocolumnar junction coincides with the GEJ; when the squamo-columnar junction is above the GEJ, there is a segment of columnar-lined esophagus.

The cardia is the small zone of proximal stomach immediately distal to the GEJ. Cardia mucosa is composed of mucus-secreting glands. Traditional teaching assigns a length of 5–30 mm for the cardia, but it has been proposed that cardia-type mucosa is *always* an acquired abnormality; that is, that the normal GEJ shows squamous mucosa immediately

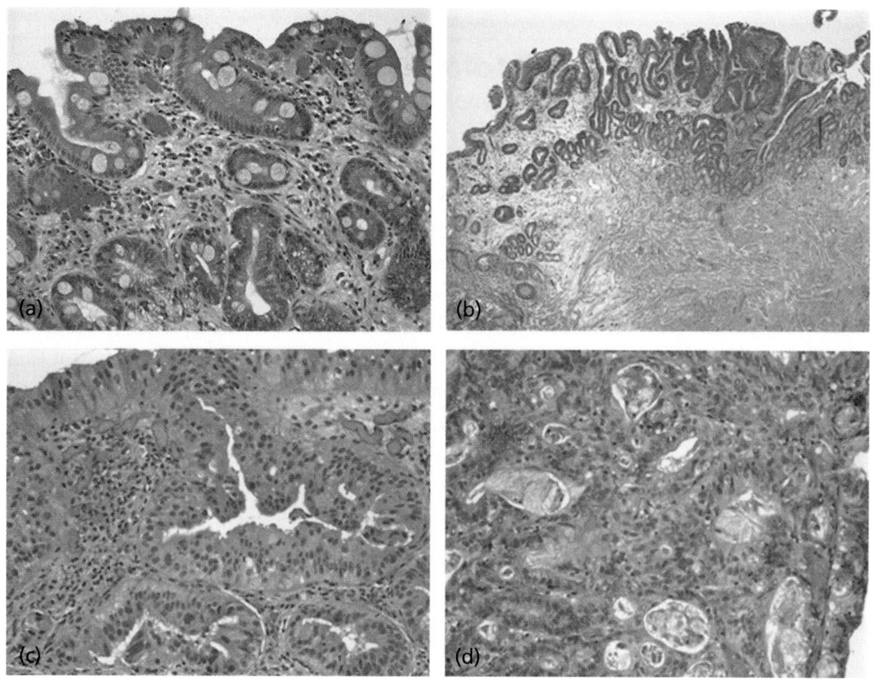

Fig. 4.6 (a) Barrett's esophagus, negative for dysplasia. Many goblet cells, indicative of intestinal metaplasia. Some deep glands have dark, crowded nuclei (particularly compared to the two cardia-type glands in the lower left corner) this is usual for Barrett's esophagus. The surface epithelium shows good maturation. (b) Low-grade dysplasia. At low power the architectural feature that stands out is the crowded, irregularly shaped glands in the upper right-center. The glands appear dark due to enlarged, hyperchromatic nuclei. The surface epithelium is also darker in this area. (c) High-grade dysplasia. Marked variability in nuclear size and shape. Loss of nuclear polarity (no longer lined up along the long axis of the cell). (d) Intramucosal adenocarcinoma. The lamina propria is effaced by fused, back-to-back glands extending from the mucosal surface (right edge) to the deep mucosal (left).

opposed to oxyntic mucosa, and that cardiac mucosa is a metaplastic epithelium secondary to reflux injury (Chandrasoma *et al.* 2000). Briefly, the hypothesis runs like this. Chronic reflux injury damages the lower esophageal sphincter, causing it to shorten. The distal esophagus, which was once above the distal border of the sphincter, is now 'sphincterless,' and dilates when the stomach dilates, allowing the mucosa to be exposed to gastric contents. The squamous lining undergoes metaplasia to cardia-type mucosa (gastricization).

Autopsy studies, however, suggest that at least some gastric cardia is present in most people at a very early age. An autopsy study in children (mean age 6.3 years) found cardiac epithelium in 30 of 30 cases, always on the gastric side of the GEJ (Kilgore *et al.* 2000). It ranged from 1 to 4 mm in length, with a mean of 1.8 mm. A similar study in 223 adult autopsies found cardiac epithelium in 99% of evaluable cases (Ormsby *et al.* 2000).

Clearly, though, cardia-type mucosa can be at least partly an acquired metaplasia. It is not unusual for biopsies from the tubular esophagus to show cardia-type mucosa. Often, the esophageal location can be confirmed histologically by the presence of submucosal esophageal glands. The gastric cardia might also expand under the influence of inflammatory stimuli; Sandick *et al.* found cardia-type mucosa in all biopsies of proximal stomach that also had intestinal metaplasia, but in only 45% of patients who did not have IM-GEJ (Sandick *et al.* 2002). Others have noted differences in the expression of mucin core polypeptides (MUCs) in 'normal' cardia vs gastric antrum, with cardia showing some expression of MUC2 and MUC3, which are commonly expressed in Barrett's esophagus (Glickman *et al.* 2003). A reasonable conclusion at this point is that a short segment (1–4 mm) of gastric cardia is normal, but that the length of cardia-type mucosa increases with age in response to inflammatory injury, either extending proximally to replace squamous epithelium or distally to replace oxyntic epithelium, or both.

Intestinal metaplasia of the esophagus (Barrett's esophagus) and esophagogastric junction (IM-GEJ)

For the pathologist, the diagnosis of Barrett's esophagus depends on identifying intestinal metaplasia. This metaplastic epithelium is characterized by a mixture of goblet, columnar, Paneth, and endocrine cells, with the goblet cell being the most useful feature for recognizing IM. It is sometimes difficult to distinguish between plump columnar cells and goblet cells; goblet cells have clear or bluish cytoplasm on H&E, while columnar cells retain a pinkish hue even when dilated (Fig. 4.7). An alcian blue stain can be useful here, as it stains goblet cells blue and leaves the goblet cell mimics unstained. (The columnar cells in BE often stain with alcian blue as well, but this does not mean that the alcian blue stain can be used to diagnose BE; the columnar cells of gastric cardia will sometimes show focal alcian blue positively. This is an abnormal finding of uncertain significance, but is not diagnostic of BE.) Because it is now recognized that not all IM near the GEJ is Barrett's esophagus, the current working definition of BE requires both the presence of goblet cells and an endoscopically abnormal segment of tubular esophagus (Sampliner *et al.* 2002) (Table 4.1).

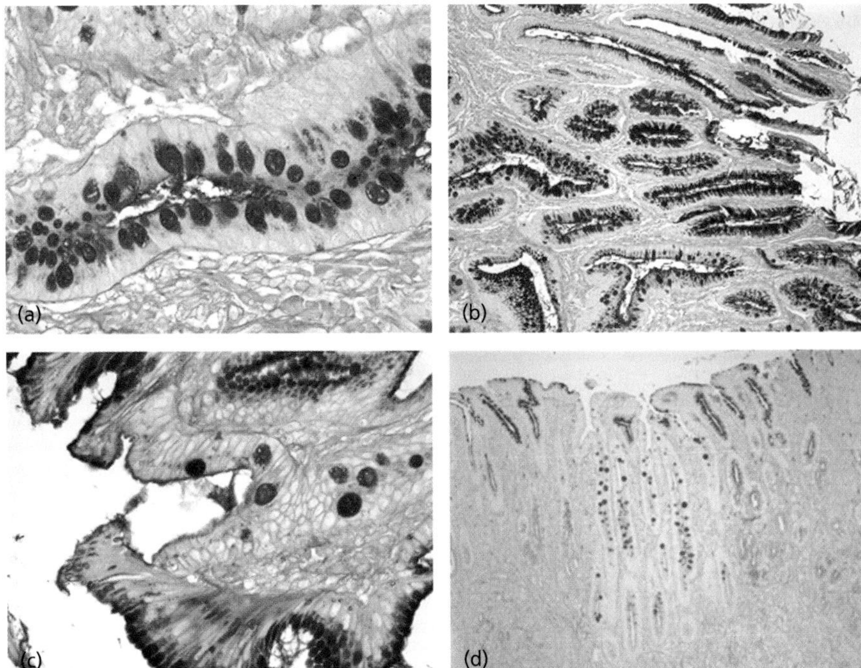

Fig 4.7 Alcian blue PAS stain. (a,b) Incomplete intestinal metaplasia (goblet cells blue, columnar cells reddish blue). (c,d) Complete intestinal metaplasia (goblet cells blue, columnar cells not staining in the metaplastic glands). Barrett's esophagus is always incomplete, intestinal metaplasia at the GE junction can be either.

Table 4.1 Changing definitions of Barrett's esophagus.

1983	At least 3 cm of columnar epithelium (any type) in distal esophagus
1992	Any intestinal metaplasia (esophagus or gastroesophageal junction)
1998	Intestinal metaplasia AND an endoscopically visible lesion (any length)

Table 4.2 Separating Barrett's esophagus (BE) from intestinal metaplasia (IM) of the gastroesophageal junction (GEJ) by histology.

Technique	BE	IM cardia
Routine histology	Band of IM at GEJ	Scattered goblets, IM in stomach, active gastritis, *Helicobacter*
Alcian blue PAS	Incomplete IM	May be incomplete or complete (goblets and columnar cells stained)
CK7/CK20	Superficial and deep glands CK7 positive	CK20 positive, CK7 negative
MUC expression	MUC1, MUC6 common	MUC1, MUC6 less common

If intestinal metaplasia is identified in biopsies from an endoscopically normal GEJ, then the presumptive diagnosis is intestinal metaplasia of the GE junction (IM-GEJ). There has been much debate in the pathology literature about whether the pathologist can separate BE from IM-GEJ independent of clinical information (Glickman *et al.* 2003). Table 4.2 lists some of the proposed techniques, none of which has achieved wide acceptance. Our opinion is that the mucin histochemistry and CK7/CK20 profiles can differentiate between BE and IM-GEJ in many instances (Fig. 4.8). Using the current definitions, the prevalences of BE and IM-GEJ are as shown in Table 4.3.

What is the etiology of IM-GEJ? Some argue that it is almost always the result of gastroesophageal reflux disease (GERD) (Oberg *et al.* 1997) while others point to *Helicobacter pylori* gastritis (Goldblum *et al.* 1998). The consensus, such as it is, seems to be that patients with IM-GEJ are different clinically from those with BE, but that both GERD and gastritis may contribute to the development of IM-GEJ. Sandick *et al.*, for example, found that patients with BE were likely to be white male smokers with a history of GERD, while those with IM-GEJ were male or female in equal proportion and had no more GERD symptoms than patients without IM-GEJ (Sandick *et al.* 2002). Gastritis was much more common in patients with

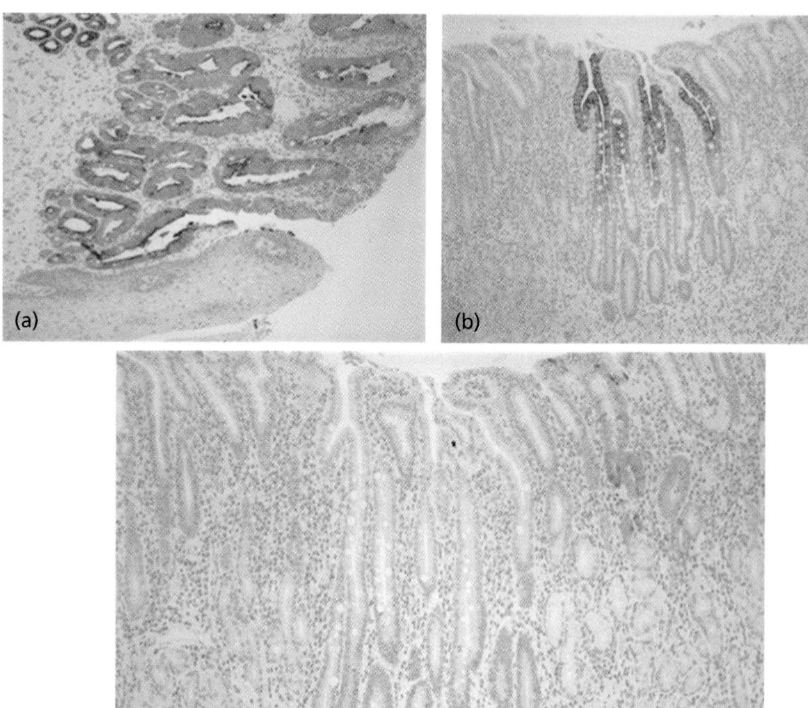

Fig 4.8 (a) CK7 staining in Barrett's esophagus, showing positive staining in superficial and deep glands. (b) CK20 in IM-GEJ, showing superficial staining. (c) CK7 in IM-GEJ, showing no staining in the metaplastic glands (the ones with goblet cells).

Table 4.3 Prevalence of Barrett's esophagus (BE) and intestinal metaplasia of the gastroesophageal junction (IM-GEJ) at endoscopy.

Reference	BE > 3 cm	BE < 3 cm	IM-GEJ
Sandick (2002)	2%	4%	9%
Spechler (1994)	1%	12%	6%
Johnston (1996)	1%	2%	7%
Morales (1997)	3%	8%	23%
Chalasani (1997)	6%	8%	10%
Hirota (1999)	2%	6%	6%
Goldblum (1998)			9%
Oberg (1997)			12%
Polkowski (2000)			12%

IM-GEJ, but the authors were not able to demonstrate differences in rates of *H. pylori* infection. Polkowski *et al.* (2000) looked at the GEJ in specimens resected for squamous carcinoma or benign conditions not associated with Barrett's esophagus. They found IM-GEJ in 9 (12%) of the specimens; 8 of the 9 also had pangastritis and the ninth was associated with carditis. Six of the 9 also had IM in the stomach. Once again, an excess of *H. pylori* infection could not be demonstrated. Hirota *et al.* (1999) found differences between patients with IM-GEF and BE, as shown in Table 4.4.

Goldstein and Karim (1999) found IM-GEJ in 27% of 150 patients undergoing elective upper endoscopy. IM was significantly associated with cardia inflammation. When patients did not have *H. pylori* infection, there was histologic evidence of

	No IM	IM-GEJ	Short-segment BE	Long-segment BE
Male : female	394 : 344	25 : 22	45 : 19	35 : 5
White	66%	66%	86%	100%
Smoker	50%	43%	69%	68%
Alcohol drinker	66%	45%	71%	80%
Helicobacter pylori	9%	21%	5%	2.5%

Table 4.4 Comparison of patients with intestinal metaplasia of the gastroesophageal junction (IM-GEJ) vs Barrett's esophagus (BE) (from Spechler *et al.* 1994).

Table 4.5 Dysplasia in short-segment Barrett's esophagus (SSBE) and intestinal metaplasia of the gastroesophageal junction (IM-GEJ).

Reference	Type	Dysplasia prevalence	Dysplasia incidence
Hirota *et al.* (1999)	SSBE	10%	–
	IM-GEJ	6.4%	–
Sharma *et al.* (2000)	SSBE	11.3%	4.6%
	IM cardia	1.3%	1.5%
Goldstein (2000)	IM cardia	0	0

esophagitis. When there was *H. pylori* infection, cardia inflammation correlated with antral inflammation. The authors conclude that cardia inflammation and intestinal metaplasia probably have multiple causes.

In a follow-up to the study described above, Goldstein found that only 7% of patients had persistent IM for up to 2 years, and that the loss of IM correlated with decreasing cardia inflammation (Goldstein 2000). Thus, IM-GEJ may be a dynamic, reversible process. Dysplasia has been described in this setting; however, as noted below, the natural history of IM-GEJ is far from settled. At present, no surveillance recommendations are made. In fact, endoscopists are discouraged from biopsing an endoscopically normal GEJ in clinical practice (Table 4.5).

Staging of esophageal cancer

Ananya Das & Amitabh Chak

The practice of dividing cancer into stages is based on the observation that patients with tumors discovered when they are localized have a better survival than those with tumors that have spread to other organs. The determination of cancer stage in each individual patient not only helps physicians assess prognosis but is important for choosing the best therapeutic plan that will benefit each patient. Cancer staging is also important for the evaluation of and enrolment into controlled clinical treatment trials and enables the accurate communication of cancer information between clinical investigators.

The American Joint Committee on Cancer and the Union Internationale Contre le Cancer agreed to develop a uniform international system for cancer staging in 1987. The TNM staging system is based on the biology of cancers: cancer develops as a primary tumor (T), then spreads to lymph nodes (N), and finally metastasizes (M) to distant organs. The development of the staging system has been a dynamic process that has changed as new information about cancer biology, new data on cancer prognosis, new surgical techniques, and new treatment approaches have become available. The 6th edition of the TNM staging system was published in 2002.

Esophageal cancers develop in the mucosal epithelial layer, at which stage they are termed carcinoma *in situ*. Sequentially, they invade in a somewhat systematic fashion, first through the lamna propria, then the muscularis mucosa, the submucosa, the muscularis propria, and finally into adjacent organs. While the primary tumor invades deeper through the esophageal wall, its risk of metastasizing also increases–first to regional nodes and then to distant nodes and to distant organs, especially the liver and the lung. Unlike other parts of the gastrointestinal tract, the esophagus does not have a serosa and this may explain why esophageal cancer is often metastatic at diagnosis. The TNM staging system for the esophagus reflects this cancer biology. The T denotes the primary tumor, N denotes the status of regional lymph nodes and M denotes metastasis to distant lymph nodes or organs. Physicians often mistakenly use the term T stage, N stage, M stage. These terms are incorrect because stage refers to the overall status of the cancer. It is recommended that the terms T category, N category, and M category be used when referring individually to the status of the primary tumor, lymph nodes, or metastases.

The TNM staging system for esophageal cancer is outlined in Table 4.6. The prefixes 'c' and 'p' can be used to designate whether the information for a given TNM stage grouping was based solely on clinical information or included surgical pathology findings. As example, a cancer with a stage of cT2 N0 M0 (stage IIA) based on computed tomography (CT) and endoscopic findings before surgery may change to pT3 N1 M0 (stage III) cancer following surgery because the resected specimen demonstrated that the cancer invaded into adventitia and was present in a lymph node. Some investigators also use a 'u' prefix to specify the use of endoscopic ultrasound (EUS) in determining the cancer stage.

Overall 5-year survival rates for esophageal cancer are very low and have not improved very much in the past three decades. The prognosis of esophageal cancer can be predicted by stage at diagnosis. Five-year survival for patients diagnosed with stage I cancer is 50%, for stage II cancer is 31%, for stage III is 20%; and stage IV is 4% (Ries *et al.* 2002). The 5-year survival for cancers confined to the mucosa (T1m N0 M0) may approach 90%. Given these statistics, patients with advanced stage disease at diagnosis are treated with palliative non-surgical approaches.

Esophageal cancer has a propensity to metastasize to regional periaortic lymph nodes, liver, and lung. Therefore, thoracoabdominal CT is typically the first step in staging esophageal cancers. In patients who do not have distant metastatic disease, EUS complements CT in the staging of esophageal cancers because the high frequency ultrasound image provides detailed structural information about the depth of the primary tumor in relation to the submucosa, muscularis propria, and adventitia. It also allows sonographic assessment of adjacent lymph nodes and EUS-guided fine needle aspiration (EUS-FNA) can also be used to sample selected regional and celiac lymph nodes. Positron emission tomography (PET) scanning using

Table 4.6 TNM staging system for esophageal cancer, 6th edn.

Primary tumor (T)	
Tx	Primary tumor cannot be assessed
T0	No evidence of primary tumor
Tis	Carcinoma *in situ*
T1	Tumor invades lamina propra or submucosa
T1m	Tumor invades through lamina propria but not through muscularis mucosa
T1sm	Tumor invades through muscularis mucosa into submucosa
T2	Tumor invades into muscularis propria but not through it
T3	Tumor invades through muscularis propria into periesophageal adventitia
T4	Tumor invades adjacent organs or vessels
Regional lymph nodes (N)	
Nx	Regional lymph nodes cannot be assessed
N0	No regional lymph node metastasis
N1	Regional lymph node metastasis present
Distant metastasis (M)	
Mx	Distant metastasis cannot be assessed
M0	No distant metastasis
M1	Distant metastasis present
M1a	Metastasis in celiac (lower thoracic) or cervical (upper thoracic) nodes
M1b	Non-regional nodes (mid thoracic) or distant metastasis
Stage grouping	
Stage 0	T0 N0 M0, Tis N0 M0
Stage I	T1 N0 M0
Stage IIA	T2 or T3 N0 M0
Stage IIB	T1 or T2 N1 M0
Stage III	T3 N1 M0, T4 Any N M0
Stage IV	Any T Any N M1
Stage IVA	Any T Any N M1a
Stage IVB	Any T Any N M1b

Table 4.7 Endoscopic ultrasound (EUS) criteria for TNM staging.

Tx	Unable to traverse cancer
T0 or Tis	Normal five-layer EUS pattern
T1	Hypoechoic mass involving first three layers
T2	Hypoechoic mass involving first four layers, smooth outer border
T3	Hypoechoic mass involving all five layers, irregular outer border
T4	Hypoechoic mass, all five layers, and loss of interface with adjacent structure
Nx	Unable to traverse cancer
N0	No regional nodes imaged or nodes are hyperechoic, elongated, diffuse borders, <1 cm in size
N1	Nodes are hypoechoic, rounded, well demarcated, ≥1 cm in size
Mx	Unable to traverse cancers
M0	EUS cannot determine M0 stage
M1a	Hypoechoic demarcated celiac node
M1b	Hypoechoic lesion in left lobe of liver

18-fluorodeoxyglucose (FDG) is increasingly being used as a third step in the staging of esophageal cancer because it may detect distant metastases that are not identified by CT.

EUS staging

EUS of normal esophagus

Ultrasonographic imaging depends on the interaction of sound waves with biologic tissue. High-frequency ultrasound waves echo from interfaces between the mucosal, submucosal, muscularis, and periesophageal adventitial tissue of the esophageal wall, giving a characteristic 'five-layer' bright–dark–bright–dark–bright EUS image of the normal esophageal wall at typical scanning frequencies of 7.5–12 MHz. The innermost first bright (hyperechoic) layer of this five-layer image is a border echo, and the second dark layer corresponds roughly to the esophageal mucosa. The third or middle bright (hyperechoic) layer corresponds to the submucosa; the fourth dark (hypoechoic) layer corresponds to the muscularis propria; and the fifth outermost thin bright (hyperechoic) layer represents the periesophageal adventitial tissue. Higher frequencies of ultrasound such as 20 MHz limit the depth of imaging to just the esophageal wall itself but separate the circular and longitudinal muscle into two dark layers separated by a thin hyperechoic layer and may be able to identify the muscularis mucosa as a thin hypoechoic layer, which may be useful for evaluating very early T1 cancers. It is primarily the ability of EUS imaging to distinguish the submucosa and the muscularis propria that makes this an important modality for staging esophageal cancer. EUS is most useful and accurate for evaluating T category, i.e. the depth of the primary cancer.

In addition to imaging the esophageal wall itself, EUS imaging also obtains high-resolution views of the celiac trunk, an important site for distant nodal metastases. Other structures seen in detail during EUS examination are the left lobe of the liver, the thoracic and proximal abdominal aorta, the azygos vein, the right and left pleura, the left atrium, and the subcarinal region. The spine and organs that contain air, such as the lungs, the bronchi, and the trachea, cannot be imaged by EUS because of the reverberations in the image.

EUS for evaluating primary tumor (T)

EUS provides a more detailed assessment of the primary tumor than any other modality. Cancers generally appear hypoechoic on EUS imaging. Criteria for assessing primary tumor status by EUS are listed in Table 4.7. Tumor penetration into the esophageal wall destroys the five-layer pattern observed in the normal esophagus. EUS accuracy for determining depth of tumor invasion (T category) is 85–90% in the hands of experienced endosonographers (Catalano *et al.* 1995; Das & Chak 2003). Overstaging may be related to the presence of inflammation and fibrosis. The tumor may also be overstaged if the tumor is scanned tangentially or the water-filled balloon around the transducer is overinflated, causing compression of the tumor into the deeper layers. Accuracy seems to be the lowest, around 80%, for assessing T2 cancers.

One-fifth to one-third of esophageal cancers are stenotic at the time of diagnosis, precluding traversal by an echoendoscope. There is controversy as to whether these cancers should be dilated to enable complete EUS examination. Some have reported a high rate of perforation when dilations were performed before EUS (Van Dam *et al.* 1993). Others have argued that this practice is safe (Pfau *et al.* 2000). Stenotic, non-traversible, cancers are invariably advanced at diagnosis. If the additional information obtained by performing a complete EUS examination does not lead to a significant change in treatment, the risk of dilating stenotic cancers may not be justified. A slim 7.9-mm caliber ultrasonic esophagoprobe equipped with a cone-shaped metal bougie-like tip has been shown to be useful in staging highly stenosing esophageal cancers (Binmoeller *et al.* 1995).

High-frequency (20- and 30-MHz) ultrasound catheter probes may have a role in differentiating T1m cancers from T1sm cancers (Binmoeller *et al.* 1995), although the reported accuracy of these probes in demarcating mucosa from the submucosa has been variable (Isenberg 2004). Early cancers that are confined to the muscularis mucosa (T1m) have a negligible rate of nodal involvement and may be amenable to endoscopic mucosal resection therapy, whereas cancers that invade the submucosa (T1sm) have a low but significant rate of nodal metastases.

EUS for evaluating lymph nodes

EUS also identifies periesophageal, perigastric, and periaortic lymph nodes. Unlike CT, which characterizes lymph nodes strictly on the basis of size, EUS criteria for malignant lymph nodes are also based on sonographic characteristics (Table 4.7). Lymph nodes that are hypoechoic, round, ≥1 cm, and have clearly demarcated borders are nearly always malignant. Lymph nodes that are elongated and hyperechoic with poorly demarcated borders are most often reactive, even when they are as large as 3 cm in size. Of course, most malignant lymph nodes do not meet all four EUS criteria for malignancy, and the EUS interpretation of nodal status is subjective and dependent on the experience of the endosonographer. The accuracy of EUS for defining the presence of nodal metastases ranges between 65 and 86% (Miyazaki *et al.* 2004).

EUS-FNA can be performed in selected lymph nodes that are not immediately adjacent to the primary tumor. To sample lymph nodes for cytology it is important to use a needle approach that does not go through the primary tumor. Even with the use of a stylet it may be difficult to avoid false positives related to contamination of the specimen with malignant cells from the primary tumor. The addition of EUS-FNA to EUS imaging may increase the accuracy of nodal assessment (Eloubeidi 2006).

Lymph nodes adjacent to the celiac trunk are imaged very nicely by EUS. They can also be easily approached by EUS-FNA. EUS assessment of celiac nodal involvement is fairly accurate based on imaging alone, and the presence of malignant disease can be confirmed by EUS-FNA (Catalano *et al.* 1999). This finding is often of importance in patient management because celiac nodal involvement in cancers that do not involve the gastroesophageal junction is considered M1a or distant metastatic disease. The classification of celiac nodal involvement and its distinction from perigastric lymph nodes may be confusing when the primary cancer involves the GEJ, and many institutions consider nodal involvement in this case to represent regional disease.

EUS for evaluating distant metastases

EUS does not image the entire liver and cannot image the lungs. Therefore, the assessment of metastatic disease by EUS is always incomplete. This is why esophageal cancer staging must include CT as well as EUS. EUS does image the left lobe of the liver and the medial portion of the right lobe with high resolution. Small metastases in the liver that are not evident on CT can occasionally be identified. The presence of cancer in hepatic metastases can also be confirmed by EUS-FNA.

Staging by computed tomography

CT scan remains an important step in the staging of esophageal cancer and is typically the initial staging modality after diagnosis is established by endoscopy and biopsy. The role of CT is most valuable in detecting metastatic disease in the liver, lungs and periaortic lymph nodes. CT scanning may give a general idea regarding T category based on CT assessment of esophageal wall thickness. However, even with newer CT scanners the different component layers of the esophageal wall cannot be differentiated for an accurate evaluation of the extent of tumor depth in terms of T category. However, CT scan has a reasonable accuracy in detecting invasion of mediastinal structures by locally advanced tumors, and accuracy rates of up to 90% in detecting aortic, tracheobronchial and pericardial invasion has been reported. Overall accuracy in assessing T category is reported as 50–60% (Harris *et al.* 1998).

Assessment of nodal disease by CT scan is not very good, with overall reported sensitivities from 50 to 79%, and specificities from 25 to 67%. The accuracy of CT scanning for periesophageal abdominal lymph nodes has been reported to be as high as 83–87%, but only 51–70% in assessment of thoracic adenopathy (Maerz *et al.* 1993). Conventional CT is insensitive for detection of metastatic involvement of celiac lymph nodes in esophageal cancer. Helical CT has theoretical advantages over 'slice' CT in this regard, although in a prospective trial, positive and negative predictive values for helical CT for assessing celiac lymph nodes in patients with esophageal cancer were only 67% and 77%, respectively, the reference standard being EUS with FNA (Romagnuolo *et al.* 2002).

Staging by magnetic resonance imaging

Although MRI with its high contrast sensitivity in delineating margins between the air-filled esophagus and mediastinal fat may have a potentially role in staging, its clinical use for this purpose has been very limited and does not offer any significant advantage over CT even with the use of experimental endoscopic MR imaging techniques (Dave *et al.* 2004).

Staging by ^{18}F-labelled fluorodeoxyglucose (FDG) positron emission tomography (PET)

PET has rapidly become a non-invasive, whole-body imaging method for the preoperative staging of a variety of cancers. The increased glucose metabolism of malignant cells is imaged by the uptake of FDG as a 'radiotracer' in oncologic PET studies. Unlike EUS, one of the basic advantages of FDG-PET is its ability to image the whole body and quantify uptake in the entire volume of the primary tumor, thus assessing the primary tumor as well as metastatic disease in a single examination. Several prospective studies have shown that FDG-PET is more sensitive than CT for revealing regional and distant metastases in patients with esophageal carcinoma. In a systemic review of the staging performance of FDG-PET, pooled sensitivity and specificity for detection of distant lymph node and hematogenous metastasis were 0.67 and 0.97, respectively (van Westreenen *et al.* 2004). However, the sensitivity and specificity of FDG-PET for the detection of locoregional disease is low and inferior to EUS. The reasons for low accuracy of FDG-PET in staging locoregional involvement may be due to limitation of spatial resolution of currently available PET scanners, masking of adjacent lymph nodes by tracer accumulation in the primary tumor, and FGD avidity which may be an issue with some poorly differentiated esophageal and junctional adenocarcinoma (Flamen *et al.* 2004).The superior sensitivity of PET for the detection of metastatic disease makes it potentially the most cost-effective method of identifying patients with occult metastases, for whom aggressive therapy such as surgical resection should not be pursued. A decision analysis study favored the strategy of initial staging of esophageal cancer by PET and EUS-FNA over a strategy based on CT and EUS-FNA in terms of higher effectiveness, although the PET-based strategy was more expensive. (Wallace *et al.* 2002). PET scanning for initial staging of esophageal cancer is covered by most insurance carriers, including Medicare.

Staging by other modalities

Endoscopic mucosal resection (EMR) is an evolving technique for resection of early superficial neoplastic lesions of the esophagus. EMR provides the resected specimen for detailed histopathologic evaluation and has been used for accurate pathologic staging of early esophageal cancer of squamous cell type as well as early adenocarcinoma complicating high-grade dysplasia in the setting of Barrett's esophagus (Noguchi *et al.* 2000; Larghi *et al.* 2005). Given the imprecise nature of the non-invasive staging modalities, a recent prospective multicenter trial evaluated the feasibility of minimally invasive surgical staging by thoracoscopy and/or laparoscopy for esophageal cancer in 113 eligible patients. Thoracoscopy and/or laparoscopy was feasible in 73% of patients and in comparison with non-invasive staging including that by EUS, in up to 30% of patients minimally invasive surgical staging identified false-negative lymph nodes or metastatic disease. No major complications or mortality was encountered and the median length of postoperative hospital stay was 3 days. Further studies are needed to assess the role and cost-effectiveness of minimal invasive surgical staging in the staging algorithm of appropriate patients with esophageal cancer (Krasna *et al.* 2001).

Recently attention has been focused on molecular biologic techniques of immunohistochemical analysis which would allow recognition of micrometastatic lesions in lymph nodes that are histologically negative. Several recent reports have highlighted the feasibility of such an approach and it remains to be seen if such sophisticated molecular techniques may lead to clinically meaningful improvement in staging accuracy of esophageal cancer, particularly in association with other staging modalities such as EUS-FNA (Jiao *et al.* 2003; Waterman *et al.* 2004).

Restaging of esophageal cancer

Given the uniformly poor results achieved with surgical intervention alone, treatment of esophageal cancer at many centers has shifted to a multimodality approach that incorporates preoperative neoadjuvant chemoradiotherapy in patients with invasive disease who are potential candidates for subsequent surgical resection (Kelsen 2005). It is known that only a subgroup of patients with esophageal cancer potentially benefit from neoadjuvant therapy and all the imaging modalities that are used for initial staging of esophageal cancer have also been used for restaging the esophageal cancer after initial neoadjuvant therapy to determine the tumor response. It is to be noted that morphologic imaging modalities such as CT and EUS are unable to distinguish between viable tumor and reactive changes such as scar tissue, necrosis, and edema. This limitation is supported by the reported suboptimal accuracy of restaging with CT and EUS after neoadjuvant therapy. For assessment of response of primary tumor to treatment by EUS, traditional T categorization is unacceptably inaccurate. A surrogate measure of tumor volume, maximal cross-sectional area, is a better parameter for assessing response. For assessment of nodal response, use of more liberal criteria for performing EUS-guided FNA could improve the nodal staging accuracy of EUS.

Several studies have assessed the role of FDG-PET in the restaging of patients with esophageal cancer after neoadjuvant therapy. It is increasingly clear that for restaging of patients with esophageal cancer who have undergone neoadjuvant treatment, EUS and FDG-PET provide complementary information. The relative advantages of FDG-PET scanning is that it is non-invasive, is feasible in most patients, provides opportunity for whole body imaging with a single test and, when integrated with CT as PET-CT, provides both structural and metabolic information. FDG-PET has high reproducibility and internal validity, can be used to assess early response, and almost all published studies of FDG-PET show its ability to clearly differentiate responders and non-responders in terms of long-term survival (Weber *et al.* 1999; Flamen *et al.* 2004). Also, unlike EUS, pre-treatment FDG-PET has been shown to correlate with response to chemoradiotherapy and is the only imaging modality that may identify *a priori* those patients who are likely to attain a major or even complete pathologic response to neoadjuvant treatment (Flamen *et al.* 2002). The disadvantages of FDG-PET are that, in the absence of tissue diagnosis, both false-positive and false-negative results are often misleading. The unique advantage of EUS relative to other imaging modalities is its ability to obtain tissue aspirate for pathologic assessment. Also, EUS is very accurate in identifying small peritumoral lymph nodes which are often below the threshold of detection of FDG-PET. Currently there is no single optimal imaging modality for assessing response in patients with locoregional and potentially resectable esophageal cancer who undergo neoadjuvant chemoradiotherapy. There are also no clear guidelines for making clinical decisions based on the results of restaging imaging tests. If postneoadjuvant assessment of response is to be used to guide subsequent therapeutic decisions, a combination of different imaging modalities may be needed. The choice will obviously vary with the local availability of resources and expertise. Ideally, if a FDG-PET integrated with CT is available, then a FDG-PET/CT may provide useful information. If PET/CT shows suspected M1a or M1b disease, which is accessible to EUS-FNA, then a EUS-FNA could help establish the diagnosis of metastatic disease. If the PET/CT shows no evidence of metastatic disease but there is suggestion of residual tumor, particularly nodal disease, then EUS with FNA of suspicious lymph nodes could also be helpful. It is not known if a repeat EUS examination should be performed in patients with a completely negative FDG-PET.

In summary, significant advances have been made in initial staging and restaging after neoadjuvant therapy of esophageal adenocarcinoma. Several imaging modalities are available and they often provide complementary information. It is expected that in the near future other evolving staging modalities including endoscopic mucosal resection and minimally invasive surgery in association with application of techniques of molecular biology will further enhance our ability to accurately stage these cancers so that stage-specific individualized treatment may be provided.

Treatment

Overview

Kenneth K. Wang

The approach to esophageal carcinoma has evolved rapidly in the recent decade due to the creation of more effective chemotherapy, minimally invasive surgical procedures, and more effective aggressive endoscopic techniques. The options for patients have expanded from a relatively simple algorithm in the past, surgery for localized cancer and chemotherapy and radiation for metastatic disease, to a wide spectrum of options depending on the degree of metastatic potential.

Surgical management of esophageal carcinoma

Daniela Molena, Fernando Herbella & Jeffrey H. Peters

The challenges of esophageal carcinoma

National Cancer Institute statistics report that approximately 15,600 people will be diagnosed with esophageal cancer in 2007, and 13,940 (or 89%) are expected to die from it (Cancer Statistics 2007). These figures increase substantially when data for cancer of the cardia are included. Clearly, curing this disease is a challenge. In fact, these rather difficult and distressing statistics have historically led many to the conclusion that therapy for esophageal cancer is largely palliative, and that the physician has little control over whether the patient is cured of his cancer or not. This historical mindset is changing however, as it is now recognized that cure is increasingly possible with surgical intervention alone, and perhaps even more so with the addition of modern adjuvant therapy.

Several important changes in the clinical biology and presentation of esophageal cancer are driving this trend favoring a curative over palliative intent. First, the detection of esophageal cancer at a stage when the disease may be confined to the mucosa or submucosa, once a decidedly rare clinical occurrence, has recently become more common (Fig. 4.9) (Oh *et al.* 2006). The clear link between Barrett's esophagus and

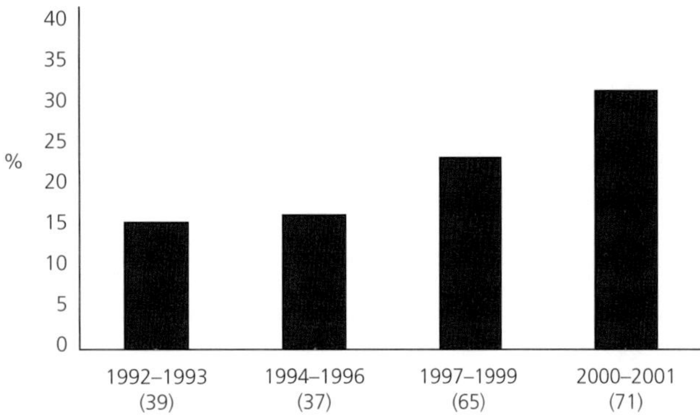

Fig. 4.9 Incidence of intramucosal esophageal carcinoma from 1992 to 2001 at the University of Southern California. Chi-square analysis for overall trend: p = 0.035. Chi-square analysis for 1992–93′ versus 2000–01′: p = 0.052.

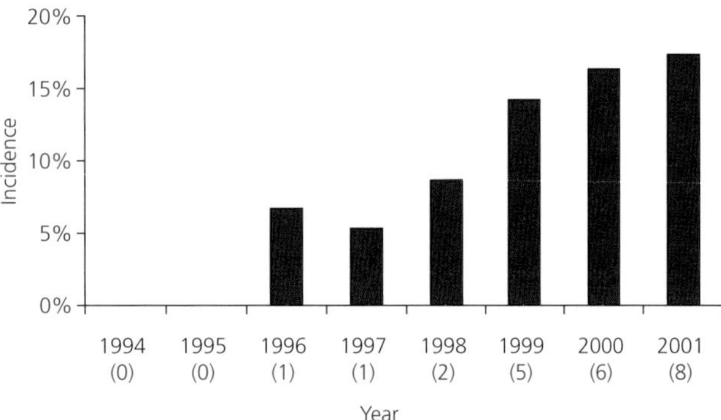

Fig. 4.10 Incidence of adenocarcinoma of the esophagus in patients less than 50 years of age. Chi-square analysis for trend: p = 0.01. Data from Portale *et al.* (2006).

esophageal adenocarcinoma, the liberal use of flexible endoscopy to investigate foregut symptoms, and the widespread adoption of surveillance programs, have all contributed to this fact. As many as 30% of patients with esophageal adenocarcinoma referred for resection at high-volume centers have been reported to have early-stage, curable disease. These changing demographics markedly increase the population of patients with curable esophageal cancer, underscoring the importance of a curative resection. Second, patients are presenting at a younger age. Significant trends documenting an increasing prevalence of adenocarcinoma of the esophagus in patients less than 50 years old have been reported (Fig. 4.10) (Portale *et al.* 2006a). It is one thing to contemplate palliation of dysphagia in an 80-year-old man with a 5-cm distal esophageal cancer, and yet another to treat a 47-year-old father of three with a barely visible lesion detected on surveillance endoscopy. Third, the morbidity and mortality associated with esophageal resection has markedly declined. Improvements in perioperative mortality increase the pool of potentially curable patients and allow for a more aggressive and extensive surgical treatment approach. Finally, the number of individuals diagnosed with this cancer in the US increases yearly (Blot *et al.* 1991; Pera *et al.* 1993). The incidence of esophageal adenocarcinoma is currently rising faster than that of any other cancer in the US. Taken together, these changes support rethinking the traditional approach of assuming palliation in all patients. Rather, the treatment of esophageal cancer has now entered into an era of individualization, each patient receiving the therapy with the best chance of eliminating all disease, or if this is not possible, eliminating debilitating symptoms.

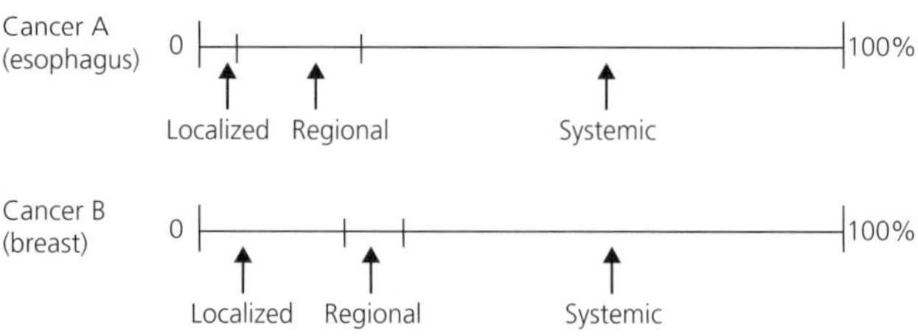

Fig. 4.11 Cartoon illustrating the relative proportions of patients with local, regional or systemic disease at the time of diagnosis. These relative proportions are different form cancer to cancer (e.g. esophageal and breast) and change over time.

As the intent of treatment shifts from palliation to cure, mechanisms that maximize the possibility of cure become paramount. Conceptually, human cancer presents itself to the clinician in three, and only three, possible forms (Fig. 4.11). It can be localized to the organ in which it originated, it may be regional, i.e. spread to regional lymph nodes but not beyond, or it may be systemic. The degree of surgical resection (i.e. lymphadenectomy) will not influence outcome in the first or last of these circumstances, but very well may do for those patients with regional disease. The controversy regarding radical lymphadenectomy lies not only in proving its benefits but also in the acceptance of the very existence of regional disease. The 'school of thought' promoting the concept that most cancer is systemic at the time of diagnosis emerged with the National Surgical Adjuvant Breast and Bowel Project studies of breast cancer in which the degree of lymphadenectomy did not influence overall survival. This observation suggested that patients who harbor nodal metastases have systemic disease at the time of diagnosis. While this may be true of breast cancer, we must be cautious in extrapolating this paradigm too far. Indeed, the multitude of Kaplan–Meier survival curves of patients with positive lymph nodes in which there exists a small but real prevalence of patients who have prolonged survival (cure) is proof of principle that regional disease, in fact, does occur. Its prevalence likely varies from cancer to cancer, and from decade to decade, but the fact that it occurs in some proportion of patients is indisputable. Once this fact is accepted, then it follows that lymphadenectomy will improve survival in the population of patients with regional disease. The challenge then becomes accurately identifying such patients before surgery.

Assessment of the extent of disease and selection of surgical options

At the initial encounter with a patient diagnosed as having carcinoma of the esophagus, a decision must be made as to whether he or she is a candidate for curative surgical therapy, palliative surgical therapy, or non-surgical palliation. The pros and cons of the use of adjuvant therapy must also be considered as well as its timing. Making these judgements can be difficult. Current methods evaluating the pretreatment stage of esophageal carcinoma are imprecise, primarily due to the difficulty of measuring the depth of tumor penetration of the esophageal wall and the inaccessibility of the organ's widespread lymphatic drainage. Even with the modern techniques of CT, MRI, PET, EUS, and laparoscopic and thoracoscopic technology, pretreatment staging remains inaccurate in many patients.

Esophageal cancer generally presents with dysphagia, although increasing numbers of relatively asymptomatic patients are now identified on surveillance endoscopy and/or with endoscopy prompted by non-specific upper gastrointestinal symptoms. Reviewing the symptomatic presentation of 213 patients referred for surgical resection over the 10 year period from 1992–2002, Portale *et al.* (2006a) found a surprisingly high proportion of patients with cancer identified before the development of dysphagia. Twenty-five per cent of the 213 patients were enrolled in a surveillance program for Barrett's esophagus or presented with a long history of GERD symptoms, and in another 30%, occult bleeding, anemia or abdominal symptoms such as pain or discomfort prompted the visit to the physician leading to a diagnosis of cancer (Table 4.8). Dysphagia usually presents late in the natural history of the disease because the lack of a serosal layer on the esophagus allows the smooth muscle to dilate with ease. As a result, the dysphagia becomes severe enough for the patient to seek medical advice only when more than 60% of the esophageal circumference is infiltrated with cancer. Consequently, the cancer is often systemic by the time dysphagia heralds its presence.

Table 4.8 Symptomatic presentation of patients with esophageal cancer. From Portale *et al.* (2006).

	n = 213
*Main symptom at presentation**	
Non-dysphagia	121 (56.8)
Barrett's surveillance or GERD	44 (24.4)
Bleeding (anemia, hematemesis)	29 (13.6)
Chest/abdominal pain, discomfort	26 (12.2)
Others	14 (6.6)
Dysphagia	92 (43.2)
Duration of dysphagia before diagnosis (months)†	2 (1–3)

Data are expressed as *n (%) and †median (interquartile range).

The characteristics of esophageal cancer that are associated with improved survival are known. Most studies suggest that only metastasis to lymph nodes and tumor penetration of the esophageal wall have significant and independent influence on prognosis. The beneficial effects of the absence of one factor persist even when the other is present. Factors known to be important in the survival of patients with advanced disease, such as cell type, degree of cellular differentiation, or location of tumor in the esophagus, have no effect on survival of patients who have undergone resection for early disease. Studies also showed that patients having five or fewer lymph node metastases have a better outcome.

Clinical factors that indicate an advanced stage of carcinoma and exclude surgery with curative intent are recurrent nerve paralysis, Horner's syndrome, persistent spinal pain, paralysis of the diaphragm, fistula formation, and malignant pleural effusion. Factors that make surgical cure unlikely include a tumor greater than 8 cm in length, abnormal axis of the esophagus on a barium radiogram, enlarged paratracheal or paraaortic lymph nodes on CT, a weight loss of more than 20%, and loss of appetite. In patients where these findings are not present, staging depends primarily on the length of the tumor as measured with endoscopy, and the degree of wall penetration and lymph node metastasis seen with EUS. Studies indicate that there are a high number of favorable parameters associated with tumors less than 4 cm in length; there are fewer with tumors between 4 and 8 cm, and favorable criteria for tumors greater than 8 cm in length are uncommon.

Upper endoscopy

Aside from symptoms, the presence or absence of an endoscopically visible lesion is the first major criterion to begin categorizing patients with esophageal cancer. Referral of patients with biopsy-proven HGD or intramucosal carcinoma is now common, and the presence of a visible lesion can predict tumor depth and nodal metastases. Patients with HGD have a significant chance (35–45%) of harboring an occult adenocarcinoma, particularly if the HGD is multifocal and a visible lesion is present at endoscopy. More recent experience suggests a less than 20% chance of occult adenocarcinoma (Tseng *et al.* 2003). Available data indicate that a biopsy showing adenocarcinoma in the absence of an endoscopically visible lesion almost always corresponds to an intramucosal tumor without nodal metastases. Nigro *et al.* (1999) reported that when there is no visible lesion on endoscopy, 88% of the tumors were intramucosal and 12 % submucosal in one recent study. Only 1 of 10 patients with no visible lesion had lymph node involvement either histologically or immunohistochemically. In contrast, patients with endoscopically visible tumors had a high prevalence of tumors that penetrated beyond the mucosa (75%) and 56% had positive nodes.

In an attempt to determine whether the combination of symptomatic and endoscopic findings of small visible lesions can accurately predict early-stage disease, Portale *et al.* (2006b) evaluated 213 consecutive patients with resectable esophageal adenocarcinoma seen from 1992 to 2002. Model-based probabilities of early-stage disease (T1 m/sm N0) were calculated for each combination of three factors (no dysphagia as main symptom at presentation, tumor length ≤2 cm, non-circumferential lesion) using a multivariable model. The data showed that utilizing combinations of the three main features, i.e. the presence of dysphagia, small visible lesions and non-circumferential lesions, correctly predicted early-stage node-negative disease 82% of the time (Table 4.9). A small but significant proportion (14%) of patients with all three of these features harbored nodal metastases however, which would preclude cure with local resection therapy alone.

Endoscopic ultrasound

EUS has gained popularity over the last 10 years as the modality of choice for pretherapeutic assessment of depth of tumor infiltration into the esophageal wall and lymph node status. While it provides us with the best information available regarding both of these important staging parameters, recent data reveal major limitations particularly in differentiating mucosal and submucosal tumors, a key branchpoint in therapeutic decision making.

Nishimaki and colleagues (1999) prospectively assessed the accuracy of preoperative staging using esophagography, esophagoscopy, EUS, and CT in 224 patients with localized esophageal cancer who underwent radical esophagectomy. The study showed that T2 tumors were poorly predicted by endoscopy or esophagography and even though EUS was shown to be the best study for predicting T2 tumors, its accuracy was only 61%, with 33% of patients being overstaged. The overall accuracy of correctly predicting stage I disease before esophagectomy was only 68% and at predicting stage III disease was 70%. The accuracy of clinical staging for predicting stage IIA or IIB disease was less than 50%.

The limits of EUS are particularly evident in the attempt to distinguish intramucosal from submucosal tumors and submucosal from intramuscular ones. In a recent study from the Cleveland Clinic Foundation, Zuccaro *et al.* (2005) directly compared clinical TNM classification with pathologic classification in 266 patients with esophageal cancer who had EUS staging followed directly by esophagectomy. EUS was confirmed to be reasonably accurate in the identification of T3 tumors (83%). T2 tumors were correctly identified by EUS in only 42% of patients; in 54% they were erroneously overstaged to T3. Even less accurate was the identification of T1 or *in situ* tumors. T1 lesions were correctly classified in 29% of patients and *in situ* tumors were never correctly identified preoperatively. T1 tumors were overstaged in 46% of cases and understaged in 24%. It is interesting to note that 16 patients with T1 tumors (20%) and 13 patients with Tis tumors (68%) were misdiagnosed as clinical T0.

Data from the Mayo Clinic suggest that preoperative locoregional lymph node staging accuracy is improved by performing EUS-guided fine needle aspiration (EUS FNA). Vazquez-Sequeiros and colleagues (2006) reported a prospective blinded study of 125 patients with newly diagnosed esophageal cancer who were candidates for surgical resection and in whom preoperative findings may have an impact on the final treatment decision. EUS FNA increased sensitivity for malignant lymph nodes (83%) compared with CT (29%) or EUS (71%), as well as overall accuracy (87%) compared with CT (51%) or EUS alone (74%). Treatment decisions were commonly altered, and although EUS FNA was more accurate than EUS alone, the impact on therapy was not significantly different.

Taken together these data reveal an unappreciated inaccuracy of EUS in correctly staging patients with esophageal cancer. Given that treatment decisions are increasingly made on the basis of whether the tumor is intramucosal or submucosal and node negative or node positive, the results of EUS must be applied with caution.

Table 4.9 Symptomatic–endoscopic–pathologic correlation. From Portale *et al.* (2006).

	n = 184	Early stage (PPV)*	Lymph-node positive*
Lack of dysphagia at diagnosis	95	51.6	42.1
Tumor length ≤ 2 cm	67	73.1	20.9
Circumferential involvement (CI) ≤ 25%	62	79	17.7
No dysphagia + tumor length ≤ 2 cm	55	80	14.5
No dysphagia + CI ≤ 25%	55	80	16.4
Tumor length ≤ 2 cm + CI ≤ 25%	56	80.4	16.1
No dysphagia + tumor length ≤ 2 cm + CI ≤ 25%	50	82	14

Data are expressed as *percentage; 29 patients with no visible lesion were excluded from the analysis. PPV, positive predictive value.

Staging aided by endoscopic mucosal resection

Endoscopic mucosal resection (EMR), initially used as a definitive resection option for early esophageal cancer and HGD, has recently been proposed as a staging tool to determine the depth of invasion of esophageal adenocarcinoma and may become the procedure of choice to reliably differentiate intramucosal from submucosal lesions. EMR consists of excision of a disc of esophageal wall down to the muscularis propria, therefore including both mucosa and submucosa. Maish and DeMeester (2004) recently published their experience with this technique in seven patients with a small visible lesion and a biopsy showing esophageal adenocarcinoma, who successively underwent esophageal resection. EMR accurately determined the depth of tumor invasion in all cases and was found to have completely excised the target lesion in 86% of patients. In particular all patients with negative margins on EMR specimens had no evidence of tumor at the pathologic assessment of the resected specimen. In one patient who had tumor present up to the cauterized lateral margin of the EMR specimen, a corresponding focus of intramucosal cancer was found after esophageal resection. Two patients that had complete removal of a visible lesion by EMR were found to have an additional adenocarcinoma within the Barrett's mucosa that was not seen on endoscopy. The limit of this procedure is in fact the need for a visible lesion to target the resection.

Positron emission tomography (PET and PET-CT)

PET, and particularly PET-CT scanning, is emerging as not only a highly useful staging modality but also as a likely provider of both prognostic and treatment-related information (predictor of response of neoadjuvant therapy).

The recent introduction of integrated PET-CT imaging has improved the ability to localize areas of increased metabolic activity by integrating the anatomical resolution of CT scan with functional images of PET. Its primary value is in the initial staging of patients with esophageal cancer, mainly because of the high sensitivity and specificity for occult distant metastasis. In addition PET-CT may have a role in the evaluation of the response after neoadjuvant treatment. Bruzzi and colleagues (2007) reported that PET-CT identified interval appearance of metastatic disease in 8% of patients. The use of PET alone detected only 2% of these lesions, which were not detected on conventional staging. In this study PET-CT was not very helpful in predicting pathologic response to neoadjuvant therapy because of a high rate of false-positive findings for residual viable tumor.

Rizk and colleagues (2006) from the Memorial Sloan-Kettering Cancer Center evaluated the significance of preoperative PET standardized uptake values (SUVs) in predicting survival of 55 patients with adenocarcinoma of the distal esophagus and gastroesophageal junction who underwent esophagectomy alone as primary treatment of their disease.

The patients were divided in two groups based on their preoperative PET SUV value. Patients with low SUV (<4.5) were more likely to have early-stage disease. Patients with low SUV were more likely to have T1–2 disease and less lymph node involvement than patients with high SUV (90% vs 60%, and 8% vs 48%). The overall survival in the low SUV group was significantly better than in the high SUV group (Fig. 4.12). Furthermore, within the subset of patients with early clinical and/or pathologic-stage disease, patients with low preoperative SUV had a significantly better survival. When the SUV was considered as a continuous variable, it correlated with the presence of lymph node metastasis, the number of nodes involved, and the risk of death. The authors concluded that PET SUV could be used to predict clinical and/or pathologic stage and overall survival in patients with esophageal cancer. High PET SUV also identifies patients with poor prognosis from within a group of patients that would otherwise be considered to have curable early-stage disease and could be potentially used to stratify patients for appropriate therapy.

PET has also been proposed as a valuable tool to predicting response to preoperative chemotherapy. While randomized, controlled studies of neoadjuvant therapy versus surgery alone have failed to prove overall survival benefit from preoperative chemotherapy, it has been shown that patients who respond to chemotherapy have a better prognosis and overall improved survival than patients with no response. Ideally only patients who respond to chemotherapy should undergo neoadjuvant treatment and several authors have suggested the use of metabolic measurement with PET scan to allow early differentiation of responding and non-responding tumors.

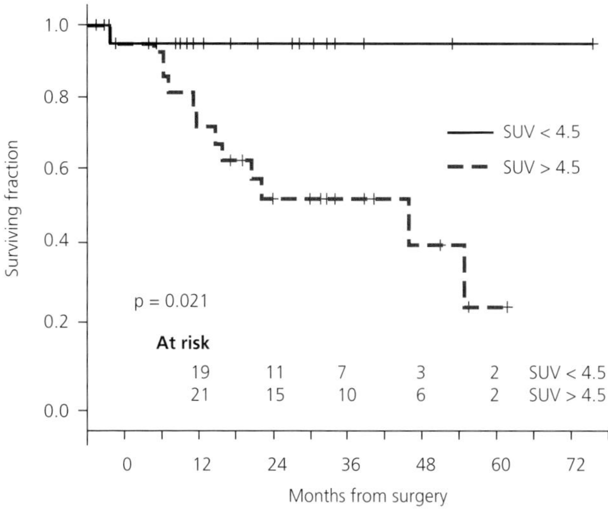

Fig. 4.12 Survival of esophageal cancer based upon standard uptake value (SUV) on positron emission tomography (PET). According to Swisher *et al.* (2004a).

Investigators from Munich, Germany (Orringer *et al.* 1993) reported on the use of ^{18}F-labeled fluorodeoxyglucose positron emission tomography (FDG-PET) as a predictor of response and patient survival in patients with locally advanced adenocarcinoma of the distal esophagus or cardia (T3 Nx M0) treated with preoperative chemotherapy. FDG is an established radiopharmaceutical for measuring exogenous glucose utilization *in vivo* and it is accumulated by the majority of malignant tumors. Responding tumors will show decrease of glucose utilization within a few days after initiation of chemotherapy. Their early data suggested that a decrease of tumor metabolic activity by more than 35% after 2 weeks of therapy predicts a high pathologic response rate (53%) and is associated with a better survival. Among 56 patients evaluated with FDG-PET at baseline and 14 days after chemotherapy was started, 18% of patients were classified as metabolic responders based on tumor uptake. Metabolic response was highly associated with clinical and histopathologic response. Overall survival of metabolic responders was significantly better than that of non-responders (Fig. 4.13). Among 50 patients who underwent surgical resection after completion of neoadjuvant chemotherapy, metabolic response remained a significant prognostic factor. Patients with metabolic response were reported to have a 3-year survival rate of 70% and a 3-year recurrence-free survival rate of 80%, compared to 35% and 38%, respectively, in non-responders.

Similarly, Swisher and colleagues (2004a) from MD Anderson Cancer Center in Houston, Texas, assessed the value of FDG-PET in predicting the pathologic response and survival of patients with esophageal carcinoma treated with preoperative chemoradiation and surgical resection. In this study, patients with postchemoradiation FDG-PET SUV <4 were found to have a significantly worse 2-year survival rate than those with an SUV <4. Furthermore, post-treatment FDG-PET was found to be the only preoperative factor that could predict survival. Even though FDG-PET was able to identify patients with large amount of residual disease after neoadjuvant treatment, the specificity was shown to be very low for low SUV, underscoring the limited ability of this test to rule out microscopic residual tumor. The use of FDG-PET could be therefore very useful for targeting personalized therapeutic strategies to patients. However it should be kept in mind that the test is limited in its ability to identify microscopic residual disease, emphasizing the need for esophagectomy even when post chemoradiation FDG-PET scan appears normal.

An individualized surgical approach

Modern treatment of esophageal cancer should be tailored to the single individual, and based on accurate clinical staging, the patient's overall health and comorbidities, and the goal of an R0 curative resection whenever possible.

As outlined above, at diagnosis cancers must be either local (confined to the mucosa or submucosa and node negative), regional (node positive without systemic metastasis), or systemic (Table 4.10). It is reasonable to conclude that the extent of operation will have little effect on survival of systemic disease but it can have a critical impact on survival for patients with isolated regional disease. The existence of a population of patients with regional disease has been debated in cancer biology, but can be proven by the extensive documentation that cure is possible with surgical resection alone in the presence of positive lymph nodes. The relatively small size of this group and the difficulty in clinically identifying these patients preoperatively account for the difficulty in establishing the benefit of a more extensive operation.

Patient with a high probability of disease confined to the mucosa (localized disease)

The detection of an esophageal adenocarcinoma at a stage where it is confined to the mucosa, once a rare clinical occurrence, is now relatively common. Current data show that as many as 37% of patients undergoing esophageal resection for adenocarcinoma have stage 1 disease (Fig. 4.14). This fact is

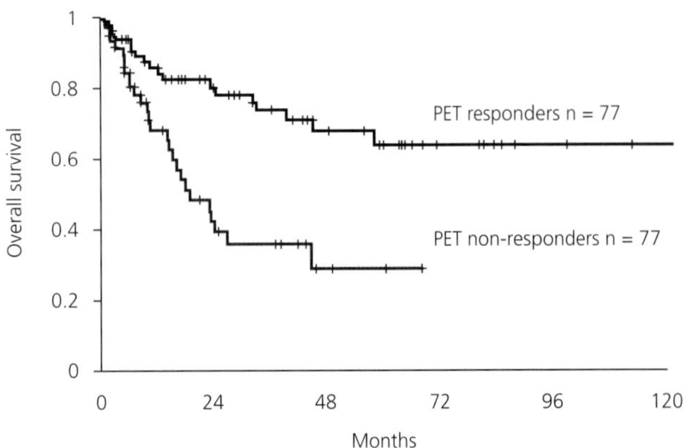

Fig. 4.13 Overall survival based on metabolic response evaluated by positron emission tomography (PET). According to Ott *et al.* (2006).

Table 4.10 Characteristics and estimated prevalence of extent of disease at presentation.

Local disease (15%)
Asymptomatic
Minimal or no visible lesion
Regional disease (25%)
Minimal symptoms (anemia)
Small (<2–3 cm), non-circumferential
Systemic disease (60%)
Dysphagia
>3-cm circumferential tumor; positive nodes on endoscopic ultrasound

largely the result of the liberal use of flexible endoscopy and the development of surveillance programs in patients with Barrett's esophagus.

A distinction between HGD, stage 1 intramucosal tumors and stage 1 submucosal tumors needs to be made. Intraepithelial tumors (carcinoma *in situ*) have a quite different biologic behavior from intramucosal tumors, which are very different than submucosal tumors (Fig. 4.15). Vessel invasion and lymph node metastasis do not occur in HGD/carcinoma *in situ* and are uncommon in intramucosal tumors, but occur in more than one-quarter of patients with submucosal lesions. As a consequence, the 5-year survival for intramucosal tumors is significantly better than for a tumor that has invaded the submucosa.

Techniques of curative resection given a high probability of local disease range from EMR to standard operative esophagectomy. There has been considerable enthusiasm for mucosal ablation, particularly photodynamic therapy (PDT) and EMR. To date the risk–benefit ratio has not been adequately evaluated.

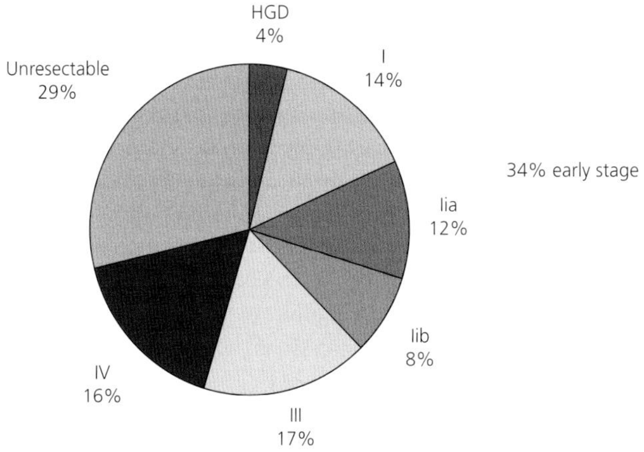

Fig. 4.14 Stage distribution of Barrett's adenocarcinoma at presentation. According to Stein and Siewert (2004).

Endoscopic treatment

EMR and PDT have both been studied in the setting of HGD. PDT suffers from incomplete ablation, a relatively high (30%) prevalence of strictures, and lack of availability and expertise in many locations, and its application is therefore becoming less common. EMR has taken its place and in the proper setting is a very viable treatment option. The primary limitation is the need to 'see' the area of interest. Further, given the well-documented 30–40% prevalence of invasive adenocarcinoma in surgical specimens of patients resected for a preoperative diagnosis of HGD, endoscopic methods used as a primary therapy have been slow to evolve. Local recurrence and/or development of metachronous lesions after EMR have been reported in 15–30% of patients. The combination of local resection and PDT has been used to reduce this possibility, especially in high-risk patients who may be precluded from undergoing esophagectomy because of multiple comorbidities.

Pacifico and colleagues (2006) from the Mayo Graduate School of Medicine reported a retrospective evaluation of 24 patients treated with EMR and PDT for early-stage Barrett's adenocarcinoma. Overall survival was 83% after a follow-up of 12 months. Persistence of adenocarcinoma was found on follow-up endoscopic biopsy in 17% of patients.

The largest experience to date has been reported by investigators in Wiesbaden Germany (Ell *et al.* 2007) in which the outcome of 100 consecutive patients with low-risk adenocarcinoma of the esophagus arising in Barrett's esophagus patients who underwent EMR was assessed. A total of 144 resections (1.47 per patient) were performed without technical problems. No major complications and only 11 minor ones (consisting of bleeding without decrease of Hb >2 g/dL; treated with injection therapy). Complete local remission was achieved in 99 of

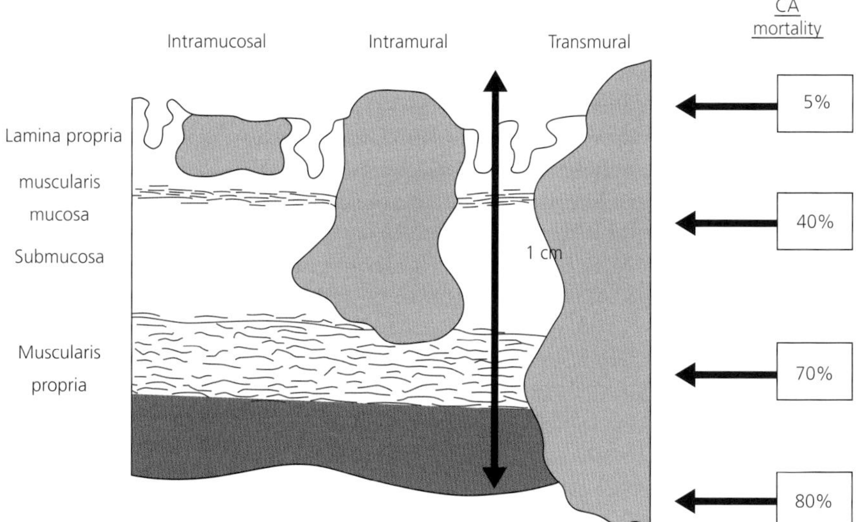

Fig. 4.15 Depth of tumor and mortality.

the 100 patients after 1.9 months (range 1–18 months) and a maximum of three resections. During a mean follow-up period of 36.7 months, recurrent or metachronous carcinomas were found in 11% of the patients, but successful repeat treatment with EMR was possible in all of these cases. The calculated 5-year survival rate was 98%. The authors have shown that EMR is a safe and efficacious treatment in highly selected patients with HGD and intramucosal adenocarcinoma.

The context of the use of EMR is critical however, and it is important that these data not be extrapolated in the treatment of patients beyond those described in this studies. It cannot be overemphasized that achieving the described outcomes requires a highly selected group of patients, which will be difficult for most centers to reproduce. The 100 patients reported from Wiesbaden were selected out of 667 possible candidates over 7 years. This equates to the referral of nearly 100 patients with very early esophageal adenocarcinoma per year. Most centers see a handful at most. All patients underwent very intensive staging, including EUS and radiographic procedures, high-resolution videoendoscopy with methylene blue chromoendoscopy, detailed morphologic assessment of the lesions according to the Japanese classification for early gastric cancer, an intense biopsy protocol (four quadrants, every 1 cm), routine assessment by two different pathologists, and high-frequency (20-MHz) ultrasound. Equally intense follow-up was required with endoscopy at 1, 2, 3, 6, 9, 12, 16, 24, 30 and 36 months with repeated high-resolution endoscopy and chromoendoscopy, a routine rigorous biopsy protocol, EUS and abdominal ultrasound, and CT. The rigor of the patient selection should be evident, as well as the difficulty most of us would have in reproducing it. The persistent neoplastic risk also needs to be recognized and emphasized. For all reports to date, the time of follow-up is short, particularly given the current prevalence of HGD and intramucosal cancer in patients with Barrett's esophagus in their 40s and 50s. The remaining Barrett's mucosa and reflux control is also a concern. Whether the advent of efficacious ablation technology and/or fundoplication for reflux control may aid this process remains unclear.

The largest experience with EMR for squamous-cell carcinoma comes from Japan. In a retrospective study of 116 consecutive patients Katada and colleagues (2005) analyzed the risk factors for local recurrence after EMR. Synchronous or metachronous lesions were found in 36% of patients. Intraepithelial carcinoma was present in 59% of cases, intramucosal tumor was found in 17% and tumor very close to or infiltrating the muscularis mucosa was found in 24% of cases. At a median follow-up of 35 months there was a local recurrence of 20% of the lesions. Median time to local recurrence after EMR was 6 months. There was no lymph node or distant recurrence. Independent risk factors for local recurrence were the presence of multicentric squamous epithelial dysplasia and piecemeal EMR. Also, patients with multicentric dysplasia had a significant shorter time to recurrence after EMR. It is interesting to note that all recurrent lesions could be treated with curative intent, mostly by a second EMR. All recurring lesions but one were shown to be mucosal cancer after the second EMR, and the overall 3-year survival was 100%.

Options for curative esophageal resection include transhiatal or transthoracic simple esophagectomy, vagal sparing or en-bloc esophagectomy. The chance of curative resection with a simple esophagectomy is critically dependent upon accurate identification of the location and depth of the tumor and/or the presence of regional nodal metastases. Since the perfect tool for preoperative staging of esophageal cancer is not yet available, the presence or absence of an endoscopically visible lesion in patients with HGD or intramucosal carcinoma has been proposed as a predictor of tumor depth and nodal metastases. The data indicate that a positive biopsy in the absence of an endoscopically visible lesion almost always corresponds to an intramucosal tumor without nodal metastases. In addition a number of studies have shown that about 40–50% of patients with the preoperative diagnosis of HGD were indeed proven to harbor occult adenocarcinoma at resection. Recently, EMR has also been used to stage the depth of invasion of small esophageal tumors. Currently patients with documented, confirmed HGD or adenocarcinoma in the absence of a visible endoscopic lesion are best treated by simple esophagectomy either transhiatal or vagal sparing. The vagal sparing approach is suitable only where there is confidence as to the absence of regional nodal disease. The mortality associated with this procedure should be less than 5%, and is minimal in centers experienced in esophageal surgery. Functional recovery is excellent, particularly in the vagal sparing group, since a significant reduction in dumping and diarrhea is observed among these patients.

Patient with a high probability of regional disease

While by no means certain, the probability of regional disease is high given a patient presenting without dysphagia (Fig. 4.16) who on endoscopy has a small (<1–2 cm) non-circumferential

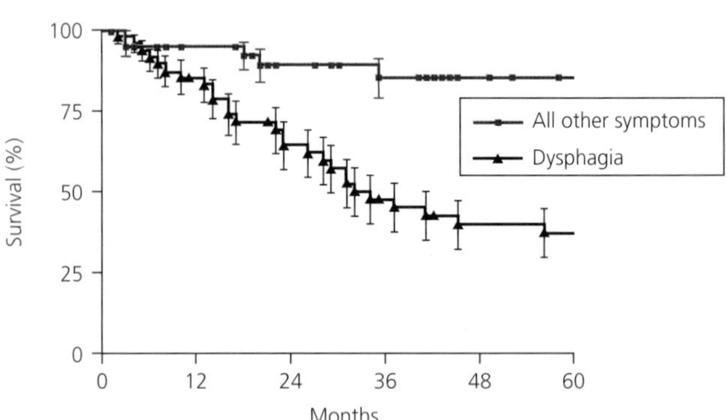

Fig. 4.16 Kaplan-Meier survival of a cohort of Los Angeles patients presenting with dysphagia compared to those with none or non-specific symptoms.

visible tumor (Fig. 4.17). It is in this setting that invasion through the muscularis mucosa into the submucosa is likely, along with its attendant 30% or more chance of lymph node metastasis but a reasonable chance of no systemic spread (Rice *et al.* 1998). These circumstances, which occur in as many as 15–25% of patients referred for surgical resection, are best approached via an en-bloc lymphadenectomy in association with esophagectomy as the treatment of choice (Fig. 4.18). Recent data indicate that where there is an early adenocarcinoma in Barrett's esophagus, nodal metastases are limited to the periesophageal location and do not involve the splenic artery, hilum greater or lesser curvature of the stomach. Thus isolated regional disease is likely and cure is possible given an appropriate resection.

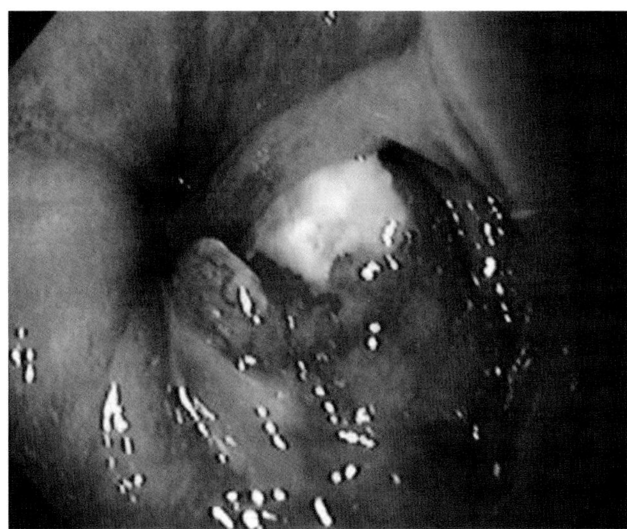

Fig. 4.17 Endoscopic view of a non-circumferential adenocarcinoma of the lower esophagus in which there is a high likelihood of regional disease.

The primary rationale for an en-bloc resection and extended lymphadenectomy is to minimize the incidence of local and regional recurrences and maximize the chances of long-term survival and cure (Table 4.11). Local recurrence has been shown to be very uncommon (<5–10%) following en-bloc resection, which contrasts with a 35% prevalence of local failure following transhiatal esophagectomy and a 15–20% prevalence after Ivor–Lewis resection (Table 4.12). These findings may be explained by the removal of unrecognized, often microscopic, disease with more extensive lymph node dissection. Involved nodes that are left behind during simple esophagectomy are likely the cause of recurrent local disease.

While it has been argued that the possibility of better survival with en-bloc esophagectomy is offset by an increased morbidity and mortality, in expert hands, the complication and mortality rates of an en-bloc esophagectomy are equivalent to simple esophagectomy. These facts, taken together with the inability to precisely predict those patients who will not gain benefit, support the use of a more extensive resection in any patient where cure is a possibility.

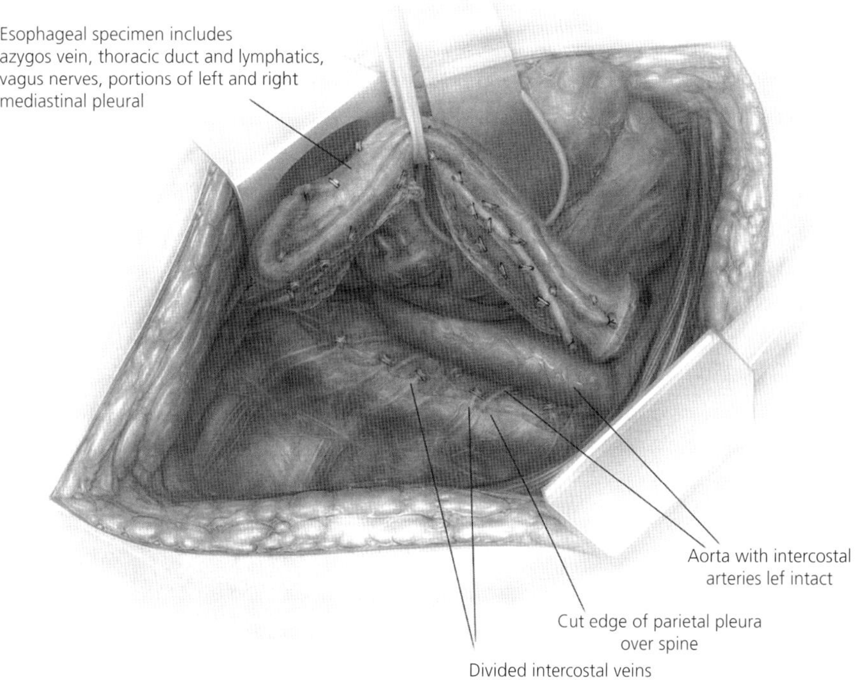

Fig. 4.18 Artist illustration of the transthoracic portion of an en-bloc esophagectomy. The aorta, pericardium. Right and left bronchi are skeletonized with a complete infracarinal posterior mediastinal lymphadenectomy. The azygous venous system and the thoracic duct are both taken in the resection specimen.

Table 4.11 Local recurrence after varied resection for cure surgical resections.

Surgical resection	n	Local recurrence within operative field (%)
En bloc*	94	1
Ivor–Lewis†	100	14
Transhiatal‡	144	35
Chemotherapy plus surgery§	124	32
Chemotherapy plus radiotherapy plus surgery¶	50	19

* Hagen *et al.* (2001)
† King *et al.* (1987)
‡ Hulscher *et al.* (2000)
§ Kelsen *et al.* (1998a)
¶ Urba *et al.* (2001)

Table 4.12 Reported ability of transthoracic en-bloc esophagectomy and transhiatal esophagectomy to control local–regional disease. From Johansson *et al.* (2004).

Reference	No. of subjects	Local recurrence (%)
Transthoracic en-bloc esophagectomy		
Matsubara *et al.* (1994)	171	10
Altorki & Skinner (2001)	111	8
Hagen *et al.* (2001)	100	1
Collard *et al.* (2001)	324	4
Swanson *et al.* (2001)	250	5.6
Range		1–10
Transhiatal esophagectomy		
Hulscher *et al.* (2000)	137	23
Becker *et al.* (1987)	35	31
Gignoux *et al.* (1987)		47
Nygaard *et al.* (1992)	186	35
Range		23–47

Patient with a high probability of systemic disease

Patients, who present with dysphagia and large (>3–5 cm) circumferential lesions on endoscopy or have five or more positive nodes on staging CT or EUS usually have a more advanced disease and a high probability of developing systemic disease after surgery. These patients are unlikely to be cured. They may benefit from neoadjuvant and /or adjuvant chemotherapy, but no definitive survival benefit has been shown to date using combined-modality therapy.

These patients, given the absence of metastatic disease, are best suited for palliative transhiatal esophagectomy (Branicki *et al.* 1998). A prospective longitudinal study from the European Organization for Research and Treatment of Cancer (EORTC) evaluating quality of life in patients after esophagectomy or other palliative procedures showed that quality-of-life scores returned to preoperative levels within 9 months after surgery (Blazeby *et al.* 2000). Dysphagia improved in both groups after treatment but the improvement was maintained until death or for the duration of the study in the surgical group whereas gradually deteriorated until death in the palliative group. Quality of life after palliative resection was shown to be comparable to that observed after curative resection in terms of quality and quantity of food intake, sleep patterns, and enjoyment of day-to-day living.

In patients with high surgical risk, systemic metastases, or unresectable local disease, promising results have been shown in palliation of symptoms with the use of coated self-expanding metal stents, which have recently become easy to use and safe for the patient.

Outcomes of surgical resection

Morbidity and mortality of resection

While esophagectomy remains a major surgical undertaking with significant morbidity and mortality, both complications and perioperative death have improved significantly over the past 15–20 years. Reasons for this include the use of epidural analgesia, improved respiratory therapy, and decreased prevalence of smoking (Table 4.13). In high-volume centers with stable and experienced teams and structured care algorithms, mortality has been reported to be as low as 0–1%. It averages 4–5% in most centers of excellence (Fig. 4.19). Also important, but often overlooked, is the fact that surgical mortality varies considerably with the type and extent of disease. It approaches zero in patients with HGD, averages 2–3% in those with adenocarcinoma, and is highest (8–10%) in patients with squamous cell carcinoma. These very different patient populations have markedly different underlying tumor burdens and comorbid conditions, and are often lumped together when reporting mortality statistics. Esophagectomy is arguably the surgical procedure most sensitive to volume–outcome relationships. With less than 4000 esophagectomies per year being performed in the US,

Table 4.13 Correlation of changes in perioperative variables with decreased hospital death rate. From Whooley *et al.* (2001).

Factor	p value
Epidural analgesia	0.0001
Bronchoscopy	0.0001
History of smoking	0.005
Blood loss < 1000 mL	0.03
P_aO_2 (kPa)	0.2
Pulmonary disease	0.3
Albumin (m/L)	0.5
Advanced stage (III/IV)	0.7
Forced expiratory volume (% predicted)	0.7

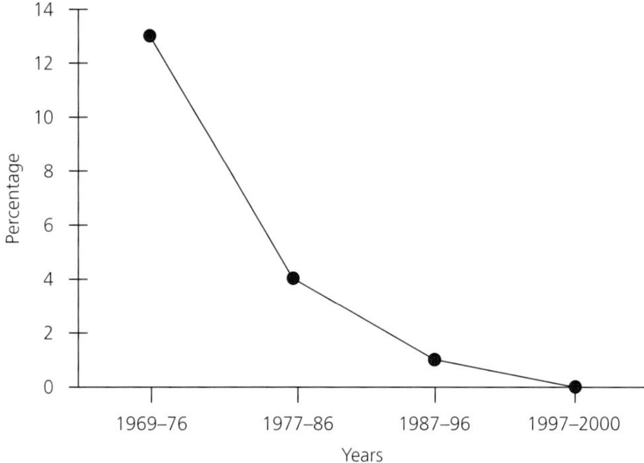

Fig. 4.19 Trends over time in 30-day operative mortality rate after esophageal cancer resection. From Ohga *et al.* (2002).

many have argued that the time has come to limit esophageal resection to high-volume centers.

Representing outcomes from a single high-volume center of expertise, Orringer (Orringer *et al.* 1999) has reported his 22-year experience with over 1000 patients who underwent transhiatal esophagectomy for either benign or malignant disease. Seventy-four per cent of the patients were treated for esophageal cancer, 69% of which was adenocarcinoma and 28% squamous cell carcinoma. The stomach was used for reconstruction in 96% of patients; the colon was used as a substitute when the stomach was not available. Mortality was 4%, significantly declining over the years. The major postoperative complication was anastomotic leak occurring in 13% and was more common after retrosternal placement of the stomach, previous radiation therapy or prior operations at the gastroesophageal junction. The leak was nearly always successfully managed conservatively; takedown of the anastomosis and cervical esophagostomy was necessary in nine patients due to necrosis of the upper stomach. Median hospital stay was 7 days, 90% of patients had no or mild dysphagia after a mean follow-up of 29 months, and only 2% had severe dysphagia requiring regular dilation. Symptoms of gastroesophageal reflux disease were present in 21% of patients but only 3.6% of them had nocturnal reflux or aspiration-related pneumonia.

Representing outcomes from multiple centers with varying volumes, Bailey *et al.* (2003) reported an analysis of 1777 esophagectomies at 109 VA medical centers entering data into the National Surgical Quality Improvement Program (NSQIP). The procedures were performed in the decade of the 1990s; 85% were for malignancy. Thirty-day mortality was 9.8% and complications occurred in 49.5% of patients. The most frequent complications were pneumonia (21%), respiratory failure (16%), and the need for more than 48-hour ventilator support (22%). The NSQIP data allow analysis of risk factors predisposing to death and complications. Predictors of mortality included neoadjuvant therapy, blood, urea, nitrogen >40, alkaline phosphatase >125 U/L, diabetes, alcohol use, decreased functional status, ascites and advanced age.

Several studies have evaluated the mortality and morbidity of en-bloc and transhiatal resections and have shown that they are similar (Table 4.14). Indeed progressive improvements in intraoperative and postoperative care have largely eliminated mortality and morbidity as a factor in the selection of patients for one procedure versus another.

Table 4.14 Mortality and morbidity as reported in the literature for transthoracic en-bloc esophagectomy and transhiatal esophagectomy. From Johansson *et al.* (2004).

Reference	n	Mortality	Morbidity	LOS
En-bloc esophagectomy				
*Putnam *et al.* (1994)	134	8%	75%	20 days
*Horstmann *et al.* (1995)	41	10%	ns	23 days
*Altorki *et al.* (1997)	78	5.1%	24%	ns
*Hulscher *et al.* (2002)	114	4%	57%	19 days
Swanson *et al.* (2001)	250	3.6%	33%	13 days
Hagen *et al.* (2001)	100	6%	71%	14 days
Range		3.6–10%	24–75%	13–23 days
Transhiatal esophagectomy				
*Putnam *et al.* (1994)	42	5%	69%	19 days
*Horstmann *et al.* (1995)	46	11%	ns	26 days
*Altorki *et al.* (1997)	50	6%	26%	ns
*Hulscher *et al.* (2002)	106	2%	27%	15 days
Orringer *et al.* (1993)	417	5%	32%	11–14 days
Rentz *et al.* (2003)	385	9.9%	49%	ns
Range		2–11%	26–69%	11–26 days

LOS, length of hospital stay.

* indicates that both en-bloc esophagectomy and transhiatal esophagectomy are included in the study.

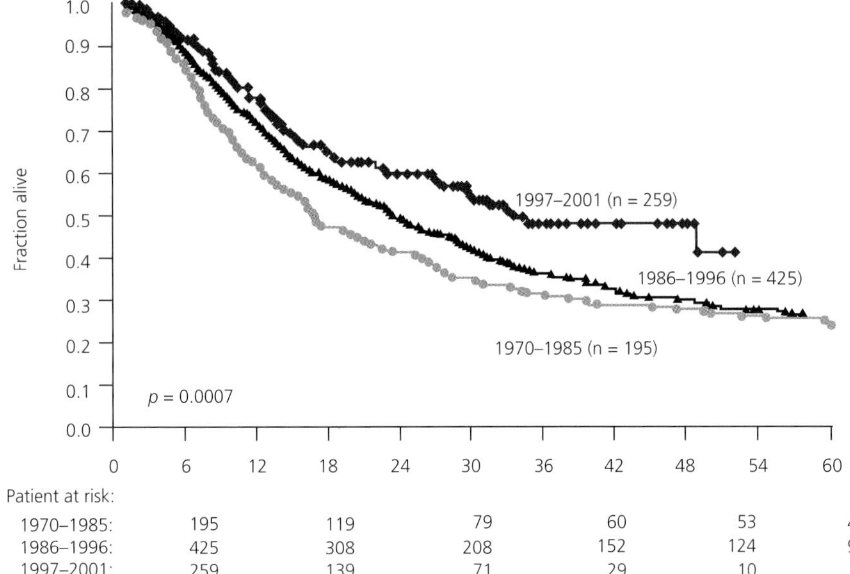

Fig. 4.20 Improved survival in esophageal cancer over 1950–2000. According to Hofstetter *et al.* (2002).

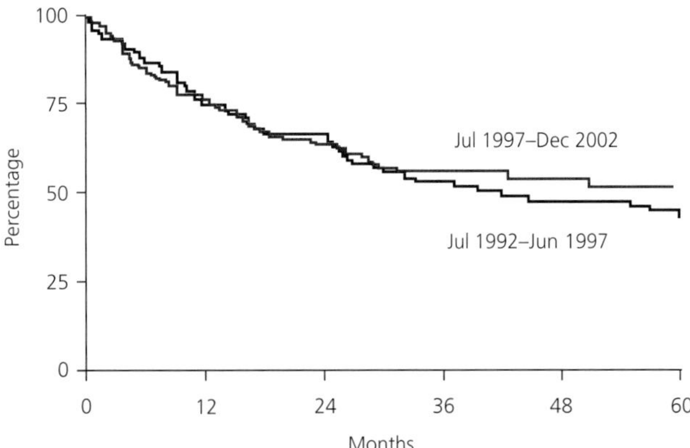

Fig. 4.21 Survival after esophagectomy for adenocarcinoma. According to Portale *et al.* (2006).

Survival data

Long-term survival following esophagectomy for cancer has improved from a dismal 10–15% in the 1960s and 70s to 20–25% in the 1980s and 90s, and to a remarkable 40–50% in recent publications utilizing an individualized approach and en-bloc resections (Fig. 4.20). Altorki and Skinner (2001) have reported a 40% 5-year survival after en-bloc resection of unselected cancers in the distal esophagus. Hagen *et al.* (2001) in a review of 100 consecutive en-bloc esophagectomies for esophageal adenocarcinoma has shown a 52% actuarial survival at 5 years. Most recently, Portale in Los Angeles (Portale *et al.* 2006a) reported an overall 5-year survival of 47% for all patients after esophagectomy, including 81% for stage I, 51% for stage II, and 14% for stage III disease (Fig. 4.21).

The evidence strongly suggests that transthoracic en-bloc resection results in better control of local–regional disease (Table 4.15). This is in contrast to the widespread practice of relying on adjuvant radiochemotherapy to improve local control which has not seen great success (Table 4.16). Johansson *et al.* (2004), examining the Los Angeles experience, reported a comparison of transthoracic en-bloc resection and transhiatal simple resection in a case–control series of patients with transmural (T3) esophageal adenocarcinomas with eight or fewer lymph nodes involved (N1). The aim was to compare survival in similar patients with pathologic T3 N1 disease. This approach removes the influence of inaccurate preoperative staging and minimizes the influence of postoperative stage migration on survival since all patients had N1 disease. The authors required that 20 or more lymph nodes were in the surgical specimen to provide confirmation that the extent of lymph node disease in both groups was comparable. As much as possible these study conditions focused the question as to which procedure was associated with a better survival. Indeed the Cox analysis identified only two independent factors that affected survival in the studied population; namely the type of resection and extent of lymph node disease categorized according to the number of involved nodes (Fig. 4.22).

Two further studies deserve mention. The first is a population-based retrospective case–control study comparing survival following transhiatal and en-bloc resection in Finland (Sihvo *et al.* 2004) and the second a prospective randomized trial of simple versus extended esophagectomy from the Netherlands (Hulscher *et al.* 2002).

Table 4.15 Comparison trials between transhiatal esophagectomy (THE) and transthoracic en-bloc esophagectomy (EBE) on long-term survival. From Johansson *et al.* (2004).

Reference	Type of trial	n	THE	EBE	p value
Hagen *et al.* (1993)	Retro	30 EBE 39 THE	14% (5 year)	41% (5 year)	<0.001
Putnam *et al.* (1994)	Retro	102 EBE 30 THE	12% (4 year)	30% (4 year)	0.02
Horstmann *et al.* (1995)	Retro	41 EBE 46 THE	18% (3 year)	17% (3 year)	ns
Altorki *et al.* (1997)	Retro	78 EBE 50 THE	11% (4 year)	35% (4 year)	0.007
Hulscher *et al.* (2002)	RCT	114 EBE 106 THE	27% (5 year)	39% (5 year)	0.08

Retro, retrospective clinical study; RCT, randomized controlled trial.

Table 4.16 Combined-modality therapy for esophageal cancer: patterns of failure.

	High dose (64.8 Gy) (n = 109)		Standard dose (50.4 Gy) (n = 109)	
	No.	%	No.	%
Alive/no failure	21	19	27	25
Any failure	88	81	82	75
Persistent local disease	36	33	37	34
Local failure	10	9	13	12
Regional failure	8	7	8	7
Distant failure	10	9	17	16
Regional and distant failure	0	0	2	2
Total local/regional persistence/failure	54	50	60	55
Treatment-related death	11	10	2	2
Second primary cancer	4	4	1	1
Cancer death/not specified	3	3	0	0
Dead of intercurrent disease	6	6	2	2

Sihvo *et al.* (2004) compared the fate of 42 patients following esophagectomy with two-field lymphadenectomy to that of 129 patients following standard esophagectomy. Slightly less than half (42.5%) of all cancers of the esophagogastric junction underwent resection. Similar to the reports outlined above, the

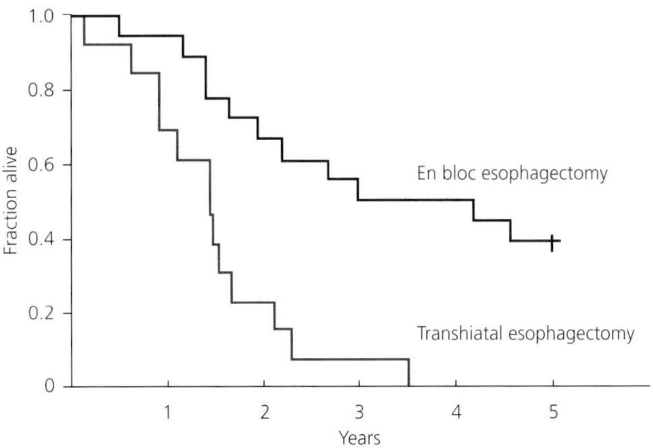

Fig. 4.22 Survival of T3N1 patients with 1–8 metastatic lymph nodes who had a transthoracic en-bloc lymph node dissection (n = 18) and those who had a transhiatal lymph node dissection (n = 13). Log rank test, statistic 10.25, df = 1, p = 0.0006. From Johansson *et al.* (2004).

5-year survival was significantly better in patients with two-field lymphadenectomy (50%) than in those with less extensive resections (23.2%, p = 0.005) (Fig. 4.23). Eight-year survival rates were also better (43% vs 21%), suggesting that the effect is longlasting. The authors concluded that in centers with experience, 'radical surgery' should be favored for patients eligible for major surgery.

The only prospective randomized controlled study was performed by Hulscher *et al.* (2002) in the Netherlands. This study showed a not quite, but nearly, significant (0.08) trend toward better survival with the en-bloc resection (Fig. 4.24). Unfortunately the study was underpowered. Their calculations for sample size were based on a survival of 30% following simple transhiatal dissection, whereas the literature would support a 25% survival rate at best. Further they estimated a 15% difference between the procedures but actually observed only a 10% difference. Given these data, the correct sample size required to detect a statistical difference would be 260 patients per arm, whereas they enrolled only 110 per arm.

An important common finding in all these studies is the correlation between survival and number of positive nodes on pathology. Survival decreased significantly with 9 or more positive nodes in Altorki and Skinner's study (2001), 80% of patients with 5 or more involved nodes developed systemic disease in Hagen's study (Hagen *et al.* 2001), and 5-year survival was significantly better when the ratio of involved nodes to the total number of nodes removed was <10% in Portale's study (Portale *et al.* 2006a). In a multivariate analysis of prognostic factors for esophageal cancer, Bollschweiler *et al.* (2006) showed that patients with fewer than 5 regional positive nodes had significant better prognosis than those with more than 5 lymph nodes involved. Also patients with negative nodes and more than 15 nodes examined showed better prognosis than those with fewer

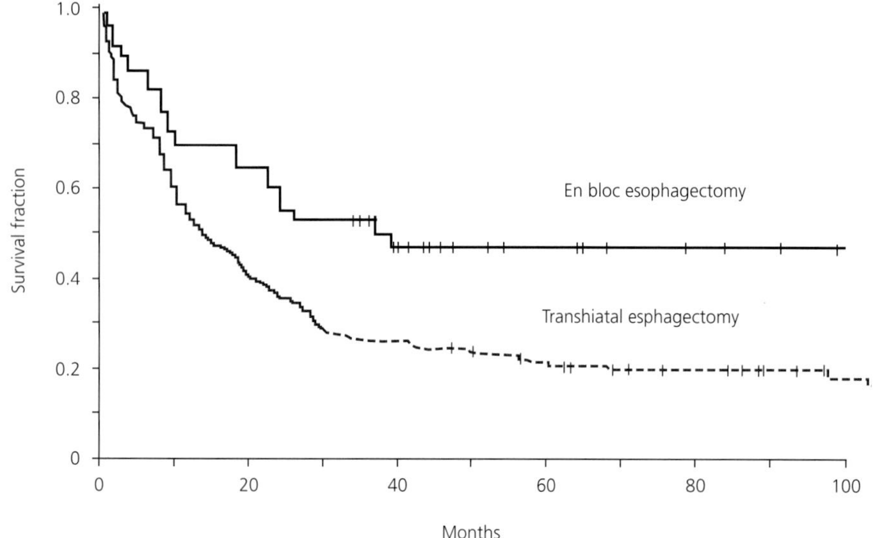

Fig. 4.23 Five-year survival of patients following esophagectomy with two-field lymphadenectomy versus standard esophagectomy. Log rank test, p = 0.005. From Sihvo *et al.* (2004).

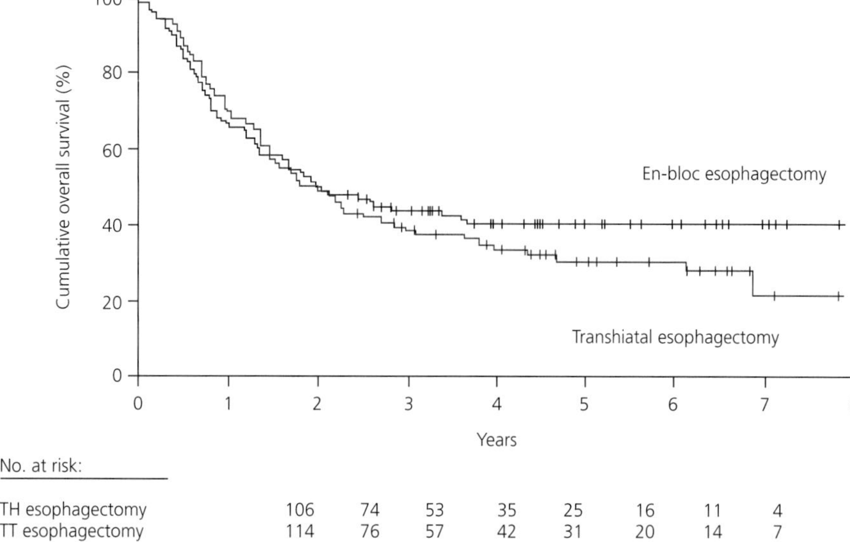

Fig. 4.24 Overall survival of patients with esophageal adenocarcinoma after transhiatal or transthoracic en-bloc esophagectomy. From Hulsher *et al.* (2002).

examined nodes. This finding again confirms the regional nature of the disease and underscores the role of lymphadenectomy for improving survival.

Taken together, these studies which encompass retrospective series, case–control studies, population-based studies and a prospective randomized trial, from around the world, strongly suggest that for early cancers of the lower esophagus and cardia, en-bloc esophagogastrectomy results in significantly better survival rates than transhiatal esophagogastrectomy. This finding is unlikely to be due to bias in the stage of disease resected, a difference in operative mortality, or death from non-tumor causes. Rather, it appears to be due to the type of operation performed.

Functional outcomes

In general the functional outcome after esophagectomy is good. Between 25 and 50% of patients suffer mild to moderate alimentary disabilities. Orringer (Orringer *et al.* 1999) evaluated alimentary outcome in 242 patients following esophagectomy and gastric pull-up. The majority (68%) were either asymptomatic or had mild symptoms which required no treatment. Sixty five per cent were free of dysphagia eating an unrestricted diet, and 60% had no regurgitation.

The most satisfactory esophageal replacement may be achieved when a vagal-sparing esophagectomy can be performed. Many of the annoyances that occur after esophageal replacement are due to the concomitant vagotomy and the loss of parasympathetic modulation of foregut function. In an elegant study by Banki *et al.* (2002), the vagal function (secretory, motor, and reservoir) after vagal-preserving esophagectomy was tested in 15 patients and compared to a control group of 23 asymptomatic normal subjects, 10 patients with standard esophagectomy and gastric pull-up, and 10 patients with esophagogastrectomy and colon interposition. The secretory function was assessed by measuring gastric acid output and serum pancreatic polypeptide after sham feeding. Gastric motor function was assessed via technetium gastric emptying scans and a symptom questionnaire to evaluate the incidence of dumping and diarrhea. Meal capacity and postoperative changes in body mass index were used as parameters to assess gastric reservoir function. The study showed that vagal-sparing esophagectomy preserves gastric secretion, gastric emptying, meal capacity, and BMI with outcomes very similar to those in normal subjects (Fig. 4.25).

Conclusion

Surgical resection is the current standard of care for the treatment of patients with curable esophageal adenocarcinoma. The extent of resection should be based on the objectives of treatment (cure vs palliation) and preoperative stage. When cure is the goal, early detection and complete removal of the tumor are the most important variables.

Novel treatment options such as the combination of en-bloc esophagectomy and systemic chemotherapy and chemotherapy tailored to the molecular aspects of the patient's tumor remain exciting prospects for the future.

Chemotherapy for metastatic cancer of the esophagus, gastroesophageal junction, and stomach

Aminah Jatoi

Cancers of the esophagus, gastroesophageal junction, and stomach comprise a worldwide health threat, particularly when the adenocarcinoma and squamous cell types are considered together. For example, esophageal cancer represents the eighth most common cause of cancer-related death, and gastric cancer the second (Devesa *et al.* 1998). Although emerging evidence suggests divergent tumor biology between the foregoing cancer types and cell types, the clinical management of patients with these cancers remains indistinguishable, particularly in the setting of metastatic disease. This chapter therefore provides an overview of the role of chemotherapy in managing these patients with metastatic disease and utilizes the term esophageal/gastric cancer to refer to the entire group of malignancies described above.

Does chemotherapy prolong life in patients with metastatic disease?

The answer to this fundamental question is 'yes.' Despite the poor prognosis associated with metastatic esophageal/gastric cancer, chemotherapy does play a pivotal role in providing a survival advantage to select patients who appear well enough to receive it. Four published trials, primarily but not exclusively in gastric cancer patients, have investigated chemotherapy versus

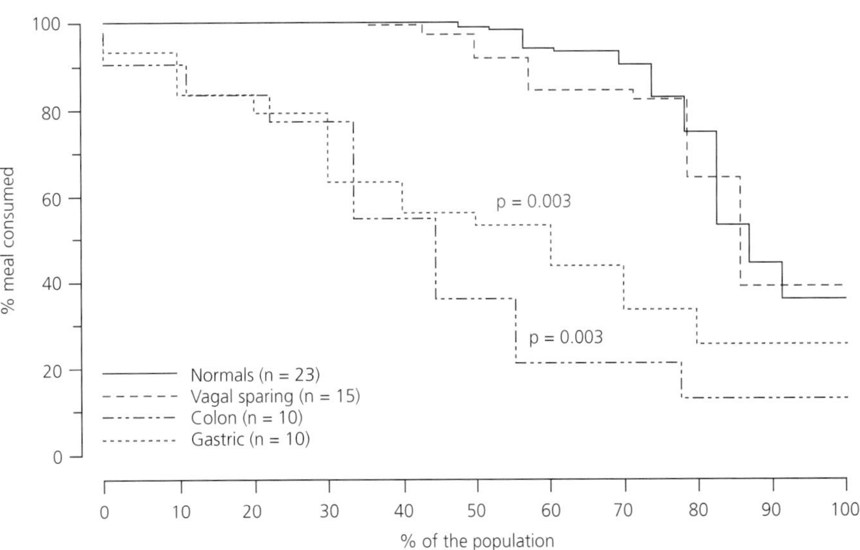

Fig. 4.25 Percentage of a standard meal consumed by normal subjects and in patients with an esophagectomy. Note that patients submitted to vagal-sparing esophagectomy have a normal eating pattern. According to Banki *et al.* 2002.

best supportive care (Murad *et al.* 1993; Pyrhonen *et al.* 1995; Scheithauer *et al.* 1995; Glimelius *et al.* 1997). Although these trials are fraught with controversial study designs, such as relatively small sample sizes and the occasional, inexplicable allowance of a treatment crossover, the fact remains that three of four showed a survival advantage of a few months with the administration of chemotherapy. All four of these trials tested multidrug regimens, but it is important to point out that the median survival with chemotherapy was consistently no greater than 1 year, despite the finding that chemotherapy appeared to gain patients a statistically significant survival advantage. Thus, although chemotherapy remains a viable option for esophageal/gastric cancer patients with metastatic disease and otherwise relatively good health, its benefits are modest and should be acknowledged as such before prescribing it.

Is there a standard chemotherapy?

This question remains highly controversial despite the completion of several phase III, comparative trials. A sizable number of trials have demonstrated no statistically significant improvement in survival with one regimen over another. Only a few exceptions exist. Most notably, Webb and others compared the regimen of epiribicin, cisplatin, and 5-fluorouracil (5-FU) versus 5-FU, doxorubicin, and methotrexate, and observed a median survival of 8.9 months and 5.7 months, respectively ($p = 0.0009$) (Webb *et al.* 1997). This trial has been criticized for two main reasons. First, it included not only patients with metastatic disease but also those with locally advanced disease. The latter was not clearly defined in the paper and ultimately nine patients who received epirubicin, cisplatin, and 5-FU went on to undergo a complete resection of their cancer. Nine patients may not appear to be a large enough number to dramatically alter the study's overall outcome. However, the fact that these nine patients were included in the trial as part of the better-performing study arm raises the possibility that the observed survival advantage might represent nothing more than an imbalance between groups. Second, the comparative regimen appears to have underperformed when one considers that in previous trials, it had helped patients attain a median survival of 7–9.5 months (Wils *et al.* 1991; Kelsen *et al.* 1992). Thus, it may not be that epiribicin, cisplatin, and 5-FU performed favorably but rather that the other regimen underperformed, thus yielding a statistically significant survival difference between groups.

But not all studies with epirubicin (E), cisplatin (C), and 5-FU (F) have consistently demonstrated a survival advantage. In a robust 580-patient study, Ross and others compared the above regimen versus mitomycin C, cisplatin, and 5-FU (Ross *et al.* 2002). In both arms, the 5-FU was given by continuous infusion throughout the duration of each cycle. Median survival was comparable between the two regimens: 9.4 months versus 8.7 months, respectively ($p = 0.32$). It was only because of improvements in global quality of life with the former regimen that the investigators concluded: 'This study confirms that the ECF regimen should be regarded as a reference treatment in advanced esophagogastric cancer.'

Much of the confusion that surrounds the 'reference treatment,' epiribicin, cisplatin, and 5-FU, promises to be settled with the REAL-2 trial (Chong & Cunningham 2005). This trial is currently ongoing in Europe as a multiarm study that compares the following four regimens: (i) epirubicin, cisplatin, 5-FU versus (ii) epirubicin, cisplatin, capecitabine versus (iii) epirubicin, oxaliplatin, 5-FU versus (iv) epirubicin, oxaliplatin, capecitabine. This 1000-patient trial is the largest ever to be conducted in patients with gastric/esophageal cancer. It promises to provide the answers to whether an oral fluoropyrimidine is just as effective as continuous-infusion 5-FU and whether the newer agent oxaliplatin, a highly valued drug in the treatment of colorectal cancer, is more effective than cisplatin. It is thought to be an important study in helping to define the new 'reference treatment' for patients with this malignancy. Results are eagerly awaited.

The REAL-2 trial will provide some important answers, but as this trial has been accruing patients and as its data have been maturing, yet other questions have emerged. The taxanes have repeatedly demonstrated antineoplastic effects in patients with gastric/esophageal cancer. Recently, Moiseyenko presented provocative preliminary data from a 445-patient study that included docetaxel in one of its treatment arms (Moisyenko *et al.* 2005). The two comparative arms included the following: (i) docetaxel, 5-FU, and cisplatin versus (ii) 5-FU and cisplatin. The former outperformed the latter with median survivals as follows: 9.2 versus 8.6 months, respectively ($p = 0.02$). Although these benefits appear modest, they nonetheless represent one of only a few studies to demonstrate survival advantage in a comparative chemotherapy trial. Thus, this study poses the following question: what will be the role of the taxanes, specifically docetaxel, in the development of future studies for patients with esophageal/gastric cancer? The study from Moiseyenko and others is notable in so far as it establishes docetaxel as a life-prolonging drug in the treatment of this malignancy.

What's next?

The number of large, definitive, phase III studies is relatively few in the treatment of patients with metastatic gastric/esophageal cancer. More commonly, single-arm phase II studies serve to explore whether a drug or a regimen might provide some preliminary evidence of efficacy to the point where a phase III trial might be considered in the future. Agents with established antineoplastic activity, such as irinotecan, merit further study to establish a better understanding of their value in treating patients with this malignancy. At the same time, an emerging number of effective agents for treating colon cancer has spawned several phase II studies that are either in development or actively recruiting patients. In the near future, clinicians will likely learn about the potential role of epidermal growth factor receptor inhibitors, such as cetuximab and panitumumab, when given in combination with other more conventional types of chemotherapy. Additionally, agents that block angiogenesis, such as bevacizumab, will continue to be tested in search of preliminary evidence of efficacy. A host of other agents not yet established in the treatment of gastrointestinal cancers, such as proteasome inhibitors and cell cycle inhibitors, are either under active investigation in patients with esophageal/gastric cancer or about to become so.

Conclusions

A sobering realization is that despite a sizable effort in drug investigation, the median survival among patients with esophageal/gastric cancer consistently falls short of 1 year. Nonetheless, there appears to be kindling hope that the median survival of patients with this disease will finally improve beyond the 1-year mark. The REAL-2 study promises to identify the better fluoropyrimidine and the better platinum agent. The survival advantage observed with docetaxel suggests that it will likely be utilized in future phase III trials. Finally, a host of relatively novel agents, some of which have already demonstrated efficacy in other gastrointestinal cancers, raise optimism that major gains in survival will finally be realized in patients with metastatic esophageal/gastric cancer.

Concurrent radiochemotherapy for esophageal cancer

Zhongxing Liao, Luka Milas, Ritsuko Komaki & Jaffer Ajani

Introduction

Over the past two decades, advances in imaging technology have allowed more accurate staging of patients with esophageal cancer and have led to better selection of patients for different treatment modalities. Also, advances in radiotherapy technique, in particular, the development of three-dimensional conformal radiotherapy (3D-CRT), which allows better strategic targeting of tumor volume and improved sparing of normal tissue, have significantly improved patient outcomes.

This section will cover definitive radiochemotherapy and preoperative radiochemotherapy in patients with esophageal cancer, the rationale for these approaches, the evidence supporting their use, side-effects, new therapeutic approaches on the horizon, and the technical details of radiotherapy delivery.

Definitive radiochemotherapy

Rationale

Radiotherapy alone as a definitive therapy for patients with inoperable esophageal cancer (those with T4 disease with tumor invading to trachea, tracheal–esophageal fistula, or most M1a nodal involvement, or those who cannot tolerate an operation for esophagectomy) produced poor long-term results. Therefore, concurrent radiotherapy and chemotherapy (radiochemotherapy) was tested in such patients. Multiple trials have established radiochemotherapy as a standard approach to the definitive treatment of local or local–regional disease.

Randomized trials of radiotherapy versus radiochemotherapy

Many trials have been performed over the past 15 years to evaluate radiochemotherapy. Most random-assignment trials comparing radiotherapy alone with radiochemotherapy (Table 4.17) have used a cisplatin- and 5-FU-based chemotherapy combination.

Perhaps the most well known of these randomized trials is the Radiation Therapeutic Oncology Group (RTOG) trial 85-01 (Herskovic *et al.* 1992; Al-Sarraf *et al.* 1997; Cooper *et al.* 1999), which compared radiation alone at a dose of 6400 cGy to radiation at a lower dose of 5000 cGy plus concurrent cisplatin- and 5-FU-based chemotherapy (Al-Sarraf *et al.* 1997). A total 126 patients were randomized until a planned interim analysis demonstrated significant difference favoring the radiochemotherapy arm that satified the early stopping rule. An additional 73 consecutive patients were treated with radiochemotherapy without randomization.

In this trial, patients received four cycles of 5-FU (1000 mg/m^2 on days 1–4) and cisplatin (75 mg/m^2 on day 1). Radiotherapy (50 Gy in 25 fractions, in 2-Gy daily fractions 5 days per week) was given concurrently with chemotherapy beginning on day 1 of cycle 1. Cycles 1 and 2 of chemotherapy (when concurrent radiotherapy was being delivered) lasted 4 weeks, whereas cycles 3 and 4 lasted 3 weeks. The radiation field encompassed bilateral supraclavicular fossae to the gastro-esophageal junction for the initial 30 Gy and 50 Gy for patients in the radiochemotherapy arm and radiotherapy-only arm, respectively, and 5-cm proximal and distal margins from the gross tumor for an additional 20 Gy and 14 Gy for patients in the radiochemotherapy arm and radiotherapy-only arm, respectively. This dose intensification in cycles 3 and 4 of chemotherapy and large target volume encompassed in the radiation fields may explain in part why patients had difficulty completing all four cycles of chemotherapy. Significant toxicity was seen in patients treated in the radiochemotherapy arm: 50% of patients experienced at least one RTOG grade III adverse event and 8% experienced life-threatening grade IV adverse events compared with 4% grade IV adverse events in the radiotherapy-only arm.

Table 4.17 Randomized trials of radiochemotherapy versus radiotherapy alone.

Study	Treatment	No. of patients	5-year survival (%)	5-year local–regional failure (%)
RTOG 85-01	RCT	61	27	45
(Herskovic *et al.* 1992; Al-Sarraf *et al.* 1997; Cooper *et al.* 1999)	RCT	69	30	54
	RT	62	0	68
ECOG 1282	RCT	59	9	Not reported
(Smith *et al.* 1998)	RT	60	7	Not reported
NCI Brazil	RCT	28	16	61
(Araujo *et al.* 1991)	RT	31	6	84
EORTC	RCT	75	12	Not reported
(Roussel *et al.* 1988)	RT	69	6	
Scandinavia	RCT	46	6	Not reported
(Nygaard *et al.* 1992)	RT	51	0	
Pretoria	RCT	34	5 months (MST)	Not reported
(Slabber *et al.* 1998)	RT	36	6 months (MST)	Not reported

ECOG, Eastern Cooperative Oncology Group; EORTC, European Organization for Research and Treatment of Cancer; MST, median survival time; NCI, National Cancer Institute; RCT, radiochemotherapy; RT, radiotherapy; RTOG, Radiation Therapy Oncology Group.

The treatment-related mortality rate in this study was 2% in the combined treatment arm compared with 0% in the radiation-only arm. Interestingly, a reduction of grade IV adverse events was noted in the non-randomized patients (4% vs 8%), and no fatal adverse event was reported, suggesting a learning curve in the administration of radiochemotherapy. Furthermore, there was no difference in late toxicity among all three groups (Cooper *et al.* 1999).

The overall survival rates were 26% and 22% at 5 and 8 years respectively for patients who received radiochemotherapy, and 0% for those who received radiotherapy alone. Persistence of disease, the most common mode of treatment failure in every group, was less common in the radiochemotherapy group (25–28%) than in the radiotherapy-alone group (37%). Distant metastasis accounted for the first site of treatment failure in 30% of patients in the radiotherapy-alone group compared with 16% of patients in the radiochemotherapy group (Al-Sarraf *et al.* 1997; Cooper *et al.* 1999).

The positive results of the RTOG trial 85-01 established radiochemotherapy rather than radiotherapy alone as the conventional non-surgical treatment for esophageal cancer. The results of this trial also established that a radiation dose of 50 Gy is appropriate for patients with esophageal cancer treated with simultaneous radiotherapy and cisplatin-based chemotherapy. However, the facts that the local failure rate in the radiochemotherapy arm was high (50% at 5 years) and that the survival rate in the radiochemotherapy arm was modest (26% at 5 years) (Fig. 4.26) indicated a need for better local–regional treatment (Al-Sarraf *et al.* 1997; Cooper *et al.* 1999).

Optimal dose of radiation

In patients with squamous cell carcinoma of the upper aerodigestive tract, it has long been recognized that radiation alone to 50 Gy at 1.8–2 Gy per fraction over 5 weeks is adequate to control more than 90% of subclinical disease. At least 60–70 Gy given at the same fractionation is needed to treat gross tumor (Withers & Peters 1980). However, the optimal dose of radiation for esophageal cancer is controversial, especially when radiation is delivered concurrently with chemotherapy as definitive treatment. Sun (1989) reported a clear association between higher radiation dose and improved 5-year survival when radiation was used as the sole therapeutic modality in patients with stage II or III esophageal cancer. The 5-year survival rates were 10.6% in patients who received 60–69 Gy and about 2% in patients who received 50–59 Gy. Coia *et al.* (1991) treated patients with clinically early-stage (stage I and II) esophageal cancer with 5-FU, mitomycin C, and 60 Gy, and found a very low 5-year local failure rate of 25%, a 5-year actuarial survival rate of 30%, and for patients with stage I disease, a 5-year actuarial local relapse-free survival rate of 70%. Of importance, this trial is the only trial of radiochemotherapy in which patients with early-stage (stage I and II) esophageal cancer were treated and analyzed separately (Coia *et al.* 1991). On the other hand, in a study of 30 patients with clinical stage I to III disease, John *et al.* (1989) reported a local failure rate of 27%, similar to that in the Coia *et al.* study, with a lower radiation dose of 40–50 Gy. The 2-year actuarial survival rate was 29%. Radiation doses of up to 66 Gy following three cycles of cisplatin and bleomycin have also been used

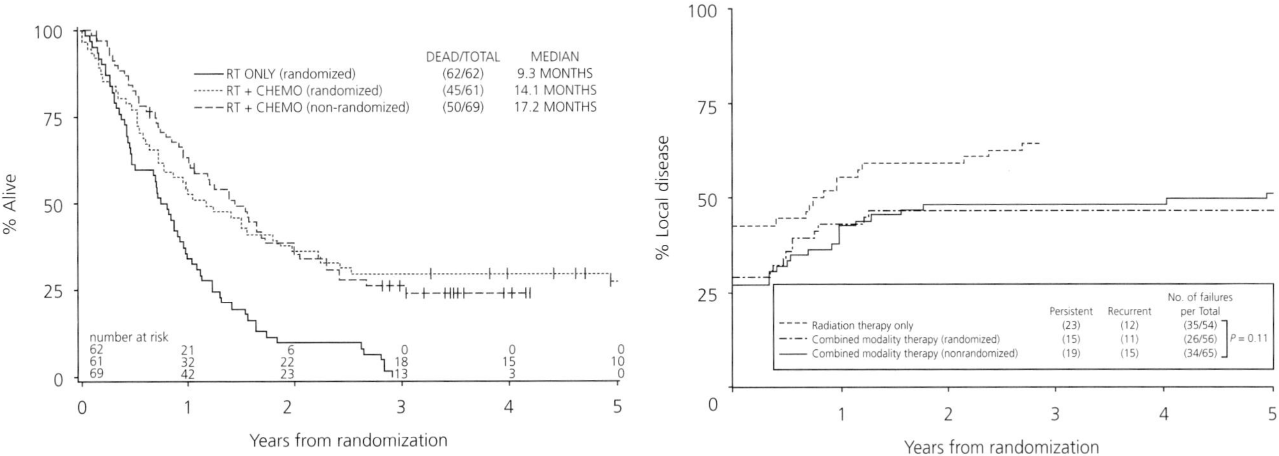

Fig. 4.26 Overall survival and local regional disease control in patients treated on RTOG 85-01, a randomized trial of radiation and concurrent chemoradiation. There was no survivor at 3 years after radiation only. The most common pattern of local failure was persistent disease. The local failure was high (50–65%) in both groups. (Graphs reproduced from Al-Sarraf *et al.* 1997 and Cooper *et al.* 1999 with permission.)

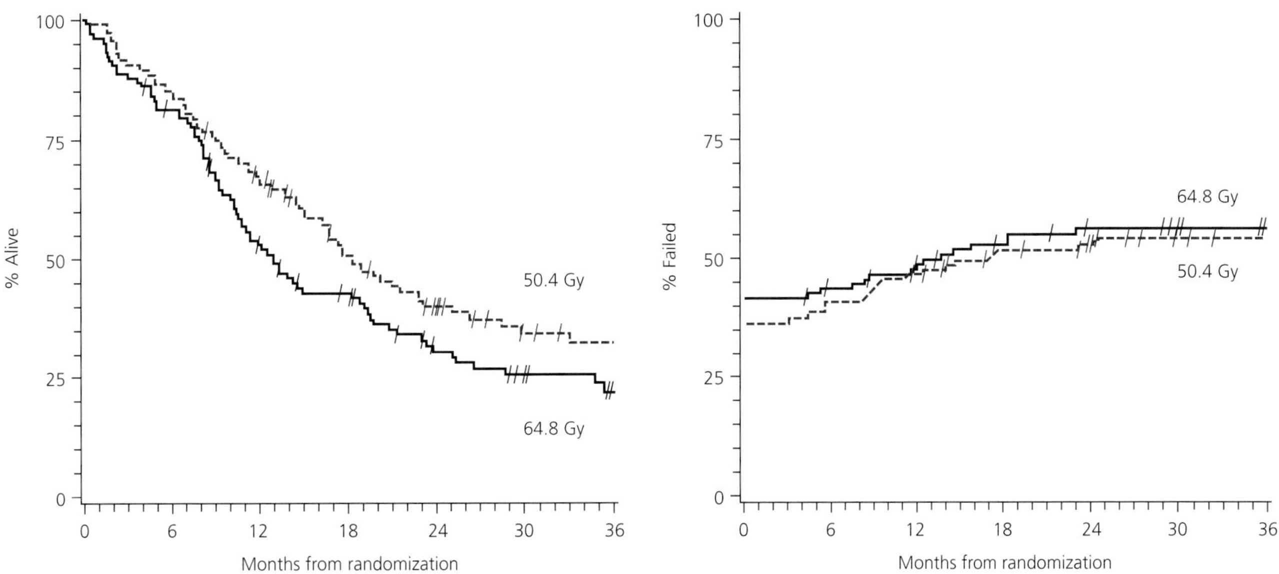

Fig. 4.27 Overall survival (left) and time to first local failure or regional persistent disease (right) in low and high radiation dose groups from RTOG 94-05. There were no differences in survival or local–regional control (reproduced from Minsky *et al.* 2002 with permission).

(Izquierdo *et al.* 1993). These non-randomized trials left open the question of whether higher-dose radiochemotherapy would be superior to standard-dose radiochemotherapy.

To address the high rates of persistent disease and local–regional recurrence after concurrent radiochemotherapy to 50 Gy, the RTOG conducted trial RTOG 94-05 (Minsky *et al.* 2002), a follow-up to the RTOG 85-01 trial, to investigate intensification of the radiation dose. In the 94-05 trial, 236 patients with cT1–4 Nx M0 squamous cell carcinoma (85%) or adenocarcinoma (15%) of the esophagus without tumor extension to within 2 cm of the stomach were randomly assigned to standard-dose radiochemotherapy using a slightly modified version of the radiochemotherapy arm of RTOG 85-01: 50.4 Gy plus concurrent 5-FU and cisplatin in weeks 1 and 4 and repeated 4 weeks after the end of radiotherapy–or high-dose radiotherapy (64.8 Gy) and the same chemotherapy. This trial failed to show any survival benefit in the high-dose arm (Fig. 4.27) (Minsky *et al.* 2002). Specifically, there were no differences between the high-dose and standard-dose arms in median survival time (13.0 and 18.1 months, respectively), 2-year survival rate (31% and 40%), or local–regional failure plus local regional disease persistence rate (52% versus 56%).

On the basis of these two well-designed prospective randomized trials (RTOG 85-01 and 94-05), 50.4 Gy at 1.8 Gy per fraction 5 days a week is currently considered standard when cisplatin-based chemotherapy is given concomitantly with radiotherapy for patients with esophageal cancer who are treated non-surgically (Herskovic *et al.* 1992; Al-Sarraf *et al.* 1997; Cooper *et al.* 1999; Minsky *et al.* 2002).

It is important to note, however, that seven of the 11 treatment-related deaths in the high-dose arm of the RTOG 94-05 trial occurred in patients who had received 50.4 Gy or less, indicating that the high death rate was not the result of radiation dose. In the high-dose arm, there was a significant prolongation of treatment time because of breaks required for recovery from side-effects, after correction for the number of radiation treatments and for the significantly lower dose of 5-FU given to patients in this arm. The authors believed that these factors might have contributed, at least in part, to the lack of benefit from high-dose versus standard-dose radiotherapy (Minsky *et al.* 2002). Therefore, a radiation dose effect in the RTOG 94-05 trial cannot be ruled out. The findings from the RTOG 94-05 trial warrant extensive research on methods to reduce treatment toxicity to allow radiation dose intensification for patients who are not considered candidates for surgery and for whom radiochemotherapy is the only treatment alternative.

It is intuitive that higher radiation doses would kill a higher fraction of clonogenic cells in tumors and result in improved local–regional control. In fact, in a retrospective study by Zhang *et al.* (2005) of radiochemotherapy in patients with stage II or III esophageal cancer, patients who had received a total dose greater than 51 Gy had significantly better local–regional control, disease-free survival, and overall survival. Of interest, there was also a trend towards better distant metastasis-free survival in the higher-dose group, indicating that elimination of local disease was important in reducing the risk of distant dissemination. The combination of increased local–regional control and decreased distant metastasis was associated with superior overall survival in patients treated with high-dose radiotherapy. This finding suggested a correlation between higher radiation dose and improved local–regional control in patients treated with radiochemotherapy, but the slope of the dose–response curve flattened in the high-dose region (Fig. 4.28) (Zhang *et al.* 2005). The shallower slope of the curve in the high-dose area suggested that there might be a threshold radiation dose beyond which further dose increases would not further improve local tumor control. A meta-analysis by Ancona *et al.* (2001) provided additional evidence of a relationship between increasing radiation dose and increased likelihood of pathologic complete response.

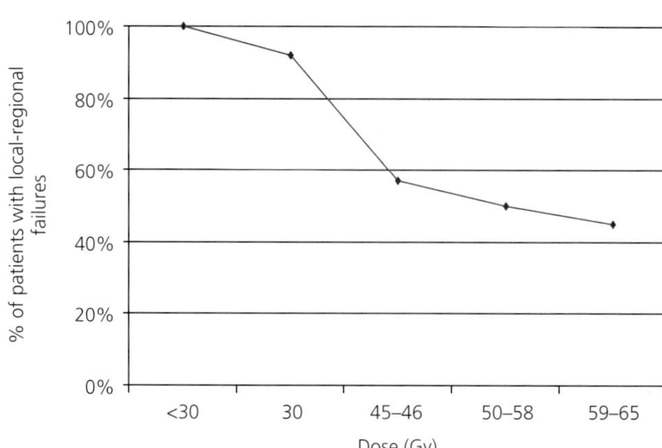

Fig. 4.28 Percentage of patients with local–regional failure 2 years after treatment as a function of radiation dose. The dose response curve seems to flatten at doses higher than 50 Gy (reproduced from Zhang *et al.* 2005 with permission).

Role of surgery after radiochemotherapy

The fact that more than 50% of patients in RTOG studies 85-01 and 95-04 had local–regional failure indicated a need for better local–regional treatment. Several groups have tried to improve outcomes by treating patients with radiochemotherapy followed by surgery. The rationale is that surgical resection would remove any residual disease and thus increase local–regional control. The evidence to date is conflicting, but results of the studies performed so far suggest that adding surgery after radiochemotherapy may improve local control but probably does not improve overall survival. Further studies are needed before definitive conclusions can be drawn about the benefits of adding surgery.

Liao *et al.* (2004) reported results from a retrospective review of 132 consecutive patients with clinical stage II or III esophageal cancer treated with radiochemotherapy, 60 of whom underwent esophagectomy 6–8 weeks after radiochemotherapy. The median radiation dose was 50 Gy (range 30–64.8 Gy) in the definitive radiochemotherapy group and 45 Gy (range 30–50.4 Gy) in the radiochemotherapy plus esophagectomy group. There were significant differences between the two groups in median age, histologic subtype, tumor location, and number of patients with T4 disease. Specifically, patients who had definitive radiochemotherapy were older ($p = 0.0004$), more likely to have squamous cell carcinoma rather than adenocarcinoma ($p < 0.000$), more likely to have upper thoracic or cervical esophageal tumors ($p < 0.000$), and more likely to have T4 tumors ($p = 0.024$). Patients treated with radiochemotherapy plus esophagectomy had significantly superior 5-year local–regional control rates (67.1% vs 22.1%; $p < 0.000$), disease-free survival rates (40.7% vs 9.9%; $p < 0.000$), and overall survival rates (52.6% vs 6.5%; $p < 0.000$), and significantly superior median overall survival time (62 months vs 12 months). However, there was no difference between the two groups in the rate of distant metastasis-free survival at 5 years (67.5% for radiochemotherapy plus esophagectomy vs 65.8% for radiochemotherapy alone; $p = 0.3$). Surgical resection of the tumor was an independent predictor of improved local–regional control and overall survival in both univariate and multivariate analyses. To reduce the effect of the selection bias on the outcome, 34 patients in each group with matched pretreatment characteristics were compared. The results showed significantly better overall survival, disease-free survival, and local–regional control rates favoring the radiochemotherapy plus esophagectomy group. There was no difference in distant metastasis-free survival in this subgroup analysis (Fig. 4.29). The authors suggested that both local–regional control and survival were improved by esophagectomy. However, this study was limited by its retrospective nature and biased patient selection (Liao *et al.* 2004).

In contrast to the findings of Liao *et al.*, the 1992–1994 patterns of care study suggested that at 4 years, there is no difference in survival between patients treated with radiochemotherapy plus surgery and those treated with definitive radiochemotherapy (Coia *et al.* 2000).

At the 2003 annual meeting of American Society of Clinical Oncology, two randomized phase III trials from Europe comparing radiochemotherapy versus radiochemotherapy followed by esophagectomy were reported in abstract form: the Fédération Francophone de Cancerologie Digestive (FFCD) 9102 trial and the German Esophageal Cancer Study Group trial (Bedenne *et al.* 2002; Stahl *et al.* 2005). Both trials enrolled patients with locally advanced but resectable esophageal cancer. The primary endpoint was overall survival, and the hypothesis was that the two treatments were equivalent. The results of both trials supported this hypothesis.

The FFCD 9102 trial (Bedenne *et al.* 2002) included patients with thoracic epidermoid or glandular T3–4 N0–1 M0 esophageal cancer. Patients underwent induction radiochemotherapy consisting of two 3-week cycles of 5-FU and cisplatin (administered on days 1–5 and 22–26) plus radiotherapy either protracted (46 Gy over 4.5 weeks) or split-course (two 15-Gy fractions on days 1–5 and 22–26). Patients who experienced at least a partial response to radiochemotherapy and had no contraindications to subsequent esophagectomy or radiochemotherapy were randomly assigned to surgery or additional radiochemotherapy (three cycles of 5-FU and cisplatin plus protracted [20 Gy] or split-course [15 Gy] radiotherapy). Between January 1993 and November 2000, 259 patients were randomly assigned out of 455 eligible patients who had started induction radiochemotherapy. There were no differences between the two groups in the 2-year survival rate (34% for surgery vs 40% for radiochemotherapy, adjusted odds ratio [OR] 0.91; p = 0.56) or median survival (17.7 months for surgery vs 19.3 months for radiochemotherapy). In the surgery arm, the mortality rate within 3 months after the start of induction radiochemotherapy appeared to be higher than that previously reported in the literature (Kelsen *et al.* 1998a) (9% vs 1%; p = 0.002). Patients in the radiochemotherapy arm had shorter hospital stays and better performance status, but they needed esophageal dilation and stent placement more frequently than did patients in the surgery arm. The authors concluded that in patients with locally advanced but operable esophageal cancer that responds to induction radiochemotherapy, continuation of radiochemotherapy is an alternative to surgery and is associated with equivalent overall survival, a lower early mortality rate, shorter hospital stays, and equivalent or better post-treatment performance status but also more frequent need for palliative procedures for. This trial was limited by its short follow-up, unconventional radiation schema, and accrual in some low volume surgical centers, which could contribute to higher operative morbidity and mortality.

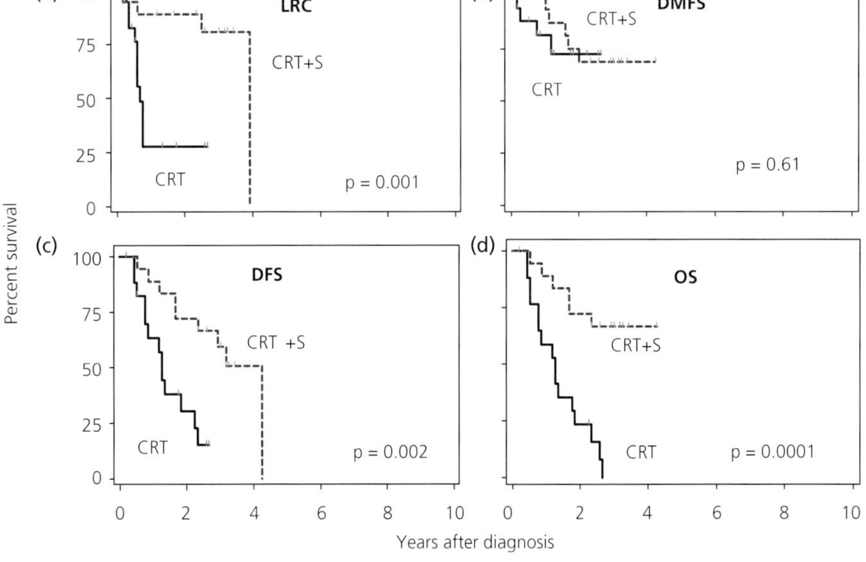

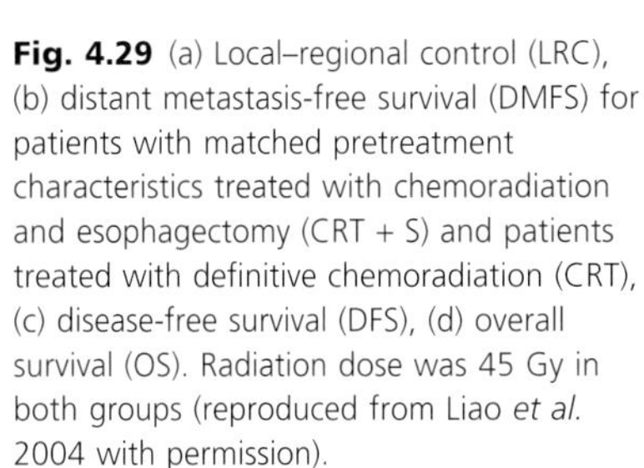

Fig. 4.29 (a) Local–regional control (LRC), (b) distant metastasis-free survival (DMFS) for patients with matched pretreatment characteristics treated with chemoradiation and esophagectomy (CRT + S) and patients treated with definitive chemoradiation (CRT), (c) disease-free survival (DFS), (d) overall survival (OS). Radiation dose was 45 Gy in both groups (reproduced from Liao *et al.* 2004 with permission).

The German esophageal cancer study group trial (Stahl *et al.* 2005) included only high-risk patients with sonograph-staged T3–4 N0–1 M0 squamous cell carcinoma of the esophagus. Patients were stratified according to center, tumor, and node status, completeness of endoscopic ultrasonography (EUS), sex, and extent of weight loss within the 8 weeks before randomization (Stahl *et al.* 2005). A total of 189 patients from 11 German institutions were enrolled. Five patients were found to be ineligible, and 12 refused randomization, leaving 172 patients in the study. Patients were randomly assigned to receive either (i) three cycles of 5-FU, leucovorin, etoposide, and cisplatin, followed by radiochemotherapy (cisplatin and etoposide and 40 Gy) and then transthoracic esophagectomy, with two-field lymphadenectomy as the standard procedure; or (ii) the same chemotherapy followed by definitive radiochemotherapy (cisplatin and etoposide and more than 65 Gy). Treatments were completed in 62% of patients in the surgery group and 85% of patients in the radiochemotherapy group. Treatment-related mortality rates were 10% in the surgery group and 3.5% in the radiochemotherapy group. The postoperative mortality rate decreased from 10.7% to 4.2% during the last 3 years of the study as surgeons gained experience. The median observation time was 6 years.

The analysis of 172 eligible, randomly assigned patients (86 per arm) showed that overall survival was equivalent in the two treatment groups (log-rank test for equivalence, $p < 0.05$). The 2-year local progression-free survival rate was better in the surgery group (64.3%; 95% CI 52.1–76.5%) than in the radiochemotherapy group (40.7%; 95% CI 28.9–52.5%; hazard ratio [HR] for radiochemotherapy versus surgery 2.1; 95% CI 1.3–3.5; $p < 0.003$). The treatment-related mortality rate was significantly higher in the surgery group (12.8% vs 3.5%; $p < 0.03$). Cox regression analysis revealed that clinical tumor response to induction chemotherapy was the single independent prognostic factor for overall survival (HR 0.30; 95% CI 0.19–0.47; $p = 0.0001$). Complete pathologic response to induction chemotherapy was experienced by 35% of the patients who underwent esophagectomy.

Tumor response to induction chemotherapy identified a favorable prognostic group among these high-risk patients–both those in the surgery group and those in the radiochemotherapy group. There was a trend toward improved local tumor control in the surgery arm: local tumor progression was the first mode of treatment failure in 64% of patients in this arm, compared to 81% of patients in the radiochemotherapy arm ($p = 0.08$). There was no difference between the surgery and radiochemotherapy arms in median survival time (16 months and 15 months, respectively) or 3-year survival rate (28% and 20%, respectively) (log rank $p = 0.22$). The 3-year survival rates among patients who responded to induction chemotherapy were 45% in the surgery arm versus 44% in the radiochemotherapy arm, and the 3-year survival rates among patients who did not respond to induction chemotherapy were 18% in the surgery arm versus 11% in the radiochemotherapy arm. The 3-year survival rate was 35% in non-responders who underwent complete tumor resection after radiochemotherapy.

The results from the FFCD study and the German Esophageal Cancer Study Group trial suggested that adding surgery to radiochemotherapy improves local tumor control but does not improve survival in patients with locally advanced squamous cell carcinoma of the esophagus (Fig. 4.30) (Stahl *et al.* 2005).

Several small phase II studies have reported that 3-year survival rates with radiochemotherapy alone among patients with operable esophageal cancer are around 28%, and long-term follow-up from the RTOG 85-01 study suggests a 20% long-term survival rate for patients with locally advanced esophageal cancer treated with radiochemotherapy (Birkmeyer *et al.* 2002). These data suggest that definitive radiochemotherapy is an acceptable alternative to surgery and may provide long-term survival equivalent to that in contemporary surgical series.

Preoperative radiochemotherapy

Preoperative radiochemotherapy has recently become a common practice in community centers and large academic centers in the US. However, on the basis of the evidence available to date, it should not at present be considered the standard of care for cancer of the esophagus.

Rationale

Traditionally, surgery was considered the standard treatment for patients with esophageal cancer who are medically fit and in whom a complete (R0) resection can be achieved (Siewert *et al.* 2000). However, with surgery alone, local–regional recurrence rates are in the range of 30–45%, and 5-year distant metastasis rates are in the range of greater than 50%. The high rates of local–regional and distant metastasis after surgery alone are a result of the aggressive behavior of esophageal tumors.

Esophageal tumors spread directly in longitudinal and radial directions, often producing 'skip metastasis' or multifocal disease. Positive resection margins resulting from longitudinal spread have been found in 4–6% of resected specimens–cancer cells have been discovered even as far as 10 cm proximal to the macroscopic tumor (Wijnhoven *et al.* 1999; Gao *et al.* 2005). Radial invasion accounts for positive lateral margin rates (R1, microscopically positive margins; R2, gross residual tumor remaining) of about 25–30% (Kelsen *et al.* 1998a; Wijnhoven *et al.* 1999; Siewert *et al.* 2000; Hullscher *et al.* 2002; MRC 2002). Regional nodal involvement is reported in 70–80% of patients who have a transmural extension of the primary tumor (Siewert *et al.* 2000; Hullscher *et al.* 2002; Lerut *et al.* 2002). The pattern of nodal dissemination appears to vary by primary site: adenocarcinomas of primary esophageal origin spread first to both mediastinal and abdominal lymph nodes, mainly along the esophageal axis; whereas adenocarcinomas of the cardia or gastroesophageal junction more often spread to abdominal lymph nodes, involving the common hepatic and splenic artery/splenic hilum stations in up to 30% and 15% of cases, respectively (de Manzoni *et al.* 1998; van de Ven *et al.* 1999; Dresner *et al.* 2001; Clarke *et al.* 2001). Rates of local–regional failure vary from 5% to 36% (Kelsen *et al.* 1998a; Wijnhoven *et al.* 1999; Siewert *et al.* 2000; Hullscher *et al.* 2002; MRC 2002; Mariette *et al.* 2003), with a median time to recurrence of about 1.5 years (Mariette *et al.* 2003). Distant failures are observed in at least 40% of patients, and patients with esophageal adenocarcinomas are estimated to have a risk of distant metastasis 2.57 times as high as that of patients with squamous cell carcinomas (Al-Sarraf *et al.* 1997).

Because further improvements in surgical outcomes are unlikely, the combination of preoperative radiochemotherapy and esophagectomy has been investigated extensively over the past two decades and has become a common practice in community and large academic centers in the US. However, the results of preoperative chemotherapy without radiotherapy have been controversial (Kelsen *et al.* 1998a; MRC 2002). The hypothesis underlying the use of preoperative radiochemotherapy for esophageal cancer is that preoperative radiochemotherapy targets both local and systemic disease, thus shrinking tumor and reducing rates of incomplete local resection and local and systemic recurrences. Many chemotherapeutic agents enhance radiosensitization, including 5-FU, platinum compounds, mitomycin C, taxanes, and topoisomerase inhibitors (Bourhis 1999). The potential benefits of preoperative radiochemotherapy for esophageal adenocarcinoma include improvement of the chances of achieving a complete resection through downstaging of the primary tumor, decreased local and systemic failure rates, and better compliance with treatment.

However, despite these potential benefits, the impact of preoperative radiochemotherapy followed by esophagectomy on survival remains controversial. Hofstetter *et al.* (2002) reviewed the University of Texas MD Anderson Cancer Center experience with 1079 consecutive esophagectomies over a 30-year period. They reported an increasing use of preoperative radiochemotherapy in the last 4 years of the study (59% of patients treated with preoperative radiochemotherapy in the most recent 4 years versus 2% treated with preoperative chemotherapy in the 1970s–1990s) accompanied by an increased complete resection rate and median survival. The authors concluded that preoperative radiochemotherapy was associated with a longer median survival and higher likelihood of complete resection. A

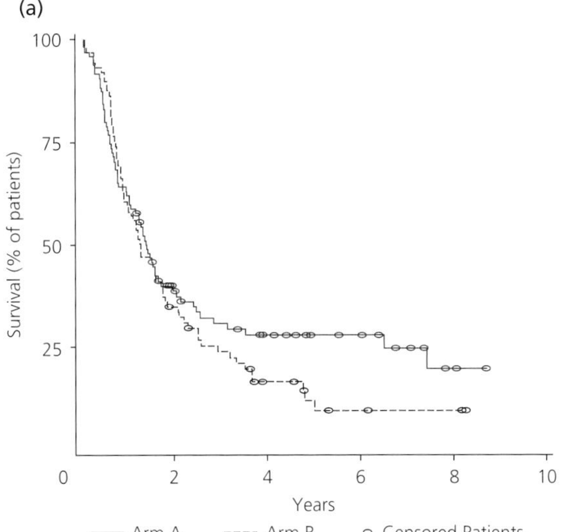

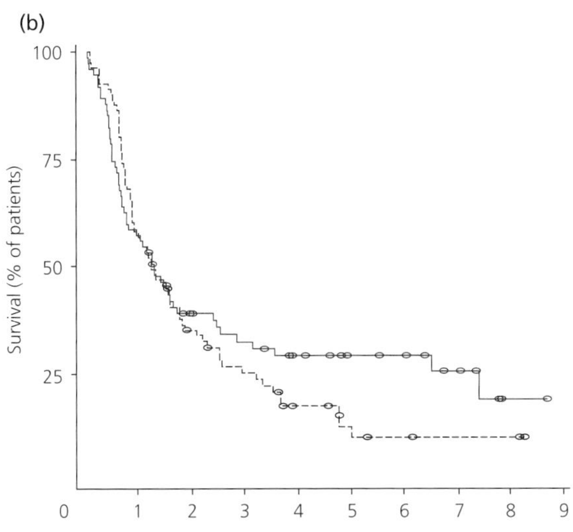

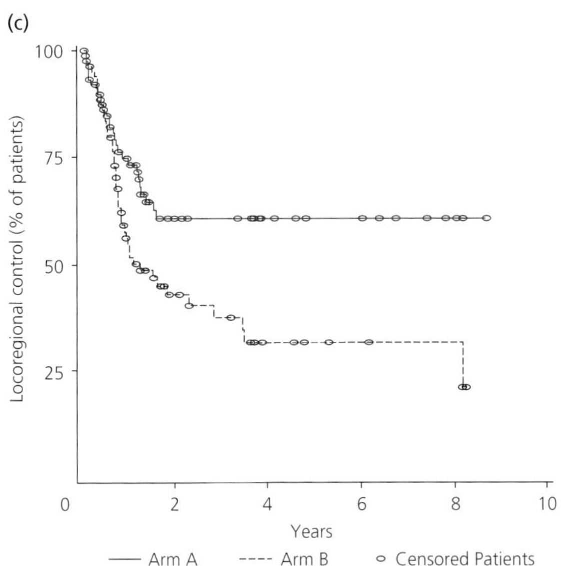

Fig. 4.30 Kaplan–Meier plots showing: (a) overall survival from the date of randomization among patients allocated to preoperative chemoradiation and surgery (arm A, n = 86) or chemoradiation without surgery (arm B, n = 86); (b) survival as randomized among patients treated according to their treatment arm excluding crossover patients (arm A, n = 75; arm B, n = 81); and (c) the freedom from locoregional progression among patients allocated to preoperative chemoradiation and surgery (arm A) or chemoradiation without surgery (arm B) (reproduced from Stahl *et al.* 2005 with permission).

recent meta-analysis of RCTs compared preoperative radiochemotherapy and surgery with surgery alone for the treatment of esophageal cancer and found an improved 3-year survival rate, reduced risk of local–regional recurrence, and improved rate of complete resection with the preoperative radiochemotherapy approach (Urschel & Vasan 2003).

Non-randomized trials

A number of prospective phase II studies (Urba *et al.* 1992; Forastiere *et al.* 1993; Keller *et al.* 1998; Adelstein *et al.* 2000; Heath *et al.* 2000; Kleinberg *et al.* 2003; Meluch *et al.* 2003; Choi *et al.* 2004) have investigated preoperative radiochemotherapy for esophageal cancer (Table 4.18). These studies have used conventional radiotherapy dose fractionation to 45 Gy over 5 weeks and platinum- and 5-FU-based chemotherapy. Preoperative radiochemotherapy was associated with generally favorable results: complete resection rates of 80–100%, complete pathologic responses in 8–49% of cases, and 2-year survival rates ranging from 27% to 62%. Patients who experienced a pathologic complete response to radiochemotherapy had 5-year survival rates of between 55% and 70%. Local recurrence rates in patients who received preoperative radiochemotherapy tended to be lower than historic local recurrence rates in patients treated with surgery alone, and patients who received preoperative radiochemotherapy were more likely to have distant metastatic recurrence than local recurrence (Urba *et al.* 1992; Forastiere *et al.* 1993; Keller *et al.* 1998; Adelstein *et al.* 2000; Heath *et al.* 2000; Kleinberg *et al.* 2003; Meluch *et al.* 2003; Choi *et al.* 2004).

These non-randomized trials have been criticized for their small numbers of patients, differences in radiation dose fractionation, and differences in chemotherapy agents. For example, split-course or accelerated regimens were used in some studies (Urba *et al.* 1992; Forastiere *et al.* 1993; Adelstein *et al.* 2000; Choi *et al.* 2004). The 2-year survival rates of 27–62% are not significantly different from the results seen with definitive radiochemotherapy (Cooper *et al.* 1999; Minsky *et al.* 2002). In three studies, paclitaxel was added to the standard platinum-based radiochemotherapy regimen, and in four studies, 5-FU was omitted from the standard radiochemotherapy regimen.

Randomized trials

At least nine randomized trials have compared preoperative radiochemotherapy followed by surgery with surgery alone (Nygaard *et al.* 1992; Apinop *et al.* 1994; Le Prise *et al.* 1994; Walsh *et al.* 1996; Bosset *et al.* 1997; Urba *et al.* 2001; Burmeister *et al.* 2002; Law *et al.* 2004; Bosset *et al.* 2005) (Table 4.19). Results of these trials are conflicting–eight of the trials did not show a survival benefit with combined therapy, but one trial did (Walsh *et al.* 1996; Urba *et al.* 2001; Bosset *et al.* 2005).

The trial showing a benefit from radiochemotherapy was the trial of Walsh *et al.* (1996) who evaluated 113 patients. In the

Table 4.18 Selected nonrandomized studies of preoperative radiochemotherapy of the esophagus.

Authors	No. of patients	Chemotherapy drugs	Radiation dose (Gy)	RO (%)	PCR (%)	2-year OS (%)	LF (%)	DM (%)
Poplin *et al.* (1987)	113	CF	30	49	16	28	–	–
Naunheim *et al.* (1992)	4	CF	30–36	72	17	40 (3 years)	–	–
Urba *et al.* (1992)	24	CF	49	100	8	–	12.5	25
Hoff *et al.* (1993)	68	CF	30		18	51	6	25
Forastiere *et al.* (1993)	43	CF	45	84	23	55	14	40
Chiappori *et al.* (1996)	87	CF	30	–	17	–	–	–
Bates *et al.* (1996)	39	CF	45	90	46	40 (3 years)	–	–
Stahl *et al.* (1996)	72	CFLE	40	67	22	33 (3 years)		
Blanke *et al.* (1997)	21	CP	30	–	16	–	–	–
Keller *et al.* (1998)	46	CF	60	72	17	27	–	–
Bedenne *et al.* (1998)	96	CF	30	82	20	40 (25% 5 years)	–	
Urba el al. (2000)	69	CP	45		19	51	–	–
Heath *et al.* (2000)	42	CF	44	83	26	62	5	43
Adelstein *et al.* (2000)	63	CP	45	93	23	30	–	–
Safran *et al.* (2001)	41	CP	39.6	–	29	42	–	–
Kleinberg *et al.* (2003)	92	CFP	44	87	33	57	8	41
Meluch *et al.* (2003)	129	CFP	45	78	49	47	2	30
Choi *et al.* (2004)	46	CFP	58.5	95	38	50	23	42

C, cisplatin; DM, distant metastasis; E, etoposide; F, 5-fluorouracil; LF, local failure; L, leucovorin; OS, overall survival; pCR, pathologic complete response; R0, complete resection.

Table 4.19 Randomized trials of preoperative radiochemotherapy with surgery versus surgery alone in patients with localized esophageal cancer.

Author and year	No. of patients	Chemotherapy drugs	Radiotherapy dose (Gy)	Median survival (month)	3-year survival (%)	p value
Nygaard *et al.* (1992)						NS
Surgery alone	41			NA	9	
Preoperative RCT	47	CB	35	NA	17	
Le Prise *et al.* (1994)						
Surgery alone	41			10	14	NS
Preoperative RCT	45	CF	20	10	19	
Apinop *et al.* (1994)						NS
Surgery alone	34			7	20	
Preoperative RCT	35	CF	40	10	26	
Walsh *et al.* (1996)						<0.01
Surgery alone	55			11	6	
Preoperative RCT	58	CF	40	16	32	
Bosset *et al.* (1997)						NS
Surgery alone	139			19	37	
Preoperative RCT	143	C	37	19	39	
Law *et al.* (1997)						NS
Surgery alone	30			27	NA	
Preoperative RCT	30	CF	40	26	NA	
Urba *et al.* (2001)						0.15
Surgery alone	50			18	16	
Preoperative RCT	50	CFV	45	17	30	
Burmeister *et al.* (2002)						0.38
Surgery alone	128			22	NA	
Preoperative RCT	128	CF	35	19	NA	
Bosset *et al.* (2005)						Ongoing study
Surgery alone	380 Planned			NA	NA	
Preoperative RCT	121 Enrolled	CF	45			

B, bleomycin, F, 5-fluorouracil; C, cisplatin; C, cisplatin; DM, distant metastasis; E, etoposide; L, fleucovorin; LF, local failure; NA, not available; OS, overall survival; pCR, pathologic complete response; RCT, radiochemotherapy; V, vinblastine.

radiochemotherapy arm, patients received 40 Gy over 3 weeks, and two courses of 5-FU and cisplatin given at weeks 1 and 6. Surgery was planned for week 8. In the radiochemotherapy arm, one patient died before surgery and four died after surgery; in the surgery-alone arm, two patients died after surgery. The 3-year survival rates were 32% and 6% in the radiochemotherapy and surgery arms, respectively ($p < 0.01$).

Urba *et al.* (2001) studied 100 patients, 75% of whom had adenocarcinoma. In the radiochemotherapy arm, patients received 45 Gy over 3 weeks (1.5-Gy fractions twice daily Monday through Friday); cisplatin and vinblastine were given at weeks 1 and 3; and 5-FU was given from day 1 to day 21. Preoperative adverse events included grade 3 or 4 neutropenia in 78% of patients, neutropenic fever in 39%, need for blood transfusions in 16%, and esophagitis necessitating feeding tube placement in 63%. Two patients in the radiochemotherapy arm and one in the surgery arm died after surgery. The 3-year survival rates in the radiochemotherapy and surgery arms were 30% and 16%, respectively ($p = 0.15$).

Burmeister *et al.* (2002) evaluated 256 patients, 157 of whom had adenocarcinoma. In the radiochemotherapy arm, patients received 35 Gy over 3 weeks and one 5-FU–cisplatin course at week 1. The median survival durations were 21.7 and 18.5 months in the radiochemotherapy and surgery arms, respectively ($p = 0.38$).

The randomized trials of preoperative radiochemotherapy versus surgery alone suffered from the same limitations as the non-randomized trials: small numbers of patients and thus limited power to detect a difference between the arms; relatively poor preoperative staging; limited characterization of clinicopathologic factors affecting prognosis; wide variation in the chemotherapy agents and radiation dose and schedule; and short follow-up duration. In the only randomized trial that reported a survival benefit from radiochemotherapy, the trial by Walsh *et al.* (1996), the 6% 3-year overall survival rate in the surgery-alone arm was significantly inferior to that in the other trials (Table 4.19). Furthermore, the survival rates of patients treated with preoperative radiochemotherapy plus surgery ranged from 25% to 35% (Walsh *et al.* 1996; Bosset *et al.* 1997; Urba *et al.* 2001), similar to the survival rates of 25–27% after radiochemotherapy alone (Cooper *et al.* 1999; Minsky *et al.* 2002), although a survival benefit from preoperative radiochemotherapy plus surgery versus surgery alone was suggested in a recent meta-analysis (Kaklamanos *et al.* 2003). A carefully designed randomized trial is needed to address the question of whether preoperative radiochemotherapy plus surgery is superior to surgery alone.

Bosset *et al.* (2005) reported in 2005 that in fact, this question is being addressed in an ongoing clinical trial conducted by the FFCD and the European Organisation for Research and Treatment of Cancer. In the trial, patients with stage IIA or IIB esophageal cancer (either squamous cell carcinoma or adenocarcinoma) are randomly assigned to preoperative radiochemotherapy (45 Gy over 5 weeks and two courses of 5-FU and cisplatin) or surgery only. The trial was designed to enrol 380 patients to be able to detect an increase in the 3-year survival rate from 35% with surgery to 50% with preoperative radiochemotherapy. At the time of Bosset *et al.*'s report, 121 patients had been enrolled (Bosset *et al.* 2005). It is hoped that this trial will more definitively address the value of preoperative radiochemotherapy.

Three-step strategies

Even with preoperative radiochemotherapy, 5-year overall survival rates are low, ranging from 25% to 36% in randomized trials (Walsh *et al.* 1996; Bosset *et al.* 1997; Urba *et al.* 2001), though local–regional control rates seem more favorable than those with surgery alone or radiochemotherapy alone (Walsh *et al.* 1996; Bosset *et al.* 1997; Urba *et al.* 2001). One important observation in patients treated with preoperative radiochemotherapy is a shift in the pattern of recurrence from local–regional persistent disease or recurrence to distant metastasis (Liao *et al.* 2002). To overcome the problem of distant metastasis, Ajani *et al.* (2004) recently proposed a three-step strategy consisting of induction chemotherapy, preoperative radiochemotherapy, and surgery. Several trials have examined this approach (Table 4.20).

Jin *et al.* (2004) reported a retrospective study comparing additional systemic chemotherapy before preoperative radiochemotherapy with preoperative radiochemotherapy alone for surgically resectable esophageal cancer. They found that patients who received induction chemotherapy before radiochemotherapy had higher rates of complete pathologic response, local–regional control, distant metastasis-free survival, disease-free survival, and overall survival. The study suggested that paclitaxel and irinotecan, two agents active against metastatic disease that increase the proportion of cells in the G2–M phase of the cell cycle, thereby enhancing radiosensitivity (Komaki *et al.* 2000), appear to be particularly promising for the three-step strategy.

Swisher *et al.* (2003) reported the long-term outcome of induction chemotherapy, radiochemotherapy, and surgery for 38 patients with local–regionally advanced esophageal cancer treated in a phase II trial. Patients initially received two cycles of paclitaxel (200 mg/m^2), 5-FU (750 mg/m^2/day for 5 days), and cisplatin (15 mg/m^2/day for 5 days). They then received radiochemotherapy consisting of 45 Gy over 5 weeks with concurrent 5-FU (300 mg/m^2/day continuous infusion) and cisplatin (15 mg/m^2/day for 5 days). Surgical resection was performed 4–6 weeks after the completion of the radiochemotherapy. Most patients had T3 tumors as revealed by EUS (87%); N1 disease (66%); and adenocarcinoma subtype (84%). Thirty-seven patients (97%) completed the planned induction chemotherapy and radiochemotherapy, and 35 patients (92%) underwent

Table 4.20 Results of three-step treatment for locally advanced esophageal cancer.

Authors	No. of patients	Induction chemotherapy drugs	Concurrent chemotherapy drugs	Radiation dose (Gy)	PCR (%)	3-year OS (%)	5-year OS (%)	Median survival time (months)
Bains *et al.* (2002)	41	C Pac	C Pac	50.4	22	NA	NA	NA
Swisher et al (2003)	38	C F Pac	C F	45	21	63	39	NA
Ajani et al (2004)	43	Irin	F Pac	50.4	28	NA	NA	22.1
Ilson et al (2003)	19	C Irin	C Irin	50.4	27	NA	NA	25.6 (pCR/pPR 18.5 (<pRP)
Pasini et al (2005)	47	Doc P F	Doc P F	50	29.8	NA	NA	NA

C, cisplatin; Doc, docetaxel; F, 5-fluorouracil; Irin, irinotecan; NA, not available; OS, overall survival; P, cisplatin; Pac, paclitaxel; PCR, pathologic complete response; pPR, pathologic partial response.

surgery. The 30-day mortality rate after surgery was 6% (two of 35 patients died). Twenty-five (71%) of the 35 patients who underwent surgery had a pathologic complete response or microscopic residual carcinoma (<10% viable) after chemotherapy, and pathologic complete response was associated with disease-free survival rates of 72% at 3 years and 51% at 5 years. On the basis of an intention-to-treat analysis and a median potential follow-up of 58 months, the 3- and 5-year overall survival rates for all 38 patients were 63% and 39%, respectively. The results of this study suggested that the three-step strategy is safe and warrants further evaluation in the treatment of patients with local–regionally advanced esophageal cancer (Swisher *et al.* 2003).

The same group (Ajani *et al.* 2004) recently reported results in 43 patients with esophageal cancer who received two cycles of induction chemotherapy with irinotecan and cisplatin followed by radiochemotherapy consisting of 45 Gy concurrent with 5-FU and paclitaxel followed by surgery. With this strategy, 50% of patients experience relief of dysphagia after induction chemotherapy. A complete (R0) resection was achieved in 36 patients who underwent surgery, and there were two postoperative deaths. The 2-year survival rate was 42%, and among patients with recurrent disease, 80% had a distant recurrence.

Similar results with the three-step strategy were reported by Bains *et al.* (2002). They treated 41 patients with two cycles of induction paclitaxel and cisplatin, followed by 50.4 Gy of radiation combined with cisplatin and paclitaxel, followed by surgery. There was improvement of dysphagia in 92% of patients after induction chemotherapy, and only 5% of patients had grade 3 esophagitis.

The addition of induction chemotherapy to preoperative radiochemotherapy is a novel approach in the treatment of esophageal cancer. The results of studies of this approach suggest that if the local effect of preoperative radiochemotherapy is sufficiently pronounced, a survival benefit may be observed (Bosset & Horiot 1999).

Adverse effects

Preoperative radiochemotherapy causes toxic effects that can make patients unable to undergo surgery and can increase the risk of perioperative death. In current clinical practice, postoperative mortality rates after esophageal resection in high-volume centers are about 2–5% (Siewert *et al.* 2000; Hulscher *et al.* 2002). Typical postoperative mortality rates after preoperative radiochemotherapy and esophagectomy are 2–8% (Forastiere *et al.* 1993; Heath *et al.* 2000; Hofstetter *et al.* 2002). The toxic effects of preoperative radiochemotherapy result from biologic effects on rapidly dividing cells both within (e.g. esophagogastric mucosa, lung) and outside (e.g. bone marrow) the irradiated volume. The severity of the toxic effects depends on the volume of critical tissues irradiated, the radiotherapy fractionation (accelerated schemes increase toxicity), and the selection of chemotherapeutic agents, including dose and method of delivery. Acute toxic effects that result in treatment interruptions may compromise the efficacy of preoperative radiochemotherapy. Late-responding tissues with slowly dividing cells (e.g. connective tissues, capillary endothelium) may exhibit late toxic effects several months or even years after completion of treatment. Late toxic effects depend on the radiation dose, the fractional dose (risk is increased for doses larger than 2 Gy), and the choice of chemotherapeutic agent (Bosset & Horiot 1999). A recent meta-analysis showed that postoperative mortality rates are higher in patients treated with radiochemotherapy plus surgery than in those treated with surgery alone (Burmeister *et al.* 2002), although this conclusion follows mainly from the increased mortality in the radiochemotherapy arm of the largest randomized trial in the analysis, in which both high radiation dose fractions and high cisplatin doses were used (Fiorica *et al.* 2004).

Adverse effects on the lung

Preoperative radiochemotherapy and esophagectomy have been associated with mortality rates of 2–18%, with deaths generally due to sepsis, pneumonia, and adult respiratory distress syndrome (Adelstein *et al.* 2000; Choi *et al.* 2004). Pulmonary complications are the most common serious adverse event after esophagectomy and the leading cause of postoperative mortality among patients treated with surgery for esophageal cancer. The incidence of pulmonary complications after esophagectomy is at least 30% (Bosset *et al.* 1997), and the associated in-hospital mortality rate in patients with pulmonary complications is 55% (Law *et al.* 2004). Poor performance status, poor lung function, and advanced age have been identified as risk factors for poor outcomes after surgery, and are used as strict patient selection criteria for surgery (Fang *et al.* 2003). Long duration of surgery and excessive blood loss have also been shown to be associated with increased morbidity and mortality after esophagectomy (Fang *et al.* 2003).

Excessive radiation doses or unconventional fractionation schemes may account for the higher mortality rates observed in selected series (Keller *et al.* 1998; Adelstein *et al.* 2000; Safran *et al.* 2001). In one study, in which patients received unconventional split-course radiotherapy with fractions of 3.5 Gy, 11 of 18 patients who survived surgical resection suffered from major radiation-induced pleural and pericardial complications (Keller *et al.* 1998). In a randomized trial conducted to evaluate preoperative radiochemotherapy for esophageal squamous cell cancer (Bosset *et al.* 1997), there was increased disease-free survival but no overall survival benefit, probably because of an excessive number of postoperative deaths (generally due to pulmonary complications) in the preoperative radiochemotherapy arm. One possible explanation was the unconventional radiotherapy scheme, which included fractional doses of 3.7 Gy. Further analysis showed that postoperative mortality was also significantly related to the number of patients treated at each participating center, with lower patient volumes associated with higher postoperative motality (Bosset *et al.* 1997).

Lee *et al.* (2003) were the first to report that postoperative pulmonary complications increased significantly when more than 40% of the lung received radiation doses higher than 10 Gy. Postoperative pulmonary complications, defined as pneumonia or adult respiratory distress syndrome that developed within 30 days after surgery and before discharge, was the clinical endpoint for this study (CDC 1989; Wang 2005). In light of the results from that study, we modified our practice to keep the volume of lung exposed to doses greater than 10 Gy below 40%, while at the same time escalating the total radiation dose from 45 Gy to 50.4 Gy.

Wang (2005) recently re-evaluated the effects of clinical and dosimetric factors on the incidence of postoperative pulmonary complications. Wang found that the volume of lung spared from doses of 5 Gy or higher was the only independent predictive factor associated with pulmonary complications in patients with esophageal cancer treated with radiochemotherapy followed by surgery. The smaller the volume of lung spared from doses of 5 Gy or higher, the higher the incidence of postoperative pulmonary complications. The results were insensitive to the use of the alpha/beta ratios and whether biologic-equivalent dose or physical doses were used (Fig. 4.31) (Wang 2005).

Findings from the Wang study suggest that the volume of remaining undamaged lung, rather than the volume of damaged

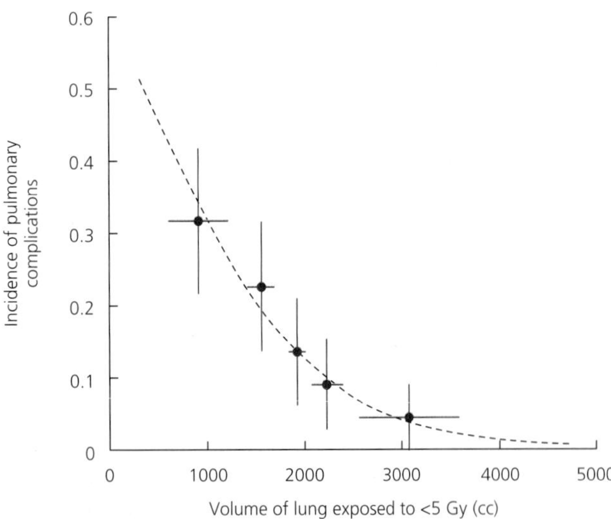

Fig. 4.31 Incidence of postoperative pulmonary complications vs lung volume spared from doses of 5 Gy or higher (VS5). The dashed curve represents the fit of the logistic model to the data (incidence of pulmonary complications vs VS5). The solid dots represent the observed incidence of pulmonary complications in each of five equal (n = 22) patient subgroups plotted at the mean value of VS5 for the group. The horizontal error bars represent ±1 standard deviation of the mean VS5 in each group. The vertical error bars represent ±1 standard deviation calculated from the observed incidence assuming binomial statistics (reproduced from Wang *et al.* 2006b with permission).

functional lung, determines postoperative pulmonary function. In other words, patients who have a small lung volume to start with may be at high risk for pulmonary complications even if their relative volume of lung receiving 5 Gy or greater is low. Strong evidence for this theory is that in the Wang study, gender was associated with the incidence of postoperative pulmonary complications on univariate but not on multivariate analysis. As noted, this outcome may have been a result of the fact that the total lung volume was smaller in females than in males, making the volume spared in females smaller than the volume spared in males despite similar lung volumes exposed to radiation. To reduce the risk of postoperative pulmonary complications, more attention may have to be paid not only to the dose–volume histogram of the lung but also to the total lung volume and non-irradiated lung volume (Wang 2005).

Tucker *et al.* (2006), applying the data set from study of Wang *et al.* to the normal tissue complication probability model, reported that the risk of postoperative pulmonary complications was most significantly associated with small absolute volumes of lung spared from doses of at least 5 Gy. However, bootstrap analysis found no significant difference in the quality of this model and fits based on other dosimetric parameters, including mean lung dose, effective dose, and relative volume of lung receiving 5 Gy or more, probably because of correlations among these factors. This study was limited by its retrospective nature and small numbers of patients and events. Therefore, the conclusions need to be substantiated with additional, preferably prospective, data.

In patients treated with radiochemotherapy alone, systemic chemotherapy before radiochemotherapy was found to be associated with increased incidence of grade 2 or greater (defined according to the National Cancer Institute Common Toxicity Criteria) treatment-related pneumonitis (Wang *et al.* 2006a).

Adverse effects on the esophagus

It is difficult to accurately assess the incidence and severity of esophagitis in esophageal cancer patients because the symptoms that are used to define esophagitis (dysphagia, odynophagia) are not specific and might be caused by the tumor itself. However, 5-FU-based chemotherapy regimens were clearly associated with adverse effects on the esophagus: severe esophagitis occurred in up to 80% of patients treated with 5-FU, and this severe esophagitis necessitated nutritional support measures and unplanned hospitalizations in half of all patients treated with 5-FU (Forastiere *et al.* 1993; Heath *et al.* 2000; Choi *et al.* 2004). In series that substituted paclitaxel for 5-FU, rates of esophagitis decreased, and there was no change in rates of complete resection or pathologic response (Blanke *et al.* 1997; Adelstein *et al.* 2000; Ulrich *et al.* 2000; Safran *et al.* 2001).

Adverse effects on the heart

There is increasing evidence that radiochemotherapy in patients with esophageal cancer has adverse effects on the heart. The most extensive evidence comes from a study by Gayed *et al.*

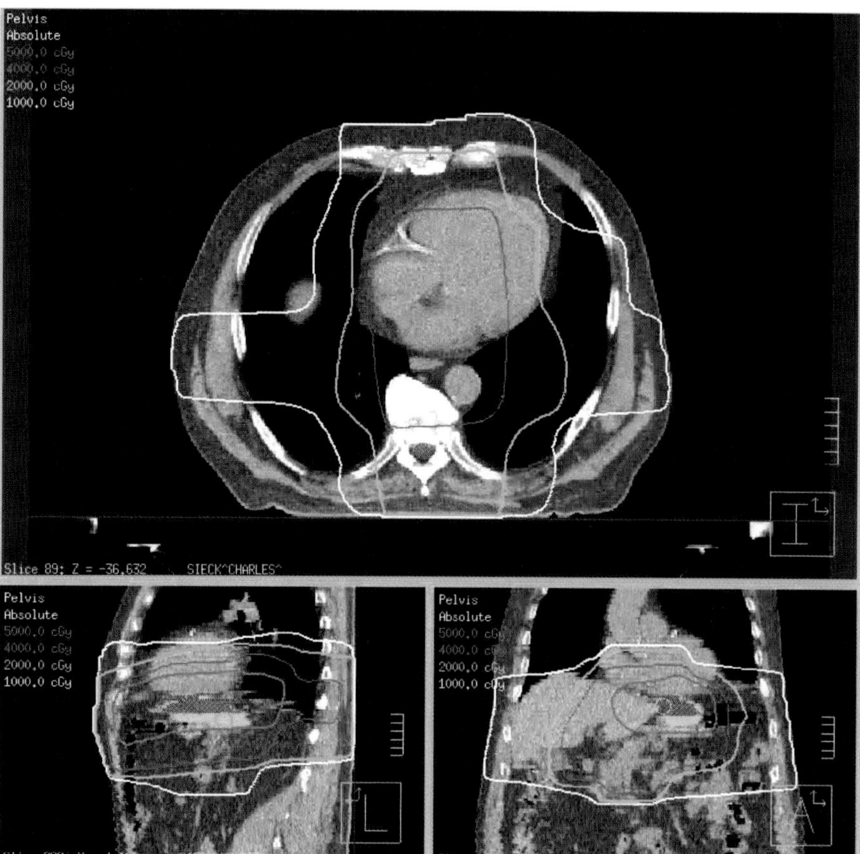

Fig. 4.32 Simulation CT slices with radiation therapy plan for treating a patient with distal esophageal cancer and the GMPI images performed 11 months after completion of radiation therapy. The area of ischemia in the inferior wall of the heart (arrow) was included in the 4000–5000 cGy isodose line (reproduced from Gayed *et al.* 2006 with permission).

(2006) who retrospectively reviewed and analyzed the records of 614 patients with esophageal cancer treated at the MD Anderson Cancer Center between 1998 and 2005. The non-surgical group comprising 101 of the patients were treated with definitive radiochemotherapy without surgery between 1998 and 2003, and the surgical group of 513 patients underwent esophagogastrectomy with (n = x; 33%) or without (n = x; 67%) radiochemotherapy between 1998 and 2005. The clinical stage distribution in the non-surgical group was I or II, 22%; III or IV, 73%. The clinical stage distribution in the surgical group was I or II, 36%; III or IV, 64%. In the non-surgical group, 35% of patients had upper or midesophageal tumors and 60% had distal tumors; in the surgical group, 11% had upper or midesophageal tumors and 88% had distal tumors. Three-dimensional conformal radiotherapy was the primary radiotherapy technique, and prescribed doses were 45 or 50.4 Gy. Patient characteristics and cardiac risk factors were matched between the non-surgical and surgical groups. Cardiac abnormality was evaluated on the basis of clinical records and perfusion imaging studies, if they were available.

In the non-surgical group, the most common cardiac adverse effects were pericardial effusion, which occurred in 27.7% of patients, and atrial fibrillation, which occurred in 7.9%. These cardiac events developed within 15 months after radiotherapy; the median time to onset was 5.3 months for pericardial effusion and 4.6 months for atrial fibrillation. The risk of pericardial effusion was associated with the mean pericardial dose ($p = 0.002$) and an array of dose–volume points for the pericardium from 5 to 45 Gy, possibly because of the correlation among the dosimetric factors. In the surgical group, atrial fibrillation occurred in 14.6% of patients within 30 days after surgery. In addition, in the surgery group, 49 patients had distal esophageal tumor located behind the heart and underwent gated myocardial perfusion single-photon emission computed tomography (SPECT) before surgery. In this subgroup (Gayed *et al.* 2006), 25 patients were treated with radiochemotherapy, and 24 patients had surgery alone. SPECT imaging revealed myocardium perfusion defects including ischemia and/or scarring in 11(42.3%) of the 25 patients treated with radiochemotherapy, but only 1 (4%) of the 24 patients treated with surgery alone ($p = 0.001$). The time to onset of myocardial perfusion defect ranged from 1 to 48 months; the mean time was 7.5 months, and the median time was 3 months (Fig. 4.32) (Gayed *et al.* 2006).

Prognostic factors in patients with esophageal cancer

Clinical experience indicates that tumors usually start responding to radiochemotherapy 2–3 weeks after treatment is initiated

Table 4.21 Prognostic factors for overall survival in esophageal cancer.

Prognostic factor	3-year OS	p value
Pretreatment celiac node positivity*	Celiac nodes negative, 54–56%; celiac nodes positive, 12%	0.03
Number of positive nodes after radiochemotherapy	0–1 positive nodes, 5-year OS 34–38%; 2 or more nodes positive, 5-year OS 6%	0.02
Postradiochemotherapy FDG-PET SUV	SUV < 4, 18-month survival 77%; SUV ≥ 4, 18-month survival 34%	0.01
R0 resection	R0, 59%; R1, 37%; R2, 4%	<0.001
Complete pathologic response†	PCR, 74%; 1–50% residual tumor, 54%; >50% residual tumor, 34%	<0.001
Clinical tumor response to induction chemotherapy‡	50% versus 17.9%	<0.0011

OS, overall survival; pCR, pathologic complete response; SUV, standard uptake value.
* Malaisrie *et al.* (2006)
† Swisher *et al.* (2005)
‡ Stahl *et al.* (2005)

and that tumor response is usually indicated by improved swallowing function. It is believed that the distinct tumor responses to radiochemotherapy reflect distinct biologic behavior of different tumors and that treatment should be individualized on the basis of the predicted response. For example, if a tumor is predicted to be relatively radioresistant, the radiation dose may need to be increased to encourage early tumor shrinkage and improve the potential for complete response and avoidance of esophagectomy. The ability to predict tumor response to radiochemotherapy before treatment is initiated would allow clinicians to individualize the intensity of therapy and the modalities delivered. The most common prognostic factors are listed in Table 4.21.

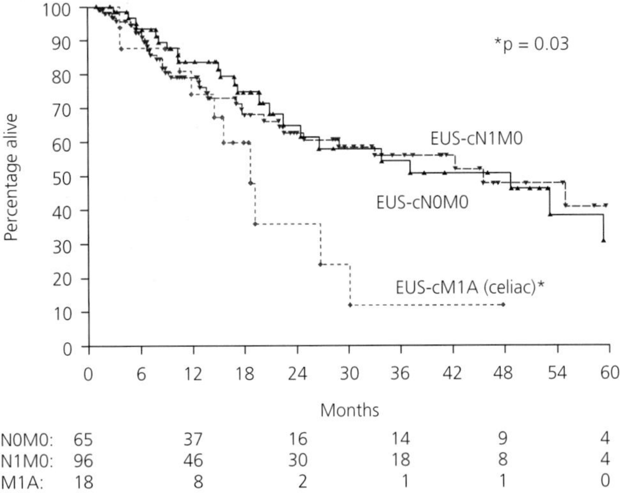

Fig. 4.33 Overall survival of patients with adenocarcinoma of the distal esophagus according to pretreatment, EUS-identified node status (cM1A vs cN0 vs M0, cN1 vs M0; p = 0.03) (reproduced from Malaisrie *et al.* 2006 with permission).

Involvement of celiac axis nodes

Celiac adenopathy is a poor prognostic factor in patients with esophageal cancer, especially those treated with surgery alone or with preoperative radiochemotherapy and surgery (Christie *et al.* 1999; Eloubeidi *et al.* 2001; Malaisrie *et al.* 2006). In fact, because the risk of relapse is high in patients with celiac axis involvement treated with surgery alone, the 2001 American Joint Committee on Cancer (2002) stage classification classifies celiac axis involvement as a form of metastatic disease (M1a) rather than a form of nodal involvement.

In a recent study, Malaisrie *et al.* (2006) retrospectively examined the impact of celiac adenopathy in a single-institutional experience that included 186 patients with adenocarcinoma of the distal esophagus who were treated with preoperative radiochemotherapy and esophagectomy, or induction chemotherapy followed by preoperative radiochemotherapy and esophagectomy. The identification of celiac adenopathy on pretreatment ultrasonography was a significant predictor of decreased long-term survival: median survival duration and 3-year survival rates were 49 months and 54% in the cN0 M0 group (n = 65), 45 months and 56% in the cN1 M0 group (n = 96), and 19 months and 12% in the cM1a (celiac adenopathy) group (n = 18) (p = 0.03). In addition, celiac adenopathy was associated with an increased risk of systemic relapse (44% vs 22% for patients without celiac nodal disease; p = 0.07). The only factor associated with increased survival in patients with celiac adenopathy (27 vs 15 months; p = 0.02) was the addition of induction chemotherapy before radiochemotherapy and surgical intervention. Celiac adenopathy also appeared to be associated with an increased risk of systemic as opposed to local–regional relapse: systemic relapse rates were 44% for patients with celiac adenopathy, 18% for patients with no lymph node involvement, and 26% for patients with periesophageal node involvement (p = 0.07) (Fig. 4.33) (Malaisrie *et al.* 2006). Local–regional relapse rates were similar between the three groups, and induction chemotherapy before radiochemotherapy was associated with long-term survival, suggesting that additional improvements in survival for patients with celiac lymph node disease will come from strategies designed to achieve better systemic control (Malaisrie *et al.* 2006). These findings also indicate that it is important to identify patients with celiac adenopathy before treatment and to evaluate the survival benefits of induction chemotherapy before radiochemotherapy in this high-risk group (Malaisrie *et al.* 2006).

Catalano *et al.* (1999) found that endoscopic ultrasonography for preoperative detection of celiac lymph node involvement, with characterization of nodes by size, shape, echogenicity, and borders, had a sensitivity of 83% and a specificity of 98%. False-positive results occurred in only 2 of 145 patients (Catalano *et al.* 1999). Another study showed that the mere detection of celiac axis lymph nodes was highly predictive of malignant involvement, and some studies have shown that 100% of celiac lymph nodes larger than 10 mm contain metastatic disease (Eloubeidi *et al.* 2001).

Pathologic response

Complete eradication of cancer cells in the surgical specimen has consistently been recognized as a favorable prognostic factor for local–regional control and overall survival in patients with esophageal cancer (Geh *et al.* 2001; Hennequin *et al.* 2001). Pathologic complete response has been reported in 2.5–5% of patients who received induction chemotherapy alone before surgery (Kelsen *et al.* 1998b; Hoffman *et al.* 1998), in 11–41% of patients who received preoperative radiochemotherapy with 5-FU and cisplatin, in 17.7–46% of patients who received preoperative radiochemotherapy including paclitaxel, and in up to 71% of patients who received induction chemotherapy before preoperative radiochemotherapy (Lynch *et al.* 1997; Weiner *et al.* 1997; Luketich *et al.* 1998; Meluch *et al.* 1999; Swisher *et al.* 2003).

Trials investigating preoperative radiochemotherapy have noted a marked local–regional control and overall survival advantage for the patients who experienced pathologic complete response (Stahl *et al.* 1996; Forastiere *et al.* 1997; Ganem *et al.* 1997; Heath *et al.* 2000). In a study of 235 consecutive patients with pretherapy clinical stage II, III, or IVA carcinoma of the esophagus or gastroesophageal junction who were treated with radiochemotherapy followed by esophagectomy, Chirieac *et al.* assessed the value of postradiochemotherapy pathologic status in predicting survival (Chirieac *et al.* 2005). Postradiochemotherapy cancer status was classified using pathologic stage and semiquantitative assessment of residual carcinoma. Clinicopathologic features, residual carcinoma status, and pretherapy and posttherapy stage were compared with disease-free and overall survival. The results showed that radiochemotherapy produced downstaging in 56% of patients. Most interesting, post-therapy pathologic stage was the strongest independent predictor of disease-free and overall survival (both p = 0.02).

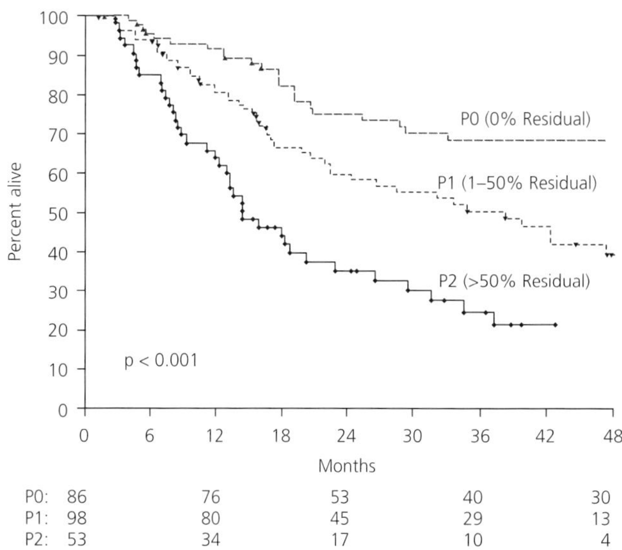

Fig. 4.34 Overall survival of patients with resected esophageal cancer treated with preoperative chemoradiation and surgery according to pathologic response at primary tumor (3 years P0 = 0%, residual = 74%; P1 = 1–50%, residual = 54%; P2 = >50%, residual = 24%; p < 0.001) (reproduced from Swisher *et al.* 2005 with permission).

Extent of residual carcinoma was also a significant predictor of overall survival (p = 0.04). On the basis of this analysis, Swisher *et al.* proposed a revision of the esophageal cancer staging system to accommodate pathologic response to preoperative radiochemotherapy (Fig. 4.34) (Swisher *et al.* 2005). These findings support the concept of downstaging by preoperative radiochemotherapy and confirm the findings of others (Walsh *et al.* 1996; Urba *et al.* 2001; Burmeister *et al.* 2002) that preoperative radiochemotherapy in local–regionally advanced esophageal cancer can produce a complete or nearly complete pathologic response in a subset of patients.

Functional imaging as a prognostic factor for radiochemotherapy

Currently, standard positron emission tomography (PET) imaging using the glucose analog fluorodeoxyglucose (FDG-PET) is widely employed for anatomic imaging and staging of esophageal cancer (Luketich *et al.* 1999; Flamen *et al.* 2000). Although tumors use glucose to provide energy for growth, they also use it to provide energy for other processes, including cellular maintenance, cellular repair, and even programmed cell death, apoptosis.

It has been hypothesized that FDG uptake on PET images reflects tumor cell metabolism and could be used as a measure of tumor response and treatment efficacy. In one study, the number of abnormalities visualized on pretreatment PET was predictive of overall survival and disease-free survival (Hong *et al.* 2005). FDG uptake on PET after preoperative chemotherapy or radiochemotherapy has correlated with patient survival and pathologic response (Swisher *et al.* 2004a). In Swisher's study, FDG-PET performed after radiotherapy but before surgery showed acceptable sensitivity for tumor viability in patients with 50–100% of viable tumor cells. Disappointingly, however, FDG-PET did not have acceptable sensitivity in detecting residual tumor with less than 50% of viable tumor (Swisher *et al.* 2004a). Downey *et al.* (2003) reported that PET could detect metastatic disease better than conventional imaging at initial evaluation but not later, and called for further studies correlating FDG-PET with survival. Flamen *et al.* (2002) performed FDG-PET before and after radiochemotherapy in 36 patients with locally advanced esophageal cancer and showed that response to radiochemotherapy as shown on the scans was strongly correlated with pathologic response and survival. Others have shown that the metabolic activity indicated by FDG-PET predicts tumor response in other types of cancer, including head and neck cancer (Brun *et al.* 2002), lung cancer (Weber *et al.* 1999, 2003), and gastric cancer (Ott *et al.* 2003).

Only a few published studies (Wieder *et al.* 2004) have attempted to measure esophageal tumor response during radiochemotherapy. Wieder *et al.* showed that early esophageal tumor response could be detected by FDG-PET. Their FDG-PET images acquired 2 and 4 weeks after the start of treatment showed continuous decrease of FDG uptake in the tumors of responding patients. More important, the change in FDG uptake seemed to level out between 4 weeks after the start of treatment and after radiation but before surgery, indicating that three sets of FDG-PET measurements may be sufficient to establish the time course of tumor response: before radiochemotherapy; during and perhaps at the midpoint of radiochemotherapy; and after radiochemotherapy, before surgery. Preliminary results from others (Weber *et al.* 2001; Wieder *et al.* 2004) have shown that it may be possible to use serial PET to track tumor response in patients with esophageal cancer. It was found that SUVs from PET were significantly decreased at midtreatment (from 9.3 ± 2.8 to 5.7 ± 1.9; $p < 0.0001$) and at post-treatment (3.3 ± 1.1) compared to baseline ($p < 0.0001$). In patients found at histopathologic examination to have responded (fewer than 10% viable cells in the specimen), the decrease in SUV between initiation and midtreatment was 44% ± 15%, but in non-responders, the decrease was only 21% ± 14% ($p = 0.0055$). Midtreatment SUVs also were significantly correlated with survival ($p = 0.011$). During the study, responders experienced a 70% reduction (±11%) in SUVs, whereas non-responders experienced only a 51% (±21%) reduction in SUVs.

Wieder *et al.* showed that inflammation of the normal esophagus was not a significant problem in measuring the tumor response, diffuse esophageal FDG uptake suggesting esophagitis was observed in only a small number of patients (15% of patients after 14 days of radiochemotherapy). The researchers concluded that the significant correlation between response and

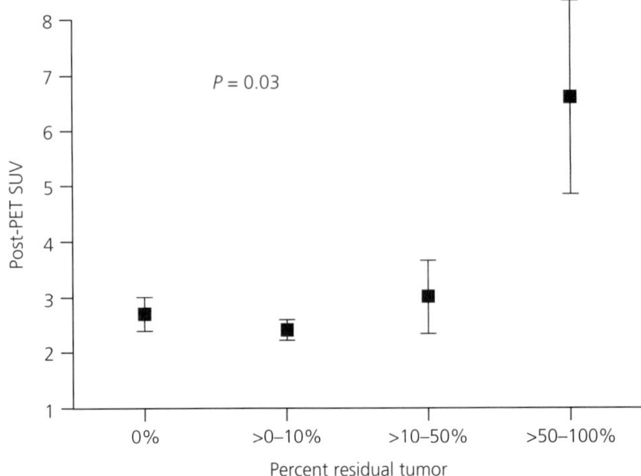

Fig. 4.35 Postchemoradiation therapy FDG-PET standardized uptake value (SUV) (mean ± the standard error of the mean) of the primary tumor as correlated with the percentage of viable cells in pathologic specimens (n = 68) at the time of esophagectomy. Patients with >50% tumor viability were found to have a significantly higher average SUV compared with the other patient groups (p = 0.03) (reproduced from Swisher *et al.* 2004a with permission).

midtreatment FDG-PET metabolic activity might be useful in stratifying patients early in treatment and appropriately modifying the therapeutic approach. Unfortunately, only a small number of patients were studied. Results from this study need further validation from other groups. The value of reduction in tumor FDG uptake on PET imaging early in the course of preoperative radiochemotherapy also warrants further investigation, as it was suggested to correlate well with tumor response to preoperative chemotherapy (Weber *et al.* 2001). Although FDG-PET imaging accurately predicts a pathologic complete response (Swisher *et al.* 2004b), at least 20% of patients with a normal preoperative PET will have residual disease in the resected specimen (Fig. 4.35) (Swisher *et al.* 2004a).

Considerations in radiotherapy

Advancement in radiotherapy technique

Radiotherapy is a critical component in the management of esophageal carcinoma. The success of radiotherapy depends on accurate delineation of the target volume and accurate delivery of the dose. The ultimate goal is to eradicate the cancer cells while sparing the normal tissue surrounding the tumor.

Traditionally, patients with esophageal cancer were treated with external-beam radiation with two-dimensional treatment planning. With this approach, however, there was great uncertainty about the dose distribution and a high probability of normal tissue toxicity. In the past decade, three-dimensional conformal radiotherapy (3D-CRT) has become the standard of care for treating esophageal cancer at MD Anderson. The dose conformality achievable with 3D-CRT minimizes irradiation of critical structures and other normal tissues and thus minimizes the toxicity of radiotherapy.

More recently, it was found that dose conformality and sparing of normal tissues could be further improved with intensity-modulated radiotherapy (IMRT). IMRT is a novel approach to the planning and delivery of radiotherapy. Unlike conventional 3D-CRT, IMRT usually involves inverse planning, whereby dose volume constraints for targets and normal tissues are defined *a priori* and then optimized with the use of a computer algorithm. Targets and normal tissues are first delineated on a CT scan. The algorithm then identifies beam orientations and patterns of intensity that optimize conformality of the prescription dose to the shape of the target in three dimensions while sparing surrounding normal tissues. Treatment is typically delivered with the help of multileaf collimators, which consist of individual motorized leaves that can move in and out of the beam's path during treatment, modulating the beam's intensity (Leibel *et al.* 2002). Numerous investigators have demonstrated the benefits of IMRT planning–normal tissue sparing (Lujan *et al.* 2003; Liu *et al.* 2004; Murshed *et al.* 2004) and delivery of higher than conventional doses (Nutting *et al.* 2002; Ahmed *et al.* 2004) in a variety of tumor sites. Preliminary clinical reports have been promising: rates of adverse events have been low (Chao *et al.* 2001; Eisbruch *et al.* 2001; Mundt *et al.* 2003), even when higher than conventional doses are delivered (Kupelian *et al.* 2002; Zelefsky *et al.* 2002).

The most cutting-edge form of radiotherapy currently being used to treat esophageal cancer is proton therapy. Protons are positively charged particles with a unique property that makes them ideal for delivering radiotherapy to sensitive structures. Protons deposit relatively little energy until they reach the end of their path, where their ionization peaks (Hall 1993). After this peak, the ionization drops to virtually zero; there is no exit dose. The length of the path of a proton beam is dependent on its initial energy, which can be tailored to the specific clinical situation. Therefore, with a proton beam, there is less radiation dose to the normal tissue in front of the tumor and hardly any dose to the normal tissue behind it. This unique property of protons predicts that proton therapy could spare more normal tissues than photon therapy and therefore increase the therapeutic ratio. In addition, the new technology of active-scanning proton beams enables the delivery of intensity-modulated proton therapy (IMPT), a method of exquisitely conforming the dose to the tumor.

Currently, there are approximately 25 proton treatment centers in the world. A variety of tumors have been treated with proton therapy An improved tumor control rate with proton therapy compared to photon therapy has been demonstrated for skull base chordomas and chondrosarcomas (Hug & Slater 2000).

The largest study of proton therapy for esophageal cancer to date is reported by Sugahara *et al.* (2005), who treated 46 patients with esophageal cancer with proton beams with or without photon irradiation between 1985 and 1998. Forty patients received a combination of photon therapy (median dose, 48 Gy) and a boost dose with proton therapy (median dose, 31.7 Gy). The median combined dose from photon and proton therapy was 76 Gy (range 69.1–87.4 Gy). The remaining six patients received only proton therapy (median dose 82 Gy; range 75–89.5 Gy). The median fraction dose was 3.0 Gy (range, 2.5–3.7 Gy), much higher than the median dose with conventional fractionation. The 5-year actuarial overall survival rates for all patients, patients with T1 tumors (n = 23), and patients with T2–4 tumors (n = 23) were 34%, 55%, and 13%, respectively. The corresponding 5-year actuarial disease-specific survival rates were 67%, 95%, and 33%, respectively, and the corresponding 5-year actuarial local–regional disease control rates were 57%, 83%, and 29%, respectively. There were 18 recurrences, 16 local–regional and 2 distant. Five patients (10%) had marginal or out-of-field recurrences. The major adverse event associated with this treatment was esophageal ulcers, which occurred in 22 patients. Seventy-five per cent of the patients who received the equivalent of 80 Gy or more developed esophageal ulcers, compared with 37% of those who received the equivalent of less than 80 Gy. The high incidence of ulcers in this study may be a result of the large fraction size and high total dose.

Target volume delineation

The success of radiotherapy, regardless of the type of radiation beam or the technique of beam delivery, depends greatly on precise positioning of the patient, accurate design of margins during treatment planning, and precise localization of the target volume during treatment delivery. Understanding the natural course of tumor dissemination is critical for accurate delineation of regions that may contain microscopic disease and accurate delineation of the clinical target volume (CTV).

Anatomic considerations

The esophagus begins in the neck at the cricoid cartilage at the level of vertebra C7, passes through the thorax in the posterior mediastinum, and extends for several centimeters past the diaphragm to the gastroesophageal junction, which is near the lower border of vertebra T11. The endoscopic distance of the esophagus is approximately 40–43 cm from the upper incisor teeth. The location of a tumor within the esophagus affects tumor classification, lymphatic drainage patterns, and appropriate treatment options.

For classifying, staging, and reporting on esophageal malignancies, the American Joint Committee on Cancer (2001) has recommended dividing the esophagus into four regions. The *cervical esophagus* extends from the lower edge of the cricoid cartilage to the thoracic inlet, approximately 18 cm from the incisors. The intrathoracic esophagus is divided into two portions: the *upper thoracic esophagus,* which extends from the thoracic inlet to the tracheal bifurcation, approximately 24 cm from the incisor teeth, and the *middle thoracic esophagus,* which extends from the tracheal bifurcation to the level of the distal esophagus just above the gastroesophageal junction, 32 cm from the incisor teeth. The *lower thoracic and abdominal esophagus* is the most distal portion of the esophagus (approximately 3 cm in length), including the gastroesophageal junction, 40–43 cm from the incisor teeth. The cervical esophagus is posterior to the trachea and bounded on both sides by the recurrent laryngeal nerve and the carotid sheath. The thoracic esophagus continues posterior to the trachea to the level of the trachea bifurcation and then courses posteriorly to the left atrium, with the azygous veins ascending on either side of the thoracic segment.

The esophagus has four layers–mucosa, submucosa, muscularis propria, and serosa. The mucosa of the esophagus consists of a non-keratinizing, stratified, squamous epithelium, the lamina propria, and the muscularis mucosa. The submucosa consists of loose connective tissue containing vessels, nerve fibers, lymphatics, and submucosal glands. The muscularis propria consists of the inner, circular, and outer longitudinal layers. The serosa lines a short segment of the thoracic and intra-abdominal esophagus (DeNardi & Riddell 1991).

The cervical esophagus is supplied mainly by branches of the inferior thyroid artery. The thoracic esophagus is supplied by branches of the bronchial arteries, intercostal arteries, and aorta. The abdominal esophagus is supplied by branches of the left gastric and inferior phrenic arteries. Branches from these arteries run within the muscularis propria and give rise to branches that course within the submucosa with extensive anastomoses.

The venous system of the esophagus consists of four layers: the radially arranged epithelial layer channels communicate with the superficial venous plexus in the upper submucosa; the latter communicates with the deep intrinsic veins in the lower submucosa. From here, perforating veins pierce the muscularis propria and connect with the adventitial veins on the esophageal surface. Branches from the upper two-thirds of the esophagus lead into the inferior thyroidal vein and the azygous system, and eventually to the superior vena cava. The lower segment drains into the systemic circulation through the branches of the azygous and left gastric veins and into the splenic vein through the short gastric veins. The caval and portal systems communicate through the veins within the submucosa (DeNardi & Riddell 1991).

A rich network of lymphatics in the lamina propria and submucosa connects with the lymphatics in the muscularis propria and adventitia. The lymphatics in the esophagus are oriented mostly in a longitudinal direction. Because of this arrangement, extensive intramucosal and submucosal spread beyond a grossly visible tumor is common. This feature becomes an important consideration in the delineation of the CTV in esophageal cancer. In general, the lymphatic network of the esophagus drains into three areas: the upper, middle, and lower lymphatic trunks. All three groups of lymphatics drain into the paraesophageal lymph nodes located immediately adjacent to the esophagus. The cervical esophagus drains into the internal jugular and upper tracheal lymph node groups; the thoracic esophagus drains into the superior, middle, and lower mediastinal lymph node groups; and the abdominal esophagus drains into the superior gastric artery, celiac axis, common hepatic artery, and splenic artery lymph nodes. However, extensive communication among the lymphatics results in a varied and unpredictable nodal involvement pattern (DeNardi & Riddell 1991).

Definition of the target volume

For radiotherapy to be successful, both the gross tumor and the microscopic disease must be encompassed in the treatment portals. Information from whichever test yields positive results–endoscopy, EUS, CT, or PET–should be used to determine the gross tumor volume (GTV). An esophageal wall thickness of more than 0.5 cm should be included in the GTV. A barium swallow procedure that images the lumen of the esophagus may be helpful in delineating the length of a primary tumor.

Coregistered PET-CT provides both anatomic and functional information in a single imaging session and also accurate registration of PET and CT data to improve the diagnosis of tumors (Beyer *et al.* 2000; Charron *et al.* 2000; Kluetz *et al.* 2000; Hany *et al.* 2002; Bar-Shalom *et al.* 2003; Lardinois *et al.* 2003; Schoder *et al.* 2003; Townsend *et al.* 2004). The impact of coregistered PET-CT imaging on planning of conformal radiotherapy for thoracic cancers has been extensively studied and reviewed (Grills *et al.* 2003; Brahme 2004; Scarfone *et al.* 2004; Ashamalla *et al.* 2005; Grosu *et al.* 2005). In a study in esophageal cancer, FDG-PET identified previously undetected distant metastatic disease and increased and decreased the GTV. Modifications of the GTV affected the planning treatment volume (PTV). Modifications of delineation of GTV and displacement of the isocenter of the PTV affected the percentage of total lung volume receiving more than 20 Gy (Moureau-Zabotto *et al.* 2005).

In esophageal cancer, accurate delineation of the CTV is more difficult than accurate delineation of the GTV. Esophageal cancer may be associated with multicentric disease or with submucosal 'skip' metastases, which are sometimes found at a considerable distance from the primary tumor (Mauer & Weichselbaum 2002). This fact supports the use of generous proximal and distal margins for treating the primary tumor. Analyses of patterns of failure after radiotherapy showed that marginal failure or failure outside the radiation field in the esophagus occurred when 5-cm longitudinal margins (Miller 1962; Elkon *et al.* 1978) were used; hence, these researchers advocated including the entire esophagus in initial treatment (Herskovic *et al.* 1992). In RTOG trial 85-01, the entire esophagus was included in the radiation portals. However, toxicity was severe, especially when chemotherapy was administered. Therefore, in the follow-up RTOG trial 94-05, 5-cm proximal and distal margins and a 2-cm lateral margin from the lateral border of the GTV were recommended.

Esophageal cancer is characterized by a high rate of nodal involvement; thus, uninvolved regional lymph nodes should also be included in the CTV. If the primary tumor is above the carina (proximal esophagus), the supraclavicular nodes should be included in the CTV. For tumors of the lower two-thirds of the esophagus, treatment of the celiac nodes should be considered. For cervical esophageal cancer, the treatment fields usually extend from the laryngopharynx to the upper two-thirds of the esophagus and encompass the lower cervical, supraclavicular, and superior mediastinal nodes. Whether to include the nodal basin of the upper jugular, subdigastric region in the treatment field is still debated. The fact that these nodes are routinely included in the CTV in treatment of oral pharyngeal or hypopharyngeal cancer supports the inclusion of these nodes in the treatment of cervical esophageal cancer.

The PTV accounts for daily set-up uncertainty and motion of the target, another critical consideration in determining target volume and treatment planning for esophageal cancer. Esophageal tumor motion can be caused by respiration and peristalsis, especially in cases of gastroesophageal junction tumors. Unfortunately, motion of esophageal cancer is severely understudied, although longitudinal respiratory motion of 2–3 cm has been reported (Konski *et al.* 2003). Bosset *et al.* (2005) proposed the definition of an initial target volume, CTV1, which includes lymph node stations with high risk (>25%) of involvement, and a second target volume, CTV2, incorporating 2-cm margins in the cephalad and caudal directions and a 1-cm margin radially from the GTV. The delineation of CTV1 and CTV2 on the CT is derived from a nodal atlas (Haustermans & Lerut 2003). The CTV1 dose is limited to 30 Gy over 3 weeks, and the CTV2 dose is 45 Gy (Bosset *et al.* 2005).

Our current standard practice includes routine use of anatomic and functional images and correction for respiratory tumor motion. Anatomic data acquisition is performed using a dedicated PET-CT scanner, and respiratory tumor motion is documented and quantified by four-dimensional CT while the patient breathes freely and quietly. Each study includes regular PET-CT followed by four-dimensional CT for radiation treatment planning. We combine information from all pretreatment evaluations for GTV definition, and we contour all the areas that were positive on these evaluations. The GTV is typically contoured on maximal intensity projection (MIP) images, which include the extremes of the tumor motion, to create a MIP-GTV. A 4.5-cm proximal and distal margin and a 1.5-cm radial margin are added to the MIP-GTV to form the internal target volume (ITV). ITV contour is individually shaved off the normal structures where subclinical involvement is unlikely, such as normal lungs, bones, and heart. The institutional standard is to deliver 100% of the prescribed dose to the GTV and 95% of the prescribed dose to the ITV (Fig. 4.36). The standard dose is 50.4 Gy at 1.8 Gy per fraction once a day. Fig. 4.37 shows a typical 3-D coronal radiation therapy plan for a distal esophageal cancer.

In an attempt to further decrease the cardiac and pulmonary toxicity of radiochemotherapy, we performed a planning study comparing IMRT and proton irradiation for esophageal cancer. A significant dosimetric advantage in proton beam therapy was demonstrated, especially in the volume of the lung receiving low-dose irradiation and the volume of heart that would have been encompassed in the radiation field. Fig. 4.38 demonstrates a actual dose volume histogram comparing an executed proton beam radiation plan with photon IMRT treatment plan in a patient with esophageal cancer. Proton beam radiation therapy significantly reduced the volume of normal lung and heart in the radiation field. We recently launched a phase I/II study using proton radiation and radiochemotherapy for unresectable esophageal cancer to test safety and efficacy. We want to guard against the possibility that treatment could cause perforation of the esophagus, grade 4 pneumonitis, or death. If we do not find an excessive rate of perforation, grade 4 pneumonitis, or death, we will enroll a maximum of 50 patients. Our target rate of perforation, grade 4 pneumonitis, or death is less than 3% within 13 weeks of initiation of treatment. We will begin by treating patients with 50 cobalt gray equivalents (CGEs) at

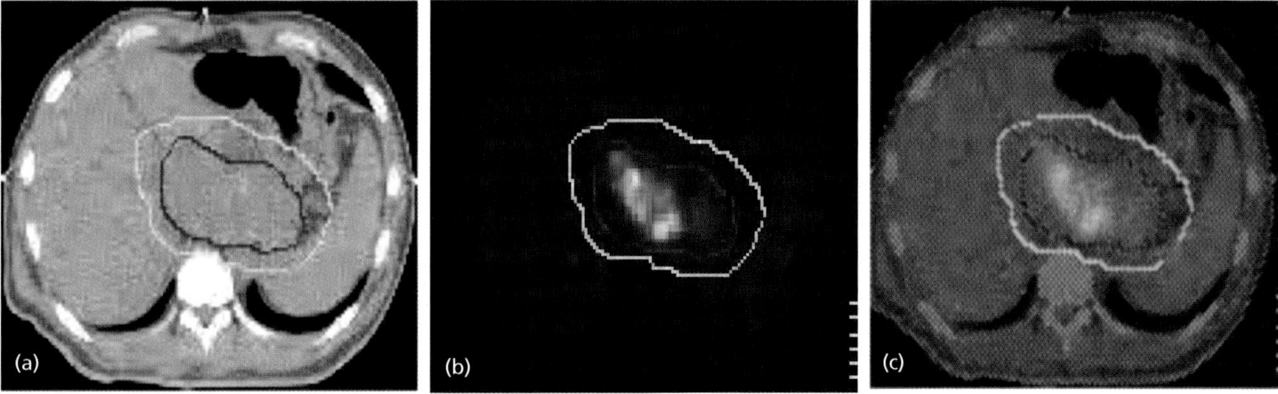

Fig. 4.36 Simulation PET-CT image is used for target volume delineation. The red line indicates MIP-GTV, the yellow line indicates ITV.

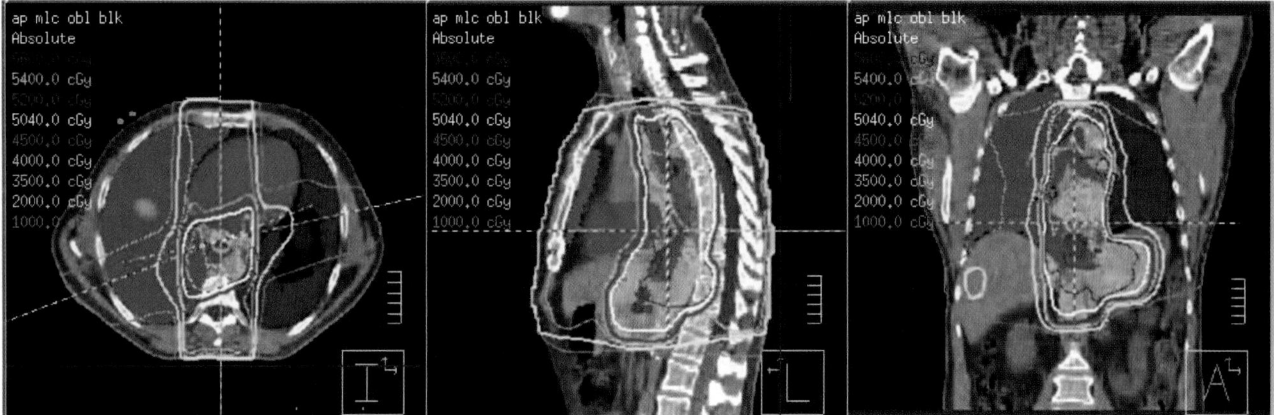

Fig. 4.37 Typical three-dimensional CRT radiation dose distribution for distal esophageal cancer.

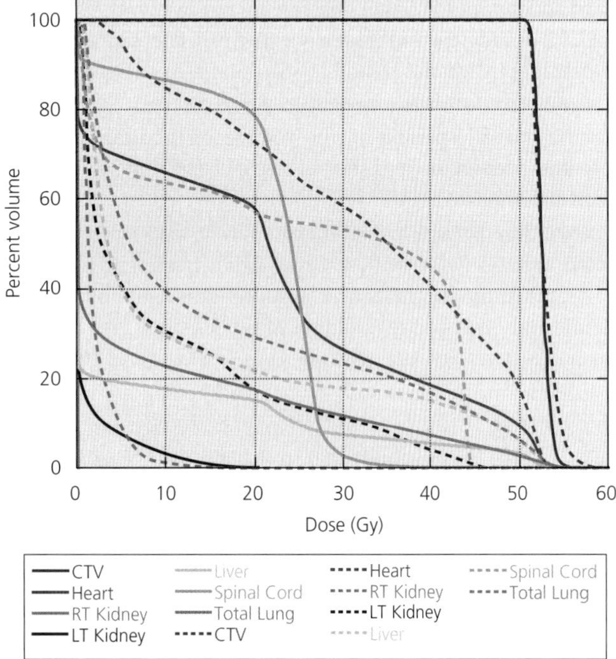

Fig. 4.38 Dose–volume histogram comparing proton beam (solid line) radiation therapy with photon IMRT radiation (dashed line).

2 CGE per fraction. If this proves safe, we will escalate the dose to 55 CGE at 2.2 CGE per fraction and then to 60 CGE at 2.4 CGE per fraction. This study has just opened to patient accrual.

Summary

In Western countries, the incidence of esophageal adenocarcinoma in the lower esophagus or gastroesophageal junction has increased 5–10% per year (Devesa *et al.* 1998; Wijnhoven *et al.*1999). It is the sixth leading cause of cancer mortality in men, causing 10,530 deaths annually (American Cancer Society 2006), or 5.1 deaths/100,000 US men and 1.2 deaths/100,000 US women. Its 5-year survival rate (<10–14.3% overall) is lower than that of 15 other cancers cited by the American Cancer Society, with only liver and pancreas cancers identified as more deadly (Capocaccia *et al.* 2003; American Cancer Society 2006). Celiac lymph node involvement at the time of diagnosis suggests an unfavorable outcome; therefore, better local–regional staging with the use of EUS, CT-PET, and newer imaging modalities may help select appropriate candidates. Approximately 50% of these patients present with local–regional disease, for which the radiochemotherapy is a critical part of the management, either as neoadjuvant or definitive measure. It is well established that radiochemotherapy is the treatment of choice for non-surgical patients with survival similar to that of surgery alone. Adding surgery to definitive radiochemotherapy has increased local regional control without clear benefit for overall survival. Preoperative radiochemotherapy has shown to downstage tumor and increase R0 resection rate. However, persistent disease after definitive radiochemotherapy remains the major pattern of local regional failure. However, this approach remains investigational because a survival benefit has not been documented. Pulmonary, cardiac and mucosal toxicity have been reported and are associated with radiation dosimetric parameters. Since different combinations of cytotoxic systemic therapy have not produced superior outcomes, it is important to incorporate biologic targeting agents such as epidermal growth factor receptor (EGFR) blockers, HER/Neu, vascular endothelial growth factor (VEGF) agents, and COX-2 in our therapeutic armamentarium to improve the dismal outlook for these patients. Preliminary results from number of small clinical trials are encouraging. Pathologic complete response is a strong indicator of favorable survival. Methods of predicting and assessing early tumor response to preoperative therapy, thus allowing individualized treatment, have attracted extensive research effort, including biomarkers and functional images.

Ablation, novel agents, and endoscopic therapy for esophageal dysplasia and carcinoma

Herbert C. Wolfsen

Introduction

This section reviews the methods of endoscopic therapy for the treatment of patients with Barrett's and squamous dysplasia, as well as early esophageal carcinoma. To provide a context for this discussion, the natural history of Barrett's esophagus and the risks associated with progression to dysplasia and invasive carcinoma are reviewed. Operative esophageal resection is traditionally recommended for patients with Barrett's high-grade dysplasia and early carcinoma, and these surgical outcomes are also reviewed. Finally, all currently approved and commercially available methods for endoscopic ablation and resection of Barrett's disease are categorized according to their application methods of ablation–focal ablation, field ablation, novel agents, mucosal resection and dissection. Clinical experience with these devices and techniques is reviewed together with the adverse events and complications associated with the use of these important technologies that hold the promise of removing or destroying esophageal dysplasia and early carcinoma in order to prevent the development of invasive carcinoma.

Barrett's esophagus represents one of the most intriguing and perplexing topics in gastrointestinal oncology and is named after a London cardiothoracic surgeon who mistakenly believed these cases represented a congenitally short esophagus associated with ulcerations of the gastric cardia (Barrett 1957). Allison and Johnstone in Leeds, however, had correctly demonstrated that this was an acquired disease of ulcerations in the distal esophagus (Allison *et al.* 1943; Allison 1946, 1948; Allison & Johnstone 1953). It was not until much later that patients with Barrett's esophagus were found to have more severe acid reflux and poorer lower esophageal sphincter function than other patients (Iascone *et al.* 1983). These findings led to the hypothesis that Barrett's esophagus develops in response to longstanding acid reflux disease and that medical or surgical antireflux therapy might prevent the development of dysplasia and invasive carcinoma. Unfortunately, there are few data that support the use of medical or surgical treatments for gastroesophageal reflux disease to prevent cancer in Barrett's esophagus patients (Blot *et al.* 1991; Wild & Hardie 2003; Triadafilopoulos *et al.* 2006) although recent studies have suggested a cancer-protective effect related to the use of anti-inflammatory medications (Vaughan *et al.* 2005). Since the early 1980s gastrointestinal endoscopy researchers have developed methods for the removal or ablation of Barrett's glandular mucosa (Eisen 2003). In order to consider the outcomes associated with the use of endoscopic therapy for Barrett's disease, it is important to establish the context of the underlying risks associated with the disease itself and non-endoscopic therapy (surgery).

Risk of dysplasia and adenocarcinoma in Barrett's esophagus

Although the natural history of Barrett's esophagus remains incompletely understood, the risk for progression to adenocarcinoma in a patient with non-dysplastic Barrett's esophagus is reported to be 0.4–1.0% per patient per year (Drewitz *et al.* 1997; O'Connor *et al.* 1999; Sharma *et al.* 2001), a risk 30–125 times higher than the general population (Reid 1991; Provenzale *et al.* 1994). According to the American Cancer Society, there were 14,520 new cases of esophageal cancer in the US in 2005 with the majority being adenocarcinoma, and 13,570 deaths associated with this disease (American Cancer Society 2005). This represents a three- to fivefold increase in the US esophageal cancer incidence over the last 30 years, an increase in incidence that surpasses that of all other cancers (Shaheen & Ransohoff 2002). One of the largest available population studies has been reported by Sharma *et al.* who studied 1376 patients from the time of their initial diagnosis of Barrett's esophagus and found that many patients had *already* developed low-grade dysplasia (7.3%), high-grade dysplasia (3.0%), or adenocarcinoma (6.0%) (Sharma *et al.* 2001, 2006b). Thereafter, 618 patients with Barrett's metaplasia were followed for a mean of 4.12 years and progression to low-grade dysplasia was found in 16.1%, to high-grade dysplasia in 3.6%, and to adenocarcinoma in 2.0%. A cancer progression rate of 0.4–0.5% annually translates into the development of invasive carcinoma in 'only' 1 in 200–250 patients with Barrett's disease each year (Sharma *et al.* 2004b). This figure is frequently cited as the number needed to treat for analysis of endoscopic therapy outcomes. However, Sharma's study and others make it clear that any number needed to treat analysis should include patients with Barrett's high-grade dysplasia *and* carcinoma in 1 in 75 patient-years of follow-up or 1.3% of Barrett's patients per year.

Risks of conventional surgical treatment

Traditionally, patients with Barrett's esophagus who are found to have high-grade dysplasia or early cancer are sent for esophageal resection surgery. Operative mortality rates are typically cited as 4–6%, although several recent reports have demonstrated that patients undergoing this operation in small, low-volume community hospitals incur a much higher mortality risk (Bartels *et al.* 2000; Urbach & Baxter 2004). A recent study evaluated the mortality associated with esophagectomy in the US in 8657 cases from 1988 to 2000. A random sample of 20% of these cases found that the overall in-hospital mortality rate was 11.3%, but was lower in high-volume surgical centers (decreasing to 7.5%) (Dimick *et al.* 2005). Additionally, several

Table 4.22 Molecular targets in esophageal cancer.

Biomarker	Alteration	Mechanism	Function	Percentage	Reference
Cyclin D1	Gene amplification	Promotes entry into S phase	Growth self-sufficiency	30–70%	Izzo *et al.* (2005); Arber *et al.* (1999); Sarbia *et al.* (1999)
Retinoblastoma	Mutation, LOH	Tumor suppressor – Blocks passage to S phase	Growth self-sufficiency	50%	Boynton *et al.* (1991); Roncalli *et al.* (1998); Sarbia *et al.* (1999)
Epidermal growth factor receptor	Gene amplification	Growth factor receptor	Growth self-sufficiency	30–90%	Wilkinson *et al.* (2004)
Her-2/neu	Gene amplification	Growth factor receptor	Growth self-sufficiency	23–52%	Safran *et al.* (2004)
Ki-67				75%	
Transforming growth factor-α	Gene amplification	Growth factor	Growth self-sufficiency	Not known	Yoshida *et al.* (1993)
Vascular endothelial growth factor (VEGF); VEGF receptor	Overexpression	Endothelial cell growth factor; receptor	Angiogenesis	30–64%	Kleespies *et al.* (2005); Saad *et al.* (2005); Driessen *et al.* (2006)
Cyclooxygenase-2	Overexpression	Angiogenesis, inhibition of apoptotic pathway, etc.	Angiogenesis, avoidance of apoptosis	75%	Sivula *et al.* (2005); Kaur *et al.* (2006)
P15	Mutation, LOH at 9p21, promoter of hypermethylation	Tumor suppressor – inhibits CD1-CDK complex	Resistance to antigrowth signal	80–90%	Wong *et al.* (1997); Klump *et al.* (1998)
P16	Mutation, LPH at 9p21, promoter of hypermethylation	Tumor suppressor – inhibits CD1-CDK complex	Resistance to antigrowth signal	52.9–81%	Chang *et al.* (2005)
P53	Mutation, LOH	Tumor suppressor, causes G1 arrest of DNA-damaged cells	Resistance to antigrowth signal	40–75%	Kaur *et al.* (2006); Chang *et al.* (2005); Huang *et al.* (2005)
Human ribosomal protein L14	LOH and down-regulation	Tumor suppressor	Resistance to antigrowth signal	43–63%	Huang *et al.* (2006)
Telomerase	Up-regulation	Maintenance of length	Unlimited DNA replication	100%	Koyanagi *et al.* (1999); Morales *et al.* (1998)
FAS; FAS ligands	Underexpression or overexpression	Death receptor and death receptor ligands	Inhibition of apoptosis in cancer cells; immune surveillance	89.7%	Chan *et al.* (2006)
E-cadherin	Down-regulation	Cell adhesion protein	Invasion and metastasis		
Periplakin	Down-regulation	Cell adhesion protein	Invasion and metastasis	44.6%	Nishimori *et al.* (2006)
Glut 1 (human erythrocyte glucose transporter)	Overexpression	Increased glucose transportation to cancer cell	Cell growth	100%	Tohma *et al.* (2005)
Chemokie and bone marrow-homing receptor (CXCR4)	Overexpression	Increased lymph node and bone marrow microinvolvement	Metastatic dissemination	55%	Kaifi *et al.* (2005)

LOH, loss of heterozygosity.

large studies have found that 30–50% of patients experienced at least one serious postoperative complication such as pneumonia, myocardial infarction, heart failure or wound infection, and the average length of hospital stay was at least 2 weeks (Lerut & Van Lanschot 2004). It is against this background of disease risk and surgical risk that the complications for endoscopic therapy of Barrett's esophagus should be considered. Further, since esophagectomy remains the standard therapy in many centers, any discussion of the potential benefits of endoscopic therapy in Barrett's patients should be based on the number of patients expected to develop high-grade dysplasia and carcinoma (not just carcinoma alone) (Puli *et al.* 2006; Spechler 2006). Recently, four large cohorts of esophagectomy patients with esophageal cancer from the USA and the Netherlands were studied with logistic regression to determine factors that could predict 30-day mortality (Steyerberg *et al.* 2006). This study developed a simple risk score based on clinical factors of patient age, comorbidities, neoadjuvant therapy, and hospital surgical volume. Combining these factors predicted the 30-day mortality of 3–18% in this analysis of 3592 esophagectomy patients. It remains to be seen whether the initial innovative results from Luketich *et al.* with a minimally invasive esophagectomy technique can be maintained over the long term and can be extrapolated to other surgical centers (Luketich *et al.* 2003).

Goals of endoscopic therapy for Barrett's esophagus

Treatment of aggressive invasive cancers such as Barrett's adenocarcinoma is difficult, expensive, and often ineffective. Therefore, the goal of endoscopic therapy for Barrett's disease is to prevent the development of invasive adenocarcinoma (Wang & Sampliner 2001). Until recently, endoscopic therapy has been most widely utilized in patients with Barrett's high-grade dysplasia or mucosal carcinoma as a minimally invasive treatment alternative to esophageal resection surgery or chemoradiation therapy (Moghissi & Dixon 2003). The development of a new generation of increasingly sophisticated endoscopic devices for mucosal ablation has reopened the question of whether a safe, effective, reliable and durable method could treat early-stage Barrett's disease to prevent the development of high-grade dysplasia and invasive neoplasia and perhaps decrease the need for surveillance endoscopy (Wolfsen 2005a). Perhaps the most significant factors in the success of endoscopic therapy are related to subjectivity and sampling error associated with disease staging (Zaninotto *et al.* 2000; Alderson 2002; Ormsby *et al.* 2002) since aggressive endoscopic therapy for high-grade disease is more likely to be associated with treatment complications while less aggressive therapy may undertreat the disease with incomplete ablation. Mucosal sampling with an aggressive biopsy protocol is frequently advocated in patients with Barrett's dysplasia, although even these methods have been shown to miss unsuspected cancers and their overall efficacy has not been established (Falk *et al.* 1999) and histopathology interpretations are notoriously variable (Montgomery *et al.* 2001). Similarly, the use of endoscopic ultrasound is routinely used to determine mucosal disease depth and evaluate adjacent structures for possible metastatic disease (Holscher *et al.* 1997; Das *et al.* 2006; Waxman *et al.* 2006). However, endosonography is not considered reliable in the setting of inflammatory disease, after previous ablation or radiation therapy, and in distinguishing high-grade dysplasia from superficial adenocarcinoma (Rice *et al.* 2003; Chak *et al.* 2005b). Assessment of lymph node involvement may also be unreliable in Barrett's early cancers even when fine needle aspiration is possible without traversing the esophageal glandular mucosa. The false-negative rate is probably much higher than the 20% figure reported in patients with advanced carcinomas (Rice *et al.* 2001; Wang 2004). Recent developments in advanced endoscopic imaging such as the use of high-resolution endoscopy with narrow-band and autofluorescence imaging have been found to better delineate areas of dysplasia and carcinoma, and targeted endoscopic biopsy detection of dysplasia and carcinoma has outperformed detection rates with time-consuming and costly extensive biopsy protocols (Bergman 2006; Kara *et al.* 2005, 2006a,b; Sharma *et al.* 2006a).

Finally, the process of mucosal regeneration is incompletely understood and the response of Barrett's mucosa to injury and subsequent healing is also quite variable between individual patients. Previous experiments have suggested that in the setting of aggressive control of gastroesophageal reflux, an acute injury to Barrett's glandular mucosa will heal with squamous regeneration that originates from pleuripotent stem cells in the distal squamous portion of the esophageal ducts or basal squamous layer (Coad *et al.* 2005). Parenthetically, some investigators have found that the neosquamous epithelium that regenerates after successful ablation has abnormal genetic characteristics (Krishnadath *et al.* 2000). Since squamous mucosal abnormalities have rarely been found in the thousands of patients who have been treated with various forms of endoscopic ablation therapy, these cytogenetic abnormalities are apparently not associated with clinical disease. After successful ablation of Barrett's mucosa it is critically important that patients understand the necessity for aggressive control of gastroesophageal reflux disease, either with antiflux surgery or high-dose drug therapy, and endoscopic surveillance to detect and destroy any recurrence of Barrett's glandular mucosa (Basu *et al.* 2002; Wolfsen *et al.* 2004c; Wehrmann *et al.* 2006).

Endoscopic therapy is frequently characterized according to the energy source (e.g. electocoagulation, thermal laser or photochemical laser). Treatment efficacy and complications seem to be related to method of energy application rather than the type of energy used. This discussion, then, will be based on the methods of energy application—focal ablation ('point and shoot') using thermal laser, multipolar electrocoagulation, or argon beam coagulation; and field ablation using photodynamic therapy, radiofrequency balloon ablation or liquid nitrogen cryotherapy. The diagnostic and therapeutic use of endoscopic mucosal resection will also be discussed.

Use of thermal focal ablation devices for esophagus dysplasia and carcinoma

The focal methods of mucosal ablation are quite similar in that thermal energy is applied to destroy the glandular mucosa of

Barrett's esophagus (Sampliner 1982, 2003, 2005). Some of these methods have been commonly used in gastrointestinal endoscopy laboratories for many years, such as multipolar electrocoagulation, heater probe, or argon beam coagulation (Sampliner 1982). After first using thermal laser ablation for Barrett's esophagus in the early 1990s (Sampliner *et al.* 1993), Sampliner went on to use multipolar electrocoagulation (MPEC) therapy since this device was readily available and relatively inexpensive to use. In the initial study in 10 patients with non-dysplastic Barrett's mucosa (Sampliner *et al.* 1996) half the circumference was treated at a time using the other side as an internal control. Patients were treated with omeprazole at a mean dose of 56 mg per day, and endoscopic complete reversal was reported in every patient. Favorable results were also reported by Kovacs who found successful reversal of Barrett's esophagus in 80% of 27 patients treated via MPEC on acid-blocker medications. However, four patients had residual islands of Barrett's glandular mucosal islands (Kovacs *et al.* 1999). Adverse effects were noted in 41% of these patients, who experienced dysphagia, odynophagia, or chest pain lasting up to 4 days. These investigators found that the success of ablation significantly decreased for Barrett's patients with 4 cm or longer segments—only 25% had eradication at this length or longer. Numerous other authors have reported similar results using MPEC for mucosal ablation with an overall success rate of 75% (Sharma *et al.* 1997; Michopoulos *et al.* 1999; Montes *et al.* 1999; Sampliner *et al.* 2001; Eisen 2003). This important work initially with thermal laser ablation and then multipolar electrocoagulation established several important points. First, it provided the proof of principle that ablation of Barrett's glandular mucosa was technically feasible. Second, it established the importance of aggressive suppression of gastric acid to enhance the successful regrowth of squamous mucosa. Finally, these studies found that this neosquamous mucosa was stable and biologically similar to normal squamous mucosa with a low cancer risk and not associated with biomarker abnormalities (Wang & Sampliner 2001).

Argon beam (or 'plasma') coagulation is a thermal cautery device that uses a high-frequency monopolar current conducted to tissue via a stream of an ionized argon gas (plasma) flowing through a catheter. Ideally, this is a non-contact method of ablation in order to prevent debris from collecting on the catheter and infusions of gas into the esophageal wall. Endoscopic application of argon plasma coagulation in the esophagus typically uses power settings of 45–90 W with gas flow of 1.0–2.0 L/min (Grade *et al.* 1999). However, complications associated with the use of argon beam coagulation include pneumatosis, pneumoperitoneum, subcutaneous emphysema, pain, ulceration, stricture, bleeding, perforation and even death. Overall occurrence of adverse effects has been reported in 24% of patients (Eisen 2003). At least 12 independent centers have evaluated 444 patients with Barrett's esophagus (Sampliner 2004). Findings of complete reversal of Barrett's esophagus are widely variable and have been reported to occur in 38–98.6%, with follow-up of 36–12 months, respectively (Schulz *et al.* 2000; Kahaleh *et al.* 2002). Subsquamous glandular epithelium has been reported to occur in 0–30% although this rate does seem to increase with the length of study follow-up (Byrne *et al.* 1998; Ginsberg *et al.* 2002; Attwood *et al.* 2003; Eisen 2003; Pinotti *et al.* 2004; Sampliner 2004; Pedrazzani *et al.* 2005). Basu *et al.* followed patients for 1 year after undergoing argon plasma treatment for Barrett's disease and studied the factors related to successful outcomes. They found that the best candidates for thermal ablation therapy would be those with shorter segments of Barrett's esophagus and good control of gastroesophageal reflux (Basu *et al.* 2002). In this study, 44% of patients still had residual Barrett's mucosa buried under squamous mucosa. One the other hand, Sharma *et al.* recently published their 'long-term' follow-up of at least 2 years in patients who had been randomized to treatment with multipolar electrocoagulation or argon plasma coagulation (60 W, 1.4–1.8 L/min gas flow) (Sharma *et al.* 2006c). These 35 patients with mostly short segments of Barrett's metaplasia (median length 3 cm, range 2–6 cm) underwent ambulatory pH testing before treatment. Interestingly, this testing confirmed that 25% of patients had positive pH testing despite twice-daily treatment with rabeprazole. These findings underscore the severity of acid reflux in patients with Barrett's metaplasia and suggest that patients with more advanced phases of dysplasia may have even higher drug requirements. Treatment complications included odynophagia and chest pain in 18 patients, while one patient treated with APC required dilation for stricture. After treatment with multiple sessions of ablation (mean 3 for APC and 4 for MPEC), histologic confirmation of complete squamous replacement of the Barrett's disease was documented in 75% of MPEC patients and 63% of APC patients, respectively. This difference in ablation success was not statistically significant. This study also found no clinical factors that were ultimately predictive of ablation success. In summary, then, these widely varying results along with the significant variation in skills that are required to use these 'point and shoot' devices suggest that these thermal ablative therapies have yet to demonstrate safety, efficacy, and durability for mucosal ablation in patients with Barrett's metaplasia or dysplasia. There are relatively few studies available that compare ablation techniques with each other in order to determine relative safety and efficacy among these methods. Recently, Dulai compared ablation using APC or MPEC in patients with Barrett's metaplasia in a randomized trial (Dulai *et al.* 2005). At 6 months after ablation, the efficacy, number of sessions to treat, and complication rates were statistically similar, although the APC treatments required a longer time to complete and the randomization was inadequate since the APC group had longer-segment Barrett's disease. In another randomized trial, Kelty and colleagues studied 68 patients with Barrett's metaplasia (median segment length 4 cm) treated with low-dose oral aminolevulinic acid photodynamic therapy (ALA-PDT) or argon plasma coagulation (Kelty *et al.* 2004). There were significantly better ablation results using argon beam coagulation compared with ALA-PDT (97% vs 50%). Further, subsquamous glandular mucosa was found more commonly in the patients treated with ALA-PDT (24% of patients) over a relatively short follow-up time compared with 21% of patients in the argon plasma-treated group. Similar problems with ALA-PDT have been noted in other trials as well (Hage *et al.* 2004; Pech *et al.* 2005; Peters *et al.* 2005; Ragunath *et al.* 2005).

These thermal treatment methods–multipolar electrocoagulation, heater probe, and argon beam coagulation–use catheters that are deployed down the working channel of an endoscope, and are extremely dependent on the experience and skill of the treating physician. Since they are used in a 'point and shoot' fashion, it is extremely difficult to maintain uniform dosimetry and depth of mucosal ablation over a large area and in patients with difficult anatomy (such as a tortuous, narrowed, angulated esophagus and large hiatal hernia). Frequently, some areas are subject to overtreatment and risk excessive mucosal damage with chest pain, dysphagia, odynophagia, stricture, bleeding, ulceration and perforation, whereas other areas may be 'skipped' or inadequately treated resulting in persistent Barrett's glandular mucosa (possibly neoplastic) that may be hidden under regenerated areas of squamous mucosa. This may be especially true when the argon plasma coagulator is used in the 'spray' mode or when using a 360° circumferential catheter where the distribution of the ablation energy is poorly controlled.

Even using modest doses of thermal energy, treatment within a limited mucosal area may generate excessive thermal damage, inflammation, edema and localized ischemia with serious consequences. This is especially true using the argon beam coagulation system where gas flow rates of 1–2 L/min will quickly distend the gut. When used in the esophagus, this gaseous distention of the stomach must be repeatedly decompressed which requires removal of the argon catheter and prolongs these procedures, as was noted in the Dulai study. Manufacturers and clinicians have suggested that mucosal overtreatment with these thermoelectric methods is not possible because the dessicated mucosa will not transit the electrical energy more deeply than 3 mm into the esophagus wall (Manner *et al.* 2006). While this may be theoretically true, clinical experiences have demonstrated that the intraluminal pressure generated from insufflated air or argon gaseous distention combined with excessive mucosal heating, edema and inflammation can readily produce gut perforation. This unfortunate lesson has been learned repeatedly using APC to treat non-dysplastic Barrett's esophagus including a recent multicenter study that used high-energy APC but achieved complete ablation in only 62% of patients (Manner *et al.* 2006). Despite treating patients with a mean Barrett's segment length of 3.6 cm, complications occurred in 17.6% of patients including two patients with serious bleeding that required transfusion and repeated endoscopic therapy. Strictures occurred in two patients who refused further participation in the trial as did another patients who suffered esophageal perforation. These well-documented risks and limitations of 'point and shoot' methods of ablation make it clear that APC is not suitable for use as primary treatment of Barrett's esophagus, especially in non-dysplastic patients who have less risk for progression to neoplasia.

The use of photothermal lasers in the gut dramatically increased during the 1980s in centers that had access to these powerful and expensive devices (Fleischer 1984), and eventually these were the first devices used for endoscopic ablation in patients with Barrett's esophagus (Brandt & Kauvar 1992; Berenson *et al.* 1993). Laser light sources were frequently used for mucosal ablation and include the neodymium yttrium aluminum garnet (Nd:YAG; 1064 nm), the potassium-titanyl-phosphate (KTP; 532 nm) and argon dye lasers (514–625 nm). Mucosal depth of ablation and injury depends on the wavelength of laser light energy used and the power settings (Van Den Boogert *et al.* 1999). In 1999, Gossner and colleagues in Germany treated 10 patients with Barrett's esophagus including four patients with high-grade dysplasia. Complete endoscopic responses were reported in all cases with a mean of 10.6 months follow-up (Gossner *et al.* 1999). While no treatment-related complications were reported, histopathologic analysis of surveillance biopsy specimens found that 20% of patients had subsquamous glandular epithelium. In England, Biddlestone treated 10 patients with Barrett's metaplasia using a KTP laser where successful squamous re-epithelialization was noted in all patients. However, follow-up endoscopy noted small superficial squamous islands in six patients and in nine cases there was surface squamous epithelium overlying glandular mucosa (or so-called subsquamous Barrett's glands) (Biddlestone *et al.* 1998). Other similar laser ablation studies have reported residual Barrett's glandular mucosa ranging from 18% to 100% with complication rates similar to that of multipolar electrocoagulation but with higher rates of esophageal stricture (Luman *et al.* 1996a,b; Barham *et al.* 1997; Salo *et al.* 1998; Gossner *et al.* 1999; Weston & Sharma 2002; Bonavina *et al.* 2003; Bowers *et al.* 2003; Eisen 2003; Fisher *et al.* 2003; Norberto *et al.* 2004; Sampliner 2004). Endoscopic technique, experience and judgment are probably more important when using lasers compared with the previously described thermal techniques. This is because most of these devices are air-cooled and thus air insufflation is problematic (as with argon beam coagulation). Most importantly, however, is the high power and very rapid tissue heating that these lasers can produce that may quickly produce full-thickness mucosal necrosis. Perhaps more importantly, the very high acquisition and servicing costs of these photothermal laser devices has largely relegated them to the archives of gastrointestinal endoscopy.

Ablation of dysplasia and carcinoma of the esophagus using field ablation devices

Field ablation devices are capable of delivering mucosal ablation over a large surface area, such as radiofrequency balloon ablation (RFA), porfimer sodium photodynamic therapy (Ps-PDT), and low-pressure liquid nitrogen cryotherapy. These devices offer several important advantages when compared with the thermal 'point and shoot' devices and they require a different set of endoscopy skills. Most importantly, field ablation devices deliver relatively uniform energy distribution that serves to minimize residual glandular dysplasia at the surface and subsquamous levels. The depth of thermal injury used with radiofrequency ablation is carefully limited to prevent deep injury and excessive tissue heating, edema and ischemic injury that can produce stricture or perforation. On the other hand, Ps-PDT and cryotherapy produce mucosal ablation not by thermal injury but rather by triggering apoptosis (programmed cell death) without destroying the collagen structure of the esophageal wall. Thus, while strictures are reported in 20–35% of patients with Ps-PDT for Barrett's high-grade dysplasia, perforations are extremely rare and usually related to dilation procedures and not the laser light treatment.

The best studied method of Barrett's ablation is photodynamic therapy using porfimer sodium which has been in clinical use in the US since at least 1982 (Mccaughan *et al.* 1996). The effectiveness of PDT depends on the photodynamic reaction that requires a chemical photosensitizing agent (such as porfimer sodium), light, and the presence of oxygen. Over the 48–72 hours after the photosensitizer is given, the drug is eliminated by normal tissues while still relatively retained in abnormal cells before light activation (Wang 2001). Photodynamic therapy requires endoscopic delivery of light of a specific wavelength to activate the photosensitizer, resulting in the formation of toxic oxygen metabolites, most likely singlet oxygen ($^1O_2$), that allows a large area of epithelium to be treated with a low risk of perforation since the submucosal collagen structure of the gut is not destroyed (Wang 2001). The potency of the photodynamic reaction seems to be most dependent on the choice of photosensitizer as sodium porfimer can produce mucosal necrosis up to 4–6 mm in depth, compared with aminolevulinic acid (ALA) PDT that produces mucosal necrosis of only 2 mm (Barr *et al.* 1990; Heier *et al.* 1995). In the case of sodium porfimer, after it enters a cell, it is distributed throughout the cytoplasm and becomes tightly bound to mitochondrial membranes but other subcellular targets include lysosomes, Golgi apparatus, and the rough endoplasmic reticulum (Kubba 1999; Webber *et al.* 1999). The literature summarizing the clinical use of PDT is not the subject of this section and has recently been published elsewhere (Overholt *et al.* 1999; Ukleja *et al.* 1999; Wang 1999; Nijhawan *et al.* 2000; Panjehpour *et al.* 2000; Chen & Yang 2001; Malhi-Chowla *et al.* 2001; Wolfsen & Ng 2002; Wolfsen *et al.* 2002; Wang & Kim 2003; Mang 2004; Wang *et al.* 2004; Wolfsen & Hemminger 2004; Wolfsen *et al.* 2004c; Wolfsen 2005b,c). While several photosensitizing agents have been developed for PDT (such as ALA and m-tetrahydroxyphenyl chlorine, mTHPC) (Javaid *et al.* 2002; Lovat *et al.* 2005), only porfimer sodium has received regulatory approval to treat patients with Barrett's esophagus with high-grade dysplasia in North America (Prosst *et al.* 2003). In a landmark publication, Overholt recently reported the results of an international, prospective, randomized controlled study using porfimer sodium PDT in 208 patients with Barrett's high-grade dysplasia using a centralized pathology laboratory. This is the only such trial ever performed in patients with Barrett's esophagus with high-grade dysplasia. These patients were randomized to treatment with omeprazole plus PDT or omeprazole alone (20 mg twice daily). At 12 months follow-up after porfimer sodium PDT, 41% of patients had complete elimination of Barrett's mucosa, and 72% of patients had high-grade dysplasia elimination that represents a statistically significant improvement compared to the omeprazole-only treatment arm. Most importantly, however, treatment with porfimer sodium PDT resulted in a twofold decrease in the development of adenocarcinoma: 13% vs 29% (Overholt *et al.* 2005). These results have been maintained at 2 years and 5 years follow-up and have led to the regulatory approval for porfimer sodium PDT in Barrett's high-grade dysplasia patients in Canada, the USA, Japan and Europe. Based on these results, this treatment has become first-line treatment for Barrett's dysplasia and carcinoma in many referral centers (Hemminger & Wolfsen 2002; Hur *et al.* 2003; Wolfsen *et al.* 2004a) (Fig. 4.39).

The success of porfimer sodium PDT is likely related to its numerous local and systemic effects including the triggering of mucosal apoptosis, the induction of ischemia, and activation of inflammatory cascades. The inflammatory response after PDT may be the most important since little if any PDT effect is seen in patients who are taking multiple anti-inflammatory medica-

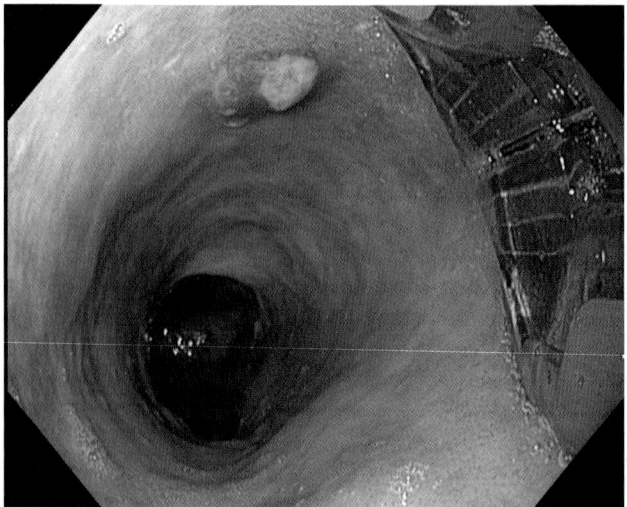

Fig. 4.39 High-resolution image taken after porfimer sodium photodynamic therapy with neosquamous lining having replaced much of the 16-cm segment of Barrett's high-grade dysplasia. At the 2 o'clock position, however, there remains an area of residual Barrett's dysplasia including an 11-mm nodular mucosal carcinoma. Note the radiofrequency focal ablation device attached to the endoscope for ablation of the residual Barrett's dysplasia before attempted mucosal resection of the mucosal carcinoma.

tions after orthotopic liver transplantation (personal observation). In the Overholt study, stricture developed after one course of PDT in 12% of patients and in 32% after two courses of PDT. This is a recurring theme in endoscopic ablation: treatment of mucosa previously treated with another ablation modality is much more likely to produce mucosal stricture. This is frequently encountered when Ps-PDT is used to treat mucosa previously treated with external beam radiation, prior PDT or even previous mucosal resection (Wolfsen & Hemminger 2006). Other common adverse events reported were chest pain (20% of patients), nausea (11% of patients), vomiting (32% of patients), constipation (13% of patients), dysphagia (19% of patients), dehydration (12% of patients), hiccups, fever and pleural effusion in 10% of patients or less, and severe sunburn-like phototoxicity reactions in 7% of patients. These adverse effects and complications may be related to direct mucosal damage with edema, inflammation and necrosis with ulceration typically producing systems of odynophagia, nausea, vomiting and dysphagia over the first 10 days of treatment. As noted above, perforation is rare since the collagen structure of the esophageal wall is not destroyed and bleeding does not occur in patients who are not anticoagulated. Significant bleeding requiring hospitalization and blood transfusion from diffuse mucosal hemorrhage after PDT has developed in patients being treated with warfarin or clopidogrel and these medications should be discontinued for PDT if at all possible. PDT-related damage to the esophageal submucosa and deeper layers has been associated with esophageal dysmotility, dysphagia, and stricture formation in 20–33% of patients. Patients who are being treated for very long Barrett's segments (more than 8 cm) or who have previously been treated with external-beam radiation or PDT have a much higher risk of stricture formation. These strictures typically manifest in 7–10 days after treatment with progressive dysphagia despite improvement in other symptoms (decreased chest and epigastric discomfort and return of appetite). These strictures require repeat dilation at short intervals (every 10–14 days) until a normal-sized, stable lumen is re-established. A recent prospective study in consecutive patients treated at our institution for endoscopic ablation for Barrett's high-grade dysplasia or mucosal carcinoma between August 2001 and May 2003 emphasized the underlying poor motility in these patients who were prospectively evaluated with esophageal manometry before and after porfimer sodium PDT. In these 41 patients, abnormal esophageal motility was found in 30% patients at study entry (diffuse esophageal spasm 6%, ineffective esophageal motility 15%, aperistalsis 9%). After undergoing porfimer sodium PDT, 11 patients experienced a change in manometric diagnosis. Three patients had an improvement in motility, seven a worsening and one changed diagnosis, but did not particularly worsen or improve. No patient developed new aperistalsis. Therefore, abnormal motility was present in 19 of 41 (46%) patients after PDT (diffuse esophageal spasm in 2, ineffective esophageal motility in 14, aperistalsis in 3). There was a statistically significant ($p = 0.016$) relationship with longer-segment Barrett's esophagus and deterioration of function. This study demonstrated that baseline abnormalities in motility were common in these patients with Barrett's high-grade dysplasia or mucosal carcinoma, and that changes in esophageal function also may occur following photodynamic therapy, but usually are not clinically significant. This worsening in function was more likely to occur in patients with longer-segment Barrett's esophagus (Shah *et al.* 2006). PDT-related effects are not limited to the esophagus and changes to structures adjacent to the esophagus include cardiac dysrhythmias (PDT used in the proximal esophagus where the left atria lies in close proximity), pleural and pericardial effusions, and transient marked lymphadenopathy. While any cardiac arrhythmia must be aggressively treated, the other conditions generally rapidly improve spontaneously with the resolution of the PDT systemic response within 7–10 days. These adverse effects associated with porfimer sodium PDT have led some European researchers to continue to use PDT with ALA for Barrett's dysplasia and carcinoma despite its limited mucosal ablation and its side-effect profile, which includes nausea, vomiting, hepatic injury and unexplained sudden death in several patients, presumably related to cardiac arrhythmias (Pech *et al.* 2005). In this study of 66 patients (mean age 61 years) there were 35 patients with Barrett's high-grade dysplasia and 31 patients with mucosal carcinoma. In all, 82 ALA-PDT procedures were performed and 34 of the 35 Barrett's high-grade dysplasia patients achieved a complete response (97%), as did all mucosal carcinoma patients (100%), over a median follow-up period of 37 months. Local recurrence of carcinoma was found in 11 patients in total (17%). Disease-free survival was 89% for patients with Barrett's high-grade dysplasia and 68% for mucosal cancer patients, with no death related to Barrett's neoplasia and no major treatment complications noted. This raises an important issue of the critical nature of the meticulous follow-up evaluations required for patients treated with endoscopic therapy, whether ablation, resection or dissection for the early detection and treatment of residual or metachronous lesions (Barr *et al.* 2005). In our program, we have found that after endoscopic ablation therapy, surveillance evaluations with upper endoscopy and chest CT were most reliable in detecting carcinoma persistence, recurrence, and metastasis. Endoscopic ultrasound, however, did not detect recurrent/persistent carcinoma that was otherwise detected by surveillance endoscopy using Seattle biopsy protocol and contrast-enhanced CT. Therefore, while considered critical for the initial evaluation of patients being considered for endoscopic ablation therapy, in our laboratory, EUS appears to have little role in the subsequent surveillance of these patients, unless discrete abnormalities are found on endoscopy or cross-sectional imaging (Savoy *et al.* 2005).

There are fewer data available regarding the use of PDT for patients with early esophageal cancer, and previous studies have not benefited from the advances in cancer staging technologies including advanced endoscopic ultrasound including use of high-frequency probes and fine needle aspirate of periesophageal lymph nodes (Sibille *et al.* 1995; Overholt *et al.* 1999). More recent single-center studies, however, have demonstrated the utility of multimodal endoscopic therapy in patients with early esophageal cancer as an alternative to esophageal resection surgery, just as for Barrett's high-grade dysplasia (Pacifico *et al.* 2003; Behrens *et al.* 2005). A prospective, multicenter cohort study of multimodal endoscopic therapy using endoscopic mucosal resection and porfimer sodium PDT in 83 patients with T1 N0 esophageal cancers has been reported from Johns Hopkins University, Duke University and Mayo Clinic, Jacksonville Florida (Canto *et al.* 2005). Over a mean follow-up of 3 years, the complete response rate for EMR and Ps-PDT therapy was similar to that of Ps-PDT alone (96% and 90%, respectively). This study used the 'bare fiber' method of Ps-PDT, without the use of a balloon fiber-centering device. Subsquamous dysplasia or cancer was found in 5 patients (6%), and strictures developed in 9 patients (11%). There were no treatment-related deaths and the 5-year survival of evaluable patients was 97%. These clinical outcomes, with a comparatively low rate of esophageal stricture, support the use of multimodal endoscopic therapy including porfimer sodium PDT as a safe and effective alternative to esophageal resection as first-line therapy for patients with early mucosal carcinoma of the esophagus and esophagogastric junction.

Attempts at minimizing the adverse effects and complications associated with porfimer sodium PDT have centered around extensive education of the patient and family so that direct sunlight exposure is avoided in the 4–6 weeks after treatment and that the medications provided are used correctly to control symptoms of nausea and epigastic discomfort while aggressively controlling acid reflux in order to optimize ablation treatment results. Other areas of research include measurement of mucosal reflectance patterns in order to optimize light dosimetry and determine mucosal concentrations of the photosensitizer (Wang 2000). The use of fiber-centering balloon devices has been investigated for the prevention of stricture, although no comparative trials have been performed and stricture rates reported from various single-center series (with or without use of a balloon for PDT) are similar (Panjehpour *et al.* 2005). These and other differences in PDT technique were the subject of a recent paper describing the treatment methodology in 10 large centers in the United States (Wolfsen 2006).

Endoscopic mucosal ablation using a balloon-based, bipolar radiofrequency ablation catheter has received governmental approval in the USA for treatment of Barrett's disease at all stages (Halo 360 device from Stellartech Research Coagulation System, manufactured for BARRx, Inc. Sunnyvale, CA). This technique requires the use of diameter-sizing balloons to determine the inner diameter of the targeted portion of the esophagus and use a standardized pressure of 0.5 atmospheres to transiently flatten the esophageal folds. Thereafter, a 3-cm length balloon-based electrode that incorporates tightly spaced, bipolar electrodes that alternate in polarity is used to deliver high power (300–350-W) short bursts of ablative energy to the target epithelium with controlled depth of ablation (Ackroyd *et al.* 1999). Ganz *et al.* have reported the use of this ablative device in a porcine model and in human patients before esophagectomy, and documented that ablation depth was related to mucosal delivery of energy density with doses of 8–12 J/cm^2 resulting in complete mucosal ablation (Ganz *et al.* 2004). As expected by this superficial ablation, the use of this technique has not been associated with stricture or perforation. This device has been used to treat patients with all phases of Barrett's disease (metaplasia and dysplasia), but not carcinoma (Ganz *et al.* 2004; Sharma *et al.* 2004a; Dunkin *et al.* 2005). Recently, the 12 month follow-up analysis of 100 patients with Barrett's metaplasia treated with this radiofrequency balloon device was presented (Fleischer *et al.* 2006). This study found no complications of bleeding, perforation or stricture associated with this device. Similar to other thermal techniques, treatment with this device was successful in completely clearing Barrett's metaplasia in 70% of patients with typically small areas of residual disease remaining in 30% of patients. No squamous or subsquamous abnormalities were found with follow-up limited to 1 year. We await publication of these results in full form (Sharma *et al.* 2007). This method of endoscopic application of radiofrequency energy circumferentially at 3-cm intervals has none of the systemic adverse effects associated with porfimer sodium photodynamic therapy. Local mucosal treatment effects appear to be limited to the expected transient nausea, vomiting, odynophagia and midepigastric pain in some patients. Since these balloons are mounted on a stiff catheter, care must be taken when inserting this catheter down the throat and proximal esophagus. Recently, a hybrid device was approved, the Halo 90. This device uses the same method of radiofrequency ablation but it not used with a balloon. Instead, the electrode array is mounted on a postage stamp-sized rectangular array (10 mm × 15 mm) that can be used as a combination focal/field ablation device used for mucosal dysplasia at energy settings of 120 W with energy density of 12 J (Fig. 4.40). Although this device may be cumbersome to use, especially during insertion and intubation, the Halo 90 provides the simplicity of use that make APC and MPEC popular while providing uniform mucosal ablation for better treatment results with fewer areas that are either over- or undertreated. Since this technology is specifically developed to destroy mucosa of limited depth based on previous studies, it remains to be seen whether there are patients with markedly glandular or polypoid dysplastic mucosa that will not be successfully or completely destroyed with this technique. Initial studies with this device in patients with Barrett's low-grade and high-grade dysplasia have been promising (Bergman *et al.* 2006; Ganz *et al.* 2006; Sharma *et al.* 2006d; Tsai *et al.* 2006).

Another newly approved ablation technique is low-pressure spray cryoablation method using liquid nitrogen that has been developed by CSA Medical, Inc. and has received FDA approval

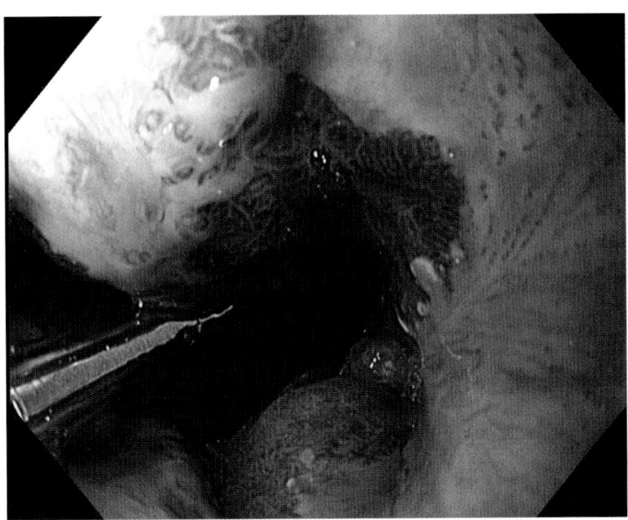

Fig. 4.40 High-resolution, narrow-band image taken during porfimer sodium photodynamic therapy procedure demonstrating a 2.5-cm 'bare laser fiber' (without utilizing a balloon fiber-centering device) for the treatment of short segment Barrett's high-grade dysplasia and mucosal carcinoma with extensive overgrowth of squamous mucosa (best seen at the 12 o'clock position).

for the CSA System (CryoSpray Ablation™ System, formally Cryo Ablator System). This class II device is an endoscopic cryosurgical tool for the destruction of unwanted tissue that uses a liquid nitrogen-cooled cryocatheter and accessories to destroy tissue during surgical procedures by applying extreme cold. This low-pressure spray cryoablation device uses a conventional liquid nitrogen tank, electronic console for monitoring and control of cryogen release, dual foot pedal for control of cryogen release and heating of the catheter, and a 7–9-Fr diameter, multilayered catheter with an open tip for spray of cooled nitrogen gas through the endoscope. The mechanism of injury appears to be distinct from other ablative injuries based on induced apoptosis and cryonecrosis resulting in transient ischemia and immune stimulation (Grana *et al.* 1981). Barrett's dysplasia and carcinoma that are resistant to ablation by other methods may be suited to this treatment. A recent publication described the results of cryoablation used in 11 patients with Barrett's metaplasia to multifocal high-grade dysplasia (glandular segments ranged from 1 to 8 cm, mean 4.6 cm) (Johnston *et al.* 2005). In 9 of the 11 patients the reversal was complete with no residual glandular mucosa found on subsequent biopsies, although further follow-up will be required to confirm these results. Like the use of radiofrequency ablation, this technology also appears to be useful in treating large areas of Barrett's mucosa without the systemic effects associated with porfimer sodium PDT. While the mucosal ablation seems to be well tolerated by patients with relatively minor symptoms of epigastric pain, nausea and painful swallowing, this technique uses liquid nitrogen that rapidly expands as its temperature increases. This has the potential of insufflating large volumes of air into the gut that must be vented using a nasogastric or orogastric tube. Gentle massage of the abdominal wall to extrude gas retrained in the stomach is used in order to decrease the risk of perforation. The study and evaluation of this ablation modality is under way at several centers in North America including the Cleveland Clinic, Fox Chase Cancer Center, National Naval Medical Center, University of Maryland and Mayo Clinic in Jacksonville, Florida (Eastone *et al.* 2001; Johnston *et al.* 1997, 1999a,b, 2000, 2003, 2005, 2006; Pasricha *et al.* 1999; Johnston 2003, 2005a,b; Kantsevoy *et al.* 2003; Raju *et al.* 2005).

Use of novel endoscopic agents for the treatment of esophageal cancer

Newer methods for treatment of patients with esophageal cancer include the use of intracavitary brachytherapy (Lah *et al.* 2005). This technique has been relatively free of harmful effects of irradiating normal tissues surrounding the cancerous lesions. The survival benefit reported with this treatment, however, has been inconsistent, although the quality of life of these patients who underwent intracavitary brachytherapy for their primary esophageal cancer was significantly improved (Araujo *et al.* 1991; Herskovic *et al.* 1992; Micaily *et al.* 1994; Sur *et al.* 1998; Gaspar *et al.* 2000; Maingon *et al.* 2000; Nemoto *et al.* 2001; Sharma *et al.* 2002). The American Brachytherapy Society guidelines suggest that intracavitary brachytherapy be used for treatment for patients with a solitary tumor of less than 10-cm length in the thoracic esophagus, without extraesophageal extension or regional lymph-node involvement (Gaspar *et al.* 1997). Currently, intracavitary brachytherapy is used in treating the primary esophageal cancers for palliation of dysphagia (Syed *et al.* 1987; Vivekanandam *et al.* 2001).

The novel use of endoscopic local administration of an antitumor agent using endoscopic ultrasound to assess tumor response and local toxicity in real time was reported at the Digestive Disease Week in Los Angeles in 2006 (Chang *et al.* 2006). This study utilized TNFerade, a second-generation replication-deficient adenovector, carrying the transgene encoding for human TNF-α, regulated by the radiation-inducible promoter Egr-1. This multicenter dose-escalating study of TNFerade with concurrent neoadjuvant chemoradiation was performed in 24 patients with resectable stage II and III esophageal cancer. The most frequent adverse events related to TNFerade were generally mild to moderate in severity and included fatigue (54%), fever (38%), and nausea (29%). Thromboembolic events occurred in 8 patients (33%). The results of this study suggest that endoscopic application of TNFerade potentially represents a new treatment paradigm in esophageal cancer treatment that may result in improved rates of clinical treatment response and optimization of surgical and long-term outcomes.

Endoscopic mucosal resection for esophageal dysplasia and cancer

Mucosal resection techniques have also been utilized to diagnose and treat high-grade dysplasia and mucosal carcinoma in Barrett's esophagus since the early 1970s when these techniques were developed in Europe (Wolfsen *et al.* 2004b; Larghi & Waxman 2005) In 1974, Deyle and colleagues in Switzerland reported the use of endoscopic mucosal resection for early gastric cancer (Deyhle *et al.* 1974). Over the next decade, EMR techniques underwent progressive refinement and improvement in the hands of researchers mostly in Japan (Inoue & Endo 1990; Inoue *et al.* 1992; Sakal *et al.* 1996). These developments coincided with that of endoscopic ultrasound and a revised classification system for esophageal cancer that distinguished between intraepithelial invasion (T1-m1), infiltration of the lamina propria (T1-m2) and infiltration of the muscularis mucosa (T1-m3) by the Japanese Society for Esophageal Diseases (Fleming *et al.* 1997). This system has been especially important as these small differences in mucosal staging are associated with significant differences in the risk for metastatic spread of cancer. This risk is very small for esophageal tumors with invasion limited to the intraepithelial layer, but increases to 10% for lesions invading the muscularis mucosa, 20% for lesion involving the superficial submucosa and at least 40% for lesions penetrating into the deeper submucosa (Makuuchi 1996). The basic techniques of EMR were developed over three decades ago, beginning with Deyle's use of the 'inject-and-cut' method followed by Martin's use of the 'lift-and-cut' technique for removing submucosal lesions using a double-channel endoscope (Martin *et al.* 1976). A third technique, the 'suck-and-cut' method, was developed by Inoue *et al.* using an overtube to create a pseudopolyp of the target lesion using suction with subsequent snare removal (Inoue & Endo 1990). Later, the development of a band ligation device for the treatment of esophageal varices was adapted for use with EMR (Inoue *et al.* 1992) that obviated the use of an overtube and permitted the rapid dissemination and use of this technique (Inoue *et al.* 1993, 1994, 1998, 1999a,b; Fleischer *et al.* 1996; Sakal *et al.* 1996; Soehendra *et al.* 1997). Currently, this method uses a commercially available cap with internal snare device or with a variceal ligation device to create a pseudopolyp followed by polypectomy, or using a monofilament snare with pure coagulation electrical current in combination with lifting of the mucosa with a biopsy forceps (Ell *et al.* 2000; Seewald *et al.* 2003; Soetikno *et al.* 2003). Generally, these resection techniques are performed after submucosal injection to separate the target mucosa from the deeper mural layers. The use of too small a volume of saline injection will allow the muscle layer to be drawn inside the cap device or band ligation device. Disruption of the muscle layer in this manner is thought to produce perforation. Similarly, when suction is applied to draw the target bleb into the cap or band ligation device, if there is no such mucosal 'lift' away from the muscularis propria then perforation might result from the mucosal resection. While many centers differ in the type of fluid used for these submucosal injections (saline, hyaluronate, or autologous blood with or without dye or epinephrine), most would agree that adequate injection volume (typically 30 cc or more) and a reliable 'lifting sign' are critically important factors in performing a safe mucosal resection (Schneider *et al.* 2006).

Mucosal resection creates a comparatively large excisional mucosal biopsy, typically with a diameter of 15–25 mm, that allows detailed histologic analysis including resection margins (Conio *et al.* 2005). EMR is indicated for superficial, well and/or moderately differentiated squamous cell carcinoma limited to the lamina propria. The role of EMR relative to other ablative techniques for the removal of Barrett's esophagus is not clearly defined given the high percentage of dysplasia noted at resection margins (Mino-Kenudson *et al.* 2005), although there are numerous publications exploring its use (Giovannini *et al.* 2004; May *et al.* 2002, 2003; Rosch *et al.* 2004). Ell *et al.* prospectively evaluated the role of EMR in 64 patients with BE: 61 with early cancer and 3 with HGD (Ell *et al.* 2000). They were divided into two groups. Group A had lesions ≤2 cm or macroscopic type I, IIA, IIB, IIC lesions ≤1 cm; well or moderately differentiated adenocarcinoma or HGD; and lesions limited to the mucosa. Group B had lesions >2 cm and limited to the mucosa and/or macroscopically type III; poorly differentiated adenocarcinoma; or infiltration of the submucosa. EMR was then performed using either the 'lift and cut' or the 'suck and ligate' technique. All patients with treated with intravenous proton pump inhibitor infusion for 48 hours. Complete local remission was achieved in 97% of the patients in group A and in 59% of those in group B. Recurrent metachronous carcinomas occurred in 17% of group A and 14% group B during a mean follow-up of 12 months. Seewald described effective ablation of Barrett's esophagus in 12 patients utilizing circumferential EMR (Seewald *et al.* 2003). Five patients had multifocal lesions and seven had none. The median number of EMR sessions was 2.5 and the median number of snare resections per EMR sessions was 5. During a follow-up of 9 months there was no recurrence of Barrett's esophagus or malignancy. However, minor bleeding occurred during 4 of the 31 EMR sessions, and two of the 12 patients developed strictures requiring dilation. These and other single-center series have reported the post-EMR incidence of major hemorrhage of 3–3.5%, minor hemorrhage reportedly 6–13%, stricture of 3.5–17% and the incidence of perforation is reportedly 0–9% (Takeshita *et al.* 1997; Nijhawan & Wang 2000; Noguchi *et al.* 2000; Buttar *et al.* 2001).

Recently, a multiband ligator with an internal hexasnare device for mucosal resection has been approved for use, with or without the use of submucosal injection. Some investigators have found that even without using submucosal injection before EMR, using multiple banded resections with this device produced larger, contiguous resection specimens (Fedi *et al.*

2006). This device, along with the traditional cap devices, were studied in a series of 303 endoscopic resections performed at the Amsterdam Medical Center between 2000 and 2005 (Peters *et al.* 2006). Mostly these were patients with Barrettt's high-grade dysplasia or early carcinoma undergoing esophageal EMR. Using the cap technique, larger specimens were resected compared with the multiband ligator snare device (mean 23 mm vs. 17 mm, respectively). However, significantly fewer complications were found after resections using the multiband ligator device (submucosal injections were used for both techniques). Acute complications were noted in 53 patients (17%) including 50 patients with bleeding that responded to endoscopic therapy but did not require transfusion. Perforation was noted in three patients, including one who required surgery. Delayed complications were found in 30 patients (10%) with stricture requiring repeated dilation and/or stent placement. Therefore, while EMR is an excellent technique for treatment of localized lesions, there are significant complications associated with its use, and serious complications (such as perforation requiring surgery) certainly may occur (Ahmad *et al.* 2002). Histopathologic analysis of resected specimens have documented totally complete resections of Barrett's disease in only a small number of cases and the vast majority of specimens feature margins involved with dysplasia or carcinoma with a high rate of tumor recurrence on follow-up (Mino-Kenudson *et al.* 2005). Therefore, after healing the post-EMR ulceration, the remainder of the residual Barrett's mucosa must also be treated with ablative therapy. In a recent study of endoscopic mucosal resection combined with argon beam coagulation in 65 patients with Barrett's high-grade dysplasia or early esophageal carcinoma over a 5-year period, recurrence of adenocarcinoma was only found in patients in whom Barrett's epithelium persisted (Wehrmann *et al.* 2006).

The development of wide-area mucosal resection (or endoscopic submucosal dissection, ESD) is emerging in the East as the primary endoscopic therapy for patients with early gastric cancer (Yamamoto *et al.* 1999, 2002; Ohkuwa *et al.* 2001; Miyamoto *et al.* 2002; Hirasaki *et al.* 2004; Yahagi *et al.* 2004) because of the limitations associated with EMR. Specifically, EMR using a cap attachment limits the size of the resected specimen to the dimension of the cap itself (around 12 mm) often leading to incomplete or piecemeal excision. This makes it very difficult to perform a complete resection with reliable lateral and deep resection margins from histologic analysis. This ambiguity regarding the completeness of resection and infiltration depth to document an R0 resection has prompted the development of ESD. Recent studies have described the use of endoscopic submucosal dissection as a new procedure that does not rely on snare techniques for dissection of submucosal tissue. This technique uses glycerin solution or sodium hyaluronate for the submucosal injection fluid followed by dissection with various devices such as an insulation-tipped needle knife (IT knife), a Hook knife, or a Flex knife (Oka *et al.* 2006). The effectiveness of en-bloc resection by ESD for large gastric cancer lesions has been described in several papers and compares favorably with the results achieved with endoscopic mucosal resection (EMR) (Wai Yan Chiu 2006). There are not yet data describing the use of ESD for esophageal cancer and much more experience will be necessary including careful prospective evaluations of complications associated with these procedures and the long-term clinical outcome and assessment of the risks for recurrent, synchronous or metachronous lesions (Rajan *et al.* 2004; Ross *et al.* 2006).

Conclusion

This section has discussed the endoscopic methods for the treatment of esophageal dysplasia and early neoplasia. To establish a clinical context for this discussion, the natural history of Barrett's esophagus is reviewed and its progression to dysplasia and invasive carcinoma. The use of conventional surgical therapy is reviewed as well. Finally, all of the currently available methods for endoscopic ablation of esophageal dysplasia and early neoplasia are categorized according to their application methods of ablation – focal ablation, field ablation, novel agents for endoscopic application and injection, mucosal resection and submucosal dissection. The clinical experience with the use of these devices is reviewed as well as their associated adverse events and complications.

As a practical matter, patients will often require evaluation and treatment with several of these techniques and devices (multimodal treatment) (Walker *et al.* 2002; Pacifico *et al.* 2003; Behrens *et al.* 2005). Patients with Barrett's high-grade dysplasia or early esophageal carcinoma will typically undergo an initial evaluation with endosonography and contrast-enhanced chest CT. Suspicious lesions (e.g. nodules) are then removed with endoscopic mucosal resection. After healing in 6–8 weeks, patients will then return for ablation of the remaining Barrett's glandular mucosa to prevent the development of metachronous disease. The method of ablation chosen requires individualization based on the anatomy of the patient and their expectations. While the use of porfimer sodium is supported by a large clinical experience, its use is associated with significant morbidity and prolonged cutaneous photosensitivity. Comparative trials will be required to determine whether these newer ablation techniques, such as radiofrequency ablation or cryotherapy, may be found to be adequate treatment alternatives that are easier to use and associated with fewer treatment-related complications. Endoscopically evident residual Barrett's glandular mucosa is not uncommon in patients who have undergone ablation therapy regardless of method. Typically, focal thermal ablation methods are required to destroy this remaining Barrett's mucosa. Caveats and concerns are discussed in order to help minimize the complications associated with the use of these technologies that hold the promise of pre-empting the development of Barrett's esophageal carcinoma.

Prognosis and follow-up

Kenneth K. Wang

Prognosis of esophageal Barrett's metaplasia and esophageal cancer

The prognosis for esophageal Barrett's metaplasia is generally good. Most patients have a very low risk of conversion to cancer, even with relatively long segments of Barrett's. The average conversion to cancer during a patient's lifetime is approximately 5–10%. For those with segments longer than 3 cm the risk is approximately 1.5 to twofold greater so therefore may be as much as a 20% lifetime risk, and for those who have a segment shorter than 1 cm the risk maybe slightly less, i.e., as low as a 2% lifetime risk.

The prognosis of patients with esophageal adenocarcinoma is poor unless invasion is caught at a mucosal stage (M1, intraepithelial neoplasia or high-grade dysplasia; M2, lamina propria; or M3, mucularis mucosa), where the prognosis remains 95% or greater. As soon as invasion preceeds past the top third of the submucosal layer, lymph nodes are often involved in the top third of the submucosal layer (Tsm1). Once the lower layer of submucosa is involved top third of the submucosal layer (Tsm3), the prognosis drops quickly to 60% or less. Once the tumour has reached muscularis propria (T2), the prognosis is less than 40% and certainly by stages 3 and 4 the overall prognosis is dismal, 20% or less, and in most cases may be as low as 8%.

Follow-up

For patients who have Barrett's esophagus the recommended length of follow-up for areas where incident cancer is high (i.e. more than 10 cancers per 100,000) the follow-up should be every 2 years. Areas where the incident cancer is low (i.e less than 10 per 100,000) follow-up can be every 3 years. The most important thing to emphasize is that the biopsy technique should be as complete as possible; the minimum recommended number of biopsies should be eight for segments of Barrett's >2 cm, but preferably a quadrantic biopsy protocol should be undertaken. Patients with low-grade dysplasia should be treated with PPI therapy and undergo endoscopic surveillance every 6 months. For patients with high-grade dysplasia the biopsy protocol should be every 3 months and adhere strictly to quadrantic biopsy protocol. If high-grade dysplasia is present at a second biopsy most investigators will now use local therapy: endoscopic mucosal resection or laser ablative therapy.

Follow-up for patients after esophagectomy whether it be endoscopic or otherwise is by upper GI endoscopy every 3 months for a year, then annually thereafter. In addition, many expert hospitals undertake CT scans at 6-monthly and 12-monthly intervals postoperatively. On some occasions where endoscopy mucosal resection has been carried out endoscopic mucosal ultrasound may be helpful, but again only in specialized centres. Where distant metastasis is suspected, such as lesions appearing in other sites, CT scanning of chest and thorax is recommended. PET is also recommended, particularly for identifying malignant pulmonary nodules and staging metastatic disease and deposits in other organs.

References

Ackroyd R, Brown NJ, Stephenson TJ, Stoddard CJ, Reed MW. (1999) Ablation treatment for Barrett oesophagus: what depth of tissue destruction is needed? *J Clin Pathol* 52: 509–12.

Adelstein D, Rice T, Rybicki L, Larto M, Ciezki J, Saxton J *et al.* (2000) Does paclitaxel improve the chemoradiotherapy of locoregionally advanced esophageal cancer? A nonrandomized comparison with fluorouracil-based therapy. *J Clin Oncol* 18: 2032–9.

Ahmad NA, Kochman ML, Long WB, Furth EE, Ginsberg GG. (2002) Efficacy, safety, and clinical outcomes of endoscopic mucosal resection: a study of 101 cases. *Gastrointest Endosc* 55: 390–6.

Ahmed R, Kim R, Duan J, Meleth S, De Los Santos J, Fiveash J. (2004) IMRT dose escalation for positive para-aortic lymph nodes in patients with locally advanced cervical cancer while reducing dose to bone marrow and other organs at risk. *Int J Radiat Oncol Biol Phys* 60: 505–12.

Ajani J, Walsh G, Komaki R *et al.* (2004) Preoperative induction of CPT-11 and cisplatin chemotherapy followed by chemoradiotherapy in patients with locoregional carcinoma of the esophagus or gastroesophageal junction. *Cancer* 100: 2347–54.

Alderson D. (2002) Observer variation in the diagnosis of superficial oesophageal adenocarcinoma: another spanner in the works? *Gut* 51: 620–1.

Allison PR. (1946) *J Thorac Surg* 15: 308.

Allison PR. (1948) Peptic ulcer of the esophagus. *Thorax* 3: 20–42.

Allison PR, Johnstone AS, Royce GB. (1943) *J Thorac Surg* 12: 432.

Allison PR, Johnstone AS. (1953) The oesophagus lined with gastric mucous membrane. *Thorax* 8: 87–101.

Al-Sarraf M, Martz K, Herskovic A *et al.* (1997) Progress report of combined chemoradiotherapy versus radiotherapy alone in patients with esophageal cancer: an intergroup study. *J Clin Oncol* 15: 277–84.

Altorki N, Skinner D. (2001) Should en bloc esophagectomy be the standard of care for esophageal carcinoma? *Ann Surg* 234(5): 581–7.

Altorki NK, Girardi L, Skinner DB. (1997) En bloc esophagectomy improves survival for stage III esophagus cancer. *J Thorac Cardiovasc Surg* 114: 948–55.

American Cancer Society (2005) *Cancer Facts and Figures 2005*. American Cancer Society, Atlanta.

American Cancer Society. (2006) *Cancer facts and figures 2006*. American Cancer Society, Atlanta.

American Joint Committee on Cancer. (2001) *Cancer Staging Manual*, 6 edn. Springer-Verlag, Chicago.

American Joint Committee on Cancer. (2002) *AJCC Cancer Staging Manual*. Springer-Verlag, New York.

Ancona E, Ruol A, Santi S *et al.* (2001) Only pathologic complete response to neoadjuvant chemotherapy improves significantly the long term survival of patients with resectable esophageal squamous cell carcinoma: final report of a randomized, controlled trial of preoperative chemotherapy versus surgery alone. *Cancer* 91: 2165–74.

Apinop C, Puttisak P, Preecha N. (1994) A prospective study of combined therapy in esophageal cancer. *Hepatogastroenterology* 41: 391–3.

Araujo C, Souhami L, Gil R *et al.* (1991) A randomized trial comparing radiation therapy versus concomitant radiation therapy and chemotherapy in carcinoma of the thoracic esophagus. *Cancer* 67: 2258–61.

Arber N, Gammon M, Hibshoosh H *et al.* (1999) Overexpression of cyclin D1 occurs in both squamous carcinomas and adenocarcinomas of the esophagus and in adenocarcinomas of the stomach. *Hum Pathol* 30: 1087–92.

Ashamalla H, Rafla S, Parikh K *et al.* (2005) The contribution of integrated PET/CT to the evolving definition of treatment volumes in radiation treatment planning in lung cancer. *Int J Radiat Oncol Biol Phys* 63: 1016–23.

Attwood SEA, Lewis CJ, Caplin S, Hemming K, Armstrong G. (2003) Argon beam plasma coagulation as therapy for high-grade dysplasia in Barrett's esophagus. *Clin Gastroenterol Hepatol* 1: 258–63.

Bailey SH, Bull DA, Harpole DH *et al.* (2003) Outcomes after esophagectomy: A ten year prospective cohort. *Ann Thorac Surg* 75: 217–22.

Bains M, Stojadinovic A, Minsky B *et al.* (2002) A phase II trial of preoperative combined-modality therapy for localized esophageal carcinoma: initial results. *J Thorac Cardiovasc Surg* 124: 270–7.

Banki F, Mason RJ, DeMeester SR *et al.* (2002) Vagal-sparing esophagectomy: a more physiologic alternative. *Ann Surg* 236: 324–35.

Barham CP, Jones RL, Biddlestone LR, Hardwick RH, Shepherd NA, Barr H. (1997) Photothermal laser ablation of Barrett's oesophagus: endoscopic and histological evidence of squamous re-epithelialisation. *Gut* 41: 281–4.

Barr H, Krasner N, Boulos PB, Chatlani P, Bown SG. (1990) Photodynamic therapy for colorectal cancer: a quantitative pilot study. *Br J Surg* 77: 93–6.

Barr H, Stone N, Rembacken B. (2005) Endoscopic therapy for Barrett's oesophagus. *Gut* 54: 875–84.

Barrett NR. (1957) The lower esophagus lined by columnar epithelium. *Surgery* 41: 881–94.

Bar-Shalom R, Yefremov N, Guralnik L *et al.* (2003) Clinical performance of PET/CT in evaluation of cancer: additional value for diagnostic imaging and patient management. *J Nucl Med* 44: 1200–9.

Bartels H, Stein HJ, Siewert JR. (2000) Risk analysis in esophageal surgery. *Recent Results Cancer Res* 155: 89–96.

Basu KK, Pick B, Bale R, West KP, De Caestecker JS. (2002) Efficacy and one year follow up of argon plasma coagulation therapy for ablation of Barrett's oesophagus: factors determining persistence and recurrence of Barrett's epithelium. *Gut* 51: 776–80.

Bates B, Detterbeck F, Bernard S, Qaqish B, Tepper J. (1996) Concurrent radiation therapy and chemotherapy followed by esophagectomy for localized esophageal carcinoma. *J Clin Oncol* 14: 156–63.

Becker CD, Barbier PA, Terrier F, Porcellini B. (1987) Patterns of recurrence of esophageal carcinoma after transhiatal esophagectomy and gastric interposition. *AJR Am J Roentgenol* 148(2): 273–7.

Bedenne L, Seitz J, Milan C *et al.* (1998) Cisplatin, 5-FU and preoperative radiotherapy in esophageal epidermoid cancer. Multicenter phase II FFCD 8804 study. *Gastroenterol Clin Biol* 22: 273–81.

Bedenne L, Michel P, Bouche O *et al.* (2002) Randomized phase III trial in locally advanced esophageal cancer: radiochemotherapy followed by surgery versus radiochemotherapy alone (FFCD 9102). *Proc Am Soc Clin Oncol* 130 (abstr).

Behrens A, May A, Gossner L *et al.* (2005) Curative treatment for high-grade intraepithelial neoplasia in Barrett's esophagus. *Endoscopy* 37: 999–1005.

Berenson MM, Johnson TD, Markowitz NR, Buchi KN, Samowitz WS. (1993) Restoration of squamous mucosa after ablation of Barrett's esophageal epithelium. *Gastroenterology* 104: 1686–91.

Bergman JJ. (2006) New developments in the endoscopic detection and treatment of early neoplasia in Barrett's oesophagus. *Scand J Gastroenterol* (Suppl): 18–24.

Bergman J, Sondermeijer C, Peters F, Ten Kate F, Fockens P. (2006) Circumferential balloon based radiofrequency ablation for Barrett's esophagus in patients with low-grade dysplasia or high-grade dysplasia with and without prior endoscopic resection using the HALO-360 ablation system. *Gastrointest Endosc* 63: AB137.

Beyer T, Townsend D, Brun T *et al.* (2000) A combined PET/CT scanner for clinical oncology. *J Nucl Med* 41: 1369–79.

Biddlestone LR, Barham CP, Wilkinson SP, Barr H, Shepherd NA. (1998) The histopathology of treated Barrett's esophagus: squamous reepithelialization after acid suppression and laser and photodynamic therapy. *Am J Surg Pathol* 22: 239–45.

Binmoeller KF, Seifert H, Seitz U, Izbicki JR, Kida M, Soehendra N. (1995) Ultrasonic esophagoprobe for TNM staging of highly stenosing esophageal carcinoma. *Gastrointest Endosc* 41(6): 547–52.

Birkmeyer JD, Siewers AE, Finlayson EVA *et al.* (2002) Hospital volume and surgical mortality in the United States. *N Engl J Med* 346: 1128–37.

Blanke C, Chiappori A, Epstein B. (1997) A phase II trial of neoajuvant paclitaxel (T) and cisplatin (P) with radiotherapy, followed by surgery (S) and postoperative T with 5-uorouracil (F) and leaucovirin (L) in patients (pts) with locally advanced esophageal cancer (LAEC). *J Clin Oncol* 16: 283 (abstr).

Blazeby JM, Farndon JR, Donovan J, Alderson D. (2000) A prospective longitudinal study examining the quality of life of patients with esophageal carcinoma. *Cancer* 88: 1781–7.

Blot WJ, Devesa SS, Kneller RW, Fraumeni JF Jr. (1991) Rising incidence of adenocarcinoma of the esophagus and gastric cardia. *JAMA* 265: 1287–9.

Bollschweiler E, Baldus SE, Schroder W, Schneider PM, Holscher AH. (2006) Staging of esophageal carcinoma: length of tumor and number of involved regional lymph nodes. Are these independent prognostic factors? *J Surg Oncol* 94(5): 355–63.

Bonavina L, Via A, Incarbone R, Saino G, Peracchia A. (2003) Results of surgical therapy in patients with Barrett's adenocarcinoma. *World J Surg* 27: 1062–6.

Borovicka J, Fischer J, Neuweiler J *et al.* (2006) Autofluorescence endoscopy in surveillance of Barrett's esophagus: a multicenter randomized trial on diagnostic efficacy. *Endoscopy* 38(9): 867–72.

Bosset J, Horiot J. (1999) Pre-operative chemoradiotherapy and total mesorectal excision surgery of rectal cancer: towards the eradication of pelvic failures? *Aust N Z J Surg* 69: 622–4.

Bosset J, Gignoux M, Triboulet J *et al.* (1997) Chemoradiotherapy followed by surgery compared with surgery alone in squamous-cell cancer of the esophagus. *N Engl J Med* 337: 161–7.

Bosset J, Lorchel F, Mantion G *et al.* (2005) Radiation and chemoradiation therapy for esophageal adenocarcinoma. *J Surg Oncol* 92: 239–45.

Bourg-Heckly G *et al.* (2000) Endoscopic ultraviolet-induced autofluorescence spectroscopy of the esophagus: tissue characterization and potential for early cancer diagnosis. *Endoscopy* 32(10): 756–65.

Bourhis JFM. (1999) The biological basis for chemoradiation. In: Mornex F, Mazeron J, Droz J, Marty M, eds. *Concomitant Chemoradiation: Current Status And Future*, pp 16–25. Elsevier, Paris.

Bowers SP, Mattar SG, Waring PJ *et al.* (2003) KTP laser ablation of Barrett's esophagus after anti-reflux surgery results in long-term loss of intestinal metaplasia. Potassium-titanyl-phosphate. *Surg Endosc* 17: 49–54.

Boynton RF, Huang Y, Blount PL *et al.* (1991) Frequent loss of heterozygosity at the retinoblastoma locus in human esophageal cancers. *Cancer Res* 51: 5766–9.

Brahme A. (2004) Recent advances in light ion radiation therapy. *Int J Radiat Oncol Biol Phys* 58: 603–13.

Brand S *et al.* (2002) Detection of high-grade dysplasia in Barrett's esophagus by spectroscopy measurement of 5-aminolevulinic acid-induced protoporphyrin IX fluorescence. *Gastrointest Endosc* 56(4): 479–87.

Brandt LJ, Kauvar DR. (1992) Laser-induced transient regression of Barrett's epithelium. *Gastrointest Endosc* 38: 619–22.

Branicki FJ, Law SY, Fok M, Poon RT, Chu KM, Wong J. (1998) Quality of life in patients with cancer of the esophagus and gastric cardia: a case for palliative resection. *Arch Surg* 133: 316–22.

Brun E, Kjellen E, Tennval J *et al.* (2002) FDG PET studies during treatment: prediction of therapy outcome in head and neck squamous cell carcinoma. *Head Neck* 24: 127–35.

Bruzzi JF, Swisher SG, Truong MT *et al.* (2007) Detection of interval distant metastases: clinical utility of integrated CT-PET imaging in patients with esophageal carcinoma after neoadjuvant therapy. *Cancer* 109(1): 125–34.

Burmeister B, Smithers B, Fitzgerald L. (2002) A randomized phase III trial of preoperative chemoradiation followed by surgery (CS-S) versus surgery alone (S) for localized resectable cancer of the esophagus. *Proc Am Soc Clin Oncol* 21: 130a (abstr).

Buttar NS, Wang KK, Lutzke LS, Krishnadath KK, Anderson MA. (2001) Combined endoscopic mucosal resection and photodynamic therapy for esophageal neoplasia within Barrett's esophagus. *Gastrointest Endosc* 54: 682–8.

Byrne JP, Armstrong GR, Attwood SE. (1998) Restoration of the normal squamous lining in Barrett's esophagus by argon beam plasma coagulation. *Am J Gastroenterol* 93: 1810–15.

Cancer Statistics 2007. (2007) *CA Cancer J Clin* 57: 43–66.

Canto MI. (2001) Methylene blue chromoendoscopy for Barrett's esophagus: coming soon to your GI unit?(comment). *Gastrointest Endosc* 54(3): 403–9.

Canto MI. (2005) Chromoendoscopy and magnifying endoscopy for Barrett's esophagus. *Clin Gastroenterol Hepatol* 3(7 Suppl 1): S12–5.

Canto MI, Gress F, Wolfsen HC. (2005) Long term outcomes of curative bare fiber porfimer sodium (Ps): photodynamic therapy (PDT) for T1N0 cancers (CA) of the esophagus and esophagogastric junction (EGJ): a multicenter prospective cohort study. *Gastrointest Endosc* 61: AB128.

Capocaccia R, Gatta G, Roazzi P *et al.* (2003) The EUROCARE-3 database: methodology of data collection, standardisation, quality control and statistical analysis. *Ann Oncol* 14: 14–27.

Catalano MF, Van Dam J, Sivak MV Jr.(1995) Malignant esophageal strictures: staging accuracy of endoscopic ultrasonography. *Gastrointest Endosc* 41(6): 535–9.

Catalano M, Alcocer E, Chak A *et al.* (1999) Evaluation of metastatic celiac axis lymph nodes in patients with esophageal carcinoma: accuracy of EUS. *Gastrointest Endosc* 50: 352–6.

Centers for Disease Control. (1989) Definitions for nosocomical infections. *Am Rev Respir Dis* 139: 1058–9.

Chak A, Wallace MB, Poneros JM. (2005a) Optical coherence tomography of Barrett's esophagus. *Endoscopy* 37(6): 587–90.

Chak A, Canto MI, Isenberg GA, Willis JE. (2005b) EUS assessment of response to chemoradiation in esophageal cancer patients. *Am J Gastroenterol* 100: 496–7; author reply 497–9.

Chalasani N *et al.* (1997) Significance of intestinal metaplasia in different areas of esophagus including esophagogastric junction. *Dig Dis Sci* 42: 603–7.

Chan KW, Lee PY, Lam AKY, Law S, Wong J, Srivastava G. (2006) Clinical relevance of Fas expression in esophageal squamous cell carcinoma. *J Clin Pathol* 59: 101–4.

Chandrasoma *et al.* (2000) Definition of histopathologic changes in gastroesophageal reflux disease. *Am J Surg Pathol* 24: 402–9.

Chang M, Lee H, Lee B, Kim Y, Lee J, Kim W. (2005) Differential protein expression between esophageal squamous cell carcinoma and dysplasia, and prognostic significance of protein markers. *Pathol Res Pract* 201: 417–25.

Chang K, Senzer N, Swisher S *et al.* (2006) Multi-center clinical trial using endoscopy (END) and endoscopic ultrasound (EUS) guided fine needle injection (FNI) of anti-tumor agent (TNFerade™) in patients with locally advanced esophageal cancer. *Gastrointest Endosc* 63: AB83.

Chao K, Majhail N, Huang C, Simpson J, Perez C, Haughey B *et al.* (2001) Intensity-modulated radiation therapy reduces late salivary toxicity without compromising tumor control in patients with oropharyngeal carcinoma: a comparison with conventional techniques. *Radiother Oncol* 61: 275–80.

Charron M, Beyer T, Bohnen N *et al.* (2000) Image analysis in patients with cancer studied with a combined PET and CT scanner. *Clin Nucl Med* 25: 905–10.

Chen X, Yang CS. (2001) Esophageal adenocarcinoma: a review and perspectives on the mechanism of carcinogenesis and chemoprevention. *Carcinogenesis* 22: 1119–29.

Chiappori A, DeVore R, Stewart J *et al.* (1996) Phase II study of neo-adjuvant cisplatin (P), 5-FU, leucovorin (LV), etoposide (E) & concurrent radiotherapy (RT) in patients with esophageal cancer. *J Clin Oncol* 15: 214.

Chirieac L, Swisher S, Ajani J *et al.* (2005) Posttherapy pathologic stage predicts survival in patients with esophageal carcinoma receiving preoperative chemoradiation. *Int J Radiat Oncol Biol Phys* 103: 1347–55.

Chobanian SJ *et al.* (1987) *In vivo* staining with toluidine blue as an adjunct to the endoscopic detection of Barrett's esophagus. *Gastrointest Endosc* 33(2): 99–101.

Choi N, Park S, Lynch T *et al.* (2004) Twice-daily radiotherapy as concurrent boost technique during two chemotherapy cycles in neoadjuvant chemoradiotherapy for resectable esophageal carcinoma: mature results of phase II study. *Int J Radiat Oncol Biol Phys* 60: 111–22.

Chong G, Cunningham D. (2005) Can cisplatin and infused 5-fluorouracil be replaced by oxaliplatin and capecitabine in the treatment of advanced oesophagogastric cancer? The REAL 2 trial. *Clin Oncol* 17: 79–80.

Christie N, Rice T, DeCamp M *et al.* (1999) M1a/M1b esophageal carcinoma: clinical relevance. *J Thorac Cardiovasc Surg* 118: 900–7.

Clark G, Peters J, Ireland A *et al.* (1994) Nodal metastasis and sites of recurrence after en-bloc esophagectomy for adenocarcinoma. *Ann Thorac Surg* 58: 646–54.

Clarke K, Smith K, Gullick W, Harris A. (2001) Mutant epidermal growth factor receptor enhances induction of vascular endothelial growth factor by hypoxia and insulin-like growth factor-1 via a PI3 kinase dependent pathway. *Br J Cancer* 84: 1322–9.

Coad RA, Woodman AC, Warner PJ, Barr H, Wright NA, Shepherd NA. (2005) On the histogenesis of Barrett's oesophagus and its associated squamous islands: a three-dimensional study of their morphological relationship with native oesophageal gland ducts. *J Pathol* 206: 388–94.

Coia L, Engstrom P, Paul A. (1991) Long term results of infusional 5-FU, mitomycin-C and radiation as primary management of esophageal cancer. *Int J Radiat Oncol Biol Phys* 20: 29–36.

Coia LR, Minsky BD, Berkey BA *et al.* (2000) Outcome of patients receiving radiation for cancer of the esophagus: results of the 1992–1994 patterns of care study. *J Clin Oncol* 18: 455–62.

Collard JM, Otte JB, Fiasse R *et al.* (2001) Skeletonizing en bloc esophagectomy for cancer. *Ann Surg* 234(1): 25–32.

Conio M, Cameron AJ, Chak A, Blanchi S, Filiberti R. (2005) Endoscopic treatment of high-grade dysplasia and early cancer in Barrett's oesophagus. *Lancet Oncol* 6: 311–21.

Cooper J, Guo M, Herskovic A *et al.* (1999) Chemoradiotherapy of locally advanced esophageal cancer: Long-term follow-up of a prospective randomized trial (RTOG 85–01). Radiation Therapy Oncology Group. *JAMA* 281: 1623–7.

Das A, Chak A. (2003) Role of endoscopic ultrasonography in the staging of esophageal cancer: a review. *Curr Opin Gastroenterol* 19(5): 474–6.

Das A, Chak A, Sivak MV, Jr., Payes J, Cooper GS. (2006) Endoscopic ultrasonography and prognosis of esophageal cancer. *Clin Gastroenterol Hepatol* 4: 695–700.

Dave UR, Williams AD, Wilson JA *et al.* (2004) Esophageal cancer staging with endoscopic MR imaging: pilot study. *Radiology* 230(1): 281–6.

DeNardi FG, Riddell RH. (1991) The normal esophagus. *Am J Surg Pathol* 15: 296–309.

Devesa S, Blot W, Fraumeni JF. (1998) Changing patterns in the incidence of esophageal and gastric carcinoma in the United States. *Cancer* 83: 2049–53.

Deyhle P, Sulser H, Sauberli H. (1974) Endoscopic snare ectomy of an early gastric cancer: A therapeutical method? *Endoscopy* 6: 195–8.

Dimick JB, Wainess RM, Upchurch GR, Jr., Iannettoni MD, Orringer MB. (2005) National trends in outcomes for esophageal resection. *Ann Thorac Surg* 79: 212–16; discussion 217–18.

Downey R, Akhurst T, Ilson D *et al.* (2003) Whole body 18FDG-PET and the response of esophageal cancer to induction therapy: results of a prospective trial. *J Clin Oncol* 21: 429–32.

Dresner S, Lamb P, Bennett M, Hayes N, Griffin S. (2001) The pattern of metastatic lymph node dissemination from adenocarcinoma of the esophagogastric junction. *Surgery* 129: 103–9.

Drewitz DJ, Sampliner RE, Garewal HS. (1997) The incidence of adenocarcinoma in Barrett's esophagus: a prospective study of 170 patients followed 4.8 years. *Am J Gastroenterol* 92: 212–15.

Driessen A, Landuyt W, Pastorekova S *et al.* (2006) Expression of carbonic anhydrase IX (CA IX), a hypoxia-related protein, rather than vascular-endothelial growth factor (VEGF), a pro-angiogenic factor, correlates with an extremely poor prognosis in esophageal and gastric adenocarcinomas. *Ann Surg* 243: 334–40.

Dulai GS, Jensen DM, Cortina G, Fontana L, Ippoliti A. (2005) Randomized trial of argon plasma coagulation vs. multipolar electrocoagulation for ablation of Barrett's esophagus. *Gastrointest Endosc* 61: 232–40.

Dunkin BJ, Martinez J, Bejarano PA, Smith CD, Chang K, Melvin WS. (2005) Thin layer ablation of human esophageal epithelium using a bipolar radiofrequency ballon device (BARRx System). *Surg Endosc* 20(1): 125–30.

Eastone JA, Horwhat JD, Haluszka O, Mathews JS, Johnston MH. (2001) Cryoablation of swine esophageal mucosa: A direct comparison to argon plasma coagulation (APC) and multipolar electrocoagulation (MPEC). *Gastrointest Endosc* 53: A3448.

Eisbruch A, Kim H, Terrell J, Marsh L, Dawson L, Ship J. (2001) Xerostomia and its predictors following parotid-sparing irradiation of head-and-neck cancer. *Int J Radiat Oncol Biol Phys* 50: 695–704.

Eisen GM. (2003) Ablation therapy for Barrett's esophagus. *Gastrointest Endosc* 58: 760–9.

Elkon D, Lee MS, Hendrickson FR. (1978) Carcinoma of the esophagus: sites of recurrence and palliative benefits after definitive radiotherapy. *Int J Radiat Oncol Biol Phys* 4: 615–20.

Ell C, May A, Gossner L *et al.* (2000) Endoscopic mucosal resection of early cancer and high-grade dysplasia in Barrett's esophagus. *Gastroenterology* 118: 670–7.

Ell C, May A, Pech O *et al.* (2007) Curative endoscopic resection of early esophageal adenocarcinomas (Barrett's cancer). *Gastrointest Endosc* 65(1): 3–10.

Eloubeidi MA. (2006) Routine EUS-guided FNA for preoperative nodal staging in patients with esophageal carcinoma: is the juice worth the squeeze? *Gastrointest Endosc* 63(2): 212–14.

Eloubeidi M, Wallace M, Hoffman B *et al.* (2001) Predictors of survival for esophageal cancer patients with and without celiac axis lymphadenopathy: impact of staging endosonography. *Ann Thorac Surg* 72: 212–20.

Endo T *et al.* (2002) Classification of Barrett's epithelium by magnifying endoscopy. *Gastrointest Endosc* 55(6): 641–7.

Falk GW, Rice TW, Goldblum JR, Richter JE. (1999) Jumbo biopsy forceps protocol still misses unsuspected cancer in Barrett's esophagus with high-grade dysplasia. *Gastrointest Endosc* 49: 170–6.

Fang W, Kato H, Tachimori Y, Igaki H, Sato H, Daiko H. (2003) Analysis of pulmonary complications after three-field lymph node dissection for esophageal cancer. *Ann Thorac Surg* 76: 903–8.

Fedi P, Abrams JA, Vakiani E, Remotti HE, Lightdale C. (2006) Endoscopic mucosal resection (E<R) in Barrett's esophagus: 'suck and cut' versus 'band and snare'. *Gastrointest Endosc* 63: AB142.

Ferguson DD *et al.* (2006) Enhanced magnification-directed biopsies do not increase the detection of intestinal metaplasia in patients with GERD. *Am J Gastroenterol* 101(7): 1611–16.

Ferlay J, Bray F, Pisani P, Parkin D. (2002) *GLOBOCAN 2002: Cancer Incidence, Mortality, and Prevalence Worldwide. IARC Cancer Base.* IARC Press, Lyon, France.

Fiorica F, Di Bona D, Schepis F *et al.* (2004) Preoperative chemoradiotherapy for oesophageal cancer: a systematic review and meta-analysis. *Gut* 53: 925–30.

Fisher RS, Bromer MQ, Thomas RM *et al.* (2003) Predictors of recurrent specialized intestinal metaplasia after complete laser ablation. *Am J Gastroenterol* 98: 1945–51.

Flamen P, Lerut A, Van Cutsem E *et al.* (2000) Utility of positron emission tomography for the staging of patients with potentially operable esophageal carcinoma. *J Clin Oncol* 18: 3202–10.

Flamen P, Van Cutsem E, Lerut A *et al.* (2002) Positron emission tomography for assessment of the response to induction radiochemotherapy in locally advanced oesopageal cancer. *Ann Oncol* 13: 361–8.

Flamen P, Lerut T, Haustermans K, Van Cutsem E, Mortelmans L. (2004) Position of positron emission tomography and other imaging diagnostic modalities in esophageal cancer. *Q J Nucl Med Mol Imaging* 48(2): 96–108.

Fleischer D. (1984) Lasers and gastroenterology. *Am J Gastroenterol* 79: 406–15.

Fleischer DE, Wang GQ, Dawsey S *et al.* (1996) Tissue band ligation followed by snare resection (band and snare): a new technique for tissue acquisition in the esophagus. *Gastrointest Endosc* 44: 68–72.

Fleischer D, Sharma VK, Reymunde A *et al.* (2006) Circumferential RF ablation for non-dysplastic Barrett's esophagus (NDBE) using the HALO360 ablation system (AIM trial): one-year follow-up of 100 patients. *Gastrointest Endosc* 63: AB127.

Fleming ID, American Joint Committee on Cancer, American Cancer Society, American College of Surgeons. (1997) *AJCC Cancer Staging Manual.* Lippincott-Raven, Philadelphia.

Forastiere A, Orringer M, Perez-Tamayo C, Urba S, Zahurak M. (1993) Preoperative chemoradiation followed by transhiatal esophagectomy for carcinoma of the esophagus: final report. *J Clin Oncol* 11: 1118–23.

Forastiere A, Heitmiller R, Lee D *et al.* (1997) Intensive chemoradiation followed by esophagectomy for squamous cell and adenocarcinoma of the esophagus. *Cancer J Sci Am* 3: 144–52.

Ganem G, Dubray B, Raoul Y *et al.* (1997) Concomitant chemoradiotherapy followed, where feasible, by surgery for cancer of the esophagus. *J Clin Oncol* 15: 701–11.

Ganz RA, Utley DS, Stern RA, Jackson J, Batts KP, Termin P. (2004) Complete ablation of esophageal epithelium with a balloon-based bipolar electrode: a phased evaluation in the porcine and in the human esophagus. *Gastrointest Endosc* 60: 1002–10.

Ganz R, Overholt B, Panjehpour M *et al.* (2006) Treatment of Barrett's esophagus and high grade dysplasia using the HALO-360 ablation system: a multi-center experience. *Gastrointest Endosc* 63: AB124.

Gao X, Qio X, Cao L *et al.* (2005) Extent of microscopic spread and lymph node metastasis in patients with esophageal and gastroesophageal junction carcinoma treated by surgical resection only. *Int J Radiat Oncol Biol Phys* 63: 277.

Gaspar LE, Nag S, Herskovic A, Mantravadi R, Speiser B. (1997) American Brachytherapy Society (ABS) consensus guidelines for brachytherapy of esophageal cancer. Clinical Research Committee, American Brachytherapy Society, Philadelphia, PA. *Int J Radiat Oncol Biol Phys* 38: 127–32.

Gaspar LE, Winter K, Kocha WI, Coia LR, Herskovic A, Graham M. (2000) A phase I/II study of external beam radiation, brachytherapy, and concurrent chemotherapy for patients with localized carcinoma of the esophagus (Radiation Therapy Oncology Group Study 9207): final report. *Cancer* 88: 988–95.

Gayed I, Liu H, Wei X. (2006) The prevalence of myocardial ischemia after concurrent chemoradiation therapy as detected by gated myocardial perfusion imaging in patients with esophageal cancer. *J Nucl Med* 47(11): 1756–62.

Geh J, Crellin A, Glynne-Jones R. (2001) Preoperative (neoadjuvant) chemoradiotherapy in esophageal cancer. *Br J Surg* 88: 338–56.

Georgakoudi I, Feld MS. (2004) The combined use of fluorescence, reflectance, and light-scattering spectroscopy for evaluating dysplasia in Barrett's esophagus. *Gastrointest Endosc Clin N Am* 14(3): 519–37.

Georgakoudi I, Van Dam J. (2003) *Characterization of dysplastic tissue morphology and biochemistry in Barrett's esophagus using diffuse reflectance and light scattering spectroscopy. Gastrointest Endosc Clin N Am* 13(2): 297–308.

Georgakoudi I *et al.*, *Fluorescence, reflectance, and light-scattering spectroscopy for evaluating dysplasia in patients with Barrett's esophagus.* Gastroenterology (2001) 120(7): 1620–9.

Gignoux M, Roussel A, Paillot B, Gillet M, Schlag P, Favre JP *et al.* The value of preoperative radiotherapy in esophageal cancer: results of a study of the E.O.R.T.C. World J Surg (1987) 11(4): 426–32.

Ginsberg GG, Barkun AN, Bosco JJ *et al.* (2002) The argon plasma coagulator: February 2002. *Gastrointest Endosc* 55: 807–10.

Giovannini M, Bories E, Pesenti C *et al.* (2004) Circumferential endoscopic mucosal resection in Barrett's esophagus with high-grade intraepithelial neoplasia or mucosal cancer. Preliminary results in 21 patients. *Endoscopy* 36: 782–7.

Glickman JN, Shahsafaei A, Odze RD. (2003) Mucin core peptide expression can help differentiate Barrett's esophagus from intestinal metaplasia of the stomach. *Am J Surg Pathol* 27: 1357–65.

Glimelius B, Ekstrom K, Hoffman K *et al.* (1997) Randomized comparison between chemotherapy plus best supportive care with best supportive care in advanced gastric cancer. *Ann Oncol* 8: 163–8.

Goldblum JR *et al.* (1998) Inflammation and intestinal metaplasia of the gastric cardia: the role of gastroesophageal reflux and *H. pylori* infection. *Gastroenterology* 114: 633–9.

Goldstein NS. (2000) Gastric cardia intestinal metaplasia: Biopsy follow-up of 85 patients. *Mod Pathol* 13: 1072–9.

Goldstein NS, Karim R. (1999) Gastric cardia inflammation and intestinal metaplasia: associations with reflux esophagitis and *Helicobacter pylori. Mod Pathol* 12: 1017–24.

Gossner L, May A, Stolte M, Seitz G, Hahn EG, Ell C. (1999) KTP laser destruction of dysplasia and early cancer in columnar-lined Barrett's esophagus. *Gastrointest Endosc* 49: 8–12.

Grade AJ, Shah IA, Medlin SM, Ramirez FC. (1999) The efficacy and safety of argon plasma coagulation therapy in Barrett's esophagus. *Gastrointest Endosc* 50: 18–22.

Grana L, Ablin RJ, Goldman S, Milhouse E Jr. (1981) Freezing of the esophagus: histological changes and immunological response. *Int Surg* 66: 295–301.

Grills I, Yan D, Martinez A, Vicini F, Wong J, Kestin L. (2003) Potential for reduced toxicity and dose escalation in the treatment of inoperable non-small-cell lung cancer: a comparison of intensity-modulated radiation therapy (IMRT), 3D conformal radiation, and elective nodal irradiation. *Int J Radiat Oncol Biol Phys* 57: 875–90.

Grosu A-L, Piert M, Weber WA, Jeremic B, Picchio M, Schratzenstaller U *et al.* (2005) Positron emission tomography for radiation treatment planning. *Strahlenther Onkol* 181: 483–99.

Guelrud M *et al.* (2001) Enhanced magnification endoscopy: a new technique to identify specialized intestinal metaplasia in Barrett's esophagus. *Gastrointest Endosc* 53(6): 559–65.

Hage M, Siersema PD, Van Dekken H *et al.* (2004) 5-aminolevulinic acid photodynamic therapy versus argon plasma coagulation for ablation of Barrett's oesophagus: a randomised trial. *Gut* 53: 785–90.

Hagen JA, Peters JH, DeMeester TR. (1993) Superiority of extended en bloc esophagogastrectomy for carcinoma of the lower esophagus and cardia. *J Thorac Cardiovasc Surg* 106(5): 850–8.

Hagen JA, DeMeester SR, Peters JH, Chandrasoma P, DeMeester TR. (2001) Curative resection for esophageal adenocarcinoma: analysis of 100 en bloc esophagectomies. *Ann Surg* 234: 520–30.

Hall E. (1993) *Radiobiology for the Radiologist*, 4th edn. Lippincott Williams & Wilkins, New York.

Hany TF, Steinert HC, Goerres GW, Buck A, von Schulthess GK. (2002) PET diagnostic accuracy: improvement with in-line PET-CT system: initial results. *Radiology* 225: 575–81.

Haringsma J. (2002) Barrett's oesophagus: new diagnostic and therapeutic techniques.(comment). *Scand J Gastroenterol* (Suppl) 236: 9–14.

Harrison R, Perry I, Haddadin W, *et al.* (2007) Detection of intestinal metaplasia in Barrett's esophagus: an observational comparator study suggests a minimum of eight biopsies. *Am J Gastroenterol* 102: 1154–61.

Harris KM, Kelly S, Berry E *et al.* (1998) Systematic review of endoscopic ultrasound in gastro-esophageal cancer. *Health Technol Assess* 2: i–iv.

Haustermans K, Lerut A. (2003) Esophageal tumors. In: Brady L, Heilmann H, Molls M, eds. *Clinical Target Volumes in Conformal and Intensity Modulated Radiation Therapy: a Clinical Guide to Cancer Treatment*, pp 107–19. Springer, New York.

Heath E, Burtness B, Heitmiller R *et al.* (2000) Phase II evaluation of preoperative chemoradiation and postoperative adjuvant chemotherapy for squamous cell and adenocarcinoma of the esophagus. *J Clin Oncol* 18: 868–76.

Heier SK, Rothman KA, Heier LM, Rosenthal WS. (1995) Photodynamic therapy for obstructing esophageal cancer: light dosimetry and randomized comparison with Nd:YAG laser therapy. *Gastroenterology* 109: 63–72.

Hemminger LL, Wolfsen HC. (2002) Photodynamic therapy for Barrett's esophagus and high grade dysplasia: results of a patient satisfaction survey. *Gastroenterol Nurs* 25: 139–41.

Hennequin C, Gayet B, Sauvanet A, Blazy A, Perniceni T, Panis Y *et al.* (2001) Impact on survival of surgery after concomitant chemoradiotherapy for locally advanced cancers of the esophagus. *Int J Radiat Oncol Biol Phys* 49: 657–64.

Herskovic A, Martz K, Al-Sarraf M *et al.* (1992) Combined chemotherapy and radiotherapy compared with radiotherapy alone in patients with cancer of the esophagus. *N Engl J Med* 326: 1593–8.

Hirasaki S, Tanimizu M, Moriwaki T *et al.* (2004) Efficacy of clinical pathway for the management of mucosal gastric carcinoma treated with endoscopic submucosal dissection using an insulated-tip diathermic knife. *Intern Med* 43: 1120–5.

Hirota WK *et al.* (1999) Specialized intestinal metaplasia; dysplasia and cancer of the esophagus and esophagogastric junction; prevalence and clinical data. *Gastroenterology* 116: 277–85.

Hoff S, Stewart J, Sawyers J *et al.* (1993) Preliminary results with neoadjuvant therapy and resection for esophageal carcinoma. *Ann Thorac Surg* 56: 282–6.

Hoffman PC, Haraf DJ, Ferguson MK, Drinkard LC, Vokes EE. (1998) Induction chemotherapy, surgery, and concomitant chemoradiotherapy for carcinoma of the esophagus: a long-term analysis. *Ann Oncol* 9: 647–51.

Hofstetter W, Swisher SG, Correa AM *et al.* (2002) Treatment outcomes of resected esophageal cancer. *Ann Surg* 236(3): 376–84.

Holscher AH, Bollschweiler E, Schneider PM, Siewert JR. (1997) Early adenocarcinoma in Barrett's oesophagus. *Br J Surg* 84: 1470–3.

Hong D, Lunagomez S, Kim E *et al.* (2005) Value of baseline positron emission tomography for predicting overall survival in patient with nonmetastatic esophageal or gastroesophageal junction carcinoma. *Cancer* 104: 1620–6.

Horstmann O, Verreet PR, Becker H, Ohmann C, Roher HD. (1995) Transhiatal oesophagectomy compared with transthoracic resection and systematic lymphadenectomy for the treatment of oesophageal cancer. *Eur J Surg* 161(8): 557–67.

Huang H, Wang L, Tian H *et al.* (2005) Expression of retinoic acid receptor-beta mRNA and p16, p53, Ki67 proteins in esophageal carcinoma and its precursor lesions. *Chinese Journal of Oncology (Zhonghua Zhong Liu Za Zhi)* 27: 152–5.

Huang X-P, Zhao C-X, Li Q-J *et al.* (2006) Alteration of RPL14 in squamous cell carcinomas and preneoplastic lesions of the esophagus. *Gene* 366: 161–8.

Hug E, Slater J. (2000) Proton radiation therapy for chordomas and chondrosarcomas of the skull base. *Neurosurg Clin N Am* 11: 627–38.

Hulscher JB, van Sandick LW, Tijssen JG. (2000) The recurrence pattern of esophageal carcinoma after transhiatal resection. *J Am Coll Surg* 191: 143–8.

Hulscher JB, van Sandick JW, de Boer AG *et al.* (2002) Extended transthoracic resection compared with limited transhiatal resection for adenocarcinoma of the esophagus. *N Engl J Med* 347(21): 1662–9.

Hur C, Nishioka NS, Gazelle GS. (2003) Cost-effectiveness of photodynamic therapy for treatment of Barrett's esophagus with high grade dysplasia. *Dig Dis Sci* 48: 1273–83.

Iascone C, Demeester TR, Little AG, Skinner DB. (1983) Barrett's esophagus. Functional assessment, proposed pathogenesis, and surgical therapy. *Arch Surg* 118: 543–9.

Ilson DH, Bains M, Kelsen DP *et al.* (2003) Phase I trial of escalating-dose irinotecan given weekly with cisplatin and concurrent radiotherapy in locally advanced esophageal cancer. *J Clin Oncol* 21: 2926–32.

Inoue H. (1998) Endoscopic mucosal resection for esophageal and gastric mucosal cancers. *Can J Gastroenterol* 12: 355–9.

Inoue H, Endo M. (1990) Endoscopic esophageal mucosal resection using a transparent tube. *Surg Endosc* 4: 198–201.

Inoue H, Endo M, Takeshita K, Yoshino K, Muraoka Y, Yoneshima H. (1992) A new simplified technique of endoscopic esophageal mucosal resection using a cap-fitted panendoscope (EMRC). *Surg Endosc* 6: 264–5.

Inoue H, Takeshita K, Hori H, Muraoka Y, Yoneshima H, Endo M. (1993) Endoscopic mucosal resection with a cap-fitted panendoscope for esophagus, stomach, and colon mucosal lesions. *Gastrointest Endosc* 39: 58–62.

Inoue H, Noguchi O, Saito N, Takeshita K, Endo M. (1994) Endoscopic mucosectomy for early cancer using a pre-looped plastic cap. *Gastrointest Endosc* 40: 263–4.

Inoue H, Kawano T, Tani M, Takeshita K, Iwai T. (1999a) Endoscopic mucosal resection using a cap: techniques for use and preventing perforation. *Can J Gastroenterol* 13: 477–80.

Inoue H, Tani M, Nagai K *et al.* (1999b) Treatment of esophageal and gastric tumors. *Endoscopy* 31: 47–55.

Inoue H *et al.* (2006) Endoscopic *in vivo* evaluation of tissue atypia in the esophagus using a newly designed integrated endocytoscope: a pilot trial. *Endoscopy* 38(9): 891–5.

Isenberg GA. (2004) Catheter-probe-assisted endoluminal US. *Gastrointest Endosc* 60(4): 608–22.

Isenberg G *et al.* (2005) Accuracy of endoscopic optical coherence tomography in the detection of dysplasia in Barrett's esophagus: a prospective, double-blinded study [see comment]. *Gastrointest Endosc* 62(6): 825–31.

Izquierdo MA, Marcuello E, Gomez de Segura G *et al.* (1993) Unresectable nonmetastatic squamous cell carcinoma of the esophagus managed by sequential chemotherapy (cisplatin and bleomycin) and radiation therapy. *Cancer* 71: 287–92.

Izzo J, Malhotra U, Wu T *et al.* (2005) Impact of cyclin D1 A870G polymorphism in esophageal adenocarcinoma tumorigenesis. *Semin Oncol* 32 (6 Suppl 9): S11–15.

Javaid B, Watt P, Krasner N. (2002) Photodynamic therapy (PDT) for oesophageal dysplasia and early carcinoma with mTHPC (m-tetrahydroxyphenyl chlorin): a preliminary study. *Lasers Med Sci* 17: 51–6.

Jiao X, Eslami A, Ioffe O *et al.* (2003) Immunohistochemistry analysis of micrometastasis in pretreatment lymph nodes from patients with esophageal cancer. *Ann Thorac Surg* 76(4): 996–9.

Jin J, Liao Z, Zhang Z *et al.* (2004) Induction chemotherapy improved outcomes of patients with resectable esophageal cancer who received chemoradiotherapy followed by surgery. *Int J Radiat Oncol Biol Phys* 60: 427–36.

Johansson J, DeMeester TR, Hagen JA *et al.* (2004) En bloc vs transhiatal esophagectomy for stage T3 N1 adenocarcinoma of the distal esophagus. *Arch Surg* 139(6): 627–31.

John M, Flam M, Mowry P *et al.* (1989) Radiotherapy alone and chemoradiation for nonmetastatic esophageal carcinoma. A critical review of chemoradiation. *Cancer* 63: 2397–2403.

Johnston MH. (2003) Cryotherapy and other newer techniques. *Gastrointest Endosc Clin N Am* 13: 491–504.

Johnston MH. (2005a) Technology insight: ablative techniques for Barrett's esophagus–current and emerging trends. *Nat Clin Pract Oncol* 2: 323–30.

Johnston MH. (2005b) Technology insight: ablative techniques for Barrett's esophagus–current and emerging trends. *Nat Clin Pract Gastroenterol Hepatol* 2: 323–30.

Johnston MH *et al.* (1996) The prevalence and clinical characteristics of short segments of specialized intestinal metaplasia in the distal esophagus on routine endoscopy. *Am J Gastroenterol* 91: 1507–11.

Johnston MH, Schoenfeld P, Mysore JV, Kita JA, Dubois A. (1997) Endoscopic cryotherapy: a new technique for tissue ablation in the esophagus. *Am J Gastroenterol* 92: A44.

Johnston CM, Schoenfeld LP, Mysore JV, Dubois A. (1999a) Endoscopic spray cryotherapy: a new technique for mucosal ablation in the esophagus. *Gastrointest Endosc* 50: 86–92.

Johnston M, Horwhat JD, Dubois A, Schoenfeld P. (1999b) Endoscopic cryotherapy in the swine esophagus: a follow-up study. *Gastrointest Endosc* 49: AB126.

Johnston MH, Horwhat JD, Haluszka O, Moses FM. (2000) Depth of injury following spray cryotherapy: EUS assisted evaluation of mucosal ablation and subsequent healing in the swine model. *Gastrointest Endosc* 51: AB98.

Johnston MH, Eastone JA, Horwhat JD. (2003) Reversal of Barrett's esophagus with cryotherapy. *Am J Gastroenterol* 98: A30, S11.

Johnston MH, Eastone JA, Horwhat JD, Cartledge J, Mathews JS, Foggy JR. (2005) Cryoablation of Barrett's esophagus: a pilot study. *Gastrointest Endosc* 62: 842–8.

Johnston MH, Cash BD, Horwhat JD, Johnston LR, Dykes CA, Mays HS. (2006) Cryoablation of Barrett's esophagus (BE). *Gastroenterology* 130: A640.

Kahaleh M, Van Laethem JL, Nagy N, Cremer M, Deviere J. (2002) Long-term follow-up and factors predictive of recurrence in Barrett's esophagus treated by argon plasma coagulation and acid suppression. *Endoscopy* 34: 950–5.

Kaifi JT, Yekebas EF, Schurr P *et al.* (2005) Tumor-cell homing to lymph nodes and bone marrow and cxcr4 expression in esophageal cancer. *J Natl Cancer Inst* 97: 1840–7.

Kaklamanos IG, Walker GR, Ferry K, Franceschi D, Livingstone AS. (2003) Neoadjuvant treatment for resectable cancer of the esophagus and the gastroesophageal junction: a meta-analysis of randomized clinical trials. *Ann Surg Oncol* 10: 754–61.

Kantsevoy SV, Cruz-Correa MR, Vaughn CA, Jagannath SB, Pasricha PJ, Kalloo AN. (2003) Endoscopic cryotherapy for the treatment of bleeding mucosal vascular lesions of the GI tract: a pilot study. *Gastrointest Endosc* 57: 403–6.

Kara MA, Bergman JJ. (2006) Autofluorescence imaging and narrow-band imaging for the detection of early neoplasia in patients with Barrett's esophagus. *Endoscopy* 38(6): 627–31.

Kara MA, Peters FP, Rosmolen WD *et al.* (2005) High-resolution endoscopy plus chromoendoscopy or narrow-band imaging in Barrett's esophagus: a prospective randomized crossover study. *Endoscopy* 37: 929–36.

Kara MA, Ennahachi M, Fockens P, Ten Kate FJ, Bergman JJ. (2006a) Detection and classification of the mucosal and vascular patterns (mucosal morphology) in Barrett's esophagus by using narrow band imaging. *Gastrointest Endosc* 64: 155–66.

Kara MA, Peters FP, Fockens P, Ten Kate FJ, Bergman JJ. (2006b) Endoscopic video-autofluorescence imaging followed by narrow band imaging for detecting early neoplasia in Barrett's esophagus. *Gastrointest Endosc* 64: 176–85.

Katada C, Muto M, Manabe T, Ohtsu A, Yoshida S. (2005) Local recurrence of squamous-cell carcinoma of the esophagus after EMR. *Gastrointest Endosc* 61(2): 219–25.

Kaur T, Khanduja K, Kaushik T *et al.* (2006) P53, COX-2, iNOS protein expression changes and their relationship with anti-oxidant enzymes in surgically and multi-modality treated esophageal carcinoma patients. *J Chemother* 18: 74–84.

Keller S, Ryan L, Coia L *et al.* (1998) High dose chemoradiotherapy followed by esophagectomy for adenocarcinoma of the esophagus and gastroesophageal junction: results of a phase II study of the Eastern Cooperative Oncology Group. *Cancer* 83: 1908–16.

Kelsen DP. (2005) Multimodality therapy of local regional esophageal cancer. *Semin Oncol* 32(6 Suppl 9): S6–10.

Kelsen D, Atiq OT, Saltz L *et al.* (1992) FAMTX versus etoposide, doxorubicin, cisplatin: a random assignment trial in gastric cancer. *J Clin Oncol* 10: 541–8.

Kelsen D, Ginsberg R, Pajak T *et al.* (1998a) Chemotherapy followed by surgery compared with surgery alone for localized esophageal cancer. *N Engl J Med* 339: 1979–84.

Kelsen D, Iison D, Minsky B, Lipton R. (1998b) Phase I trial of combined modality therapy for localized esophagel cancer: Radiation therapy + concurrent cisplatin and escalating doses of 96 hour infusional paclitaxel. *Proc Am Soc Clin Oncol* 17: 260a (abstr).

Kelty CJ, Ackroyd R, Brown NJ, Stephenson TJ, Stoddard CJ, Reed MW. (2004) Endoscopic ablation of Barrett's oesophagus: a randomized-controlled trial of photodynamic therapy vs. argon plasma coagulation. *Aliment Pharmacol Ther* 20: 1289–96.

Kendall C *et al.* (2003) Raman spectroscopy, a potential tool for the objective identification and classification of neoplasia in Barrett's oesophagus. *J Pathol* 200(5): 602–9.

Kiesslich R, Neurath MF. (2006) Chromoendoscopy in Barrett's oesophagus: is cresyl violet the magic bullet?(comment). *Dig Liver Dis* 38(5): 301–2.

Kiesslich R *et al.* (2005) Confocal laser endomicroscopy. *Gastrointest Endosc Clin N Am* 15(4): 715–31.

Kiesslich R *et al.* (2006) *In vivo* histology of Barrett's esophagus and associated neoplasia by confocal laser endomicroscopy. *Clin Gastroenterol Hepatol* 4(8): 979–87.

Kilgore SP, Ormsby AH, Gramlich TL *et al.* (2000) The gastric cardia: fact or fiction? *Am J Gastroenterol* 95: 921–4.

King RM, Pairolero PC, Trastek VF, Payne WS, Bernatz PE. (1987) Ivor Lewis esophagogastrectomy for carcinoma of the esophagus: early and late functional results. *Ann Thorac Surg* 44: 119–22.

Kleespies A, Bruns C, Jauch K. (2005) Clinical significance of VEGF-A, -C and -D expression in esophageal malignancies. *Onkologie* 28: 281–8.

Kleinberg L, Knisely J, Heitmiller R *et al.* (2003) Mature survival results with preoperative cisplatin, protracted infusion 5-fluorouracil, and 44-Gy radiotherapy for esophageal cancer. *Int J Radiat Oncol Biol Phys* 60: 427–36.

Kluetz P, Meltzer C, Villemagne V *et al.* (2000) Combined PET/CT imaging in oncology. impact on patient management. *Clin Positron Imaging* 3: 223–30.

Klump B, Hsieh C, Holzmann K, Gregor M, Porschen R. (1998) Hypermethylation of the CDKN2/p16 promoter during neoplastic progression in Barrett's esophagus. *Gastroenterology* 115: 1381–6.

Komaki R, Janjan N, Ajani J *et al.* (2000) Phase I study of irinotecan and concurrent radiation therapy for upper GI tumors. *Oncology* 14: 34–7.

Konski A, Chen L, Doss M, Palacio E, Milestone B, Freedman G. (2003) *Preliminary analysis of incorporating PET and MRI scans into the treatment planning process for esophageal carcinoma.* American Radium Society 85th Annual Meeting, Houston, Texas.

Kovacs BJ, Chen YK, Lewis TD, Deguzman LJ, Thompson KS. (1999) Successful reversal of Barrett's esophagus with multipolar electrocoagulation despite inadequate acid suppression. *Gastrointest Endosc* 49: 547–53.

Koyanagi K, Ozawa S, Ando N, Takeuchi H, Ueda M, Kitajima M. (1999) Clinical significance of telomerase activity in the non-cancerous epithelial region of oesophageal squamous cell carcinoma. *Br J Surg* 86: 674–9.

Krasna MJ, Reed CE, Nedzwiecki D *et al.*; CALGB Thoracic Surgeons. (2001) CALGB 9380: a prospective trial of the feasibility of thoracoscopy/laparoscopy in staging esophageal cancer. *Ann Thorac Surg* 71(4): 1073–9.

Krishnadath KK, Wang KK, Taniguchi K *et al.* (2000) Persistent genetic abnormalities in Barrett's esophagus after photodynamic therapy. *Gastroenterology* 119: 624–30.

Kubba AK. (1999) Role of photodynamic therapy in the management of gastrointestinal cancer. *Digestion* 60: 1–10.

Kumagai Y, Monma K, Kawada K. (2004) Magnifying chromoendoscopy of the esophagus: in-vivo pathological diagnosis using an endocytoscopy system. *Endoscopy* 36(7): 590–4.

Kupelian P, Reddy C, Carlson T, Altsman K, Willoughby T. (2002) Preliminary observations on biochemical relapse-free survival rates after short-course intensity-modulated radiotherapy (70 Gy at 2.5 Gy/fraction) for localized prostate cancer. *Int J Radiat Oncol Biol Phys* 53: 904–12.

Lah JJ, Kuo JV, Chang KJ, Nguyen PT. (2005) EUS-guided brachytherapy. *Gastrointest Endosc* 62: 805–8.

Lardinois D, Weder W, Hany TF, Kamel EM, Korom S, Seifert B *et al.* (2003) Staging of non-small-cell lung cancer with integrated positron-emission tomography and computed tomography. *N Engl J Med* 348: 2500–7.

Larghi A, Waxman I. (2005) Endoscopic mucosal resection: treatment of neoplasia. *Gastrointest Endosc Clin N Am* 15: 431–54, viii.

Larghi A, Lightdale CJ, Memeo L, Bhagat G, Okpara N, Rotterdam H. (2005) EUS followed by EMR for staging of high-grade dysplasia and early cancer in Barrett's esophagus. *Gastrointest Endosc* 62(1): 16–23.

Law S, Fok M, Chow S, Chu K, Wong J. (1997) Preoperative chemotherapy versus surgical therapy alone for squamous cell carcinoma of the esophagus: a prospective randomized trial. *J Thorac Cardiovasc Surg* 114: 210–17.

Law S, Wong K, Kwok K, Chu K, Wong J. (2004) Predictive factors for postoperative pulmonary complications and mortality after esophagectomy for cancer. *Ann Surg* 240: 791–800.

Le Prise E, Etienne P, Meunier B *et al.* (1994) A randomized study of chemotherapy, radiation therapy, and surgery versus surgery for localized squamous cell carcinoma of the esophagus. *Cancer* 73: 1779–84.

Lee H, Vaporciyan A, Cox J *et al.* (2003) Postoperative pulmonary complications after preoperative chemoradiation for esophageal carcinoma: correlation with pulmonary dose–volume histogram parameters. *Int J Radiat Oncol Biol Phys* 57: 1317–22.

Leibel S, Fuks Z, Zelefsky M *et al.* (2002) Intensity-modulated radiotherapy. *Cancer J* 8: 164–76.

Lerut TE, Van Lanschot JJ. (2004) Chronic symptoms after subtotal or partial oesophagectomy: diagnosis and treatment. *Best Pract Res Clin Gastroenterol* 18: 901–15.

Lerut T, De Leyn P, Coosemans W, Van Raemdonck D, Scheys I, LeSaffre E. (1992) Surgical strategies in esophageal carcinoma with emphasis on radical lymphadenectomy. *Ann Surg* 216: 583–90.

Liao Z, Jin J, Zhang Z *et al.* (2002) Does surgical resection in addition to concurrent chemoradiation increase survival in patients with clinical stage II - III esophageal cancer? 84th Annual Meeting of American Radium Society, Puerto Rico. *The Cancer Journal* 8(6).

Liao Z, Zhang Z, Jin J *et al.* (2004) Esophagectomy after concurrent chemoradiotherapy improves locoregional control in clinical stage II or III esophageal cancer patients. *Int J Radiat Oncol Biol Phys* 60: 1484–93.

Liao Z, Liu H, Swisher SG *et al.* (2006) Polymorphism at the 3'-UTR of the thymidylate synthase gene: A potential predictor for outcomes in Caucasian patients with esophageal adenocarcinoma treated with preoperative chemoradiation. *Int J Radiat Oncol Biol Phys* 64: 700–8.

Liu H, Wang X, Dong L *et al.* (2004) Feasibility of sparing lung and other thoracic structures with intensity-modulated radiotherapy for non-small-cell lung cancer. *Int J Radiat Oncol Biol Phys* 58: 1268–79.

Lovat L, Bown S. (2004) Elastic scattering spectroscopy for detection of dysplasia in Barrett's esophagus. *Gastrointest Endosc Clin N Am* 14(3): 507–17.

Lovat LB, Jamieson NF, Novelli MR *et al.* (2005) Photodynamic therapy with m-tetrahydroxyphenyl chlorin for high-grade dysplasia and early cancer in Barrett's columnar lined esophagus. *Gastrointest Endosc* 62: 617–23.

Lovat LB *et al.* (2006) Elastic scattering spectroscopy accurately detects high grade dysplasia and cancer in Barrett's oesophagus. *Gut* 55(8): 1078–83.

Lujan A, Mundt A, Yamada S, Rotmensch J, Roeske J. (2003) Intensity-modulated radiotherapy as a means of reducing dose to bone marrow in gynecologic patients receiving whole pelvic radiotherapy. *Int J Radiat Oncol Biol Phys* 57: 516–21.

Luketich J, Nguyen N, Ramanathan R *et al.* (1998) Induction and post-operative chemotherapy with paclitaxel, 5-fluorourcial and cisplatin regimen for carcinoma of the esophagus. *Proc Am Soc Clin Oncol* 17: 295a.

Luketich JD, Friedman DM, Weigel TL *et al.* (1999) Evaluation of distant metastases in esophageal cancer: 100 consecutive positron emission tomography scans. *Ann Thorac Surg* 68: 1133–6.

Luketich JD, Alvelo-Rivera M, Buenaventura PO *et al.* (2003) Minimally invasive esophagectomy: outcomes in 222 patients. *Ann Surg* 238: 486–94; discussion 494–485.

Luman W, Lessels AM, Palmer KR. (1996a) Failure of Nd-YAG photocoagulation therapy as treatment for Barrett's oesophagus–a pilot study. *Eur J Gastroenterol Hepatol* 8: 619–21.

Luman W, Lessels AM, Palmer KR. (1996b) Failure of Nd-YAG photocoagulation therapy as treatment for Barrett's oesophagus–a pilot study. *Eur J Gastroenterol Hepatol* 8: 627–30.

Luthra R, Wu T-T, Luthra MG *et al.* (2006) Gene expression profiling of localized esophageal carcinomas: association with pathologic response to preoperative chemoradiation. *J Clin Oncol* 24: 259–67.

Lynch T, Choi N, Wright M *et al.* (1997) A phase I/II trial of preoperative taxol (T), 5-FU (F) and concurrent boost radiation (XRT) in esophageal cancer. *Proc Am Soc Clin Oncol* 16: 261a.

Ma BBY, Bristow RG, Kim J, Siu LL. (2003) Combined-modality treatment of solid tumors using radiotherapy and molecular targeted agents. *J Clin Oncol* 21: 2760–6.

Maerz LL, Deveney CW, Lopez RR, McConnell DB. (1993) Role of computed tomographic scans in the staging of esophageal and proximal gastric malignancies. *Am J Surg* 165(5): 558–60.

Maingon P, D'hombres A, Truc G *et al.* (2000) High dose rate brachytherapy for superficial cancer of the esophagus. *Int J Radiat Oncol Biol Phys* 46: 71–6.

Maish MS, DeMeester SR. (2004) Endoscopic mucosal resection as a staging technique to determine the depth of invasion of esophageal adenocarcinoma. *Ann Thorac Surg* 78(5): 1777–82.

Makuuchi H. (1996) Esophageal endoscopic mucosal resection (EEMR) tube. *Surg Laparosc Endosc* 6: 160–1.

Malaisrie S, Hofstetter W, Correa A *et al.* (2006) Endoscopic ultrasonography-identified celiac adenopathy remains a poor prognostic factor despite preoperative chemoradiotherapy in esophageal adenocarcinoma. *J Thorac Cardiovasc Surg* 131: 65–72.

Malhi-Chowla N, Wolfsen HC, Devault KR. (2001) Esophageal dysmotility in patients undergoing photodynamic therapy. *Mayo Clin Proc* 76: 987–9.

Mang TS. (2004) Laser and light sources for PDT. *Photodiag Photodyn Ther*: 1: 43–8.

Manner H, May A, Miehlke S *et al.* (2006) Ablation of nonneoplastic Barrett's mucosa using argon plasma coagulation with concomitant esomeprazole therapy (APBANEX): a prospective multicenter evaluation. *Am J Gastroenterol* 101: 1762–9.

de Manzoni G, Morgagni P, Roviello F *et al.* (1998) Nodal abdominal spread in adenocarcinoma of the cardia. Results of a multicenter prospective study. *Gastric Cancer* 1: 146–51.

Mariette C, Balon J, Piessen G, Fabre S, Van Seuningen I, Triboulet J. (2003) Pattern of recurrence following complete resection of esophageal carcinoma and factors predictive of recurrent disease. *Cancer* 97: 1616–23.

Martin TR, Onstad GR, Silvis SE, Vennes JA. (1976) Lift and cut biopsy technique for submucosal sampling. *Gastrointest Endosc* 23: 29–30.

Matsubara T, Ueda M, Yanagida O, Nakajima T, Nishi M. (1994) How extensive should lymph node dissection be for cancer of the thoracic esophagus? *J Thorac Cardiovasc Surg* 107(4): 1073–8.

Mauer AM, Weichselbaum RR. (2002) Multimodality therapy for carcinoma of the esophagus. In: Steele GD, Phillips TL, Chabner BA, eds. *American Cancer Society Atlas of Clinical Oncology. Cancer of the Upper Gastrointestinal Tract*, pp 157–83. BC Decker Inc., Chicago.

May A, Gossner L, Pech O *et al.* (2002) Local endoscopic therapy for intraepithelial high-grade neoplasia and early adenocarcinoma in Barrett's oesophagus: acute-phase and intermediate results of a new treatment approach. *Eur J Gastroenterol Hepatol* 14: 1085–91.

May A, Gossner L, Behrens A *et al.* (2003) A prospective randomized trial of two different endoscopic resection techniques for early stage cancer of the esophagus. *Gastrointest Endosc* 58: 167–75.

McCaughan JS Jr, Ellison EC, Guy JT *et al.* (1996) Photodynamic therapy for esophageal malignancy: a prospective twelve-year study. *Ann Thorac Surg* 62: 1005–9.

Meluch A, Hainsworth J, Gray J *et al.* (1999) Preoperative combined modality therapy with paclitaxel, carboplatin, prolonged infusion 5-fluorouracil, and radiation therapy in localized esophageal cancer: preliminary results of a Minnie Pearl Cancer Research Network phase II trial. *Cancer J Sci Am* 5: 84–91.

Meluch A, Greco F, Gray J *et al.* (2003) Preoperative therapy with concurrent paclitaxel/carboplatin/infusional 5-FU and radiation therapy in locoregional esophageal cancer: final results of a Minnie Pearl Cancer Research Network phase II trial. *Cancer J* 9: 251–60.

Micaily B, Miyamoto C, Valicenti RK, Brady LW. (1994) Intracavitary brachytherapy for squamous cell carcinoma of the esophagus. *Am J Clin Oncol* 17: 170–4.

Michopoulos S, Tsibouris P, Bouzakis H, Sotiropoulou M, Kralios N. (1999) Complete regression of Barrett's esophagus with heat probe thermocoagulation: mid-term results. *Gastrointest Endosc* 50: 165–72.

Miller C. (1962) Carcinoma of the esophagus and gastric cardia. *Br J Surg* 49: 507–22.

Mino-Kenudson M, Brugge WR, Puricelli WP *et al.* (2005) Management of superficial Barrett's epithelium-related neoplasms by endoscopic mucosal resection: clinicopathologic analysis of 27 cases. *Am J Surg Pathol* 29: 680–6.

Minsky B, Pajak T, Ginsberg R *et al.* (2002) INT 0123 (Radiation Therapy Oncology Group 94–05) phase III trial of combined-modality therapy for esophageal cancer: high-dose versus standard-dose radiation therapy. *J Clin Oncol* 20: 1167–74.

Miyamoto S, Muto M, Hamamoto Y *et al.* (2002) A new technique for endoscopic mucosal resection with an insulated-tip electrosurgical knife improves the completeness of resection of intramucosal gastric neoplasms. *Gastrointest Endosc* 55: 576–81.

Miyazaki T, Kato H, Kuwano H. (2004) Usefulness and limitations of endoscopic ultrasonography for detection of lymph node metastasis in esophageal cancer. *J Gastroenterol* 239(1): 90–1.

Moghissi K, Dixon K. (2003) Photodynamic therapy (PDT) in esophageal cancer: a surgical view of its indications based on 14 years experience. *Technol Cancer Res Treat* 2: 319–26.

Moisyenko J, Ajani J, Tjulandin SA *et al.* (2005) Final results of a randomized controlled phase III trial comparing docetaxel combined with cisplatin and 5-fluorouracil to CF in patients with metastatic gastric cancer. *Proc Soc Clin Oncol*: 4022.

Montes CG, Brandalise NA, Deliza R, Novais De Magalhaes AF, Ferraz JG. (1999) Antireflux surgery followed by bipolar electrocoagulation in the treatment of Barrett's esophagus. *Gastrointest Endosc* 50: 173–7.

Montgomery E, Bronner MP, Goldblum JR *et al.* (2001) Reproducibility of the diagnosis of dysplasia in Barrett esophagus: a reaffirmation. *Hum Pathol* 32: 368–78.

Morales TG *et al.* (1997) Intestinal metaplasia of the gastric cardia. *Am J Gastroenterol* 92: 414–18.

Morales C, Lee C, Shay J. (1998) In situ hybridization for the detection of telomerase RNA in the progression from Barrett's esophagus to esophageal adenocarcinoma. *Cancer* 83: 652–9.

Moureau-Zabotto L, Touboul E, Lerouge D *et al.* (2005) Impact of CT and 18F-deoxyglucose positron emission tomography image fusion for conformal radiotherapy in esophageal carcinoma. *Int J Radiat Oncol Biol Phys* 63: 340–5.

Medical Research Council Oesophageal Cancer Working Party (MRC). (2002) Surgical resection with or without properative chemotherapy in oesophageal cancer: a randomised controlled trial. *Lancet* 359: 1727–33.

Mundt A, Mell L, Roeske J. (2003) Preliminary analysis of chronic gastrointestinal toxicity in gynecology patients treated with intensity-modulated whole pelvic radiation therapy. *Int J Radiat Oncol Biol Phys* 56: 1354–60.

Murad AM, Santiago FF, Petroianu A *et al.* (1993) Modified therapy with 5-fluorouracil, doxorubicin, and methotrexate in advanced gastric cancer. *Cancer* 72: 37–41.

Murshed H, Liu H, Liao Z *et al.* (2004) Dose and volume reduction for normal lung using intensity-modulated radiotherapy for advanced-stage non-small-cell lung cancer. *Int J Radiat Oncol Biol Phys* 58: 1258–67.

Naunheim K, Petruska P, Roy T *et al.* (1992) Preoperative chemotherapy and radiotherapy for esophageal carcinoma. *J Thorac Cardiovasc Surg* 103: 887–93.

Nemoto K, Yamada S, Hareyama M, Nagakura H, Hirokawa Y. (2001) Radiation therapy for superficial esophageal cancer: a comparison of radiotherapy methods. *Int J Radiat Oncol Biol Phys* 50: 639–44.

Nigro JJ, Hagen JA, DeMeester TR *et al.* (1999) Occult esophageal adenocarcinoma extent of disease and implications for effective therapy. *Ann Surg* 230(3): 433–40.

Nijhawan PK, Wang KK. (2000) Endoscopic mucosal resection for lesions with endoscopic features suggestive of malignancy and high-grade dysplasia within Barrett's esophagus. *Gastrointest Endosc Clin N Am* 10: 421–37.

Nijhawan PK, Wolfsen HC, Wang KK, Buttar NS, Lutzke L, Anderson M. (2000) Cutaneous photosensitivity after photodynamic therapy: Is it really more common in sunny climates? [abstract]. *Gastroenterology* 118: A227.

Nishimaki T, Tanaka O, Ando N *et al.* (1999) Evaluation of the accuracy of preoperative staging in thoracic esophageal cancer. *Ann Thorac Surg* 68(6): 2059–64.

Nishimori T, Tomonaga T, Matsushita K *et al.* (2006) Proteomic analysis of primary esophageal squamous cell carcinoma reveals downregulation of a cell adhesion protein, periplakin. *Proteomics* 6: 1011–18.

Noguchi H, Naomoto Y, Kondo H *et al.* (2000) Evaluation of endoscopic mucosal resection for superficial esophageal carcinoma. *Surg Laparosc Endosc Percutan Tech* 10: 343–50.

Norberto L, Polese L, Angriman I, Erroi F, Cecchetto A, D'amico DF. (2004) High-energy laser therapy of Barrett's esophagus: preliminary results. *World J Surg* 28: 350–4.

Nutting CM, Corbishley CM, Sanchez-Nieto B, Cosgrove VP, Webb S, Dearnaley DP. (2002) Potential improvements in the therapeutic ratio of prostate cancer irradiation: dose escalation of pathologically identified tumour nodules using intensity modulated radiotherapy. *Br J Radiol* 75: 151–61.

Nygaard K, Hagen S, Hansen H *et al.* (1992) Pre-operative radiotherapy prolongs survival in operable esophageal carcinoma: a randomized, multicenter study of pre-operative radiotherapy and chemotherapy. The second Scandinavian trial in esophageal cancer. *World J Surg* 16: 1104–10.

Oberg S *et al.* (1997) Inflammation and specialized intestinal metaplasia of cardiac mucosa is a manifestation of gastroesophageal reflux disease. *Ann Surg* 226: 522–32.

O'Connor JB, Falk GW, Richter JE. (1999) The incidence of adenocarcinoma and dysplasia in Barrett's esophagus: report on the Cleveland Clinic Barrett's Esophagus Registry. *Am J Gastroenterol* 94: 2037–42.

Oh DS, Hagen JA, Chandrasoma PT *et al.* (2006) Clinical biology and surgical therapy of intramucosal adenocarcinoma of the esophagus. *J Am Coll Surg* 203(2): 152–61.

Ohga E, Kimura Y, Futatsugi M, Miyazaki M, Saeki H, Nozoe T. (2002) Surgical and oncological advances in the treatment of esophageal cancer. *Surgery* 131: S28–S34.

Ohkuwa M, Hosokawa K, Boku N, Ohtu A, Tajiri H, Yoshida S. (2001) New endoscopic treatment for intramucosal gastric tumors using an insulated-tip diathermic knife. *Endoscopy* 33: 221–6.

Oka S, Tanaka S, Kaneko I *et al.* (2006) Advantage of endoscopic submucosal dissection compared with EMR for early gastric cancer. *Gastrointest Endosc* 64(6): 877–83.

Ormsby AH, Goldblum JR, Kilgore SP *et al.* (2000) The frequency and nature of cardiac musoa and intestinal metplasia of the esophagogastric junction: a population based study of 223 consecutive autopsies: implications for patient treatment and preventive strategies in Barrett's esophagus. *Mod Pathol* 13: 614–20.

Ormsby AH, Petras RE, Henricks WH *et al.* (2002) Observer variation in the diagnosis of superficial oesophageal adenocarcinoma. *Gut* 51: 671–6.

Orringer MB, Marshall B, Stirling MC. (1993) Transhiatal esophagectomy for benign and malignant disease. *J Thorac Cardiovasc Surg* 105(2): 265–76.

Orringer MB, Marshall B, Iannettoni MD. (1999) Transhiatal esophagectomy: Clinical experience and refinements *Ann Surg* 230(3): 392–403.

Ortner MA *et al.* (2003) Time gated fluorescence spectroscopy in Barrett's oesophagus. *Gut* 52(1): 28–33.

Ott K, Weber W, Fink U *et al.* (2003) Fluorodeosyglucos-positron emission tomography in adenocarcinomas of the distal esophagus and cardia. *World J Surg* 27: 1035–9.

Ott K, Weber WA, Lordick F *et al.* (2006) Metabolic imaging predicts response, survival, and recurrence in adenocarcinomas of the esophagogastric junction. *J Clin Oncol* 24(29): 4692–8.

Overholt BF, Panjehpour M, Haydek JM. (1999) Photodynamic therapy for Barrett's esophagus: follow-up in 100 patients. *Gastrointest Endosc* 49: 1–7.

Overholt BF, Lightdale CJ, Wang KK *et al.* (2005) Photodynamic therapy with porfimer sodium for ablation of high-grade dysplasia in Barrett's esophagus. *Gastrointest Endosc* 62: 488–98.

Pacifico RJ, Wang KK, Wongkeesong LM, Buttar NS, Lutzke LS. (2003) Combined endoscopic mucosal resection and photodynamic therapy versus esophagectomy for management of early adenocarcinoma in Barrett's esophagus. *Clin Gastroenterol Hepatol* 1(4): 252–7.

Panjehpour M *et al.* (1996) Endoscopic fluorescence detection of high-grade dysplasia in Barrett's esophagus [see comment]. *Gastroenterology* 111(1): 93–101.

Panjehpour M, Overholt BF, Haydek JM, Lee SG. (2000) Results of photodynamic therapy for ablation of dysplasia and early cancer in Barrett's esophagus and effect of oral steroids on stricture formation. *Am J Gastroenterol* 95: 2177–84.

Panjehpour M, Overholt BF, Phan MN, Haydek JM. (2005) Optimization of light dosimetry for photodynamic therapy of Barrett's esophagus: efficacy vs. incidence of stricture after treatment. *Gastrointest Endosc* 61: 13–18.

Pasini F, de Manzoni G, Pedrazzani C, Grandinetti A, Durante E, Gabbani M *et al.* (2005) High pathological response rate in locally advanced esophageal cancer after neoadjuvant combined modality therapy: dose finding of a weekly chemotherapy schedule with protracted venous infusion of 5-fluorouracil and dose escalation of cisplatin, docetaxel and concurrent radiotherapy. *Ann Oncol* 16: 1133–9.

Pasricha PJ, Hill S, Wadwa KS *et al.* (1999) Endoscopic cryotherapy: experimental results and first clinical use. *Gastrointest Endosc* 49: 627–31.

Pech O *et al.* (2006) The impact of endoscopic ultrasound and computed tomography on the TNM staging of early cancer in Barrett's esophagus. *Am J Gastroenterol* 101(10): 2223–9.

Pech O, Gossner L, May A *et al.* (2005) Long-term results of photodynamic therapy with 5-aminolevulinic acid for superficial Barrett's cancer and high-grade intraepithelial neoplasia. *Gastrointest Endosc* 62: 24–30.

Pedrazzani C, Catalano F, Festini M *et al.* (2005) Endoscopic ablation of Barrett's esophagus using high power setting argon plasma coagulation: a prospective study. *World J Gastroenterol* 11: 1872–5.

Pera M, Cameron AJ, Trastek VF, Carpenter HA, Zinsmeister AR. (1993) Increasing incidence of adenocarcinoma of the esophagus and esophagogastric junction. *Gastroenterology* 104: 510–13.

Peters F, Kara M, Rosmolen W *et al.* (2005) Poor results of 5-aminolevulinic acid-photodynamic therapy for residual high-grade dysplasia and early cancer in barrett esophagus after endoscopic resection. *Endoscopy* 37: 418–24.

Peters F, Brakendhoff LP, Curvers WL *et al.* (2006) Endoscopic resection in esophagus and stomach is safe: a prospective analysis of 303 procedures. *Gastrointest Endosc* 63: AB97.

Pfau PR, Ginsberg GG, Lew RJ, Faigel DO, Smith DB, Kochman ML. (2000) Esophageal dilation for endosonographic evaluation of malignant esophageal strictures is safe and effective. *Am J Gastroenterol* 95(10): 2813–15.

Pfefer TJ *et al.* (2003) Temporally and spectrally resolved fluorescence spectroscopy for the detection of high grade dysplasia in Barrett's esophagus. *Lasers Surg Med* 32(1): 10–16.

Pinotti AC, Cecconello I, Filho FM, Sakai P, Gama-Rodrigues JJ, Pinotti HW. (2004) Endoscopic ablation of Barrett's esophagus using argon plasma coagulation: a prospective study after fundoplication. *Dis Esophagus* 17(3): 243–6.

Polkowski W *et al.* (2000) Intestinal and pancreatic metaplasia at the esophagagogastric junction in patients without Barrett's esophagus. *Am J Gastroenterol* 95: 617–25.

Poneros JM *et al.* (2001) Diagnosis of specialized intestinal metaplasia by optical coherence tomography. *Gastroenterology* 120(1): 7–12.

Poneros J. (2005) Optical coherence tomography and the detection of dysplasia in Barrett's esophagus [comment]. *Gastrointest Endosc* 62(6): 832–3.

Poneros JM. (2004) Diagnosis of Barrett's esophagus using optical coherence tomography. *Gastrointest Endosc Clin N Am* 14(3): 573–88.

Poplin E, Fleming T, Leichman L *et al.* (1987) Combined therapies for squamous-cell carcinoma of the esophagus, a Southwest Oncology Group Study (SWOG-8037). *J Clin Oncol* 5: 622–8.

Portale G, Hagen JA, Peters JH *et al.* (2006a) Modern 5-year survival of resectable esophageal adenocarcinoma: single institution experience with 263 patients. *J Am Coll Surg* 202: 588–96.

Portale G, Peters JH, Hsieh CC *et al.* (2006b) Can clinical and endoscopic findings accurately predict early-stage adenocarcinoma? *Surg Endosc* 20(2): 294–7.

Prosst RL, Wolfsen HC, Gahlen J. (2003) Photodynamic therapy for esophageal diseases: a clinical update. *Endoscopy* 35: 1059–68.

Provenzale D, Kemp JA, Arora S, Wong JB. (1994) A guide for surveillance of patients with Barrett's esophagus. *Am J Gastroenterol* 89: 670–80.

Puli SR, Rostogi A, Mathur S, Bansal J, Sharma P. (2006) Development of esophageal adenocarcinoma in patients with Barrett's esophagus and high grade dysplasia undergoing surveillance: a meta-analysis and systematic review. *Gastrointest Endosc* 63: AB82.

Putnam JB Jr, Suell DM, McMurtrey MJ *et al.* (1994) Comparison of three techniques of esophagectomy within a residency training program. *Ann Thorac Surg* 57(2): 319–25.

Pyrhonen S, Kuitunen T, Nyandoto P, Kouri M. (1995) Randomized comparison of fluorouracil, epidoxorubicin and methotrexate plus supportive care aloine in patients with non-resectable gastric cancer. *Br J Cancer* 71: 587–91.

Qi X, Sivak MV, Isenberg G *et al.* (2006) Computer-aided diagnosis of dysplasia in Barrett's esophagus using endoscopic optical coherence tomography. *J Biomed Opt* 11(4): 044010.

Ragunath K, Krasner N, Raman VS, Haqqani MT, Phillips CJ, Cheung I. (2005) Endoscopic ablation of dysplastic Barrett's oesophagus comparing argon plasma coagulation and photodynamic therapy: a randomized prospective trial assessing efficacy and cost-effectiveness. *Scand J Gastroenterol* 40: 750–8.

Rajan E, Gostout CJ, Feitoza AB *et al.* (2004) Widespread EMR: A new technique for removal of large areas of mucosa. *Gastrointest Endosc* 60: 623–7.

Raju GS, Ahmed I, Xiao SY, Brining D, Bhutani MS, Pasricha PJ. (2005) Graded esophageal mucosal ablation with cryotherapy, and the protective effects of submucosal saline. *Endoscopy* 37: 523–6.

Ramirez FC, Shaukat MS, Young MA, Johnson DA, Akins R. (2005) Feasibility and safety of string, wireless capsule endoscopy in the diagnosis of Barrett's esophagus. *Gastrointest Endosc* 61(6): 741–6.

Reid BJ. (1991) Barrett's esophagus and esophageal adenocarcinoma. *Gastroenterol Clin North Am* 20: 817–34.

Rentz J, Bull D, Harpole D *et al.* (2003) Transthoracic versus transhiatal esophagectomy: a prospective study of 945 patients. *J Thorac Cardiovasc Surg* 125(5): 1114–20.

Rice TW, Zuccaro G Jr, Adelstein DJ, Rybicki LA, Blackstone EH, Goldblum JR. (1998) Esophageal carcinoma: depth of tumor invasion is predictive of regional lymph node status. *Ann Thorac Surg* 65: 787–92.

Rice TW, Blackstone EH, Adelstein DJ *et al.* (2001) N1 esophageal carcinoma: the importance of staging and downstaging. *J Thorac Cardiovasc Surg* 121: 454–64.

Rice TW, Blackstone EH, Adelstein DJ *et al.* (2003) Role of clinically determined depth of tumor invasion in the treatment of esophageal carcinoma. *J Thorac Cardiovasc Surg* 125: 1091–1102.

Ries LAG, Eisner MP, Kosary C *et al.* (2002) *SEER Cancer Statistics Review, 1973–1999.* National Cancer Institute, Bethesda (MD).

Rizk N, Downey RJ, Akhurst T *et al.* (2006) Preoperative 18[F]-fluorodeoxyglucose positron emission tomography standardized uptake values predict survival after esophageal adenocarcinoma resection. *Ann Thorac Surg* 81(3): 1076–81.

Romagnuolo J, Scott J, Hawes RH *et al.* (2002) Helical CT versus EUS with fine needle aspiration for celiac nodal assessment in patients with esophageal cancer. *Gastrointest Endosc* 55(6): 648–54.

Roncalli M, Bosari S, Marchetti A *et al.* (1998) Cell cycle-related gene abnormalities and product expression in esophageal carcinoma. *Lab Invest* 78: 1049–57.

Rosch T, Sarbia M, Schumacher B *et al.* (2004) Attempted endoscopic en bloc resection of mucosal and submucosal tumors using insulated-tip knives: a pilot series. *Endoscopy* 36: 788–801.

Ross P, Nicolson M, Cunningham D *et al.* (2002) Prospective randomized trial comparing mitomycin, cisplatin, and protracted venous infusion fluorouracil with epirubicin, cisplatin, and PVI 5-FU in advanced esophagogastric cancer. *J Clin Oncol* 20: 1996–2004.

Ross A, Larghi A, Stearns L *et al.* (2006) Complete Barrett's eradication endoscopic mucosal resection as a treatment for high grade dysplasia or intramucosal adenocarcinoma arising from Barrett's epithelium: a viable alternative to esophagectomy. *Gastrointest Endosc* 63: AB126.

Roussel A, Jacob J, Haegele P *et al.* (1988) Controlled clinical trial for the treatmnt of patietns with inoperable esophageal carcinoma: a study of EORTC gastrointestinal tract cancer cooperative group. *Recent Results Cancer Res* 110: 21–9.

Saad RS, El-Gohary Y, Memari E, Liu YL, Silverman JF. (2005) Endoglin (CD105) and vascular endothelial growth factor as prognostic markers in esophageal adenocarcinoma. *Hum Pathol* 36: 955–61.

Safran H, Gaissert H, Akerman P *et al.* (2001) Paclitaxel, cisplatin, and concurrent radiation for esophageal cancer. *Cancer Invest* 19: 1–7.

Safran H, DiPetrillo T, Nadeem A *et al.* (2004) Trastuzumab, paclitaxel, cisplatin, and radiation for adenocarcinoma of the esophagus: a phase I study. *Cancer Invest* 22: 670–7.

Sakal P, Maluf Filho F, Iryia K *et al.* (1996) An endoscopic technique for resection of small gastrointestinal carcinomas. *Gastrointest Endosc* 44: 65–8.

Salo JA, Salminen JT, Kiviluoto TA *et al.* (1998) Treatment of Barrett's esophagus by endoscopic laser ablation and antireflux surgery. *Ann Surg* 227: 40–4.

Sampliner RE. (1982) Management of premalignant esophagogastric lesions. *Ariz Med* 39: 312–13.

Sampliner RE. (2003) Prevention of adenocarcinoma by reversing Barrett's esophagus with mucosal ablation. *World J Surg* 27: 1026–9.

Sampliner RE. (2004) Endoscopic ablative therapy for Barrett's esophagus: current status. *Gastrointest Endosc* 59: 66–9.

Sampliner RE. (2005) Epidemiology, pathophysiology, and treatment of Barrett's esophagus: reducing mortality from esophageal adenocarcinoma. *Med Clin North Am* 89: 293–312.

Sampliner RE, ACG Practice Parameters Committee. (2002) Updated guidelines for the diagnosis, surveillance, and therapy of Barrett's esophagus. *Am J Gastroenterol* 97: 1888–95.

Sampliner RE, Hixson LJ, Fennerty MB, Garewal HS. (1993) Regression of Barrett's esophagus by laser ablation in an acid environment. *Dig Dis Sci* 38: 365–8.

Sampliner RE, Fennerty B, Garewal HS. (1996) Reversal of Barrett's esophagus with acid suppression and multipolar electrocoagulation: preliminary results. *Gastrointest Endosc* 44: 532–5.

Sampliner RE, Faigel D, Fennerty MB *et al.* (2001) Effective and safe endoscopic reversal of nondysplastic Barrett's esophagus with thermal electrocoagulation combined with high-dose acid inhibition: a multicenter study. *Gastrointest Endosc* 53: 554–8.

Sandick JW *et al.* (2002) Intestinal metaplasia of the esophagus or esophagogastric junction. *Am J Clin Pathol* 117: 117–25.

Saporiti MR *et al.* (2003) Methylene blue chromoendoscopy for Barrett's esophagus diagnosis [see comment]. *Arq Gastroenterol* 40(3): 139–47.

Sarbia M, Stahl M, Fink U *et al.* (1999) Prognostic significance of cyclin D1 in esophageal squamous cell carcinoma patients treated with surgery alone or combined therapy modalities. *Int J Cancer* 84: 86–91.

Savoy AD, Wolfsen HC, Raimondo M, Noh KW, Pungpapong S, Wallace MB. (2005) Surveillance after endoscopic ablation for Barrett's dysplasia? *Gastrointest Endosc* 61: AB300.

Scarfone C, Lavely WC, Cmelak AJ *et al.* (2004) Prospective feasibility trial of radiotherapy target definition for head and neck cancer using 3-dimensional PET and CT imaging. *J Nucl Med* 45: 543–52.

Scheithauer W. Kornek G, Zeh B *et al.* (1995) *Palliative chemotherapy versus best supportive care in patients with metastatic gastric cancer: a randomized trial.* Proceedings of the Second International Conference on Biology, Prevention and Treatment of GI Malignancy, Koln, Germany, p. 68.

Schneider AR, Kriener S, Hoepffner N, Shastri Y, Caspary WF. (2006) Submucosal injection of autolgous blood before endoscopic resection —an option to NaCl and hyaluronate? Results of an ex-vivo pilot study. *Gastrointest Endosc* 63: AB80.

Schoder H, Erdi Y, Larson S, Yeung H. (2003) PET/CT: a new imaging technology in nuclear medicine. *Eur J Nucl Med Mol Imaging* 30: 1419–37.

Schulz H, Miehlke S, Antos D *et al.* (2000) Ablation of Barrett's epithelium by endoscopic argon plasma coagulation in combination with high-dose omeprazole. *Gastrointest Endosc* 51: 659–63.

Seewald S, Akaraviputh T, Seitz U *et al.* (2003) Circumferential EMR and complete removal of Barrett's epithelium: a new approach to management of Barrett's esophagus containing high-grade intraepithelial neoplasia and intramucosal carcinoma. *Gastrointest Endosc* 57: 854–9.

Shah AK, Wolfsen HC, Hemminger LL, Shah AA, Devault KR. (2006) Changes in esophageal motility after porfimer sodium photodynamic therapy for Barrett's dysplasia and mucosal carcinoma. *Dis Esophagus* 19: 335–9.

Shaheen N, Ransohoff DF. (2002) Gastroesophageal reflux, Barrett esophagus, and esophageal cancer: scientific review. *JAMA* 287: 1972–81.

Sharma P. (2005) Narrow band imaging in Barrett's esophagus. *Clin Gastroenterol Hepatol* 3(7 Suppl 1): S21–2.

Sharma P, Sampliner RE, Camargo E. (1997) Normalization of esophageal pH with high-dose proton pump inhibitor therapy does not result in regression of Barrett's esophagus. *Am J Gastroenterol* 92: 582–5.

Sharma P *et al.* (2000) Relative risk of dysplasia for patients with intestinal metaplasia in the distal oesophagus and in the gastric cardia. *Gut* 46: 9–13.

Sharma P, Reker D, Falk G, Al E. (2001) Progression of Barrett's esophagus to high-grade dysplasia and cancer: preliminary results of the BEST trial. *Gastroenterology* 120: A16.

Sharma V, Mahantshetty U, Dinshaw KA, Deshpande R, Sharma S. (2002) Palliation of advanced/recurrent esophageal carcinoma with high-dose-rate brachytherapy. *Int J Radiat Oncol Biol Phys* 52: 310–15.

Sharma P *et al.* (2003) Magnification chromoendoscopy for the detection of intestinal metaplasia and dysplasia in Barrett's oesophagus [see comment]. *Gut* 52(1): 24–7.

Sharma VK, Fleisher DE, Wang KK, Overholt B, Fennerty B. (2004a) A randomized trial of radio-frequency ablation of specialized intestinal metaplasia of the esophagus. *Gastrointest Endosc* 59: AB113.

Sharma P, McQuaid K, Dent J *et al.* (2004b) A critical review of the diagnosis and management of Barrett's esophagus: the AGA Chicago Workshop. *Gastroenterology* 127: 310–30.

Sharma P, Bansal A, Mathur S *et al.* (2006a) The utility of a novel narrow band imaging endoscopy system in patients with Barrett's esophagus. *Gastrointest Endosc* 64: 167–75.

Sharma P, Falk GW, Weston AP, Reker D, Johnston M, Sampliner RE. (2006b) Dysplasia and cancer in a large multicenter cohort of patients with Barrett's esophagus. *Clin Gastroenterol Hepatol* 4: 566–72.

Sharma P, Wani S, Weston AP *et al.* (2006c) A randomised controlled trial of ablation of Barrett's oesophagus with multipolar electrocoagulation versus argon plasma coagulation in combination with acid suppression: long term results. *Gut* 55: 1233–9.

Sharma VK, Kim HJ, McLaughlin R *et al.* (2006d) Successful circumferential ablation of Barrett's esophagus with low grade dysplasia using the HALO-360 ablation system: one-year follow-up of the AIM-LGD pilot trial. *Gastrointest Endosc* 63: AB127.

Sharma VK, Wang KK, Overholt BF *et al.* (2007) Balloon-based, circumferential endoscopic ablation of Barrett's esophagus: 1-year follow-up of 100 patients. *Gastrointest Endosc* 65: 185–95.

Sibille A, Lambert R, Souquet JC, Sabben G, Descos F. (1995) Long-term survival after photodynamic therapy for esophageal cancer. *Gastroenterology* 108: 337–44.

Siewert J, Feith M, Werner M, Stein H. (2000) Adenocarcinoma of the esophagogastric junction: results of surgical therapy based on anatomical/topographic classification in 1,002 consecutive patients. *Ann Surg* 232: 353–61.

Sihvo EI, Luostarinen ME, Salo JA. (2004) Fate of patients with adenocarcinoma of the esophagus and the esophagogastric junction: a population-based analysis. *Am J Gastroenterol* 99(3): 419–24.

Sivula A, Buskens C, van Rees B *et al.* (2005) Prognostic role of cyclooxygenase-2 in neoadjuvant-treated patients with squamous cell carcinoma of the esophagus. *Int J Cancer* 116: 903–8.

Slabber C, Nel J, Schoeman L, Burger W, Falkson G, Falkson C. (1998) A randomized study of radiotherapy alone versus radiotherapy plus 5-fluorouracil and platinum in patients with inoperable, locally advanced squamous cancer of the esophagus. *Am J Clin Oncol* 21: 462–5.

Smith T, Ryan L, Douglass HJ *et al.* (1998) Combined chemoradiotherapy vs. radiotherapy alone for early stage squamous cell carcinoma of the esophagus: A study of the Eastern Cooperative Oncology Group. *Int J Radiat Oncol Biol Phys* 42: 269–76.

Soehendra N, Binmoeller KF, Bohnacker S *et al.* (1997) Endoscopic snare mucosectomy in the esophagus without any additional equipment: a simple technique for resection of flat early cancer. *Endoscopy* 29: 380–3.

Soetikno RM, Gotoda T, Nakanishi Y, Soehendra N. (2003) Endoscopic mucosal resection. *Gastrointest Endosc* 57: 567–79.

Spechler SJ. (2006) Thermal ablation of Barrett's Esophagus: a heated debate. *Am J Gastroenterol* 101: 1770–2.

Spechler SJ. (2002) Barrett's esophagus and esophageal adenocarcinoma: pathogenesis, diagnosis, and therapy. *Med Clin North Am* 86(6): 1423–45.

Spechler SJ *et al.* (1994) Prevalence of metaplasia at the gastro-oesophageal junction. *Lancet* 344: 1533–6.

Stahl M, Wilke H, Fink U *et al.* (1996) Combined preoperative chemotherapy and radiotherapy in patients with locally advanced esophageal cancer: Interim analysis of a phase III trial. *J Clin Oncol* 14: 829–37.

Stahl M, Stuschke M, Lehmann N *et al.* (2005) Chemoradiation with and without surgery in patients with locally advanced squamous cell carcinoma of the esophagus. *J Clin Oncol* 23: 2310–17.

Stein HJ, Siewert JR. (2004) Improved prognosis of resected esophageal cancer. *World J Surg* 28(6): 520–5.

Stevens PD *et al.* (1994) Combined magnification endoscopy with chromoendoscopy for the evaluation of Barrett's esophagus. *Gastrointest Endosc* 40(6): 747–9.

Steyerberg EW, Neville BA, Koppert LB *et al.* (2006) Surgical mortality in patients with esophageal cancer: development and validation of a simple risk score. *J Clin Oncol* 24: 4277–84.

Sugahara S, Tokuuye K, Okumura T *et al.* (2005) Clinical results of proton beam therapy for cancer of the esophagus. *Int J Radiat Oncol Biol Phys* 61: 76–84.

Sun D. (1989) Ten-year follow-up of esophageal cancer treated by radical radiation therapy: analysis of 869 patients. *Int J Radiat Oncol Biol Phys* 16: 329–34.

Sur RK, Donde B, Levin VC, Mannell A. (1998) Fractionated high dose rate intraluminal brachytherapy in palliation of advanced esophageal cancer. *Int J Radiat Oncol Biol Phys* 40: 447–53.

Swanson SJ, Batirel HF, Bueno R *et al.* (2001) Transthoracic esophagectomy with radical mediastinal and abdominal lymph node dissection and cervical esophagogastrostomy for esophageal carcinoma. *Ann Thorac Surg* 72(6): 1918–24.

Swisher S, Ajani J, Komaki R *et al.* (2003) Long-term outcome of phase II trial evaluating chemotherapy, chemoradiotherpy, and surgery for locoregionally advanced esophageal cancer. *Int J Radiat Oncol Biol Phys* 57: 120–7.

Swisher S, Erasmus J, Maish M *et al.* (2004a) 2-fluoro-2-deoxy-d-glucose positron emission tomographyimaging is predictive of pathologic response and survival after preoperative chemoradiation in patients with esophageal carcinoma. *Cancer* 101: 1776–85.

Swisher S, Maish M, Erasmus J *et al.* (2004b) Utility of PET, CT, and EUS to identify pathologic responders in esophageal cancer. *Ann Thorac Surg* 78: 1152–60.

Swisher S, Hofstetter W, Wu T *et al.* (2005) Proposed revision of the esophageal cancer staging system to accommodate pathologic response (pP) following preoperative chemoradiation (CRT). *Ann Surg* 241: 810–17; discussion.

Syed A, Puthawala A, Severance S. (1987) Intraluminal irradiation in the treatment of esophageal cancer. *Endocurietherapy/Hyperthermia Oncology* 3: 105–13.

Takeshita K, Tani M, Inoue H *et al.* (1997) Endoscopic treatment of early oesophageal or gastric cancer. *Gut* 40: 123–7.

Tohma T, Okazumi S, Makino H *et al.* (2005) Overexpression of glucose transporter 1 in esophageal squamous cell carcinomas: a marker for poor prognosis. *Dis Esophagus* 18: 185–9.

Townsend DW, Carney JP.J., Yap JT, Hall NC. (2004) PET/CT today and tomorrow. *J Nucl Med* 45: 4S–14.

Triadafilopoulos G, Kaur B, Sood S, Traxler B, Levine D, Weston A. (2006) The effects of esomeprazole combined with aspirin or rofecoxib on prostaglandin E2 production in patients with Barrett's oesophagus. *Aliment Pharmacol Ther* 23: 997–1005.

Tsai F, Vosoghi M, Khoshini R *et al.* (2006) Preliminary results of BARRx ablation trial in patients with non-dysplastic intestinal metaplasia versus low or high grade dysplasia. *Gastrointest Endosc* 63: AB142.

Tseng EE, Wu TT, Yeo CF, Heitmiller RF. (2003) Barrett's esophagus with high-grade dysplasia: surgical results and long-term outcome – an update. *J Gastrointest Surg* 7: 164–71.

Tucker S, Liu H, Wang S *et al.* (2006) Dose-volume modeling of the risk of postoperative pulmonary complications among esophageal cancer patients treated with concurrent chemoradiotherapy followed by surgery. *Int J Radiat Oncol Biol Phys* 66(3): 754–61.

Ukleja A, Scolapio JS, Wolfsen HC. (1999) Endoscopic ultrasonography (EUS) and endoscopic mucosal resection (EMR) for staging and treatment of high-grade dysplasia (HGD) and early adenocarcinoma (EAC) in Barrett's esophagus (BE) [abstract]. *Gastroenterology* 116: A-582.

Ulrich CM, Bigler J, Velicer CM, Greene EA, Farin FM, Potter JD. (2000) Searching expressed sequence tag databases: discovery and confirmation of a common polymorphism in the thymidylate synthase gene. *Cancer Epidemiol Biomarkers Prev* 9: 1381–5.

Urba SG, Orringer MB, Turrisi A, Iannettoni M, Forastiere A, Strawderman M. (2001) Randomized trial of preoperative chemoradiation versus surgery alone in patients with locoregional esophageal carcinoma. *J Clin Oncol* 19: 305–13.

Urba S, Orringer M, Perez-Tamayo C, Bromberg J, Forastiere A. (1992) Concurrent preoperative chemotherapy and radiation therapy in localized esophageal adenocarcinoma. *Cancer* 69: 285–91.

Urba S, Orringer M, Iannettoni M. (2000) A phase II trial of preoperative cisplatin, paclitaxel, and radiation therapy XRT before trans-hiatal esophagectomy (THE) in patients (pts) with locoregional esophageal cancer (CA). *J Clin Oncol* 19: 248a.

Urba S, Orringer M, Turrisi A, Iannettoni M, Forastiere A, Strawderman M. (2001) Randomized trial of preoperative chemoradiation versus surgery alone in patients with locoregional esophageal carcinoma. *J Clin Oncol* 19: 305–13.

Urbach DR, Baxter NN. (2004) Does it matter what a hospital is 'high volume' for? Specificity of hospital volume-outcome associations for surgical procedures: analysis of administrative data. *BMJ* 328: 737–40.

Urschel J, Vasan H. (2003) A meta-analysis of randomized controlled trials that compared neoadjuvant chemoradiation and surgery to surgery alone for resectable esophageal cancer. *Am J Surg* 185: 538–43.

Van Dam J, Rice TW, Catalano MF, Kirby T, Sivak MV Jr. (1993) High-grade malignant stricture is predictive of esophageal tumor stage. Risks of endosonographic evaluation.*Cancer* 71(10): 2910–7.

Van Den Boogert J, Van Hillegersberg R, Siersema PD, De Bruin RW, Tilanus HW. (1999) Endoscopic ablation therapy for Barrett's esophagus with high-grade dysplasia: a review. *Am J Gastroenterol* 94: 1153–60.

Vaughan TL, Dong LM, Blount PL *et al.* (2005) Non-steroidal anti-inflammatory drugs and risk of neoplastic progression in Barrett's oesophagus: a prospective study. *Lancet Oncol* 6: 945–52.

Vazquez-Sequeiros E, Levy MJ, Clain JE *et al.* (2006) Routine vs. selective EUS-guided FNA approach for preoperative nodal staging of esophageal carcinoma. *Gastrointest Endosc* 63(2): 204–11.

van de Ven C, De Leyn P, Coosemans W, Van Raemdonck D, Lerut T. (1999) Three-field lymphadenectomy and pattern of lymph node spread in T3 adenocarcinoma of the distal esophagus and the gastro-esophageal junction. *Eur J Cardiothorac Surg* 15: 769–73.

Vivekanandam S, Reddy KS, Velavan K *et al.* (2001) External beam radiotherapy and intraluminal brachytherapy in advanced inoperable esophageal cancer: JIPMER experience. *Am J Clin Oncol* 24: 128–30.

Wai Yan Chiu P. (2006) Endoscopic submucosal dissection—bigger piece, better outcome! *Gastrointest Endosc* 64(6): 884–5.

Walker SJ, Selvasekar CR, Birbeck N. (2002) Mucosal ablation in Barrett's esophagus. *Dis Esophagus* 15: 22–9.

Wallace MB. (2006) Detecting dysplasia with optical coherence tomography [comment]. *Clin Gastroenterol Hepatol* 4(1): 36–7.

Wallace MB *et al.* (2000) Endoscopic detection of dysplasia in patients with Barrett's esophagus using light-scattering spectroscopy. *Gastroenterology* 119(3): 677–82.

Wallace MB, Nietert PJ, Earle C *et al.* (2002) An analysis of multiple staging management strategies for carcinoma of the esophagus: computed tomography, endoscopic ultrasound, positron emission tomography, and thoracoscopy/laparoscopy. *Ann Thorac Surg* 74(4): 1026–32.

Wallace MB *et al.* (2006) Advanced imaging and technology in gastrointestinal neoplasia: summary of the AGA-NCI Symposium October 4–5, 2004. *Gastroenterology* 130(4): 1333–42.

Walsh T, Noonan N, Hollywood D, Kelly A, Keeling N, Hennessy T. (1996) A comparison of multimodal therapy and surgery for esophageal adenocarcinoma. *N Engl J Med* 335: 462–7.

Wang KK. (1999) Current status of photodynamic therapy of Barrett's esophagus. *Gastrointest Endosc* 49: S20–23.

Wang KK. (2000) Photodynamic therapy of Barrett's esophagus. *Gastrointest Endosc Clin N Am* 10: 409–19.

Wang K. (2001) Photodynamic therapy made simple. *Clin Perspect Gastroenterol* March/April: 90–100.

Wang KK. (2004) Detection and staging of esophageal cancers. *Curr Opin Gastroenterol* 20: 381–5.

Wang Z. (2005) The role of COX-2 in oral cancer development, and chemoprevention/ treatment of oral cancer by selective COX-2 inhibitors. *Curr Pharm Des* 11: 1771–7.

Wang KK, Kim JY. (2003) Photodynamic therapy in Barrett's esophagus. *Gastrointest Endosc Clin N Am* 13: 483–9, vii.

Wang KK, Sampliner RE. (2001) Mucosal ablation therapy of barrett esophagus. *Mayo Clin Proc* 76: 433–7.

Wang KK, Wong Kee Song LM, Buttar NS, Papenfuss S, Lutzke L. (2004) Barrett's esophagus after photodynamic therapy: risk of cancer development during long term follow up [abstract]. *Gastroenterology* 126 (suppl 2): A-50.

Wang KK, Wongkeesong M, Buttar NS. (2005) American Gastroenterological Association technical review on the role of the gastroenterologist in the management of esophageal carcinoma. *Gastroenterology* 128(5): 1471–505.

Wang S, Liao Z, Wei X *et al.* (2006a) Association between induction chemotherapy and increased risk of treatment related pneumonitis in esophageal cancer patients treated with concurrent chemoradiotherapy. *Int J Radiat Oncol Biol Phys* 66(5): 1399–407.

Wang S, Liao Z, Vaporciyan A *et al.* (2006b) Investigation of clinical and dosimetric factors associated with postoperative pulmonary complications in esophageal cancer patients treated with concurrent chemoradiotherapy followed by surgery. *Int J Radiat Oncol Biol Phys* 64: 692–9.

Waterman TA, Hagen JA, Peters JH, DeMeester SR, Taylor CR, Demeester TR. (2004) The prognostic importance of immunohistochemically detected node metastases in resected esophageal adenocarcinoma. *Ann Thorac Surg* 78(4): 1161–9.

Waxman I, Raju GS, Critchlow J, Antonioli DA, Spechler SJ. (2006) High-frequency probe ultrasonography has limited accuracy for detecting invasive adenocarcinoma in patients with Barrett's esophagus and high-grade dysplasia or intramucosal carcinoma: a case series. *Am J Gastroenterol* 101(8): 1773–9.

Webb A, Cunningham D, Scarffe H *et al.* (1997) Randomized trial comparing epirubicin, cisplatin, and fluorouracil versus fluoruouracil, doxorubicin, and methotrexate in advanced esophagogastric cancer. *J Clin Oncol* 15: 261–7.

Webber J, Herman M, Kessel D, Fromm D. (1999) Current concepts in gastrointestinal photodynamic therapy. *Ann Surg* 230: 12–23.

Weber W, Ziegler S, Thodtmann R, Hanauske A, Schwaiger M. (1999) Reproducibility of metabolic measurements in malignant tumors using FDG PET. *J Nucl Med* 40: 1771–7.

Weber WA, Ott K, Becker K *et al.* (2001) Prediction of response to preoperative chemotherapy in adenocarcinomas of the esophagogastric junction by metabolic imaging. *J Clin Oncol* 19: 3058–65.

Weber W, Petersen V, Schmidt B *et al.* (2003) Positron emission tomography in non-small-cell lung cancer: prediction of response to chemotherapy by quantitative assessment of glucose use. *J Clin Oncol* 21: 2651–7.

Wehrmann T, Frenz MB, Stergiou N, Riphaus A. (2006) Frequency of recurrence of pre-malignant esophageal lesions and early stage esophageal cancer after endoscopic resection. *Gastrointest Endosc* 63: AB120.

Weiner L, Colarusso P, Goldberg M, Dresler C, Coia L. (1997) Conbined modality therapy for esophageal cancer: Phase I trail of escalating doses of pacitaxel in combination with cisplatin, 5-fluorouracil, and high-dose radiation before esophagectomy. *Semin Oncol* 24: S19-93–S19-95.

Weston AP, Sharma P. (2002) Neodymium:yttrium-aluminum garnet contact laser ablation of Barrett's high grade dysplasia and early adenocarcinoma. *Am J Gastroenterol* 97: 2998–3006.

van Westreenen HL, Westerterp M, Bossuyt PM *et al.* (2004) Systematic review of the staging performance of 18F fluorodeoxyglucose positron emission tomography in esophageal cancer. *J Clin Oncol* 22(18): 3805–12.

Whooley BP, Law S, Murthy SC, Alexandrou A, Wong J. (2001) Analysis of reduced death and complication rates after esophageal resection. *Ann Surg* 233(3): 338–44.

Wieder H, Brucher B, Zimmermann F *et al.* (2004) Time course of tumor metabolic activity during chemoradiotherapy of esophageal squamous cell carcinoma and response to treatment. *J Clin Oncol* 22: 900–8.

Wijnhoven B, Siersema P, Hop W, van Dekken H, Tilanus H. (1999) Adenocarcinomas of the distal esophagus and gastric cardia are one clinical entity. *Br J Surg* 86: 529–35.

Wild CP, Hardie LJ. (2003) Reflux, Barrett's oesophagus and adenocarcinoma: burning questions. *Nat Rev Cancer* 3: 676–84.

Wilkinson N, Black J, Roukhadze E *et al.* (2004) Epidermal growth factor receptor expression correlates with histologic grade in resected esophageal adenocarcinoma. *J Gastrointest Surg* 8: 448–53.

Wils O, Klein HO, Wagener DJT *et al.* (1991) Sequential high-dose methotrexate and fluorouracil combined with doxorubicin: a step ahead in the treatment of gastric cancer. a trial of the European Organization for Research and Treatment of Cancer of the Gastrointestinal Tract Co-operative Group. *J Clin Oncol* 9: 827–31.

Withers HR, Peters LJ. (1980) Basic principles of radiotherapy: basic clinical parameters. In: Fletcher GA, ed. *Textbook of Radiotherapy*, 3rd edn. Lea & Febiger, Philadelphia.

Wo JM *et al.* (2001) Comparison of methylene blue-directed biopsies and conventional biopsies in the detection of intestinal metaplasia and dysplasia in Barrett's esophagus: a preliminary study [see comment]. *Gastrointest Endosc* 54(3): 294–301.

Wolfsen HC. (2002) Photodynamic therapy for mucosal esophageal adenocarcinoma and dysplastic Barrett's esophagus. *Dig Dis* 20: 5–17.

Wolfsen HC. (2005a) Endoprevention of esophageal cancer: endoscopic ablation of Barrett's metaplasia and dysplasia. *Expert Rev Med Devices* 2: 713–23.

Wolfsen HC. (2005b) Photodynamic therapy for Barrett's esophagus with high-grade dysplasia. *Compr Ther* 31: 137–44.

Wolfsen HC. (2005c) Present status of photodynamic therapy for high-grade dysplasia in Barrett's esophagus. *J Clin Gastroenterol* 39: 189–202.

Wolfsen HC. (2006) Bare fiber photodynamic therapy using porfimer sodium for esophageal disease. *Photodiag Photodyn Ther* 3(2): 87–92.

Wolfsen HC, Hemminger LL. (2004) Photodynamic therapy for dysplastic Barrett's esophagus and mucosal adenocarcinoma (abstr). *Gastrointest Endosc* 59: AB251.

Wolfsen HC, Hemminger LL. (2006) Salvage photodynamic therapy for persistent oesophageal cancer after chemoradiation therapy. *Photodiag Photodyn Ther* 3: 11–14.

Wolfsen HC, Ng CS. (2002) Cutaneous consequences of photodynamic therapy. *Cutis* 69: 140–2.

Wolfsen HC, Woodward TA, Raimondo M. (2002) Photodynamic therapy for dysplastic Barrett esophagus and early esophageal adenocarcinoma. *Mayo Clin Proc* 77: 1176–81.

Wolfsen HC, Hemminger LL, Devault KR. (2004a) Barrett's dysplasia and mucosal carcinoma patients referred for photodynamic therapy—

do they come from surveillance programs? (abstr). *Gastrointest Endosc* 59: AB265.

Wolfsen HC, Hemminger LL, Raimondo M, Woodward TA. (2004b) Photodynamic therapy and endoscopic mucosal resection for Barrett's dysplasia and early esophageal adenocarcinoma. *South Med J* 97: 827–30.

Wolfsen HC, Hemminger LL, Wallace MB, Devault KR. (2004c) Clinical experience of patients undergoing photodynamic therapy for Barrett's dysplasia or cancer. *Aliment Pharmacol Ther* 20: 1125–31.

Wong Kee Song LM. (2005) Optical spectroscopy for the detection of dysplasia in Barrett's esophagus. Clin Gastroenterol Hepatol 3(7 Suppl 1): S2–7.

Wong Kee Song LM, Marcon NE. (2003) Fluorescence and Raman spectroscopy. *Gastrointest Endosc Clin N Am* 13(2): 279–96.

Wong D, Barrett M, Stoger R, Emond M, Reid B. (1997) p16INK4a promoter is hypermethylated at a high frequency in esophageal adenocarcinomas. *Cancer Res* 57: 2619–22.

Yahagi N, Fujishiro M, Kakushima N. (2004) Endoscopic submucosal dissection for early gastric cancer using the tip of an electrosurgical snare (thin type). *Dig Endosc* 16: 34–8.

Yamamoto H, Yube T, Isoda N *et al.* (1999) A novel method of endoscopic mucosal resection using sodium hyaluronate. *Gastrointest Endosc* 50: 251–6.

Yamamoto H, Kawata H, Sunada K *et al.* (2002) Success rate of curative endoscopic mucosal resection with circumferential mucosal incision assisted by submucosal injection of sodium hyaluronate. *Gastrointest Endosc* 56: 507–12.

Yoshida K, Kuniyasu H, Yasui W, Kitadai Y, Toge T, Tahara E. (1993) Expression of growth factors and their receptors in human esophageal carcinomas: regulation of expression by epidermal growth factor and transforming growth factor alpha. *J Cancer Res Clin Oncol* 119: 401–7.

Zaninotto G, Parenti AR, Ruol A, Costantini M, Merigliano S, Ancona E. (2000) Oesophageal resection for high-grade dysplasia in Barrett's oesophagus. *Br J Surg* 87: 1102–5.

Zelefsky M, Fuks Z, Hunt M *et al.* (2002) High-dose intensity modulated radiation therapy for prostate cancer: early toxicity and biochemical outcome in 772 patients. *Int J Radiat Oncol Biol Phys* 52: 1111–16.

Zhang Z, Liao Z, Jin J *et al.* (2005) Dose–response relationship in locoregional control for patients with stage II-III esophageal cancer treated with concurrent chemotherapy and radiotherapy. *Int J Radiat Oncol Biol Phys* 61: 656–64.

Zuccaro G Jr, Rice TW, Vargo JJ *et al.* (2005) Endoscopic ultrasound errors in esophageal cancer. *Am J Gastroenterol* 100(3): 601–6.

5 Squamous Cancer of the Esophagus

Edited by Hugh Barr

Diagnosis

History and etiology

Alastair Sammon & Mark Vipond

As with many cancers there is a marked geographic and ethnic variation in the incidence of squamous cell cancer of the esophagus. In most countries of the world the incidence of squamous esophageal cancer is in single or low double figures per 100,000, and it occurs predominantly in men between the ages of 35 and 64. The incidence per 100,000 is 5.8 in the United States of America (white population), 4.8 in the UK, and 2.5 in the Netherlands. There are a few areas of moderately high occurrence, including parts of France (25.5 per 100,000), among the black population of southern USA (20.5 per 100,000), and Jamaica in the Caribbean (26.6 per 100,000). In many of the low-incidence countries, adenocarcinoma of the gastroesophageal junction is much more common and is rising in incidence, and again there is a male predominance (Cotton & Sammon 1989; Wang *et al.* 2005; Cancer Research UK 2006). Research from the Netherlands has looked at socioeconomic status, defined as the average net yearly income, and the incidence of both adenocarcinoma and squamous cancer. Adenocarcinoma appears to be a disease of the more affluent, whereas those of lower socioeconomic status are more prone to squamous carcinoma (van Vliet *et al.* 2006). Similarly, in a multivariate model looking at the risk factors in a high-incidence region in Linzhou (China), higher household income was also associated with a lower risk of developing squamous dysplasia, a risk factor for subsequent development of invasive cancer (Wei *et al.* 2005). Other factors associated with an increase in the incidence of dysplasia were a family history, heating the home without a chimney, and having lost more of your teeth.

Gastrointestinal Oncology: A Critical Multidisciplinary Team Approach.
Edited by J. Jankowski, R. Sampliner, D. Kerr, and Y. Fong.

Overall, squamous cell cancer predominates around the world. The incidence rate achieves almost endemic proportions in several regions of the world. Around the Caspian littoral region and in Kazakhstan the recorded incidence reaches 547.2 per 100,000 for males aged 35–64; in the Transkei region of South Africa it is 357.2 per 100,000; and in Linxian Province China it is 379 per 100,000 (Cotton & Sammon 1989; Wang *et al.* 2005). In Linxian, esophageal cancer accounts for 20% of total deaths. In these 'endemic' regions around 97% of esophageal malignancies are squamous. The marked geographical variation is a remarkable feature in China and also in Africa. This is illustrated by the high incidence being limited to only one part of the Transkei region of South Africa. Within these high-incidence areas in Southern Africa, there is also considerable local variation.

In low- and medium-incidence areas, tobacco and alcohol have a close and dose-related association with the disease, and the evidence supports these as major etiologic factors. Attempts to find general genetic factors have failed to reveal a significant or useful relationship. The following are the major etiologic factors.

- Patients with the hereditary condition tylosis (autosomal dominant), which is associated with hyperkeratosis of the palms and soles, have a 70% chance of developing squamous cell carcinoma (SCC) of the esophagus. The condition was first described in two Liverpool families in the UK, and is referred to as the Howell-Evans syndrome (Howell-Evans *et al.* 1958). The genetic basis for the development of squamous cell cancer is now understood, with the tylosis esophageal cancer locus mapped to 17q25. It is now become apparent that this locus is commonly deleted in sporadic cases of squamous esophageal cancer (Iwaya *et al.* 1999).
- Patients with achalasia of the cardia of more than 25 years' duration have approximately a 7% chance of developing SCC in the esophagus. This is possibly related to prolonged exposure to carcinogens in the stagnant food.
- Patients with previous head or neck or upper aerodigestive tract SCC are more prone to further cancers in the region, including the esophagus (cumulative risk 25% at 5 years). This

has led to the suggestion that these patients may require repeated endoscopic inspection to identify dysplastic lesions which can be treated in a minimally invasive fashion. Another at-risk group are those who have received radiotherapy to the thorax to treat lymphoma or other thoracic conditions.

- Paterson–Brown–Kelly (Plummer–Vinson) syndrome (iron-deficiency anemia, glossitis and postcricoid esophageal web) is associated with a 10% incidence of esophageal or pharyngeal cancer, and is more common in women.
- The human papillomavirus, part of a group of DNA viruses which infects skin and mucous membranes, is implicated in several forms of squamous cancer. If the viral sequences are incorporated into host cellular DNA they can act as oncogenes and promote malignant transformation. Recently, oncogenic types of human papillomavirus have been detected by polymerase chain reaction analysis in esophageal cancers in patients from Japan.

Environmental etiology in endemic areas

In the endemic areas of China, the Caspian Littoral region and South Africa, there is as yet no agreement on causation. The two common threads are dependence on a single staple, either of wheat or maize (Sammon & Alderson 1998), and an otherwise vitamin-poor diet. Tobacco has a proven association in some endemic areas, but in these areas tobacco exposure is not exceptionally high and more than a quarter of the victims of the disease are non-smokers. Single environmental and ingested causes of the disease, such as fumonisin (a fungal toxin which grows on maize), nitrosamines and aflatoxins have been proposed. Predisposition followed by an environmental carcinogen appears to be a possible pathway.

It is a consistent observation that in Africa, there is a strong association with consumption of maize. This diet has deficiencies, particularly in vitamins and trace elements, and it is high in unbalanced fatty acids. Although a clear etiologic mechanism has not been described, van Rensburg (1985) has consistently pointed out the deficiency in maize of zinc, magnesium, riboflavin and nicotinic acid, arguing that these predispose the esophagus to malignant transformation. Sammon's research leads us to believe that the critical factor in predisposition is the fatty acid content of maize. Maize is high in linoleic acid, an omega-6 polyunsaturated fatty acid. It is very low in omega-3 fatty acid, with an N-6 to N-3 ratio of 70 : 1 or more. This type of imbalance is known to favor production of prostaglandin E2 (PGE2). Availability of other dietary fats reduces this tendency. However, in those on a maize-based diet, prostaglandin E2 in the saliva falls as other fats in the diet rise. Riboflavin deficiency, a common accompaniment of a maize-based diet, also increases PGE2 biosynthesis. This type of maize has been shown to have a strong association with esophageal cancer both in South Africa and in Veneto, a medium-incidence area of Italy. Specifically, feeding human subjects a diet high in linoleic acid results in an increase in intragastric PGE2 production (van Rensburg *et al.* 1985; Sammon & Alderson 1998; Sammon & Morgan 2002). Prostaglandin E2's effects include gastric acid suppression, and loss of tone of pyloric and cardiac sphincters. The high intragastric pH and reflux one would expect from excess intragastric PGE2 production have been documented to be present in more than 50% of a high-risk population in Transkei with an intragastric pH above 4. The high pH is associated with frequency of maize consumption; 60% of a sample of Transkeians suffered from diet-associated heartburn, and a significant number of those reported regurgitation of bile (Grant *et al.* 1988; Sammon *et al.* 2003). There is therefore an evidence trail leading from a heavily maize-based diet, to gastric acid suppression and reflux into the esophagus, that reflux containing much PGE2 and little or no acid. The situation bears comparison with the chronic achlorhydria of pernicious anemia and partial gastrectomy. It therefore appears that in African endemic areas there is a mechanism for a dietary predisposition. The same mechanism may apply in maize-growing areas of China. Wheat is the staple in the areas around the Caspian Sea, and there is as yet no mechanism described to link it to esophageal cancer there. Alcohol has no association in the endemic areas of the world.

Clinical

Alastair Sammon & Mark Vipond

The disease occurs predominantly among the rural population (predominantly poor) of developing countries. For them medical facilities are often out of reach both geographically and financially. Thus early detection is unlikely and patients present late when local and/or lymphatic spread has already occurred; some present with the symptoms of metastatic spread. The history may be of a minor change in sensation when swallowing, or of non-specific dyspepsia. This is followed by impairment of the ability to swallow, occasionally also pain on swallowing. Meat and bread are often the first foods to stick or to be regurgitated, this progressing over weeks to an inability to swallow thin soups and even saliva. Some patients present with dribbling saliva (sialorrhea), when even water cannot be swallowed. The patient can often identify accurately the level of the obstruction. Cough and dyspnea are present in some due to regurgitation and aspiration into the trachea. A small number of patients will present with chest infection or a lung abscess. Weight loss is usual, and associated with that, weakness and lethargy. Many rural patients do not present until this stage (72%).

Screening

The detection of early disease by population screening is an important issue in endemic areas. In China, screening for SCC is based on cytology of cells from the esophagus obtained by *lawang*, in which a balloon covered with a fine mesh is swallowed, inflated and pulled up the esophagus. Individuals found to have malignant cells undergo endoscopy and biopsy. The sensitivity of detection is 80% and surgical cure is possible in 90% of patients with early asymptomatic cancer. In the high-risk rural population in Linxian, China early diagnosis with endoscopy has resulted in the detection of premalignant conditions of dysplasia and carcinoma *in situ* (Wang *et al.* 2005; Wei *et al.* 2005). In Western countries, esophageal cancer screening is unlikely to become a priority and no major trend towards earlier diagnosis in asymptomatic patients can be expected. Certain patients with previous squamous cancers, particularly in the head and neck, are being increasingly monitored and the dysplasia detected (Fig. 5.1) and treated endoscopically (Radu *et al.* 2000).

Thus, in the developed world, it is apparent that most patients with esophageal cancer still present with difficulty in swallowing, as is the case in the developing world. The esophagus can distend to a remarkable degree without conscious sensation; a malignant tumor of the esophagus must be almost circumferential before the residual, uninvolved esophageal muscle can no longer accommodate swallowed food. The lumen diameter has been shown to be reduced to less than 12 mm before dysphagia occurs, and this is therefore a late symptom. Occasionally, patients present with hematemesis, enlarged cervical lymph node or esophageal pain. Even in late presentations, weight loss or cachexia may be the only clinical sign. Dehydration is common. Laryngeal palsy may be present. Enlarged neck nodes may be palpable. All of these are indicators of poor prognosis.

The disease may occur anywhere from pharynx to cardia. The middle third of the esophagus is the commonest site. The sequence for the development of a cancer has been clarified in large Chinese series. A cohort of 682 patients were followed with endoscopy and biopsy for 13.5 years, with 114 (16.7%) developing a squamous cell cancer. The relative risk was assessed according to the initial histologic diagnosis. It was 1 if normal, 0.8 if esophagitis was present, 1.9 for basal cell hyperplasia, and 2.9–9.8 for mild to moderate dysplasia. The major risk was an initial diagnosis of severe dysplasia (28.3) and carcinoma *in situ* (34.4). There also appeared to be no clinically relevant difference between high-grade dysplasia and carcinoma *in situ* (Wang *et al.* 2005; Wei *et al.* 2005).

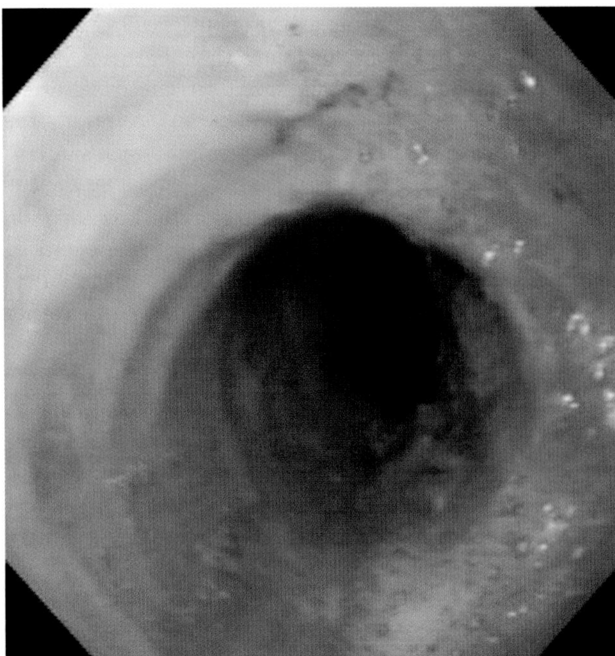

Fig. 5.1 Endoscopic picture of squamous dysplasia in an asymptomatic patient.

Histopathology and staging

Salim Anjarwalla, David Hewin & Neil Shepherd

The pathologist plays two important roles in the upper gastrointestinal multidisciplinary team (MDT): to present the findings from the endoscopic biopsy and to present the pathologic stage of the resection specimen.

Biopsy pathology of squamous neoplasia (Fig. 5.2)

The main concerns for the pathologist are the identification of squamous dysplasia, the grading of the severity of dysplasia and,

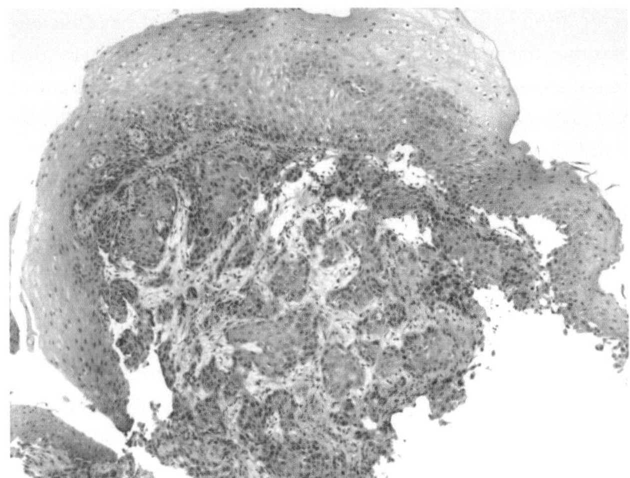

Fig. 5.2 Squamous cell carcinoma of the esophagus on biopsy. The surface shows non-neoplastic squamous epithelium with infiltrating moderately differentiated squamous cell carcinoma beneath. The morphologic similarity between the surface mucosa and the tumor is clearly evident.

most importantly, the diagnosis of invasive carcinoma. The pathologic diagnosis of dysplasia and carcinoma is not always a straightforward one and is subject to observer variation. One of the reasons for this, in the UK at least, is the relative lack of experience with esophageal squamous dysplasia compared to dysplasia in Barrett's esophagus and its associated adenocarcinoma. In Eastern countries, in particular China, esophageal squamous dysplasia is much more commonly encountered pathologically. In fact, criteria for the diagnosis of intraepithelial neoplasia and dysplasia differ widely between Eastern and Western pathologists, especially with regard to the distinction between severe dysplasia and invasive carcinoma (Takubo 2000). Whilst this distinction is of obvious importance, it is our experience that severe dysplasia is often associated with underlying carcinoma, although this observation may simply reflect the fact that most patients present with dysphagia due to established invasive malignancy. Furthermore, in the UK at least, there is still considerable controversy as to whether the three-tier classification (mild, moderate and severe) or the simpler and more reproducible two-tier system (low grade and high grade) should be used, the latter is now fully accepted as the appropriate classification for glandular neoplasia in the columnar-lined esophagus.

Another diagnostic challenge for pathologists is to distinguish neoplasia from the various mimics of malignancy and pseudoneoplastic conditions. One prime example is the inflammatory polyp typically located at the esophagogastric junction. In this situation the combination of marked squamous proliferation and bizarre stromal cells can mislead a pathologist into making a diagnosis of invasive SCC (Carr & Sobin 1999; Gill *et al.* 2003).

Given these difficulties, it is clear that the pathologic findings must be interpreted in the context of the clinical, endoscopic and radiologic findings: herein lies the importance of thorough discussion at the MDT meeting (Manek & Warren 2006). It is good practice for there to be a full review of the pathologic diagnosis at the meeting before management decisions are undertaken, and this should include review of any biopsies that have been carried out at a different institution. The pathologist presenting the biopsy findings must confirm whether or not a definitive histologic diagnosis of malignancy is appropriate for a suitable management plan to be formulated. In equivocal cases, the pathologist should stress the degree of uncertainty so that repeat endoscopy and biopsy may be considered if appropriate. For instance, in the example given above of the 'inflammatory polyp of the esophagogastric junction' the pathologist, at the MDT meeting, will have full knowledge of the clinical and endoscopic features. If that pathologist is told that there is a small polypoid lesion at the esophagogastric junction, then that would allow a better understanding of the clinical circumstances and indicate that the pathologic changes merely represent mimicry of malignancy.

In order to further limit the occurrence of errors, we firmly believe that two pathologists should confirm the diagnosis of severe dysplasia and carcinoma in the esophagus as this has such major implications for the patient.

Resection specimens of esophageal squamous neoplasia

The TNM classification (2002) of malignant tumors is the most widely used method for the pathologic staging of the resection specimen. Meticulous macroscopic examination and dissection by the pathologist, combined with comprehensive microscopic analysis, is of fundamental importance in accurately staging resected tumors.

Discussion at the MDT meeting is again essential in order to review the pathologic stage of the resection specimen and arrive at a decision regarding the role of adjuvant therapy and follow-up of patients. In addition to the stage, the pathologist must highlight important prognostic factors which may not have been incorporated into staging but influence the choice of management. The MDT meeting also provides an excellent opportunity to correlate pathologic staging with radiologic staging, to assess tumor response in cases given preoperative adjuvant therapy, and to provide surgeons with feedback on the quality of surgery and adequacy of resection margins. There is now evidence that discussion at the MDT meeting is associated with improved patient outcomes after surgery for esophageal carcinoma (Stephens *et al.* 2006).

Relevant anatomy and microanatomy

The discussion of pathologic staging cannot begin without a brief revision of basic anatomic and histologic concepts. Unlike other parts of the gastrointestinal tract, most of the esophagus lacks a serosal covering. The absence of this protective barrier of mesothelial cells and associated basement membrane is thought to contribute to the early involvement of mediastinal structures often seen in esophageal cancers. The outermost layer of much of the esophagus is hence the subserosa, better termed the 'adventitia' since there is no overlying serosa. This lies immediately deep to the longitudinal layer of the bowel wall and represents a much thicker tissue layer, consisting of loose fibrous connective tissues rich in blood vessels and lymphatics.

The short distal intraperitoneal portion of the esophagus is invested in a serosa. In the thorax, the lateral surfaces of the esophagus are closely applied to the pleural surfaces of the lungs. This creates potential for pleural involvement in esophageal carcinoma, and a radical esophagectomy will always include a bilateral medial pleurectomy. Like the serosa, the pleural surface is also composed of a mesothelial layer with a basement membrane (as are the pericardial and peritoneal surfaces). Technically, therefore, the pleura and serosa are synonymous terms. The impact of involvement of either on pathologic staging is, however, different.

T staging: the extent of spread of the primary tumor (Tables 5.1 & 5.2)

The depth of invasion of the tumor through the wall of the esophagus is the most important prognostic indicator, with considerable independent prognostic significance. The pathologist identifies areas of the tumor that show the greatest depth of invasion macroscopically in multiple blocks and this can then be confirmed microscopically.

As previously mentioned, a bilateral medial pleurectomy is also included in radical esophagectomy specimens. The pleura must be identified and distinguished from the adventitial or circumferential resection margin as the implications of involvement are quite different. Pleural infiltration reflects on local tumor extent and increases the stage to pT4 (Ludeman & Shepherd 2005). It must be stated that, to date, there has been no large series assessing the significance of pleural involvement, in terms of locoregional recurrence and prognostic implication.

Table 5.1 TNM staging classification of esophageal cancer.

T1	Tumor involves lamina propria and/or submucosa
T2	Tumor involves muscularis propria
T3	Tumor involves adventitial tissues
T4	Tumor involves adjacent structures
N1	Regional nodes involved
M1	Distant metastases
For tumor of lower thoracic esophagus	
M1a	Celiac nodes involved
M1b	Other distant metastasis
For tumor of upper thoracic esophagus	
M1a	Cervical nodes involved
M1b	Other distant metastasis
For tumor of midthoracic esophagus	
M1b	Distant metastasis including non-regional lymph nodes

Table 5.2 Stages groupings and TNM classification.

Stage 0	Tis	N0	M0
Stage I	T1	N0	M0
Stage IIA	T2	N0	M0
	T3	N0	M0
Stage IIB	T1	N1	M0
	T2	N1	M0
Stage III	T3	N1	M0
	T4	Any N	M0
Stage IV	Any T	Any N	M1
Stage IVA	Any T	Any N	M1a
Stage IVB	Any T	Any N	M1b

However, it has been shown that positive pleural lavage cytology may be predictive of local recurrence (Jiao *et al.* 2000).

N staging: the presence or absence of lymph node metastases

The importance of a thorough and accurate lymph node harvest from all parts of the specimen cannot be overemphasized. The presence or absence of lymph node metastases is a significant and independent indicator of prognosis and, according to some studies, the most important one. The number of nodes involved has also frequently been found to be significant. Both involvement of more than four or five nodes and a ratio of positive to resected nodes of more than 50% have been associated with a very poor outcome.

M staging: the presence or absence of distant metastatic disease

In the TNM staging system, celiac, cervical and non-regional lymph node involvement are considered as distant metastases. Metastases in other organs, however, are not staged pathologically unless biopsies or resections of these are submitted.

Other prognostic parameters

Resection margins

Completeness of resection is not included in the TNM staging system, despite being shown to be a strong prognostic factor after surgical resection (Hofstetter *et al.* 2002). Residual tumor, after resection with curative intent, can be categorized by the R classification, as shown below.

- R0 for complete tumor resection with all margins negative
- R1 for incomplete tumor resection with microscopic involvement of a margin
- R2 for incomplete tumor resection with macroscopic residual tumor not resected.

Proximal margin involvement has been shown to increase the likelihood of tumor recurrence, attributable to the risk of discontinuous foci of carcinoma in the proximal esophagus. Evidence of the significance of involvement of the distal margin is less convincing.

The importance of involvement of the adventitial or circumferential margin (i.e. the margin not covered by pleura or intraperitoneal serosa) is now established. There is good evidence that, as in the rectum, this margin should be regarded as involved (R1) if tumor extends to 1 mm or less of the margin as these tumors have been shown to have an increased risk for local recurrence (Dexter *et al.* 2001). The advantage of a clear circumferential margin appears to be confined to cases with a low metastatic nodal burden (less than 25% of nodes involved).

Serosal/peritoneal involvement (other than pleural)

There are few studies assessing the prognostic importance of involvement of this margin for eventual outcome, although there is one paper that describes a high incidence of death due to peritoneal carcinomatosis in esophageal cancer (Katayama *et al.* 2003).

T1 subclassification

One major disadvantage of the basic TNM staging system (2005) is its failure to differentiate between tumors confined to the mucosa and those involving the submucosa (both regarded as T1 although a recent supplement has advocated dividing these two categories into T1a and T1b respectively). This distinction has been shown to be of considerable prognostic significance, especially for SCC (Goseki *et al.* 1992). Whereas intramucosal carcinomas have very low rates of lymph node metastatic disease, 30–40% of patients with submucosal spread have lymph node metastasis.

Vascular invasion

Venous/lymphatic invasion is not included in the TNM system but has been shown to be an important prognostic factor on univariate analysis.

Squamous cell carcinoma vs. adenocarcinoma – key differences that affect staging (Day *et al.* 2003)

• Squamous cell carcinoma tends to spread linearly via the submucosa. Whilst this is also seen in adenocarcinoma, more commonly these tumors show transverse spread through the wall.
• There is a greater risk of discontinuous foci of tumor with SCC than with adenocarcinoma, particularly in the proximal esophagus. This, coupled with the high incidence of submucosal extension, stresses the need for histologic sampling of the resection margins.
• Squamous cell carcinoma may show a very different pattern of lymph node involvement to adenocarcinoma, with the latter most often showing involvement of lower periesophageal and upper gastric lymph nodes (Matsubara *et al.* 1999). This is because the lymphatic drainage of the upper esophagus is to the deep cervical lymph nodes, while the lower two-thirds are drained by the posterior mediastinal (periesophageal) and upper gastric lymph nodes.
• Because of the complex lymphatic network communicating with the thoracic duct at multiple levels, there is often involvement of lymph nodes not directly draining the site of the tumor. This phenomenon of 'jumping' nodal metastases is now well recognized and is particularly true for early-stage SCC.

Imaging and clinical staging

David Hewin, Neil Shepherd & Salim Anjarwalla

In some poorly resourced rural situations a clinical diagnosis may be all that is possible. A straight chest X-ray may show a fluid level in the mediastinum. Referral to a secondary or tertiary facility will allow diagnosis by barium swallow or endoscopy with or without a tissue biopsy. Barium swallow, even a single view, unscreened, can provide evidence of tumor position, length, axial deviation and fistula formation. The typical ragged stricture deformity may be seen. A histologic diagnosis is important whenever possible, and vital whenever any form of local treatment is to be carried out.

In the developed world esophageal cancer is usually diagnosed at upper gastrointestinal endoscopy and biopsy. Occasionally a barium swallow is the first investigation but it must be followed by endoscopic biopsy to confirm diagnosis. The preferred approach for patients with suspected cancer or dysphagia is an early endoscopy and biopsy. There has been concern that early endoscopy in dysphagic patients carries a risk of perforation of an unsuspected pharyngeal pouch. This risk is minimal if endoscopy is performed under direct vision by an experienced endoscopist. Care must be exercised in patients who have a long history of regurgitation, in whom a pharyngeal pouch may be present. Figures 5.1 and 5.3 show endoscopic pictures of squamous dysplasia and an early T1 cancer of the esophagus, and illustrate that the changes can be subtle. Chromoendoscopy with dye spraying using Lugol's iodine can enhance the con-

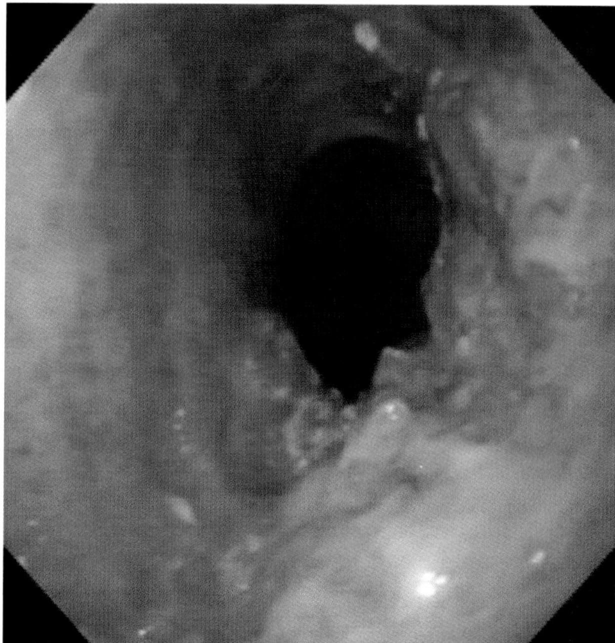

Fig. 5.3 Endoscopic picture of an early T1 cancer of the esophagus.

trast, since dysplasia and cancer may not take up the dye due to depletion in glycogen. This practice is not widespread and predominantly used for patients suspected to have or being screened for synchronous or metachronous lesions.

Assessing the length of the tumor is not only important for resection but can provide prognostic information. Lymph node metastases are present in about 50% of patients with tumors less than 5 cm long, and in more than 80% of those with longer tumors.

Patients with a diagnosis of esophageal SCC are discussed at the upper GI cancer MDT meeting and a management plan is developed, based upon clinical staging and patient fitness. Clinical staging involves clinical examination and a range of investigations which give an estimation of clinical stage, enabling appropriate management decisions. Frequently investigation for staging is combined with assessment of fitness before definitive MDT discussion.

It is important to arrange the order of investigations to obtain accurate staging as early as possible in order to distinguish patients for whom management will be palliative from those who will be treated with curative intent and so avoid unnecessary tests. Thus investigation for metastatic disease should be completed before tests designed to inform strategy for curative treatment. The various staging modalities are described in the sequence in which they are usually performed.

Endoscopic ultrasonography is particularly useful in staging the extent of tumor in the esophageal wall and in the detection of enlarged lymph nodes. Ultrasonography, CT and chest radiography are necessary to exclude metastatic disease. However, use of CT and MRI has failed to improve the local preoperative staging of esophageal cancer, because they do not accurately assess depth of invasion and lymph node involvement. Even when the tumor is detected early and is limited to the mucosa, up to 40% of patients have lymph node metastasis. Metastases from SCC may be very extensive: nodal metastases are found in the upper gastric area in one-third of patients with tumors in the upper esophagus. Conversely, superior mediastinal lymph node metastasis is found in 10% of tumors of the lower esophagus. In most solid tumors, the presence of histologic lymph node metastasis is associated with reduced survival.

Staging at diagnosis

The majority of patients present with dysphagia caused by esophageal stricture at the site of the tumor. Such presentation usually implies a locally advanced tumor and may be associated with other symptoms such as odynophagia and weight loss. Patients with already established metastatic disease or invasion of local structures may, in addition, present with more unusual symptoms, such as constant back pain, hoarse voice, neck or abdominal swellings, bony pain or pathologic fracture.

At the other end of the scale, a small proportion of patients may be asymptomatic, having the carcinoma identified during endoscopy or barium swallow for unrelated symptoms. Tumors identified in this way are frequently at an early stage and may therefore be suitable for local therapy such as endoscopic mucosal resection (May & Ell 2006). Definitive diagnosis is made by endoscopy and biopsy, although a significant number of patients will have had barium studies organized by primary-care practitioners before referral. Endoscopic biopsy may be combined with brush cytology and occasionally endoscopic mucosal resection. The visual appearance of the tumor at endoscopy gives an early indication of the predicted clinical stage, since tumors presenting with impassable stricture are nearly always stage T3 (Vickers & Alderson 1998).

Computed tomography (CT)

CT scanning is most useful for identifying hematogenous metastases, typically lung or liver (Lerut *et al.* 2006). The scan should include the neck, thorax and abdomen, and be performed with both oral and intravenous contrast agents. Modern spiral scanners allow multiplane and three-dimensional reconstruction which can be of great benefit in planning surgical resection. The high definition of scans now also allows more accurate primary tumor and nodal staging, although these parameters may be more accurately defined by endoscopic ultrasound.

Endoscopic ultrasound (EUS) (Fig. 5.4)

EUS allows very accurate primary tumor and nodal staging. Standard radial ultrasound may distinguish early tumors suitable for endoscopic resection from more invasive lesions which require more radical therapy. Management strategies with intent to cure may involve primary chemoradiotherapy,

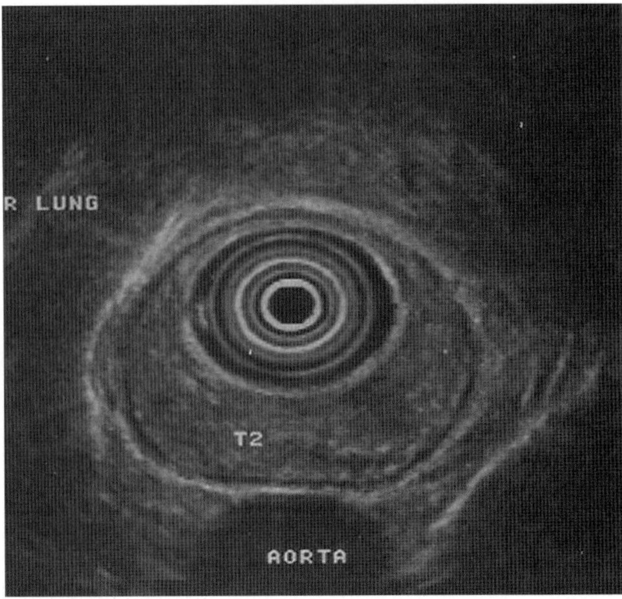

Fig. 5.4 Endoscopic ultrasound scan of T2 esophageal carcinoma.

neoadjuvant therapy followed by surgery, or surgery alone. Accurate staging of the primary tumor and locoregional lymph nodes by EUS can be used to inform decisions on curative therapy. Occasionally EUS may identify criteria that make tumor unresectable. Local invasion of adjacent structures (airway, aorta, pericardium) or the presence of metastatic disease (liver, celiac lymph nodes) are examples.

Advancements in the technology of linear endoscopic ultrasound scanners, together with refinement of fine needle biopsy techniques now allows biopsy of structures adjacent to the esophagus, typically lymph nodes. This technique results in more accurate lymph node staging which may in turn influence the management strategy (Mariette *et al.* 2004). A randomized clinical trial is currently being performed by the British National Health Service for the assessment of EUS in the management of esophagogastric cancer.

Positron emission tomography/computed tomography (PET-CT) (Fig. 5.5)

Positron emission tomography (PET) makes use of the high rate of glucose metabolism within carcinomas which enables their detection with ^{18}F-labeled fluoro-2-deoxy-D-glucose (FDG). The development of PET-CT provides fused PET and CT data. The combination of functional imaging and accurate anatomic localization is a powerful technique, especially in the assessment of secondary tumor.

Ideally PET-CT would replace standard CT for staging esophageal SCC, because the added functional imaging of PET may help to clarify the nature of lesions which are indeterminate on CT (typically small nodules in the lung or liver) (Bruzzi *et al.* 2007). In practical terms, the limited availability and cost of PET-CT demand a rational approach where PET-CT is used as a final control to rule out metastatic disease before treatment for patients in whom all other staging tests would support treatment with curative intent. Even in these restricted circumstances PET-CT scanning may change treatment strategy from curative to palliative in up to 20% of patients (Cerfolio *et al.* 2005).

Other staging techniques

In addition to the techniques already described, a variety of specific diagnostic and imaging modalities may be recommended by the MDT for tumor staging depending on the presentation, site of the primary tumor or suspicion of metastatic disease.

Theses include transabdominal ultrasound scan for hepatic metastases, MRI scanning of the neck together with percutaneous fine needle aspiration biopsy for assessment of lymphadenopathy, and bronchoscopy if direct invasion of airways is suspected or if pathologic assessment of biopsies suggests a possible bronchogenic origin.

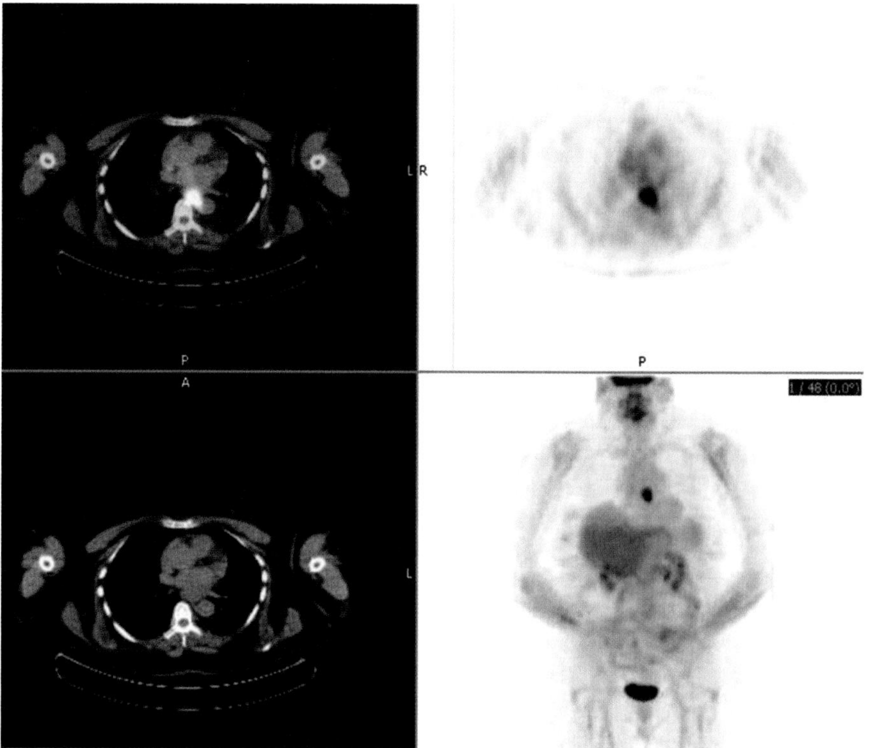

Fig. 5.5 PET-CT scan of midesophageal carcinoma. The uptake is clearly seen in the esophagus.

Most staging algorithms also include laparoscopy in the assessment of lower-third tumors. This allows both the visualization and biopsy of small peritoneal or liver surface metastases which may not be apparent on other imaging modalities. It also allows direct anesthetic assessment of patients who may be recommended to have surgical resection as part of definitive treatment. Similarly, staging thoracoscopy and mediastinoscopy are sometimes recommended.

The esophageal cancer MDT should have a complete range of investigations which can be called upon to provide timely, accurate clinical staging of tumors. The initial MDT discussion should result in an individualized care pathway which will produce enough information to plan appropriate management whilst avoiding unnecessary investigation. A pragmatic approach will often combine staging tests and fitness assessment in the shortest possible time to allow initiation of curative treatment where possible, and effective palliative treatment where cure is not an option.

Treatment

Overview

Hugh Barr

Squamous cell carcinoma presents usually at an advanced stage and radical therapy offers the best chance of control and cure. Worldwide each year 462,000 people are diagnosed with esophageal cancer and 386,000 people die from it. Population-based 5-year relative survival rates for all patients diagnosed with esophageal cancer (both squamous and adenocarcinoma) in 2000–01 in England and Wales were 8% for both men and women (30% for men and 27% for women at 1 year after diagnosis) (Cancer Research UK 2006). The mean age of diagnosis is the seventh decade, and mortality is clearly associated with increasing age and associated comorbidity. There is intense interest in areas of high incidence to detect and manage premalignant lesions with endoscopic or chemopreventative therapy. In Linxian, China the impetus is to address nutritional deficiencies. In particular, selenium is seen as being an important food additive in this region (Blot *et al.* 1993; Mark *et al.* 2002). Case–control studies have consistently demonstrated the importance of diet and drugs, in particular aspirin, in cancer prevention. Aspirin is a synthetic agent of a naturally occurring phytochemical class (salicylates). These are commonly found in fruit and vegetables, but may be destroyed by overprocessing food such that supplements are required. The role of non-steroidal drugs and aspirin appear to be pleomorphic, and their use is associated with gastrointestinal morbidity, in particular bleeding (Jankowski & Hawk 2006).

In the Western world the problem of metchronous squamous lesions in patient who have had a previous cancer is becoming a major problem. These patients may have received radiotherapy, chemotherapy or surgery and further intervention is complex and difficult.

There are patient and service imperatives to ensure timely access to diagnosis and treatment. The data as to whether delay adversely affects outcome remain a subject of debate. A retrospective series of 632 patients treated with curative intent who were stratified into groups who received esophagectomy within 3 weeks, at 3–6 weeks, at 6–9 weeks or after 9 weeks has demonstrated no adverse outcome by delay. It appears that patients with a longer delay had a higher rate of complete tumor resection, suggesting that they were more appropriately selected for surgery (Kotz *et al.* 2006).

Surgery

Ferdinandos Skoulidis, Yu Jo Chua & David Cunningham

Anatomic considerations

The esophagus is divided into cervical portion, extending from the lower border of the cricoid cartilage to the thoracic inlet, the surface marking of which is the jugular notch. On entering the thorax the esophagus is divided into an upper part extending to the carina, and a middle part extending to an arbitrary point halfway between the bifurcation of the trachea and the esophagogastric junction. The lower esophagus extends into the abdomen to join the stomach. Accurate location of this junction is very dependent on the endoscopist clearly identifying the site of the biopsy as being in the gastric cardia, hiatal hernia, or the esophagus. The endoscopic problem is that the anatomy and position of the gastroesophageal junction are difficult to define. There is a lack of a universally accepted and reproducible set of criteria to endoscopically distinguish the cardia of the stomach from the distal esophagus. During endoscopy, it is important to identify certain key anatomic landmarks to allow some delineation of the position of the tumor. The squamocolumnar junction is usually visible where the pale squamous epithelium merges into redder columnar mucosa. The precise location of the gastroesophageal junction is hard to identify clinically. At present, it is defined endoscopically as the level of the most proximal gastric fold. Some patients with a hiatal hernia have defective and weak lower esophageal sphincters, and there is therefore no clear-cut demarcation as the clinician enters the stomach with the endoscope. The proximal margin of the gastric folds must be determined when the distal esophagus is minimally inflated. Overinflation will flatten and obscure all the gastric folds. If the squamocolumnar and gastroesophageal junction coincide, the entire esophagus is lined with squamous mucosa. When the squamocolumnar junction is proximal to the gastroesophageal junction, there is a columnar-lined segment or Barrett's esophagus. Pathology can offer a clear indication of esophageal origin when an esophageal gland or, more usually (in a biopsy sample), a duct from these glands is seen. The depth of biopsy required makes these findings unusual as the endoscopic biopsy is usually too shallow.

Lymphatic drainage

The lymphatics in the squamous esophagus are located in an extensive, highly interconnected submucosal plexus. They drain through the muscularis propria to a paraesophageal plexus and a group of lymph nodes situated on the outer wall, then to the periesophageal nodes close by, and finally to lateral esophageal nodes. Sequential drainage may not occur with connections direct from the periesophageal nodes to lateral lymph nodes. The Japanese Society (1976) published the original and detailed lymph node maps allowing classification and defining radical surgical excision (Akiyama *et al.* 1994; Griffen 2006).

The extent of lymphadenectomy

The Japanese data have demonstrated that at least 80% of patients with SCC have lymph node metastases at the time of resection, and it would seem appropriate therefore to recommend that surgery should attempt to eradicate these foci of disease. The problem is that these data were collected before the widespread use of neoadjuvant chemotherapy, with the benefits of eradicating or downstaging regional nodal disease. Radical formal lymphadenectomy has not been widely practised for esophageal SCC by most surgeons in the West. The concept is gaining increasing support, however, and there are data to suggest that some patients may benefit from radical lymph node dissection. The technique is now evolving with the concept of tailored resection dependent on intraoperative staging with sentinel node assessment (Lamb *et al.* 2005).

Preoperative assessment

Accurate staging and assessment of the patient remain essential before surgery. Only curative resection with excision of all involved tissue allows a worthwhile period of survival with good quality of life. It is now clear that unless the patient survives 2 years the quality of life benefit is not sufficient to warrant the morbidity and mortality of surgery (Blazeby *et al.* 2001, 2005). Careful assessment with formal respiratory, cardiac and nutritional testing is essential. Use of a rigorous scoring system to allow appropriate patient selection can reduce the operative mortality significantly, but must be applied with caution for the individual patient. Their general condition, nutritional status, respiratory function and cardiac function should be optimized before resection.

Principles of resection

Resection margin

The great challenge for esophageal surgeons is that of extensive submucosal spread (Fig. 5.2) of the tumor longitudinally within the esophageal wall. A radical resection which leaves behind microscopically positive margins is of great surgical concern, and defeats the primary objective of surgery. It is advocated that a minimum of 10 cm (from the edge of the macroscopic tumor) of esophageal wall should be removed. This didactic statement must be interpreted with caution since it fails to take into account anatomic location, the nature of the primary tumor, and individual patient characteristics. Current data suggest that a 4-cm margin is associated with an anastomotic recurrence rate below 15%. This can be reduced if radiotherapy is given postoperatively. The lateral or circumferential margin in the esophagus remains a challenge, but again positive margins are associated with local recurrence. It should be an aspiration to remove tumor en bloc without resecting through it. The anatomic location clearly determines whether this is possible.

Lymphadenectomy

Since at least 80% of cancers will have lymph node metastases at the time of surgery the resection level is vital. In addition, 25% of lower third squamous cancers have cervical lymph nodal involvement. It is clear that a formal lymphadenectomy should be part of the resection. The extent is again dependent on the position of the cancer. A one-field resection would only encompass the para- and periesophageal nodes, a two-field resection will include these nodes together with the thoracic duct, the left and right pulmonary hilar nodes, and the paratracheal and tracheal bifurcation nodes. A radical three-field dissection includes the nodes around the right and left recurrent laryngeal nerve, the deep lateral and external cervical chain, and those around the brachiocephalic vein. In addition, an abdominal dissection of the diaphragmatic, right and left paracardiac, diaphragmatic, perigastric and celiac nodes is required. A small trial has shown that an extended lymphadenectomy was associated with a trend to less recurrence and increased survival. The data are incomplete because of the addition of radiotherapy and chemotherapy after surgery. The current literature has not shown a difference in 1-year survival between a two-field and three-field lymphadenectomy (Griffen 2006).

Types of esophageal resection and reconstruction

The nature of the resection is again very dependent on the site of the primary tumor. Tumors in the upper third/cervical esophagus may require removal of the pharynx, larynx and trachea. Reconstruction can be by a free jejunal graft with microvascular anastomosis, or more usually total gastric interposition with removal of the entire esophagus. A lesion in the thoracic esophagus can be removed using the McKeown three-stage esophagectomy. Following a right-sided thoractomy the tumor and the whole esophagus is mobilized. The patient is then laid supine and the stomach is mobilized to act as a conduit, brought to the neck and anastomosed to the cervical esophagus. Colon can also be used as a new conduit if there are problems with the stomach. Lower-third tumors and some middle-third tumors can be removed using an initial abdominal approach to free the stomach followed by a right thoracotomy with intrathoracic anastomosis (the Ivor Lewis operation). Some surgeons prefer a left-sided approach with a thoracoabdominal incision. Fears of the possible hazards of intrathoracic surgery have lead to a transhiatal approach with transposition of the stomach to the neck with a cervical anastomosis. Increasingly laparoscopic and thoracoscopic techniques are being used to reduce trauma to normal tissue and are proving to be very effective. The principles of surgery are the same, but the overall insult to the patient is reduced. Many surgical units are moving to this approach and large series are now being reported with no mortality. This surgery was initially reserved for patients with dysplasia (Nguyen *et al.* 2000).

Complications of surgery

This type of surgery still has among the highest morbidity and mortality rates of all operations. It is essential that surgeons and units performing it concentrate their expertise and demonstrate mortality rates below 5%. Studies have revealed an overall 11% mortality, and morbidity rates remain between 20 and 40%. The main complications are infective, respiratory, and cardiac. Specific dangers are anastomotic dehiscence, ischemia of the transposed colon, jejunum or stomach, chylothorax, recurrent laryngeal nerve palsy and thromboembolic disease. Late complications include anastomosis, stricture, biliary reflux and vomiting (Muller *et al.* 1990; Bachmann *et al.* 2002). Minimally invasive esophagectomy is still associated with major morbidity in 27% of patients with respiratory complications and an anastomotic leak rate of 9% (Nguyen *et al.* 2000).

Palliative surgery

Surgery will relieve dysphagia and prevent aspiration and fistula formation, and was used in the past for palliative relief of these symptoms. It is now clear that it is associated with such high morbidity, mortality and poor survival with decreased quality of life that it should not be advocated. Relief of symptoms of dysphagia is now possible using less invasive endoscopic therapy (Blazeby & Alderson 2006). These approaches are discussed in a later section.

Chemotherapy

Ferdinandos Skoulidis, Yu Jo Chua & David Cunningham

Chemotherapy represents one of the cornerstones of the management of SCC of the esophagus (SSCE). It is the treatment of choice for patients of good performance status with metastatic disease, where it is offered with the intent of prolonging survival, improving and maintaining quality of life and ameliorating disease-related symptoms. It is also given concurrently with radiotherapy as part of a combined modality approach; the use of chemoradiotherapy will be discussed in a separate section. As less than 50% of all patients present with potentially resectable tumors and the majority of them will eventually develop metastatic disease, there is a strong rationale for the use of systemic treatment as a component of both palliative and radical therapeutic strategies. This chapter will focus on established regimens as well as current trends in the use of chemotherapy for patients with both advanced and potentially operable SCCE.

Chemotherapy for advanced disease

Drugs with single-agent activity leading to response rates of at least 15% in previously untreated patients include cisplatin, 5-fluorouracil (5-FU), the vinca alkaloids vinorelbine and vindesine, mitomycin, bleomycin, doxorubicin, methotrexate, mitoguazone, and most recently the taxanes and irinotecan. The most widely studied of these is cisplatin, which has been in use since the early 1980s and forms the basis of many of the combination regimens used in this disease. Pooled data from six phase 2 trials resulted in a cumulative response rate of 20% in 161 patients (95% confidence interval [CI] 14–26%), which was, however, short lived and associated with a median survival of not more than 7 months (Sheithauer 2004). The addition of 5-FU quickly became favored over previously attempted combination regimens due to its superior toxicity profile and preclinical synergy with cisplatin. This combination (CF), typically administered at doses of 100 mg/m^2 for cisplatin and 1000 mg/m^2/24 h as a continuous infusion for 96–120 h for 5-FU, repeated every 3–4 weeks, yielded response rates of 35% and was established as the reference regimen for advanced disease for almost two decades. It should, however, be noted that the obtained responses were, on average, of brief duration (3–6 months) and translated to only modest survival benefit at the cost of substantial toxicity (Sheithauer 2004).

Attempts at improving on the reported efficacy of cisplatin/5-FU included use of the biomodulator interferon alpha-2a, as well as schedules incorporating etoposide or vinorelbine. Despite evidence of anti-tumor activity, none of these regimens proved to be superior.

The triplet combination of epirubicin, cisplatin and protracted venous infusion (PVI) 5-FU (ECF) was first developed in the UK in the late 1980s. Initially tested in a randomized comparison in patients with adenocarcinoma or undifferentiated carcinoma, ECF proved superior in all parameters of efficacy to FAMTX (5-FU, doxorubicin, methotrexate), a reference regimen for gastric adenocarcinoma at the time (Webb *et al.* 1997). A subsequent randomized trial which included 40 patients with SCCE out of a total of 580 patients found that the efficacy of the combination was not improved by substituting epirubicin with mitomycin (MCF) (Ross *et al.* 2002). In both trials, ECF was well tolerated. Data are also available from an earlier report of 21 patients with SCCE treated with ECF in which an objective response rate of 57%, progression-free survival of 7 months and overall survival of 8.4 months were observed (Andreyev *et al.* 1995). Despite the paucity of randomized trial data specifically addressing the use of ECF in patients with squamous histology, this regimen has been widely accepted in the UK, parts of Europe, and Australia, and represents the current standard regimen for patients with advanced disease in these regions (Scottish Intercollegiate Guidelines Network 2006).

The substitution of cisplatin with oxaliplatin and of 5-FU with capecitabine in ECF has been examined in the recently reported REAL2 trial in which 1002 patients with previously untreated locally advanced or metastatic carcinoma of the esophagus, gastroesophageal junction and stomach (mostly adenocarcinomas) were randomized into one of four treatment arms in a 2 × 2 factorial fashion (Cunningham *et al.* 2006). The primary objective of the study, which was to demonstrate non-inferiority for survival for both substitutions, was achieved. Furthermore, the EOX regimen (epirubicin, oxaliplatin and capecitabine) proved superior to ECF in terms of overall survival in the planned comparison for superiority of the individual treatment arms (Table 5.3). Again, treatment was well tolerated in all four arms. The results of this trial suggest that oxaliplatin can be used instead of cisplatin, and capecitabine instead of infusional 5-FU. Certainly, the latter may obviate the need for indwelling intravenous access catheters, making treatment more convenient and acceptable to patients.

More recently, the use of taxanes has generated considerable interest. Paclitaxel is one of the most active single agents in SCCE with a response rate of 32% (28% for the subset of patients with SCC); however granulocyte colony-stimulating factor (GCSF) support was required (Sheithauer 2004). The two-drug combination with cisplatin, following preclinical demonstration of schedule-dependent synergy, also proved active, with response rates between 43% and 52%, albeit at the expense of considerable treatment-related morbidity (Schull *et al.* 2003; Sheithauer 2004). Myelosuppression, neurotoxicity in the form of sensory neuropathy, and fatigue are the main limiting factors and they appear at least partially schedule dependent, with shorter infusions (3 h) associated with less hematologic and more neurologic toxicity. The further addition of 5-FU in a phase II trial of 61 patients led to a comparable overall response rate of 48% including complete responses in 20% of patients with squamous histology, which is a striking result for a patient group with a high incidence of metastatic disease (Sheithauer 2004). Although toxicity was substantial in this trial, indicating that the optimal schedule and dose of paclitaxel in combination chemotherapy regimens for esophageal cancer has not yet been determined, results are clearly encouraging. Carboplatin, which is less nephrotoxic, neurotoxic and emetogenic than cisplatin, has also been used in conjunction with paclitaxel (El-Rayes *et al.* 2004). A semisynthetic taxane, docetaxel, also has single-agent activity and has been tested in combination regimens with cisplatin and the oral fluoropyrimidine carbamate capecitabine with encouraging efficacy, even in patients who are not chemonaive (Table 5.1) (Schull *et al.* 2003; Muro *et al.* 2004; Lorenzen *et al.* 2005). However, considerable toxicity was encountered and remains a problem.

Irinotecan is a semisynthetic camptothecin analog already established in the first- and second-line management of metastatic colorectal cancer. More recently, its use has been assessed in upper gastrointestinal tumors. Although single-agent activity is modest (Muhr-Wilkenshoff *et al.* 2003), a 6-week schedule in combination with cisplatin developed at the Memorial Sloan-Kettering Cancer Centre produced major objective responses in 57% of patients, including complete responses in 6%. The median duration of response was 4.2 months and the median actuarial overall survival 14.6 months. Effective palliation of dysphagia and pain was achieved and global quality of life was enhanced. Crucially, the treatment was tolerated well and grade 3/4 toxicities other than myelosuppression were uncommon. As 66% of patients experienced a delay in treatment, an alternative 2-week 'on', 1-week 'off' schedule was also explored in the same institution, and demonstrated reduced myelosuppression with maintained anti-tumor activity. Irinotecan has further been combined with the taxanes (Lordick *et al.* 2003) but these schedules, though active, have not yet been optimized, as evidenced by their at times excessive toxicities. Evidence of efficacy has been demonstrated even in the setting of primary refractory disease, where a clinically meaningful overall disease control rate was achieved with the combination of irinotecan and 5-FU/Leucovorin in a recent phase II trial (Assersohn *et al.* 2004).

Finally, note should be made of the emerging role of gemcitabine, a potent and specific deoxycytidine analog, in the treatment of upper gastrointestinal tumors, including esophageal cancer. A representative study of its combination with cisplatin is included in Table 5.1 (Millar *et al.* 2005).

In conclusion, the historical standard of cisplatin/5-FU for the palliative treatment of inoperable SCCE, has been expanded over the last 10–15 years with the development of novel two- or three-drug regimens with considerable activity. Despite the absence of a direct randomized comparison to CF, the ECF regimen is currently used extensively in the UK and is likely to be replaced by ECX in the near future, based on the results of recent trials. Furthermore, the combination of irinotecan and cisplatin is effective and tolerable, and warrants further investigation, while the optimal therapeutic index for taxane-based schedules has not been established. Following failure of first-line chemotherapy, there is a paucity of established second-line treatments, although preliminary evidence suggests activity for irinotecan/5-FU/leucovorin, oxaliplatin/5-FU (Mauer *et al.* 2005) or docetaxel-based combinations in this setting.

Table 5.3 Selected clinical trials of chemotherapy in advanced carcinoma of the esophagus, including patients with squamous histology.

Study	Patient group	n (evaluable)	Regimen	Histology	ORR	m PFS (months)	mOS (months)	Comments
Cisplatin/5-FU								
Bleiberg *et al.* (1997) (Phase II)	Locally advanced/ metastatic (inoperable)	44	Cisplatin 100 mg/m^2 5-FU 1000 mg/m^2/d continuous infusion vs	SCC	35%		7.7	Excessive toxicity with 16% TRM in the combination arm
		44	Cisplatin 100 mg/m^2		19%		6.5	
Webb *et al.* (1997) (Phase III)	Locally advanced/ metastatic (inoperable)	126	Epirubicin 50 mg/m^2 Cisplatin 60 mg/m^2 5-FU PVI 200 mg/m^2/24 h (ECF) vs	AC/UC	45% (*)	7.4 (*)	8.9 (*)	ECF: —improved global QoL at 24 weeks —less G3/4 neutropenia infection —more G2 alopecia, G3/4 nausea/vomiting, G1/2 mucositis
		130	Metastatic 1500/mg/m^2 5-FU 1500 mg/m^2 Doxorubicin 30 mg/m^2		21%	3.4	5.7	
Ross *et al.* (2002) (Phase III)	Locally advanced/ metastatic (inoperable)	289	ECF vs	Mostly AC SCC 7%	42.4%	7	9.4	Better QoL scores at 3 and 6 months with ECF
			Cisplatin 60 mg/m^2 Mitomycin C 7 mg/m^2 (max 14 mg) 5-FU PVI 300 mg/m^2/24 h		44.1%	7	8.7	
Taxanes								
Paclitaxel								
Ajani *et al.* (2004) (Phase II)	Locally advanced/ metastatic (inoperable)	50	Paclitaxel 250 mg/m^2 (24 h infusion) (median dose, range 150–280)	SCC (36%) AC (64%)	32% overall (28% for SCC)	4	13.2 (actuarial)	GCSF support as part of protocol. Treatment well tolerated
van der Gaast *et al.* (1999) (Phase I)	Locally advanced/ metastatic (inoperable)	59	Cisplatin 60 mg/m^2 Paclitaxel 100–200 mg/m^2 (3 h infusion)	SCC (47%) AC (52%) UC (1%)	52% (3% CR)			180 mg/m^2 MTD (DLT: neurotoxicity)
Polee *et al.* (2002) (Phase II)	Locally advanced/ metastatic (inoperable) Esophagus/GEJ	51	Cisplatin 60 mg/m^2 Paclitaxel 180 mg/m^2 (3 h infusion)	SCC (31%) AC (61%) UC (98%)	43% (4% CR)	8	9	70% G3-4 neutropenia but no neutropenic fever. No TRM

Ilson *et al.* (2000) (Phase II)	Advanced disease Esophagus/GEJ	32	Paclitaxel 200–250 mg/m^2 (24 h infusion) Cisplatin 75 mg/m^2	Mostly AC	44%	3.9	6.9	Excessive toxicity 11% TRM
Ilson *et al.* (1998) (Phase II)	Locally advanced/ metastatic (inoperable)	60	Cisplatin 20 mg/m^2 Paclitaxel 175 mg/m^2 (3 h infusion) 5-FU 1000 mg/m^2/d reduced to 750 mg/m^2/d after first 10 patients Dose of cisplatin reduced after 3rd cycle	SCC 52%	48% 20% CR in SCC	5.7	10.8	48% hospitalized 46% required dose attenuation 18% neutropenic fever 18% G3 neurotoxicity
El-Rayes *et al.* (2004) (Phase II)	Stage IIA or higher 57% metastatic disease	33	Paclitaxel 200 mg/m^2 (3 h infusion) Carboplatin 5 mg/h/mL	SCC(37%) AC(63%)	43%	2.8	9	Tolerable regimen
Docetaxel								
Muro *et al.* (2004) (Phase II)	Metastatic (chemonaive or pretreated)	49	Docetaxel 70 mg/m^2	SCC 94%	20% 36% in untreated	4.7	8.1	88% G3–4 neutropenia 18% febrile neutropenia 37% dose reduction 57% received G-CSF
Schull *et al.* (2003) (Phase II)	Metastatic	37	Cisplatin 50 mg/m^2 Docetaxel 50 mg/m^2 G-CSF allowed depending on ANC		66% (11% CR)	7	11	Tolerable
Lorenzen *et al.* (2005) (Phase II)	Metastatic (including pretreated) Esophagus/GEJ	24	Docetaxel 75 mg/m^2 Capecitabine 1000 mg/m^2 bd d1–14	SCC 71%	46% (56% in untreated) (25% in previously treated)	6.1	15.8	8% febrile neutropenia 29% G3/4 hand–foot syndrome 41% of patients had dose adjustments
Irinotecan								
Muhr-Wilkenshoff *et al.* (2003) (Phase II)	Metastatic/Locally advanced (inoperable)	9	Irinotecan 125 mg/m^2 weekly for 4 w followed by 2 w rest (6-week cycle)	SCC 77%	22%	3.8 (mean)	6.1 (mean)	
Ilson *et al.* (1999) (Phase II)	Metastatic (97%)/ locally advanced (inoperable)	35	Cisplatin 30 mg/m^2 Irinotecan 65 mg/m^2 weekly for 4 w followed by 2 w gap (6-week cycle)	SCC 34% AC 66%	57 (6% CR)	4.2 (mDOR)	14.6 (actuarial)	Well tolerated Improved dysphagia Improved QoL 66% treatment delay

continued on p. 128

Table 5.3 *Continued*

Study	Patient group	n (evaluable)	Regimen	Histology	ORR	m PFS (months)	mOS (months)	Comments
Ilson (2004) (Phase II)	Metastatic (87%)/ locally advanced (inoperable)	32	Cisplatin 30 mg/m^2 Irinotecan 65 mg/m^2	SCC (26%) AC (74%)	36%			Well tolerated and feasible 22% G3/4 fatigue
Lordick *et al.* (2003) (Phase II)	Refractory/relapsed	24	Docetaxel 25 mg/m^2 Irinotecan 55 mg/m^2	SCC 46% AC 54%	12.5%	2.1	6.0	33.3% disease stabilization 20.8% G3/4 asthenia
Assersohn *et al.* (2004) (Phase II)	Primary refractory	38	Irinotecan 180 mg/m^2 5-FU 400 mg/m^2/LV 125 mg/m^2 bolus Followed by 5-FU 1200 mg/m^2 infusion over 48 h	SCC 7% AC 93%	29%	3.7	6.4	Good palliation of symptoms
Gemcitabine								
Millar *et al.* (2005) (Phase II)	Metastatic (93%)/ locally advanced (inoperable)	32	Cisplatin 75 mg/m^2 d1 Gemcitabine 1250 mg/m^2 Subsequently reduced to 1000 mg/m^2	SCC (33%) AC (64%)	45% (9% CR) 71% in SCC ($p = 0.036$)		11	Unacceptable toxicity at initial dose level 31% G3/4 fatigue 37% G3/4 nausea/ vomiting at lower dose but less myelosuppression
Oxaliplatin								
Mauer *et al.* (2005) (Phase III)	Metastatic (97%)/ recurrent 11% prior chemotherapy	34	Oxaliplatin 85 mg/m^2 LV 500 mg/m^2/5-FU 400 mg/ m^2 bolus followed by 5-FU 600 mg/m^2	SCC 9% AC (82%) UC (9%)	40% (3% CR) 45% (chemonaive) 0% (pretreated)	4.6 4.9 (*) 1.7	7.1 7.6 (*) 2.1	26% G2/3 peripheral neuropathy
Cunningham *et al.* (2006) (Phase III)	Locally advanced/ metastatic (inoperable) (esophageal, GEJ, gastric)	249	ECF	SCC 10%/AC (overal)	40.7%	6.2	9.9	
		241	ECX (capecitabine 625 mg/m^2 bd)		46.4%	6.7	9.9	
		235	EOF (oxaliplatin 130 mg/m^2)		42.4%	6.5	9.3	
		239	EOX		47.9%	7.0	11.2 (*)	
			All regimens					

* denotes statistically significant result ($p < 0.05$)

5-FU, 5-fluorouracil; AC, adenocarcinoma; ANC, absolute neutrophil count; bd, twice daily; CR, complete response; DLT, dose-limiting toxicity; G-CSF, granulocyte colongy-stimulating factor; GEJ, gastroesophageal junction; LV, leucovorin; mDOR, median duration of response; mOS, median overall survival; mPFS, median progression-free survival; MTD, maximal tolerated dose; QoL, quality of life; ORR, overall response rate; PVI, protracted venous infusion; SCC, squamous cell carcinoma; TRM, treatment-related mortality; UC, undifferentiated carcinoma.

Preoperative chemotherapy

Based on the dismal long-term survival rates following potentially curative resection and the observed patterns of failure, including both locoregional and distant recurrences, a strategy featuring preoperative use of chemotherapy for potentially resectable disease appears well reasoned. The conceptual basis for this approach is dual: downsizing or downstaging the primary tumor, therefore enhancing the microscopic complete (R0) resection rate; and sterilizing occult micrometastatic sites, thus improving systemic control, and with it, overall and disease-free survival. Potential drawbacks include a delay in definitive surgical management for the subset of patients with chemoresistant disease, the possible early emergence of drug-resistant clones, and the morbidity and mortality associated with the side-effects of chemotherapy in an already undernourished patient population scheduled to undergo a major surgical procedure.

A number of randomized clinical trials (RCTs) of preoperative chemotherapy for SCCE were conducted in the late 1980s and throughout the 1990s. A variety of drugs and schedules were used which typically included cisplatin in combination with vinca alkaloids, bleomycin or etoposide early on and subsequently 5-FU. Unfortunately, most of these comparisons included a limited number of patients and were thus underpowered to detect a difference in outcome between the prescribed treatments. In order to obtain more definitive data, two large-scale, multi-institutional phase III trials were launched on either side of the Atlantic (Table 5.4). These included patients with both adenocarcinoma and SCC in order to reflect the evolving epidemiology of the disease. The US Intergroup-0113 trial randomized 440 patients to three cycles of preoperative chemotherapy with cisplatin and infusional 5-FU followed by surgery, versus immediate surgery (Kelsen *et al.* 1998). Patients with stable or responding disease and R0 resection were offered two further cycles of chemotherapy with a reduced dose of cisplatin (75 mg/m^2) postoperatively. In the intention-to-treat analysis, median overall survival, disease-free survival (DFS) and the pattern of first failure did not differ significantly between the two arms, although a slightly higher incidence of distant failure ($p = 0.21$) was noted for the surgery-only arm. Chemotherapy did not affect the rate of R0 resection; however, a significantly higher rate of R1 resections was evident for the surgery-only group ($p = 0.001$). Treatment-related mortality was similar in both arms (7% vs 6%). Subgroup analysis did not reveal any significant effect of histology on outcome. Based on the results of this study, preoperative chemotherapy has not been adopted as standard therapy in the US, where impetus has shifted towards the investigation of preoperative or definitive chemoradiation options (Ajani *et al.* 2006).

On the contrary, the more recent multi-institutional MRC OEO2 study established preoperative chemotherapy as a treatment option for operable esophageal cancer in the UK and parts of Europe. This is the largest randomized study to date, with 802 eligible patients randomized to two cycles of preoperative chemotherapy with cisplatin and 5-FU followed by surgery, versus immediate surgery. The use of preoperative radiotherapy was allowed; however, only 9% of patients in each group received this treatment. Contrary to the Intergroup-0113 trial results, a statistically significant improvement in overall survival in favor of preoperative chemotherapy was noted (hazard ratio [HR] 0.79; 95% CI 0.67–0.93; $p = 0.004$; median survival 16.8 months vs 13.3 months), with an absolute survival benefit of 9% at 2 years. DFS was also significantly longer in the preoperative chemotherapy group ($p = 0.0014$) and these patients had smaller tumors with less heavy involvement of regional lymph nodes and were more likely to undergo a curative resection. R1 resection rates were, however, not different (MRC Oesophageal Working Group 2002). Again, no effect of tumor histology on outcomes could be detected, although it should be emphasized that the trial was not powered to detect a difference in the primary endpoint within subgroups. A limitation of both studies is the inadequate (by current standards) preoperative staging which prohibited accurate assessment of the effect of treatment in the group of patients with early-stage disease. The reasons for the discordant results in these two major phase III trials are unclear and have been the subject of ongoing debate.

In a further attempt to define the role of preoperative chemotherapy, a number of meta-analyses of RCTs were conducted. In the most recent update of their initial report, Malthamer *et al.* (2006) concluded, based on the analysis of eight RCTs including 1729 patients, that there was some evidence of a survival benefit with the use of neoadjuvant chemotherapy; however, this was not unequivocal (HR 0.88; 95% CI 0.75–1.04). Neither improved DFS (RR for tumor recurrence 0.81; 95% CI 0.54–1.22) nor improved resectability (RR 0.96; 95% CI 0.92–1.01) or improved R0 resection rate (RR 1.05; 95% CI 0.97–1.15) could account for the apparent effect (Malthaner *et al.* 2006). This conclusion was at odds with the outcome of the initial meta-analyis by the same authors as well as one reported subsequently by Urschel, whereas the systematic review by Kaklamanos supported the use of preoperative chemotherapy (Chong & Cunningham 2004). Contrary to all previous studies, the 2006 update by Malthamer employed hazard ratios instead of relative risks at fixed time points as the primary measure of effect on survival in order to avoid the potential confounding effect of the inclusion of different clinical trials in the assessment of survival at specific time points. One methodologic flaw inherent in all the above meta-analyses is that they do not rely on updated individual patients' data in order to draw their conclusions, which inevitably limits their validity.

A consistent finding across neoadjuvant studies is that response to preoperative chemotherapy, especially pathologic complete response (pCR), is a strong predictor of survival. As a result, newer chemotherapeutic agents with promising activity in the setting of advanced disease have been incorporated in preoperative regimens with the aim of improving the pCR rate and with it, long-term outcome. Selected clinical trials of some

Table 5.4 Selected clinical trials of preoperative chemotherapy for esophageal cancer, including patients with squamous histology.

Study	n	Histology	Regimen	RR	Surgical resection	R0	pCR	mOS	Comments
Kelsen *et al.* (1998) (Phase III)	233	SCC(46%) AC(54%)	Cisplatin 100 mg/m² d1 5-FU 1000 mg/m²/24 h d1–5 continuous infusion for 3 cycles followed by surgery vs		80%	59%	2.5%	14.9 m (2 y survival 35%) p = 0.53	Two further cycles with reduced dose of cisplation offered to patients with stable or responding disease.
	234		Immediate surgery		96%	62%	NA	16.1 m (2 y survival 37%)	TRM comparable between arms (7% vs 6%)
MRC Oesophageal Cancer Working Party (OEO2 phase III study) (2002)	400	SCC (31%) AC (66%)	Cisplatin 80 mg/m² d1 5-FU 1000 mg/m²/24 h d1–4 continuous infusion for 2 cycles followed by surgery vs		92%		4%	16.8 m (2 y survival 43%) p = 0.0004	9% in both arms received preoperative radiotherapy
	402		Immediate surgery		97%		NA	13.3 m (2 y survival 34%)	
Polee *et al.* (2003) (Phase II)	50	SCC	Cisplatin 60 mg/m² d1 Paclitaxel 180 mg/m² d1 for 3–6 cycles prior to surgery	59% (14% CR)	90%	84%	16%	20 m	Longer survival in responders (32 m vs 11 m, p = 0.009) G3/4 neutropenia in 71% but only 4% neutropenic fever
Keresztes *et al.* (2003) (Phase II)	26	SCC (42%) AC (58%)	Carboplatin Paclitaxel 200 mg/m² d1 for 2 cycles prior to surgery	61% (19% CR)	77%	69%	11%	48% actuarial 3-year survival	pCR noted only in patients with SCC
Darnton *et al.* (2003) (pooled data from two phase II trials)	66	SCC	Cisplatin 50 mg/m² Ifosfamide 3 g/m² Mitomycin C 6 mg/m² for 2–4 cycles prior to surgery	61% (27% CR)	79%		14%	12.4 m	Survival correlated with response to treatment

5-FU, 5-fluorouracil; AC, adenocarcinoma; CR, complete response; mOS, median overall survival; pCR, pathologic complete response; R0, curative resection; PR, relative risk; SCC, squamous cell carcinoma; TRM, treatment-related nortality.

of these agents are summarized in Table 5.2 (Chong & Cunningham 2004).

The routine use of postoperative adjuvant chemotherapy for SCCE has also been appraised and, based on the lack of a survival benefit in a review of two RCTs, is currently not recommended (Scottish Intercollegiate Guidelines Network 2006).

Radiotherapy

Ferdinandos Skoulidis, Yu Jo Chua & David Cunningham

Despite recent advances in perioperative management and refinement of surgical technique, the outlook for patients who undergo surgical resection as single treatment modality for esophageal cancer remains poor, with 20–25% 5-year survival. Both locoregional and systemic failure contribute to this outcome. Radiotherapy is active against esophageal cancer and its role has been investigated either as single-modality treatment or in conjunction with surgery, in an attempt to improve local disease control. More recently, with the incorporation of active chemotherapeutic regimens in treatment algorithms, chemoradiotherapy has emerged as a particularly attractive option, both as definitive treatment and in the neoadjuvant setting.

Radiotherapy alone has a modest role in the radical management of locally advanced SCCE and is usually reserved for patients who are not considered good candidates for surgery or chemotherapy. Historical data indicate 5-year survival rates of 0–10% for conventional radiotherapy (Ajani *et al.* 2006) and this was confirmed in the large RTOG 85-01 trial (Herskovic *et al.* 1992). However, Sykes *et al.*, reporting on a cohort of 101 carefully selected patients (89% SCC) with short tumors (≤5 cm in length) treated with radical radiotherapy at doses of between 45 and 52.5 Gy in 15–16 fractions over 3 weeks, indicated a 5-year survival rate of 21% with a plateau in the survival curve after approximately 4 years (Sykes *et al.* 1998). These data compare favorably with those reported for surgery alone, and indicate that for a subgroup of patients who are unfit for a combined modality approach, radiotherapy alone may still be an option (Schull *et al.* 2003). The use of external-beam radiotherapy is further established in the setting of inoperable disease where, at doses of 20 Gy in 5 fractions or 30 Gy in 10 fractions, it can effectively palliate dysphagia and pain. In the same context, endoluminal brachytherapy with cesium or iridium pellets constitutes an acceptable alternative (The Royal College of Radiologists 2006).

The neoadjuvant or adjuvant use of radiotherapy has not yielded satisfactory results. In a recently published update of a meta-analysis from the Oesophageal Cancer Collaborative Group, preoperative radiotherapy failed to provide clear evidence for a survival benefit (Arnott *et al.* 2005). Similarly, no survival advantage could be demonstrated in two RCTs of postoperative radiotherapy; nonetheless, this approach may retain a role in the case of positive resection margins following definitive surgery (Scottish Intercollegiate Guidelines Network 2006).

The preoperative combination of chemotherapy and radiotherapy aims to achieve improved local and systemic disease control, while exploiting the potent radiosensitizing properties of several chemotherapy agents. The feasibility and efficacy of this approach was demonstrated in several non-randomized trials, although toxicities were increased. In the randomized trials literature, a number of studies have evaluated preoperative chemoradiotherapy compared to surgery alone with conflicting results (Table 5.5) (Walsh *et al.* 1996; Urba 2004; Tepper *et al.* 2006). Until recently, the only positive trial was reported by Walsh *et al.* (2006) which established preoperative chemoradiotherapy as an acceptable pathway for the radical treatment of esophageal carcinoma in the US. However, this trial included only patients with adenocarcinoma and was criticized for inadequate (by current standards) staging and poor survival in the surgery-only arm. In June 2006, Tepper *et al.* reported on a prematurely closed phase III CALGB trial comparing preoperative chemoradiotherapy with cisplatin/5-FU to surgery alone. Despite the poor accrual (56 patients out of a total 475 planned), trimodality therapy was associated with significantly longer median and 5-year survival, and treatment was well tolerated. Three recently reported meta-analyses also reached incongruous conclusions. Urschel and Fiorica, reporting on analyses of nine and six RCTs with 1116 and 764 patients respectively, observed a survival advantage for preoperative chemoradiotherapy which reached statistical significance at 3 years but occurred at the expense of increased operative mortality (Urba 2004). On the contrary, Greer *et al.* could not demonstrate a significant difference in outcome between the two groups (Greer *et al.* 2005). Due to methodologic limitations and the observed heterogeneity in the above studies, preoperative chemoradiation remains an investigational approach in the UK and parts of Europe, despite its wide acceptance as a treatment option in North America (Scottish Intercollegiate Guidelines Network 2006).

In the above trials of neoadjuvant chemoradiotherapy, the rate of pathological complete response (pCR) consistently correlated with prolonged survival, suggesting it may be useful as a surrogate endpoint for the evaluation of new treatments. Two emerging strategies aiming to improve the pCR rate are the addition of novel chemotherapy drugs (taxanes, irinotecan, oxaliplatin, and capecitabine) to preoperative combined modality regimens, and the introduction of a three-step approach to treatment, which employs a distinct phase of induction chemotherapy before chemoradiation and eventual surgery (Table 5.6) (Ilson *et al.* 2003; Swisher *et al.* 2003; Ajani *et al.* 2004; Barnes *et al.* 2006; Meluch *et al.* 2006). Despite sometimes impressive results, with rates of pCR exceeding 50%, these schedules remain for the present investigational, as none have outperformed conventional chemoradiotherapy in the setting of a randomized trial.

Definitive chemoradiation has been the mainstay for the non-operative management of localized esophageal cancer after

Table 5.5 Selected clinical trials of neoadjuvant chemoradiotherapy for esophageal cancer, including patients with squamous histology.

Trial	Regimen	Patient group	Histology	n	Mortality	pCR	mOS	3-year survival	Comments
Neoadjuvant chemoradiotherapy versus surgery alone									
Walsh *et al.* (1996)	5-FU 15 mg/m^2 for 16 h daily d1–5 Cisplatin 75mg/m^2 d7 Cycle repeated in week 6 RT 40Gy in 15 fractions d1–5,d8–12,d15–19 Surgery planned 8w from start of treatment	Non-metastatic Non-cervical	AC	58	8.6%	25%	16 m p = 0.01	32% p = 0.01	Established preoperative chemoradiation in the US. Criticized for inadequate staging, non-specific definition of resectability, poor survival in surgery-only arm.
	vs Surgery alone			55	3.6%	na	11 m	6%	Only patients with AC included
Bosset *et al.* (1997)	Cisplatin 80mg/m^2 0–2 d prior to RT RT 18.5 Gy in 5 fractions Schedule repeated with 2w gap Followed by surgery 4w later	Stage 1–2 Tumors within first 4 cm excluded	SCC	143	12.3% p = 0.012	26%	18.6 m	~39%	Improved DFS in combined modality arm offset by higher treatment-related mortality.
	vs Immediate surgery			139	3.6%	na	18.6 m	~37%	Criticized for unconventional chemotherapy/ radiotherapy schedules
Urba *et al.* (2001)	Cisplatin 20 mg/m^2 d1–5 and d17–21 as continuous infusion 5-FU 300 mg/m^2/24h d1–21 as continuous infusion Vinblastine 1 mg/m^2/d d1–4 and d17–20 RT 1.5 Gy twice daily d1–5,d8–12,d15–19 (total dose 45 Gy) followed by surgery ~d42	No metastatic disease or invasion of airways	SCC 25% AC 75%	50 50	2.0%	28%	16.9 m	30% p = 0.15	Power calculation based on large expected survival benefit. Multivariate analysis revealed a p value of 0.09 for effect of treatment on survial
	vs Immediate surgery				4.0%	na	17.6 m	16%	

Burmeister *et al.* (2005)	Cisplatin 80 mg/m^2 d1 5-FU 800 mg/m^2/24 h d1–4 RT 35 Gy in 15 fractions Followed by surgery		SCC 39% AC 61%	128	4.6% overall		21.7 m ns		SCC associated with better PFS following preoperative chemoradiotherapy
	vs Immediate surgery			128			18.5m		
Tepper *et al.* (2006)	Cisplatin 100 mg/m^2 d1 5-FU 1000 mg/m^2/24 h d1–4 Cycle repeated in week 5 RT 50.4 Gy in 28 fractions (1.8 Gy/fraction) Followed by surgery		SCC 39% ACC 75%	30	0%	40%	4.5 y p = 0.02	39% (5-year) p = 0.005	Closed early due to poor accrual
	vs Immediate surgery			26	7.7%		1.8 y	16% (5-year)	
Trials of novel chemotherapeutic drugs									
Taxanes									
Swisher *et al.* (2003) (Phase II)	*Induction chemotherapy with:* 5-FU 750 mg/m^2/d d1–5 Cisplatin 15 mg/m^2/d d1–5 Paclitaxel 200 mg/m^2 d1 as 24 h infusion q28d for up to 2 cycles *Followed by concurrent chemoradiotherapy with:* RT 45 Gy in 25 fractions (1.8 Gy/fraction) 5-FU 300 mg/m^2/d 5 days per week as continuous infusion Cisplatin 15 mg/m^2/d d1–5 *Followed by surgery 4–6 w later*	Locally advanced (excluding unresectable and early T1 N0 tumors)	SCC 16% AC 84%	38	6.0%	23%	57.5 m	63%	Feasible regimen, acceptable morbidity/mortality. 71% pCR and microscopic residual carcinoma (≤10% cells viable)
Meluch *et al.* (2006) (phase II, pooled)	Paclitaxel 200 mg/m^2 d1,22 Carboplatin AUC6 d1,22 5-FU 225 mg/m^2/d d1–42 as continuous infusion RT 45 Gy at 1.8 Gy/d Followed by surgery 6–10 w later.	Stage I–III	SCC 26% AC 74%	226	6.0%	45%	26.3 m	40%	33% 5-year survival Moderate acute toxicity 58% G3/4 leucopenia 43% G3/4 mucositis

continued on p. 134

Table 5.5 *Continued*

Trial	Regimen	Patient group	Histology	n	Mortality	pCR	mOS	3-year survival	Comments
Barbes *et al.* (2006) (Phase I–II)	Oxaliplatin 40 mg/m^2 weekly w1–5 Docetaxel 20 mg/m^2 weekly w1–5 Capecitabine 1000 mg/m^2 bd d1–7, 15–21, 29–35 RT 45 Gy, 1.8 Gy/fraction, 5 days/week Followed by surgery 4–8 w later	Stage I-III	SCC 22% AC 78%	24		67%	Not reached		Tolerable. 79% 1-year actuarial survival
Irinotecan									
Ajani *et al.* (2004) (Phase II)	*Induction chemotherapy with:* Irinotecan 70 mg/m^2 d1,7,21,28 (6-week cycle) Cisplatin 20 mg/m^2 d1,7,21,28 (6-week cycle) Repeated for two cycles *Followed by concurrent chemoradiation with:* RT 45 Gy, 1.8 Gy/fraction, 5 days/week Paclitaxel 45 mg/m^2 once a week (max 5 doses) 5-FU 300 mg/m^2/d, 5 days/week as a continuous infusion *Followed by surgery 5–6 w later.*	T1 N0/T4 excluded	SCC 14% AC 86%	43	5.0%	28%	22.1 m	42% (2-year)	
Ilson *et al.* (2003) (Phase I)	*Induction chemotherapy with:* Irinotecan 65 mg/m^2 once a week, weeks 1,2,4,5 Cisplatin 30 mg/m^2 once a week, weeks 1,2,4,5 *Followed by concurrent chemoradiotherapy with:* RT 50.4 Gy, 1.8 Gy per fraction, weeks 8–13 Cisplatin 30 mg/m^2 d1,8,22,29 Irinotecan escalating doses d1,8,22,29	Stage II/III	SCC 17% AC 83%	19	5.0%	27%	25 m		Well tolerated. 20% pulmonary embolism; low-dose warfarin given to remaining patients

5-FU, 5-fluorouracil; AC, adenocarcinoma; DFS, disease-free survival; mOS, median overall survival; pCR, pathologic complete response; PFS, progression-free survival; RT, radiotherapy; SCC, squamous cell carcinoma.

Table 5.6 Chemoradiotherapy with and without surgery for esophageal cancer (including patients with squamous histology).

Trial	Regimen	Patient group	Histology	n	TRM	R0	pCR	2yFFP	mOS*
Stahl *et al.* (2005) (Phase III)	*Induction chemotherapy with:*	T3/T4	SCC	86	12.8%	82%	35%	39.9%	16.4 m
	5-FU 500 mg/m^2 d1–3 bolus	No airway invasion							
	Leucovorin 300 mg/m^2 d1–3								
	Etoposide 100 mg/m^2 d1–3								
	Cisplatin 30 mg/m^2 d1–3 q3w for three courses								
	Followed by chemoradiotherapy with:								
	RT 40 Gy in 20 fractions, 2 Gy per fraction, 5 days/week							p = 0.003	
	Cisplatin 50 mg/m^2 d2–8								
	Etoposide 80 mg/m^2 d3–5								
	Followed by surgery (TTE), 3–4 w later								
	vs								
	Same induction chemotherapy			86	3.5%			35.4%	14.9 m
	Followed by:								
	a) Chemoradiotherapy with 50 Gy at 2 Gy per fraction and HF-EBRT 1.5 Gy bd for 5 days (total dose 65 Gy) (Chemotherapy identical to first arm) if T4/obstructing T3 tumor								
	b) Chemoradiotherapy with 60 Gy at 2 Gy per fraction and HDR-AL 4 Gy in a depth of 5 mm for T3 tumors with no or traversable stenosis								
Bedenne *et al.* (2002) (Phase III) FFCD 9102	5-FU/cisplatin d1–5 and d22–26 and RT 46 Gy in 5.5 w or 2 × 15 Gy d1–5 and d22–26 (split course)	T3/T4,N0/1,M0	SCC/AC	455					
	Responding patients were then randomized to:			259					
	Surgery				9.0%				
	vs				p = 0.002			34%	17.7 m
	Further chemoradiotherapy: 3 course of 5-FU/cisplatin and RT—either protracted (20 Gy) or split course (15 Gy)				1.0%			40%	19.3 m

HDR-AL, high dose rate afterloading therapy; HF-EBRT, hyperfractionated external-beam radiotherapy; mOS, median overall survival; pCR, pathologic complete response; R0, curative resection; RT, radiotherapy; TRM, treatment-related mortality; TTE, transthoracic esophagectomy.

several RCTs revealed its superiority to radiation alone, and it represents a standard of care in both Europe and the US. Furthermore, it constitutes the treatment of choice for tumors (usually SCC) of the cervical esophagus, where radical surgery requires concomitant removal of the larynx and is associated with a chronically elevated risk of aspiration (Allum *et al.* 2002). The pivotal trial comparing definitive chemoradiation to radiation alone was the Intergroup RTOG 85-01 trial in which 123 patients (88% with squamous histology) with T1–3 tumors were randomized to receive either concurrent chemoradiation or radiotherapy alone. Patients in the treatment arm received cisplatin at a dose of 75 mg/m^2 on day 1 and infusional 5-FU at a dose of 1000 mg/m^2/24 h on days 1–4 repeated in weeks 1, 5, 8, 11 (four courses), with radiation therapy commencing on day 1 and consisting of a total dose of 50 Gy in 25 fractions (5 fractions per week, 2 Gy per fraction) (Herskovic *et al.* 1992). The radiotherapy in the control arm of the study consisted of a total dose of 64 Gy, delivered in doses of 2 Gy per fraction. Randomization was suspended after a preplanned interim analysis revealed a statistically significant survival advantage for the combined modality arm; however, a further cohort of 73 consecutive patients was treated according to the combined modality protocol, in order to validate the initial results. In the most recent update (Cooper *et al.* 1999), with minimum follow-up of 5 years, the median survival for the chemoradiation arm was 14.1 months compared to 9.3 months for patients treated with radiotherapy only. Five-year overall survival was 26% (95% CI 15–37%) and 0% respectively ($p < 0.0001$ by the log-rank test), with no patients in the control arm surviving 3 years. More importantly, there was clear evidence of a plateau in the survival curve for the combined treatment, with no deaths beyond 5 years attributed to esophageal cancer, indicating that these patients were truly cured of their disease. These results were confirmed in the prospectively studied cohort, in which chemoradiotherapy produced a 5-year survival rate of 14% (95% CI 6–23%) and a median survival of 16.7 months, which need to be viewed in the light of a higher proportion of T3 tumors in this group. Combined modality treatment further resulted in superior local and distant disease control. This improved outcome occurred at the cost of increased acute life-threatening (grade 4–5) toxicity which occurred in 10% (one death) and 2% (no deaths) of the study and control arms respectively, although this high rate was not corroborated in the non-randomized cohort, where grade 4 toxicity occurred in 4% of patients. More recently, a Cochrane systematic review of chemoradiotherapy versus radiotherapy alone for localized carcinoma of the esophagus confirmed the benefit from dual-modality therapy with an estimated absolute survival benefit of 9% at 1 year and 4% at 2 years, and an absolute reduction in local recurrence rate of 12% (Wong & Malthaner 2006).

The high rates of local recurrence reported in the RTOG 85-01 trial prompted attempts at treatment intensification. The Intergroup 0123 phase III trial assessed the impact of increasing the total dose of radiation to 64.8 Gy, while maintaining almost the same chemotherapy regimen as the RTOG 85-01 trial. Analysis of the results revealed no benefit for the intensified arm in terms of local control or overall survival (Minsky 2006). The use of a brachytherapy boost as an adjunct to chemoradiation was evaluated in the multi-institutional RTOG 92-07 phase I–II trial; however a preliminary toxicity report raised concerns about the incidence of potentially fatal tracheoesophageal fistulas (Minsky 2006). In an alternative approach to treatment intensification, late-course accelerated hyperfractionated radiotherapy (LCAF) with or without concurrent chemotherapy for patients with locally advanced ESCC resulted in a median survival of 30.8 months versus 23.9 months, and a 5-year survival of 40% versus 28% respectively, although this did not reach statistical significance ($p = 0.310$). The 6% rate of treatment-related mortality in the combined modality arm indicated that this strategy, though interesting, remains investigational at present (Zhao *et al.* 2005). Finally, both irinotecan and the taxanes have been utilized in chemoradiation regimens, but again, there is insufficient evidence to recommend a specific schedule outside a clinical trial. As an additional strategy, induction chemotherapy with ECX before radical chemoradiation is the subject of an ongoing phase II clinical trial.

The RTOG 85-01 trial unequivocally demonstrated the superiority of chemoradiotherapy over radiation therapy alone in the management of esophageal cancer. However, two fundamental questions remain: (i) how does definitive chemoradiotherapy, delivered optimally, compare to surgery alone; and (ii) what is the role of surgery following radical chemoradiation? An unequivocal answer to the first question would require a large number of patients and recruitment may be difficult; however, some early data can be drawn from a prospective Chinese trial in which 80 patients with potentially operable SCC of the mid- or lower esophagus were randomized to definitive chemoradiotherapy with cisplatin/5-FU or surgery. Patients with inadequate response to chemoradiotherapy could then undergo salvage surgery. With a median follow-up of 16.9 months no difference in DFS or early cumulative overall survival could be detected.

The question of the role of surgery following chemoradiation has recently been addressed by two groups. Stahl *et al.* (2005) reported on the results of a phase III RCT on behalf of the German Oesophageal Cancer Study Group. In this study, 172 eligible patients with locally advanced SCCE (T3/T4 but with no invasion of the tracheobronchial tree) were randomized to receive either (i) induction chemotherapy followed by chemoradiation and surgery or (ii) induction chemotherapy followed by definitive chemoradiation to a higher overall dose (65 Gy vs 40 Gy).The primary endpoint was overall survival, and the alternative hypothesis was equivalence between the two groups. With a median follow-up of 6 years, both median and 2-year overall survival were comparable between the two arms. Two-year freedom from locoregional progression favored the surgical arm (40.7% vs 64.3%, $p = 0.003$), indicating improved local control with the addition of surgery. This effect was, however, probably offset by the higher treatment-related mortality in the surgical arm. Of note, at the 3-year time point there was evidence of divergence in the survival curves in favor of the surgical arm; however, this failed to attain statistical significance. An important outcome from this trial was that it highlighted response to induction chemotherapy as the most important independent prognostic factor for the entire group of patients, regardless of treatment allocation. Responders had a 3-year survival of more than 50%, whereas lack of response to induction chemotherapy heralded a poor outcome, with 3-year survival rates of 17.9% for patients who received surgery and 9.4% for patients in the definitive chemoradiotherapy arm. This could be partially reversed if curative (R0) resection could be achieved, leading to 3-year survival of up to 32%. This finding ultimately raises the question of the role of salvage surgery in patients who do not respond to definitive chemoradiation and suggests that treatment can be individualized based on the response to induction chemotherapy. This issue was further explored in the FFCD 9102 trial (Fédération Francophone de Cancerologie Digestive) in which responders to chemoradiation were randomized to surgery or further chemoradiation. There was no significant difference in outcome between the two groups, although patients randomized to surgery had a significantly greater decrease in their quality of life in the initial postoperative period (Bedenne *et al.* 2002). By restricting the analysis of the effect of surgery to chemoradiotherapy responders, this trial may have failed to reveal the true potential of surgery in the subset of patients who are most likely to benefit from it.

In conclusion, radiotherapy has an established role in the treatment of patients with esophageal cancer, particularly in those with squamous histology. In the potentially curative setting, the superiority of chemoradiotherapy compared to radiation alone has been established, although no conclusive RCT evidence has demonstrated the superiority of this approach compared to surgery. For SCCE, definitive chemoradiotherapy seems to be associated with equivalent overall survival with improved toxicity when compared with preoperative chemotherapy followed by surgery, especially for the group of patients who respond to induction chemotherapy. Following incomplete response to radical chemoradiotherapy there is a role for salvage surgical resection, which, if complete, is associated with significantly improved overall survival.

Ablation of early cancer

Hugh Barr

If disease is localized to the mucosa or remains at the level of microscopic dysplasia then endoscopic therapy may well be a realistic and possibly curative option in certain patients. There is variation between the Western and Eastern (Japanese) classification of invasive and preinvasive neoplastic lesions. This may in part be because many Western pathologists are reluctant to call a dysplastic lesion a cancer in case the patient is subjected to massive surgery for microscopic disease. There are currently several methods used to ablate mucosal disease at endoscopy.

Photodynamic, thermal and laser therapy

Endoscopic photodynamic therapy for both early SCC and adenocarcinoma has been followed by prolonged survival, in one trial. Patients with T1 and T2 cancers, staged using endoscopic ultrasound, who were considered unsuitable for surgical treatment received endoscopic photodynamic therapy. The disease-specific 5-year survival was unaffected by the addition of chemotherapy or radiotherapy, and was 74% (Sibille *et al.* 1995; Barr *et al.* 2003) (Table 5.7). Thus these patients' outcomes resulted predominantly from local therapy. This indicates that if the disease is local then local therapy can eradicate it. The depth of damage is so predictable that it is only suitable for early disease penetrating up to 5 mm. The detection of these early lesions must be matched with methods to stage them accurately. Other laser and thermal methods, such as argon plasma coagulation (APC), may produce similar results. However, the effect is often very superficial and limited once the surface has been charred. It is clear that APC is less efficient than laser coagulation and more treatments are required to produce the desired effect. Treatment with thermal laser therapy alone has resulted in prolonged survival, with 4% of 211 patients surviving 2 years (Savage *et al.* 1997).

Endoscopic mucosal resection (Fig. 5.6)

It is now clear that endoscopic mucosal resection is highly effective, with a complete remission rate of 82.5% in a series of 350 patients with carcinoma and high-grade dysplasia (predominantly adenocarcinoma with a mean follow-up of 12 months). The best results occurred in patients with high-grade dysplasia and small (<20 mm) well or moderately differentiated cancers (97%) (Pech *et al.* 2003). A combination of methods is often necessary to fully eradicate the disease in many patients. The major concern is that metachronous tumors can occur in up to 14% of patients. Patients must therefore continue to have endoscopic surveillance. These patients may need treatment with photodynamic therapy to prevent development of further cancers in this unstable epithelium, particularly those who may have multifocal dysplastic disease. The overall complication rate for both the major complications of bleeding and stricture formation and other milder complications is 12.5%, and most can be managed endoscopically. It is important to have suitable devices available for the endoscopic control of hemorrhage. In order to avoid perforation great care should be taken to ensure that the lesion lifts with submuosal injection, or suction into the cap and will form a pseudopolyp following suction ligation. Large lesions can be treated with multistep piecemeal resection.

Table 5.7 Patients with early squamous cell cancers of the esophagus treated with photodynamic therapy with a curative intent. Photosensitizers were Photofrin and tetra(m-hydroxyphenyl)chlorin (Barr *et al.* 2003).

Patients	Stage of cancer (clinical and EUS)	Complete response (%)	Follow-up (median months or range)	Recurrence (+ time in months of detection)	Complications
24	Tis 10	41	15	–	Skin 5% Stricture 10%
11	Early	55	4	–	Skin 18% Perforation 18%
96	T1 51 T2 24	88	24	29% (12–18)	Skin 13% Stricture 35%
21	Tis 5 T1 16	74	36	13% (14–96)	Skin 4% Stricture 9%
33	Early	93	–	9%	–
18	Tis	37	32	48% (30–95)	Skin 8% Stricture 7% Fistula 2.5%
68	Early	67	1–47	–	Stricture 2% Fistula 2%
31	Early	84	3–36	–	Fistula 6% Perforation 6%
35	Early	77	3–38	–	Fistula 5% Perforation 11%

Tis, carcinoma *in situ*; T1, tumor confined to the mucosa; T2, tumor penetrating into the submucosa.

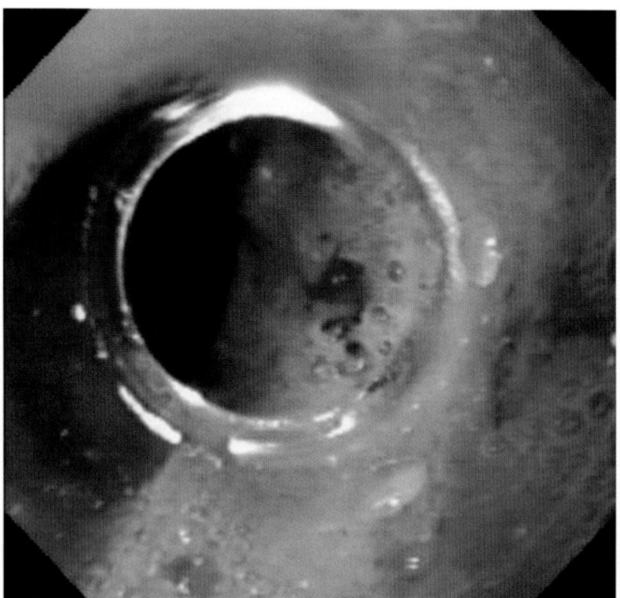

Fig. 5.6 Area of squamous dysplasia viewed through the endoscope with a suction cap before endoscopic mucosal resection. This technique is very useful for a deep staging biopsy to exclude invasive cancer.

Submucosal endoscopic dissection can be performed in a single endoscopic session for large superficially spreading lesions. Repeat injection is necessary to ensure lifting and polyp formation.

Palliation and endoscopic therapy

(Table 5.8)

Hugh Barr

For many years the main role of endoscopic therapy has been in the palliation of advanced esophageal cancer. Dysphagia is found to occur in approximately 90% of patients with esophageal cancer. At the time of diagnosis many cancers are not curable and aggressive therapy is futile. Indeed, medical palliative care regimens are effective for the relief of dysphagia without recourse to endoscopic intervention and are usually appropriate for those in the late stages of their disease. The concept of a single approach to palliation has been replaced by a multidisciplinary approach (Blazeby & Alderson 2006).

Dilatation

Endoscopic dilatation may be necessary to assess the extent of

Table 5.8 Comparison of the palliation methods for advanced inoperable esophageal cancer (Barr *et al.* 2003).

Method of palliation	Average symptom/ dysphagia-free interval and need for repeat therapy	Procedure-related mortality (%)
Endoscopic dilatation	8–10 days	1
Injection therapy	<4 weeks	0
Nd YAG laser therapy	4–6 weeks	2–3
Nd YAG laser therapy and brachytherapy	9–14 weeks	0
Photofrin photodynamic therapy	9–14 weeks	<1
	Recurrent dysphagia (%)	**Mortality (%)**
Semirigid stent	14–20	6–16
Self-expanding stent	20	5

a tumor and also at the diagnostic endoscopy, and to allow endoscopic ultrasound assessment. This also improves swallowing. Some patients with large exophytic fleshy tumors often have early reocclusion. Overall the effect of dilatation is only short, lasting 8–11 days, and repeated dilatations are usually necessary if the patient survives for any length of time. Perforation is the most worrying complication; it occurs following 1–5% of dilatations, and carries a mortality of 1%.

Thermal, laser and injection therapy

Thermal recanalization using a laser or APC is highly effective at restoring a lumen to the esophagus. Most patients can be restored to swallowing a near-normal diet. Repeated treatments need to be performed at 4–6-weekly intervals to prevent recurrent dysphagia. Treatment is on an outpatient basis under conscious sedation. Complications occur in approximately 5%, with an overall procedure-related mortality of 1%. The commonest complication is esophageal perforation (2.5%), followed by fistulation (1%), hemorrhage (0.75%), and sepsis (0.5%). Many of the perforations are caused by the preliminary dilatation rather than the subsequent laser treatment. Perforation is usually best managed with immediate intubation with a covered self-expanding stent, and aggressive conservative therapy with antibiotics and intravenous feeding. APC is cheaper, but generally felt to be less efficient than the laser, and more treatments are required to produce the same effect (Gossner & Ell 1998). Endoscopic laser therapy with intraluminal radiotherapy has been used in an attempt to prolong the dysphagia-free interval with the time to repeat treatment increasing to 11 weeks. There is a worrying incidence of recurrent dysphagia due to either radiotherapy-induced fibrous stricture (34%) or a combination of intraluminal tumor with fibrous stricture (37%), and only 29% of patients require no further intervention (Bown 1996; Shumeli *et al.* 1996).

Photodynamic therapy

Photodynamic therapy (PDT) is perceived as being a complex technique, involving the administration of a photosensitizer followed by activation with light. The laser and optical devices are not readily available in many endoscopy departments. Thus simple expediency dictates that other methods are used. In addition, clinicians have concerns regarding the possible side-effects and the precautions required to avoid skin photosensitization. Photodynamic therapy may be particularly useful for patients with completely obstructing, very long tortuous tumors, an overgrown or blocked stent, and high cervical esophageal tumors. A large randomized comparison (236 patients) of thermal neodymium, yttrium, aluminium, garnet (Nd YAG) laser versus PDT showed that both were equally effective. PDT was associated with temporary photosensitivity but was easier to perform and associated with fewer perforations (PDT 1%, thermal laser 7%) (Lightdale *et al.* 1995). Injection of alcohol and intratumoral chemotherapy can also be very useful. As with PDT and thermal therapy treatment, it has to be repeated.

Endoscopic intubation

It is apparent that self-expanding stents are safer than the rigid prostheses, and may be associated with a longer dysphagia-free interval with greater improvement in dysphagia score. The ease of insertion, initial effectiveness, and safety in patients with advanced disease are highly attractive features. The advantage is that this is generally regarded as a single procedure that may not need to be repeated; unfortunately reintervention is frequently necessary. The use of covered prosthesis is vital for the treatment of tracheoesophageal fistula since they occlude the defect. Randomized comparison of endoscopic laser therapy and self-expanding metal prosthesis insertion reveals very similar overall results, although the laser therapy was repeated at monthly intervals until death to maintain esophageal patency (Barr *et al.* 2003).

Novel agents

Ferdinandos Skoulidis, Yu Jo Chua & David Cunningham

Over the last decade, our growing understanding of tumor biology has led to the identification of key components of malignant signal transduction pathways as possible molecular targets, and a panoply of biologic agents have entered clinical development. Despite several high-profile success stories, most notably in the fields of colorectal, lung, breast, and head and neck cancer, their integration into esophageal cancer treatment has been slow. This section will focus on the current and possible future roles and future perspectives of targeted therapies in the management of SCCE, with particular emphasis on compounds targeting members of the epidermal growth factor receptor family, inhibitors of angiogenesis, cell-cycle progression and apoptosis, and regulators of the inflammatory response.

The epidermal growth factor receptor (EGFR, ERBB1) is a member of the ERBB family of receptor tyrosine kinases. It consists of an extracellular ligand-binding domain, a transmembrane region that anchors the receptor to the cell membrane, and an endodomain with tyrosine kinase activity. Ligand binding (EGF or TGF-α) triggers a conformational change, allowing receptor homo- or heterodimerization, which culminates in activation of the tyrosine kinase domain through autophosphorylation at several tyrosine residues. Downward initiation of intracellular signal transduction cascades ensues, affecting and regulating cell proliferation, evasion of apoptosis, angiogenesis, invasion, metastasis, and resistance to chemo/radiotherapy Valverde *et al.* 2006).

Overexpression of EGFR is a common feature in SCCE (50% as determined by immunohistochemistry in a recent study) and correlates with poor prognosis. Correspondingly, EGFR gene amplification is noted in up to 28% of primary tumors (Hanawa *et al.* 2006). These data provide a rationale for targeting EGFR in an attempt to improve outcomes.

There are currently two major approaches to targeting EGFR: monoclonal antibodies (mAbs) that bind to the extracellular domain; and small molecule receptor tyrosine kinase inhibitors (TKIs), which occupy the ATP-binding site in the tyrosine kinase domain of the receptor, thus inhibiting autophosphorylation and blocking downstream signal transduction.

Gefitinib ('Iressa', ZD1839) and erlotinib ('Tarceva', OSI-774) are the most extensively studied small-molecule TKIs in gastrointestinal malignancies and preclinical data support their activity in SCCE. In cell culture experiments, erlotinib potently induced growth inhibition and cell-cycle arrest at the G1/S checkpoint, without triggering apoptosis or cytotoxicity (Sutter *et al.* 2006). In the case of gefitinib, the drug inhibited proliferation of SCCE cell lines in a dose-dependent manner and caused G1/S arrest and induction of apoptosis. This effect was translated into prolonged survival in murine xenograft models (Hara *et al.* 2005). Three phase II clinical trials of TKIs in esophageal cancer including patients with squamous histology have been reported to date in abstract form. Tew *et al.* (2005) examined the effect of erlotinib at a dose of 150 mg once daily in 22 patients with metastatic esophageal cancer, nine of whom had SCC. The patients had received up to one systemic treatment before inclusion in the study. The objective response rate to erlotinib was 9%, with two patients achieving partial response to treatment, both of whom had squamous histology, EGFR overexpression and nodal limited disease (Valverde *et al.* 2006). In a phase II study from the Netherlands, gefitinib at a dose of 500 mg once daily was given to patients with advanced esophageal cancer after failure of one previous chemotherapy regimen. Of the 26 evaluable patients, three had a partial response to treatment (Valverde *et al.* 2006). Comparable efficacy with a dose of 250 mg once daily was reported however, only one patient with SCC was included in this phase II study (Valverde *et al.* 2006). Current ongoing clinical trials are further exploring the role of gefitinib preoperatively, either alone or in combination with cisplatin/irinotecan/radiotherapy as well as in the adjuvant setting, following radical therapy with surgery, radiotherapy, chemotherapy or combined modality approaches. In the setting of metastatic or recurrent (unresectable) disease gefitinib is being assessed as a single agent or in combination with chemotherapy (cisplatin and irinotecan). Other small-molecule TKIs (lapatinib, CI-1033) are undergoing preclinical and early-phase clinical development in patients with solid tumors, including patients with esophageal cancer.

Compared to small-molecule tyrosine kinase inhibitors (TKIs), the evaluation of mAbs against EGFR in esophageal cancer is lagging. Cetuximab ('Erbitux', C225) is a mouse–human chimeric IgG1 mAb licensed for the treatment of irinotecan-refractory colorectal cancer. Cetuximab binds to the ectodomain of EGFR, competing with its natural ligands and triggering receptor internalization. In the field of head and neck cancer its addition to radiotherapy resulted in a significant improvement in median overall survival, highlighting its radiosensitizing properties, and this has been corroborated by the preliminary results of a phase II trial assessing the safety and efficacy of cetuximab in combination with paclitaxel, carboplatin and radiation in esophageal/gastric cancer, which reported a 43% pCR rate (Tew *et al.* 2005). Despite the limited published data, ongoing phase II clinical trials are assessing its use in esophageal cancer in a variety of settings, including: (i) metastatic disease, either as monotherapy or as an adjunct to three different chemotherapy schedules; (ii) locally advanced, inoperable esophageal cancer in combination with chemoradiotherapy (cisplatin/irinotecan); and (iii) preoperatively in combination with radiotherapy. Other mAbs with a similar mechanism of action include the genetically engineered humanized IgG1 mAb matuzumab (EMD72000), and the fully human IgG2 mAb panitumumab (ABX-EGF). In the phase I trial of matuzumab, one patient with metastatic SCCE previously treated with 5-fluorouracil, cisplatin and irinotecan showed a partial response to treatment with a time to tumor progression of 6 months. Matuzumab has been further used with promising results in patients with esophageal and gastric adenocarcinoma, but no phase II trials in patients with squamous histology have yet been launched. Panitumumab has shown preliminary evidence of efficacy in colorectal cancer, but it has not yet been evaluated in patients with esophageal cancer.

Targeting the ERBB2 (HER-2/Neu) receptor is also an appealing strategy in SCCE given the reported rate of HER-2/Neu overexpression in this malignancy (mean 23%, range 0–52%), and its association with extramural invasion and poor response to neoadjuvant chemotherapy. Trastuzumab ('Herceptin') is a humanized IgG1 mAb against the ERBB2 receptor which has gained regulatory approval for the treatment of HER-2/Neu-positive breast carcinoma. In SCCE cell lines, the addition of trastuzumab resulted in antibody-dependent cell-mediated cytotoxicity against HER-2-expressing cells and enhanced sensitivity to ionizing radiation (Mimura *et al.* 2005). The feasibility of combining trastuzumab with cisplatin, paclitaxel and radiotherapy has been established in a phase I study in patients with esophageal adenocarcinoma, although this has yet not been shown in cases with squamous histology. Beyond trastuzumab, pertuzumab, the first member in a novel class of agents termed HER dimerization inhibitors, has entered early-phase clinical trials, although no reports of its use in patients with esophageal cancer have yet emerged (Valverde *et al.* 2006).

A cardinal component of the malignant phenotype is the ability to generate adequate tumor blood supply through the induction of angiogenesis. Among the many mediators of this process, vascular endothelial growth factor (VEGF) has emerged as the key player. There are three isoforms of this soluble factor which exert their pleiotropic effects through attachment to two different cellular receptors (Flt-1 and Flk-1/KDR). VEGF over-expression occurs in 24–93% of SCCE cases in various series, and correlates with poor survival (Kleespies *et al.* 2004). As is the case with EGFR, inhibition of the VEGF pathway can be achieved either by using mAbs to target soluble VEGF or its receptors or by means of low molecular weight TKIs. Bevacizumab ('Avastin'), a recombinant humanized mAb active against all isoforms of VEGF, is by far the most advanced amongst angiogenesis inhibitors, having gained regulatory approval for use with any 5-fluorouracil-containing regimen in the first-line treatment of metastatic colorectal cancer in the US. Bevacizumab normalizes tumor vasculature and reduces tumor interstitial pressure, facilitating delivery of chemotherapy, and there is further evidence to support a radiosensitizing effect (Tew *et al.* 2005). Preliminary data support efficacy in combination with chemotherapy in gastric and gastroesophageal junction adenocarcinoma, but clinical trials in SCCE are so far lacking, partly due to concerns about a high reported incidence of life-threatening hemoptysis associated with the use of bevacizumab in bronchial SCC trials. Small-molecule TKIs against angiogenic receptors are the focus of intense research effort, but none have as yet entered the clinical field in this disease.

Agents that interfere with cell-cycle progression have recently generated a lot of interest in the fields of both solid tumors and hematologic oncology. Flavopiridol, a pan-cyclin-dependent-kinase inhibitor (inhibiting CDK-1, CDK-3, CDK-4, and CDK-6), is the first member of this class to enter clinical trials. *In vitro*, it induces cell-cycle arrest in G1/S and G2/M, and triggers p53-independent apoptosis in a variety of cell lines. When combined with chemotherapy, it potentiates its ability to induce apoptosis in a schedule-dependent manner and, at low doses, a potent radiosensitizing role has recently been recognized in SCCE cell lines (Sato *et al.* 2004). Despite lack of single-agent activity, two phase I trials revealed promising activity for the combination with cisplatin/irinotecan and docetaxel respectively. Further investigation of the role of flavopiridol as a chemotherapy and radiotherapy modulator is ongoing.

Bortezomib ('Velcade', PS-341) is a potent and selective proteasome inhibitor that exerts its antineoplastic activity by blocking NF-κB signalling, inducing apoptosis and inhibiting angiogenesis and cell-cycle progression (Valverde *et al.* 2006). It has an established role in the management of relapsed multiple myeloma and is undergoing clinical evaluation in a wide range of solid tumors, including gastroesophageal carcinomas. Promising activity was recently demonstrated in combination with irinotecan in the first-line management of inoperable gastric adenocarcinoma, with a response rate of 33%, and a further phase II trial including patients with esophageal adenocarcinoma is currently accruing. Its efficacy, however, in patients with squamous histology remains undetermined.

Invasion and metastasis involves active remodeling of the extracellular matrix by a class of zinc-dependent proteases known as matrix metalloproteinases (MMPs). Members of this group are frequently overexpressed in cancer and have emerged as plausible targets for pharmacologic inhibition. Marimastat, an orally active MMP inhibitor, demonstrated a trend towards improved median overall survival compared to placebo in a phase III trial in patients with gastric and gastroesophageal junction adenocarcinoma (Valverde *et al.* 2006). Up to now MMP inhibitors have not been tested in patients with esophageal cancer.

Finally, inhibition of cyclooxygenase-2 (cox-2), a key enzyme in prostaglandin synthesis, has long been evaluated as both a chemoprevention and treatment strategy in gastrointestinal malignancies, including esophageal cancer (Tew *et al.* 2005). A meta-analysis of observational studies supported the protective effect of aspirin/non-steroidal anti-inflammatory inhibitors against both adenocarcinoma and SCC of the esophagus. Further clinical assessment of the selective cox-2 inhibitors was, however, suspended pending further research into an increased risk of thrombotic events associated with their use. Encouraging activity has been documented in combined-modality approaches for potentially resectable disease; these findings are, however, far from conclusive and need to be validated in larger, randomized comparisons.

In conclusion, despite the advent of a wealth of novel biologic agents in the field of esophageal cancer, none has yet convincingly demonstrated superiority in large randomized phase III clinical trials as an adjunct or alternative to conventional treatment approaches. Intense preclinical and clinical effort is, however, ongoing and will hopefully clarify their role in future treatment algorithms. There is a pressing and widely acknowledged need to identify molecular predictors of response to targeted agents, and transcriptional profiling endpoints should form an integral component of future clinical trials.

Prognosis and follow-up

Hugh Barr

The prognosis of symptomatic SCC of the esophagus is bad. It remains one of the most lethal cancers, with poor outcomes worldwide. The incidence and mortality currently run closely in parallel, with few patients surviving the disease. Many patients are identified at an advanced stage or have advanced age and fragility, making resection and radical therapy difficult.

Survival

Large, but somewhat dated, reviews have revealed that following resection 56% will survive to 1 year, with 34% and 25% surviving to the second and third year respectively (Muller *et al.* 1990; Griffin 2006). These data showed no real improvement in the 10 years since a previous review (Earlam & Cunha Melo 1980). The long-term outlook is little changed. As with most cancers the overall outcome is very stage dependent. There are some recent data from expert centres that reveal excellent 5-year survival for early disease: stage 0/1, 90%; stage 2a, 60%; stage 2b, 16%; stage 3, 13% (Dresner & Griffin 2000). These data do not distinguish SCC from adenocarcinoma of the esophagus.

Follow-up

The optimal follow-up and supervision of patients treated for cancer is surprisingly controversial. Patients naturally feel that early detection of any recurrent disease will allow therapy and prolongation of quality of life. Certainly, with second-line chemotherapy there are options for treatment. However, it remains unclear as to whether asymptomatic detection and treatment is better than responding when there is a symptomatic relapse. Several clinical trials are addressing these issues.

Clearly patients with early disease who have had therapy may be offered screening of the rest of the aerodigestive tract to detect mucosal relapse and institute therapy. There is intense work on identifying biomarkers and methods of growth arrest in patients with early tumors. Enormous hope has been placed on defining a biomarker, but so far the promise has not been realized since very large and validated data sets from randomized trials are required (Ransohoff 2004; Jankowski & Hawk 2006). Nevertheless, several tissue biomarkers have been evaluated, the main example being p53, a protein that controls transcription of other proteins responsible for regulating cell proliferation into the S phase. Persistent inactivation of the p53 tumor suppressor pathway is required for tumor maintenance (Ventura *et al.* 2007). This may be a target for future therapy.

Squamous cell carcinoma remains an enormously challenging disease; most patients will not survive for long. The future remains early detection, chemoprevention and addressing the environmental etiologic factors.

It is, however, becoming increasingly apparent that specialization and the multidisciplinary approach offer the best outcome for patients. High surgeon volume and specialist approaches are associated with better results, but high hospital volume being of limited benefit (Choudhury *et al.* 2007).

References

Ajani JA, Walsh G, Komaki R *et al.* (2004) Preoperative induction of CPT-11 and cisplatin chemotherapy followed by chemoradiotherapy in patients with locoregional carcinoma of the esophagus or gastroesophageal junction. *Cancer* 100(11): 2347–54.

Ajani J, Bekaii-Saab T, D'Amico TA *et al.* (2006) Esophageal cancer clinical practice guidelines. *J Natl Compr Canc Netw* 4(4): 328–47.

Akiyama H, Tsurumaru M, Udagawa H *et al.* (1994) Radical lymph node dissection for cancer of the thoracic esophagus. *Ann Surg* 22: 364–373.

Allum WH, Griffin SM, Watson A, Colin-Jones D. (2002) Association of Upper Gastrointestinal Surgeons of Great Britain and Ireland; British Society of Gastroenterology; British Association of Surgical Oncology. Guidelines for the management of oesophageal and gastric cancer. *Gut* 50 (Suppl 5): v1–23.

Andreyev HJ, Norman AR, Cunningham D *et al.* (1995) Squamous oesophageal cancer can be downstaged using protracted venous infusion of 5-fluorouracil with epirubicin and cisplatin [ECF]. *Eur J Cancer* 31a: 2209–14.

Arnott SJ, Duncan W, Gignoux M *et al.* (2005) Oesophageal Cancer Collaborative Group. Preoperative radiotherapy for esophageal carcinoma. *Cochrane Database Syst Rev* 2; 19(4): CD001799.

Assersohn L, Brown G, Cunningham D *et al.* (2004) Phase II study of irinotecan and 5-fluorouracil/leucovorin in patients with primary refractory or relapsed advanced oesophageal and gastric carcinoma. *Ann Oncol* 15: 64–9.

Bachmann MO, Alderson D, Edwards D *et al.* (2002) Cohort study in South and West England of the influence of specialization on the management and outcome of patients with oesophageal and gastric cancers. *Br J Surg* 89: 914–922.

Barnes EK, Spigel DR, Greco FA *et al.* (2006) Preoperative oxaliplatin (O), docetaxel (D), capecitabine, and concurrent radiation therapy (RT) for patients (pts) with localized esophageal cancer: A phase I/II trial of the Minnie Pearl Cancer Research Network. *Proc Am Soc Clin Oncol* 24 (abstr 4058).

Barr H, Kendall C, Stone N. (2003) Photodynamic therapy for oesophageal cancer. A realistic and useful option. *TCRT* 2: 65–75.

Bedenne L, Michel P, Bouche O *et al.* (2002) Randomized phase III trial in locally advanced esophageal cancer: radiochemotherapy followed by surgery versus radiochemotherapy alone (FFCD 9102). *Proc Am Soc Clin Oncol* 21 (abstr 519).

Blazeby JM, Alderson D. (2006) Palliative treatments of carcinoma of the oesophagus and stomach. In: Griffin SM, Raimes SS, eds. *A Companion To Specialist Surgical Practice: Oesophagogastric Surgery*, 3rd edn, pp. 213–230. Elsevier Saunders, Netherlands.

Blazeby JM, Brooks ST, Alderson D. (2001) The prognostic value of quality of life scores during treatment for oesophageal cancer. *Gut* 49: 227–30.

Blazeby JM, Metcalfe C, Nicklin J, Donovan J, Alderson D. (2005) The prognostic value of quality of life scores for short term outcomes after surgery for oesophageal and gastric cancer. *Br J Surg* 92: 1502–7.

Bleiburg H, Conroy T, Palliott B. (1997) Randomized phase II study of cisplatin and S-fluorouracil (SFU) versus cisplatin alone in advanced squamous cell oesophageal cancer. *Eur J Cancer* 33(8): 1216–20.

Blot WJ, Li JY, Taylor PR *et al.* (1993) Nutrition intervention trials in Linxian, China: supplementation with specific vitamin/mineral combinations, cancer incidence, and disease-specific mortality in the general population. *J Natl Cancer Inst* 85: 1483–92.

Bosset JF, Gignoux M, Triboulet JP *et al.* (1997) Chemoradiotherapy followed by surgery compared with surgery alone in squamous-cell cancer of the esophagus. *N Engl J Med* 337: 161–7.

Bown SG. (1996) Laser and brachytherapy in the palliation of adenocarcinoma of the oesophagus and cardia. *Gut* 39: 726–31.

Bruzzi JF, Swisher SG, Truong MT *et al.* (2007) Detection of interval distant metastases: clinical utility of integrated CT-PET imaging in patients with oesophageal carcinoma after neoadjuvant therapy. *Cancer* 109(1): 125–34.

Burmeister B, Smithers B, Gebski V *et al.* (2005) Surgery alone versus chemoradiotherapy followed by surgery for resectable cancers of the oesophagus: a randomised antrolled phase III trial. *Lancet Oncology* 6: 659–68.

Carr NG, Sobin LH. (1999)Gastrointestinal tract. In: Al-Sam SZ, Lakhani SR, Davies JD, eds. *Practical Atlas of Pseudomalignancy: Benign Lesions Mimicking Malignancy*, pp. 204–205. Arnold, London.

Cerfolio RJ, Bryant AS, Ohja ,. Bartolucci AA, Eloubeidi MA. (2005) The accuracy of endoscopic ultrasonography with fine-needle aspiration, integrated positron emission tomography with computed tomography, and computed tomography in restaging patients with oesophageal cancer after neoadjuvant chemoradiotherapy. *J Thorac Cardiovasc Surg* 129(6): 1232–41.

Chong G, Cunningham D. (2004) Oesophageal cancer: preoperative chemotherapy. *Ann Oncol* 15 (Suppl 4): iv87–91.

Choudhury MM, Dagash H, Pierro A. (2007) A systematic review of the impact of volume of surgery and specialization on patient outcome. *Br J Surg* 94: 145–61.

Cooper JS,Guo MD, Herskovic A *et al.* (1999) Chemoradiotherapy of locally advanced esophageal cancer. Long-term follow up of a prospective randomized trial (RTOG 85-01). *JAMA* 281(17): 1623–7.

Cotton MH, Sammon AM. (1989) Carcinoma of the oesophagus in Transkei: treatment by intubation. *Thorax* 44: 42–47.

Cunningham D, Rao S, Starling N *et al.* (2006) Randomised multicentre phase II study comparing capecitabine with fluorouracil and oxaliplatin with cisplatin in patients with advanced oesophagogastric cancer: the REAL 2 trial. *J Clin Oncol 2006 ASCO Annual Meeting Proceedings* Part 1, Vol 24, no. 18S (June 20 Supplement): LBA 4017.

Darton SJ, Archer VR, Stocken DD *et al.* (2007) Preoperative mitomycin, isosfamide, and cisplatin followed by esophagectomy in squamous cell carcinoma. *J Clin Oncol* 21: 4009–15.

Day DW, Jass JR, Price AB *et al.* (2003) Tumours and tumour-like lesions of the oesophagus. In: Day DW, *et al.* eds. *Morson & Dawson's Gastrointestinal Pathology*, pp 59–84. Blackwell Scientific Publications, Oxford.

Dexter SP, Sue-Ling H, McMahon MJ, Quirke P, Mapstone N, Martin IG. (2001) Circumferential resection margin involvement: an independent predictor of survival following surgery for oesophageal cancer. *Gut* 48: 667–70.

Dresner SM, Griffin SM. (2000) Pattern of recurrence following radical oesophagectomy with two field lymphadenectomy *Br J Surg* 87: 1426–33.

Earlam R, Cunha Melo JR (1980) Oesophageal squamous cell carcinoma 1: A critical review of surgery. *Br J Surg* 67: 381–90.

El-Rayes BF, Shields A, Zalupski M *et al.* (2004) A phase II study of carboplatin and paclitaxel in esophageal cancer. *Ann Oncol* 15(6): 960–5.

van der Gaast A, Kok TC, Kerkhofs L *et al.* (1999) Phase I study of a biweekly schedule of a fixed dose of cisplat with increasing doses of paclitaxel in patients with advanced oesophageal cancer. *Br J Cancer* 80(7): 1052–7.

Gill P, Piris J, Warren BF. (2003) Bizarre stromal cells in the oesophagus. *Histopathology* 42: 88–90.

Goseki N, Koike M, Yoshida M. (1992) Histopathologic characteristics of early stage esophageal carcinoma. A comparative study with gastric carcinoma. *Cancer* 69: 1088–93.

Gossner L, Ell C. (1998) Malignant stricture thermal treatment. *Gastrointest Endosc Clin N Am* 8: 493–501.

Grant HW, Palmer KR, Kelly RW, Wilson NH, Misiewicz JJ. (1988) Dietary linoleic acid, gastric acid, and prostaglandin secretion. *Gastroenterology* 94: 955–9.

Greer SE, Goodney PP, Sutton JE, Birkmeyer JD. (2005) Neoadjuvant chemoradiotherapy for esophageal carcinoma: a meta-analysis. *Surgery* 137(2): 172–7.

Griffen SM. (2006) Surgery for cancer of the oesophagus. In: Griffin SM, Raimes SS, eds. *A Companion To Specialist Surgical Practice: Oesophagogastric Surgery*, 3rd edn, pp. 129–53. Elsevier Saunders, Netherlands.

Hanawa M, Suzuki S, Dobashi Y *et al.* (2006) EGFR protein overexpression and gene amplification in squamous cell carcinoma of the esophagus. *Int J Cancer* 118(5): 1173–80.

Hara F, Aoe M, Doihara H *et al.* (2005)Antitumor effect of gefitinib ('Iressa') on esophageal squamous cell lines in vitro and in vivo. *Cancer Lett* 226(1): 37–47.

Herskovic A, Martz K, al-Sarraf M *et al.* (1992) Combined chemotherapy and radiotherapy compared with radiotherapy alone in patients with cancer of the esophagus. *N Engl J Med* 326(24): 1593–8.

Hofstetter W, Swisher SG, Correa AM *et al.* (2002) Treatment outcomes of resected esophageal cancer. *Ann Surg* 236: 376–84; discussion 384–5.

Howell-Evans W, McConnell RB, Clarke CA, Sheppard PM. (1958) Carcinoma of the oesophagus with keratosis palmaris et plantaris (tylosis): a study of two families. *Q J Med* 27: 413–29.

Ilson DH, Ajani J, Bhalla K *et al.* (1998) Phase II trial of paclitaxel, fluorouracil, and cisplatin in patients with advanced carcinoma of the esophagus. *J Clin Oncol* 16: 1826–34.

Ilson DH, Saltz L, Enzinger P *et al.* (1999) Phase II trial of weekly irinotecan plus cisplatin in advanced esophageal cancer. *J Clin Oncol* 17: 3270–5.

Ilson DH, Forastiere A, Arquette M *et al.* (2000) A phase II trial of paclitaxel and cisplatin in patients with advanced carcinoma of the esophagus. *Cancer J* 6(5): 316–23.

Ilson DH, Bains M, Kelsen DP *et al.* (2003) Phase I trial of escalating-dose irinotecan given weekly with cisplatin and concurrent radiotherapy in locally advanced esophageal cancer. *J Clin Oncol* 21(15): 2926–32.

Iwaya T, Maesawa C, Ogasawara S, Tamura G. (1999) Tylosis esophageal cancer locus on chromosome 17q25.1 is commonly deleted in sporadic human esophageal cancer. *Gastroenterology* 114: 1206–10.

Jankowski J. Cancer Research UK (2006) *UK Oesophageal Cancer Mortality Statistics* [www document]. http://info.cancerresearchuk.org/cancerstats/types/oesophagus/mortality/ [accessed 2007]

Jankowski JA, Hawk ET. (2006) A methodological analysis of chemoprevention and cancer prevention strategies for gastrointestinal cancer. *Nat Clin Pract Gastroenterol Hepatol* 3: 1–11.

Japanese Society for Oesophageal Diseases. (1976) Guidelines for the clinical and pathological studies on carcinoma of the oesophagus. Part 1: clinical classification. *Jpn J Surg* 6: 64–78.

Jiao X, Zhang M, Wen Z, Krasna MJ. (2000) Pleural lavage cytology in esophageal cancer without pleural effusions: clinicopathologic analysis. *Eur J Cardiothorac Surg* 17: 575–9.

Katayama A, Mafune K, Tanaka Y, Takubo K, Makuuchi M, Kaminishi M. (2003) Autopsy findings in patients after curative esophagectomy for esophageal carcinoma. *J Am Coll Surg* 196: 866–73.

Kelsen DP, Ginsberg R, Pajak TF *et al.* (1998) Chemotherapy followed by surgery compared with surgery alone for localised esophageal cancer. *N Engl J Med* 339: 1979–84.

Keresztes RS, Port JL, Pasmantier, MW, Korst RJ, Altorki NK. (2003) Preoperative chemotherapy for esophageal cancer with paclitaxel and carboplatin: results of a phase II trial. *J Thoracic Cardiovasc Surg* 126: 1603–8.

Kleespies A, Guba M, Jauch KW, Bruns CJ. (2004) Vascular endothelial growth factor in esophageal cancer. *J Surg Oncol* 87(2): 95–104.

Kotz BS, Croft S, Ferry DR. (2006) Do delays between diagnosis and surgery in resectable oesophageal cancer affect survival? A study based on West Midlands cancer registration data. *Br J Cancer* 95: 835–40.

Lamb PJ, Griffin SM, Burt AD *et al.* (2005) Sentinel node biopsy to evaluate the metastatic dissemination of oesophageal adenoarcinoma. *Br J Surg* 92: 60–67.

Lerut T, Coosemans W, Decker G *et al.* (2006) Diagnosis and therapy in advanced cancer of the esophagus and the gastroesophageal junction. *Curr Opin Gastroenterol* 22(4): 437–41.

Lightdale CJ, Heier SK, Marcon NE *et al.* (1995) Photodynamic therapy with porfimer sodium versus thermal ablation therapy with Nd:YAG laser for palliation of esophageal cancer: a multicentre randomized trial. *Gastrointest Endosc* 42: 507–12.

Lordick F, von Schilling C, Bernhard H, Hennig M, Bredenkamp R, Peschel C. (2003) Phase II trial of irinotecan plus docetaxel in cisplatin-pretreated relapsed or refractory oesophageal cancer. *Br J Cancer* 18; 89(4): 630–3.

Lorenzen S, Duyster J, Lersch C *et al.* (2005) Capecitabine plus docetaxel every 3 weeks in first- and second-line metastatic oesophageal cancer: final results of a phase II trial. *Br J Cancer* 92(12): 2129–33.

Ludeman L, Shepherd NA. (2005) Serosal involvement in gastrointestinal cancer: its assessment and significance. *Histopathology* 47: 123–31.

Malthaner RA, Collin S, Fenlon D. (2006) Preoperative chemotherapy for resectable thoracic esophageal cancer. *Cochrane Database Syst Rev* 19; 3: CD001556.

Manek S, Warren BF. (2007) The multidisciplinary team (MDT) meeting and the role of pathology. In: Kirkham N, Shepherd NA, eds. *Progress in Pathology* Volume 7, pp. 235–46. Cambridge University Press, Cambridge.

Mariette C, Taillier G, Van Seuningen I, Triboulet JP (2004) Factors affecting postoperative course and survival after en bloc resection for esophageal carcinoma. *Ann Thorac Surg* 78(4): 1177–83.

Mark SD, Qiao Y-L, Dawsey SM *et al.* (2002) Prospective study of serum selenium levels and incident esophageal and gastric cancers. *J Natl Cancer Inst* 92: 1753–63.

Matsubara T, Ueda M, Abe T, Akimori T, Kokudo N, Takahashi T. (1999) Unique distribution patterns of metastatic lymph nodes in patients with superficial carcinoma of the thoracic oesophagus. *Br J Surg* 86: 669–73.

Mauer AM, Kraut EH, Krauss SA *et al.* (2005) Phase II trial of oxaliplatin, leucovorin and fluorouracil in patients with advanced carcinoma of the esophagus. *Ann Oncol* 16: 1320–5.

May A, Ell C. (2006) Diagnosis and treatment of early oesophageal cancer. *Curr Opin Gastroenterol* 22(4): 433–6.

Meluch AA, Greco FA, Spigel DR *et al.* (2006) Long-term follow up and compilation of two trials utilising concurrent paclitaxel/carboplatin/infusional 5-FU/radiation therapy (RT) in patients with localised esophageal cancer involved in the Minnie Pearl Cancer Research Network. *Proc Am Soc Clin Oncol* 24 (abstr 4028).

Millar J, Scullin P, Morrison A *et al.* (2005) Phase II study of gemcitabine and cisplatin in locally advanced/metastatic oesophageal cancer. *Br J Cancer* 93(10): 1112–6.

Mimura K, Kono K, Hanawa M *et al.* (2005) Trastuzumab-mediated antibody-dependent cellular cytotoxicity against esophageal squamous cell cancer. *Clin Cancer Res* 1; 11(13): 4898–904.

Minsky BD. (2006) Primary combined-modality therapy for esophageal cancer. *Oncology (Williston Park)* 20(5): 497–505.

MRC Oesophageal Working Group. (2002) Surgical resection with or without preoperative chemotherapy in esophageal cancer: a randomised controlled trial. *Lancet* 359: 1727–33.

Muhr-Wilkenshoff F, Hinkelbein W, Ohnesorge J *et al.* (2003) A pilot study of irinotecan (CPT-11) as single agent therapy in patients with locally advanced or metastatic esophageal carcinoma. *Int J Colorectal Dis* 18(4): 330–4.

Muller JM, Erasmus TT, Stelzner M. (1990) Surgical therapy of oesophageal cancer. *Br J Surg* 77: 845–57.

Muro K, Hamaguchi T, Ohtsu A *et al.* (2004) A phase II study of single-agent docetaxel in patients with metastatic esophageal cancer. *Ann Oncol* 15(6): 955–9.

Nguyen NT, Schauer P, Luketich JD. (2000) Minimally invasive esophagectomy for Barrett's esophagus with high-grade dysplasia. *Surgery* 127: 284–90.

Pech O, May A, Gossner L, Ell C. (2003) Barrett's esophagus: endoscopic resection. *Gastrointest Endosc Clin N Am* 13: 505–12.

Polee MB, Eskens FA, van der Burg ME *et al.* (2002) Phase II study of bi-weekly administration of paclitaxel and cisplatin in patients with advanced oesophageal cancer. *Br J Cancer* 86(5): 669–73.

Polee MB, Hop WCJ, Kok TC *et al.* (2003) Prognostic factors for survival in patients with advanced oesophageal cancer treated with cisplatin-based combination therapy. *Br J Cancer* 89: 2045–50.

Radu A, Wagnieres G, van den Berg H, Monnier P. (2000) Photodynamic therapy of early squamous cell cancers of the esophagus. *Gastrointest Endosc Clin N Am* 10: 439–60.

Ransohoff D. (2004) Rules of evidence for cancer molecular-marker discovery and validation. *Nat Rev Cancer* 93: 309–14.

Ross P, Nicolson M, Cunningham D *et al.* (2002) Prospective randomized trial comparing mitomycin, cisplatin, and protracted venous infusion fluorouracil (PVI 5-FU) with epirubicin, cisplatin and PVI 5-FU in advanced esophagogastric cancer. *J Clin Oncol* 20(8): 1996–2004.

Sammon AM, Alderson D. (1998) Diet, reflux and the development of squamous cell carcinoma of the oesophagus in Africa. *Br J Surg* 85: 891–2.

Sammon AM, Morgan A. (2002) Dietary fat and salivary prostaglandin E2. *Prostaglandins Other Lipid Mediat* 67: 137–41.

Sammon AM, Mguni M, Mapele L, Awotedu KO, Iputo JE. (2003) Bimodal distribution of fasting gastric acidity in a rural African population. *S Afr Med J* 93: 786–8.

Sato S, Kajiyama Y, Sugano M, Iwanuma Y, Tsurumaru M. (2004) Flavopiridol as a radio-sensitizer for esophageal cancer cell lines. *Dis Esophagus* 17(4): 338–44.

Savage AP, Baigre RJ, Cobb RA, Barr H, Kettlewell MGW. (1997) Palliation of malignant dysphagia by laser therapy. *Dis Esophagus* 10: 243–6.

Schull B, Kornek GV, Schmid K *et al.* (2003) Effective combination chemotherapy with bimonthly docetaxel and cisplatin with or without hematopoietic growth factor support in patients with advanced gastroesophageal cancer. *Oncology* 65(3): 211–7.

Scottish Intercollegiate Guidelines Network. (2006) *Management of Oesophageal and Gastric Cancer. A National Clinical Guideline*. Sign, Edinburgh.

Sheithauer W. (2004) Esophageal cancer: chemotherapy as palliative therapy. *Ann Oncol* 15 (Suppl 4): iv97–100.

Shumeli E, Srivastava, Dawes PJ, Claque M, Matthewson K, Record CO. (1996) Combination of laser treatment and intraluminal radiotherapy for malignant dysphagia. *Gut* 38: 803–5.

Sibille A, Lambert R, Souquet J-P, Sabben G, Descos F. (1995) Long-term survival after photodynamic therapy for esophageal cancer. *Gastroenterology* 108: 337–44.

Stahl M, Stuschke M, Lehmann N *et al.* (2005) Chemoradiation with and without surgery in patients with locally advanced squamous cell carcinoma of the esophagus. *J Clin Oncol* 23(10): 2310–17.

Stephens MR, Lewis WG, Brewster AE *et al.*(2006) Multidisciplinary team management is associated with improved outcomes after surgery for esophageal cancer. *Dis Esophagus* 19: 164–71.

Sutter AP, Hopfner M, Huether A, Maser K, Scherubl H. (2006) Targeting the epidermal growth factor receptor by erlotinib (Tarceva^{TM}) for the treatment of esophageal cancer. *Int J Cancer* 118: 1814–22.

Swisher SG, Ajani JA, Komaki R *et al.* (2003) Long term outcome of phase II trial evaluating chemotherapy, chemoradiotherapy, and surgery for locoregionally advanced esophageal cancer. *Int J Radiat Oncol Biol Phys* 57(1): 120–7.

Sykes AJ, Burt PA, Slevin NJ, Stout R, Marrs JE. (1998) Radical radiotherapy for carcinoma of the oesophagus: an effective alternative to surgery. *Radiother Oncol* 48(1): 15–21.

Takubo K. (2000) *Pathology of the Esophagus*. Educa Inc., Tokyo.

Tepper JE, Krasna M, Niedzwiecki D *et al.* (2006) Superiority of trimodality therapy to surgery alone in esophageal cancer: Results of CALGB 9781. *Proc Am Soc Clin Oncol* 24: 18S (abstr 4012).

Tew WP, Kelsen DP, Ilson DH. (2005) Targeted therapies for esophageal cancer. *Oncologist* 10(8): 590–601.

The Royal College of Radiologists. (2006) *Board of the Faculty of Clinical Oncology. Radiotherapy Dose-Fractionation*. The Royal College of Radiologists, London. Available from url:http://www.rcr.ac.uk/index.asp?PageID = 149

UICC (2002) *TNM Classification of Malignant Tumours*, 6th edn. Wiley-Liss, New York.

UICC (2005) *TNM Classification of Malignant Tumours*, 6th edn, Supplement. Wiley-Liss, New York.

Urba SG, Orringer MB, Turrisi A *et al.* (2001) Randomized trial of preoperative chemoradiation versus surgery alone in patients with locoregional esophageal carcinoma. *J Clin Oncol* 19: 305–13.

Urba S. (2004) Esophageal cancer: preoperative or definitive chemoradiation. *Ann Oncol* 15 (Suppl 4): iv93–6.

Valverde CM, Maraculla T, Casado E, Ramos FJ, Martinelli E, Tabernero J. (2006) Novel targets in gastric and esophageal cancer. *Crit Rev Oncol Hematol* 59(2): 128–38.

van Rensburg SJ, Bradshaw ES, Bradshaw D, Rose EF. (1985) Oesophageal cancer in Zulu men, South Africa: a case–control study. *Br J Cancer* 51: 399–405.

van Vliet EPM, Eijkemans MJC, Steyerberg EW *et al.* (2006) The role of socio-economic status in the decision making on diagnosis and treatment of oesophageal cancer in The Netherlands. *Br J Cancer* 95: 1180–5.

Ventura A, Kirsch DG, McLaughlin ME *et al.* (2007) Restoration of p53 function leads to tumour regression in vivo. *Nature* 445: 661–5.

Vickers J, Alderson D. (1998) Influence of luminal obstruction on oesophageal cancer staging using endoscopic ultrasonography. *Br J Surg* 85(7): 999–1001.

Walsh TN, Noonan N, Hollywood D *et al.* (1996) A comparison of multimodal therapy and surgery for esophageal carcinoma. *N Engl J Med* 335(7): 462–7.

Wang G-Q, Abnet CC, Shen Q *et al.* (2005) Histological precursors of oesophageal squamous cell carcinoma: results from a 13 year prospective follow up study in a high risk population. *Gut* 54: 187–92.

Webb A, Cunningham D, Scarrfe JC *et al.* (1997) Randomized trial comparing epirubicin,cisplatin and fluorouracil versus fluorouracil, doxorubicin and methotrexate in advanced esophagogastric cancer. *J Clin Oncol* 15(1): 261–7.

Wei W-Q, Abnet CC, Lu N *et al.* (2005)Risk factors for oesophageal squamous dysplasia in adult inhabitants of a high risk region of China. *Gut* 54: 759–63.

Wong R, Malthaner R. (2006) Combined chemotherapy and radiotherapy (without surgery) compared with radiotherapy alone in localised carcinoma of the esophagus. *Cochrane Database Syst Rev* 25 (1): CD002092.

Zhao KL, Shi XH, Jiang GL *et al.* (2005) Late course accelerated hyperfractionated radiotherapy plus concurrent chemotherapy for squamous cell carcinoma of the esophagus: a phase III randomized study. *Int J Radiat Oncol Biol Phys* 15; 62(4): 1014–20.

6 Diffuse Gastric Cancer

Edited by Ilfet Songun & Cornelius van de Velde

Diagnosis

History

Ilfet Songun & Cornelius van de Velde

Introduction

Today, gastric cancer is still the fourth most common cancer and the second leading cause of cancer-related mortality worldwide (Jemal *et al.* 2004). Over the last few decades, there has been a decline in gastric cancer-related mortality, associated with a declining incidence worldwide and not due to improving cure rates.

Because of the morphologic heterogeneity of gastric carcinomas, many classification systems were designed to cover different aspects of this tumor. Of these, the Laurén classification (Laurén 1965), which is based on epidemiology, morphology and growth pattern, has clinicopathologic importance but no unequivocal prognostic value. The decreasing incidence rate is a result of environmental awareness (e.g. better food preservation) and is mainly observed in the intestinal-type gastric cancer (according to the Laurén classification) and not the diffuse-type gastric cancer. The latter type has shown a relative increase in incidence over the last few decades.

History

The acknowledged known risk factors for developing gastric cancer are summarized in Table 6.1. Initial symptoms are usually vague and non-specific, resulting in dyspeptic complaints sometimes mimicking ulcer disease. Because gastric cancer causes symptoms late in the course of the disease and symptoms respond to antiacid medication, H_2-blocking agents or proton pump inhibitors (PPIs), the diagnosis is usually made at an advanced stage. The lack of screening programs—not cost-effective in Western countries because of the low incidence—also contributes to diagnosis being mostly at an advanced stage. As the disease progresses, the symptoms become more specific: pain in the (epi)gastric region, dysphagia (obstructing proximal tumors), loss of appetite, fatigue, weight loss, vomiting (gastric outlet obstruction), indigestion, heartburn, rectal blood loss (melena), hematemesis, and epigastric/abdominal mass. If the disease has progressed even further with distant metastases, patients can present with an enlarged left supraclavicular nodule or mass (Virchow's nodule), an abdominal mass as a sign of metastasis to the ovaries (Krukenberg tumor) or a periumbilical mass (Sister Mary Joseph nodule), all signs of incurable (stage IV) disease stage. However, discrimination between diffuse- and intestinal-type gastric cancer cannot be made on the basis of history-taking.

Gastrointestinal Oncology: A Critical Multidisciplinary Team Approach.
Edited by J. Jankowski, R. Sampliner, D. Kerr, and Y. Fong.

Clinical

Annemieke Cats

A meticulous history and physical examination are unlikely to aid the early detection of gastric cancer, as the clinical features are generally vague and non-specific. This means that up to 50% of patients in Western countries are diagnosed with advanced gastric cancer, and less than about 25% present with early-stage gastric cancer. In Asia, and especially in Japan, gastric cancer is detected much earlier: more than 50% of all newly diagnosed gastric cancers are early-stage cancers (Inoue & Tsugame 2005). This difference may be explained by a higher prevalence of gastric cancer, a more liberal use of gastroduodenoscopy, and possibly by the existence of population-based screening programs and better endoscopic techniques.

Table 6.1 Risk factors for gastric cancer (partly derived from Lynch *et al.* 2005).

Age
Mainly > 60 years
Sex
Male : female = 2 : 1
Sporadic
Chronic atrophic gastritis (CAG)
Hereditary
10% of gastric carcinomas are familial, while only 5% show a classical hereditary etiology
Family history of gastric cancer
Hereditary diffuse gastric cancer (HDGC): associated with CDH1 (E-cadherin) germline mutations in one-third of the families. Mutation carriers have a > 70% lifetime risk of developing diffuse-type gastric cancer; when symptomatic it is lethal in 80% of cases
Other autosomal dominant inherited gastric cancer predisposition syndromes
Hereditary non-polyposis colon cancer syndrome (HNPCC): gastric cancers arise in 11% of HNPCC families and 79% of gastric carcinoma is of the intestinal type
Lynch syndrome: increased risk of gastric cancer in endemic regions (Korea, Japan); not in the West
Peutz–Jeghers syndrome (PJS)
Familial adenomatous polyposis (FAP): gastric cancer occurs in excess in Japanese FAP families, but no increased risk is demonstrated in Western countries
Cowden syndrome
Li–Fraumeni syndrome (LFS): gastric cancers are both intestinal and diffuse type
Blood group type A: conflicting reports in literature concerning the association with gastric cancer
Geographic
More frequent in the far east (e.g. Japan, Korea) and South America
Environmental
Dietary: salted and smoked food (fish, meat); protective are fresh fruit, vegetables and milk
Helicobacter pylori: associated with both types of gastric cancer
Epstein–Barr virus (EBV): association with EBV may in fact be a reflection of epidemiologic factors and/or dietary habits
Tobacco smoking
Alcohol
Stress

Physical examination in relation to spreading

When patients present with gastric cancer, 40% already have liver and lung metastases and about 10% have bone metastases and peritoneal carcinomatosis. A palpable abdominal mass may be felt only after extensive enlargement of the liver, ventral peritoneal implants or the primary tumor.

In the diffuse type of gastric cancer, malignant cells that infiltrate the gastric wall can rapidly spread through the extensive intramural lymphatics and the stomach's rich blood supply, and into the subserosal layers. Although not unique to this type of cancer, this gives rise to a characteristic locoregional spreading pattern. Lateral local extension into the esophagus and duodenum is principally through direct penetration and submucosal lymphatic spread, and this may subsequently give rise to intraluminal obstruction.

Peritoneal carcinomatosis primarily originates from subserosal infiltration with subsequent cell shedding and distant peritoneal attachment, but may also occur without demonstrable histologic serosal involvement as a result of hematogenous spread. It is difficult to detect peritoneal tumor deposits either by physical examination or through currently available imaging techniques such as (endoscopic) ultrasonography and CT scan. However, the presence of ascites suggests such a diagnosis. Small amounts of ascites, however, can easily be missed as well. Peritoneal carcinomatosis often becomes apparent only during surgery or after cytologic evaluation of peroperative washings of the abdominal cavity. As peritoneal carcinomatosis progresses, slow colonic transit with symptoms of constipation develops, and eventually tumor obstruction of small and large bowel segments may occur. Large peritoneal implants beyond the abdominal wall may be palpated during physical examination, and drop metastases in the pouch of Douglas may be encountered during digital pelvic or rectal examination (Blumer's shelf).

Local extension of the primary tumor into adjacent structures may cause several problems. Proximal gastric cancer may directly penetrate the splenic hilum, pancreas, diaphragm, and lateral segment of the left lobe of the liver. Extensive diffuse infiltration into the porta hepatis, or enlarged hepatic hilar or peripancreatic lymph nodes—and to a lesser extent intrahepatic metastases—may cause jaundice. Distal gastric tumors may spread through the gastrocolic ligament and can lead to extraluminal impression or tumor growth into the transverse colon, and thus may cause obstruction or formation of a gastrocolic fistula. Ingrowth may be mistaken for primary transverse colon cancer. Transperitoneal or hematogenous spread in the ovaries is also known as a Krukenberg tumor and typically consists of mucinous, signet-ring carcinoma cells surrounded by non-neoplastic ovarian stroma. These tumors are usually quite bulky, and therefore may give rise to symptoms before the primary tumor has been detected. They often affect both ovaries but a unilateral presentation is possible as well. Besides extensive intramural lymphatics, a widespread locoregional perigastric lymph node system also exists. Clinically manifest metastatic lymph nodes in the left supraclavicular fossa (Virchow's node) and left axilla (Irish's node) are the result of extensive spread through intrathoracic lymph channels. A subcutaneous periumbilical tumor implant, the so-called Sister Mary Joseph's node, probably originates from the lymphatics in the hepatoduodenal ligament that extend into the falciform ligament alongside the obliterated umbilical vein, although transperitoneal spread has also been described.

Subcutaneous or dermal nodules may occur at other sites on the trunk, and also on the scalp and extremities. They are usually non-tender, firm and sometimes ulcerated. A more cellulite-like lesion that presents as a warm, erythematous, edematous and slightly infiltrating plaque is rare, and preferentially associated with the diffuse type of gastric cancer (Fig. 6.1). Histologic examination reveals signet-ring cells diffusely infiltrating in the dermis, both with and without occlusion of dilated lymphatics by tumor cells (Han *et al.* 2000; Navarro *et al.* 2002). The pleura and pericardium may be involved via abdominal tumor implants penetrating the thorax, the lymphatics and, more rarely, the blood. This may lead to pleural effusion and cardiac tamponade.

Gastric cancer is occasionally associated with paraneoplastic conditions. Acanthosis nigrans is a patchy velvety dark-brown hyperpigmentation and thickening that usually occurs in intertriginous zones and areas subjected to trauma such as knees and elbows. The Leser–Trélat sign (seborrheic keratoses) may occur in association with acanthosis nigrans in 35% of cases. Thrombophlebitis migrans (Trousseau's syndrome) is a prothrombotic state with poorly understood pathophysiology. It is best managed by anticancer treatment and the administration of low-molecular-weight heparins. Other rare paraneoplastic conditions associated with gastric cancer are membranous nephropathy, microangiopathic hemolytic anemia, dermatomyositis, palmar fasciitis and polyarthritis (flexion contractures of both hands and thickening of palmar fascia), and cerebellar degeneration.

Laboratory investigations

Anemia occurs in 50% of patients with gastric cancer and is usually microcytic, although it can be megaloblastic or mixed. Liver enzymes may be elevated in the presence of liver metastases. Several proteins and carbohydrates have been tested as diagnostic and prognostic markers for cancer. Carcinoembryonic antigen (CEA) is elevated in 15–30% of patients with gastric cancer and tends to indicate disseminated disease or, in the case of poorly differentiated or signet-ring cell carcinoma, massive local infiltration (Horrie *et al.* 1996). Its sensitivity and specificity for advanced disease increases when used in combination with other antigens, such as carbohydrate antigen 19-9 (CA 19-9) and CA 72-4, but it is still too low to merit routine clinical use for (early) detection of gastric cancer.

Endoscopy

The gold standard for the diagnosis of gastric cancer is endoscopy with biopsy specimens from areas suspected of tumor growth. The number of biopsies correlates with its diagnostic yield. In diffuse gastric cancer, however, it is less accurate. Endoscopy is not a suitable instrument for staging. Irrespective

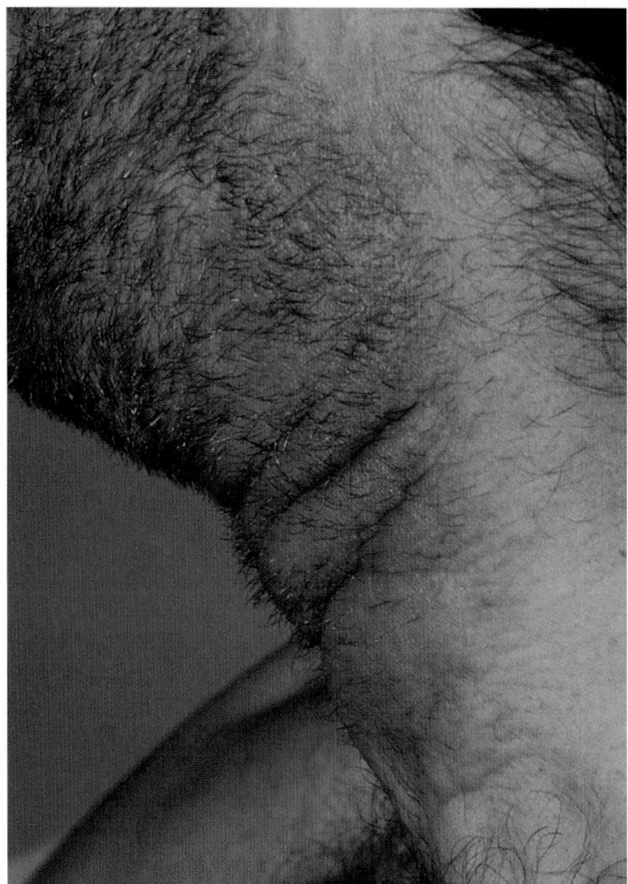

(a)

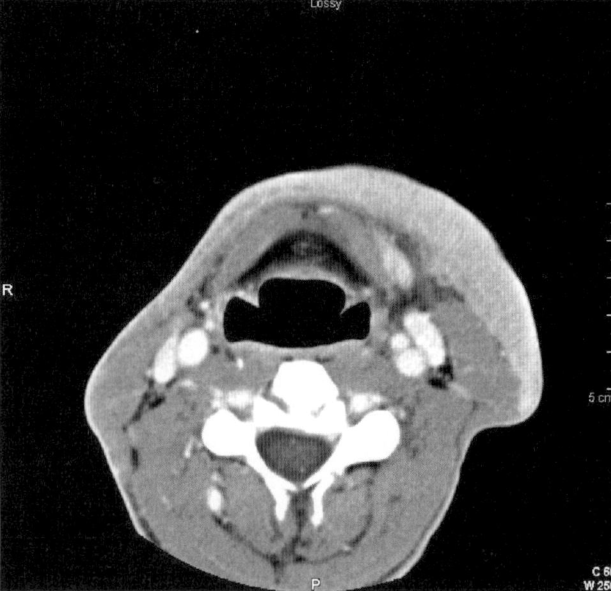

(b)

Fig. 6.1 A 35-year-old male patient with pT3 N2 diffuse-type gastric cancer. Seven months after total gastrectomy with splenectomy he developed focal erythematous infiltration of the skin in his neck, which cytology showed to contain adenocarcinoma cells (a). As can be seen on the CT scan tumor infiltration was limited to the skin, without evidence of lymph node infiltration (b).

of this, determination of the location of the tumor within the stomach is essential for further surgical or palliative treatment planning.

Gastric cancers can be endoscopically classified according to the macroscopic presentation of their growth pattern. The Japanese classification divides early gastric cancer into three types: protruded (type I), superficial (type II), and excavated (type III). Type II is further subdivided into type IIa (elevated), type IIb (flat), and type IIc (depressed). Diffuse gastric cancers are usually types IIc and III, and account for less than 15% of early gastric cancers. Borrmann's classification for more advanced gastric cancers consists of four types: polypoid (type I), ulceration (type II), ulceration with border infiltration (type III), and diffuse infiltration (type IV). The latter represents about 50% of cases. Its superficial spread through the mucosa and submucosa produces thickening of the mucosal folds that develop into flat, plaque-like lesions with or without shallow ulcerations. When infiltration further progresses and involves the entire stomach, this results in linitis plastica or so-called 'leather bottle' stomach. This situation frequently coincides with retention of food due to decreased gastric peristalsis or gastric outlet obstruction, and is, therefore, often accompanied with endoscopic signs of reflux esophagitis. Further signs are diminished distensibility of the stomach and pain during air insufflation.

Even in early-stage gastric cancer, 5–15% of cancers are multifocal. However, the presence of satellite lesions is often only recognized after histopathologic examination of the resected stomach.

Both the importance of and the technical difficulties with early detection of diffuse gastric cancer are illustrated by the autosomal dominant predisposition to gastric cancer known as hereditary diffuse gastric cancer (HDGC). Patients with HDGC have a germline mutation in the *CDH1* gene, which causes impaired production and function of E-cadherin. This protein belongs to the family of cell–cell adhesion molecules and plays an important role in maintaining the normal architecture of epithelial tissues. Patients with HDGC develop diffuse, poorly differentiated infiltrative adenocarcinomas, often associated with signet-ring cells, at an early age (median age 37 years). A prophylactic total gastrectomy is currently the treatment of choice in patients with established *CDH1* gene mutations. Histopathologic examination of postgastrectomy specimens reveals tens to hundreds of intramucosal foci of malignant cells that cannot be recognized endoscopically (Shaw *et al.* 2005). Therefore, endoscopy does not seem to be a reliable tool for the detection of precursor lesions. Additional techniques such as chromoendoscopy have been tested to overcome this diagnostic shortcoming. Shaw *et al.* (2005) reintroduced a slightly modified chromodye enhanced endoscopy with methylene blue and congo red in 33 *CDH1* gene mutation carriers for whom total gastrectomy was not an acceptable treatment. In 24 of 93 chromoendoscopies 1–6 pale areas of 2–10 mm were detected per stomach. In 41% of biopsies taken from these lesions signet-ring cell carcinoma was detected. In patients subsequently undergoing surgery many more malignant foci were observed, and foci less than 4 mm in particular were missed during endoscopy. The technique may thus facilitate surveillance endoscopy in mutation carriers who decline gastrectomy or in subjects in whom a familial predisposition is suspected, but a genetic defect has not been demonstrated. In conjunction with chromoendoscopy, newly developed magnification and high-resolution endoscopes may offer better imaging. Other diagnostic modalities, such as (auto)fluorescence spectroscopy, narrow-band imaging and confocal endoscopy have also been tested. Their role remains to be established in the near future as well.

Histopathology and molecular pathology

Cen Si, Nicole C.T. van Grieken & Gerrit A. Meijer

Several classification systems for gastric cancer have been described, of which the most widely accepted are the classifications by the World Health Organization (WHO) (Table 6.2) and Laurén (Laurén 1965; Hamilton & Aaltonen 2000). Gastric adenocarcinomas can be subdivided into intestinal-type and diffuse-type adenocarcinomas (Laurén 1965). These tumor types differ with respect to epidemiologic and clinicopathologic characteristics as well as the involvement of certain molecular pathways, such as E-cadherin (Carvalho *et al.* 2006).

For the intestinal-type adenocarcinoma a clear sequence of precursor lesions has been described by Correa: long-term *Helicobacter pylori* infection leads to chronic gastritis, mucosal atrophy, intestinal metaplasia, dysplasia, and finally adenocarcinoma (Correa *et al.* 1976). Macroscopically, intestinal-type adenocarcinomas form well-circumscribed tumor masses, sometimes with a central ulcer. The definitive diagnosis,

Table 6.2 World Health Organization classification of epithelial neoplasms of the stomach.

Intraepithelial neoplasia – adenoma
Carcinoma
Adenocarcinoma
Papillary adenocarcinoma
Tubular adenocarcinoma
Mucinous adenocarcinoma
Signet-ring cell carcinoma
Adenosquamous carcinoma
Squamous cell carcinoma
Small cell carcinoma
Undifferentiated carcinoma
Others
Carcinoid

however, should be made on histologic examination. Intestinal-type tumors consist of well-defined ducts or cords, surrounded by newly formed desmoplastic stroma, containing various amounts of a mixed inflammatory infiltrate. The tumor cells are large and have variable sizes and shapes. Nuclei are often hyperchromatic, with coarse chromatin, and mitotic figures are easy to find. Intestinal-type tumors are usually well or moderately differentiated (Fig. 6.2a,b).

In contrast to intestinal-type adenocarcinoma, there is no clear sequence of precursor lesions leading to diffuse-type adenocarcinomas. The only precursor described so far is carcinoma *in situ*. Carneiro *et al.* systematically screened complete prophylactic gastrectomy specimens from subjects with an E-cadherin germline mutation for foci of invasive adenocarcinoma and potential precursor lesions (Carneiro *et al.* 2006). In 7 out of 10 cases they found small foci of signet-ring cells lining foveolae and glands, sometimes forming two layers: an inner layer of benign cells and an outer layer of neoplastic cells. Intestinal metaplasia was found in none of the specimens. Macroscopically, the stomachs of patients with diffuse gastric adenocarcinomas often show a diffuse thickening of the gastric wall due to an extensive stroma reaction surrounding the diffusely invaded tumor cells, leading to a rigid gastric wall. This rigidity, also known as 'linitis plastica', often results in obstruction at the side of the pyloris. Malignant cells may extend submucosally under the normal-appearing mucosa, making it difficult for the clinician or endoscopist to establish the extent of the tumor. This is of clinical importance when making decisions about treatment options. Histologic type according to the Laurén classification is also a prognostic marker. Diffuse-type adenocarcinomas are associated with a significantly worse prognosis compared to the intestinal-type tumors. However, a paper by Kattan *et al.* (2003) weighted several survival-related parameters and showed that the number of positive lymph nodes and depth of invasion are far more important in predicting patient survival (Zhao *et al.* 2005). Diffuse-type tumors, however, are often associated with positive lymph nodes and deeper invasion.

The macroscopic appearances of diffuse adenocarcinomas are reflected microscopically in the typical discohesive growth pattern of this tumor, with solitary or small groups of tumor cells infiltrating the gastric wall. There is extensive formation of new stroma, often to such an extent that it is difficult to recognize the actual tumor cells on a standard H&E section, and the true numbers of tumor cells are only revealed by cytokeratin stains. Glandular formations are absent. Diffuse adenocarcinomas typically exist of cells with relatively uniform size and shape. They have round to oval nuclei with coarse chromatin (Fig. 6.2c). In some cases intracytoplasmic vacuoles can be seen. These mucus-containing vacuoles push the nucleus to the periphery of the cell, giving it a signet-ring appearance (Fig. 6.2d). If a tumor predominantly exists of such signet-ring cells, it should be classified as a signet-ring cell carcinoma (WHO). Although diffuse carcinomas often show less cytonuclear atypia, they should always be graded as poorly differentiated, because of their discohesive growth pattern. In some cases Indian files

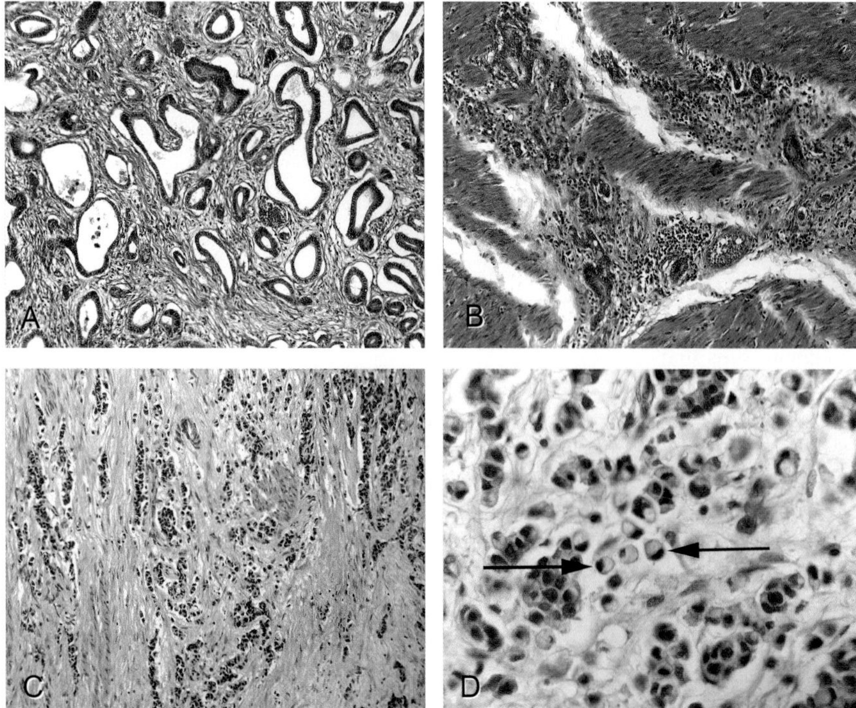

Fig. 6.2 Intestinal-type adenocarcinoma with irregularly shaped glandular structures surrounded by desmoplastic stroma (A). (B) shows the same intestinal-type tumor with neoplastic glands infiltrating the muscularis propria. Diffuse-type adenocarcinomas often show cords and small groups of tumor cells surrounded by extensive fibrosis (C). In some cases signet-ring cells can be detected (D, arrows).

can be seen. This growth pattern can also be seen in lobular carcinoma of the breast, a tumor that shares a particular biologic characteristic with diffuse gastric cancers, i.e. loss of function of the E-cadherin gene.

Histopathologically, gastric adenocarcinoma is usually diagnosed on endoscopically obtained biopsy specimens. Such biopsies are often small, and especially in the case of ulceration and extensive inflammation, it may be difficult to recognise single tumor cells infiltrating the lamina propria. For this reason, additional stainings can be used to detect tumor cells. Epithelial markers give a clear architectural overview, and mucin stains can be helpful in detecting single signet-ring cells that otherwise can be mistaken for histiocytes.

In the case of a mucin-producing tumor outside the stomach, such as in lymph nodes, ovary, mesenterium, omentum or peritoneum, immunohistochemistry may reveal the primary tumor of origin. Markers that are positive in up to 100% of gastric adenocarcinomas (irrespective of tumor type) are epithelial membrane antigen (EMA) and carcinoembryonic antigen (CEA). The majority of cases show cytokeratin 7 positivity, while a minority are positive for cytokeratin 20. A subset of cases, however, are positive for both CK7 and CK20. A combination of both these keratin markers may often differentiate between gastric and colorectal cancer, since the latter are usually CK20+ and CK7–. However, with immunohistochemical markers also, 100% specificity cannot be achieved. Loss of membranous E-cadherin expression, a cell–cell adhesion molecule, is seen more commonly but not exclusively in diffuse-type carcinomas as compared to intestinal-type carcinomas (Guilford *et al.* 1998).

Pathologic staging

Whereas preoperative clinical staging is based on physical examination, imaging, endoscopy and/or surgical exploration, pathologic staging is based on macroscopic and microscopic examination of a surgical gastrectomy specimen. For this purpose the most recent edition of the UICC pTNM classification is used (Sobin & Wittekind 2002). This classification includes depth of invasion (T), lymph node status (N) and presence of distant metastases (M).

Primary tumors restricted to the mucosa (lamina propria) or submucosa are T1. Tumors invading the muscularis propria or subserosa are T2a and T2b, respectively. If there is invasion of the visceral peritoneum the tumor is T3, and if adjacent structures are invaded by the tumor it is T4. Adjacent structures include the spleen, transverse colon, liver, diaphragm, pancreas, abdominal wall, adrenal gland, kidney, small intestine, and retroperitoneum.

Gastric adenocarcinomas primarily metastasize to the paragastric lymph nodes along the lesser and greater curvatures, the lymph nodes along the left gastric, common hepatic, splenic, and celiac arteries, and the hepatoduodenal lymph nodes. If the primary tumor is located at the gastroesophageal junction, regional lymph nodes include the paracardial, left gastric, celiac, diaphragmatic, and lower mediastinal paraesophageal lymph nodes. Lymph node metastases are scored from N0 to N3: N0 means no lymph node involvement, N1 involvement of 1–6 lymph nodes, N2 involvement of 7–15 lymph nodes and N3 involvement of more than 15 lymph nodes. Usually at least 15 lymph nodes can be found in a gastrectomy specimen. However, it should be noted that neoadjuvant therapy may decrease the number of lymph nodes.

The presence of pathologically confirmed distant metastases of the tumor is M1. However, distant metastases cannot usually be determined by the pathologist. In this case, the M stage should be reported as MX. As already mentioned, involvement of the adjacent organs does not influence M stage. On the other hand, metastases in distant intra-abdominal lymph nodes, such as retropancreatic, mesenteric and para-aortic lymph nodes, are classified as M1.

Molecular pathology

Most gastric adenocarcinomas are sporadic, i.e. non-hereditary, while about 10% of gastric cancers show familial clustering. This familial clustering can in part be explained by environmental factors, but germline mutations in several tumor suppressor genes have been associated with hereditary gastric cancer. As one allele is already missing or malfunctioning at birth, secondary loss or hypermethylation of the other allele results in gene silencing in a gastric epithelial cell, leading to cancer early in life. About 30% of hereditary gastric cancers are associated with germline mutations of E-cadherin, and consequently are diffuse gastric cancers. Other known germline mutations include mutation of *p53*, which is part of the Li–Fraumeni syndrome, and mutations of mismatch repair genes like *hMLH1*, *hMSH2*, *hMSH6*, and *hPMS2*. Li–Fraumeni syndrome is characterized by sarcomas of the soft tissues, bone and miscellaneous tumors of juvenile onset, and frequent occurrence of metachronous tumors. Germline mutations of mismatch repair genes are seen in hereditary non-polyposis colorectal cancer (HNPCC/Lynch syndrome). These patients have an increased risk of developing colorectal cancers, endometrial carcinoma, and gastric adenocarcinomas.

Sporadic gastric adenocarcinomas arise through a multistep process, in which accumulation of (epi)genetic changes that affect key biologic processes such as proliferation, apoptosis, cell cycle control, etc. ultimately lead to invasive cancer. For the necessary genetic alterations to be acquired, some form of genomic instability needs to occur. This can be genomic instability at the DNA level, such as failing DNA mismatch repair resulting in microsatellite instability, but most gastric carcinomas show genomic instability at the chromosomal level resulting in coarse genomic changes, like translocations, inversions and gains and losses of complete or parts of chromosome arms. A minority of sporadic gastric carcinomas show microsatellite instability (MSI); in a study by Vauhkonen *et al.* (2005)

MSI was found in 28% of sporadic diffuse gastric cancers. Loss of function of these genes leads to accumulation of mutations. In the following paragraphs some of the known genomic changes that occur frequently in gastric cancer are discussed. Given the enormous amount of reports and the rapid new developments in the field of molecular pathology, we obviously cannot give a complete overview.

E-cadherin (*CDH1*) is a protein involved in cellular adhesion. Loss of function of this gene, results in epithelial cells losing their adhesive properties so that they may easily migrate to and infiltrate other tissues. Germline mutations in this gene, mentioned above, account for 30% of hereditary gastric cancers, leading to diffuse-type carcinomas (Richards *et al.* 1999). Sporadic diffuse-type gastric cancers also show reduced or absent E-cadherin expression in about 50% of cases. In sporadic cases, the gene is silenced by somatic mutation and/or promoter hypermethylation (Guilford *et al.* 1998; Grady *et al.* 2000; Machado *et al.* 2001).

Another gene that is frequently involved in gastric carcinogenesis is *p53*. *p53* plays a critical role in cellular response to DNA damage, leading to cell cycle arrest in G1 or apoptosis. Loss of this gene, or loss of the short arm of chromosome 17 (locus of *p53*), is associated with 50% of gastric cancers of both types (Grieken *et al.* 2000). Accumulation of (mutated) *p53* has been found by immunohistochemical means in about 60% of diffuse-type gastric cancers without E-cadherin alterations (Fricke *et al.* 2003). Intestinal-type carcinomas show p53 expression in up to 60 % (Vollmers *et al.* 1997).

SMAD proteins play a role in signal transduction via the transforming growth factor beta (TGFβ) pathway. This pathway is involved in many cellular functions, including cell growth and differentiation, adhesion, migration, extracellular matrix formation, and immune function. In a series of 88 gastric adenocarcinomas (diffuse type, n = 39; intestinal type, n = 49), expression of *SMAD4* was significantly reduced in the diffuse-type carcinomas as compared to the intestinal-type tumors and gastric adenomas (Kim *et al.* 2005a). Furthermore, *SMAD4* expression has been claimed by some authors to have prognostic significance in advanced gastric carcinomas (without stratification for histologic type) (Xiangming *et al.* 2001).

Mutations of *APC*, known for its association with the development of colorectal adenomas in both familial adenomatous polyposis (FAP) and sporadic adenomas, have also been studied in gastric cancer. Absence of *APC* expression has been seen in up to 80% of gastric adenocarcinomas, independent of tumor type (Grace *et al.* 2002). Previously, only 4% of adenocarcinomas were found to harbor somatic mutations (Lee *et al.* 2002). However, the high frequency of absent expression can now be explained by frequent promoter hypermethylation (Sarbia *et al.* 2004).

About 70% of gastric carcinomas show loss of expression of fragile histidine triad (*FHIT*), more often in difuse-type (82%) than in intestinal-type (66%) carcinomas (Bragantini *et al.* 2006). Although in univariate analysis *FHIT* has been associated with higher clinical stage and poorer survival, multivariate analysis has shown that it is not an independent marker of prognosis (Zhao *et al.* 2005; Bragantini *et al.* 2006).

$p16^{INK4A}$ is a cell-cycle regulatory gene involved in G1–S arrest. Germline mutations of this gene confer susceptibility to melanomas. Downregulation of *p16* by either mutation or loss of heterozygosity has previously been found in a small subset of diffuse-type adenocarcinomas (Gunther *et al.* 1998). However, recently hypermethylation of *p16* has been detected in about 30% of cases, irrespective of histologic type (Vo *et al.* 2002).

Her2/Neu overexpression by gene amplification has proven its clinical importance in breast carcinomas. Recently, in a large series of 131 cases, about 12% of gastric adenocarcinomas showed mutations of c-erbB-2, but in diffuse gastric cancers this was only 2% (Tanner *et al.* 2005). In other studies, however, no correlation between overexpression and histologic type could be detected.

K-ras mutations have been shown to occur not as frequently in gastric carcinomas as compared to colorectal carcinomas (10% vs 40%, respectively). However, it has been reported repeatedly that *K-ras* mutations in gastric cancer are mainly associated with the diffuse-type gastric adenocarcinomas (Kim *et al.* 1997; Arber *et al.* 2000).

Imaging and staging of gastric cancer

Regina G.H. Beets-Tan & Cornelius van de Velde

In patients who have suspected gastric cancer, early detection and accurate preoperative staging are important for determining the most suitable therapy modality. The delineation of tumor extent and local spread will influence the extent of surgery performed. The extent of nodal dissection is a major determining factor in staging and can influence stage-related outcome. Preoperative staging by imaging is necessary to determine the proportion of stomach involved by tumor, to assist in deciding the extent of gastric resection, to identify the presence of locoregional and distant nodal enlargement for determining the extent of lymphadenectomy, and to identify metastatic disease in the liver and peritoneum, including ovarian deposits.

The therapeutic spectrum for gastric cancer has been widely enlarged by both the introduction of preoperative chemotherapy and the possibility of endoscopic resection. Because treatment of gastric cancer is no longer exclusively surgical, precise preoperative staging by imaging has also become more important for selection of patients for different treatment strategies.

Tumor detection

Endoscopic examination is more reliable than double-contrast barium upper GI (UGI) studies in the diagnosis of gastric cancer, for it allows biopsies to be taken. However, for type IV advanced gastric cancer—the diffuse-type infiltrating adenocarcinoma or scirrhous-type gastric carcinoma—endoscopy has been reported to have a sensitivity of only 33–73% (Levine *et al.* 1990), and UGI studies are known to be superior (Levine *et al.* 1990; Park *et al.* 2004). The main reason for the poor sensitivity of endoscopy is that these tumors are predominantly located in the submucosa, with the overlying mucosa often appearing normal. Therefore, the tumor extent is easily underestimated. On UGI studies, however, the presence of this diffuse-type gastric cancer can be suspected when there is typical loss of gastric distensibility, thickened or irregular folds and/or obliteration of the gastric folds.

Tumor staging

Endoscopic ultrasonography (EUS)

EUS is the most accurate method for evaluation of the depth of tumor ingrowth into the gastric wall. Furthermore, it has been reported that EUS can predict resectability with high sensitivity and specificity (Willis *et al.* 2000). Therefore EUS is valuable for selection of patients with early gastric cancer for local excision or (immediate) surgery.

The high accuracy of EUS for preoperative staging of T1 lesions has been reported in many studies (Botet *et al.* 1991) and was confirmed in a recent publication where the authors found an accuracy of 83% for T1, 60% for T2 and 100% for T3 respectively (Tsendsuren *et al.* 2006). Nevertheless, one must be aware of the relatively high rate of overstaging for the T1 and T2 stages, with 20–25% overstaging failures for T1 and 30% for T2 (Willis *et al.* 2000; Tsendsuren *et al.* 2006). Main reasons for overstaging are thickening of the gastric wall due to peritumoral inflammation and absence of the serosal layer in certain areas of the stomach. A systematic review of 13 EUS studies in gastric cancer showed a very high overall T staging performance, with an area under the receiver operating characteristic curve of 0.93 (Kelly *et al.* 2001). The articles included in this review, which compared EUS with CT, all suggested that the T staging performance of EUS was superior to that of conventional CT. Botet *et al.* for example, found an accuracy for T staging of 92% for EUS versus 42% for CT (Botet *et al.* 1991). Unlike CT, EUS can distinguish five layers within the gastric wall. Invasion of any of these layers by tumor can be more accurately assessed by EUS than by conventional CT.

The downside of EUS however is that, due to its limited range of view, EUS cannot provide information on distant staging.

Computed tomography (CT)

CT is a powerful tool in that it provides local and distant staging in one single examination. Conventional CT techniques, however, have been poor for T-stage determination. Although initial studies found good agreement between T stage as determined by CT and pathology (Balfe *et al.* 1981), many subsequent studies reported disappointing results. One of these studies involving 75 patients reported an accuracy of only 47% for conventional CT, with understaging in 31% and overstaging in 16% (Sussman *et al.* 1988). Recently, an advanced CT technique, multidetector row CT (MDCT), has been used for more accurate staging of gastric cancer (Fig. 6.3). MDCT has been reported to show promising results for T staging, comparable to those of EUS (D'Elia *et al.* 2000; Bhandari *et al.* 2004; Kim *et al.* 2005c). Bhandari *et al.* reported an overall accuracy for MDCT for detection of gastric lesions of 94%, with an accuracy of 97% for the detection of early gastric cancer and of 100% for the detection of advanced tumors. The overall accuracies for EUS and MDCT in the preoperative determination of depth of invasion (T stage) were similar at 88% and 82%, respectively; their sensitivities were 96% and 83%, respectively, and their specificities 69% and 94%, respectively (Bhandari *et al.* 2004). MDCT allows for thinner slices and faster scanning, and enables rapid and easy handling of image reconstruction to generate cross-sectional transverse and multiplanar reformation (MPR) images, which may contribute to the markedly improved results.

Nevertheless, some studies of MDCT have been less positive (D'Elia *et al.* 2000; Fukuya *et al.* 1997). According to Fukuya *et al.* CT with MPR images does not improve T staging (66%). D'Elia *et al.* also reported disappointing results for MDCT, with a far lower accuracy for the detection of early gastric cancer (20%) as compared to that of advanced gastric cancer (87%), and a tendency to overstage T1 tumors as T2 (D'Elia *et al.* 2000).

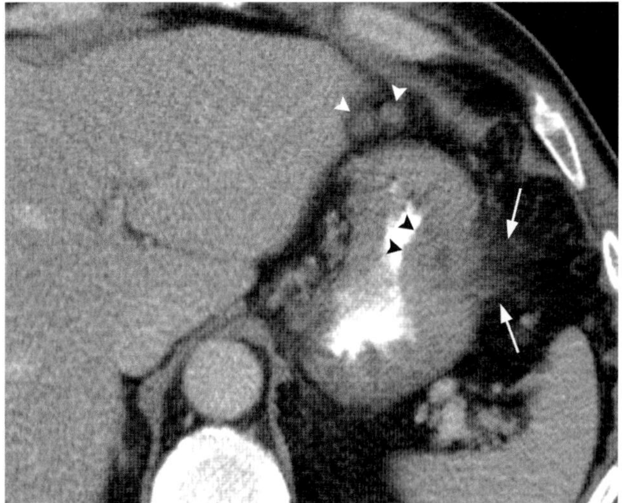

Fig. 6.3 Axial contrast-enhanced CT shows obliteration of the gastric folds and diffuse thickening of the wall of the gastric body (black arrowheads), blurring of the serosal contour, and tissue strands (white arrows) extending into the perigastric fat, due to a T3 gastric cancer. Two 8-mm large nodes are also seen in the perigastric fat, suspected to be involved nodes in compartment I (white arrowheads).

They found that the main causes of overstaging are due to the difficulty in observing the multilayered pattern of the gastric wall in the areas where the gastric wall is thinner (prepylorus) and where the obliquely scanned area (gastric angle) causes confounding partial volume effects.

Clearly there is a need for further improvement of planar imaging methods in the preoperative staging of stomach cancer. To improve tumor staging, exact tumor detection and location is essential. The detection of early gastric cancer in the absence of a thickened gastric wall remains very difficult even with MDCT. MDCT using volumetric data analysis might provide the solution. This so-called 'virtual gastroscopy' technique has been reported in some studies to increase the detection rate of early gastric cancer from 65 to 94% (Kim *et al.* 2005b). This technique, however, is limited to expert single centers and certainly not ready yet for general use.

Positron emission tomography (PET)

PET with 2-[fluorine-18]fluoro-2-deoxy-D-glucose (FDG) has been recognized as a useful diagnostic technique in clinical oncology (Rohren *et al.* 2004), but experience of its use in evaluating stomach cancer is limited. FDG PET appears to be very accurate in detecting distant metastatic disease at the time of initial diagnosis, but it may be of limited use in locoregional staging (Kole *et al.* 1998). PET is not helpful in T staging because the FDG uptake can vary according to the histologic type of gastric cancer. Gastric adenocarcinomas, such as mucinous carcinoma, signet ring cell carcinoma and poorly differentiated adenocarcinomas, have been reported to show significantly lower FDG uptake than other histologic types of gastric cancer. PET, however, could play a significant role in monitoring treatment response. Recent reports involving patients with gastric cancer have demonstrated that response to preoperative chemotherapy can be predicted with FDG PET early in the course of therapy (Ott *et al.* 2003). Although further studies are needed to determine its efficacy, it is hoped that response to treatment will be apparent much earlier at PET than at CT, allowing early alteration of management in non-responders.

Nodal staging

The systematic review by Kelly *et al.* shows that EUS is not as effective for lymph node staging as it is for T staging, with an area under the receiver operating characteristic curve of 0.79 (Kelly *et al.* 2001). But a more accurate assessment of nodal disease can be obtained with EUS than with CT. An additional useful role of EUS in gastric nodal staging is the ability to take biopsies of suspected nodes. In the literature the accuracy figures of EUS for the determination of gastric nodal disease range from 66 to 77% (Botet *et al.* 1991; Willis *et al.* 2000; Tsendsuren *et al.* 2006).

N stage determination by EUS is not optimal and there are several reasons for this. Although the EUS criteria for malignant node prediction are very sensitive (size, shape, border, echogenicity and echo texture), they are less specific. Furthermore the para-aortic and celiac regions are often beyond the scope of the endosonography probe; consequently distant node metastases at these locations cannot be detected with EUS.

As already mentioned, alternative methods such as CT do not perform any better. Accuracies previously reported for prediction of gastric nodal metastases with CT have ranged between 51% and 76% (Kim *et al.* 2001). Although the use of MPR and volumetric imaging was expected to improve N staging, the results remained unsatisfactory. Kim *et al.* reported no improvement for nodal staging using these advanced CT tools, with an overall accuracy of only 64% (Kim *et al.* 2005c). These poor results are considered to be due to the lack of reliable CT criteria for metastatic lymph nodes. Regional lymph nodes are considered to be involved when the short-axis diameter is larger than 6 mm for perigastric lymph nodes and larger than 8 mm for extraperigastric lymph nodes (Balfe *et al.* 1981). Although there is a clear correlation between lymph node size and cancer involvement, CT, which is inherently low in contrast resolution, has significant limitations in nodal staging based on size criteria because of the high frequency of microscopic nodal invasion (involvement of normal-size nodes) and the poor differentiation between reactive and metastatic nodal enlargement. The wide ranges of sensitivity (48–91%) in the literature demonstrate this problem of CT in nodal staging (Sussman *et al.* 1988).

MRI with lymph node-specific iron oxide contrast agent has been reported by several investigators to be very effective for the detection of metastatic lymph nodes in various pelvic cancers. So far only one study has confirmed its efficacy in gastric cancer nodes, with 100% sensitivity, 93% specificity, 86% positive predictive value, and 100% negative predictive value (Tatsumi *et al.* 2006). It remains unclear though whether iron oxide MRI will work in gastric cancer because MRI of the gastric area is very susceptible to motion artefacts and because the contrast agent is not yet commercially available.

FDG PET as a metabolic imaging method could theoretically be used to overcome this limitation of anatomic imaging. PET is less sensitive than CT in the detection of locoregional lymph node metastasis mainly due to its poor spatial resolution, which makes it very difficult to distinguish between lymph nodes and the primary tumor (McAteer *et al.* 1999). However, the presence of these regional nodes may not be important in planning surgical extent, since these nodes would be removed at the time of surgery. Detection of nodal metastases distant from the tumor can change the extent of lymph node dissection or may preclude unnecessary surgery. Nodes at distant sites would theoretically be easier to identify at PET because they are remote from the hot spot of the primary tumor. Two recent studies on FDG PET have indeed shown its usefulness in nodal staging of gastric cancer (Yun *et al.* 2005; Kim *et al.* 2006). CT was superior to PET in terms of sensitivity but PET was superior to CT in terms of specificity for staging distant nodes in gastric cancer (Kim *et al.* 2006). PET seems to complement CT and vice versa. Therefore the value of combined functional–anatomical techniques such as PET-CT should be further investigated for nodal staging.

Staging for distant metastasis

Hematogenous metastases from gastric cancer most commonly involve the liver. The optimal CT strategy is helical scanning during the portal venous phase of enhancement, because hepatic metastatic lesions are usually hypovascular. This technique improves lesion conspicuity by increasing the attenuation of normal liver tissue. CT staging for liver metastases is superior to abdominal ultrasound staging. Reported sensitivities for the CT detection of lesions larger than 9 mm vary between 64 and 85%, with the best results obtained by the newest-generation helical CT (Bipat *et al.* 2005). CT is therefore the preferred method for detection of liver metastases.

The advantage of helical CT is the 'one-stop shop' imaging evaluation of local and distant tumor spread in one single examination. Diffuse gastric carcinoma in particular tends to spread over the peritoneum with rapid growth and early metastasis. CT allows the determination of the presence of peritoneal metastases (Fig. 6.4) or Krukenberg tumors. Krukenberg tumors are readily detected on CT as often large and bilateral adnexal solid masses with heterogeneous contrast enhancement.

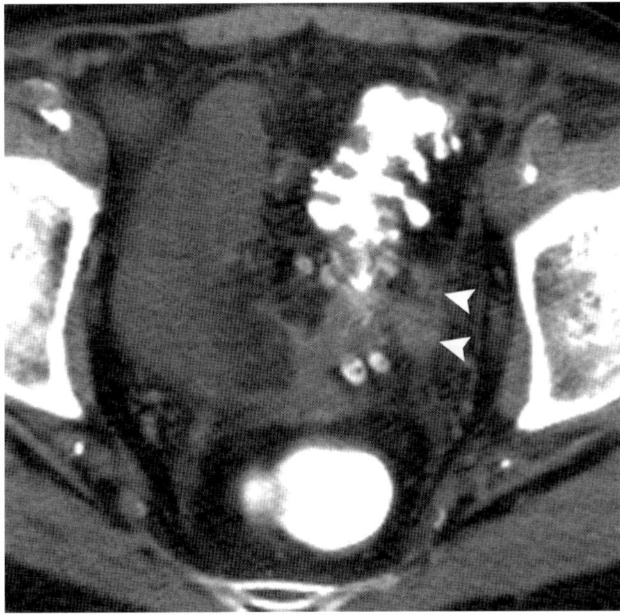

Fig. 6.4 Axial contrast-enhanced CT through the pelvis of a patient with advanced gastric cancer. Nodular deposits are seen on a thickened peritoneal surface (white arrowheads), suspicious of peritoneal metastases. Peritonitis carcinomatosa caused by the stomach cancer was confirmed at laparoscopy.

CT, although superior to all other imaging modalities, is not optimal for the preoperative diagnosis of peritoneal carcinomatosis, because it has a limited sensitivity for the detection of peritoneal nodules smaller than 1 cm, with reported figures ranging between 30 and 50% (D'Elia *et al.* 2000; Coakley *et al.* 2002). The identification of peritoneal metastases on CT strongly depends on factors such as size, location, the presence of ascites, the paucity of intra-abdominal fat and the adequacy of bowel enhancement.

FDG PET has been reported to be more sensitive than CT in the evaluation of peritoneal carcinomatosis. One report showed a sensitivities of 57% for PET, 42% for CT, and 78% for PET plus CT (Turlakow *et al.* 2003). A specific pattern of diffuse FDG uptake has been described to be a strong predictor for peritoneal carcinomatosis (Turlakow *et al.* 2003). However, the utility of PET for detection of peritoneal metastases remains controversial. Small peritoneal nodules may be missed because of the low spatial resolution of PET.

The major advantage of FDG PET in screening for distant metastases and peritoneal metastases is that it helps the CT radiologist to focus on and increase lesion conspicuity. Peritoneal deposits on bowel walls or small metastases in bones, adrenal glands, lungs, and ovaries can be easily overlooked on CT, but when suggested by PET are often detected on CT in retrospect. PET, which has low anatomic resolution but powerful contrast, undoubtedly helps CT, which has powerful anatomic resolution, to improve lesion detection. This valuable role of PET and CT being complementary tools to one another was confirmed by Turlakow's study where the combined use of PET and CT led to a major improvement in the detection rate (Turlakow *et al.* 2003).

Follow-up

CT is the primary tool for the investigation of a suspected recurrence and for evaluation of response to non-surgical treatment of recurrent disease. CT detection of recurrences is usually based on morphologic changes such as wall thickening and focal enhancement. However, treatment-induced bowel wall thickening caused by inflammation or fibrosis cannot be easily distinguished from wall thickening caused by residual tumor. These potential sources of erroneous interpretation are the reasons why it can be very difficult to detect early tumor recurrence on CT. For this reason CT at 3 months following surgery has been recommended as a baseline for further assessment. Equivocal CT findings that are suggestive of tumor recurrence can be further characterized with FDG PET, because tumor tissue shows uptake of FDG while scar tissue lacks uptake. However, PET is limited as a first-line screening tool in the follow-up of recurrent tumors because FDG PET may give false negative results in poorly differentiated gastric adenocarcinoma, and gastric cancer of the signet ring cell and mucinous types. Furthermore, the detection of recurrent gastric cancer may be difficult with PET imaging alone, because of its lack of adequate spatial resolution (De Potter *et al.* 2002).

Conclusions

CT is the imaging modality of first choice for both the preoperative locoregional and the distant staging of gastric cancer. However, nodal staging remains a difficult issue, even with advanced MDCT techniques.

EUS is the most accurate method for evaluation of the exact depth of tumor growth into the gastric wall and therefore is preferred over CT when early gastric cancer has to be selected for local excision. Nodal staging with EUS, although better than with CT, remains suboptimal.

FDG PET is limited for locoregional staging but complementary to CT for accurate distant staging.

For *follow-up* CT is the modality of choice for the investigation of a suspected recurrence. Where CT findings are equivocal, FDG PET can be of value in distinguishing benign from malignant masses.

Treatment

Overview

Ilfet Songun & Cornelius van de Velde

In the 19th century, gastric cancer was the leading cause of cancer-related death, and many patients died of upper gastrointestinal obstruction. The first pylorus resection in a human being was performed by the French surgeon Péan in 1879 without success. The Polish surgeon Rydygier also operated unsuccessfully in 1880 (Polak & Vojtisek 1959). In 1881, Billroth was the first to perform a successful gastric resection. In fact, as he removed several enlarged lymph nodes, he performed a lymph node dissection as well (Wolfler 1881). The patient died 14 months later of recurrent disease. In 1898 Mikulicz advocated lymph node dissection in addition to gastrectomy, with removal of the tail of the pancreas if necessary (Mikulicz 1898).

After reviewing reports of 298 total gastrectomies, Pack and McNeer (1943) found a postoperative mortality rate of 37.6% and therefore rejected the use of total gastrectomy. From that time on, discussion was ongoing about what type of resection should be performed to achieve the best survival with the least morbidity and postoperative mortality. In a review of articles published in English since 1970, the proportion of patients undergoing resection (resectability rate), was found to increase from 37% in the series ending before 1970 to 48% in those ending before 1990 (Macintyre & Akoh 1991; Akoh & Macintyre 1992). The 5-year survival rate after all resections increased significantly from 21% in the series ending before 1970 to 28% in those ending before 1990, and the 5-year survival rate after curative resection rose from 38% to 55% over the same period (Akoh & Macintyre 1992). Reports from Japanese institutions have shown an even better prognosis: they have demonstrated an improvement in 5-year survival rates exceeding the decline in incidence, resulting in an improved overall cure rate (Kajitani 1981).

Surgery

The mainstay of treatment for both the diffuse and intestinal types of gastric cancer still consists of curative surgery (R0), because it is still at present the only treatment modality that offers the chance of a cure. A curative resection consists of gastrectomy with lymph node dissection. The extent of the gastrectomy (total or subtotal) depends on the extent of the tumor and its location in the stomach. In locally advanced disease with invasion of adjacent organs (T4), such as the colon, spleen, and pancreas, an en-bloc resection of the stomach with the invaded organ should be performed in addition to adequate lymph node dissection if the tumor is resectable. The most important current surgical controversy is the extent of lymphadenectomy (D classification), which the Japanese believe to be the most important explanation for the improved outlook for patients with gastric cancer. In 1997 the D classification was redefined according to the number of lymph nodes dissected, instead of their location.

The outcome of surgery depends on the quality of the resection performed. This means not only carefully selecting patients for surgery, but also performing radical surgery depending on the extent of the disease, because the outcome of inadequate surgery can never be compensated completely by additional radiotherapy and/or chemotherapy. Maruyama *et al.* (1987) have compiled a computer-based database which can be used to identify nodal stations at risk (pre- or peroperatively) to customize lymphadenectomy in order to perform an operation with a low MI (Maruyama Index), which is associated with better outcome. Since there is also substantial heterogeneity of risk within stages, there is also a validated gastric carcinoma nomogram available, which can be used for individual patient counseling and adjuvant therapy decision-making (Peeters *et al.* 2005b).

Surgical prognostic factors

As well as the issue of the extent of lymphadenectomy (D1 versus D2 dissections), other aspects of gastric surgery have generated controversies. These include the type of gastrectomy (subtotal vs total), pancreatectomy and/or splenectomy, patient selection, stage and stage migration, and the experience of the surgeon as a prognostic factor. The extent of the operation, in particular, has an influence on surgical complications and mortality and a number of studies have addressed this topic. In particular, the resection of spleen or pancreas, or both, plays an important role in surgical complications. Most studies find a significant increase in morbidity and hospital mortality if a pancreaticosplenectomy is performed, without any beneficial effect on survival. The spleen should also preferably be spared as this may reduce concomitant morbidity, such as an increase in anastomotic leakage due to division of the vascularization, and immunologic factors associated with resection of the spleen itself and with immune suppression induced by blood transfusions.

Radiotherapy and chemotherapy

Gastric cancer is still mostly diagnosed at an advanced disease stage, except in some countries in the East, e.g. Japan. With surgery being the only curative treatment modality, the need has been felt to increase the number of patients having a curative resection (resectability rate). Screening has proven to be an option in Japan, where the incidence of gastric cancer is high. In Western countries, however, screening is not an option because of the relatively high cost involved because of the low incidence. Even though gastric cancer used to be known as a cancer notoriously resistant to radiation and chemotherapy, various (neo)adjuvant treatment regimens have been studied extensively. The MAGIC trial from the British Medical Research Council compared surgery alone with perioperative chemotherapy consisting of three courses of ECF (epirubicin, cisplatin, and 5-FU) preoperatively and three courses postoperatively in 503 randomized patients in the period between 1994 and 2002. This regimen resulted in downstaging, downsizing and an improved overall survival rate of 13% (Cunningham *et al.* 2006a). The other randomized trial comparing surgery alone with surgery and preoperative chemotherapy, the FAMTX (5-FU, adriamycin and methotrexate) trial from the Netherlands, was closed prematurely due to low accrual rate after 56 patients in the period between 1993 and 1996. There was no significant difference in overall survival rate (Hartgrink *et al.* 2004a). These two studies illustrate the importance of developing effective combination chemotherapy regimens.

Radiotherapy can be applied as palliative treatment for uncontrolled gastric bleeding and for irresectable tumors. In these cases radiation as a single modality did not result in a survival benefit, but locoregional control rates of 70% were reported. Due to the high incidence of locoregional failures after surgical treatment, radiotherapy has always been considered as an attractive modality in curative treatment of these tumors. Radiotherapy can be applied intra-, pre-, or postoperatively (with or without concurrent chemotherapy) using external-beam radiotherapy.

The US Intergroup study (INT 0116) in which 556 patients with completely resected stage IB–IV adenocarcinoma of the stomach or esophagogastric junction were randomized to either postoperative chemoradiotherapy or standard postoperative surveillance only, showed an improvement in overall and relapse-free survival (MacDonald *et al.* 2001). This study changed practise in most of the US. However, the majority of the benefit came from a reduction in the proportion of those with a locoregional relapse. As 54% of trial participants had a D0 dissection and only 10% had a D2 dissection, many have argued that the principal reason for an improvement in the survival was a countering of the effect of an inadequate operation. While the question of whether a D2 dissection is better than a D1 dissection is debated, most agree that a D0 procedure is inadequate. This study is a good example of the importance of interpreting data, before changing practise.

Considering both the MAGIC and the INT 0116 trials, the question that remains to be answered is whether postoperative radiochemotherapy improves survival and/or locoregional control in patients receiving neoadjuvant chemotherapy followed by D1+ gastric resection. Therefore, the so-called CRITICS trial (ChemoRadiotherapy after Induction chemotherapy In Cancer of the Stomach) has been launched in the Netherlands. In this trial, quality control will be prospectively applied to standardize treatment and measured using the Maruyama Index of unresected lymph nodes.

Surgery

Ilfet Songun & Cornelius van de Velde

Introduction and background

As previously mentioned, the mainstay of treatment for gastric cancer is still curative surgery (R0). However, there have been changing trends in the treatment for gastric cancer, such as endoscopic mucosal or submucosal resection and minimally invasive surgery because the incidence of early-stage gastric cancer has greatly increased in Japan (Aikou *et al.* 2006). While standard uniform lymphadenectomy (D2) has been well accepted in Japan, in Western countries there is still no evidence that a D2 resection should be the standard. On the other hand, in Japan minimally invasive surgery has become the most common approach in early gastric cancer. The determination of the extent of lymphadenectomy in early gastric cancer has been controversial, because the incidence of micrometastasis in lymph nodes was nearly 20%, even if no lymph node metastasis was detected by routine histologic examination (Aikou *et al.* 2001).

The standard treatment of gastric cancer in the Western world for many years was a total or subtotal gastrectomy, with more or less complete removal of omentum and perigastric lymph nodes (D1 dissection; see Fig. 6.5). Hospital mortality, most often defined as death within 30 days postoperatively, has decreased over the years. Before the 1970s a median mortality rate of 15% was reported, but in the decade before 1990 this rate had decreased to 4.6% (Macintyre & Akoh 1991). The 5-year survival rate in curative resections also improved from 38% before 1970 to 55% in the decade before 1990 (Macintyre & Akoh 1991; Akoh & Macintyre 1992). A survey by the American College of Surgeons showed a 77.1% resection rate in 18,365 patients, with a postoperative mortality of 7.2%, and a 5-year survival rate of 19%. Only 4.7% of these were D2 dissections (lymph node dissection of the N1 and the N2 tier; see Fig. 6.5). Stage-related 5-year survival was 50% for stage I, 29% for stage II, 13% for stage III, and 3% for stage IV (Wanebo *et al.* 1993). Japanese centers report 5-year overall survival rates above 50%, and above 70% for curative resections with hospital mortality rates of approximately 2% (Soga *et al.* 1979; Akoh & Macintyre 1992; Kinoshita *et al.* 1993). Japanese national stage-related 5-year survival is reported at 96.6% for stage I disease, 72% for stage II, 44.8% for stage III, and 7.7% for stage IV (Kinoshita *et al.* 1993). Differences in surgical techniques may in part be responsible for these better outcomes. In Japan a total gastrectomy in combination with en-bloc resection of adjacent organs, as well as a standard D2, is performed more often than in Western countries. This aggressive approach is thought by the Japanese to be the main explanation for the difference in stage-specific survival (Cuschieri 1989; Bonenkamp *et al.* 1993, 1999). Other factors may also contribute, however, such as the younger age of Japanese patients, the lower rates of systemic (such as cardiovascular) disease and obesity among gastric cancer patients, earlier diagnosis due to screening programs, stage migration, and the more aggressive chemotherapy policy in Japan. In a study by Schlemper *et al.* (1997) it was demonstrated that for high-grade adenoma/dysplasia according to most western pathologists, the Japanese gave the diagnosis of definite carcinoma. Therefore they concluded that this may also contintute to the relatively high incidence and good prognosis of gastric carcinoma in Japan as compoved to western countries (Schlemper *et al.* 1997). In the last decade D2 dissections have become more popular in Western countries as well. Non-randomized gastric cancer studies from Germany, England, Norway, and the United States have reported postoperative mortality of between 4% and 5%, morbidity of between 22% and 30.6%, and 5-year survival between 26.3% and 55% for patients undergoing D2 dissections (Siewert *et al.* 1993; Sue-Ling *et al.* 1993; Arak & Kull 1994; Wanebo *et al.* 1996). The variation in outcomes is substantial, because of the different definitions of D2 dissections in most series. Comparison (usually historical) of outcomes between a limited (D1) and D2 lymph node dissection showed better results for D2 dissection, although morbidity rates seemed to be higher. D2 dissection thus appears to improve survival even in Western countries, but results are still not near those reported by the Japanese.

Curative surgery (in intent)

A curative resection in intent (R0) consists of gastrectomy with lymph node dissection. The extent of the gastrectomy (total or subtotal) depends on the extent of the tumor and its location in the stomach. During resection a proximal tumor-free margin of 5 cm is required, and the perigastric lymph nodes, the N1 tier (D1 resection) should be dissected. In 1997 the D classification was redefined according to the number of lymph nodes dissected, instead of their location (Sobin & Wittekind 1997).

In locally advanced disease with invasion of adjacent organs (T4) such as the colon, spleen, and pancreas, an en-bloc resection of the stomach with the invaded organ should be performed in addition to adequate lymph node dissection if the tumor is resectable.

Based on retrospective data, four randomized studies comparing D1 and D2 dissections have been conducted. The first was by Dent *et al.* (1988), who described a selected group of only 43 patients. In 21 D2 dissections no hospital mortality was seen, but morbidity, hospital stay, and blood transfusion requirements were significantly higher than for those in the D1 dissection group. No difference in survival was noted between the two groups. A randomized study by Robertson *et al.* (1994) in 55 patients was set up to determine the difference in out-

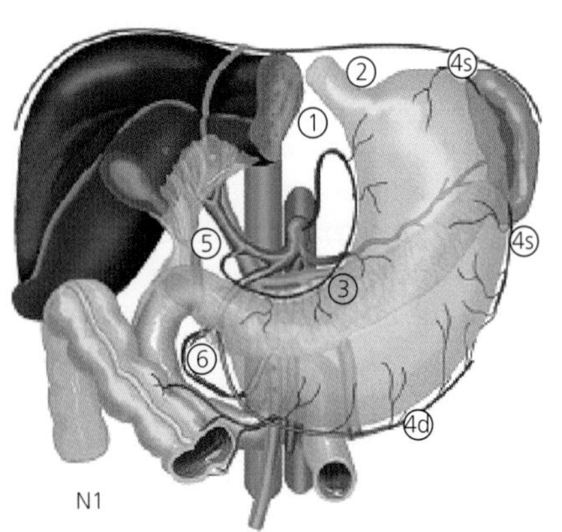

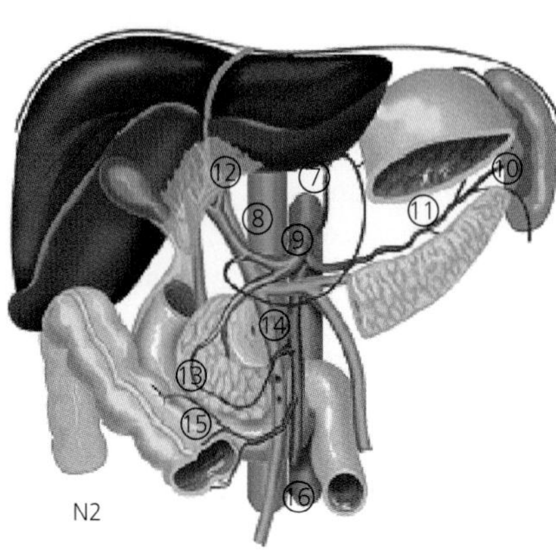

Fig. 6.5 Lymphatic drainage of the stomach (Japanese classification). 1, right cardial nodes; 2, left cardial nodes; 3, nodes along the lesser curvature; 4, nodes along the greater curvature; 5, suprapyloric nodes; 6, infrapyloric nodes; 7, nodes along the left gastric artery; 8, nodes along the common hepatic artery; 9, nodes along the celiac axis; 10, nodes at the splenic hilus; 11, nodes along the splenic artery; 12, nodes in the hepatoduodenal ligament; 13, nodes at the posterior aspect of the pancreas head; 14, nodes at the root of the mesentery; 15, nodes along middle colic vessels; 16, para-aortic nodes. N1, perigastric lymph nodes. N2, extra-perigastric regional lymph nodes.

comes between a D1 subtotal gastrectomy with omentectomy (n = 25) and a D3 total gastric resection including pancreaticosplenectomy (n = 30) in patients with adenocarcinoma of the gastric antrum. Postoperative death occurred only in one patient in the D3 group due to abdominal sepsis. Morbidity was significantly increased in patients undergoing extended resections, as half of the patients who had D3 dissections developed a subphrenic abscess. Survival was significantly better among patients undergoing a D1 dissection compared with those having D3 resection. In both studies no benefit was seen from more extended resections.

In the first large multicenter randomized study from the Netherlands (Dutch Gastric Cancer Trial, DGCT), 80 hospitals participated to compare morbidity, hospital mortality, survival, and cumulative relapse risk after D1 or D2 lymph node dissection for gastric cancer. Between 1989 and 1993, 996 patients were randomized; 711 patients underwent the allocated treatment (D1 or D2 resection defined according to the guidelines of the JRSGC) with curative intent, and 285 patients required palliative treatment. Continuous quality control was implemented to maintain the appropriate level of lymph node dissection. After curative resection, patients in the D2 arm had higher postoperative mortality compared with the D1 arm (10% vs 4%; p = 0.004), significantly more complications (43% vs 25%; p < 0.001) and significantly prolonged hospital stay. Hemorrhage (5% vs 2%), anastomotic leakage (9% vs 4%), and intraabdominal infection (17% vs 8%) were the most frequent complications (Bonenkamp *et al.* 1993). In the most recent evaluation with a median follow-up of 11 years for all eligible patients (range 6.8 to 13.1 years), survival rates were 30% and 35% for D1 and D2, respectively (p = 0.53). The risk of relapse is 70% for D1 and 65% for D2 (p = 0.43). When hospital deaths are excluded, survival rates are 32% for D1 (n = 365) and 39% for D2 (n = 299, p = 0.10). The relapse risk of these patients (n = 664) is in favor of the D2 dissection group (p = 0.07) (Hartgrink *et al.* 2004b).

In a univariate analysis of all 711 patients, no significant impact on survival rates was found for any of the subgroups based on the selected prognostic variables between D1 and D2 dissection. The only subgroup with a trend to benefit is the N2 tumor-positive group. When hospital mortality is excluded, there is a significant survival and relapse advantage for patients with N2 disease who had a D2 dissection (p = 0.01). Other stages show no significant difference. Furthermore, there is no difference in survival at 11 years whether fewer than 15 lymph nodes, between 15 and 25 lymph nodes, or more than 25 lymph nodes are harvested.

In the second large prospectively randomized multicenter trial, conducted by the British Medical Research Council (MRC), D1 dissection was compared with D2 dissection. Central randomization to treatment groups followed a staging laparotomy. Out of 737 patients with histologically proven gastric adenocarcinoma registered, 337 patients were judged ineligible by staging laparotomy because of advanced disease and 400 were randomly assigned to treatment (200 to D1 and 200 to D2 dissection). Postoperative mortality (13% vs 6.5%; p = 0.04) and postoperative complications were significantly higher in the D2 group (46% vs 28%; p < 0.001). In this study anastomotic leakage (26% for D2 vs 11% for D1), cardiac complications (8% for D2 vs 2% for D1), and respiratory complications (8% for D2 vs 5% for D1) were the most frequent complications. The 5-year survival rates were 35% and 33% for D1 and D2, respectively (Cuschieri *et al.* 1999).

These the only two major randomized studies, the MRC trial and the DGCT, obviously show the same tendency. The postoperative mortality and morbidity rates in both trials were significantly higher in the group undergoing D2 dissection, without a 5-year survival advantage for D2 dissections. The conclusion from these randomized studies was that generally no support exists for the standard use of D2 lymph node dissection in patients with gastric cancer in the West. There is also recent evidence from Japan that extending resection (beyond D2) with para-aortic lymph node dissection even in clinically M0 advanced gastric cancer (linitis plastica was excluded in this study) does not further improve survival (Sasako *et al.* 2006). The only study demonstrating a survival benefit from extended lymphadenectomy (D3) has recently been published by Wu *et al.* (2006). In this single-institution study from Taiwan, 221 patients were randomized: 110 were allocated to D1 and 111 to D3 surgery; 215 of them had an R0 resection. With a median follow-up of 94.5 months (range 62.9–135.1), the overall 5-year survival was significantly higher in patients having D3 resection compared with those having D1 resection (59.5% vs 53.6%; p = 0.041). At 5 years the recurrence rates were 50.6% for D1 and 40.3% for D1 (p = 0.197). They conclude that D3 offers a survival benefit over D1 surgery for patients with gastric cancer when done by well trained, experienced surgeons. This single-institution study reports an absolute overall survival advantage of 5.9%, which is statistically significant. However, it does not mean that this difference is clinically relevant and cannot be generalized. Moreover, there is no logical explanation for the survival advantage, which is not supported by, for example, significantly lower recurrence rates.

The success (outcome) of surgery depends on the quality of the resection performed, mandating surgery 'de necessité' instead of surgery 'de principe'. This means not only carefully selecting patients for surgery, but also performing radical surgery depending on the extent of the disease. Maruyama (1987) has compiled a computer-based database containing the pathologic data from 3040 patients. With the knowledge of tumor size, position, and depth of invasion (judged preoperatively by endoscopy and double-contrast barium meal or by endosonography), the likelihood of lymph node metastasis in each of the 16 lymph node stations can be predicted accurately. The applicability of this program to Western patients is shown by Peeters *et al.* (2005a) in a blinded, retrospective analysis of the DGCT data. Results indicate that low Maruyama Index (MI) surgery is associated with significantly increased survival.

Therefore we advocate using the Maruyama Program, a computerized tool based on patient experience, to identify nodal stations at risk (pre- or intraoperatively) in order to customize surgical lymphadenectomy and routinely generate a low MI operation, because the outcome of inadequate surgery can never be compensated for by additional radiotherapy and/or chemotherapy. Since there is also substantial heterogeneity of risk within stages, there is also a validated gastric carcinoma nomogram available, which can be used for individual patient counseling and adjuvant therapy decision-making. This nomogram provides a better prediction of outcome compared to the AJCC, regardless of the extent of lymphadenectomy (Peeters *et al.* 2005b).

Sentinel node mapping in gastric cancer

The sentinel lymph node (SLN) is defined as the first draining node from the primary lesion and has proven to be a good indicator of the metastatic status of regional lymph nodes in solid tumors. For gastric cancer, the combined method with dye and radio-guided method with lymphoscintigraphy using radioisotope (RI)-labeled colloid is recommended for stable and accurate sampling of SLNs in the laparoscopic setting for early-stage gastric cancer. Using a dual tracer method as the optimal procedure, the radio-guided method allows confirmation of the complete harvest of SLNs by gamma probing, while the dye procedure enables real-time observation of the lymphatic vessels. Clinically staged T1 N0 gastric cancer seems to be appropriate to try a therapy based on SN biopsy. At present, two large-scale prospective multicenter trials are ongoing in Japan. To overcome some remaining issues, such as limited sensitivity of intraoperative diagnosis of metastasis, and technical difficulty in laparoscopic SLN detection, further technical and instrumental developments will be required. The most common cause of a false-negative result from SLN mapping for gastric cancer is an obstructed lymphatic vessel caused by cancer invasion. In these cases, the tracer cannot migrate into the initial SLNs and will escape into the second echelon or false SLNs. Clinically positive node status and advanced tumors should therefore be excluded from SN procedures. Five to 10% of the SLNs in gastric cancer are located in the second compartment without distribution in the perigastric nodes (skip metastases). According to Kitagawa *et al.* (2005), during this transitional phase, focused lymph node dissection targeted to sentinel lymphatic basins and modified resection of the stomach is an acceptable approach.

Palliative surgery

In incurable cases, which usually need to be determined definitely by laparotomy, a palliative resection is indicated whenever the condition of the patient allows this, because resection offers the best palliative results. If there are gastric outlet obstruction symptoms (distal tumors) a gastroenterostomy should be performed; in cases of obstruction due to ingrowth of proximal tumors into the cardia and/or esophagus, palliative radiation therapy or endoscopic stent placement can be considered.

In a fit patient, chemotherapy should be considered: if there is an adequate response with significant tumor reduction, surgery could still be an option and deserves consideration.

Prophylactic surgery

Prophylactic gastrectomy is recommended in patients who are germline CDH1 mutation carriers. In a review Lynch *et al.* (2005) report that all prophylactic gastrectomies revealed multiple intramucosal diffuse gastric cancer, which were not visible at endoscopy. They recommend a total gastrectomy without lymphadenectomy when endoscopy is negative. If the surgical option is not taken, endoscopy with random biopsies every 6 months should be performed, because when diffuse gastric cancers (DGCs) become symptomatic, they will be lethal in 80% and mutation carriers have a greater than 70% chance of developing a clinically detectable DGC.

Chemotherapy

Christopher Jackson, Naureen Starling & David Cunningham

Early clinical trials which demonstrated that gastric cancer is sensitive to chemotherapy have led to research into the best regimen, the timing of chemotherapy with respect to surgery in resectable disease, and combination with radiotherapy, making the management of gastric cancer a model of the multidisciplinary approach.

Chemotherapy versus best supportive care in advanced gastric cancer

Four randomized controlled trials (Glimelius *et al.* 1997) and one meta-analysis (Wagner *et al.* 2006) address the issue of chemotherapy versus best supportive care (BSC) in metastatic gastric cancer. The regimens initially tested were FAMTX (5-fluorouracil [5-FU], adriamycin [doxorubicin], methotrexate), FEMTX (5-FU, epirubicin, methotrexate), and ELF (etoposide, leucovorin, 5-FU).

Median survival was increased in all of the studies in favor of treatment with chemotherapy by 3 to 9 months. Chemotherapy was generally well tolerated, and quality-of-life data reported in one trial favored the chemotherapy group. Response rates to chemotherapy were between 23 and 50%. The most common grade 3/4 side-effects were alopecia, hematological effects, nausea/vomiting (40% with FEMTX), stomatitis and diarrhea. The trial designs were flawed, with early termination or crossover from treatment to BSC arms.

Allowing for the design flaws, significant benefit is seen from the chemotherapy. This shifted the debate from whether chemotherapy is beneficial in the metastatic setting to which chemotherapy is most beneficial.

Selection of the most active regimen in advanced disease

The experimental arms of the chemotherapy versus BSC were adopted as the comparator arms in further trials in advanced disease. The European Organisation for Research and Treatment of Cancer (EORTC) group randomized 399 patients to 5-fluorouracil and cisplatin, ELF or FEMTX (Vanhoefer *et al.* 2000) (Table 6.3). With the broader inclusion criteria associated with a phase III trial compared to early phase trials, the results were disappointing. Progression-free survival was only 3.3 to 4.1 months. Median survival was 6.7 to 7.2 months, and was not significantly different between groups. In their final report the trialists concluded that none of these regimens should be the reference treatment.

In the 1990s the ECF regimen (epirubicin, cisplatin, and continuous intravenous infusion 5-FU) was developed. In phase II evaluation, response rates of 71% were seen, with 12% obtaining a complete response. Median survival was 8.2 months, and toxicity was not notably greater than with other regimens in historical trials. These results were sufficient to warrant direct comparison to other regimens in phase III trials.

In a head-to-head trial, 274 patients were randomized to receive either ECF or FAMTX (Webb *et al.* 1997). ECF outperformed FAMTX with a response rate (RR) of 45% versus 21%, and median survival of 8.9 versus 5.7 months ($p = 0.0002$).

Table 6.3 Summary of trials in advanced disease.

Author	Regimen	n	RR (%)	TTP (months)	MS (months)	1 year OS (%)	p (for OS)
Glimelius	ELF	31	23	5	8	NR	
et al. (1997)	BSC	30	–	2	5	NR	0.12
Murad *et al.*	FAMTX	30	50	NR	9	40	
(1993)	BSC	10	–	NR	3	0	0.001
Webb *et al.*	ECF	126	45	7.4*	8.9	36	
(1997)	FAMTX	130	21	3.4	5.7	21	
Vanhoefer	FAMTX	133	12	3.3†	6.7	28	
et al. (2000)	ELF	132	9	3.3	7.2	25	
	FUP	134	20	4.1	7.2	27	NS
Thuss-Patience	DF	45	37.8	5.5	9.5	NR	
et al. (2005)	ECF	45	35.6	5.3	9.7	NR	
Moiseyenko	TCF	227	36.7	5.6	9.2	40.2	
et al. (2005)	CF	230	25.4	3.7	8.6	31.6	0.0201
Dank *et al.*	IF	170	31.8	5.0	9.0	–	
(2005)	CF	163	25.8	4.2	8.7	–	
Cunningham	ECF	249	40.7	6.2†	9.9	37.3	
et al. (2006)	EOF	245	42.4	6.5	9.3		
	ECX	241	46.4	6.7	9.9		
	EOX	244	47.9	7.0	11.2	46.8	0.020
Kang *et al.*	XP	160	41	5.6†	10.5	–	0.003‡
(2006)	FP	156	29	5.0	9.3	–	
Al-Batran	FLO	112	34	5.7	–	–	
et al. (2006)	FLP	108	25	3.8	–	–	

* Failure-free survival.

† Progression-free survival.

‡ of non-inferiority for median survival.

A, adriamycin (doxorubicin); BSC, best supportive care; C/P, cisplatin; D/T, docetaxel (Taxotere); E, epirubicin; F/FU, 5-fluorouracil; I, irinotecan; L, leucovorin; MS, median survival; MTX, methotrexate; O, oxaliplatin; OS, overall survival; RR, relative risk; TTP, time to progression; X, Xeloda (capecitabine).

Quality-of-life data and improvement in symptoms all favored ECF. Line complications necessitated removal in 19% of trial patients. Patients in the ECF arm had more alopecia and nausea and vomiting, but less neutropenia and infection. Other toxicities were comparable between groups. In a separate randomized comparison between ECF and MCF, efficacy was similar but quality of life was greater with ECF.

Anthracyclines

In Europe cisplatin with 5-FU (CF) is used as the reference regimen and the value of adding an anthracycline is questioned. Two small trials have examined CF with and without an anthracycline and although each showed no additional benefit in terms of either median or overall survival, these were underpowered and the trends favored the anthracycline-based regimens. The recent Cochrane meta-analysis combined the data from these and one further trial. It concluded that there was a significant benefit in favor of the anthracycline/platinum-containing regimen in the order of an additional 2-month average survival, and that of the available regimens ECF appeared to be the best tolerated.

Taxanes

A randomized phase III trial presented at ASCO 2005 reported a study comparing CF to docetaxel (Taxotere, T) combined with CF (Moiseyenko *et al.* 2005): 457 patients were randomized to either CF or to TCF. Time to progression (TTP) was 5.6 versus 3.7 months favoring TCF ($p = 0.004$); RR was 36.7% compared to 25.4% ($p = 0.01$); median survival was 9.2 versus 8.6 months ($p = 0.02$); and 1-year overall survival was 40.2% compared to 31.6%, all in favor of TCF. However grade 3/4 neutropenia for TCF was 82.3% compared to 56.0%, and the rate of febrile neutropenia was 30 versus 13.5%, which highlights the intense myelotoxicity of this regimen. Taxanes are clearly active and further investigation is under way to identify the best-tolerated regimen.

Irinotecan

Irinotecan is highly active in advanced colorectal cancer, and has been trialled in gastric cancer. In a phase III study presented at the ASCO annual meeting in 2005, 337 patients were randomized to a regimen of either irinotecan, folinic acid and a 22-hour infusion of 5-FU (IF), or to cisplatin and a 5-day continuous infusion of 5-FU (Dank *et al.* 2005). The primary endpoint was TTP, and there was a non-significant trend in favor of the IF regimen (5.0 vs 4.2 months). Grade 3/4 diarrhea was higher in the IF group (21.6% vs 7.2%), but grade 3/4 stomatitis (2.4% vs 16.9%), neutropenia (25% vs 52%), and febrile neutropenia (4.8% vs 10.2%) were all lower in the IF compared to the CF group. This shows that the activity of the regimen is preserved when compared to CF, with a more favorable side-effect profile presenting an alternative regimen in selected patients.

Substitution of agents in the ECF regimen

The incidence of line complications as well as the inconvenience to the patient of protracted infusions of 5-FU have been noted. Additionally, cisplatin is contraindicated in patients with renal dysfunction or with hearing loss, both of which are common in the population affected by gastric cancer. In the REAL-2 trial presented at ASCO 2006 (Cunningham *et al.* 2006b), cisplatin and 5-FU were replaced with either oxaliplatin (O) or capecitabine (Xeloda, X), or both (Fig. 6.6). This trial included patients with advanced/non-resectable esophagogastric cancers.

The study randomized 1002 patients with advanced gastroesophageal cancer (40% with gastric cancer), had a two by two factorial design, and tested for non-inferiority of capecitabine over infusional 5-FU, and of oxaliplatin over cisplatin. Non-inferiority was demonstrated for both these agents, and in the individual arm comparisons 1-year and median survivals were highest for EOX (46.8% and 11.2 months) compared to ECF (37.7% and 9.9 months). Treatment was generally well tolerated in all the arms, with grade 3/4 peripheral neuropathy higher in the oxaliplatin arms and a slight increase in grade 3/4 diarrhea. Thrombotic events were highest in the ECF arm, significantly lower in the oxaliplatin arms, and mainly related to line thromboses. There were no significant differences in quality of life.

A further phase III trial presented at the same meeting randomized 316 chemotherapy-naive patients with advanced gastric cancer to receive either cisplatin and infused 5-FU (FP) or capecitabine with cisplatin (XP) (Kang *et al.* 2006). The study tested for non-inferiority in progression-free survival. With a median progression-free survival of 5.6 months with XP and 5.0 months for FP, non-inferiority was demonstrated. Objective response rates were greater with XP, but 1-year overall survival

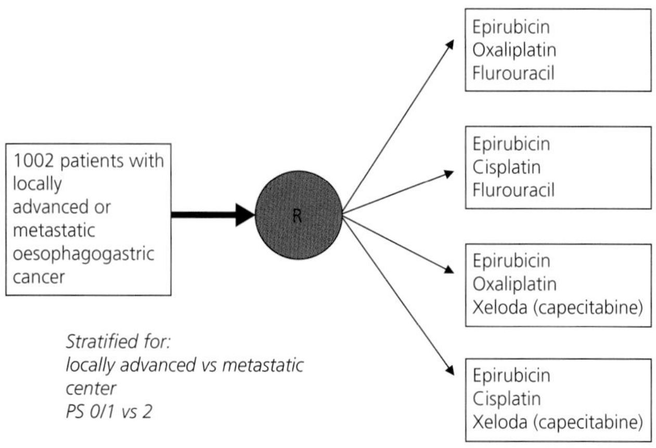

Fig. 6.6 The design of the REAL-2 trial. R, randomization; PS, performance scale/score.

was similar. Toxicities were comparable, with the exception of greater hand–foot syndrome in the XP group (22% vs 4%). Another trial that randomized 220 patients to receive either 5-FU, leucovorin and oxaliplatin (FLO), or 5-FU, leucovorin and cisplatin (FLP) showed a longer but non-significant TTP with FLO than with FLP (5.7 vs 3.8 months; $p = 0.081$) (Al-Batran *et al.* 2006). Other measures of efficacy such as time to treatment failure and response rates favored FLO, and severe toxicities were fewer. These two trials corroborate the findings of the REAL-2 trial.

Summary of advanced disease

ECF is a standard reference regimen in much of Europe, and recent data support the substitution of capecitabine over infused 5-FU. EOX has comparable, if not better, efficacy and is currently used in selected populations. Taxane-based regimens represent another promising area of investigation with superior efficacy compared to CF, another worldwide reference.

Localized disease

Several randomized controlled trials and five meta-analyses have examined the use of adjuvant chemotherapy, few showing a positive effect. In general, the trials are thwarted by small sample sizes, failure to specify a standard surgical technique, inclusion of patients with positive surgical margins, and lack of adequate randomization.

The first meta-analysis which found no benefit of adjuvant chemotherapy included trials with regimens including intraperitoneal chemotherapy, and older regimens such as semustine (MeCCNU), and FAM. The largest trial analysed included 281 patients, but most had under 90 patients in each arm. This analysis points out that to detect an increase in survival from 30% to 40% requires 500 patients in each arm—a hurdle not overcome by any of the included trials. A later meta-analysis found an overall survival benefit of approximately 4% in favor of adjuvant chemotherapy. When they analysed trials where more than two-thirds of the patients included were node positive, they found a non-significant trend towards greater benefit (Earle & Maroun 1999). A further meta-analysis confirmed this benefit, whist a fourth failed to do so.

Intraperitoneal chemotherapy regimens with 5-FU, mitomycin, and cisplatin individually or in combination have been trialled and have had no impact on recurrence, with one trial showing a greater number of postoperative complications.

Two recent trials have informed the current standards for the treatment of localized resectable disease. The first was a US Intergroup study where 556 patients with completely resected stage IB–IV adenocarcinoma of the stomach or esophagogastric junction were randomized to either postoperative chemoradiotherapy or standard postoperative surveillance only (MacDonald *et al.* 2001). The type of surgical procedure or degree of lymph node dissection (D0, D1, or D2) was not specified, although a D2 procedure was recommended (achieved in only 10% of participants).

Patients randomized to chemoradiotherapy had one cycle of 5-FU chemotherapy followed by chemoradiotherapy, then two further cycles of chemotherapy. With a median follow-up period of 5 years, the median survival was 36 months in the chemoradiotherapy group compared to 27 months in the surgery-only group. Relapse-free survival was 30 months versus 19 months respectively ($p < 0.001$), and 3-year overall survival was 50% versus 41% in favor of the adjuvant treatment arm ($p = 0.005$). Toxicity consisted of three (1%) treatment-related deaths, 54% grade 3–4 hematologic toxicity, and grade 3–4 gastrointestinal toxicity in 33%. These results were preserved when the 7-year follow-up was presented in 2004.

This impressive improvement in overall and relapse-free survival changed practice in most of the US, where the pattern of referral is postsurgical. However, the majority of the benefit came from a reduction in the proportion of those with a locoregional relapse. As 54% of trial participants had a D0 dissection, many have argued that the principal reason for an improvement in the survival was a countering of the effect of an inadequate operation. The data on whether a D2 operation is better than a D1 procedure are debated, but most agree that a D0 procedure is inadequate.

Another problem facing surgeons is that gastric cancers are often bulky and have margins that are difficult to clear. For this and other reasons, interest in a neoadjuvant approach has been stimulated. In the 2006 MRC 'MAGIC' trial, 503 patients with resectable adenocarcinoma of the stomach, esophagogastric junction or lower-third esophagus were randomized to either three cycles of preoperative ECF followed by surgery then three postoperative cycles, or to surgery alone (Cunningham *et al.* 2006c).

With a median follow-up of 4 years, the 5-year overall survival was 36.3% for the ECF group versus 23.0% for the surgery-only group ($HR = 0.75$, $p < 0.001$). Local recurrence was also less with chemotherapy (14.4% vs 20.6%) and tumors were smaller in the resected specimens of patients undergoing perioperative chemotherapy. Surgical complications were comparable (45.7% vs 45.3% in the surgery-only group). No patient had a D0 dissection, but a D1 versus D2 procedure was at the discretion of the surgeon.

Of those randomized to receive perioperative chemotherapy 54.8% received postoperative chemotherapy. The reasons for this included disease progression or early death (37 patients), patient choice (11), postoperative complications (10), and Hickman catheter problems (4). Only 5 patients did not complete treatment because of previous toxic effects or lack of response to preoperative treatment.

These results have introduced another standard of care into the UK and other parts of Europe. Subsequent research on this systemic approach has focused on replacing infusional 5-FU with the oral prodrug capecitabine, on substituting cisplatin with oxaliplatin, and incorporating targeted drugs.

The cross-study comparisons between the Intergroup and MAGIC trials are difficult as the patient populations are not comparable. The Intergroup patients were preselected to a degree by virtue of their ability to survive an operation, and the fact that complete resection had to be obtained before randomization into the trial, both factors biasing towards better outcome. MAGIC also contained a small number of patients with esophageal tumors, although their outcomes were similar. A current US Intergroup study is examining the issue of postoperative ECF with radiotherapy versus 5-FU with radiotherapy, but does not include any preoperative arm.

In summary, the pattern of referral essentially determines the type of treatment. When a patient has already received an operation at the time of referral, the US Intergroup study will have greater influence. However the MAGIC study and perioperative chemotherapy has gained greater influence in parts of the world where treatment decisions are made at the time of diagnosis and there is a greater MDT approach to the management of gastric cancer.

Radiotherapy

Edwin P.M. Jansen & Marcel Verheij

Radiotherapy can be applied as palliative treatment for uncontrolled gastric bleeding and for irresectable tumors. In such cases radiation as a single modality did not result in a survival benefit, but locoregional control rates of 70% were reported (Moertel *et al.* 1969; Henning *et al.* 2000a). Because of the high incidence of locoregional failures after surgical treatment, radiotherapy has always been considered as an attractive modality in curative treatment of these tumors (Gunderson & Sosin 1982; Landry *et al.* 1990; Henning *et al.* 2000a; Smalley *et al.* 2002; Jansen *et al.* 2005). Radiotherapy can be applied intraoperatively (intraoperative radiotherapy, IORT) or pre- or postoperatively (with or without concurrent chemotherapy) using external-beam radiotherapy (EBRT).

Intraoperative radiotherapy

In a prospective randomized trial by the National Cancer Institute 41 patients with non-metastatic disease at surgery were randomized to receive 20 Gy to the gastric bed intraoperatively or postoperative 50 Gy in 25 fractions in locally advanced cases (Sindelar *et al.* 1993). Median survival was the same in both groups, but locoregional disease failures were significantly less in the IORT group (44% and 92%, respectively), without a difference in toxicity. Although IORT has shown to favorably affect locoregional control, this technique has not gained wide acceptance in the radiation oncology community. This is most likely due to logistic reasons, an anticipated increased risk of late neurologic sequelae and because other, more conformal external-beam techniques have emerged.

Postoperative radiotherapy

Adjuvant radiotherapy in operable gastric cancer has been evaluated in several studies. In the British Stomach Cancer group study, 436 stage II and III patients were randomized to receive surgery only, surgery followed by 45–50-Gy radiotherapy or surgery plus eight courses of FAM (5-fluorouracil, adriamycin and mitomycin C) chemotherapy (Allum *et al.* 1989; Hallissey *et al.* 1994). Only 58% of patients in the chemotherapy group completed the recommended eight cycles, while 24% of patients failed to start radiotherapy. This phenomenon of noncompliance is frequently encountered after surgery of the upper abdomen and stresses the importance of less toxic adjuvant strategies, careful patient selection, and intensive clinical support. The differences in 5-year survival were statistically non-significant in the three arms, with 20% for surgery alone, 12% for surgery plus radiotherapy, and 19% for surgery plus chemotherapy. The EORTC randomized 115 patients after surgery into four arms: 55.5-Gy radiotherapy only; radiotherapy with short-term concurrent 5-FU chemotherapy; radiotherapy with long-term (1–18 months postoperatively) 5-FU; and combined short- and long-term chemotherapy (Bleiberg *et al.* 1989). After correction for prognostic factors such as T stage, age, and type of surgery, no differences between the four arms were found. In a retrospective study from Thomas Jefferson University, 70 patients were treated with surgery alone, while 50 had adjuvant therapy (chemotherapy in 17, radiotherapy in 13, both in 20). Patients with T3–4 N1–2 stage disease had a 5-year survival of 4% with surgery alone and 22% with adjuvant therapy ($p < 0.03$). In the surgery-alone group 45% developed a locoregional relapse, while this was only 19% after adjuvant chemotherapy and radiotherapy (Regine & Mohiuddin 1992). In summary, although postoperative radiotherapy seems to have a modest favorable impact on locoregional control, a survival benefit only appears achievable when concurrent chemotherapy is added.

Preoperative radiotherapy

Theoretically, preoperative radiotherapy is an interesting concept because: (i) no patients are lost to protracted postoperative recovery; (ii) the target volume is much easier to delineate because the tumor and stomach are still *in situ*; and (iii) tumor downsizing facilitates surgery. A disadvantage is that no pretreatment pathologic staging is available. However, since the majority of gastric cancer cases in the Western world present at advanced stages, overtreatment will occur in a minority, especially as pretreatment staging with modern CT scanning and endoscopic ultrasound is used. In Russia two trials have been performed since the 1970s in which 152 patients were randomized between surgery alone, or 20-Gy radiotherapy (5 fractions) using a cobalt source in the week before surgery, or the same regimen combined with radiosensitizing metronidazole (Skoropad *et al.* 2002, 2003). In the evaluable patients,

5-year overall survival was 39% after radiotherapy and surgery and 30% after surgery alone, which was not statistically significant. In the metronidazole arm 5-year overall survival was 46%. No increase in postoperative complications was found, but total radiation doses were rather modest. In China a large prospective trial was performed which randomized 370 patients between surgery only and surgery with preoperative 40-Gy radiotherapy (20 fractions in 4 weeks) (Zhang *et al.* 1998). Five-year overall survival was 19.8% with surgery only, and 30.1% with preoperative radiotherapy ($p < 0.01$). Resectability (79.4 vs 89.5%) and radical resection rates (61.8 vs 80.1%) also increased after preoperative radiotherapy. Perioperative mortality and anastomotic leakage rates were not significantly different between both arms. While this study demonstrates an advantage of this neoadjuvant strategy, a confirmatory study is unlikely to be conducted, because all efforts are currently directed towards perioperative chemotherapy and chemoradiotherapy (see below).

Postoperative chemoradiotherapy

Since the 1960s reports of randomized studies comparing surgery with surgery plus 5-FU-based chemoradiotherapy have appeared. The Gastrointestinal Tumor Study Group (GITSG) and Eastern Cooperative Oncology Group (ECOG) were among the first to randomize patients with residual or unresectable gastric cancer between chemotherapy and 5-FU-based chemoradiotherapy (GITSG 1982; Klaassen *et al.* 1985). Both studies showed no clear survival advantage but an increase in toxicity with chemoradiotherapy. These studies demonstrate the feasibility of concurrent chemoradiotherapy, but lack homogeneous treatment schedules and sufficient patient numbers (Dent *et al.* 1979; Moertel *et al.* 1984). A retrospective study from the Mayo Clinic showed that after 50.4-Gy radiotherapy combined with 5-FU, survival and locoregional control were greater in patients without residual disease (Henning *et al.* 2000b). In another study from Italy, postoperative 55-Gy radiation in 50 fractions of 1.1 Gy twice a day with continuous 5-FU infusion resulted in 36% 5-year overall survival and 43% cause-specific survival (Arcangeli *et al.* 2002). In 2001 the landmark SWOG/Intergroup 0116 trial was published, in which 556 patients were prospectively randomized between surgery only and surgery plus postoperative chemoradiotherapy (Macdonald *et al.* 2001). The adjuvant treatment consisted of 5-FU (425 mg/m^2) and leucovorin (20 mg/m^2) for 5 days, followed by 45 Gy of radiation at 1.8 Gy per day, given 5 days per week for 5 weeks, with modified doses of 5-FU and leucovorin on the first 4 and the last 3 days of radiotherapy. One month after the completion of radiotherapy, two 5-day cycles of 5-FU (425 mg/m^2) plus leucovorin (20 mg/m^2) were given 1 month apart. Although there was significant acute toxicity observed in the chemoradiotherapy arm (41% grade III; 4% grade IV), median overall survival was 27 months in the surgery-only group and 36 months after chemoradiotherapy ($p = 0.005$). Furthermore, relapse-free survival was prolonged from 19 months in the surgery-only arm to 30 months in the chemoradiotherapy arm ($p < 0.001$). Since the publication of these results, postoperative chemoradiotherapy has become standard treatment in the US. Nevertheless, many have criticized this study, mainly focusing on the suboptimal surgery. Indeed, 54% of all patients underwent a D0, instead of the prescribed D2 lymph node dissection, which could be a factor in undermining survival (Hundahl *et al.* 2002). However, an observational study from Korea showed that 544 patients who received chemoradiotherapy after a D2 resection had a 5-year overall survival of 57.1%, compared to 51.0% ($p = 0.02$) in 446 patients who did not receive adjuvant chemoradiotherapy. Locoregional failure rates in the radiation field were 14.9% and 21.7% respectively ($p = 0.005$) (Kim *et al.* 2005d). No details on late toxicity of combined treatment have been provided yet. Nevertheless, late progressive renal toxicity after chemoradiotherapy for gastric cancer with the use of common straightforward radiation techniques has been described. It can also be demonstrated that modern, sophisticated image-guided or intensity-modulated radiotherapy (IGRT/IMRT) techniques are able to spare the kidneys and prevent renal damage (Fig. 6.7) (Jansen *et al.* 2006; Verheij *et al.* 2006). However, a retrospective study from the Princess Margaret hospital showed that even with 5-field three-dimensional conformal radiotherapy and concurrent chemotherapy according to the Intergroup 0116 study, grade III or greater acute toxicity occurred in 57% of their patients. It is suggested that when individualized target volumes are defined, based on T and N stage and tumor location in the stomach, treatment volumes can be reduced and normal tissue toxicity minimized (Tepper & Gunderson 2002).

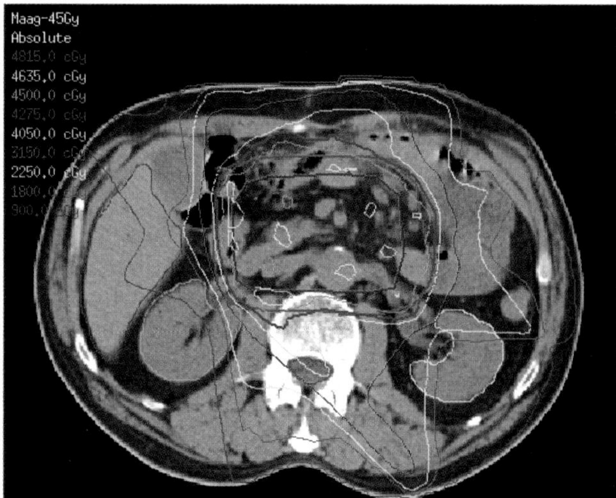

Fig. 6.7 Typical dose distribution of an intensity-modulated radiotherapy (IMRT) treatment plan in postoperative chemoradiotherapy for gastric cancer. It is clearly visible that IMRT is able to spare both kidneys. Green, right kidney; yellow, left kidney; purple, the planned target volume (PTV); blue, 95% isodose.

The Intergroup study was initiated at the beginning of the 1990s, when the concept of concurrent chemoradiotherapy was not yet widely accepted. Nowadays, regimens in which patients are exposed to radiation and radiosensitizing chemotherapy (cisplatin) on a daily and thus prolonged basis seem to have a beneficial effect. Paclitaxel is also reported to have favorable radiosensitizing properties, and when given concurrently with 45-Gy radiotherapy in inoperable gastric cancer, resulted in an overall response of 56% and complete resection rate of 40% (Safran *et al.* 2000). Postoperative chemoradiation has improved locoregional control, but the high incidence of systemic failures highlights the need for more effective systemic treatment. Studies that combine chemoradiation with epirubicin and paclitaxel-based chemotherapy show that these regimens are feasible, but effects on survival have to be awaited (Leong *et al.* 2003; Kollmannsberger *et al.* 2005). In conclusion, for the first time in the history of gastric cancer treatment, a survival benefit was demonstrated with adjuvant therapy in a prospective randomized trial. Although there are issues such as optimization of radiotherapy and chemotherapy and the value of chemoradiotherapy after an extended lymph node dissection that have to be resolved, postoperative chemoradiotherapy is a very promising concept that deserves further study.

Preoperative chemoradiotherapy

Since preoperative combined chemoradiotherapy has been shown to have a beneficial effect on surgical outcome in esophageal and rectal cancer, this is an attractive approach to explore in operable gastric cancer as well. The MD Anderson Cancer Center has reported a study in which 33 patients completed a preoperative regimen that started with two series of continuous infusion of 5-FU for 21 days, followed by 45-Gy radiotherapy in 25 fractions during 5 weeks which was combined on radiation days with continuous intravenous 5-FU (Ajani *et al.* 2004). In 28 (85%) of the patients a gastrectomy was performed and a D2 lymph node dissection was attempted. The median number of removed nodes was 16. Resection of spleen or other organs was performed only in cases of tumor invasion. Pathologic complete and partial response (pathCR; pathPR) was found in 54% of all operated patients. These patients showed a significant longer median survival of 64 months in comparison with 13 months in patients who did not reach pathCR or PR. In a study from the same center 41 patients with operable gastric cancer received two cycles of continuous 5-FU, paclitaxel and cisplatin followed by 45-Gy radiotherapy with concurrent 5-FU and paclitaxel (Ajani *et al.* 2005). An R0 resection was achieved in 78% of patients; pathCR and pathPR were found in 20% and 15% respectively. Median overall survival was more than 36 months. Pathologic response, R0 resection and postoperative T and N stage were correlated with overall and disease-free survival. In a Swiss study also, promising results with preoperative cisplatin and 5-FU-based chemoradiotherapy and hyperfractionated radiotherapy in doses of 31.2–45.6 Gy were found (Allal *et al.* 2005). Five-year locoregional control and overall survival were 85% and 35%, respectively. Thus, preoperative chemoradiotherapy theoretically combines the proven benefit of chemoradiotherapy with the advantages of a neoadjuvant approach, and therefore deserves further exploration in clinical trials.

Future developments

Further improvements in the treatment of gastric cancer are expected from technologic advances in radiotherapy allowing high-dose and high-precision irradiation, and from more effective systemic treatment, including novel biologic response modifiers. By applying several beams from different angles, each consisting of multiple smaller segments (IMRT), even complicated treatment volumes like the stomach and adjacent nodal areas can be irradiated with high precision. Consequently, this also allows delivery of the higher radiation doses necessary to obtain locoregional control of this relatively radioresistant tumor type, without an increase in normal tissue complications. In addition, better imaging techniques used both before and also during treatment (IGRT) contribute to improved tumor/target delineation and smaller treatment volumes.

More effective chemotherapy can be given sequentially or concurrently with radiation. In the latter setting the chemotherapeutic agents are used as radiosensitizers, mainly enhancing the locoregional cytotoxic effect of radiotherapy. 5-FU (and its oral derivative capecitabine) and cisplatin are well known potent radiosensitizers used in the treatment of a variety of gastrointestinal malignancies. Newer-generation cytotoxic agents such as oxaliplatin, irinotecan and the taxanes show also promising activity, and are combined with radiation on a limited scale (Safran *et al.* 2000; Ilson & Minsky 2003; Ajani *et al.* 2005). Recently, a variety of novel biologic agents with specific modes of action have become available for clinical use, including monoclonal antibodies, angiogenesis inhibitors and tyrosine kinase inhibitors. It is expected that these molecularly targeted agents will be incorporated into (neo)adjuvant treatment strategies for gastric cancer as well. In fact, accumulating data indicate that the anti-EGFR monoclonal antibody cetuximab can be safely combined with concurrent chemoradiation in gastric and esophageal cancer (Suntharalingam *et al.* 2006).

Novel agents

Annemieke Cats

Advances in combination chemotherapy have led to improved survival in patients with advanced gastric cancer. However, survival is still poor, with median progression-free survival and overall survival not exceeding 7 months and 11 months, respectively, in phase III studies. Therefore, new treatment strategies with better outcomes, but without increased toxicity, are urgently required.

Over the last decade, major advances in molecular biology technology have identified many signal transduction pathways that regulate cellular processes essential for cell growth, proliferation, differentiation, migration, and apoptosis. Biologically based or targeted therapy aims to disrupt critical components in signal transduction networks unique to cancer cells and simultaneously leave normal cells unharmed, thus avoiding the toxic effects common with conventional chemotherapy and radiotherapy.

Such novel targeted agents have recently become available and their exploitation in clinical trials has now become a reality. While clinical data in gastric cancer patients are still limited, an overview will be given here focusing mainly on the epidermal growth factor receptor (EGFR) and vascular endothelial growth factor (VEGF) pathways.

Epidermal growth factor receptor inhibitors

EGFR is a receptor tyrosine kinase of the erbB family that is abnormally activated in many epithelial tumors, including gastric cancer. This aberrant activation of EGFR occurs through its natural ligands and leads to homo- or heterodimerization of the receptor. As a consequence, the intracellular tyrosine kinase domain is autophosphorylated, and signal transduction cascades are initiated, leading to enhanced proliferation, cell motility and angiogenesis, and reduced apoptosis. EGFR levels have been found to be elevated in gastric carcinomas relative to adjacent mucosa. Such elevated EGFR levels have been found especially in more invasive T3–4 carcinomas, lymph node-positive tumors, and undifferentiated and diffuse-type carcinomas, and have been associated with poor prognosis (Kopp *et al.* 2002). Two classes of EGFR inhibitors exist: monoclonal antibodies (mAbs) that are directed at the extracellular receptor domain, and small molecules that compete with adenosine triphosphate binding to the intracellular tyrosine kinase domain of the receptor.

Monoclonal antibodies directed at the EGFR

Trastuzumab (Herceptin), a humanized mAb directed at the erbB2/HER-neu receptor, was the first anti-EGFR agent approved for use in solid tumors, i.e. breast cancer. Its use in gastric cancer has been discouraged because of an extremely low erbB2/HER-neu expression in distal gastric cancer.

Cetuximab (Erbitux) is a chimeric IgG2 mAb directed at erbB1/EGFR, and has been approved for the treatment of metastasized colorectal cancer. Cetuximab has been demonstrated to act in synergy with irinotecan, cisplatin, oxaliplatin and taxanes, which are all cytotoxic drugs with confirmed activity in advanced gastric cancer. Preliminary results in 25 patients with EGFR-positive, advanced gastric cancer have shown an objective response of 56% after treatment with weekly cetuximab in combination with biweekly irinotecan, 5-FU, and folinic acid (Pinto *et al.* 2006). In a small feasibility study, heavily pretreated metastasized gastric cancer patients received weekly cetuximab and irinotecan, and an impressive 5 out of 13 patients (38%) showed a partial response (Stein *et al.* 2007). These results should, of course, be confirmed in larger, randomized phase II and phase III studies. Cetuximab has demonstrated encouraging efficacy as a radiation sensitizer in esophageal cancer as well. In these studies gastric cancer patients were treated too, but their numbers were too small to draw any conclusion.

Another humanized EGFR mAb, matuzumab (EMD 72000), has been tested as first-line treatment in combination with fixed doses of epirubicine, cisplatin and capecitabine in 17 patients with EGFR-positive and advanced esophagogastric cancer (Rao *et al.* 2005). In this ongoing phase I study, the preliminary efficacy data are promising, with 7 partial responses.

Small molecule tyrosine kinase inhibitors

The number of agents of this class under development is rapidly increasing. They are differentiated mainly on their ability and potency in binding to and inhibiting the various erbB and other tyrosine kinase receptors. Probably due to their success in the treatment of patients with non-small-cell lung cancer (NSCLC), gefitinib (Iressa) and erlotinib (Tarceva) are the most extensively studied compounds in gastric cancer treatment as well.

In a randomized multicenter phase II study, gefitinib 250 mg/day or 500 mg/day was administered orally in 75 Japanese and non-Japanese patients with metastasized adenocarcinoma of the stomach (n = 54) and esophagogastric junction (n = 15). Patients were stratified according to ethnicity, and all patients had received prior chemotherapy. The preliminary safety and efficacy results showed good tolerability (grade 3/4 toxicity: rash 5.4%, diarrhea 4.1%, and anorexia 2.7%), but unfortunately only modest clinical activity (1 partial response and 12 stable disease) (Doi *et al.* 2003). In a pharmacodynamic side study, the biologic activity of gefitinib was investigated in available gastric tumor biopsy samples obtained at baseline and during therapy (Rojo *et al.* 2006). EGFR was detected in about 60% of baseline samples, and the degree of EGFR inhibition, measured as the amount of phosphorylated EGFR (pEGFR), was almost complete in these tumors during gefitinib treatment. However, reduction of pEGFR was not accompanied by abolition of the downstream signalling pathways, such as the mitogen-activated protein kinase (MAPK) and phosphatidyl-inositol-3-kinase (PI3K)/Akt survival pathways, although a subpopulation may benefit from EGFR inhibition as demonstrated by a decrease in proliferation and increase of apoptosis in some tumors. No differences in outcomes were detected according to ethnicity and efficacy parameters.

In a second multicenter phase II study, patients without prior chemotherapy for advanced or metastasized adenocarcinoma of the esophagogastric junction (n = 47) or stomach (n = 25) received 150 mg/day erlotinib orally as monotherapy

(Dragovich *et al.* 2006). Four patients in the esophagogastric junction cohort experienced a confirmed objective response (1 complete response, 3 PR), and although baseline characteristics were similar in the gastric cancer patients, none of these patients perceived any clinical benefit. Moreover, four of the gastric cancer patients discontinued erlotinib treatment because of toxicity or death (one each of anemia, fatigue, CNS hemorrhage, hepatic failure). Median overall survival was 6.7 months in the esophagogastric junction cohort and 3.5 months in the gastric cancer group.

Recently, somatic EGFR mutations in the region encoding for the tyrosine kinase domain (exons 18–21) and also EGFR amplification have been linked to responsiveness to monotherapy gefitinib and erlotinib in NSCLC. The fact that no such mutations and EGFR amplification have been detected in gastric cancer (Dragovich *et al.* 2006) may explain the disappointing results in the above-mentioned studies.

Angiogenesis inhibitors

The vascular endothelial growth factor (VEGF) pathway plays a critical role in the process of new blood vessel formation under normal and pathologic conditions, such as tumor growth and dissemination. Activation of the VEGF family of proteins and receptors triggers multiple signaling networks that result in endothelial cell survival, proliferation, invasion, migration, and vessel permeability. Overexpression of VEGF in gastric cancer has been associated with tumor progression, relapse following resection and poor clinical outcome (Maeda *et al.* 1996; Takahashi *et al.* 1996; Yoshikawa *et al.* 2000; Juttner *et al.* 2006). Such and other findings have stimulated interest in and efforts to develop drugs that may induce suppression or disruption of the VEGF/VEGFR axis. Several strategies have been developed for this, including neutralizing antibodies against VEGFs and VEGFRs, and VEGFR tyrosine kinase domain inhibitors. The humanized anti-VEGF antibody bevacizumab (Avastin) has been approved for fluoropyrimidine-based colorectal cancer therapy, and it has demonstrated efficacy in other tumor types as well.

In a recently published phase II study, the efficacy and safety of bevacizumab in combination with irinotecan and cisplatin in patients with advanced adenocarcinoma of the esophagogastric junction (n = 23) and stomach (n = 24) was tested (Shah *et al.* 2006). Prior adjuvant or neoadjuvant chemotherapy was allowed, as long as it did not consist of irinotecan or cisplatin. Results were compared with historical findings of three pooled studies with irinotecan- and cisplatin-containing regimens in gastric and esophageal cancer patients. The primary tumor was unresected in 40 patients. In 13 patients the tumor was assessable, but not measurable. The primary endpoint of the study was TTP, which was met at the number of 47 patients. In patients with measurable disease TTP was 9.2 months, whereas in patients with non-measurable disease this was 6.4 months, with an overall TTP of 8.3 months, which proves to be an increase of 75% over historical controls. Median overall survival was 12.3 months, and thus far is the highest ever reported. In 12 patients (26%) a thromboembolic (TE) event occurred; of these, eight pulmonary emboli were found incidentally during protocol-specified CT scans. The authors reported that the incidence of TE events was not higher than in the previously re-evaluated historical controls (30%) (Shah *et al.* 2005). After TE diagnosis, eight patients—all with their primary *in situ*—continued treatment while receiving anticoagulant agents. One of these patients subsequently had an episode of GI bleeding. Grade 3 hemorrhage was observed in one other patient. Other toxicities, possibly related to bevacizumab, consisted of grade 3 hypertension (28%), myocardial infarction (2%), and GI perforation (6%). The incidence of GI perforations in colorectal cancer patients while on fluoropyrimidine-based therapy with bevacizumab is about 1–2%. It has been suggested that in these patients GI perforations are related to the presence of the primary tumor, non-steroidal anti-inflammatory drug use, and peritoneal carcinomatosis. Notwithstanding the encouraging results of this study, larger randomized phase II and III studies are needed to confirm these findings and to evaluate its toxicity in this fragile patient population.

Other anti-angiogenetic agents targeting the VEGFR tyrosine domain have been tested in preclinical experimental and xenograft models, and these studies report a reduced proliferation and microvasculature density, and increased apoptosis. Clinical data are still awaited.

Besides the combination of targeted agents and conventional cytotoxic agents in these malignancies, another treatment strategy for the near future is the combination of multiple targeted agents in order to simultaneously inhibit multiple and 'cross-talking' pathways responsible for tumor growth and dissemination. Preclinical studies underscore this approach.

Gene therapy is another innovative therapeutic approach for cancer. Although few gene therapeutic approaches have demonstrated promising anti-tumor effects in preclinical studies, clinical trials have been disappointing. A major breakthrough is still needed. Hopefully, the introduction of new powerful molecular techniques such as RNA interference (RNAi) and detection of new target genes may improve gastric cancer therapy in the near future.

Conclusion

Clinical data on targeted therapy in advanced gastric cancer are limited. Despite the rational basis for these novel treatments, their identification and validation remains a challenge. For example, the inhibition of key processes in carcinogenesis has not always proved effective; nor have rationally assumed predictive markers helped to distinguish patients who are more or less likely to respond to targeted therapy.

In light of the rapidly changing landscape for cancer treatment, we are faced with the ongoing challenge of choosing from an ever-changing variety of agents, and identifying appropriate combinations and sequences of application, which may one day substantially improve survival rates.

Prognosis and follow-up

Ilfet Songun & Cornelius van de Velde

Cancer stage

Tumor stage is an important prognostic factor for survival in gastric cancer. A clear relation is seen between increasing depth of invasion and survival (Bonenkamp *et al.* 1993). With increasing depth of invasion a steady increase is seen in lymph node metastasis, from 45.7% when the tumor invades the muscularis propria, to 79.6% when adjacent organs are directly invaded. Also, the frequency with which the more distant tiers of nodes (second, third, and fourth) are involved rises steadily with depth of invasion (Sasako *et al.* 1995).

The incidence of metastasis and 5-year survival rate show a strong correlation. Moreover, with increasing distance between involved node and the primary tumor, the 5-year survival rate decreases. Involvement of node station 13 is associated with a zero 5-year survival rate. In the DGCT, surgery with an involved N4 node was regarded as a non-curative operation. Benefit from extended dissections (stations 7 to 12 and 16) in Japanese studies is estimated to be between 0% and 10.5% (Sasako *et al.* 1995), although this benefit was not found in randomized studies in the West (Cuschieri *et al.* 1996; Bonenkamp *et al.* 1999). In Japan, dissections even beyond the D2 level are now being studied in two randomized studies; one of them shows no survival benefit (Sasako *et al.* 2006) and the results of the second study are not expected before 2008 (Sano *et al.* 2004).

A survey by the American College of Surgeons showed a 77.1% resection rate in 18,365 patients, with a postoperative mortality of 7.2%, and 5-year survival of 19%. Only 4.7% of these were D2 dissections. Stage-related 5-year survival was 50% for stage I, 29% for stage II, 13% for stage III, and 3% for stage IV (Wanebo *et al.* 1993). Japanese national stage-related 5-year survival is reported at 96.6% for stage I disease, 72% for stage II, 44.8% for stage III, and 7.7% for stage IV (Kinoshita *et al.* 1993). Differences in surgical techniques may in part be responsible for these better outcomes. Non-randomized gastric cancer studies from Germany, England, Norway, and the United States have reported 5-year survival at between 26.3% and 55% for patients undergoing D2 dissections (Siewert *et al.* 1993; Sue-Ling *et al.* 1993; Arak & Kull 1994; Wanebo *et al.* 1996). The variability in outcomes is substantial, likely because of the different definitions of D2 dissections in most series.

Patterns of spread and recurrence

Understanding the patterns of spread of gastric cancer can help to direct therapeutic approaches, particularly those using systemic or regional (intraperitoneal) chemotherapy and radiation. Especially in more advanced stages in which the propensity for systemic metastasis is high, surgery alone (or any local treatment modality alone) is unlikely to offer long-term benefit.

Gastric cancer shows several patterns of recurrence: local recurrence in the gastric bed or regional lymph nodes, peritoneal metastasis, liver metastasis and distant metastasis. The pattern of spread has been evaluated both in patients with newly diagnosed cancer and in patients undergoing potentially curative surgical resection. In the West, the pattern of recurrence tends to be mainly local. In a study by Gunderson and Sosin (1982) of planned relaparotomy following curative resection, distant metastasis alone was found in 25.6%. Local recurrence and/or regional lymph node metastasis occurred as the only failure in 53.7% of the failure group if localized peritoneal failures were included, and as any component of failure in 87.8%. A similar high rate of local failure (54%) was reported by the British Stomach Cancer Group in patients undergoing operation alone (Allum *et al.* 1989). In an Italian study by Roviello *et al.* (2003) in 441 patients after curative resections for gastric cancer, recurrence was seen in 215 (49%) patients: peritoneal recurrence in 36%, locoregional recurrence in 45%, hepatic recurrence in 27%, and distant metastases in 9%. In the DGCT involving 1078 patients, death from recurrent disease was noted in a total of 289 patients: 30% of the patients had locoregional recurrence only, and 51% had locoregional and distant disease (Bonenkamp *et al.* 1999). In summary, patients with gastric cancer frequently have intraabdominal metastasis, even at the time of diagnosis. Sunderland and colleagues evaluated lymph node metastasis for proximal versus distal lesions (Sunderland 1967). Proximal tumors were much more likely to have lymph node involvement than were distal lesions. The extent of spread within the stomach also varies widely. Tumor invasion of intramural lymphatics may extend into the distal esophagus or the proximal duodenum. As mentioned earlier, inadequate resection margins resulting in an R1 resection (with a concomitant high likelihood of local failure) may occur because of lymphatic vessel invasion. Deep penetration of primary lesions may increase the risk of intraperitoneal contamination. Positive findings on cytologic examination of abdominal lavage fluid in gastric cancer are associated with a poor prognosis (Nakajima *et al.* 1978). In the DGCT, cytologic examination was performed in 535 patients: 457 (85%) after curative resection and 78 (15%) after palliative resection. A clear association was seen between positive cytologic findings and serosal invasion (12.4% positive cytology) and lymph node invasion (7.5% positive cytology). Survival was significantly lower in patients with positive cytology findings compared with those with negative cytology findings, irrespective of the procedure used (curative or palliative).

Some studies, especially those from Japan, have evaluated the lymph node drainage from various portions of the stomach to direct the extent of resection for tumors in relatively early stages. Maruyama *et al.* (1989) have extensively studied the incidence of metastasis to different lymph node groups. In their study, lymph node metastases were seen in 49% of patients. The likelihood of metastasis was analysed based on the location of the primary tumor within the stomach (proximal, middle, or distal third) and its location on the lesser or greater curvature and anterior or posterior wall. Not surprisingly, metastases were considerably more likely in lymph node groups closest to the primary tumor and in the nodal chain immediately adjacent. The risk of metastasis to more distant lymph node sites could be predicted using this database. This type of data might direct the extent of resection. In a series from Korea examining 508 patients with recurrent gastric cancer from an initial 2328 operated patients, 425 had recurrence at only one site, 23% had local recurrence, 40% had peritoneal recurrence, 18% had hepatic metastasis and 19% had distant metastasis (Yoo *et al.* 2000). The lower local recurrence rates in the East seem to be related to the routine performance of D2 resection.

Because peritoneal recurrence is common, these data might influence the design of clinical trials by, for example, supporting the use of intraperitoneal chemotherapy in selected patients.

The type of adjuvant therapy that might be proposed (systemic vs locoregional) also depends, as noted above, on recurrence sites after potentially curative (R0) resection. Treatment failure patterns in patients who have undergone resection for primary gastric cancer have been evaluated by autopsy series, second-look laparotomy, and clinical evaluation. In one early study, McNeer and colleagues (1951) reviewed the autopsy results of 92 patients who had undergone potentially curative resections. In 50% of patients, local failure was noted, either in the gastric remnant or at the gastroenterostomy. An additional 21% of patients had recurrence in the gastric bed. Thirteen per cent of patients had distant failure only without any local component. Wisbeck *et al.* (1986) reviewed the autopsy data for 85 patients with primary gastric cancer. Only 16 of these patients had undergone potentially curative resections. For the group as a whole, peritoneal involvement was seen in 47% of patients. Hepatic metastases were also common, occurring in 39% of patients. Lung metastases occurred in 34% of patients.

Surgical prognostic factors

Besides the issue of the extent of lymph node dissection, other aspects of gastric cancer surgery have generated controversies. These include type of gastrectomy (subtotal vs total), pancreatectomy and/or splenectomy, patient selection, stage and stage migration, and the experience of the surgeon as a prognostic factor.

Surgical complications are influenced by the extent of the operation, and a number of studies have addressed this topic. In a Norwegian study (Viste *et al.* 1988) morbidity was significantly lower after subtotal resection (28%) than after total gastrectomy (38%), while proximal gastrectomy had the highest morbidity (52%). In a German study (Bottcher *et al.* 1994) these differences in morbidity were also found (23% for subtotal vs 48% for total gastrectomy). Gennari *et al.* (1986) also found a decreased morbidity for subtotal resections without any significant influence on survival. Comparison of their results with those of previous studies led to the conclusion that subtotal gastrectomy should be standard, provided that a safe proximal margin is guaranteed. In the DGCT and MRC trials, hospital mortality in the groups undergoing D1 dissection and D2 dissection was significantly lower for subtotal gastrectomy (3% and 7%, respectively) than for total gastrectomy (5% and 14%, respectively) (Cuschieri *et al.* 1996; Sasako 1997; Hartgrink *et al.* 2004). In both trials the complication rate was also lower after subtotal resections. In the DGCT this difference was statistically significant. The prognostic value of microscopic resection-line involvement in the DGCT was studied by Songun *et al.* (1996). Tumor-positive resection lines were seen in 5.9% of evaluable patients. Resection-line involvement was significantly associated with T stage, N stage, tumor location, and tumor differentiation. Presence of resection-line involvement was also associated with significantly worse survival. The conclusion from this study was that peroperative frozen-section examination is mandatory in patients undergoing a curative resection for gastric cancer, especially in those with poorly differentiated, signet-ring cell, or anaplastic tumors. In this context arguments can be made for performing a total gastrectomy in all patients with poor tumor differentiation.

Pancreatectomy and splenectomy

Resection of spleen or pancreas or both plays an important role in surgical complications. Most studies find a significant increase of morbidity and hospital mortality if a pancreaticosplenectomy is performed (Arak & Kull 1994; Griffith *et al.* 1995; Degliulie *et al.* 1997). Two studies in Japan did not show any beneficial effect on survival if pancreaticosplenectomy was combined with total gastrectomy, whereas morbidity was increased in these patients (Kodera *et al.* 1997; Kitamura *et al.* 1999). In the DGCT pancreatectomy and type of gastrectomy were the only factors significantly influencing the occurrence of major surgical complications. Although the number of dissected lymph nodes increases, septic complications occur more often due to anastomotic leakage, intraabdominal infections, and pancreatic fistula (Siewert *et al.* 1995).

The spleen should also preferably be spared as this may reduce concomitant morbidity (Brady *et al.* 1991; Sasako 1997). An increase of anastomotic leakage was seen, especially in subtotal D2 gastrectomies. The most likely explanation for this finding is that in D2 dissections the left gastric artery is divided at its origin and the rest of the stomach is dependent on the blood supply of its short gastric arteries. In D1 dissections, in which the left gastric artery is divided more peripherally, the vascularization of the rest of the stomach is probably less compromised. Immunologic factors may play a role in this as well, associated both with resection of the spleen itself (Meyers *et al.* 1987; Aldridge & Williamson 1991) and also with the immunosuppression induced by blood transfusions, which may be needed for increased hemorrhage (Kaneda *et al.* 1987; Kampschoer *et al.* 1989; Sugezawa *et al.* 1989).

Timeline of recurrence

With regard to the timeline over which the disease recurs, over two-thirds of recurrences are in the first 3 years and fewer than 10% occur after 5 years (Katai *et al.* 1994; Shiraishi *et al.* 2000; Kodera *et al.* 2003). Early gastric cancer (EGC) carries a very favorable prognosis, with a 1.4% recurrence rate in 1475 patients with EGC (Sano 1993). This study from NCC Tokyo reported that 40% of the deaths from recurrence occurred within the first 3 years and 23% after 5 years.

Adjuvant treatment after gastrectomy may alter patterns of recurrence; adjuvant chemoradiation reduced the proportion of local recurrences from 29% to 19% and regional recurrences from 72% to 65% as the first site of relapse compared with surgery alone (Macdonald *et al.* 2001).

Follow-up

Today, CT is the primary tool for the investigation of a suspected recurrence and for evaluation of response to non-surgical treatment of recurrent disease. CT detection of recurrences is usually based on morphologic changes such as wall thickening and focal enhancement. However treatment-induced bowel wall thickening caused by inflammation or fibrosis cannot be easily distinguished from wall thickening caused by residual tumor. For this reason a CT at 3 months following surgery has been recommended as a baseline for further assessment. However, PET is limited as a first-line screening tool in the follow-up of recurrent tumors because FDG PET may give false negative results in poorly differentiated gastric adenocarcinoma, and gastric cancers of the signet-ring cell and mucinous types. Furthermore the detection of recurrent gastric cancer may be difficult with PET imaging only.

Although there is broad agreement as to staging, classification, and surgery for gastric cancer, there is no consensus regarding follow-up after gastrectomy. Follow-up varies from investigations on the basis of clinical suspicion of relapse to intensive investigations to detect recurrences early, on the assumption that this improves survival and quality of life. For early gastric cancers, endoscopy can detect new primaries, but the incidence of these tumors is low, and many thousands of procedures are required to detect each operable case.

Advanced gastric cancers recur mainly locoregionally or as distant metastasis. Local recurrences detected at endoscopy or on CT are mainly incurable. CT is much better at detecting liver metastases, and although these are usually multiple and unresectable, there are several reports of good survival following liver resection for isolated metastasis.

Tumor markers have been used with some success to detect subclinical recurrences and could be used to target more invasive or expensive procedures. In chemotherapy, many newer agents are promising significantly improved survival, but again, the evidence for greater benefit when administered before the patient becomes symptomatic is lacking. Overall, it appears that follow-up policy is as much decided by the wealth and facilities of the institution as by any significant evidence base (Whiting *et al.* 2006). Although the early detection of recurrent cancer is an emotive issue for both patients and surgeons, considering the amount of time and money invested in follow-up, and the lack of evidence of efficacy, a randomized controlled trial of intensive follow-up is not cost-effective.

References

Aikou T, Higashi A, Notsugoe S, Hokita S *et al.* (2001) Can sentinel node navigation surgery reduce the extent of lymph node dissection in gastric cancer? *Ann Surg Oncol* 4 (Suppl): 90–3.

Aikou T, Kitagawa Y, Kitajima M, Uenosuno Y *et al.* (2006) Sentinel lymph node mapping with GI cancer. *Cancer Metastasis Rev* 25: 269–77.

Ajani JA, Mansfield PF, Janjan N *et al.* (2004) Multi-institutional trial of preoperative chemoradiotherapy in patients with potentially resectable gastric carcinoma. *J Clin Oncol* 22(14): 2774–80.

Ajani JA, Mansfield PF, Crane CH *et al.* (2005) Paclitaxel-based chemoradiotherapy in localized gastric carcinoma: degree of pathologic response and not clinical parameters dictated patient outcome. *J Clin Oncol* 23(6): 1237–44.

Akoh JA, Macintyre IM. (1992) Improving survival in gastric cancer: review of 5-year survival rates in English language publications from 1970. *Br J Surg* 79(4): 293–9.

Al-Batran S, Hartmann J, Probst S *et al.* (2006) A randomized phase III trial in patients with advanced adenocarcinoma of the stomach receiving first-line chemotherapy with fluorouracil, leucovorin and oxaliplatin (FLO) versus fluorouracil, leucovorin and cisplatin (FLP). *J Clin Oncol 2006 ASCO Annual Meeting Proceedings* Part I, Vol 24, no. 18S (June 20 Supplement): LBA4016.

Aldridge MC, Williamson RC. (1991) Distal pancreatectomy with and without splenectomy. *Br J Surg* 78(8): 976–9.

Allal AS, Zwahlen D, Brundler MA *et al.* (2005) Neoadjuvant radiochemotherapy for locally advanced gastric cancer: long-term results of a phase I trial. *Int J Radiat Oncol Biol Phys* 63(5): 1286–9.

Allum WH, Hallissey MT, Ward LC, Hockey MS. (1989) A controlled, prospective, randomised trial of adjuvant chemotherapy or radiotherapy in resectable gastric cancer: interim report. British Stomach Cancer Group. *Br J Cancer* 60: 739–44.

Arak A, Kull K. (1994) Factors influencing survival of patients after radical surgery for gastric cancer. A regional study of 406 patients over a 10-year period. *Acta Oncol* 33(8): 913–20.

Arber N, Shapira I, Ratan J *et al.* (2000) Activation of c-K-ras mutations in gastrointestinal tumors. *Gastroenterology* 118(6): 1045–50.

Arcangeli G, Saracino B, Arcangeli G *et al.* (2002) Postoperative adjuvant chemoradiation in completely resected locally advanced gastric cancer. *Int J Radiat Oncol Biol Phys* 54(4): 1069–75.

Balfe DM, Koehler RE, Karstaedt N *et al.* (1981) Computed tomography of gastric neoplasms. *Radiology* 140(2): 431–6.

Bhandari S, Shim CS, Kim JH *et al.* (2004) Usefulness of three-dimensional, multidetector row CT (virtual gastroscopy and multiplanar reconstruction) in the evaluation of gastric cancer: a comparison with conventional endoscopy, EUS, and histopathology. *Gastrointest Endosc* 59(6): 619–26.

Bipat S, van Leeuwen MS, Comans EF *et al.* (2005) Colorectal liver metastases: CT, MR imaging, and PET for diagnosis—meta-analysis. *Radiology* 237(1): 123–31.

Bleiberg H, Goffin JC, Dalesio O *et al.* (1989) Adjuvant radiotherapy and chemotherapy in resectable gastric cancer. A randomized trial of the gastro-intestinal tract cancer cooperative group of the EORTC. *Eur J Surg Oncol* 15(6): 535–43.

Bonenkamp JJ, van de Velde CJ, Kampschoer GH *et al.* (1993) Comparison of factors influencing the prognosis of Japanese, German, and Dutch gastric cancer patients. *World J Surg* 17(3): 410–14.

Bonenkamp JJ, Hermans J, Sasako M, van de Velde CJ. (1999) Extended lymph-node dissection for gastric cancer. Dutch Gastric Cancer Group. *N Engl J Med* 340(12): 908–14.

Botet JF, Lightdale CJ, Zauber AG *et al.* (1991) Preoperative staging of gastric cancer: comparison of endoscopic US and dynamic CT. *Radiology* 181(2): 426–32.

Bottcher K, Siewert JR, Roder JD, Busch R, Hermanek P, Meyer HJ. (1994) Risk of surgical therapy of stomach cancer in Germany. Results of the German 1992 Stomach Cancer Study. *Chirurg* 65(4): 298–306.

Brady MS, Rogatko A, Dent LL, Shiu MH. (1991) Effect of splenectomy on morbidity and survival following curative gastrectomy for carcinoma. *Arch Surg* 126: 359–64.

Bragantini E, Barbi S, Beghelli S *et al.* (2006) Loss of Fhit expression is associated with poorer survival in gastric cancer but is not an independent prognostic marker. *J Cancer Res Clin Oncol* 132(1): 45–50.

Carneiro F, Huntsman DG, Smyrk TC *et al.* (2006) Model of the early development of diffuse gastric cancer in E-cadherin mutation carriers and its implications for patient screening. *J Pathol* 203: 681–7.

Carvalho B, Buffart TE, Reis RM *et al.* (2006) Mixed gastric carcinomas show similar chromosomal aberrations in both their diffuse and glandular components. *Cell Oncol* 28(56): 283–94.

Coakley FV, Choi PH, Gougoutas CA *et al.* (2002) Peritoneal metastases: detection with spiral CT in patients with ovarian cancer. *Radiology* 223(2): 495–9.

Correa, P. Cuello C, Duque E *et al.* (1976) Gastric cancer in Colombia. III. Natural history of precursor lesions. *J Natl Cancer Inst* 57: 1027–35.

Cunningham D, Allum WH, Stenning SP *et al.* MAGIC trial Participants. (2006a) Perioperative chemotherapy versus surgery alone for resectable gastroesophageal cancer. *N Engl J Med* 355(1): 11–20.

Cunningham D, Rao S, Starling N *et al.* (2006b) Randomised multicentre phase III study comparing capecitabine with fluorouracil and oxaliplatin with cisplatin in patients with advanced oesophagogastric (OG) Cancer: the REAL 2 trial. *J Clin Oncol 2006 ASCO Annual Meeting Proceedings* Part I, Vol 24, no. 18S (June 20 Supplement): LBA4017.

Cunningham D, Allum WH, Stenning SP *et al.* (2006c) Periooperative chemotherapy versus surgery alone for resectable gastroesophageal cancer. *N Engl J Med* 355(1): 11–20.

Cuschieri A. (1989) Recent advances in gastrointestinal malignancy. *Ann Chir Gynaecol* 78(3): 228–37.

Cuschieri A, Fayers P, Fielding J *et al.* (1996) Postoperative morbidity and mortality after D1 and D2 resection for gastric cancer: preliminary results of the MRC randomized controlled surgical trial. *Lancet* 347: 995–9.

Cuschieri A, Weeden S, Fielding J *et al.* (1999) Patient survival after D1 and D2 resections for gastric cancer: long-term results of the MRC randomized surgical trial. Surgical Cooperative group. *Br J Cancer* 79(9–10): 1522–30.

Dank, Zaluski J, Barone C *et al.* (2005) Randomized phase 3 trial of irinotecan (CPT-11) + 5FU/folinic acid (FA) vs CDDP + 5FU in 1st-line advanced gastric cancer patients. *J Clin Oncol 2005 ASCO Annual Meeting Proceedings* Part I, Vol 23, no. 16S (June 1 Supplement): 4003.

De Potter T, Flamen P, van Cutsem E *et al.* (2002) Whole-body PET with FDG for the diagnosis of recurrent gastric cancer. *Eur J Nucl Med Mol Imaging* 29(4): 525–9.

Degliulie M, Sasako M, Ponzetti A *et al.* (1997) Extended lymph node dissection for gastric cancer: results of a prospective, multi-centre analysis of morbidity and mortality in 118 consecutive cases. *Eur J Surg Oncol* 23: 310–14.

D'Elia F, Zingarelli A, Palli D, Grani M (2000) Hydro-dynamic CT preoperative staging of gastric cancer: correlation with pathological findings. A prospective study of 107 cases. *Eur Radiol* 10(12): 1877–85.

Dent DM, Werner ID, Novis B, Cheverton P, Brice P. (1979) Prospective randomized trial of combined oncological therapy for gastric carcinoma. *Cancer* 44(2): 385–91.

Dent DM, Madden MV, Price SK. (1988) Randomized comparison of R1 and R2 gastrectomy for gastric carcinoma. *Br J Surg* 75(2): 110–12.

Doi T, Koizumi W, Siena S *et al.* (2003) Efficacy, tolerability, and pharmacokinetics of gefitinib (ZD1839) in pretreated patients with metastatic gastric cancer. *J Clin Oncol* 22: A1036.

Dragovich T, McCoy S, Fenoglio-Preiser CM *et al.* (2006) Phase II trial of erlotinib in gastroesophageal junction and gastric adenocarcinomas: SWOG 0127. *J Clin Oncol* 24: 4922–7.

Earle CC, Maroun JA. (1999) Adjuvant chemotherapy after curative resection for gastric cancer in non-Asian patients: revisiting a meta-analysis of randomised trials. *Eur J Cancer* 35(7): 1059–64.

Fricke E, Keller G, Becker I *et al.* (2003) Relationship between E-cadherin gene mutation and p53 gene mutation, p53 accumulation, Bcl-2 expression and Ki-67 staining in diffuse-type gastric carcinoma. *Int J Cancer* 104(1): 60–5.

Fukuya T, Honda H, Kaneko K *et al.* (1997) Efficacy of helical CT in T-staging of gastric cancer. *J Comput Assist Tomogr* 21(1): 73–81.

Gastrointestinal Tumor Study Group (GITSG) (1982) A comparison of combination chemotherapy and combined modality therapy for locally advanced gastric carcinoma. Gastrointestinal Tumor Study Group. *Cancer* 49(9): 1771–7.

Gennari L, Bozzetti F, Bonfanti G *et al.* (1986) Subtotal versus total gastrectomy for cancer of the lower two- thirds of the stomach: a new approach to an old problem. *Br J Surg* 73: 534–8.

Glimelius B, Ekström K, Hoffman K *et al.* (1997) Randomized comparison between chemotherapy plus best supportive care with best supportive care in advanced gastric cancer. *Ann Oncol* 8: 1–6.

Grace A, Butler D, Gallagher M *et al.* (2002) APC gene expression in gastric carcinoma: an immunohistochemical study. *Appl Immunohistochem Mol Morphol* 10(3): 221–4.

Grady WM, Willis J, Guilford PJ *et al.* (2000) Methylation of the CDH1 promoter as the second genetic hit in hereditary diffuse gastric cancer. *Nat Genet* 26(1): 16–7.

van Grieken NCT, Weiss MM, Meijer GA *et al.* (2000) *Helicobacter pylori*-related and -non-related gastric cancers do not differ with respect to chromosomal aberrations. *J Pathol* 192(3): 301–6.

Griffith J, Sue-Ling HM, Dixon MF, McMahon MJ, Axon AT, Johnston D. (1995) Preservation of the spleen improves survival after radical surgery for gastric cancer. *Gut* 36(5): 684–90.

Guilford P, Hopkins J, Harraway J *et al.* (1998) E-cadherin germ line mutations in familial gastric cancer. *Nature* 392: 402–5.

Gunderson LL, Sosin H. (1982) Adenocarcinoma of the stomach: areas of failure in a re-operation series (second or symptomatic look) clinicopathologic correlation and implications for adjuvant therapy. *Int J Radiat Oncol Biol Phys* 8(1): 1–11.

Gunther T, Schneider-Stock R, Pross M *et al.* (1998) Alterations of the p16/MTS1-tumor suppressor gene in gastric cancer. *Pathol Res Pract* 194(12): 809–13.

Hallissey MT, Dunn JA, Ward LC, Allum WH. (1994) The second British Stomach Cancer Group trial of adjuvant radiotherapy or chemotherapy in resectable gastric cancer: five-year follow-up. *Lancet* 343(8909): 1309–12.

Hamilton SR, Aaltonen LA. (2000) Pathology and genetics of tumours of the digestive system. In: Hamilton SR, Aaltonen LA, eds. *World Health Organization. Classification of Tumours.* IARC press, Lyon, France.

Han MH, Koh GJ, Choi JH, Sung KJ, Koh JK, Moon KC. (2000) Carcinoma erysipelatoides originating from stomach adenocarcinoma. *J Dermatol* 27: 471–4.

Hartgrink HH, van de Velde CJ, Putter H *et al.* (2004a) Neo-adjuvant chemotherapy for operable gastric cancer: long term results of the Dutch randomised FAMTX trial. *Eur J Surg Oncol* 30(6): 643–9.

Hartgrink HH, van de Velde CJ, Putter H *et al.* (2004b) Extended lymph node dissection for gastric cancer: who may benefit? Final results of the randomized Dutch gastric cancer group trial. *J Clin Oncol* 22(11): 2069–77.

Henning GT, Schild SE, Stafford SL *et al.* (2000a) Results of irradiation or chemoirradiation for primary unresectable, locally recurrent, or grossly incomplete resection of gastric adenocarcinoma. *Int J Radiat Oncol Biol Phys* 46(1): 109–18.

Henning GT, Schild SE, Stafford SL *et al.* (2000b) Results of irradiation or chemoirradiation following resection of gastric adenocarcinoma. *Int J Radiat Oncol Biol Phys* 46(3): 589–98.

Horie Y, Miura K, Matsui K *et al.* (1996) Marked elevation of plasma carcinoembryonic antigen and stomach carcinoma. *Cancer* 77: 1991–7.

Hundahl SA, Macdonald JS, Benedetti J, Fitzsimmons T. (2002) Surgical treatment variation in a prospective, randomized trial of chemoradiotherapy in gastric cancer: the effect of undertreatment. *Ann Surg Oncol* 9(3): 278–86.

Ilson DH, Minsky B. (2003) Irinotecan in esophageal cancer. *Oncology (Williston Park)* 17(9 Suppl 8): 32–6.

Inoue M, Tsugane S. (2005) Epidemiology of gastric cancer in Japan. *Postgrad Med J* 81: 419–24.

Jansen E, Boot H, Verheij M, van de Velde C. (2005) Optimal locoregional treatment in gastric cancer. *J Clin Oncol* 23(20): 4509–17.

Jansen E, Saunders M, Boot H *et al.* (2007) A prospective study on late renal toxicity following postoperative chemoradiotherapy in gastric cancer. *Int J Radiat Oncol Biol Phys* 67(3): 781–5.

Jemal A, Tiwari RC, Murray T *et al.* (2004) Cancer statistics 2004. *CA Cancer J Clin* 54: 8–29.

Juttner S, Wissmann C, Jons T *et al.* (2006) Vascular endothelial growth factor-D and its receptor VEGFR-3: two novel independent prognostic markers in gastric adenocarcinoma. *J Clin Oncol* 24: 228–40.

Kajitani T. (1981) The general rules for the gastric cancer study in surgery and pathology. Part I. Clinical classification. *Jpn J Surg* 11(2): 127–39.

Kampschoer GH, Maruyama K, Sasako M, Kinoshita T, van de Velde CJ. (1989) The effects of blood transfusion on the prognosis of patients with gastric cancer. *World J Surg* 13: 637–43.

Kaneda M, Horimi T, Ninomiya M *et al.* (1987) Adverse effect of blood transfusions on survival of patients with gastric cancer. *Transfusion* 27: 375–7.

Kang Y, Kang WK, Shin DB *et al.* (2006) Randomized phase III trial of capecitabine/cisplatin (XP) vs. continuous infusion of 5-FU/cisplatin (FP) as first-line therapy in patients with advanced gastric cancer (AGC): efficacy and safety results. *J Clin Oncol 2006 ASCO Annual Meeting Proceedings* Part I, Vol 24, no. 18S (June 20 Supplement): LBA4018.

Katai H, Maruyama K, Sasako M *et al.* (1994) Mode of recurrence after gastric cancer surgery. *Dig Surg* 11: 99–103.

Kattan MW, Karpeh MS, Mazumdar M *et al.* (2003) Postoperative nomogram for disease-specific survival after an R0 resection for gastric carcinoma. *J Clin Oncol* 21(19): 3647–50.

Kelly S, Harris KM, Berry E *et al.* (2001) A systematic review of the staging performance of endoscopic ultrasound in gastro-oesophageal carcinoma. *Gut* 49(4): 534–9.

Kim TY, Bang YJ, Kim WS *et al.* (1997) Mutation of ras oncogene in gastric adenocarcinoma: association with histological phenotype. *Anticancer Res* 17(2B): 1335–9.

Kim HS, Han HY, Choi JA *et al.* (2001) Preoperative evaluation of gastric cancer: value of spiral CT during gastric arteriography (CTGA). *Abdom Imaging* 26(2): 123–30.

Kim JY, Park DY, Kim GH *et al.* (2005a) Smad4 expression in gastric adenoma and adenocarcinoma: frequent loss of expression in diffuse type of gastric adenocarcinoma. *Histol Histopathol* 20: 543–9.

Kim AY, Kim HJ, Ha HK (2005b) Gastric cancer by multidetector row CT: preoperative staging. *Abdom Imaging* 30(4): 465–72.

Kim HJ, Kim AY, Oh ST *et al.* (2005c) Gastric cancer staging at multidetector row CT gastrography: comparison of transverse and volumetric CT scanning. *Radiology* 236(3): 879–85.

Kim S, Lim do H, Lee J *et al.* (2005d) An observational study suggesting clinical benefit for adjuvant postoperative chemoradiation in a population of over 500 cases after gastric resection with D2 nodal dissection for adenocarcinoma of the stomach. *Int J Radiat Oncol Biol Phys* 63(5): 1279–85.

Kim SK, Kang KW, Lee JS *et al.* (2006) Assessment of lymph node metastases using 18F-FDG PET in patients with advanced gastric cancer. *Eur J Nucl Med Mol Imaging* 33(2): 148–55.

Kinoshita T, Maruyama K, Sasako M *et al.* (1993) Treatment results of gastric cancer patients: Japanese experience. In: Nishi M, Ichakawa H, Nakajima T *et al.*, eds. *Gastric Cancer*, pp. 319–30. Springer-Verlag, Tokyo.

Kitagawa Y, Fujii H, Kumai K *et al.* (2005) Recent advances in sentinel node navigation for gastric cancer: A paradigm shift of surgical management. *J Surg Oncol (Seminars)* 90: 147–52.

Kitamura K, Nishida S, Ichikawa D *et al.* (1999) No survival benefit from combined pancreaticosplenectomy and total gastrectomy for gastric cancer. *Br J Surg* 86(1): 119–22.

Klaassen DJ, MacIntyre JM, Catton GE, Engstrom PF, Moertel CG. (1985) Treatment of locally unresectable cancer of the stomach and pancreas: a randomized comparison of 5-fluorouracil alone with radiation plus concurrent and maintenance 5-fluorouracil—an Eastern Cooperative Oncology Group study. *J Clin Oncol* 3(3): 373–8.

Kodera Y, Yamamura Y, Shimizu Y *et al.* (1997) Lack of benefit of combined pancreaticosplenectomy in D2 resection for proximal-third gastric carcinoma. *World J Surg* 21(6): 622–7.

Kodera Y, Ito S, Yamamura Y *et al.* (2003) Follow-up surveillance for recurrence after curative gastric cancer surgery lacks survival benefit. *Ann Surg Oncol* 10(8): 898–902.

Kole AC, Plukker JT, Nieweg OE, Vaalburg W *et al.* (1998) Positron emission tomography for staging of oesophageal and gastroesophageal malignancy. *Br J Cancer* 78(4): 521–7.

Kollmannsberger C, Budach W, Stahl M *et al.* (2005) Adjuvant chemoradiation using 5-fluorouracil/folinic acid/cisplatin with or without paclitaxel and radiation in patients with completely resected high-risk gastric cancer: two cooperative phase II studies of the AIO/ARO/ACO. *Ann Oncol* 16(8): 1326–33.

Kopp R, Ruge M, Rothbauer E *et al.* (2002) Impact of epidermal growth factor (EGF) radioreceptor analysis on long-term survival of gastric cancer patients. *Anticancer Res* 22: 1161–7.

Landry J, Tepper JE, Wood WC, Moulton EO, Koerner F, Sullinger J. (1990) Patterns of failure following curative resection of gastric carcinoma. *Int J Radiat Oncol Biol Phys* 19(6): 1357–62.

Laurén P. (1965) The two histological main types of gastric carcinoma: diffuse and so-called intestinal-type carcinoma. An attempt at a histoclinical classification. *Acta Pathol Microbiol Scand* 64: 31–49.

Lee JH, Abraham SC, Kim HS *et al.* (2002) Inverse relationship between APC gene mutation in gastric adenomas and development of adenocarcinoma. *Am J Pathol* 161(2): 611–18.

Leong T, Michael M, Foo K *et al.* (2003) Adjuvant and neoadjuvant therapy for gastric cancer using epirubicin/cisplatin/5-fluorouracil (ECF) and alternative regimens before and after chemoradiation. *Br J Cancer* 89(8): 1433–8.

Levine MS *et al.* (1990) Scirrhous carcinoma of the stomach: radiologic and endoscopic diagnosis. *Radiology* 175(1): 151–4.

Lynch HT, Grady W, Suriano G, Huntsman D. (2005) *Gastric Cancer*: new genetic developments. *J Surg Oncol (Seminars)* 90: 114–33.

Macdonald JS, Smalley SR, Benedetti J *et al.* (2001) Chemoradiotherapy after surgery compared with surgery alone for adenocarcinoma of the stomach or gastroesophageal junction. *N Engl J Med* 345(10): 725–30.

Machado JC, Oliveira C, Carvalho R *et al.* (2001) E-cadherin gene (CDH1) promoter methylation as the second hit in sporadic diffuse gastric carcinoma. *Oncogene* 20(12): 1525–8.

Macintyre IM, Akoh JA. (1991) Improving survival in gastric cancer: review of operative mortality in English language publications from 1970. *Br J Surg* 78: 771–6.

Maeda K, Chung YS, Ogawa Y *et al.* (1996) Prognostic value of vascular endothelial growth factor expression in gastric carcinoma. *Cancer* 77: 858–63.

Maruyama K. (1987) The most important prognostic factors for gastric cancer patients: a study using univariate and multivariate analysis. *Scand J Gastroenterol* 22 (Suppl 133): 63–8.

Maruyama K, Okabayashi K, Kinoshita T. (1987) Progress in gastric cancer surgery in Japan and its limits of radicality. *World J Surg* 11: 418–25.

Maruyama K, Gunven P, Okabayashi K, Sasako M, Kinoshita T. (1989) Lymph node metastases of gastric cancer. General pattern in 1931 patients. *Ann Surg* 210: 596–602.

McNeer G, Vandenberg H Jr, Donn FY, Bowden L. (1951) A critical evaluation of subtotal gastrectomy for the cure of cancer of the stomach. *Ann Surg* 134(1): 2–7.

McAteer D, Wallis F, Couper G *et al.* (1999) Evaluation of 18F-FDG positron emission tomography in gastric and oesophageal carcinoma. *Br J Radiol* 72(858): 525–9.

Meyers WC, Damiano RJ Jr, Rotolo FS, Postlethwait RW. (1987) Adenocarcinoma of the stomach. Changing patterns over the last 4 decades. *Ann Surg* 205: 1–8.

Mikulicz J. (1898) Beitrage zur Technik der Operation des Magenkarzinoms. *Arch Clin Chir Berl* 1(vii): 524–32.

Moertel CG, Childs DS Jr, Reitemeier RJ, Colby MY Jr, Holbrook MA. (1969) Combined 5-fluorouracil and supervoltage radiation therapy of locally unresectable gastrointestinal cancer. *Lancet* 2(7626): 865–7.

Moertel CG, Childs DS, O'Fallon JR, Holbrook MA, Schutt AJ, Reitemeier RJ. (1984) Combined 5-fluorouracil and radiation therapy as a surgical adjuvant for poor prognosis gastric carcinoma. *J Clin Oncol* 2(11): 1249–54.

Moiseyenko VM, Ajani JA, Tjulandin SA *et al.* (2005) Final results of a randomized controlled phase III trial (TAX325) comparing docetaxel (T) combined with cisplatin (C) and 5-fluorouracil (F) to CF in patients (pts) with metastatic gastric adenocarcinoma (MGC). *J Clin Oncol 2005 ASCO Annual Meeting Proceedings* Part I, Vol 23, no. 16S (June 1 Supplement): 4002.

Nakajima T, Harashima S, Hirata M, Kajitani T. (1978) Prognostic and therapeutic values of peritoneal cytology in gastric cancer. *Acta Cytol* 22(4): 225–9.

Navarro V, Ramon D, Calduch L, Llombart B, Monteagudo C, Jorda E. (2002) Cutaneous metastasis of gastric adenocarcinoma: an unusual clinical presentation. *Eur J Dermatol* 12: 85–7.

Ott K, Fink U, Becker K *et al.* (2003) Prediction of response to preoperative chemotherapy in gastric carcinoma by metabolic imaging: results of a prospective trial. *J Clin Oncol* 21(24): 4604–10.

Pack GT, McNeer GP. (1943) Total gastrectomy for cancer: a collective review of the literature and an original report on 20 cases. *Internat Abstr Surg* 77: 265–99.

Park MS, Ha HK, Choi BS *et al.* (2004) Scirrhous gastric carcinoma: endoscopy versus upper gastrointestinal radiography. *Radiology* 231(2): 421–6.

Peeters KC, Hundahl SA, Kranenbarg EK, Hartgrink H, van de Velde CJ. (2005a) Low Maruyama index surgery for gastric cancer: blinded reanalysis of the Dutch D1-D2 trial. *World J Surg* 29(12): 1576–84.

Peeters KC, Kattan MW, Hartgrink HH *et al.* (2005b) Validation of a nomogram for predicting disease-specific survival after an R0 resection for gastric carcinoma. *Cancer* 103(4): 702–7.

Pinto C, Di Fabio F, Siena S *et al.* (2006) Phase II study of cetuximab plus FOLFIRI as first-line treatment in patients with unresectable/metastatic gastric or gastroesophageal junction (GEJ) adenocarcinoma (FOLCETUX study): preliminary results. *J Clin Oncol* 24(18S): A4031.

Polak E, Vojtisek V. (1959) Experience with gastric resection by the Péan-Rydygier-Billroth I method. *Ann Surg* 149(4): 475–80.

Rao S, Starling N, Benson M *et al.* (2005) Phase I study of the humanised epidermal growth factor receptor (EGFR) antibody EMD 72000 (matuzumab) in combination with ECX (epirubicin, cisplatin and capecitabine) as first-line treatment for advanced oesophagogastric (OG) adenocarcinoma. *J Clin Oncol* 23(16S): A4028.

Regine WF, Mohiuddin M. (1992) Impact of adjuvant therapy on locally advanced adenocarcinoma of the stomach. *Int J Radiat Oncol Biol Phys* 24(5): 921–7.

Richards FM, McKee SA, Rajpar MH, *et al.* (1999) Germline E-cadherin gene (CDH1) mutations predispose to familial gastric cancer and colorectal cancer. *Hum Mol Genet* 8: 607–10.

Robertson CS, Chung SC, Wood SD *et al.* (1994) A prospective randomized trial comparing R1 subtotal gastrectomy with R3 total gastrectomy for antral cancer. *Ann Surg* 220(2): 176–82.

Rohren EM, Turkington TG, Coleman RE. (2004) Clinical applications of PET in oncology. *Radiology* 231(2): 305–32.

Rojo F, Tabernero J, Albanell J *et al.* (2006) Pharmacodynamic studies of gefitinib in tumor biopsy specimens from patients with advanced gastric carcinoma. *J Clin Oncol* 24(26): 4309–16.

Roviello F, Marelli D, de Manzoni G *et al.* (2003) Prospective study of peritoneal recurrence after curative surgery for gastric cancer. *Br J Surg* 90: 1113–9.

Safran H, Wanebo HJ, Hesketh PJ *et al.* (2000b) Paclitaxel and concurrent radiation for gastric cancer. *Int J Radiat Oncol Biol Phys* 46(4): 889–94.

Sano T, Sasako M, Kinoshita T, Maruyama K. (1993) Recurrence of early gastric cancer. follow-up of 1475 patients and review of the Japanese literature. *Cancer* 72(11): 3174–8.

Sano T, Sasako M, Yamamoto S *et al.* (2004) Gastric cancer surgery: morbidity and mortality results from a prospective randomized controlled trial comparing D2 and extended para-aortic lymphadenectomy. *J Clin Oncol* 22(14): 2767–73.

Sarbia M, Gedert H, Klump B *et al.* (2004) Hypermethylation of tumor suppressor genes (p16INK4A, p14ARF and APC) in adenocarcinomas of the upper gastrointestinal tract. *Int J Cancer* 111(2): 224–8.

Sasako M. (1997) Risk factors for surgical treatment in the Dutch gastric cancer trial. *Br J Surg* 84(11): 1567–71.

Sasako M, McCulloch P, Kinoshita T, Maruyama K. (1995) New method to evaluate the therapeutic value of lymph node dissection for gastric cancer. *Br J Surg* 82(3): 346–51.

Sasako M, Sano T, Yamamoto S *et al.* (2006) Randomized phase III trial of standard D2 versus D2 + para-aortic lymph node (PAN) dissection (D) for clinically M0 advanced gastric cancer. JCOG9501 Abstract number: LBA 4015.

Schlemper RJ, Itabashi M, Kato M *et al.* (1997) Differences in diagnostic criteria for gastric carcinoma between Japanese and western pathologists. *Lancet* 349(9067): 1725–9.

Shah MA, Ilson D, Kelsen DP. (2005) Thromboembolic events in gastric cancer: high incidence in patients receiving irinotecan- and bevacizumab-based therapy. *J Clin Oncol* 23: 2574–6.

Shah MA, Ramanathan RK, Ilson DH *et al.* (2006) Multicenter phase II study of irinotecan, cisplatin, and bevacizumab in patients with metastatic gastric or gastroesophageal junction adenocarcinoma. *J Clin Oncol* 24: 5201–6.

Shaw D, Blair V, Framp A *et al.* (2005) Chromoendoscopic surveillance in hereditary diffuse gastric cancer: an alternative to prophylactic gastrectomy? *Gut* 54: 461–8.

Shiraishi N, Inomata M, Osawa N, Yasuda K, Adachi Y, Kitano S. (2000) Early and late recurrence after gastrectomy for gastric carcinoma. Univariate and multivariate analyses. *Cancer* 89: 255–61.

Siewert JR, Bottcher K, Roder JD *et al.* (1993) Prognostic relevance of systemic lymph node dissection in gastric carcinoma. *Br J Surg* 80: 1015–8.

Siewert JR, Bottcher K, Stein HJ, Roder JD, Busch R. (1995) Problem of proximal third gastric carcinoma. *World J Surg* 19(4): 523–31.

Sindelar WF, Kinsella TJ, Tepper JE *et al.* (1993) Randomized trial of intraoperative radiotherapy in carcinoma of the stomach. *Am J Surg* 165(1): 178–86.

Skoropad V, Berdov B, Zagrebin V. (2002) Concentrated preoperative radiotherapy for resectable gastric cancer: 20-years follow-up of a randomized trial. *J Surg Oncol* 80(2): 72–8.

Skoropad VY, Berdov BA, Zagrebin VM. (2003) Preoperative radiotherapy in combination with metronidazole for resectable gastric cancer: long-term results of a phase 2 study. *Eur J Surg Oncol* 29(2): 166–70.

Smalley SR, Gunderson L, Tepper J *et al.* (2002) Gastric surgical adjuvant radiotherapy consensus report: rationale and treatment implementation. *Int J Radiat Oncol Biol Phys* 52(2): 283–93.

Sobin LH, Wittekind C. (1997) *International Union Against Cancer: TNM Classification of Malignant Tumors.* Wiley-Liss, New York.

Sobin LH, Wittekind C. (2002) *International Union Against Cancer: TNM Classification of Malignant Tumours*, 6th edn. Wiley-Liss, New York.

Soga J, Kobayashi K, Saito J, Fujimaki M, Muto T. (1979) The role of lymphadenectomy in curative surgery for gastric cancer. *World J Surg* 3(6): 701–8.

Songun I, Bonenkamp JJ, Hermans J, van Krieken JH, van de Velde CJ. (1996) Prognostic value of resection-line involvement in patients undergoing curative resections for gastric cancer. *Eur J Cancer* 32A(3): 433–7.

Stein A, Al-Batran SE, Arnold D, Peinert S, Siewczynski R, Schmoll HJ. (2007) Cetuximab with irinotecan as salvage therapy in heavily pretreated patients with metastatic gastric cancer. Gastrointestinal Cancers Symposium 2007, Abstract 47.

Sue-Ling HM, Johnston D, Martin IG *et al.* (1993) Gastric cancer: a curable disease in Britain. *BMJ* 307(6904): 591–6.

Sugezawa A, Kaibara N, Sumi K *et al.* (1989) Blood transfusion and the prognosis of patients with gastric cancer. *J Surg Oncol* 42: 113–6.

Sunderland D. (1967) The lymphatic spread of gastric cancer. In: McNeer G, Pack G, eds. *Neoplasms of the Stomach*, p. 408. Lippincott, Philadelphia.

Suntharalingam M, Dipetrello T, Akerman P *et al.* (2006) Cetuximab, paclitaxel, carboplatin and radiation for esophageal and gastric cancer. *Proc Am Soc Clin Oncol* Part 1, Vol 24, no. 18S: abstract 4029.

Sussman SK, Halvorsen RA Jr, Illescas FF *et al.* (1988) Gastric adenocarcinoma: CT versus surgical staging. *Radiology* 167(2): 335–40.

Takahashi Y, Cleary KR, Mai M, Kitadai Y, Bucana CD, Ellis LM. (1996) Significance of vessel count and vascular endothelial growth factor and its receptor (KDR) in intestinal-type gastric cancer. *Clin Cancer Res* 2: 1679–84.

Tanner M, Hollmen M, Junttila TT *et al.* (2005) Amplification of HER-2 in gastric carcinoma: association with topoisomerase II alpha gene amplification, intestinal type, poor prognosis and sensitivity to trastuzumab. *Ann Oncol* 16(2): 273–8.

Tatsumi Y, Tanigawa N, Nishimura H *et al.* (2006) Preoperative diagnosis of lymph node metastases in gastric cancer by magnetic resonance imaging with ferumoxtran-10. *Gastric Cancer* 9(2): 120–8.

Tepper JE, Gunderson LL. (2002) Radiation treatment parameters in the adjuvant postoperative therapy of gastric cancer. *Semin Radiat Oncol* 12(2): 187–95.

Thuss-Patience PC, Kretzschmar A, Repp M *et al.* (2005) Docetaxel and continuous-infusion fluorouracil versus epirubicin, cisplatin, and fluorouracil for advanced gastric adenocarcinoma: a randomized phase II study. *J Clin Oncol* 23(3): 494–501.

Tsendsuren T, Jun SM, Mian XH. (2006) Usefulness of endoscopic ultrasonography in preoperative TNM staging of gastric cancer. *World J Gastroenterol* 12(1): 43–7.

Turlakow A, Yeung HW, Salmon AS *et al.* (2003) Peritoneal carcinomatosis: role of (18)F-FDG PET. *J Nucl Med* 44(9): 1407–12.

Vanhoefer U, Rougier P, Wilke H *et al.* (2000) Final results of a randomized phase III trial of sequential high-dose methotrexate, flurouracil, and doxorubicin versus etoposide, leucovorin, and flurouracil versus infusional flurouracil and cisplatin in advanced gastric cancer: a trial of the European Organization for Research and Treatment of Cancer Gastrointestinal Tract Cancer Cooperative Group. *J Clin Oncol* 18(14): 2648–57.

Vauhkonen M, Vauhkonen H, Sajantila A *et al.* (2005) Differences in genomic instability between intestinal-type and diffuse-type gastric cancer. *Gastric Cancer* 8(4): 238–44.

Verheij M, Oppedijk V, Boot H *et al.* (2006) Late renal toxicity following post-operative chemoradiotherapy in gastric cancer. *Proc Am Soc*

Clin Oncol Gastrointestinal Cancers Symposium, Miami, 2006, abstract 2.

Viste A, Haugstvedt T, Eide GE, Soreide O. (1988) Postoperative complications and mortality after surgery for gastric cancer. *Ann Surg* 207: 7–13.

Vo QN, Geradts J, Boudreau EA *et al.* (2002) CDKN2A promoter methylation in gastric adenocarcinomas: clinical variables. *Hum Pathol* 33(12): 1200–4.

Vollmers HP, Dammrich J, Hensel F *et al.* (1997) Differential expression of apoptosis receptors on diffuse and intestinal type stomach carcinoma. *Cancer* 79(3): 433–40.

Wagner AD, Grothe W, Haerting J *et al.* (2006) Chemotherapy in advanced gastric cancer: a systematic review and meta-analysis based on aggregate data. *J Clin Oncol* 24(18): 2903–9.

Wanebo H, Kennedy BJ, Chmiel J, Steele G, Winchester D, Osteen R. (1993) Cancer of the stomach. A patient care study by the American College of Surgeons. *Ann Surg* 218(5): 583–92.

Wanebo HJ, Kennedy BJ, Winchester DP *et al.* (1996) Gastric carcinoma: does lymph node dissection alter survival? *J Am Coll Surg* 183(6): 616–24.

Webb A, Cunningham D, Scarffe JH *et al.* (1997) Randomized trial comparing epirubicin, cisplatin, and flurouracil versus flurouracil, doxorubicin, and methotrexate in advanced esophagogastric cancer. *J Clin Oncol* 15(1): 261–7.

Whiting J, Sano T, Saka M, Fukagawa T, Katai H, Sasako M. (2006) Follow-up of gastric cancer: a review. *Gastric Cancer* 9: 74–81.

Willis S, Truong S, Gribnitz S *et al.* (2000) Endoscopic ultrasonography in the preoperative staging of gastric cancer: accuracy and impact on surgical therapy. *Surg Endosc* 14(10): 951–4.

Wisbeck W, Becher E, Russel A. (1986) Adenocarcinoma of the stomach: autopsy observations with therapeutic implications for the radiation oncologist. *Radiother Oncol* 7(1): 13–18.

Wolfler A. (1881) Über die von Herrn Professor Billroth ausgeführten Resektionen des karzinomatösen Pylorus. *Zblt Chir* 8: 359.

Wu CW, Hsiung CA, Lo SS *et al.* (2006) Nodal dissection for patients with gastric cancer: a randomised controlled trial. *Lancet Oncol* 7(4): 309–15.

Xiangming C, Natsugoe S, Takaho S *et al.* (2001) Preserved Smad4 expression in the transforming growth factor beta signaling pathway is a favorable prognostic factor in patients with advanced gastric cancer. *Clin Cancer Res* 7(2): 277–82.

Yoo CH, Noh SH, Shin DW, Choi SH, Min JS. (2000) Recurrence following curative resection for gastric carcinoma. *Br J Surg* 87: 236–42.

Yoshikawa T, Tsuburaya A, Kobayashi O *et al.* (2000) Plasma concentrations of VEGF and bFGF in patients with gastric carcinoma. *Cancer Lett* 153: 7–12.

Yun M, Lim JS, Noh SH *et al.* (2005) Lymph node staging of gastric cancer using (18)F-FDG PET: a comparison study with CT. *J Nucl Med* 46(10): 1582–8.

Zhang ZX, Gu XZ, Yin WB, Huang GJ, Zhang DW, Zhang RG. (1998) Randomized clinical trial on the combination of preoperative irradiation and surgery in the treatment of adenocarcinoma of gastric cardia (AGC)—report on 370 patients. *Int J Radiat Oncol Biol Phys* 42(5): 929–34.

Zhao P, Liu W, Lu YL *et al.* (2005) Clinicopathological significance of FHIT protein expression in gastric adenocarcinoma patients. *World J Gastroenterol* 11(36): 5735–8.

7 Intestinal Gastric Cancer

Edited by Benjamin C.Y. Wong

Diagnosis: history, clinical and histopathology

Annie On On Chan & Asif Rashid

Introduction

For over 100 years, gastric cancer has remained one of the most important malignant diseases with significant geographical, ethnic, and socioeconomic differences in distribution. Globally, gastric cancer is still currently the second commonest cancer with approximately 900,000 incident cases each year (Pisani *et al.* 1997), accounting for 9.9% of new cancers (Parkin 1998). Gastric cancer used to be the leading cause of cancer deaths of the world until recently (the overall mortality incidence ratio is around 85–90%), when it was overtaken by lung cancer (Pisani *et al.* 1993). With the rapid decline in the global incidence of gastric cancer from the 1930s to the 1970s, the discovery of *Helicobacter pylori*, and the advancement in molecular biology, the view towards gastric cancer has been changing. This chapter focuses on the intestinal type of gastric cancer, the staging system, treatment, prognosis and follow-up.

Intestinal gastric cancer

Lauren classified gastric cancer into intestinal and diffuse types, according to glandular formation (Lauren 1965). These two biological entities are different with regard to epidemiology, etiology, pathogenesis and behavior. Intestinal gastric cancer is commoner in males and older age groups and is likely linked to environmental factors. A recent decline in the incidence of the intestinal type in the past few decades worldwide that parallels the overall decline in the incidence of gastric cancer has been observed. The precursor lesions and environmental factors are summarized in the following section.

Gastrointestinal Oncology: A Critical Multidisciplinary Team Approach.
Edited by J. Jankowski, R. Sampliner, D. Kerr, and Y. Fong.

Precursor lesions and environmental factors

Helicobacter pylori and the Correa's cascade

Studies of gastric cancer among migrants have shown that emigrants from high-incidence countries to low-incidence locations often experience a decreased risk of developing gastric carcinoma. This reduction in the risk was seen in subsequent generations and to a lesser degree in the first generation (Haenszel 1982). Such findings strongly suggest that environmental factors play an important role in the etiology of gastric cancer and that exposure to risk factors occurs early in life.

The intestinal-type gastric cancer typically arises through the Correa's cascade, progressing from chronic gastritis to chronic atrophic gastritis, intestinal metaplasia, dysplasia, and eventually to adenocarcinomas (Correa 1982, 1983, 1988; Correa *et al.* 1975). The commonest cause of gastritis is *Helicobacter pylori*. *H. pylori* infection may trigger inflammation of the corpus mucosa that results in atrophy and intestinal metaplasia. This association has been demonstrated in large epidemiology studies (Parsonnet *et al.* 1991a, b; Kikuchi *et al.* 1995; Wong *et al.* 1999). The World Health Organization's International Agency for Research on Cancer has now classified *Helicobacter pylori* as a Group 1 or definite carcinogen (IARC 1994). *H. pylori* is a Gram-negative rod bacterium that localizes beneath the mucous layer of the mucosa from stomach, metaplastic esophagus, duodenum, and even Meckel's diverticulum. The *Helicobacter* genus also includes *mustelae*, *muridarum*, and *nemestrinae*, which are ureasepositive but appear to be limited to stomachs of other mammals (Blaser 1992). The ability of the bacterium to survive in the acidic environment of the stomach relies on the presence of a high molecularweight urease. This enzyme catalyzes the transformation of urea to ammonium and bicarbonate, which alkalinizes the environment and protects the bacteria from gastric acid. The organism's production of proteases, lipases, phospholipases, and cytotoxins, combined with its ability to attach to epithelial cells via adherence proteins, contributes to its pathogenicity (Fennerty 1994).

Elder pointed out that 10% of patients with chronic atrophic gastritis would eventually develop gastric cancer within a period of 15 years (Elder 1995). In atrophic gastritis, there is progressive atrophy of the glandular epithelium with loss of parietal and chief cells. The loss of the normal exocrine glands of the gastric mucosa causes hypochlorhydria and a resultant increase in gastric pH. An abnormally high pH in the stomach allows microbial colonization, some of which possess nitrate reductase, allowing nitrosation that is genotoxic. In addition, there is a loss of endocrine cells which normally secrete epidermal and transforming growth factors, which aid the stomach in regenerating damaged tissue (Elder 1995). Finally, populations with a high prevalence of atrophic gastritis also have a high prevalence of gastric cancer, and vice versa (Genta 1998).

Metaplasia is a potentially reversible change from a fully differentiated cell type to another cell type, a process in adaptation to environmental stimuli. In the stomach, intestinal-type metaplasia is commonest. This occurs as a result of *Helicobacter pylori* infection, or bile reflux (Sobala *et al.* 1993), or can be induced experimentally by irradiation (Watanabe 1978). Intestinal metaplasia is more frequent in countries with a higher incidence of gastric carcinoma (Correa *et al.* 1970), and has been shown to precede gastric carcinoma (Sasajima *et al.* 1979). Within the gastric cancer risk index, the presence of intestinal metaplasia was the only criterion associated with the development of intestinal-type gastric cancer in Japan (Shimoyama *et al.* 2000). Atrophy and intestinal metaplasia occur significantly more often in the antrum of carcinoma patients. The odds ratio for gastric carcinoma was 8.85 for high-grade corpus gastritis and 8.04 when atrophy in the antrum was present (Miehlke *et al.* 1998). In China, intestinal metaplasia was found in 33% of the population in a high-prevalence area of gastric cancer; and dysplasia, common in the lesser curvature of the body and in the incisura, was found in 20% (You *et al.* 1993).

Most patients diagnosed with high-grade dysplasia of the gastric mucosa will either already have or soon develop gastric cancer. In gastrectomy specimens for gastric cancer 20–40% of patients had associated dysplasia, and progression of dysplasia to gastric cancer has been estimated at 21%, 33%, and 57% of cases of mild, moderate, and severe dysplasia, respectively (Rugge *et al.* 1994). Epidemiologic studies have shown that intestinal metaplasia and dysplasia in the stomach have a high cancer risk. For example, in a study carried out in two provinces in China with high and low cancer risk, the prevalence of intestinal metaplasia and dysplasia were much higher in the area with high risk for gastric cancer (You *et al.* 1998).

Follow-up data from mass screening by endoscopy helped to clarify the natural history of gastritis. Kato *et al.* (1992) found that if baseline endoscopic findings indicated the presence of atrophic gastritis, the risk of developing gastric cancer during 4.4 years of average follow-up period was increased 5.7-fold, compared with no atrophic gastritis at the baseline. Tatsuta *et al.* (1993) reported a similar risk (5.76-fold) in patients with severe fundal atrophic gastritis diagnosed by the endoscopic Congo red test.

H. pylori is associated with adenocarcinomas distal to the cardia, including both intestinal and diffuse types. *H. pylori* infection has been estimated to increase the risk of gastric cancer by sixfold (Forman 1991). Three sources of evidence support the association of *H. pylori* infection and gastric cancer: epidemiologic studies comparing gastric cancer and *H. pylori* infection prevalence rates, crosssectional studies evaluating *H. pylori* infection in cancer patients, and prospective studies associating *H. pylori* with gastric cancer (Forman 1991; Nomura *et al.* 1991; Parsonnet *et al.* 1991a, b; Talley *et al.* 1991; Eurogast 1993; Parsonnet 1993). Epidemiologically, the incidences of both *H. pylori* infection and gastric cancer follow similar geographic and temporal trends (Parsonnet 1993). Cross-sectional studies investigating *H. pylori* infection in gastric cancer patients have revealed that *H. pylori* is more likely to infect populations of gastric cancer patients than normal populations, with rates of infection ranging from 50% to 100% in patients with gastric adenocarcinoma (Parsonnet *et al.* 1991; Parsonnet 1993) Paradoxically, histologic association of the bacteria with tumor can be difficult to determine because *H. pylori* has an affinity for normal gastric mucosa but not metaplastic, dysplastic, or malignant tissue (Hazell *et al.* 1987). Prospective studies of *H. pylori* and cancer reveal that *H. pylori* infection increases the risk of developing gastric cancer in later life, although most people infected with *H. pylori* do not develop gastric carcinoma (Forman *et al.* 1991; Nomura *et al.* 1991; Parsonnet *et al.* 1991). One study suggested that 35–55% of all gastric cancer might be attributable to *H. pylori* infection (Forman *et al.* 1991). However, a paradox in *H. pylori* infection is that divergent clinical outcomes occur: patients may develop duodenal ulcer or gastric cancer, while the majority of them develop no significant clinical symptoms. Bacterial virulence factors have failed to explain why the ulcer or the gastric cancer phenotype develops. This has highlighted the need to explore host genetic factors as determinants of clinical outcome of the infection, including gastric cancer.

The host: blood group, genetic polymorphisms, germline mutation

The role of genetic factors was first suggested by the study of blood groups and determinants of chronic gastritis (Langman 1988). Individuals of blood group A have been known for decades to show approximately 20% higher rates of gastric cancer than those of group O, B or AB. They also show a similar increase of pernicious anaemia. Some data suggest that group A may be particularly associated with the diffuse type of gastric cancer (Langman 1988). A genetic etiology has been reported for chronic atrophic gastritis (Bonney *et al.* 1986). The genetic segregation analysis showed Mendelian transmission of a recessive autosomal gene with penetrance dependent on age and the status of chronic atrophic gastritis in the mother. Of individuals with affected mothers 48% were affected as compared to only 7% of those who mother did not have chronic atrophic gastritis. A familial tendency to stomach cancer has long been suspected and repeatedly confirmed (Langman 1988; Palli *et al.* 1994; Zhao *et al.* 1994).

The human interleukin-1 beta (IL-1B) gene is the most important candidate gene in the host that could affect the clinical outcome of *H. pylori* infection, because it is upregulated by infection, is profoundly proinflammatory, and is the most powerful acid inhibitor known. Polymorphisms in the IL-1B gene (carriers of IL-1B-511*T) and in the IL-1 receptor antagonist gene (IL-1RN*2/*2) were found to be associated with an increased risk of gastric cancer (El-Omar *et al.* 2000). Figueiredo *et al.* (2002) had further suggested I L-1B-511*T carriers (IL-1B-511*T/*T or IL-1B-511*T/*C) homozygous for the short allele of IL-1RN (IL-1RN*2/*2) in the prescence of vacAs1-, vacAm1-, and cagA-positive strains of *H. pylori* had an increased gastric carcinoma risk. The presence of several cytokine polymorphisms also leads to a multiplied risk of cancer.

The IFNGR1 gene encodes chain 1 of the interferon-gamma (IFN-gamma) receptor. Sequencing of IFNGR1 revealed -56C→T, H318P, and L450P variants, which were found to be associated with high *H. pylori* antibody concentrations. The variants were more prevalent in Africans than in whites. These findings indicate that IFN-gamma signaling plays an essential role in human *H. pylori* infection, and they might in part explain the observations of high prevalences and relatively low pathogenicity of *H. pylori* in Africa (Thye *et al.* 2003).

A germline mutation in the E-cadherin gene was identified in a New Zealand family with gastric cancer (Guilford *et al.* 1998) and in several UK families in 1999 (Richards *et al.* 1999). Thereafter, in two kindreds with familial gastric cancer and germline E-cadherin mutation, promoter CpG hypermethylation was found to be the second 'genetic hit' in abrogating E-cadherin expression (Grady *et al.* 2000). These results show that E-cadherin is an important putative tumour suppressor gene involved in gastric carcinogenesis.

Interplay between environmental factors, the organism and the host

Tsugane *et al.* have found that in a Japanese population, higher salt intake correlates with higher prevalence of *H. pylori* infection (Tsugane *et al.* 1994). It was postulated that gastric mucosal damage caused by high salt intake facilitated *H. pylori* infection. The resultant hypochlorhydria and bacterial overgrowth, with the subsequent conversion of nitrites to the mutagenic N-nitrosamines, were postulated to be the instigating events that led to metaplasia, dysplasia, and cancer. Gastric juice of *H. pylori*-positive individuals had a lower concentration of vitamin C than *H. pylori*-negative individuals, but the concentration returned to normal when *H. pylori* was eradicated (Schorah *et al.* 1991). Therefore, vitamin C could play an important role in preventing the damage caused by *H. pylori* through its antioxidant effect (Schorah *et al.* 1991). In addition, through their antinitrosation and antioxidant effects, beta-carotene and ascorbic acid are believed to halt this progression to cancer and thus act as protective factors (Parsonnet 1993). However, this dogma has been supplanted by the hypothesis that *H. pylori* infection in early life leads to the formation of chronic atrophic gastritis, and the resultant transformation to metaplasia, dysplasia and, ultimately, malignancy. The most convincing hypothesis is that chronic inflammation, with the resultant inflammation-related mutagenesis, may lead to genetic mutations culminating in malignant transformation. In addition, the resulting cellular proliferation may increase the likelihood of mitotic error and invoke a role for genotoxicity. This model also acknowledges the role of dietary factors in gastric carcinogenesis. While dietary mutagens may increase the risk of mutation, dietary antioxidants may act as protective factors. Because some DNA damage can be self-corrected, *H. pylori*-related mutations may only rarely lead to malignant transformation. Thus, longer duration of infection, especially infection acquired during childhood and continuing until old age, increases the risk of significant DNA damage with subsequent malignant transformation (Parsonnet 1993). In addition, both *H. pylori* genotype and host genetic polymorphisms play a role in determining the clinical consequences of *H. pylori* infection and hence the risk of developing gastric cancer. It has been suggested that combined bacterial/host genotyping may provide an important tool in defining disease risk and targeting *H. pylori* eradication to high-risk individuals.

Despite the proposal of dietary, environmental factors and the identification of *H. pylori*, the rapid global decline in gastric cancer is still not fully explained. An interesting hypothesis is that the introduction of refrigeration marks a pivotal point for the decline (Coggon *et al.* 1989; La Vecchia *et al.* 1990). Refrigerators improved the storage of food, thereby reducing salting for preserving food and preventing bacterial and fungal contamination of food. Refrigeration also enables fresh food and vegetables to be more readily available, which may be a valuable source of antioxidants important for cancer prevention.

Diet

Large epidemiology studies demonstrating the association between diet and gastric cancer were mainly based on the amount of food imported and produced rather than actual food consumption (Howson *et al.* 1986). This takes no account of the losses during storage, distribution, and consumption of food, nor any ethnic dietary differences. Nonetheless, the information provides important insights into environmental causes of gastric cancer. The association between N-nitroso compounds and gastric cancer has been summarized by Bartsch *et al.* (1987). The risk of gastric cancer induced by N-nitroso compounds has been demonstrated in animal experiments (Drukrey 1975; Magee *et al.* 1976; Bulay *et al.* 1979). An increase in gastric nitrite was observed in patients with intestinal metaplasia, dysplasia, and gastric cancer (Stewart 1967; Jones *et al.* 1978; Ruddell *et al.* 1978). The use of nitrate-based fertilizers (Jones *et al.* 1978; Frazer *et al.* 1980; Schlag *et al.* 1980) and consumption of pickled foods that contain nitrosated products (Sato *et al.* 1959; Haenszel *et al.* 1972) have been shown to positively correlate with gastric cancer. Diets low in vegetables, fruits, milk, and vitamin A, and high in fried food, processed meat, and fish and alcohol have been associated with an increased risk of gastric carcinoma in several cohort studies (Graham *et al.* 1990). Diets low in citrus fruit show the strongest association with gastric carcinoma. The protection afforded by vegetables and fruits is most likely related to their vitamin C content, which is thought to reduce the formation of carcinogenic N-nitroso compounds inside the stomach. Cooked vegetables, however, do not show the same protective effect as uncooked vegetables (Buiatti *et al.* 1989). High salt intake has been shown to damage stomach mucosa and increase the susceptibility to carcinogenesis in rodents (Tatematsu *et al.* 1975; Hanawa *et al.* 1980; Takahashi *et al.* 1984). The positive correlation between nitrate intake, salt excretion and gastric cancer has recently been shown in the Intersalt study involving 24 countries from 39 populations (Joossens *et al.* 1996). Although no consistent association has been found between alcohol and tobacco consumption and an increased risk of gastric carcinoma (Buiatti *et al.* 1989), a number of prospective studies have linked cigarette smoking with an increased risk of this cancer (Hammond 1966).

Socioeconomic status

Risk of gastric cancer is associated with socioeconomic status. Subjects from lower socioeconomic classes had approximately twice as high a risk of developing intestinal-type gastric cancer as subjects from higher socioeconomic groups (Haenszel 1958; Wynder *et al.* 1963; Berndt *et al.* 1968; Barker *et al.* 1990). On the contrary, proximal gastric cancers were associated with higher socioeconomic class (Powell & McConkey 1990).

Gastric surgery

There is an increased risk of gastric cancer after gastric surgery, with the risk being greatest 15–20 years after surgery and then increasing with time (Neugut *et al.* 1996; Nomura 1996). The Bilroth II procedure (gastrojejunostomy) carries a higher risk than the Bilroth I (gastroduodenostomy). It is thought this is due to the greater regurgitation of bile and pancreatic juice in the former procedure, leading to postoperative gastritis. Although still controversial, in the majority of cases gastric ulcers are not related to the eventual formation of gastric cancer.

Epstein–Barr virus

The Epstein–Barr virus (EBV) is associated with a number of malignancies, especially nasopharyngeal carcinoma. It has been suggested that it might play a role in the development of gastric cancer also. In a study conducted in Korea (Shin *et al.* 1996), evidence of EBV was found in the tumor cells of 12 of 89 (13.5%) gastric carcinoma patients, whereas EBV was found in none of the gastric tissues of 37 controls with benign ulcer disease, nor in any of the benign tissues of the cases. Some of the tumor cells had a histologic appearance similar to nasopharyngeal carcinoma.

Imaging and staging

Annie On On Chan & Benjamin C.Y. Wong

Imaging

Computed tomography (CT) of the abdomen, chest X-ray, esophagogastroduodenoscopy, and, in female patients, CT or ultrasound of the pelvis have been recommended as the minimal required preoperative tests for gastric cancer by the National Comprehensive Cancer Network (NCCN 1998). The major limitations of CT as a staging study are in the evaluation of small lesions, including early gastric tumors and peritoneal or liver metastases smaller than 5 mm (Davies *et al.* 1997). The overall accuracy of CT in assessing tumor stage is reported to be 66–77% (Minami *et al.* 1992; Rossi *et al.* 1997). Node classification using CT is based primarily on lymph node size and is accurately assigned in 25–86% of patients (Fukuya *et al.* 1995, Halvorsen *et al.* 1996). Endoscopic ultrasound (EUS) is an investigation used increasingly in the preoperative work-up of patients with gastric cancers. However, EUS does not reliably define T2 from T3 and T3 from T4 tumors. Lymph nodes may be detectable when they are greater than 3 mm (Kuntz & Herfarth 1999). According to Kuntz and Herfarth, the T category and node involvement can be staged with 60–90% and 50–80% accuracy, respectively, with the use of EUS. The accuracy of node staging is as low as 50%, but technical improvements and experience have improved the accuracy of nodal evaluation to about 65% for N1 disease (de Manzoni *et al.* 1999). EUS staging has demonstrated an overall staging accuracy of 75% (Fockens 1998). Laparoscopy is also being recommended prior to a major resection. The use of laparoscopy may be supported by the fact that an R0 resection cannot be performed in 30–40% of patients undergoing surgery. Distant metastasis has been detected in patients in whom CT did not reveal signs of unresectability (O'Brien *et al.* 1995; Lowy *et al.* 1996). Laparoscopy identifies CT-occult metastatic disease in 23–37% of patients (Possik *et al.* 1986; Stell *et al.* 1996; Burke *et al.* 1997; D'Ugo *et al.* 1997; Charukhchyan & Lucas 1998;

Feussner *et al.* 1999). Moreover, fewer than 2% of the patients in these reports required subsequent laparotomy for palliation. Limitations of laparoscopy in the staging of gastric cancer include the following: (i) the technique allows for only two-dimensional inspection of the surface of the liver and peritoneal cavity; (ii) it does not allow palpation, limiting the identification of small intraparenchymal hepatic metastases and perigastric lymph nodes; and (iii) laparoscopic inspection of the peritoneal surfaces does not allow critical tumor–vessel relationships to be accurately evaluated. Laparoscopic ultrasonography has been proposed as a means of overcoming some of these limitations and improving the diagnostic yield (Conlon & Karpeh 1996). Magnetic resonance imaging (MRI) probably has the potential to be at least as accurate as EUS, but comparative studies are lacking at the moment.

Staging

The two main staging systems for gastric cancer are the TNM staging system of the International Union Against Cancer (UICC), and the Japanese Classification of Gastric Carcinoma by the Japanese Gastric Cancer Association (JGCA). The two systems are similar in that staging is dependent on the extent of the primary tumor, the extent of lymph node involvement, and the presence or absence of distant metastasis. But the difference between the two systems lies in the classification of regional lymph node spread. The UICC/TNM staging system divides N stage on the basis of the number of metastatic lymph nodes, while the Japanese classification stresses the location of involved nodes. The current main classification systems for gastric cancer are the 6th edition of the UICC/TNM classification (2002) (Table 7.1) (Sobin & Wittekind 2002), and the 13th edition of the Japanese classification of gastric carcinoma (2nd English edition 1998) (JGCA 1998).

Based on TNM staging criteria, the depth of invasion (T), presence of lymph node metastases, and number of lymph nodes involved (N) predict the risk of relapse. This was confirmed in a large German multicenter trial published by Siewert et al (1998). The study involved 1654 patients undergoing surgical resection of gastric tumors. By contrast, the JGCA classification is much more than a staging system. It provides comprehensive and meticulous guidance to surgeons because it describes in detail the anatomical involvement of lymph nodes.

Table 7.1 TNM classification of carcinoma of the stomach.

Category	Criteria
Primary tumor (T)	
TX	Primary tumor cannot be assessed
T0	No evidence of primary tumor
Tis	Carcinoma in situ; intraepithelial tumor without invasion of the lamina propria
T1	Tumor invades lamina propria or submucosa
T2	Tumor invades muscularis propria or subserosa
T2a	Tumor invades muscularis propria
T2b	Tumor invades subserosa
T3	Tumor penetrates serosa (visceral peritoneum) without invasion of adjacent structures
T4	Tumor invades adjacent structures
Regional lymph nodes (N)	
NX	Regional lymph nodes cannot be assessed
N0	No regional lymph node metastasis
N1	Metastases in 1–6 lymph nodes
N2	Metastases in 7–15 lymph nodes
N3	Metastases in >15 lymph nodes
Distant metastasis (M)	
MX	Distant metastasis cannot be assessed
M0	No distant metastasis
M1	Distant metastasis

Stage grouping				*5-year overall survival rate*
Stage 0	Tis	N0	M0	Stage 0: 89%
Stage IA	T1	N0	M0	Stage IA: 78%
Stage IB	T1	N1	M0	Stage IB: 58%
	T2a–b	N0	M0	
Stage II	T1	N2	M0	
	T2a–b	N1	M0	Stage II: 34%
	T3	N0	M0	
	T2a–b	N2	M0	
Stage IIIA	T3	N1	M0	Stage IIIA: 20%
	T4	N0	M0	
Stage IIIB	T3	N2	M0	Stage IIIB: 8%
	T4	N1–3	M0	
Stage IV	T1–3	N3	M0	Stage IV: 7%
	Any T	Any N	M1	

Treatment

Annie On On Chan & Benjamin C.Y. Wong

Endoscopic mucosal resection (EMR)

Therapeutic endoscopy in gastric cancer offers minimally invasive procedures that aim at complete cancer removal in early gastric cancer. Endoscopic mucosal resection proposed by Tada (Tada *et al.* 1994) has been performed in patients with early gastric cancer. For differentiated-type T1 mucosal cancers, EMR is often successful, as metastasis does not generally occur (Gotoda *et al.* 2000). The Japanese Gastric Cancer Treatment Guideline indicates the criteria for EMR as follows: mucosal cancer of intestinal type, no ulcer nor ulcer scar in the lesion, and size smaller than 21 mm (Nakajima 2002). Complications of EMR include pain, bleeding, perforation, and stricture formation. Bleeding is the most common complication and is typically minor and treatable with endoscopy.

Laparoscopic gastrectomy

Laparoscopic gastrectomy is intermediate between EMR and conventional surgery in terms of invasiveness. With the advances in instruments and techniques, lymph node dissection becomes possible laparoscopically and thus enables curative resection even when there is lymph node involvement. Compared with conventional open surgery, laparoscopic gastrectomy is reported to have several benefits for patients, including less pain, less inflammatory response, faster recovery of gastrointestinal function, preserved postoperative immune function, shorter hospital stay, reduced medical costs, and better QOL (Adachi *et al.* 1999, 2000a, 2002; Shimizu *et al.* 2000; Asao *et al.* 2001; Mochiki *et al.* 2002; Fujii *et al.* 2003; Migoh *et al.* 2003; Weber *et al.* 2003). Huscher et al (2005) reported in a 5-year prospective randomized trial that laparoscopic gastrectomy and open surgery did not differ in the mean number of lymph nodes resected, or in the morbidity and mortality rates.

Surgery with intent to cure: R0 resection

R0 resection refers to surgery with intent to cure, and R1 resection to surgery with microscopic positive resection margin. A number of controversies exist over the surgical management of gastric cancer. First, there is controversy over the partial or total gastrectomy approaches for distal cancer. The two approaches have been compared in two multicenter randomized controlled trials (RCTs) (Gouzi *et al.* 1989; Bozzetti *et al.* 1999). Both studies did not demonstrate any significant difference between the two approaches. Thus the conclusion is that subtotal gastrectomy is adequate for patients with gastric cancer located in the distal half of the stomach, allowing a proximal resection margin of 6 cm. The margin has to be verified by frozen section. However, the debate continues for proximal gastric cancer. When the resection requires supradiaphragmatic anastomosis, some groups favor proximal gastrectomy, and others feel that either total gastrectomy or esophagectomy with proximal cervical anastomosis is the procedure of choice (Harrison 1998; Bonenkamp 2004).

The second and more important controversy is the extent of lymph node dissection. A D1 resection entails a gastrectomy with the removal of all perigastric nodes and the removal of the greater and lesser omenta. In addition to these structures, for a D2 dissection the surgeon removes the omental bursa portion of the transverse mesocolon and the nodes along the left gastric, celiac, and splenic arteries. For a D3 dissection, in addition to the standard D2 dissection, lymph nodes in the hepatoduodenal ligament, along the superior mesenteric vein, posterior to the common hepatic artery, and on the posterior surface of the pancreatic head are also removed. A D4 dissection involves the removal of lymph nodes around the abdominal aorta, in addition to all of the structures mentioned above.

The surgical strategy of the Japanese Research Society for Gastric Cancer (JRSGC) is based on the gastric lymphatic drainage. D2 radical gastrectomy has been advocated and has been practiced as standard surgery in Japan for the past 30 years. All the lymph nodes are retrieved from the resection specimen and examined for micrometastasis, which may sometimes be difficult to see intraoperatively. This is in contrast to the Western world where conventional limited D1 radical gastrectomy is more commonly performed due to the lower mortality rate. Japanese series demonstrated a survival benefit using D2 resection (Maruyama *et al.* 1987). Non-randomized studies have further supported the concept that an adaptation of the Japanese surgical technique could improve the results of gastric cancer surgery in the West (Siewert *et al.* 1993, 1996). However, this was not proven in other studies from the Western world. In a prospective RCT, D2 resections were associated with significantly higher mortality and morbidity and may nullify the survival benefits from D2 procedures (Cuschieri *et al.* 1996). In addition, in a long-term follow-up study, there was no difference observed in the tumor recurrence rate in the two groups (Cushieri *et al.* 1999). Similar findings were also reported in a Dutch study (Bonenkamp *et al.* 1999). Further, the difference could also be accounted for partially by understaging in the Western world where fewer regional lymph nodes were resected (Bunt 1995). In addition, the Japanese tumors could have been overstaged as some of the stage I carcinomas were reported to be dysplasia by Western pathologists (Schlemper *et al.* 1997).

Palliative treatment

The goal of palliative care is the achievement of the best quality of life for patients and their families (WHO 1990). R2 resection refers to non-curative gastrectomy. Total gastrectomy was not suggested to be worthwhile as a palliative surgery in the old days for patients with non-curative disease because of the perioperative morbidity (Lawrence & McNeer 1958; Remine 1979). However, the current view is that total palliative gastrectomy and esophagogastrectomy is justified in selected patients, based on observations that total gastrectomy provided better symptom relief and improved survival without increasing complication rates (Welvaart & de Jong 1986; Bozzetti *et al.* 1987; Monson *et al.* 1991; Geoghegan *et al.* 1993; Ouchi *et al.* 1998).

Therapy for palliation can be achieved endoscopically by recanalization or hemostasis of cancer bleeding. Endoscopic laser ablation technique is very effective in treating deeper invasive cancers. Endoscopic placement of expandable metal stents has been proposed as an alternative technique for palliation in patients not suitable for surgery.

Chemotherapy

The role of adjuvant chemotherapy after curative surgery was evaluated in seven meta-analysis studies (Hermans *et al.* 1993; Nakjima *et al.* 1994; Earle & Maroun 1999; Mari *et al.* 2000; Hu *et al.* 2002; Janunger *et al.* 2002; Panzini *et al.* 2002). Despite these meta-analysis studies, the beneficial role of adjuvant systemic chemotherapy after curative surgery is still controversial. Most of the meta-analysis studies were able to show marginal survival benefits. However, when Western and Asian studies were analyzed separately, no survival benefit was observed in the Western groups, thus emphasizing the apparent difference in the biology of gastric cancers arising in Western and Asian populations.

Neoadjuvant chemotherapy aims at reducing tumor bulk, thus downstaging the primary tumor to increase resectability rates. Recently, the MAGIC study, performed by the British Medical Research Council (MRC), randomly allocated 503 cases of potentially resectable gastric cancer to either preoperative and postoperative ECF (epirubicin, cisplatin, and 5-fluorouracil) chemotherapy, or surgery alone (Allum *et al.* 2003). Preoperative chemotherapy resulted in a statistically significant improvement in disease-free survival. There was an increased rate of overall survival at 2 years (48% vs 40%) with preoperative chemotherapy, but this improvement was not statistically significant. The curative resection rate was increased by neoadjuvant therapy because of a significant downstaging of tumor stage (surgery only, T3 = 64%; neoadjuvant therapy T3 = 49%; p = 0.011). The results demonstrated that there are some potentially important clinical benefits for neoadjuvant chemotherapy. A disadvantage of neoadjuvant therapy is that it obscures accurate pathologic staging because neoadjuvant chemotherapy causes an alteration of information regarding lymph node status prior to surgery.

Adjuvant chemoradiation therapy may also have a role in resected gastric cancer. A US gastrointestinal cancer Intergroup study was initiated in early 1991 to test whether the combination of 5-FU leucovorin plus radiation therapy after surgical resection would be of value to patients with resected gastric carcinoma. This study enrolled a total of 603 patients in 7 years of accrual. Compared to observation alone, patients treated with adjuvant chemoradiotherapy had a significantly improved chance of 3-year disease-free survival (48% vs 31%, p = 0.001). The median survival in the adjuvant group was 42 months, compared with 27 months among controls (p = 0.03). These figures represent a 44% improvement in relapse-free survival and a 28% improvement in overall survival; however, the survival gains are comparable to survival figures reported with D1 resection in the literature (Macdonald *et al.* 2001). Combining neoadjuvant and postoperative chemoradiation may well result in further improvement in outcomes for patients with resectable gastric cancer.

Intraperitoneal chemotherapy has also been investigated to attempt improve locoregional control. However, different studies have shown that there was no significant benefit (Schiessel *et al.* 1989; Hagiwara *et al.* 1992; Sautner *et al.* 1994; Rosen *et al.* 1998; Yu *et al.* 1998).

It has been shown that, in RCTs, systemic chemotherapy improves survival and quality of life compared to the best supportive treatment in advanced disease (Glimelius *et al.* 1997; Hill & Cunningham 1998). There is no clear standard of treatment of chemotherapy in gastric cancer. Many single-agent or combination chemotherapy regimens have been used. The drug 5-FU remains one of the most frequently used chemotherapy agents for gastric cancer.

Prognosis and follow-up

Annie On On Chan & Benjamin C.Y. Wong

Prognosis

The survival rates in gastric cancer have been shown to be improving in both Asian and Western countries. It has been reported that, in a British study, the survival improved from 15% to 41% over a period of 20 years (Desai *et al.* 2004). The number of curative resections increased from 33% to 73%, and similar results have been reported from Germany (Siewert *et al.* 1998), the United States (Brennan & Karpeh 1996), with data beginning to approximate that of Asia. The 5-year survival rate for the total population of patients with gastric cancer was estimated to be 15–25% (Janunger *et al.* 2002).

The pathologic stage has consistently been shown to be of prognostic significance for both 5-year survival and local recurrence rates (Roder *et al.* 1998; Siewert *et al.* 1998, Adachi *et al.* 2000b; Yokota *et al.* 2000). Siewert *et al.* has shown that lymph node ratio and lymph node status are the most important prognostic factors in patients with resected gastric cancer in a prospective multicenter observation trial. The data confirmed the therapeutic value of D_2 lymphadenectomy in patients with stage II disease. He also reported that in experienced centers, extended lymph node dissection does not increase the mortality or morbidity rate of resection for gastric cancer but markedly improves long-term survival in patients with stage II tumors. This effect appears to be independent of the phenomenon of stage migration. Size of the tumor is another important prognostic factor. The evidence comes from a prospective, randomized trial that demonstrated tumor size to be an independent prognostic factor in a multivariate analysis (p = 0.0002) in patients with tumor-free margins (Siewert *et al.* 1998). Vascular and lymphatic permeation are both important potential independent prognostic factors. Studies have demonstrated that lymph node involvement is a statistically significant predictor of survival, and the presence of tumor emboli significantly influences tumor recurrence and death after curative resection (Yokota *et al.*

1999, 2000; Maehara *et al.* 2002). These findings were recently supported by Hyung *et al.* (2002), who reported a poor prognosis associated with advanced T stage and the presence of vascular invasion. Kooby et al (2003) similarly demonstrated, in adequately staged node-negative patients, that vascular invasion was an independent negative prognostic factor and may be a predictor of biologic aggressiveness. On the other hand, tumor differentiation, age and sex have not been persistently shown to be valid prognostic factors.

Patterns of recurrence have been analyzed (Ikeda *et al.* 2005). Of 1172 patients undergoing R0 resection, 42% recurred (n = 496). Complete data on 367 (74%), showed that 79% of the documented recurrences occurred within 2 years. Recurrence was local in 54%, metastatic in 51%, and peritoneal in 29%. Median time to death after recurrence was 6 months. Recurrence of a second primary tumor has been studied (Ikeda *et al.* 2005) after treatment for early gastric cancer. Examining 1070 patients, risk factors for recurrence were presence of lymph node metastases and older age.

Prognostic markers

The most frequently used tumor markers in gastric cancer are carcinoembryonic antigen (CEA) and CA19-9, but only a modest proportion of patients have elevated levels of these markers (Kim *et al.* 1995; Pectasides *et al.* 1997; Ohkura 1999; Yamo *et al.* 1999; Ychou *et al.* 2000). In a recent large prospective study by Takahashi et al (2003), it was found that preoperative positivities for CEA and/or CA19-9 or both were 28.3% and 45.0%, respectively, among 321 patients with gastric cancer. In addition, the sensitivities of CEA and either CEA or CA19-9, or both, for recurrence were 65.8% and 85.0%, respectively, among the 120 patients who had recurrence (Takahashi *et al.* 2003). Soluble E-cadherin has also been reported to have significant prognostic value (Chan *et al.* 2003) and to predict recurrence (Chan *et al.* 2005).

References

Adachi Y, Suematsu T, Shiraishi N, Katsuta T, Morimoto A, Kitano S *et al.* (1999) Quality of life after laparoscopy-assisted Billroth I gastrectomy. *Ann Surg* 229: 49–54.

Adachi Y, Shiraishi N, Shiromizu A, Bandoh T, Aramaki M, Kitano S. (2000a) Laparoscopy-assisted Billroth I gastrectomy compared with conventional open gastrectomy. *Arch Surg* 135: 806–10.

Adachi Y, Shiraishi N, Suematsu T *et al.* (2000b) Most important lymph node information in gastric cancer: multivariate prognostic study. *Ann Surg Oncol* 7: 503–7.

Adachi Y, Shiraishi N, Kitano S. (2002) Modern treatment of early gastric cancer: Review of the Japanese experience. *Dig Surg* 19: 333–9.

Allum W, Cunningham D, Weeden S *et al.* (2003) Perioperative chemotherapy in operable gastric and lower oesophageal cancer: A randomized, controlled trial (the MAGIC trial, ISRCTN 9379(3971) [Abstract #998]. *Proc ASCO* 22: 249a.

Asao T, Hosouchi Y, Nakabayashi T, Haga N, Mochiki E, Kuwano H. (2001) Laparoscopically assisted total or distal gastrectomy with lymph node dissection for early gastric cancer. *Br J Surg* 88: 128–32.

Barker DJ, Coggon D, Osmond C, Wickham C. (1990) Poor housing in childhood and high rates of stomach cancer in England and Wales. *Br J Cancer* 61: 575–8.

Bartsch H, O'Neill I, Hermann R. (1987) *The Relevance of N-nitroso Compounds to Human Cancer. Exposures and Mechanisms. IARC Scientific Publications No 84.* International Agency for Research on Cancer, Lyon, France.

Berndt H, Wildner GP, Klein K. (1968) Regional and social differences in cancer incidence of the digestive tract in the German Democratic Republic. *Neoplasm* 15: 501–15.

Blaser MJ. (1992) *Helicobacter pylori*: its role in disease. *Clin Infect Dis* 15: 386–91.

Bonenkamp JJ, Hermans J, Sasako M, van de Velde JC. (1999) Extended lymph-node dissection for gastric cancer. Dutch Gastric Cancer Group. *N Engl J Med* 340: 908–14.

Bonekamp JJ. (2004) Surgery for upper gastrointestinal malignancies. *Semin Oncol* 31: 542–53.

Bonney GE, Elston RC, Correa P *et al.* (1986) Genetic association of gastric carcinoma: I. Chronic atrophic gastritis. *Genet Epidemiol* 3: 213–24.

Bozzetti F, Bonfanti G, Audisio RA *et al.* (1987) Prognosis of patients after palliative surgical procedures for carcinoma of the stomach. *Surg Gynecol Obstet* 164: 151–4.

Bozzetti F, Marubini E, Bonfanti G, Miceli R, Piano C, Gennari L. (1999) Subtotal versus total gastrectomy for gastric cancer: Five-year survival rates in a multicenter randomized Italian trial. Italian Gastrointestinal Tumor Study Group. *Ann Surg* 230: 170–8.

Brennan MF, Karpeh MS Jr. (1996) Surgery for gastric cancer: the American view. *Semin Oncol* 23: 352–9.

Buiatti E, Palli D, Decarli A *et al.* (1989) A case-control study of gastric cancer and diet in Italy. *Int J Cancer* 44: 611–6.

Bulay O, Mirvish SS, Garcia H *et al.* (1979) Carcinogenicity test of six nitrosamides and a nitro-cyanamide administered orally to rats. *J Natl Cancer Inst* 62: 1523–8.

Burke E, Karpeh M, Conlon K. (1997) Laparoscopy in the management of gastric adenocarcinoma. *Ann Surg* 225: 262–7.

Bunt AM, Hermans J, Smit VT *et al.* (1995) Surgical/pathology stage migration confounds comparisons of gastric cancer survival rates between Japan and Western countries. *J Clin Oncol* 13: 19–25.

Chan AO, Chu KM, Lam SK *et al.* (2003) Soluble E-cadherin is an independent pretherapeutic factor for long-term survival in gastric cancer. *J Clin Oncol* 21: 2288–93.

Chan AO, Chu KM, Lam SK *et al.* (2005) Early prediction of tumor recurrence after curative resection of gastric carcinoma by measuring soluble E-cadherin. *Cancer* 104: 740–6.

Charukhchyan S, Lucas G. (1998) Laparoscopy and lesser sac endoscopy in gastric carcinoma operability assessment. *Am Surg* 64: 160–4.

Coggon D, Barker DJ, Cole RB, Nelson M. (1989) Stomach cancer and food storage. *J Natl Cancer Inst* 81: 1178–82.

Conlon K, Karpeh M Jr. (1996) Laparoscopy and laparoscopic ultrasound in the staging of gastric cancer. *Semin Oncol* 23: 347–51.

Correa P. (1982) Precursors of gastric and esophageal cancer. *Cancer* 50: 2554–65.

Correa P. (1983) The gastric precancerous process. *Cancer Surv* 2: 437–50.

Correa P. (1988) A human model of gastric carcinogenesis. *Cancer Res* 48: 3554–60.

Correa P, Cuello C, Duque E. (1970) Carcinoma and intestinal metaplasia of the stomach in Colombian migrants. *J Natl Cancer Inst* 44: 297–306.

Correa P, Haenszel W, Cuello C, Arder M, Tannenbaum SR. (1975) A model for gastric cancer epidemiology. *Lancet* 2: 58–60.

Correa P, Haenszel W, Tannenbaum S. (1982) Epidemiology of gastric carcinoma: review and future prospects. *Natl Cancer Inst Monogr* 62: 129–34.

Cuschieri A, Fayers P, Fielding J *et al.* (1996) Postoperative morbidity and mortality after D_1 and D_2 resections for gastric cancer: preliminary results of the MRC randomized controlled surgical trial. The Surgical Cooperative Group. *Lancet* 13: 995–9.

Cuschieri A, Weeden S, Fielding J *et al.* (1999) Patient survival after D1 and D2 resections for gastric cancer: long-term results of the MRC randomized surgical trial. Surgical Co-operative Group. *Br J Cancer* 79: 1522–30.

D'Ugo D, Persiani R, Caracciolo F. (1997) Selection of locally advanced gastric carcinoma by preoperative staging laparoscopy. *Surg Endosc* 11: 1159–62.

Davies J, Chalmers A, Sue-Ling H. (1997) Spiral computed tomography and operative staging of gastric carcinoma: A comparison with histopathological staging. *Gut* 41: 314–9.

Desai AM, Pareek M, Nightingale PG, Fielding JW. (2004) Improving outcomes in gastric cancer over 20 years. *Gastric Cancer* 7: 196–201.

Druckrey H. (1975) Chemical carcinogenesis on N-nitroso derivatives. *Gann Monogr* 17: 107–32.

Earle CC, Maroun JA. (1999) Adjuvant chemotherapy after curative resection for gastric cancer in non-Asian patients: Revisiting a meta-analysis of randomised trials. *Eur J Cancer* 35: 1059–64.

Elder JB. (1995) Carcinoma of the stomach. In: Haubrich WS, Schaffner F, Berk JE, eds. *Bockus Gastroenterology*, 5th edn, vol. I, pp. 805–815. WB Saunders Co., Philadelphia.

El-Omar EM, Carrington M, Chow WH *et al.* (2000) Interleukin-1 polymorphisms associated with increased risk of gastric cancer. *Nature* 404: 398–402.

Eurogast Study Group. (1993) An international association between *Helicobacter pylori* infection and gastric cancer. *Lancet* 341: 1359–62.

Fennerty MB. (1994) *Helicobacter pylori. Arch Intern Med* 154: 721–7.

Feussner H, Omote K, Fink U. (1999) Pre-therapeutic laparoscopic staging in advanced gastric carcinoma. *Endoscopy* 31: 342–7.

Figueiredo C, Machado JC, Pharoah P *et al.* (2002) *Helicobacter pylori* and interleukin 1 genotyping: an opportunity to identify high-risk individuals for gastric carcinoma. *J Natl Cancer Inst* 94: 1680–7.

Fockens P. (1998) Gastrointestinal cancer staging by endoscopic ultrasonography. *Abdom Imaging* 23: 543–5.

Forman D. (1991) *Helicobacter pylori* infection: a novel risk factor in the etiology of gastric cancer. *J Natl Cancer Inst* 83: 1702–3.

Forman D, Newell DG, Fullerton F *et al.* (1991) Association between infection with *Helicobacter pylori* and risk of gastric cancer: evidence from a prospective investigation. *BMJ* 302: 1302–5.

Frazer P, Chilvers C, Beral V *et al.* (1980) Nitrate and human cancer: a review of the evidence. *Int J Epidemiol* 9: 3–11.

Fujii K, Sonoda K, Izumi K. (2003) T lymphocyte subsets and Th1/Th2 balance after laparoscopy-assisted distal gastrectomy. *Surg Endosc* 9: 1440–4.

Fukuya T, Honda H, Hayashi T. (1995) Lymph-node metastases: efficacy for detection with helical CT in patients with gastric cancer. *Radiology* 197: 705–11.

Genta RM. (1998) Acid suppression and gastric atrophy: sifting fact from fiction. *Gut* 43 (Suppl 1): S35–38.

Geoghegan JG, Keane TE, Rosenberg IL *et al.*(1993) Gastric cancer. The case for a selective policy in surgical management. *J R Coll Surg Edinb* 38: 1863–8.

Glimelius B, Ekstrom K, Hoffman K *et al.* (1997) Randomized comparison between chemotherapy plus best supportive care with best supportive care in advanced gastric cancer. *Ann Oncol* 8: 163–8.

Gotoda T, Yanagisawa A, Sasako M *et al.* (2000) Incidence of lymph node metastasis from early gastric cancer: estimation with a large number of cases at two large centers. *Gastric Cancer* 3: 219–25.

Gouzi JL, Huguier M, Fagniez PL *et al.* (1989) Total versus subtotal gastrectomy for adenocarcinoma of the gastric antrum. A French prospective controlled study. *Ann Surg* 209: 162–6.

Grady WM, Willis J, Guilford PJ *et al.* (2000) Methylation of the CDH1 promoter as the second genetic hit in hereditary diffuse gastric cancer. *Nat Genet* 26: 16–17.

Graham S, Haughey B, Marshall J *et al.* (1990) Diet in the epidemiology of gastric cancer. *Nutr Cancer* 13: 19–34.

Guilford P, Hopkins J, Harraway J *et al.* (1998) E-cadherin germline mutations in familial gastric cancer. *Nature* 392: 402–5.

Haenszel W. (1958) Variation in incidence of and mortality from stomach cancer, with particular reference to the United States. *J Natl Cancer Inst* 21: 213–62.

Haenszel W. (1982) Migrant studies. In: Schottenfeld D, Fraumeni JF, eds. *Cancer Epidemiology and Prevention*, pp 194–207. WB Saunders, Philadelphia.

Haenszel W, Kurihara M, Segi M *et al.* (1972) Stomach cancer among Japanese in Hawaii. *J Natl Cancer Inst* 49: 969–88.

Hagiwara A, Takahashi T, Kojima O *et al.* (1992) Prophylaxis with carbon-adsorbed mitomycin against peritoneal recurrence of gastric cancer. *Lancet* 339: 629–31.

Halvorsen R Jr, Yee J, McCormick V. (1996) Diagnosis and staging of gastric cancer. *Semin Oncol* 23: 325–35.

Hammond EC. (1966) Smoking in relation to the death rates of 1 million men and women. *Natl Cancer Inst Monogr* 19: 127–204.

Hanawa K, Yamada S, Suzuki H *et al.* (1980) Effects of sodium chloride on gastric cancer induction by N-methyl-N-nitro-N-nitrogoguanidine (MNNG) in rats. In: Proceedings of the Thirty-ninth Annual Meeting of the Japanese Cancer Association, p. 49. Japanese Cancer Association, Tokyo.

Harrison LE, Karpeh MS, Brennan MF. (1998) Total gastrectomy is not necessary for proximal gastric cancer. *Surgery* 123: 127–30.

Hazell SL, Hennessy WB, Borody TJ *et al.* (1987) Campylobacter pyloridis gastritis II: distribution of bacteria and associated inflammation in the gastroduodenal environment. *Am J Gastroenterol* 82: 297–301.

Hermans J, Bonenkamp JJ, Boon MC *et al.* (1993) Adjuvant therapy after curative resection for gastric cancer: meta-analysis of randomised trials. *J Clin Oncol* 11: 1441–7.

Hill ME, Cunningham D. (1998) Medical management of advanced gastric cancer. *Cancer Treat Rev* 248: 113–8.

Howson CP, Hiyama T, Wynder EL. (1986) The decline in gastric cancer: epidemiology of an unplanned triumph. *Epidemiol Rev* 8: 1–27.

Hu JK, Chen ZX, Zhou ZG *et al.* (2002) Intravenous chemotherapy for resected gastric cancer: meta-analysis of randomized controlled trials. *World J Gastroenterol* 8: 1023–8.

Huscher CG, Mingoli A, Sgarzini G *et al.* (2005) Laparoscopic versus open subtotal gastrectomy for distal gastric cancer: five-year results of randomized prospective trial. *Ann Surg* 241: 232–7.

Hyung WJ, Lee JH, Choi SH *et al.* (2002) Prognostic impact of lymphatic and/or blood vessel invasion in patients with node-negative advanced gastric cancer. *Ann Surg Oncol* 9: 562–7.

IARC Working Group on the Evaluation of Carcinogenic Risks to Humans, Schistosomes, Liver Flukes and *Helicobacter pylori.* (1994) Vol 61 of IARC monographs on the evaluation of carcinogenic risks to humans. International Agency for Research on Cancer, Lyon.

Ikeda Y, Saku M, Kishihara F, Maehara Y. (2005) Effective follow-up for recurrence or a second primary cancer in patients with early gastric cancer. *Br J Surg* 92: 235–9.

Janunger KG, Hafstrom L, Glimelius B. (2002) Chemotherapy in gastric cancer: A review and updated meta-analysis. *Eur J Surg* 168: 597–608.

Japanese Gastric Cancer Association. (1998) Japanese classification of gastric carcinoma: 2nd English edition. *Gastric Cancer* 1: 10–24.

Jones SM, Davies PW, Savage A. (1978) Gastric-juice nitrite and gastric cancer. *Lancet* 1: 1355.

Joossens JV, Hill MJ, Elliott P. (1996) Dietary salt, nitrate and stomach cancer mortality in 24 countries. *Int J Epidemiol* 25: 494–504.

Kato I, Tominager S, Ito Y *et al.* (1992) A prospective study of atrophic gastritis and stomach cancer rosk. *Jpn J Cancer* 83: 1137–42.

Kikuchi S, Wada O, Nakajima T *et al.* (1995) Serum anti-*Helicobacter pylori* antibody and gastric carcinoma among young adults. *Cancer* 75: 2789–93.

Kim YH, Ajani JA, Ota DM, Lynch P, Roth JA. (1995) Value of serial carcinoembryonic antigen levels in patients with resectable adenocarcinoma of the esophagus and stomach. *Cancer* 75: 451–6.

Kooby DA, Suriawinata A, Klimstra DS *et al.* (2003) Biologic predictors of survival in node-negative gastric cancer. *Ann Surg* 237: 828–835; discussion 835–7.

Kuntz C, Herfarth C. (1999) Imaging diagnosis for staging of gastric cancer. *Semin Surg Oncol* 17: 96–102.

La Vecchia C, Negri E, D'Avanzo E, Franceschi S. (1990) Electric refrigerator use and gastric cancer risk. *Br J Cancer* 62: 136–7.

Langman MJS. (1988) Genetic influences upon gastric cancer frequency. In: Reed PI, Hill MJ, eds. *Gastric Carcinogenesis*, pp. 81–6. Excerpta Medica, Amsterdam.

Lauren P. (1965) The two histological main types of gastric carcinoma: diffuse and so-called intestinal-type carcinoma. *Acta Pathol Microbiol Scand* 64: 31–49.

Lawrence W, McNeer G. (1958) The effectiveness of surgery for palliation of incurable gastric cancer. *Cancer* 1: 23–32.

Lowy AM, Mansfield PF, Leach SD, Ajani J. (1996) Laparoscopic staging for gastric cancer. *Surgery* 119: 611–4.

Macdonald JS, Smalley SR, Benedetti J *et al.* (2001) Chemoradiotherapy after surgery compared with surgery alone for adenocarcinoma of the stomach or gastroesophageal junction. *N Engl J Med* 345: 725–30.

Maehara Y, Kakeji Y, Koga T *et al.* (2002) Therapeutic value of lymph node dissection and the clinical outcome for patients with gastric cancer. *Surgery* 131 (Suppl): S85–91.

Magee PN, Montesano R, Preussmann R. (1976) N-Nitroso compounds and related carcinogens. In: Searle CE, ed. *Chemical Carcinogens*, Am Chem Soc Monogr 173, pp. 491–625. American Chemical Society, Washington, DC.

de Manzoni G, Pedrazzani C, Di Leo A. (1999) Experience of endoscopic ultrasound in staging adenocarcinoma of the cardia. *Eur J Surg Oncol* 25: 595–8.

Mari E, Floriani I, Tinazzi A *et al.* (2000): Efficacy of adjuvant chemotherapy after curative resection for gastric cancer: A meta-analysis of published randomised trials. A study of the GISCAD (Gruppo Italiano per lo Studio dei Carcinomi dell'Apparato Digerente). *Ann Oncol* 11: 837–43.

Maruyama K, Okabayashi K, Kinoshita T. (1987) Progress in gastric cancer surgery in Japan and its limits of radicality. *World J Surg* 11: 418–25.

Miehlke S, Hackelsberger A, Meining A *et al.* (1998) Severe expression of corpus gastritis is characteristic in gastric cancer patients infected with *Helicobacter pylori. Br J Cancer* 78: 263–6.

Migoh S, Hasuda K, Nakashima K, Anai H. (2003) The benefit of laparoscopy-assisted distal gastrectomy compared with conventional open distal gastrectomy: a case-matched control study. *Hepatogastroenterology* 50: 2241–54.

Minami M, Kawauchi N, Itai Y. (1992) Gastric tumors: radiologic–pathologic correlation and accuracy of T staging with dynamic CT. *Radiology* 185: 173–8.

Mochiki E, Nakabayashi T, Kamimura H, Haga N, Asao T, Kuwano H. (2002) Gastrointestinal recovery and outcome after laparoscopy-assisted versus conventional open distal gastrectomy for early gastric cancer. *World J Surg* 26: 45–9.

Monson JR, Donoue JH,McIlrath DC *et al.* (1991) Total gastrectomy for advanced cancer. A worthwhile palliative procedure. *Cancer* 68: 1863–8.

Nakajima T. (2002) Gastric cancer treatment guidelines in Japan. *Gastric Cancer* 5: 1–5.

Nakajima T, Ota K, Ishihara S *et al.* (1994): Meta-analysis of 10 post-operative adjuvant chemotherapies for gastric cancer in CIH. *Jpn J Cancer Chemother* 21: 1800–5.

Neugut AI, Hayek M, Howe G. (1996) Epidemiology of gastric cancer. *Semin Oncol* 23: 281–91.

NCCN (1998) www.ncn.org

Nomura A. (1996) Stomach cancer. In: Scottenfeld D, Fraumeni JF Jr, eds. *Cancer Epidemiology and Prevention*, 2nd edn. Oxford University Press, NY.

Nomura A, Stemmermann GN, Chyou PH *et al.* (1991) *Helicobacter pylori* infection and gastric carcinoma among Japanese Americans in Hawaii. *N Engl J Med* 325: 1132–6.

O'Brien M, Fitzgerald E, Lee G. (1995) A prospective comparison of laparoscopy and imaging in the staging of esophagogastric cancer before surgery. *Am J Gastroenterol* 90: 2191–4.

Ohkura H. (1999) Tumor markers in monitoring response to chemotherapy for patients with gastric cancer. *Jpn J Clin Oncol* 29: 525–6.

Ouchi K, Sugawara T,Ono H *et al.* (1998) Therapeutic significance of palliative operations for gastric cancer for survival and quality of life. *J Surg Oncol* 69: 41–4.

Palli D, Galli M, Caporaso NE *et al.* (1994) Family history and risk of stomach cancer in Italy. *Cancer Epidemiol Biomarkers Prev* 3: 15–18.

Panzini I, Gianni L, Fattori PP *et al.* (2002) Adjuvant chemotherapy in gastric cancer: A meta-analysis of randomized trials and a comparison with previous meta-analyses. *Tumori* 88: 21–27.

Parkin DM. (1998) Epidemiology of cancer: global patterns and trends. *Toxicol Lett* 102: 227–34.

Parsonnet J. (1993) *Helicobacter pylori* and gastric cancer. *Gastroenterol Clin North Am* 22: 89–104.

Parsonnet J, Friedman GD, Vandersteen DP *et al.* (1991a) *Helicobacter pylori* infection and the risk of gastric carcinoma. *N Engl J Med* 325: 1127–31.

Parsonnet J, Vandersteen D, Goates J *et al.* (1991b) *Helicobacter pylori* infection in intestinal- and diffuse-type gastric adenocarcinomas. *J Natl Cancer Inst* 83: 640–3.

Pectasides D, Mylonakis A, Kostopoulou M *et al.* (1997) CEA, CA 19–9, and CA-50 in monitoring gastric carcinoma. *Am J Clin Oncol* 20: 348–53.

Pisani P, Parkin DM, Ferlay J. (1993) Estimates of the worldwide mortality from eighteen major cancers in 1985. Implications for prevention and projections of future burden. *Int J Cancer* 55: 891–903.

Pisani P, Parkin DM, Munoz N, Ferlay J. (1997) Cancer and infection: estimates of the attributable fraction in 1990. *Cancer Epidemiol Biomarkers Prev* 6: 387–400.

Possik R, Franco E, Pires D. (1986) Sensitivity, specificity, and predictive value of laparoscopy for the staging of gastric cancer and for the detection of liver metastases. *Cancer* 58: 1–6.

Powell J, McConkey CC. (1990) Increasing incidence of adenocarcinoma of the gastric cardia and adjacent sites. *Br J Cancer* 62: 440–3.

Remine WH. (1979) Palliative operations for incurable gastric cancer. *World J Surg* 3: 721–9.

Richards FM, McKee SA, Rajpar MH *et al.* (1999) Germ-line E-cadherin gene (CDH1) mutations predispose to familial gastric and colorectal cancer. *Hum Mol Genet* 4: 607–10.

Roder JD, Bottcher K, Busch R *et al.* (1998) Classification of regional lymph node metastasis from gastric carcinoma. German Gastric Cancer Study Group. *Cancer* 82: 621–31.

Rosen HR, Jatzko G, Repse S *et al.* (1998) Adjuvant intraperitoneal chemotherapy with carbon-adsorbed mitomycin in patients with gastric cancer: Results of a randomized multicenter trial of the Austrian Working Group for Surgical Oncology. *J Clin Oncol* 16: 2733–8.

Rossi M, Broglia L, Maccioni F. (1997) Hydro-CT in patients with gastric cancer: Preoperative radiologic staging. *Eur Radiol* 7: 659–64.

Ruddell WS, Bone ES, Hill MJ *et al.* (1978) Pathogenesis of gastric cancer in pernicious anaemia. *Lancet* 1: 521–3.

Rugge M, Farinati F, Baffa R *et al.* (1994) Gastric epithelial dysplasia in the natural history of gastric cancer: a multicenter prospective follow-up study. Interdisciplinary Group on Gastric Epithelial Dysplasia. *Gastroenterology* 107: 1288–96.

Sasajima K, Kawachi T, Matsukura N *et al.* (1979) Intestinal metaplasia and adenocarcinoma induced in the stomach of rats by N-propyl-N-nitro-N-nitrosoguanidine. *J Cancer Res Clin Oncol* 94: 201–6.

Sato T, Fukuyama T, Suzuki T *et al.* (1959) Studies of the causation of gastric cancer. 2. The relation between gastric cancer mortality rate and salted food intake in several places in Japan. *Bull Inst Public Health (Japan)* 8: 187–98.

Sautner T, Hofbauer F, Depisch D *et al.* (1994) Adjuvant intraperitoneal cisplatin chemotherapy does not improve long-term survival after surgery for advanced gastric cancer. *J Clin Oncol* 12: 970–4.

Schlemper RJ, Itabashi M, Kato Y *et al.* (1997) Differences in diagnostic criteria for gastric carcinoma between Japanese and western pathologists. *Lancet* 349: 1725–9.

Schiessel R, Funovics J, Schick B *et al.* (1989) Adjuvant intraperitoneal cisplatin therapy in patients with operated gastric carcinoma: Results of a randomized trial. *Acta Med Austriaca* 16: 68–9.

Schlag P, Bockler R, Ulrich H *et al.* (1980) Are nitrite and N-nitroso compounds in gastric juice risk factors for carcinoma in the operated stomach? *Lancet* 1: 727–9.

Schorah CJ, Sobala GM, Sanderson M, Collis N, Primrose JN. (1991) Gastric juice ascorbic acid: effects of disease and implications for gastric carcinogenesis. *Am J Clin Nutr* 53 (Suppl): 287–293S.

Shimizu S, Uchiyama A, Mizumoto K *et al.* (2000) Laparoscopically assisted distal gastrectomy for early gastric cancer. *Surg Endosc* 14: 27–31.

Shimoyama T, Fukuda S, Tanaka M, Nakaji S, Munakata A. (2000) Evaluation of the applicability of the gastric carcinoma risk index for intestinal type cancer in Japanese patients infected with *Helicobacter pylori*. *Virchows Arch* 436: 585–7.

Shin WS, Kang MW, Kang JH *et al.* (1996) Epstein–Barr virus-associated gastric adenocarcinomas among Koreans. *Am J Clin Pathol* 105: 174–81.

Siewert JR, Bottcher K, Roder JD, Busch R, Hermanek P, Meyer HJ. (1993) Prognostic relevance of systematic lymph node dissection in gastric carcinoma. German Gastric Carcinoma Study Group. *Br J Surg* 80: 1015–8.

Siewert JR, Kestlmeier R, Busch R *et al.* (1996) Benefits of D2 lymph node dissection for patients with gastric cancer and pN0 and pN1 lymph node metastases. *Br J Surg* 83: 1144–7.

Siewert JR, Bottcher K, Stein HJ, Roder JD. (1998) Relevant prognostic factors in gastric cancer: ten-year results of the German Gastric Cancer Study. *Ann Surg* 228: 449–61.

Sobala GM, O'Connor HJ, Dewar EP, King RF, Axon AT, Dixon MF. (1993) Bile reflux and intestinal metaplasia in gastric mucosa. *J Clin Pathol* 46: 235–40.

Sobin LH, Wittekind CH, eds. (2002) *TNM Classification Of Malignant Tumors*, 6th edn. Wiley-Liss, New York.

Stell D, Carter C, Stewart I. (1996) Prospective comparison of laparoscopy, ultrasonography and computed tomography in the staging of gastric cancer. *Br J Surg* 83: 1260–2.

Stewart HL. (1967) Experimental alimentary tract cancer. *NCI Monogr* 25: 199–217.

Tada M, Murata M, Takemoto T *et al.* (1994) Development of 'strip-off' biopsy. *Gastroenterol Endosc* 26: 833–9.

Takahashi M, Kokubo T, Furukawa F *et al.* (1984) Effects of sodium chloride, saccharin, phenobarbital and aspirin on gastric carcinogenesis by N-methyl-N-Nitro-N-nitrogoguanidine. *Gann* 75: 494–501.

Takahashi Y, Takeuchi T, Sakamoto J *et al.* Tumor Marker Committee. (2003) The usefulness of CEA and/or CA19-9 in monitoring for recurrence in gastric cancer patients: a prospective clinical study. *Gastric Cancer* 6: 142–5.

Talley NJ, Zinsmeister AR, Weaver A *et al.* (1991) Gastric adenocarcinoma and *Helicobacter pylori* infection. *J Natl Cancer Inst* 83: 1734–9.

Tatematsu M, Takahashi M, Hanaouchi M, Shirai T. (1975) Effects in rats of sodium chloride on experimental gastric cancers induced by N-methyl-N-nitro-N-nitrogoguanidine or 4-nitroquinoline-1-oxide. *J Natl Cancer Inst* 55: 101–6.

Tatsuta M, Lishi H, Nakaizumi A *et al.* (1993) Fundal atrophic gastritis as a risk factor for gastric cancer. *Int J Cancer* 53: 70–4.

Thye T, Burchard GD, Nilius M, Muller-Myhsok B, Horstmann RD. (2003) Genomewide linkage analysis identifies polymorphism in the human interferon-gamma receptor affecting *Helicobacter pylori* infection. *Am J Hum Genet* 72: 448–53.

Tsugane ZS, Tei Y, Takahashi T, Watanabe S, Sugano K. (1994) Salty food intake and risk of *Helicobacter pylori* infection. *Jpn J Cancer Res* 85: 474–8.

Watanabe H. (1978) Experimentally induced intestinal metaplasia in Wistar rats by X-ray irradiation. *Gastroenterology* 75: 796–9.

Weber KJ, Reyes CD, Gagner M, Divino CM. (2003) Comparison of laparoscopic and open gastrectomy for malignant disease. *Surg Endosc* 17: 968–71.

Welvaart K, de Jong PL. (1986) Palliation of patients with carcinoma of the lower esophagus and cardia: the question of quality of life. *J Surg Oncol* 32: 197–9.

Wong BCY, Lam SK, Ching CK *et al.* (1999) Differential *Helicobacter pylori* infection rates in two contrasting gastric cancer risk regions of South China. *J Gastroenterol Hepatol* 14: 120–5.

World Health Organization. (1990) *Cancer pain relief and palliative care: report of a WHO expert committee.* Technical Report Series no. 804. World Health Organization, Geneva, Switzerland.

Wynder EL, Kmet J, Dungal N *et al.* (1963) An epidemiologic investigation of gastric cancer. *Cancer* 16: 1461–96.

Yamao T, Kai S, Kazami A *et al.* (1999) Tumor markers CEA, CA19-9 and CA125 in monitoring of response to systemic chemotherapy in patients with advanced gastric cancer. *Jpn J Clin Oncol* 29: 550–5.

Ychou M, Duffour J, Kramar A, Gourgou S, Grenier J. (2000) Clinical significance and prognostic value of CA72-4 compared with CEA and CA19-9 in patients with gastric cancer. *Dis Markers* 16: 105–10.

Yokota T, Kunii Y, Teshima S *et al.* (1999) Significant prognostic factors in patients with node-negative gastric cancer. *Int Surg* 84: 331–6.

Yokota T, Kunii Y, Teshima S *et al.* (2000) Significant prognostic factors in patients with early gastric cancer. *Int Surg* 85: 286–90.

You WC, Blot WJ, Li JY. (1993) Precancerous gastric lesions in a population at high risk of stomach cancer. *Cancer Res* 53: 1317–21.

You WC, Zhang L, Gail MH *et al.* (1998) Precancerous lesions in two counties of China with contrasting gastric cancer risk. *Int J Epidemiol* 27: 945–8.

Yu W, Whang I, Suh I *et al.* (1998) Prospective randomized trial of early postoperative intraperitoneal chemotherapy as an adjuvant to resectable gastric cancer. *Ann Surg* 228: 347–54.

Zhao L, Blot WJ, Liu W-D *et al.* (1994) Familial predisposition to precancerous gastric lesions in a high-risk area of China. *Cancer Epidemiol Biomarkers Prev* 3: 461–4.

8 Small Bowel Tumors

Edited by Nadir Arber

Diagnosis

Epidemiology

Kerin Adelson, Eyal Sagiv, Nadir Arber & Alfred I. Neugut

Introduction

Relative to other cancers of the gastrointestinal tract, small bowel cancers are extremely rare. They make up only 2% of all gastrointestinal malignancies and only 0.39% of all cancers in the US (Ries *et al.* 2006; Jemal *et al.* 2007). It is estimated that in 2007 there will be 5640 new cases and 1090 deaths due to cancer of the small intestine in the United States, making it one of the rarest types of cancer (Ries *et al.* 2006; Jemal *et al.* 2007). Its low incidence is especially interesting when one considers that the small bowel contains 90% of the mucosal surface area of the alimentary tract, 75% of its length, and lies between the stomach and large bowel, two organs whose cancer incidence and mortality significantly impact the worldwide cancer burden (Lowenfels 1973; Weiss & Yang 1987; Ross *et al.* 1991; Schottenfeld 1996; Neugut *et al.* 1997, 1998). Its importance, therefore, is specifically related to its infrequency. By determining the specific molecular, genetic, and biologic processes that lead to its low incidence and mortality, new preventive strategies could theoretically be devised and applied to other cancers.

However, disappointingly little has been done to study this potentially important tumor. The reasons for this are multifactorial. Because small bowel adenocarcinoma is so rare, it is difficult to amass enough cases to study. In addition epidemiologic researchers and molecular biologists have often failed to see the valuable information such a rare tumor could provide in terms of cancer prevention and processes of carcinogenesis.

Gastrointestinal Oncology: A Critical Multidisciplinary Team Approach.
Edited by J. Jankowski, R. Sampliner, D. Kerr, and Y. Fong.
© 2008 Blackwell Publishing, ISBN: 978-1-4501-2783-7

Descriptive epidemiology

According to recent data from the National Cancer Institute's Surveillance, Epidemiology and End-Results (SEER) registries, the annual age-adjusted incidence rate of small bowel cancer in the US is 1.8/100,000 men and women per year based on cases diagnosed between 2000 and 2003 in 17 SEER geographic areas (Ries *et al.* 2006). The median age of death from cancer of the small intestine is 72 years, with an age-adjusted death rate of 0.4/100,000. It affects males slightly more often than females and the mean age at diagnosis is 57 years with a median age of 67 years (Ries *et al.* 2006). As stated in the Introduction, it is estimated that in 2007 there will be 5640 new cases of small bowel cancer in the US, and 1090 deaths (Jemal *et al.* 2007). This can be contrasted with 21,260 new cases of gastric cancer and 153,760 new cases of colorectal cancer during the same period (Jemal *et al.* 2007).

To summarize briefly, small bowel cancer has four major histologic subtypes: adenocarcinoma, neuroendocrine tumor, gastrointestinal stromal tumor (GIST), and lymphoma. The incidence of small bowel adenocarcinoma tends to be higher in industrialized Western countries than in non-industrialized developing world countries. The average major medical center can expect to see two to four cases of small bowel adenocarcinoma per year (Neugut *et al.* 1998). A predominance of the descriptive and analytic epidemiology that has been published regarding small bowel cancer has not been categorized by histologic subtype. Consequently, data have been mingled for a variety of tumors that may or may not share common features. Because certain tumors are more likely to arise in certain anatomic designations, some reviews have been divided by subsite. While it is true that adenocarcinomas are often found in the duodenum, particularly in proximity to the ampulla of Vater, carcinoids and lymphomas tend to arise in the ileum or jejunum, and sarcomas are evenly spread throughout the small bowel.

An important paper by Lowenfels in 1973 showed a strong association between the international distributions of small bowel and large bowel cancer (Lowenfels 1973), but data from the 1990s suggest a much weaker association (Neugut *et al.*

1998). Several North American population studies provide most of the data on small bowel cancer rates (see Table 8.1). From 1965 to the 1990s, the overall incidence of small bowel cancer was approximately 10–14 cases per million people per year, with adenocarcinoma being the predominant subtype. According to these registries, the incidence ranges from 3.0 cases per million to 6.5 cases per million per year, and mortality rates have generally been about one-fourth of the incidence rates. In their experience with the German Cancer Registry, Stang *et al.* (1999) found the age-standardized incidence rate of small bowel cancer to be 3.3–6.2 cases per million per year.

Adenocarcinoma makes up 40–50% of small bowel cancers in North America and Europe, making it the most common subtype in industrialized countries. The tumor originates from small bowel enterocytes (Weiss & Yang 1987; Ross *et al.* 1991; Chow *et al.* 1993; Gabos *et al.* 1993; DiSario *et al.* 1994; Severson *et al.* 1996; Neugut *et al.* 1998; Stang *et al.* 1999).

Table 8.1 Population-based studies of small bowel cancer incidence and histology.

Population, period (reference)	Histology	n (%)	Incidence per million per year
Los Angeles County, 1972–1985 (Ross *et al.* 1991)	Adenocarcinoma	446 (37.5)	
	Carcinoid	503 (42.3)	
	Sarcoma	152 (12.8)	
	Lymphoma	89 (7.5)	
	Total*	1190	
Nine SEER Registries, 1973–1982 (Weiss & Yang 1987)	Adenocarcinoma	732 (40.0)	3.9
	Carcinoid	542 (29.6)	2.9
	Sarcoma	232 (12.7)	1.2
	Lymphoma	312 (17.0)	1.6
	Total*	1832	9.6
Cancer Registries of Western Canada, 1966–1990 (Gabos *et al.* 1993)	Adenocarcinoma	521 (41.9)	
	Carcinoid	334 (26.8)	
	Sarcoma	140 (11.3)	
	Lymphoma	244 (19.6)	
	Total*	1244	11.0
Utah Cancer Registry, 1966–1990 (DiSario *et al.* 1994)	Adenocarcinoma	80 (24.4)	3.0
	Carcinoid	136 (41.3)	6.5
	Sarcoma	36 (11.0)	1.5
	Lymphoma	72 (22.0)	2.5
	Total*	328	14.0
Nine SEER Registries, 1973–1991 (Severson *et al.* 1996)	Adenocarcinoma	1609	6.5
	Carcinoid	1683	6.5
	Total*	†3292	13.0

* Total includes other histologies.
† Excludes lymphomas and sarcomas.

Epidemiology of adenocarcinoma

Adenocarcinoma of the small bowel occurs most frequently within the duodenum (49% of cases), particularly around the ampulla of Vater, and with decreasing frequency in the jejunum (21%), and ileum (15%) (Dabaja *et al.* 2004; Haselkorn *et al.* 2005). One exception is in Crohn's-associated cases, where 70% present in the ileum.

We have previously noted an overlap in the epidemiology of adenocarcinomas of the large and small bowel (see Table 8.2) (Neugut *et al.* 1998). The risk of both small and large bowel cancers is increased in the setting of Crohn's disease and familial adenomatous polyposis (FAP). Here, they tend to present at a younger age than in the general population. People with a history of adenoma are at increased risk of small bowel adenocarcinoma. In addition, there is an elevated risk of small bowel adenocarcinoma in large bowel cancer survivors and vice versa. Small bowel adenocarcinomas occur at 1/50th the rate of large bowel adenocarcinomas, but share the same geographic and international distribution, occurring with greater frequency in Western countries and much less often in the developing world (Lowenfels 1973). Finally, both tumors seem to arise from adenomatous polyps and evolve into carcinoma (Sellner 1990), though this is still under study in the small bowel.

Given the shared epidemiology of small and large bowel carcinoma, it is odd that small bowel adenocarcinomas tend to arise from the proximal, gastric end of the small intestine rather than the distal, large bowel end. This pattern has triggered much speculation in the literature, particularly by Lowenfels, about the role that bile and/or its metabolites may play in the development of small bowel carcinoma (Lowenfels 1978; Ross *et al.* 1991; Chen *et al.* 1994).

Sex differences

Most studies have demonstrated that males have higher small

Table 8.2 Risk factors for adenocarcinoma of the small bowel and large bowel (modified from Neugut *et al.* 1998).

Risk factor	Small bowel	Large bowel
Adenomas	+++	+++
FAP	++	++++
Crohn's disease	++++	+/++
Other GI tract cancer	+++	+++
Animal fat intake	+	++
Smoking	++	+/++
Alcohol use	+/++	?
Radiation exposure	+	?
Cholecystectomy	+	+

Number of plus signs refers to strength and/or consistency of association.

bowel cancer incidence rates than females (Weiss & Yang 1987; Ross *et al.* 1991; Chow *et al.* 1993; Gabos *et al.* 1993; DiSario *et al.* 1994; Severson *et al.* 1996; Neugut *et al.* 1998; Stang *et al.* 1999) (see Table 8.3). For the most part, this gender distribution has been similar in international studies (Parkin *et al.* 1993; Neugut *et al.* 1997), and holds true for colorectal and gastric cancer (Ries *et al.* 1996) as well. Our own study of small bowel cancer incidence (Chow *et al.* 1996) utilizing SEER data found similar results. Interestingly, when studied, males appear to have a higher incidence of all four of the main histological subgroups of small bowel cancer.

Racial differences

Black people have almost twice the incidence of small bowel adenocarcinoma as white people. Haselkorn's group reports that there were 10.6 cases per million among black people compared to 5.6 per million among white people (Haselkorn *et al.* 2005). There have been no large-scale studies that break down the incidence of small bowel cancer by race. Blacks may have a somewhat higher incidence than whites according to US population-based studies (see Table 8.3). Specifically, the Los Angeles County Cancer Surveillance Program found age-adjusted small bowel cancer incidence rates of 1.5/100,000/year for black males as compared to 0.9/100,000/year for white males, and a similar ratio of 1.0/100,000/year for black females as compared to 0.6/100,000/year for white females. When they looked specifically at adenocarcinoma rates, they found a similar pattern (Ross *et al.* 1991).

Time trends

Four studies have used SEER data spanning 1973 until the present to study the time trends for small bowel malignancies (Weiss & Yang 1987; Chow *et al.* 1996; Severson *et al.* 1996). From 1973 through 1982, the rates of small bowel cancer, and specifically adenocarcinoma, were stable. From 1983 to 1993, the incidence rate increased from 1.2 to 1.6/100,000 among white males, from 0.8 to 1.1/100,000 among white females, from 1.8 to 2.4 among black males, and from 1.3 to 2.0/100,000 among black females (see Table 8.3). The SEER data for 2000–2003 showed still increasing incidence rates of 2.0/100,000 among white males, and 1.4/100,000 among white females, and 3.9/100,000 among black males and 2.6/100,000 among black females. SEER data show an increase of 2.6% in the total joinpoint trend with associated annual percentage change for incidence of small cancer of the small intestine from 1975 to 2003 (Ries *et al.* 2006). This was the same for all races, and both males and females. Among all groups the mortality rate increased from 1975 to 1995, but subsequently decreased from 1995 to 2003.

Table 8.3 Age-adjusted incidence rate of small bowel cancer per 100,000 population by race and sex, SEER, 1973–2003 (Uppaputhangkule *et al.* 1976; Neugut *et al.* 1998; Ries *et al.* 2006).

	1973	1983	1993	2003
White males	0.9	1.2	1.6	2
White females	0.7	0.8	1.1	1.4
Black males	1.8	1.8	2.4	3.9
Black females	1.2	1.3	2.0	2.6

Haselkorn's group using SEER data from 1973 to 2000 reports average annual small bowel adenocarcinoma rates adjusted to the US population in 2000: 6.9/1,000,000 among white males, 4.7/1,000,000 among white females, 12.1/1,000,000 among black males, and 9.5/1,000,000 among black females (Haselkorn *et al.* 2005). The incidence of all types of small bowel cancer has increased most rapidly in black people, by 120% over the 28-year period (Haselkorn *et al.* 2005).

Age distribution

In most studies the mean age at diagnosis of small bowel carcinoma has been approximately 60 years of age (Schottenfeld 1996; Neugut *et al.* 1997, 1998). Recent SEER data report a median age of diagnosis of 67 years (Ries *et al.* 2006). Like most cancers, the incidence increases with age. In population studies that break down incidence by histologic subtypes, it appears that adenocarcinomas present at a somewhat older age than the other subtypes (Weiss & Yang 1987; Ross *et al.* 1991; Gabos *et al.* 1993; DiSario *et al.* 1994; Severson *et al.* 1996).

Crohn's disease

Since 1956, when Crohn's disease was first identified as a risk factor for small bowel adenocarcinoma, over 100 cases have been reported in the medical literature (Ginzburg *et al.* 1956, Michelassi *et al.* 1993). While most small bowel adenocarcinomas occur in the duodenum, Crohn's-associated adenocarcinomas tend to occur in the ileum (Michelassi *et al.* 1993). These generally arise after a latency period of about 20 years from the initial Crohn's diagnosis. Interestingly, this is similar to the latency period from the diagnosis of ulcerative colitis to the development of large bowel adenocarcinoma.

A Danish cohort study of 373 patients diagnosed with Crohn's disease between 1962 and 1987 and followed for 10–15 years found two cases of small bowel cancer in the ileum (Munkholm *et al.* 1993). According to this study, 0.04 cases would have been expected using general population incidence rates. Thus, they found that people with Crohn's had a relative risk of 50 (95% CI 37.1–65.9) for small bowel adenocarcinoma. A retrospective cohort study from Stockholm (Persson *et al.* 1994) found a relative risk of 15.6 (95% CI 4.3–40.1) for development of small bowel adenocarcinoma among patients with Crohn's disease. A study by Darke concluded that there is a 0.3% probability of

Crohn's disease and small bowel cancer occurring in the same individual (Darke *et al.* 1973).

In a small case–control study at Columbia Presbyterian Medical Center in New York, we compared 19 small bowel adenocarcinoma cases from 1980 to 1987 to 52 control patients undergoing benign non-GI surgical procedures, like herniorrhaphy and transurethral resection of the prostate (Chen *et al.* 1994). Of the 19 adenocarcinoma cases, four were in the ileum and, of these, three were associated with previous Crohn's disease. Looking at 17 carcinoid tumors, we found that 14 of 17 were in the ileum but none occurred in the context of previous Crohn's disease. Comparing 7 patients with Crohn's disease that progressed to adenocarcinoma to 28 age- and sex-matched Crohn's patients who did not develop a malignancy, Lashner identified several risk factors including treatment with 6-mercaptopurine, and occupational exposure to aromatic compounds or other potential carcinogens (OR 20.3, 95% CI 2.7–150.5) (Lashner 1992).

A multicenter European study, which compared 70 histologically confirmed cases of small bowel adenocarcinoma to 2070 controls, identified two cases associated with Crohn's disease (OR 53.6, 95% CI 6–477) (Kaerlev *et al.* 2001).

Adenomas

Similar to the adenoma–carcinoma sequence that characterizes the development of large bowel adenocarcinoma, Sellner (1990) has found circumstantial evidence suggesting an adenoma–carcinoma sequence for cancer of the small intestine. For both large and small bowel cancers: the average age of patients with carcinoma is several years older than those with adenomas; carcinoma is often found in physical proximity to adenomatous tissue; the risk of invasive carcinoma correlates with the site, size, and villous histology of small bowel adenomas; there are similar male/female ratios for the incidence of small bowel adenomas and adenocarcinomas; small bowel adenomas and carcinomas have similar international prevalence variations. There are three case reports that describe small bowel adenomas which were pathologically diagnosed and subsequently left *in situ*. One of these progressed to adenocarcinoma (Greenwald *et al.* 1962; Uppaputhangkule *et al.* 1976; Hessler & Braunstein 1978). A 1999 Finnish study looked at 98 patients with familial adenomatous polyposis (FAP) who underwent upper endoscopy (Heiskanen *et al.* 1999). They detected duodenal adenomas in 78 patients (80%). In 71 patients who underwent repeat endoscopy, the stage of adenomatosis progressed in 52 (73%).

Cancer syndromes

Small bowel adenocarcinoma is one of the malignancies associated with FAP syndrome (Jagelman *et al.* 1988; Spigelman *et al.* 1989, 1990, 1994; Offerhaus *et al.* 1992; Nugent *et al.* 1994). Similar to the large bowel mucosa, these patients tend to develop multiple adenomas in the small bowel, and these tend to cluster in the duodenum. In the Finnish study mentioned previously, the cumulative risks of stage IV adenomatosis and duodenal carcinoma were 30% and 4%, respectively (Heiskanen *et al.* 1999). A 1988 study showed that 2.9% of FAP patients developed periampullary carcinoma of the small intestine, making it the most common extracolonic malignancy among these patients (Jagelman *et al.* 1988). Among 1262 FAP patients followed at St. Mark's Hospital in London, 47 (3.7%) developed duodenal cancer. Periampullary carcinoma was the most common cause of death among these patients (Spigelman *et al.* 1994). Interestingly, one study found that bile from 29 patients with FAP was more mutagenic than bile from 24 patients without FAP (Spigelman *et al.* 1990).

Offerhaus and his colleagues at Johns Hopkins (Baltimore, MD) followed FAP patients for 18,679 person-years and found 11 cases of duodenal and ampullary adenocarcinoma (Offerhaus *et al.* 1992). In their population, there was a relative risk for duodenal adenocarcinoma of >300, a relative risk for ampullary adenocarcinoma of 123.7 (95% CI 33.7–316.7), and no elevation in risk for gastric or non-duodenal small bowel cancers.

As with FAP, an increased risk of small bowel adenocarcinoma is seen in other genetic cancer syndromes, including hereditary non-polyposis colorectal cancer (HNPCC) (Spigelman *et al.* 1990; Offerhaus *et al.* 1992) and Peutz–Jeghers syndrome (Schottenfeld *et al.* 1996). Studies have suggested that HNPCC patients have a lifetime risk of 1% for small bowel adenocarcinoma.

Prior colon cancer

Patients in the general population with a history of prior colorectal cancer have a higher risk of small bowel adenocarcinoma. Specifically, Neugut and Santos found a standardized incidence ratio of 7.1 (95% CI 4.7–10.3) in males and 9.0 (95% CI 6.0–12.9) in females (Neugut & Santos 1993). Interestingly, the reverse scenario is also true: patients with a history of small bowel adenocarcinoma have an elevated risk of developing colorectal cancer. The risk ratios are similar. Patients with small bowel carcinoids did not have a higher risk of colorectal cancer or other malignancies. These data reinforce the finding that adenocarcinoma of the small and large bowel have similar epidemiology.

Other medical conditions

As already mentioned, some studies have suggested that bile concentrated in the periampullary region of the duodenum contributes to the development of small bowel adenocarcinoma (Lowenfels 1978; Ross *et al.* 1991). Three of 19 adenocarcinoma cases in a small case–control trial by Chen *et al.* (1994) occurred in patients with a previous cholecystectomy, while none of the 52 patients in the control group had a cholecystectomy ($p = 0.004$). The same investigators found that 2 of the 19 adenocarcinoma cases had a prior history of peptic ulcer disease, while none of the 52 controls did ($p = 0.02$) (Chen *et al.* 1994). Twelve years before the findings of that case–control study, Lightdale *et al.* (1982) speculated that the alkaline environment of the small bowel as compared to the stomach and other portions of the GI tract account for its low cancer rates.

Cystic fibrosis has also been associated with small bowel adenocarcinoma. Several case reports have suggested that it increases the risk of ileal adenocarcinoma. A cohort study looked at 412 cystic fibrosis patients and found one case of small bowel adenocarcinoma. Only 0.001 cases would have been expected in the general population ($p = 0.003$) (Sheldon *et al.* 1993). Conversely, a larger retrospective cohort study followed 28,511 cystic fibrosis patients for 7 years and found only two small bowel cancers (Neglia *et al.* 1995).

Celiac sprue has also been associated with small bowel cancer (Begos *et al.* 1995; Kaerlev *et al.* 2001).

Radiation therapy

One large cohort study compared close to 50,000 women treated for cervical cancer with radiation therapy, to 16,713 women treated for cervical cancer without radiation therapy. Among those who received radiation, they found a relative risk of 1.8 for small bowel cancer (95% CI 1.1–2.0). The study did not define the histologic subtypes of small bowel cancer (Kleinerman *et al.* 1995).

Diet

One study, by Chow *et al.* (1993) compared dietary and other lifestyle habits reported by the next of kin of 430 patients who died of small bowel adenocarcinoma to 921 controls who died of other causes . They found a statistically significant odds ratios of 2–3 for diets heavy in red meat and salt-cured/smoked foods. They derived their data from the 1986 National Mortality Follow-Back Survey of the National Center for Health Statistics, a survey which used a probability sample of 1% of US deaths for 1986. Unfortunately, this large small bowel cancer study did not break down the small bowel cancer cases into histologic subtypes.

In a population-based case–control study (Wu *et al.* 1997), Wu compared 36 small bowel adenocarcinoma cases with 998 population controls. They used interviews to obtain information on dietary risk factors and found a non-statistically significant association between small bowel cancer and the intake of fried, smoked, or barbecued meat and fish. They also found an increased risk of small bowel cancer with intake of sugar in the form of non-alcoholic beverages (OR 3.3, 95% CI 1.2–9.4).

Another report describes the results of two case–control studies from six Italian centers between 1985 and 1996 (Negri *et al.* 1999) designed to identify risk factors for small bowel adenocarcinoma. These investigators compared 23 small bowel adenocarcinoma patients to 230 controls and found an increased risk with diets high in bread, pasta or rice (OR 3.8), sugar (OR 2.9) and red meat (OR 4.6), and decreased risk with diets high in coffee (OR 0.4), fish (OR 0.3), vegetables (OR 0.3) and fruit (OR 0.6). Interestingly, these are risk factors similar to those that have often been associated with carcinoma of the large bowel.

An ecologic study of small bowel cancer mortality found a correlation coefficient of 0.61 ($p < 0.005$) with per capita daily animal fat consumption, and 0.75 ($p < 0.001$) with per capita daily animal protein consumption (Lowenfels & Sonni 1977).

Obesity

Obesity may be associated with an increased risk of small bowel adenocarcinoma. A cohort study looked at cancer rates among 4 million obese veterans in the US. They found an overall RR of 1.6 (95% CI 1.2–2.1) of small bowel cancer among obese white men compared to non-obese white men, and a non-significant increased risk among obese black men (Samanic *et al.* 2004).

Tobacco and alcohol

Chow and her colleagues (1993) did not find an increased risk of small bowel cancer among alcohol and tobacco users. As already stated, this study did not break down analysis by histologic subtype. Similarly, the Italian case–control study (Negri *et al.* 1999) did not find an association between tobacco and alcohol use and the development of small bowel adenocarcinoma. Conversely, a small case–control medical record review study by Chen *et al.* (1994) found that smoking (OR 6.2, 95% CI 1.5–26.7) and alcohol consumption (OR 5.5, 95% CI 1.4–21.4) both increased risk of small bowel adenocarcinoma. Similar results were obtained by Wu *et al.* (1997) who found an odds ratio of 2.9 (95% CI 1.2–7.1) with ethanol intake, and a non-significant association with smoking (OR 2.1, 95% CI 0.8–5.1). A European multicenter case–control study published in 2000 looked at 70 cases of pathologically confirmed small bowel adenocarcinoma and compared them to 2070 age, sex, and geographically matched controls (Kaerlev *et al.* 2000). They found that a high intake of beer (OR 3.5, 95% CI 1.5–8) or strong alcohol (OR 3.4, 95% CI 1.3–9.2) were associated with small bowel adenocarcinoma. Interestingly, there was no association with wine intake and small bowel adenocarcinoma. The authors speculated that wine may have protective benefits that counterbalanced the carcinogenic effects of the alcohol. They did not find a statistically significant association between tobacco use and small bowel adenocarcinoma.

Occupational exposure

A European case–control study compared 107 cases of small bowel adenocarcinoma to 3915 controls and correlated risk with occupation (Wu *et al.* 1997). Among women, they found a higher risk for general farmers, dry cleaners and launderers, textile workers, dockers, and housekeeping service workers. Among men, they found building caretakers and welders had significantly increased risk.

Gastrointestinal stromal tumors (GISTs)

GISTs are the mesenchymal tumors of the gut, commonly located in the stomach or small intestine, and are thus usually small, hard, and well circumscribed, with central ulceration. They may be benign or malignant. In nearly 90–95% of cases, GISTs express a mutant c-KIT (CD117) protein (Miettinen *et al.* 2006b; Ferrucci & Zucca 2007). Before recent advances in immunohistochemistry that have allowed the molecular characterization of mutant c-KIT, the tumor was often hard to definitively diagnose. Consequently, the epidemiologic data describing its incidence and geographic distribution were, until recently, relatively uncharacterized. However, modern innovations in diagnostic techniques have led to several recent studies that better characterize this tumor.

In a population-based study of 1458 malignant GISTs in the US, Tran *et al.* (2005) using SEER data, calculated an age-adjusted yearly incidence rate of 0.68 cases per 100,000 people per year. A study by Kindblom (2003) suggests that the incidence rate is higher in Sweden (1.3 cases per 100,000 people per year). In the Tran study, there were significant racial differences in GIST incidence rates. African-Americans had the highest incidence rate at 1.16/100,000, compared to only 0.6/100,000 among Caucasian Americans. It is slightly less common in women than men (Tran *et al.* 2005; Miettinen *et al.* 2006a). The mean reported age at presentation is 62.9. GIST is rare before the age of 50 (Tran *et al.* 2005; Miettinen *et al.* 2006a), although the disease is found in any age group including children and young adults. The Tran study reported that 51% of GIST cases were diagnosed in the stomach, 36% in the small intestine, 7% in the colon, 5% in the rectum, and 1% in the esophagus. Other studies have reported similar regional prevalences, with the majority of cases arising in the stomach, and an additional 25–36% arising in the small intestine (DeMatteo *et al.* 2000; Kindblom 2003).

Nearly all GIST cases are sporadic. Increased incidence was seen in patients with neurofibromatosis type 1 (NF1), and about 5% of GIST cases are multiple. Out of 906 patients with jejunoileal GISTs, 38 patients had NF1 (Ferrucci & Zucca 2007). Twenty-three of them (60%) developed multiple small tumors. Rare familial forms of GIST are associated with a germline mutation in KIT (Ginzburg *et al.* 1956) or rarely PDGFR-α (Chompret *et al.* 2004).

Primary lymphomas

Lymphomas, primary or secondary, account for 5–20% of all small bowel malignancies. A doubling in its incidence rate has been seen in the last two decades in the US due to an increase in predisposing conditions such as immune-compromised state. Up to 40% of lymphomas arise in sites other than the lymph nodes and the gut is the most common extralymphatic site. The genotype of these tumors differs from the genotype of lymphomas arising in lymph node tissue. Four different types of lymphoma may be found in the small bowel: celiac-associated T-cell high-grade lymphoma, Burkitt-type lymphoma, maltoma and Mediterranean lymphoma.

Celiac-associated T-cell high-grade lymphoma

Enteropathy-associated T-cell lymphoma (EATL) is a rare form of high-grade, T-cell non-Hodgkin's lymphoma (NHL) of the upper small intestine that is associated with celiac disease. In approximately 80% of refractory celiac disease cases, an abnormal clonal IEL (intraepithelial lymphocyte) cell population is diffusely present throughout the gastrointestinal tract. These cells are characterized by a low ratio of CD8+/CD3+ and TCR-γ gene rearrangement (Catassi *et al.* 2005).

The mechanisms responsible for the development of malignancies in patients with celiac disease are not known. The following inciting factors have been suggested:

1 increased intestinal permeability to environmental carcinogens
2 chronic inflammation
3 chronic antigenic stimulation
4 release of proinflammatory cytokines
5 immune surveillance problems
6 nutritional deficiencies caused by the disease or the gluten-free diet.

Refractory celiac disease is strongly associated with partial trisomy of the 1q region (Verkarre *et al.* 2003).

Burkitt-type lymphoma of the small intestine

Burkitt's lymphoma is an aggressive type of B-cell lymphoma characterized by a high rate of malignant cell proliferation (indicated by ki-67 expression) and by morphologic features that are distinct from diffuse large B-cell lymphoma. It has both endemic and sporadic types, and can be seen in the setting of AIDS or chronic immunosuppression. Because their treatment differs, it is critical to differentiate Burkitt's lymphoma from other B-cell malignancies. Burkitt's lymphoma requires higher doses of chemotherapy. In addition, because Burkitt's lymphoma has a high rate of CNS involvement, it requires agents that can cross the blood–brain barrier.

More than 90% of Burkitt's lymphoma have translocations involving the *c-myc* oncogene. In the well known 8,14 chromosome translocation, *c-myc* is juxtaposed to the immunoglobulin heavy-chain loci. This leads to deregulation and overactivation of the *c-myc* gene (Dalla-Favera *et al.* 1983).

Maltoma

In 1983, Isaacson and Wright (Isaacson & Wright 1983) introduced the term 'maltoma' to characterize primary low-grade gastric B-cell lymphoma and immunoproliferative small intestinal disease. Subsequently, the definition of maltoma was extended to include several other extranodal low-grade B-cell non-Hodgkin's lymphomas. These displayed a similar histology to Payer's patches of the salivary gland, lung, thyroid, and stomach. The gastric form is the most common and best characterized maltoma (Lee *et al.* 2004). The cells are small, and characterized by condensed nuclear chromatin and a low proliferative rate. They tend to stay localized in the mucosal wall without involvement of regional lymph nodes. A more recent study by Parsonnet and Isaacson (2004) ties this type of malignancy with the response to bacterial infections.

Mediterranean lymphoma

Mediterranean lymphoma is also named immunoproliferative small intestinal disease. It is an unusual intestinal B-cell lymphoma that occurs in children and young adults of Mediterranean ancestry. It is the only lymphoproliferative disease associated with a single protein abnormality (Salem & Estephan 2005). The mucosal IgA alpha heavy chain has a deletion in its variable region. Treatment with antibiotics can lead to a remission (Parsonnet & Isaacson 2004; Salem & Estephan 2005), suggesting that the proliferative burst is due to an abberant immunogenic response to bacterial infection. Lecuit *et al.* (2004) suggest that *C. jejuni* may play the same part in immunoproliferative small intestinal disease as *H. pylori* plays in gastric MALT lymphoma.

Neuroendocrine tumors

The overall incidence of all neuroendocrine tumors have been estimated to be 1–2 per 100,000 people, although in a Swedish-based study the incidence was as high as 8.4 per 100,000 people (Hemminki & Li 2001). The small intestine is the most common site for these tumors (Modlin *et al.* 2003; Maggard *et al.* 2004). They occur six times more frequently in the distal ileum (mostly located within 60 cm of the ileocecal valve) than in the jejunum. Carcinoids are slightly more prevalent in men and in particular in black males (Modlin *et al.* 2003).

Why are small bowel tumors so rare?

The small intestine is remarkably resistant to carcinogenesis. When gastric carcinoma patients who have undergone gastrojejunostomy have a recurrence, it is five times more likely to be of gastric than of jejunal origin. Conversely, when peptic ulcer patients who have undergone gastrojejunostomy have a recurrence, it is nearly always jejunal (Martin 1985). Similarly, the terminal ileum is highly resistant to tumor invasion from the proximal colon. Only 0.7% of colon cancers have a local recurrence after an ileocolic anastamosis, compared to 14% after colocolic anastamosis (Martin 1985). Differences in prevalence of changes in oncogenes and tumor suppressor genes were observed and are summarized in Table 8.5.

Several speculative theories attempt to explain the low incidence of small bowel cancer.

1 Because small intestinal mucosal cells are lost and replaced very rapidly at a rate of 1 g of intestinal mucosa every 16 minutes (Kim *et al.* 1993; Boyle & Brenner 1995), mutated cells may be shed into the intestinal lumen before a tumor develops.

2 Through apoptosis of cells that have been exposed to carcinogens, genetic mutations are quickly removed (Kim *et al.* 1993).

3 The well-developed immune network of lymphoid tissues and secretory IgA may offer protection from carcinogens. Deficiency of IgA has been associated with increased incidence of small bowel cancer (Kim *et al.* 1993).

4 The lower anaerobic and total bacterial counts in the small bowel may prevent conversion of bile acids into carcinogens (Laqueur & Matsumoto 1966; Hill *et al.* 1971; Lowenfels 1973).

5 The alkaline pH of the small bowel prevents formation of nitrosamines that appear to be carcinogenic in the acidic stomach environment (Lightdale *et al.* 1982; Potten 1984).

6 Liquified chyme may increase transit, reduce mechanical trauma, and minimize exposure to carcinogens (Lowenfels 1973; Potten 1984).

7 The small bowel has fewer stem cells that can be affected by carcinogens than the colon or the stomach (Potten 1984). Furthermore, these stem cells lie deep within the small bowel crypts where they are protected from carcinogens by layers of mucosal cells (Potten 1992).

8 The duodenum contains a water-soluble tumor-inhibiting component (Arbuna 1996).

9 The small bowel contains low levels of precarcinogen-activating enzymes (Wattenberg 1966).

None of these hypotheses has been well studied at the molecular level. For example, while the rapid turnover of small bowel mucosal cells has been put forward as an explanation for the low cancer rate, most experts feel that a high proliferation and turnover rate is directly correlated with carcinogenesis. Lipkin and others (Lipkin & Higgins 1988) have suggested that the higher cell proliferation rate in the large bowel is an inciting factor, or at least a marker for increased cancer risk.

Table 8.5 Comparison of small and large bowel tumors (Arber *et al.* 1999).

	Small bowel tumors		Large bowel tumors	
	Polyp	Adenocarcinoma	Polyp	Adenocarcinoma
Allelic loss of 5q	0	5%	40%	40%
K-*ras*	35%	40%	40%	40–50%
Allelic loss of 18q	10%	5%	40%	60%
p53	33%	47%	30%	50%
MSI	–	13%	–	15%

Endoscopy in the diagnosis of small bowel tumors

Ian M. Gralnek & Rami Eliakim

Introduction

The development of flexible endoscopy has facilitated the diagnosis, evaluation and treatment of diseases of the esophagus, stomach, duodenum, proximal jejunum, and colon. However, the small bowel, beyond the proximal jejunum, has remained an elusive anatomic location that endoscopic methods have only recently been able to begin to fully evaluate. This chapter will detail currently available endoscopic techniques, including push enteroscopy, video capsule endoscopy, double-balloon enteroscopy, and intraoperative enteroscopy for diagnosing small bowel tumors and surveillance of hereditary polyposis syndromes.

Push enteroscopy

Push enteroscopy (PE) permits evaluation of the proximal one-third of the small intestine, to a distance that is approximately 50–100 cm beyond the ligament of Treitz. Dedicated videoenteroscopes (160–220 cm in length) are commercially available, but if these instruments are not in the possession of a specific endoscopy site, then a pediatric or standard adult colonoscope can be used instead. The use of an overtube, backloaded onto the endoscope shaft, may help limit looping of the enteroscope within the stomach and facilitate deeper small bowel intubation. The diagnostic yield with PE is reported to increase with a greater depth of scope insertion. For example, using a pediatric or adult colonoscope, the reported diagnostic yields in the evaluation of obscure GI bleeding range between 13% and 38%. With the use of a dedicated videoenteroscope, reported diagnostic yield rates increase, and range between 26% and 80% (Chak *et al.* 1998; Eisen *et al.* 2001; Pennazio 2004; Gralnek 2005). Data regarding the diagnostic yield of small bowel tumors and polyps using PE are limited to studies investigating PE in the context of obscure GI bleeding, and range from 1 to 5% (Marmo *et al.* 2005; Triester *et al.* 2005). With the development of endoscopic accessories for dedicated videoenteroscopes, such as biopsy forceps, snares, thermal probes (contact and noncontact), and injection needles, PE may be preferred over alternative radiologic diagnostic modalities because of the ability to obtain tissue, perform polypectomy or hemostasis if necessary, and mark lesion sites with India ink tattoo (Pennazio 2004; Chak *et al.* 1998). PE, however, does not allow for the visualization of the entire small bowel, and severe complications, including perforation and mucosal laceration, have been reported with the use of an overtube.

Video capsule endoscopy

Video capsule endoscopy (CE) is a relatively new technology, approved by the US Food and Drug Administration in 2001, that is able to obtain endoscopic images from the entire small bowel (Lewis & Swain 2002; Lewis & Goldfarb 2003). Capsule endoscopy is safe, easy, minimally invasive, and patient-friendly, and has become a first-line tool in imaging and managing small bowel pathologies. Consequently there has been rapid uptake and wide acceptance of this revolutionary endoscopic technology for detecting small bowel abnormalities (ASGE 2006).

The Pillcam SB video capsule endoscope (Given Imaging Ltd., Yoqneam, Israel) is a wireless capsule (measuring 11 mm × 26 mm) composed of a light source, lens, complementary metal oxide semiconductor imager, battery, and a wireless transmitter (Fig. 8.1a,b). The Pillcam SB has a battery life of approximately 7–8 hours over which time the capsule captures two images per second (approximately 60,000 total images per examination) in a 140° field of view and 8 : 1 magnification (Eliakim 2006). The smooth outer coating of the capsule allows easy ingestion and prevents adhesion of intestinal contents, while the capsule moves via natural peristalsis from the mouth to the anus. Endoscopic images are transmitted via sensor arrays to a recording device worn as a belt by the patient. The recorded images are downloaded into a Reporting and Processing of Images and Data (RAPID) computer workstation, and then reviewed as a continuous video by the physician. Recently, Olympus (Olympus Corporation, Tokyo, Japan) has introduced a wireless capsule endoscope (EndoCapsule) with similar features.

The utility of CE has more than doubled the rate of detection of small bowel tumors from the precapsule endoscopy era of approximately 3% to today's 6–9% prevalence rate, when the procedure is done for obscure GI bleeding (Eliakim 2006). Small bowel tumors found in patients undergoing CE for evaluation of obscure GI bleeding are malignant in more than 50% of such cases (Bailey *et al.* 2004; DeFranchis *et al.* 2004) (Fig. 8.2a–d). Additional studies in this population are needed to better evaluate patient management and outcomes, especially survival, based upon CE findings. Capsule endoscopy is also used as a screening tool in patients with hereditary polyposis syndromes (familial adenomatous polyposis, Peutz–Jegher etc.) in which patients have increased risk for developing gastric, ampullary, and small bowel polyps and/or tumors (Barkay *et al.* 2004; Schulman *et al.* 2005; Wong *et al.* 2006) (Fig. 8.3a,b).

There are limitations with CE, including that at the present time neither biopsy, therapy, nor endoscopic marking (e.g. India ink tattooing) is possible. In addition, not all CE examinations make it to the cecum (complete small bowel examination occurs approximately 80% of the time) and in some patients, luminal debris and bubbles interfere with viewing. This has led some physicians to use PEG-based preparations, prokinetic agents, simethicone, or a combination of these products before capsule ingestion. Other limitations are that the capsule's imaging

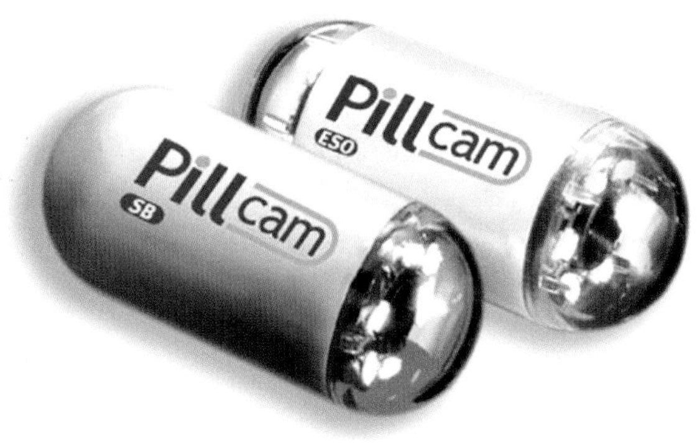

(a)

M2A
4
1
2
3
6
6
8
4
1
2
3
4
5
6
7
8
INSIDE THE M2A™ CAPSULE
1. Optical dome
2. Lens holder
3. Lens
4. Illuminating LEDs (Light Emitting Diode)
5. CMOS (Complementary Metal Oxide Semiconductor) imager
6. Battery
7. ASIC (Application Specific Integrated Circuit) transmitter
8. Antenna

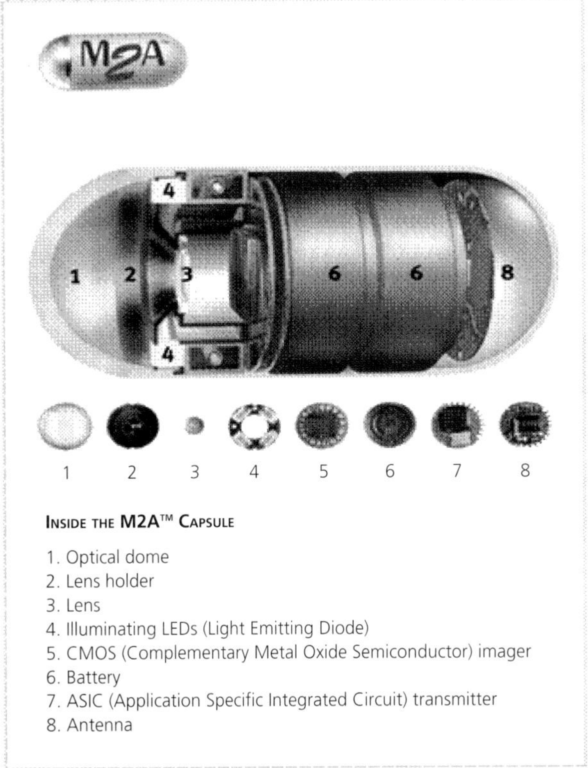

(b)

Fig. 8.1 (a,b) The Pillcam™ SB video capsule endoscope (Given Imaging Ltd, Yoqneam, Israel) is a wireless capsule (measuring 11 mm × 26 mm) composed of a light source, lens, complementary metal oxide semiconductor imager, battery, and wireless transmitter.

cannot be controlled/localized and therefore images are not viewed in real time, and some patients may not be suitable candidates for CE, including those with cardiac pacemakers, defibrillators, or suspected small bowel obstruction. Capsule retention is the major, and for all practical purposes, the only complication of CE. The reported incidence of capsule retention ranges from 0% in healthy volunteers, to up to 2% in obscure GI hemorrhage, and up to 21% in persons with suspected small bowel obstruction (Yamamoto *et al.* 2001). The retention rate in patients with small bowel tumors may be in the range of 10%.

Double-balloon enteroscopy

Double-balloon enteroscopy (DBE), initially described and reported by Yamamoto and colleagues, is a novel endoscopic insertion technique that attempts to improve upon currently available endoscopic insertion methods to evaluate the entire length of the small bowel (Yamamoto *et al.* 2001). The DBE system (Fujinon-Toshiba ES System Co., Tokyo, Japan), uses a high-resolution, dedicated video endoscope that has a working length of 200 cm and two soft, latex balloons: one balloon is attached to the tip of the endoscope and the other to the distal end of a soft, flexible overtube (Fig. 8.4a,b). The balloons can be inflated and deflated using an air pump that is controlled by the endoscopist while monitoring air pressure (Akahoshi *et al.* 2006). The balloons grip the wall of the bowel, thus allowing the endoscope to be advanced without looping. The procedure can be performed via an oral and/or transanal approach with or without fluoroscopic guidance. Choice of oral or transanal approach may be dictated by suspicion for the location of a possible tumor(s) as determined by preceding small bowel capsule endoscopy or other non-endoscopic small bowel imaging technique (Gerson 2005; Manabe *et al.* 2006).

In a peroral approach, when the two balloons reach the duodenum, the overtube balloon is inflated to fix the overtube to the small bowel wall. The overtube is thus held in place as the endoscope is inserted further. Once the tip of the endoscope is maximally inserted, the balloon on the tip of the endoscope is inflated, the balloon on the overtube is deflated, and the overtube is then advanced over the shaft of the endoscope. When the distal end of the overtube reaches the tip of the endoscope, the overtube balloon is then re-inflated, once again fixing the overtube to a second point on the small bowel wall. This sequence is repeated until the entire small bowel is evaluated or further advancement of the endoscope is difficult (Hsu *et al.* 2007).

There are two types of double balloon enteroscope available, one for general diagnostic use (EN-450P5) and one for therapeutic use (EN-450T5). The EN-450P5 is a thinner endoscope with an external diameter of 8.5 mm and maximum working channel diameter of 2.2 mm. The EN-450T5 has an external diameter of 9.4 mm and working channel of 2.8 mm (Akahoshi *et al.* 2006). DBE has been shown to be able to visualize the entire length of the small bowel and allows for biopsy, marking of lesions for subsequent surgical resection (e.g. India ink tattoo), and therapeutics.

In a recent reported retrospective case series of 152 patients evaluated by DBE for obscure GI bleeding, DBE demonstrated a bleeding site in 115 patients (75.7%), of which 45 (39.1%) were small bowel tumors (Sun *et al.* 2006). Double-balloon enteroscopy findings impacted patient management, with 39 (86.6%) of these small bowel tumor patients undergoing surgical resection of the tumor. In a prospective study evaluating

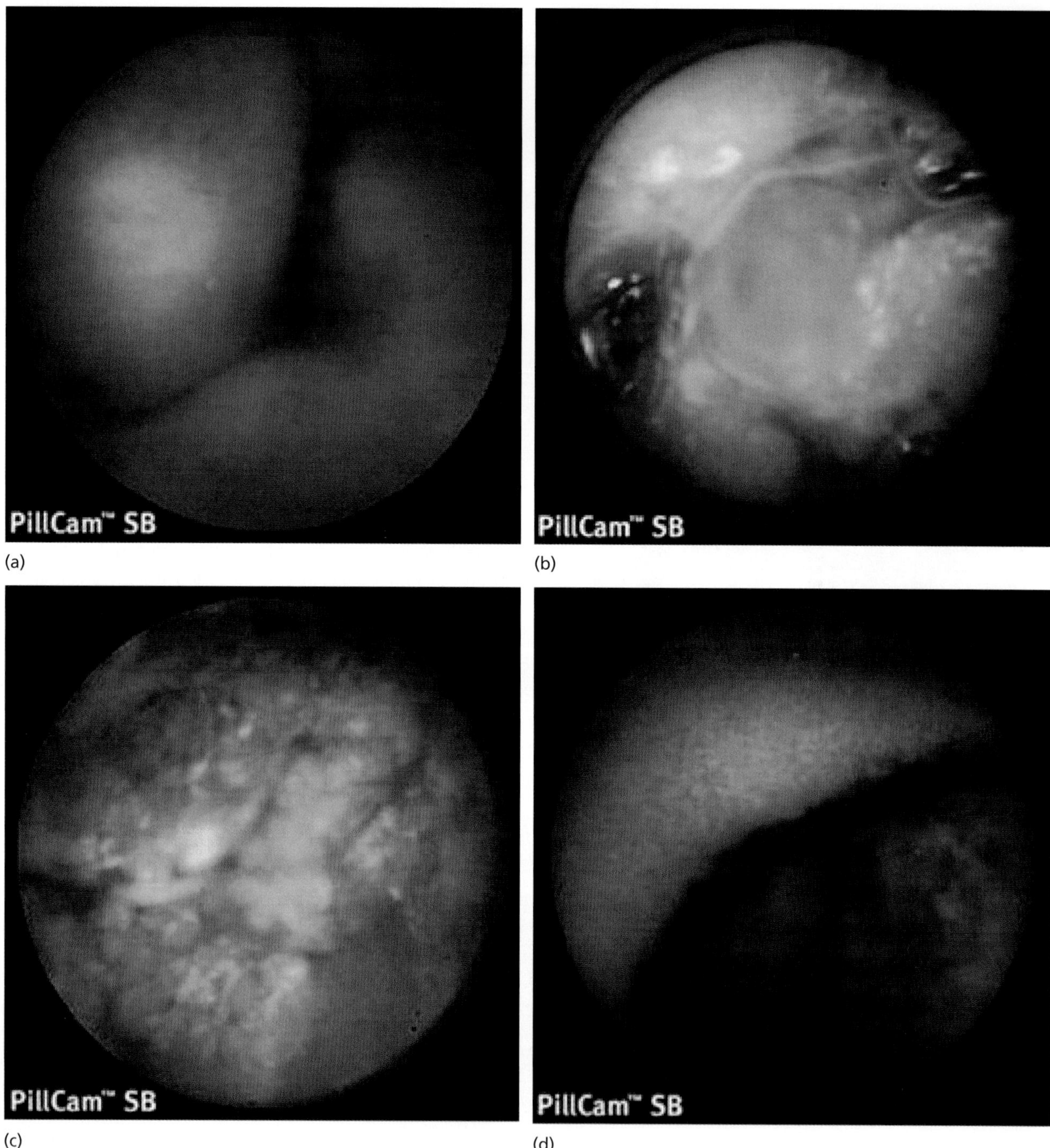

(a) (b) (c) (d)

Fig. 8.2 (a–d) Various small bowel tumors found in patients undergoing capsule endoscopy for evaluation of obscure GI bleeding.

DBE in 137 patients with suspected small bowel disease, most of whom (66%) had obscure GI bleeding, May and colleagues reported that tumors and polyps accounted for 25% of the total lesions found (May *et al.* 2005).

There are, however, limitations of DBE, including concerns about the endoscopic learning curve, common need for endoscopy on two separate days (transoral and then transanal approaches), limitations in visualization of the entire small bowel, miss rates for subepithelial lesions due to insufflation issues, a time-consuming procedure that also requires a high level of ancillary staffing, increased moderate sedation requirements, and patient tolerance and preferences. In addition, although uncommon, the reported incidence of severe complications associated with DBE has ranged from 0% to 2.5%, and has included pancreatitis, perforations, bleeding, abdominal pain, and fever (Akahoshi *et al.* 2006).

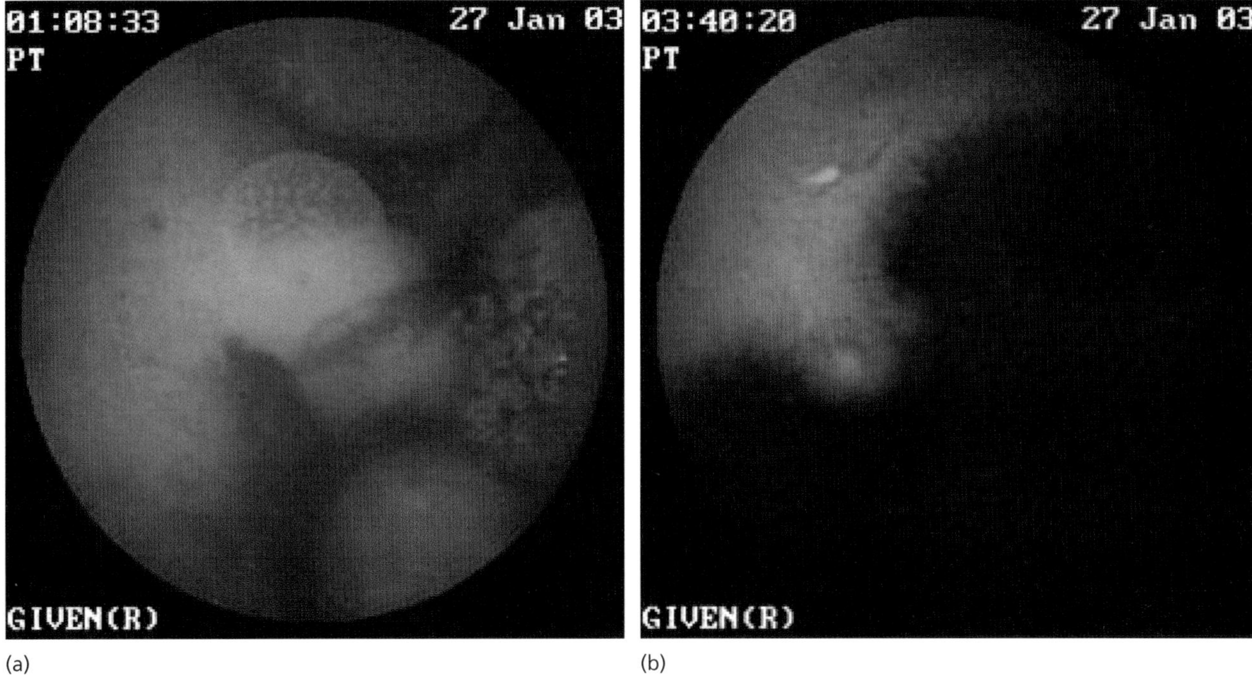

(a) (b)

Fig. 8.3 (a,b) Small bowel hamartomatous polyps from a patient with Peutz–Jegher syndrome.

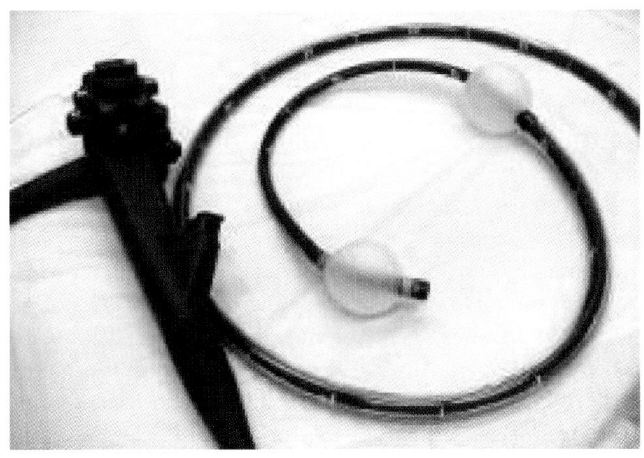

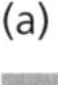
(a)

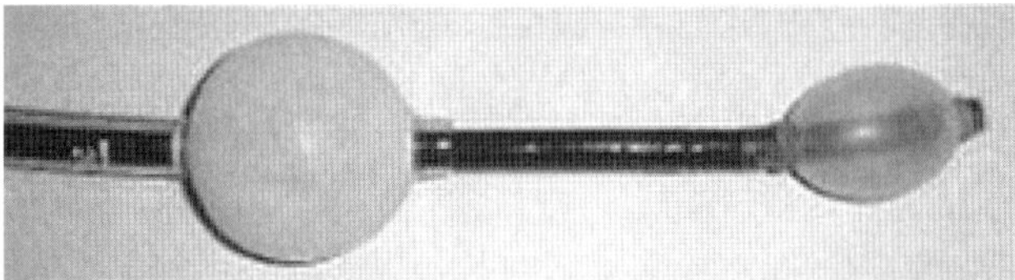

(b)

Fig. 8.4 (a,b) The double balloon enteroscopy system (Fujinon-Toshiba ES System Co., Tokyo, Japan) uses a high-resolution, dedicated video enteroscope that has a working length of 200 cm and two soft, latex balloons.

Intraoperative enteroscopy

Exploratory laparotomy with intraoperative enteroscopy has been utilized since the 1980s and is an important diagnostic and potentially therapeutic endoscopic modality in suspected small bowel disease, including small bowel polyps and tumors (Zaman *et al.* 1999; Kovacs & Jensen 2002). It is considered to be the ultimate endoscopic evaluation of the small bowel. In addition to being able to diagnose small bowel sources of obscure bleeding, intraoperative enteroscopy allows for identification of lesions for definitive surgical resection.

Using an *orally passed* colonoscope, or more optimally, a dedicated small bowel videoenteroscope, the endoscope is advanced beyond the ligament of Treitz into the proximal jejunum. At that point, the surgeon gently telescopes the small bowel over the shaft of the endoscope, allowing for careful inspection of the mucosa. Inspection of the small bowel mucosa should be performed in an anterograde manner. Dimming the operating room lights facilitates endoscopic visualization, as well as extrinsic inspection of the bowel by the surgeons. Lesions identified endoscopically can be marked for resection by the surgeon with a suture placed on the serosal aspect of the bowel. After completion of the enteroscopy and withdrawal of the endoscope, the marked site(s) can be resected. An alternative approach to intraoperative enteroscopy involves insertion of a sterilized endoscope through a single enterotomy or multiple, surgically created enterotomies, rectal insertion, or laparoscopy-assisted enteroscopy.

Reported complications associated with intraoperative enteroscopy include mucosal lacerations, perforations, prolonged ileus, abdominal abscess, and bowel ischemia (Zaman *et al.* 1999; Kovacs & Jensen 2002). Therefore, due to its invasive nature and potential for complications, the decision to perform intraoperative enteroscopy must not be taken lightly. All risks and benefits need to be fully considered and well explained to the patient, and only experienced endoscopists and surgeons should perform this procedure.

Molecular biology of small bowel tumors

Eyal Sagiv, Kerin Adelson, Alfred I. Neugut & Nadir Arber

One of the major advances in cancer research in the past 10–15 years has been the elucidation of the molecular genetics of colorectal cancer. Elegant studies by Vogelstein and others have explored the somatic genetic changes that take place in the course of colorectal carcinogenesis (Cho & Volgelstein 1992; Vogelstein & Kinzler 1994; Real & Fearon 1996). The result is that we now have a clearer perception of the process of colorectal carcinogenesis on a molecular genetic level than for any other solid tumor. Clinical benefits from these discoveries have included the identification of germ-line mutations and predisposing factors. Research efforts are currently underway to take advantage of these new findings in the development of new screening tools for colon cancer (Sidransky *et al.* 1992; Wargovich 1996), and of pharmacologic agents that capitalize on the new genetic discoveries to treat colorectal cancer (Schulz & Nyce 1991; Dansei *et al.* 1995). In contrast, very little research has been carried out in the investigation of molecular markers in small bowel cancer. Even those few studies that have been done have been limited in size.

Adenocarcinomas

Vogelstein and coworkers have described the genetic changes contributing to the adenoma–carcinoma sequence at various steps (Bos *et al.* 1987; Vogelstein *et al.* 1988). A morphological adenoma–carcinoma sequence has been described in the small intestine (Kozuka *et al.* 1981; Perzin & Bridge 1981; Hermanek 1987; Sellner 1990; Seifert *et al.* 1992), and the adenoma–carcinoma sequence was noted in those tumors as well. Thus, studies have been conducted to demonstrate the molecular similarities between carcinogenesis in the large and small intestines (Hallak & Arber 2003).

APC and allelic loss of *5q*

The initial genetic alteration in the transformation from normal epithelial tissue to adenoma in the colon is most likely the loss of function of the *APC* (adenomatous polyposis coli) gene. Thus, familial adenomatous polyposis (FAP) patients, who carry a germline APC mutation have multiple colonic adenomas and carcinomas, and also often have multiple tumors in the small bowel (Spigelman *et al.* 1990; Offerhaus *et al.* 1993). Both malignancies tend to occur in the same individuals. The APC protein forms a complex with β-catenin, leading to the degradation of β-catenin. In the absence of the APC protein, there is an excess of β-catenin in the nucleus that binds to TCF-4 to form a transcription factor complex that activates the transcription of several genes, e.g. *cyclin-D1*, *COX-2*, *c-myc*, *survivin* and *VEGF* (Connacci-Sorrel *et al.* 2002), that ultimately results in increased cell proliferation and inhibition of apoptosis.

The APC gene is located in the 5q chromosome. A deletion in the long arm of chromosome 5 is less common than in colon cancer as it was noted in only three out of 17 (17.6%) sporadic cases of small intestine adenocarcinomas (Blaker *et al.* 2002). One should keep in mind that the most common mutations in the *APC* gene are due to truncating mutations, and not to allelic loss. Nevertheless, mutations at the APC gene are rarely present in the small intestine, in contrast to the large intestine. Interestingly, Liberman *et al.* searched for nucleotide polymorphisms in locations 1307 and 1317 on the *APC* gene in 40 patients with small bowel adenocarcinoma and found no such changes from the wild type gene. This differed from their findings in the colon, where mutations in I1307K and E1317Q are significantly related to predisposition to cancer (Liberman *et al.* in press).

c-K-*ras*

Ras proteins act as molecular switches of signaling pathways that modulate many aspects of cell proliferation, differentiation, survival, motility and phagocytosis through activation of the MAP kinases. The mutated *ras* gene is found in about 30% of all human cancers (Bos 1989). The mutated protein is constitutively active (Giehl 2005). Arber *et al.* (1997) have shown the importance of *ras* as an oncogene in small bowel tumorigenesis. This group transfected normal enterocytes (IEC 18 cells) with human mutant K-*ras* and these cells became transformed (Arber *et al.* 1996). In a large study on 262 paraffin-embedded sections from the entire GI tract, point mutations at codon 12 of the K-*ras* gene were detected in 8 out of 20 small bowel adenomas (40%), and in 10 out of 28 adenocarcinomas (36%) (Arber *et al.* 2000). Nishiyama *et al.* (2002) and Rashid and Hamilton (1997) observed similar percentages of ras mutations.

p53

p53 is the classical tumor suppressor protein. It acts as a transcription factor for normal regulation of the cell cycle (Li *et al.* 1997). Its binding to DNA stimulates the production of p21 that leads to arrest in the cell cycle. Mutant p53 cannot bind DNA effectively, and consequently the p21 protein is not made available to act as the 'stop signal' for cell division. Thus, cells divide uncontrollably, and form tumors.

Similar to CRC, Rashid and Hamilton (1997) found increased expression of mutant p53 protein in 30% of adenomas and in about half the cases of sporadic and Crohn's associated adenocarcinoma. Arber *et al.* (1999) observed a similar trend: increased expression of mutant p53 protein in 47% of the adenomas and in 65% of the adenocarcinoma, suggesting a significant increase with tumor progression. Increased p53 levels were more prevalent in females than males (71% vs. 37%, $p < 0.05$) and were associated with a poorer prognosis. Nishiyama *et al.* (2002) found that 14 out of 35 cases showed overexpression of p53 (40%), and p53 tended to be expressed more frequently in poorly differentiated tumors.

Cell cycle proteins

Genetic alterations affecting the G1 phase of the cell cycle are so frequent in human cancers that abnormalities in this pathway may actually be necessary for tumor development (Hunter & Pines 1994; Hall & Peters 1996). During the G1 phase, cells respond to extracellular signals by either advancing towards the S phase and cell division or withdrawing from the cycle into a resting state or they undergo apoptosis (Harn *et al.* 1995; Ghazizadeh *et al.* 2005). Cyclins and cyclin-dependent kinases (CDKs) are important regulators of the cell cycle progression during the G1 phase of the cell cycle. The levels of cyclin D1, cyclin E, p16, p21, p27 and p53 proteins were determined by immunohistochemistry in normal (n = 16), adenomas (n = 20) and small bowel adenocarcinomas (n = 24) (Arber *et al.* 1999) (Table 8.6). Normal-appearing small bowel mucosa expressed $p27^{kip1}$ protein, whereas $p16^{ink4a}$, $p21^{cip1}$, cyclin D1 or cyclin E were not seen in normal mucosa. The most common alteration involved an increase in $p16^{ink4a}$, which was overexpressed in 92% of the adenomas and 91% of the adenocarcinomas. It may serve as a protective mechanism from malignant transformation of small intestine epithelial cells. There was also increased expression of cyclin D1, cyclin E and $p21^{cip1}$ proteins in both adenomas and adenocarcinoma. The $p27^{kip1}$ protein, which was seen in all the normal mucosal samples, was not detected in 17% of the adenomas and 23% of the adenocarcinomas. Increased expressions of cyclin D1 or p53 were associated with a significantly decreased 3-year survival (Arber *et al.* 1999). Similar results were obtained in 25 Israeli patients with small bowel adenomas and adenocarcinomas (unpublished data).

Table 8.6 Cell cycle abnormalities in small bowel tumors (Arber *et al.* 1999).

	Cyclin D1	*Cyclin E*	p16	p21	p27	p53
Adenomas	31%*	31%	92%	50%	83%	47%
Adenocarcinomas	30%	38%	91%	46%	77%	65%

* Percentage of patients with detectable levels of the protein.

18q loss of heterozygosity (LOH) and mutations in SMAD4

SMAD4 (DPC4) is a tumor suppressor gene that mediates the TGF-β signaling pathway, suppressing epithelial cell growth. The intracellular proteins SMAD-2 and 3 are phosphorylated by TGFβ receptor-I and are then able to form a complex with SMAD4 that translocates into the nucleus and regulates gene transcription. The tumor suppressor DCC and SMAD4 genes are located on 18q LOH; however, the malignant potential is related to SMAD4, since mutations in this gene were frequently found while none were found in DCC. Germline mutations in SMAD4 are believed to account for 25–60% of the cases of juvenile polyposis, which usually manifest with small bowel polyps (Miyaki & Kuroki 2003). Therefore 18q LOH and mutations in SMAD4 are believed to contribute to intestinal malignant transformation.

*erb*B-2-*neu* (HER-2)

*erb*B-2-*neu* encodes a trans-membrane glycoprotein that has tyrosine-specific kinase activity. Increased expression of NEU protein was detected in about 60% of small bowel tumors and was associated with a poorer prognosis (Zhu *et al.* 1996). A point mutation in the *neu* gene, leading to a single amino acid substitution (valine to glutamine at residue 664), may be responsible for the transforming phenotype.

TGFα

Transforming growth factor-α (TGFα) competes with epidermal growth factor (EGF) for the EGFR that transmits a proproliferative signal. TGF-α levels were evaluated in one study using immunohistochemistry: 9 out of 15 tumors were positively stained. TGF-α levels were not associated with the patient's survival, tumor stage, or grade. Mitomi *et al.* (2003) have found a strong expression of TGF-α in 5 out of 7 high-grade sporadic adenocarcinomas of the small intestine, while only one tumor showed a weak staining for EGF and none was stained for VEGF.

Other genetic changes

Disruptions in DNA mismatch repair genes that cause microsatellite instability (MSI) play an important role in the pathogenesis of intestinal tumor formation. Replication errors were found in about 15% and above of small bowel tumors (Planck *et al.* 2003). Moreover, HNPCC patients are at a higher risk to develop small intestinal tumors. Recently, Planck *et al.* (2003) found MSI in 16 out of 89 sporadic cases of small intestine adenocarcinomas (18%), similar to what is found in CRC (Miyaki & Kuroki 2003).

Gastrointestinal stromal tumors (GISTs)

Benign or malignant tumors arise from the mesenchyme of the GI tract, and from the interstitial cell of Cajal (ICC), which are the pacemaker cells of the gut.

c-KIT

c-KIT is a transmembrane receptor for stem cell factor with an intracytoplasmic portion functioning as a tyrosine kinase (Rubin *et al.* 2001; De Giorgi & Verweij 2005). GISTs are characterized by gain-of-function mutations in this proto-oncogene, most commonly in exon 11, but may also involve exons 9, 13, and 17; GISTs with KIT exon 11 mutations are associated with a poorer prognosis (De Giorgi & Verweij 2005). In the rare cases of GISTs without KIT mutations, the gain of function is obtained in mutations in the platelet-derived growth factor receptor α (PDGFR α), that seems to be an alternative oncogenetic mechanism (De Giorgi & Verweij 2005). Imatinib mesylate (Gleevec), a small-molecule inhibitor, is a recent major breakthrough in cancer therapy. It inhibits several tyrosine kinase receptors, including KIT, PDGFR α and BCR-ABL. It has a major therapeutic benefit for GISTs, both via KIT and via unknown mechanisms (Tarn *et al.* 2006).

Neurofibromatosis type 1

NF1 is a syndrome that conveys a higher risk for several tumors, including GISTs, and is caused by a mutation in the NF1 gene that encodes for the tumor supressor gene, neurofibromin, a Ras GTPase activating protein. Patients with this mutation are at a higher risk of developing GISTs. Recently, among 45 cases of NF1 patients with GISTs, Miettinen *et al.* (2006) have found that 38 of the tumors were located in the small intestine. Associated Cajal cell hyperplasia was common. Maertens *et al.* (2006) analyzed 7 NF1-related GIST tumors and found that they do not share the common pathogenesis of KIT and PDGFRα mutations, but transformation is the result of the loss of the wild-type NF1 allele.

Other genetic and epigenetic alterations

In 20 GIST cases of the small bowel, Feakins (2005) has shown mutation in p53 in 40% of the cases. BCL-2 was overexpressed in 90% of the cases, and TGF-α in six out of six GISTs (Cai *et al.* 1999). A loss of $p16^{INK4a}$ and $p14^{ARF}$ mRNA expression was demonstrated in 41% and 24% respectively, mostly through chromosomal deletion in 9q12 (Perrone *et al.* 2005).

Neuroendocrine tumors

These tumors arise from endocrine cells of the intestinal mucosa and are characterized by presenting neurosecretory granules seen in elctron microscopy. They are often secretory and release exessive levels of a specific hormone: serotonin (causing carcinoid syndrome), somatostatin, glucagon (Verner–Morrison syndrome), histamine, gastrin (Zollinger–Ellison syndrome) or enterochromaffin.

Multiple endocrine neoplasia type 1 (MEN1)

Although the vast majority of these tumors occur sporadically, a subset of tumors is associated with inherited syndromes, among which MEN1 is the most significant one (Gortz *et al.* 1999). The MEN1 gene encodes a tumor suppressor gene and is located on chromosome 11q13. It is a ubiquitously expressed nuclear protein of an unknown function, which acts as a transcriptional repressor. LOH at 11q13, deletions or point mutations in the wild-type allele of MEN1 in these patients is responsible for tumor formation. Furthermore, Jakobovitz *et al.* (1996) demonstrated that loss of 11q13 is also encountered in 100% of sporadic neuroendocrine tumors of the jejunum and ileum, suggesting that somatic mutations of the MEN1 gene might also contribute to the pathogenesis of these tumors. The tumors often overexpress β-catenin and p53 Ki67 and E-cadherin (Barshack *et al.* 2002).

Primary lymphomas

Up to 40% of lymphomas arise in sites other than lymph nodes and the gut is the most common site. The genotype of these tumors differs from the nodal ones. Four different types of lymphomas may be found in the small bowel:

1 celiac-associated T-cell high-grade lymphoma
2 Burkitt-type lymphoma
3 maltoma
4 Mediterranean lymphoma.

Celiac-associated T-cell high-grade lymphoma

Refractory celiac disease is strongly associated with partial trisomy of the 1q region. Gain of chromosome 1q was recently found in 16% of EATL (Verkarre *et al.* 2003). The loss of heterozygosity at chromosome 9p21 is frequent in enteropathy associated T-cell lymphoma (EATL), especially in tumors with large cell morphology. Deletions at chromosome 9p21, which harbors the tumor suppressor genes p14/ARF, p15/INK4b, and p16/INK4a, and 17p13, where p53 is located, are associated with the development and progression of intestinal lymphomas (Verkarre *et al.* 2003).

Burkitt-type lymphoma of the small intestine

The molecular characteristic of this type of cancer is t(8;14)(q24,q32) translocation that leads to deregulation and activation of the *c-myc* gene (Dalla-Favera *et al.* 1983). The translocation juxtaposes the oncogene and an immunoglobulin heavy-chain loci, leading to elevation in *c-myc* transcription level, respective to that of the Ig. Translocations (2;8) and (8;22) that position *myc* under *IgK* and *Igλ* respectively are also known. This genetic alteration, however, is not specific for this type of cancer, as it presents in 5–10% of diffuse large B-cell lymphoma. Other biomarkers that characterize the tumor cells are CD20+, BCL6+, CD10+, BCL2– and CD5–.

Maltoma

MALT lymphoma is specifically associated with t(11;18)(q21;q21), t(1;14)(p22;q32) and t(14;18)(q32;q21). t(11;18) fuses the *API2* downstream to the C-terminus of the *MALT1* gene which generates a functional API2-MALT1 product. t(1;14) and t(14;18) bring the BCL10 and MALT1 genes respectively to the *IgH* locus and deregulate their expression (Lee *et al.* 2004). The oncogenic activity of the three chromosomal translocations is linked by the physiologic role of BCL10 and MALT1 in antigen receptor-mediated NFkappa B activation; Ye *et al.* (2005) defined the prevalence of these three translocations as 15.8%, 3% and 2% of the cases. In a sample of 33 MALT-type lymphoma tissues and 28 diffuse large B-cell lymphomas from stomach and small intestine, Ki-67 expression in more than 30% of tumor cells was detected in 42 (68.6%), bcl-2 expression in 20 (32.8%), and p53 in 16 (26.2%) of lymphomas (Krugmann *et al.* 2001).

Mediterranean lymphoma

The alpha heavy chain for the mucosal IgA antibodies is abnormal due to a deletion in the variable portion which leads to hyperactivation of the immune system in bowel due to aberrant antibacterial response. No other molecular abnormalities are known.

Imaging and staging

Yulia Bronstein & Ronelle Dubrow

Small bowel (SB) neoplasms account for only 1.4% of gastrointestinal cancers but are responsible for 75% of the symptomatic small bowel lesions that require surgery (Hara *et al.* 2005).

The detection of tumors by traditional imaging modalities is often compromised by overlapping bowel loops and suboptimal bowel distention. There are some newer techniques described below, which address these factors and may improve the diagnostic accuracy of imaging for these tumors and therefore decrease delays in diagnosis. These have yet to be evaluated systematically.

Imaging modalities

Small bowel follow-through (SBFT)

SBFT is the oldest barium study traditionally used for evaluation of the small bowel. There is a questionable role for this non-invasive test due to a reported wide range of sensitivities for tumor detection (30–90%). In the study of Bessette in 1989 SBFT detected 61% of tumors (Bessette *et al.* 1989).

Enteroclysis

Enteroclysis is more sensitive than SBFT, but is a more difficult examination for both the radiologist and the patient, requiring nasojejunal intubation and oral administration of large volumes of contrast material. The sensitivity of enteroclysis is as high as 95% with 90% correct estimation of the actual size of the tumor (Bessette *et al.* 1989).

Computed tomography

With the development of multidetector scanners and their widespread use in evaluating abdominal symptomatology, CT is beginning to play a more important role in the detection of SB tumors. Most modern multidetector scanners allow excellent spatial resolution due to thin collimation (from 0.625 mm). Future generations of scanners with increased number of detector rows will allow volumetric imaging with multiplanar reconstructions, which is a very helpful tool in analysis of small bowel anatomy. The lumen of the small bowel must be distended with orally administered contrast to demonstrate the wall thickening that characterizes small bowel tumors on CT.

Multidetector CT enteroclysis (MDCT enteroclysis)

MDCT enteroclysis shares advantages of both conventional enteroclysis and cross-sectional imaging. This relatively new technique seems to be more sensitive than conventional barium studies and less invasive than enteroscopy. Lesions as small as 5 mm can be identified (Lappas *et al.* 2003).

The enteroclysis catheter is placed in the distal horizontal duodenum under fluoroscopy. Neutral luminal contrast (either water or 0.5% methylcellulose) is used. MDCT acquisition is obtained after 120–130 mL of intravenous contrast medium. Images are reconstructed every 0.625–3 mm. Post-processing and multiplanar reformatting and interpretation are performed on dedicated workstations (Romano *et al.* 2005; Rajesh & Maglinte 2006).

In the study of Orjollet *et al.* (2000) 48 MDCT-E studies revealed 22 small bowel tumors with 3 false-positive results. This corresponds with almost 100% sensitivity and 85% concordance with enteroscopy.

Boudiaf *et al.* (2004) in a group of 107 patients with inflammatory and neoplastic small bowel abnormalities (including 8 tumors) report 100% sensitivity, 95% specificity, 97% accuracy, 94% positive predictive value, and 100% negative predictive value of multidetector row helical CT enteroclysis for detection of small bowel disease abnormality.

MDCT enterography

MDCT enterography is a non-invasive technique of cross-sectional imaging which achieves good or excellent SB distention with negative oral contrast without nasojejunal cannulation. Wold in his study on patients with Crohn's disease demonstrated no advantage of CT enteroclysis over non-invasive CT-enterography (Wold *et al.* 2003).

In addition to water, lactulose (Arslan *et al.* 2005) or mannitol (Zhang *et al.* 2005) is used to achieve luminal distention. Thin CT collimation (2.5 mm with 0.625–2.0 mm reconstructions) along with the negative oral contrast and a good intravenous contrast bolus improves the sensitivity of CT for detecting SB tumors. The lumen of the SB appears hypodense compared with the contrast-enhanced wall, producing excellent delineation of abnormal wall thickening.

In their study on 51 patients, Zhang *et al.* (2005) scanned 16 patients with SB tumors, both primary and secondary. CT images were obtained during two phases: arterial (20–30 s) and venous (50–70 s). Accurate assessment of tumor location and size was possible, as well as evaluation for calcification or necrosis, and demonstration of arterial supply and venous drainage. Post-processed three-dimensional images (3D CT) are usually not necessary for radiologists for diagnostic purposes, but are valuable for clinicians and surgeons for surgical planning and more comprehensible demonstration to the patient.

MRI and magnetic resonance enteroclysis

Many investigators have assessed the potential of magnetic resonance imaging (MRI) in examining the SB. Advantages of MRI over CT include superb soft-tissue contrast, absence of radiation exposure and iodine contrast exposure, and multiple contrast sources.

SB tumors are demonstrable on MR images (Semelka *et al.* 1996). High-resolution images of the entire SB free from susceptibility, ghosts, and motion artifacts can be acquired during comfortable breath-hold times (less than 20 s) on new MRI units (Papanikolaou *et al.* 2002).

MR enteroclysis, a combined functional and morphologic imaging method, was introduced only recently into clinical practice (Reiber *et al.* 2000; Gourtsoyiannis *et al.* 2001). Comprehensive MR enteroclysis examination protocol includes SB intubation, administration of a biphasic contrast agent (i.e. an iso-osmotic water solution), heavily T2-weighted single-shot spin echo images for MR fluoroscopy and for monitoring the infusion process, T2-weighted imaging using half-Fourier acquisition single-shot turbo spin echo and true fast imaging with steady-state precession sequences, and dynamic T1-weighted imaging using a postgadolinium 3D fast low-angle shot sequence with fat suppression or fast spoiled gradient echo. This protocol can provide anatomic demonstration of the normal intestinal wall, identification of wall thickening or tumorous lesions, lesion characterization or evaluation of disease activity and assessment of exoenteric/mesenteric disease extension.

PET

The role of PET in the initial diagnosis of SB malignant tumors is not yet established. However there are indications for the utility of PET in monitoring response to treatment, manifested as change in metabolic activity of the tumor.

^{18}F-labeled FDG PET is highly sensitive and specific for evaluation of the treatment response of nodal and extranodal diseases in patients with malignant lymphomas. A positive ^{18}F-FDG PET scan after the completion of chemotherapy in patients with lymphomas with GI tract involvement is a strong predictor of relapse. In the study of Kumar *et al.* (2004) on 19 patients with lymphoma involving the GI tract, including 13 patients with SB involvement, ^{18}F-FDG PET showed higher diagnostic accuracy than CT in the detection of residual disease after therapy. The sensitivity and specificity of post-therapy ^{18}F-FDG PET were 86% and 100%. The corresponding values for CT were 67% and 75%, respectively. Patients with positive ^{18}F-FDG PET results had statistically significant lower disease-free survival than did those with positive CT results.

Despite the mild physiologic ^{18}F-FDG uptake in the GIT, ^{18}F-FDG PET has potential value in monitoring the response to treatment in patients with GIT lymphomas, particularly when pretreatment PET results are positive.

Gastrointestinal stromal tumors (GISTs) are gaining the interest of researchers because of impressive metabolic response to the targeted molecular therapeutic drug imatinib mesylate. Initial reports suggest an important role for ^{18}F-FDG PET in the follow-up of therapy for these tumors.

Gayed *et al.* (2004) in a series of 49 patients with GIST found that the performances of ^{18}F-FDG PET and CT were comparable in staging GISTs before initiation of imatinib mesylate therapy. However, ^{18}F-FDG PET was superior to CT in predicting early response to therapy. Thus, ^{18}F-FDG PET is a better guide for imatinib mesylate therapy.

In a series of 10 patients with malignant GIST tumors, six of which were in the SB, Goldstein *et al.* (2005) found ^{18}F-FDG

PET to be a useful modality to monitor treatment response to imatinib. ^{18}F-FDG PET studies demonstrated changes preceding CT findings in all patients with subsequent concordant improvement.

FDG PET is sensitive and specific for evaluating tumor response but cannot be used in patients whose baseline FDG PET results are negative for tumors (Choi *et al.* 2004).

PET was also shown to be more sensitive and specific than CT for detection of melanoma metastasis (Swetter *et al.* 2002).

Primary malignant tumors of the small bowel

Adenocarcinoma

Adenocarcinoma is the most common primary malignancy of the SB, accounting for 40% of primary SB neoplasms (Horton & Fishman 2004). Sporadic adenocarcinoma of the SB is most common within 30 cm of the duodenojejunal junction. A concentric soft tissue mass commonly produces obstruction of the proximal jejunum. On barium studies (SBFT and enteroclysis) the tumor is seen as a short circumferentially narrowed segment with overhanging borders known as an 'apple core' lesion (Fig. 8.5).

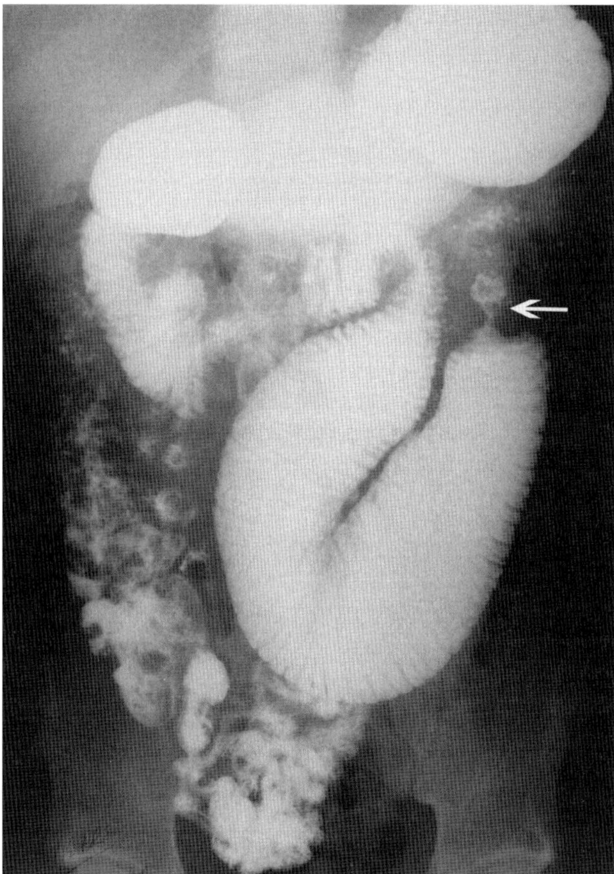

Fig. 8.5 Adenocarcinoma of the jejunum. SBFT demonstrates classic obstructing 'apple core' lesion suggestive of malignancy.

On CT adenocarcinomas typically will appear as a focal areas of wall thickening causing luminal narrowing (Fig. 8.6). However, polypoid masses or infiltrative lesions without narrowing have also been reported. These tumors are often rigid and fibrotic and can therefore result in early obstruction. Ulceration of tumors has also been reported in up to 40% of cases. Ulcers are not always well visualized on CT scans. CT can aid in staging (Table 8.4) by detecting local extension, adenopathy, or distant metastasis. Typically, SB adenocarcinoma metastatic to the liver will appear as low attenuation masses, which are best visualized during the portal venous phase of enhancement.

Adenocarcinoma complicating longstanding Crohn's disease is most common in the distal ileum. This tumor is difficult to detect because of preexisting abnormality of the involved bowel segment.

Carcinoid

Carcinoid is the next most common SB malignancy, representing approximately 25% of all primary SB tumors. Carcinoid tumors are more common in the ileum. These are slow-growing tumors, which first appear as submucosal nodules. In the past, at this stage, the SBFT series or enteroclysis would be much more sensitive for detection. However, given improvements in CT scanning and technique, occasionally the submucosal carcinoid tumor can be identified with CT (Horton & Fishman 2004). It appears as an intramural mass demonstrating increased enhancement due to hyperemia. Because approximately 30% of carcinoid tumors are multicentric, multiple nodules may be identified. As the tumor grows, it will usually extend into the adjacent mesentery. At this point, the CT appearance is fairly characteristic. On CT, the mesenteric extension from carcinoid will usually appear as a spiculated soft tissue-density, a mesenteric mass due to desmoplastic reaction (Fig. 8.7). Calcification within the mesenteric extension can be seen in up to 70% of cases (Fig. 8.7b). Although the mesenteric mass is typically soft tissue density, cystic carcinoid tumors have been described.

Metastasis from carcinoid tumors typically involves the liver. The lesions are best demonstrated on late arterial phase imaging, and may become isodense in the portal venous phase. Dual phase CT or MRI of the liver should be performed to detect subtle hypervascular liver metastasis.

Lymphoma

The third most common SB malignancy is non-Hodgkin's lymphoma, representing 10%–15% of SB malignancies. Primary

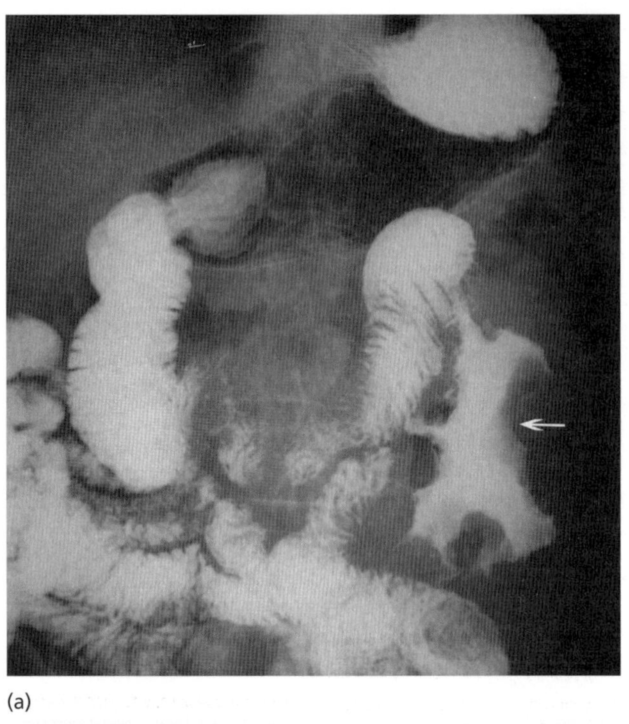

(a)

(b)

Fig. 8.6 (a) Adenocarcinoma of the jejunum. SBFT radiograph demonstrates an irregular mass (arrow) in the loop of jejunum distal to the ligament of Tretz. (b) Adenocarcinoma of the jejunum. CT confirms large concentric non-obstructive mass.

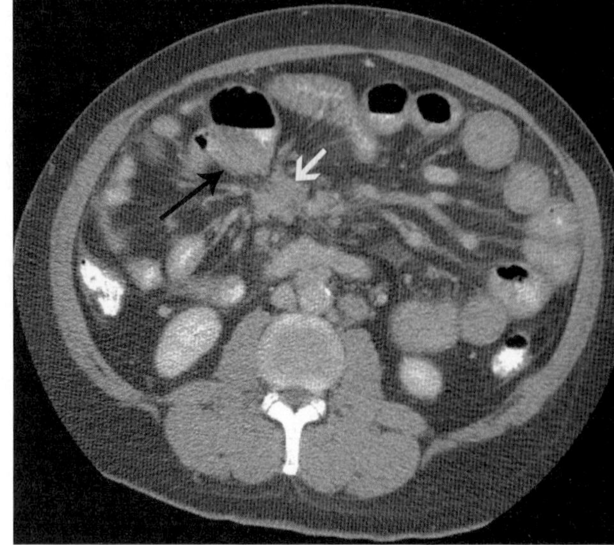

(a)

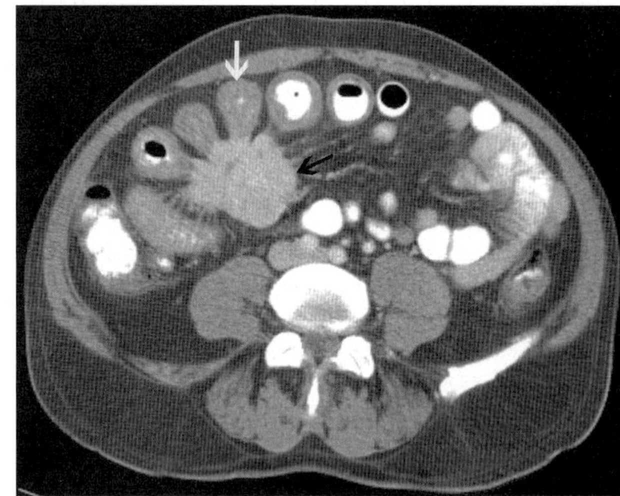

(b)

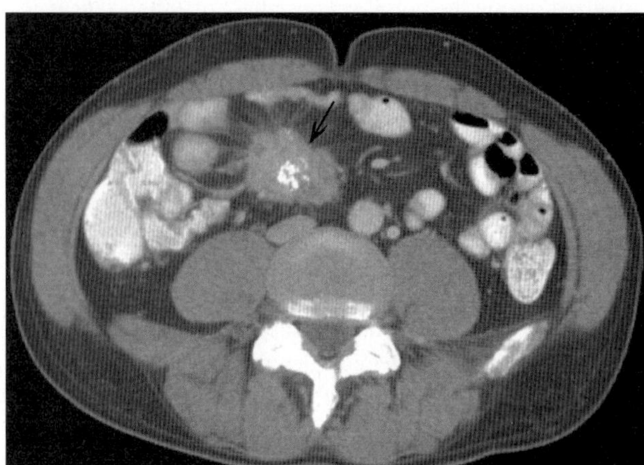

(c)

Fig. 8.7 Three different patients with carcinoid. (a) Patient 1. CT shows small primary mass in the ileum (black arrow) with mesenteric metastasis (white arrow). (b) Patient 2. Classic spiculated mesenteric mass (black arrow) with retraction of ileal loops due to desmoplastic reaction. Diffuse thickening of ileal wall (white arrow) is commonly seen preoperatively with no definite tumorous mass in the bowel. (c) Patient 3. Calcification is present in 70% of metastatic mesentery mass (arrow).

Table 8.4 Staging of small bowel carcinoma according to the American Joint Committee on Cancer staging system (Greene *et al.* 2002).

Primary tumor (T)
TX: Primary tumor cannot be assessed
T0: No evidence of primary tumor is present
Tis: Carcinoma in situ is present
T1: Tumor invades the lamina propria or submucosa
T2: Tumor invades the muscularis propria
T3: Tumor invades through the muscularis propria into subserosa or into non-peritonealized perimuscular tissue (mesentery or retroperitoneum), with extension of less than 2 cm
T4: Tumor penetrates the visceral peritoneum or directly invades other organs or structures

Regional lymph nodes (N)
NX: Regional lymph nodes cannot be assessed
N0: No regional lymph node metastasis is present
N1: Regional lymph node metastasis has occurred

Distant metastases (M)
MX: Presence of distant metastasis cannot be assessed
M0: No distant metastasis is present
M1: Distant metastasis has occurred

Stage grouping
Stage 0: Tis, N0, M0
Stage I: T1–2, N0, M0
Stage II: T3–4, N0, M0
Stage III: Any T, N1, M0
Stage IV: Any T, any N, M1

small bowel lymphomas have a better prognosis than carcinomas.

Four major patterns of SB lymphoma have been identified on radiographic studies (Horton & Fishman 2004).

1 Infiltrating pattern which appears as wall thickening with destruction of the normal SB folds. Because the tumor infiltrates the muscular layer of the wall, it can inhibit peristalsis and, therefore, result in aneurysmal dilatation of the affected bowel loop. As a result, the lumen is dilated with focal bulging of the wall, which is commonly excentric. On CT this mass appear homogeneously hypodense with minimal contrast enhancement (Fig. 8.8a,b).

2 Exophytic mass, which can ulcerate. This pattern can simulate an adenocarcinoma or gastrointestinal stromal tumor. Ulceration may result in localized perforation into a sealed-off mesenteric space.

3 Multifocal submucosal nodules within the SB. This appearance is often better appreciated on a SB series or enteroclysis as 'bull's eye' or 'target' lesions because the nodules can be very small.

4 Single-mass lesion, which can lead to intussusception (Fig. 8.8c,d), but rarely will result in obstruction because the masses are typically pliable and soft.

PET-CT scan is highly sensitive for detection of nodal and extranodal involvement of lymphoma, including small bowel involvement. PET plays a crucial role in monitoring response to treatment (Kumar *et al.* 2004).

Gastrointestinal stromal tumors (GISTs)

Gastrointestinal stromal cell tumors (GIST) are the 4th most common malignant SB tumors (9%). These rare lesions occur anywhere within the gastrointestinal tract, but are most common in the stomach (60–70%). 20–25% of GISTs occur in the SB. GISTs smaller than 2 cm are generally considered benign, with a very low risk of recurrence.

Because of the exophytic growth of these tumors CT is the imaging modality of choice. Small tumors tend to appear homogeneous on CT.

Larger tumors (>6 cm) frequently show central areas of necrosis or hemorrhage. These tumors may be so large that it may be difficult to appreciate the communication of the tumor with the intestinal wall (Fig. 8.9a). If intraluminal contrast is seen in the tumor, bowel origin is confirmed (Fig. 8.9b,c). Large size, significant necrosis and cavitation are signs suggestive of malignancy. However it is often difficult to distinguish benign from malignant GIST based on the radiographic appearance unless obvious metastases are present.

Nearly 50% of patients with GISTs present with metastasis. The most common site for GIST metastasis is the liver, followed by the peritoneum. Liver metastasis appears isointense or hypointense to normal liver parenchyma on non-contrast images and usually has a lesser degree of enhancement than normal liver parenchyma on portal phase contrast images. It can also appear cystic and can be difficult to differentiate from other cystic hepatic lesions, like amebic abscess (Zonios *et al.* 2003).

Peritoneal metastasis may also be seen as separate nodules not causing direct invasion of parenchymal organs (sarcomatous pattern of peritoneal spread). Ascites is rarely seen.

Recurrent tumors after surgical resection can also appear hypodense and should not be mistaken for postoperative fluid collections.

CT is the imaging modality of choice for diagnosis and staging of GISTs at initial presentation and for monitoring the disease during and after treatment (Choi *et al.* 2004; Horton *et al.* 2004; Hong *et al.* 2006). A response to imatinib is characterized by rapid transition from a heterogeneously hyperattenuating pattern to a homogeneously hypoattenuating pattern with resolution of the enhancing tumor nodules. Overall tumor attenuation decreases dramatically with the development of myxoid degeneration and, occasionally, hemorrhage or necrosis. Tumor size was found to have decreased significantly 2 months after treatment. However, in 75% of the patients, the disease was stable according to the traditional tumor response criteria of Response Evaluation Criteria in Solid Tumors. Development of a nodule within the treated tumor is unique to GISTs and indicates recurrence regardless of changes in tumor size (Hong *et al.* 2006).

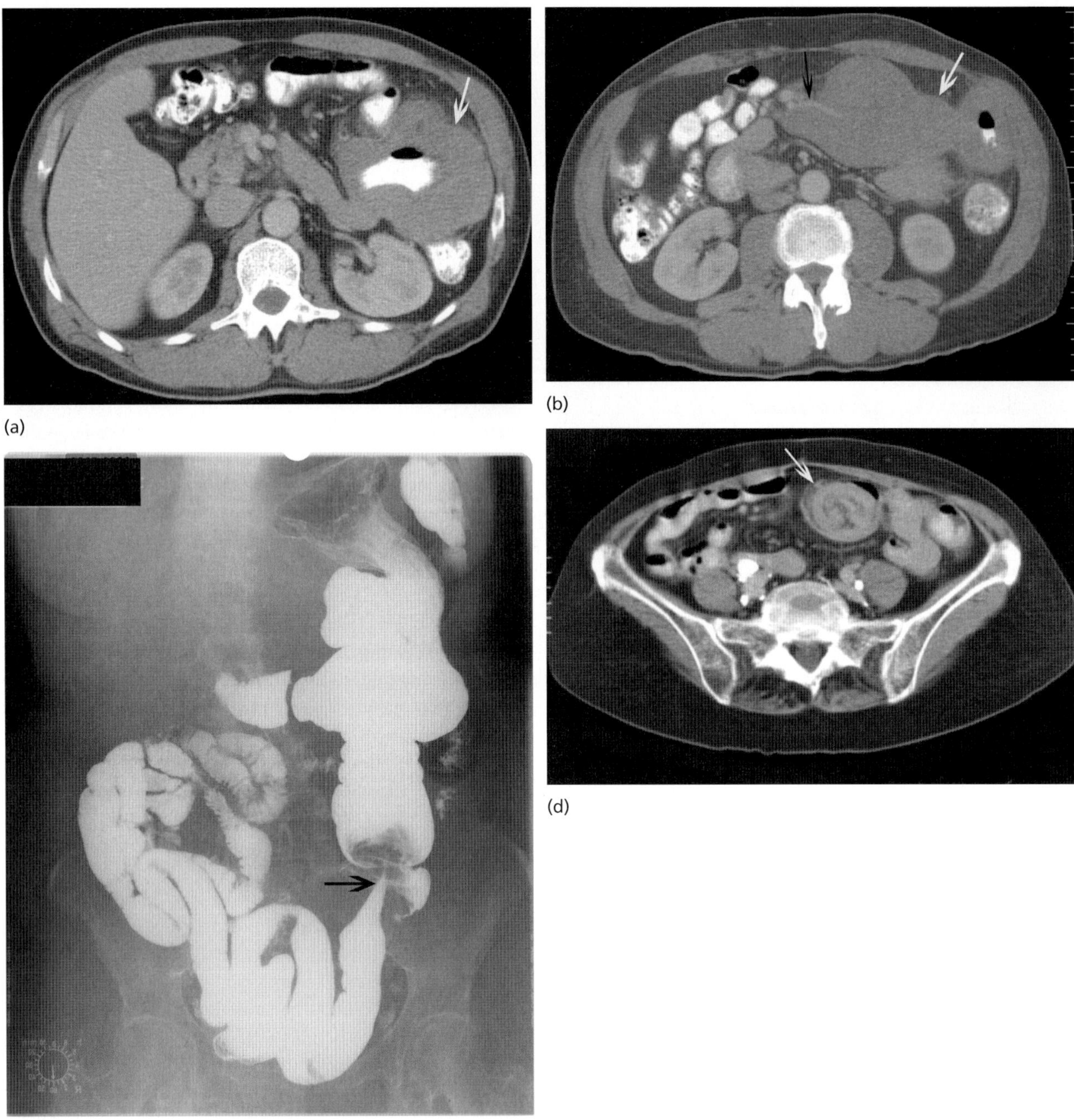

Fig. 8.8 Lymphoma of the jejunum. (a) Patient 1. Large non-obstructing mass in the jejunum (arrow) is very homogeneous and minimally enhancing with contrast. (b) Patient 1. Bulky hypodense mesenteric mass (white arrow) surrounds jejunal vessels (black arrow) and is typical of lymphomatous mesenteric involvement. (c) Patient 2. SBFT demonstrates smooth narrowing of the distal ileum (arrow) with an associated 'swirl' filling defect within the distal bowel suggestive of intussusception. (d) Patient 2. CT shows concentric mass (arrow) in the small bowel containing layers of mesenteric fat consistent with intussusception.

When CT findings are inconclusive or inconsistent with the clinical presentation, FDG PET should be performed (Hong *et al.* 2006). PET exceeds CT in monitoring tumor response to chemotherapy (Choi *et al.* 2004; Gayed *et al.* 2004; Goldstein *et al.* 2005). Dramatic decrease in FDG uptake within GIST tumors is noted within a short interval after initiation of imatinib therapy. In a study of Choi *et al.* (2004) on 29 patients a good qualitative correlation was shown between decrease in metabolic activity of the tumor and CT evidence of response after 2 months of imatinib therapy. No quantitative concordance was demonstrated between Hounsfield Units measured on CT as a single criterion and standardized uptake value as a measure of FDG uptake, because of the difference in measurement methods.

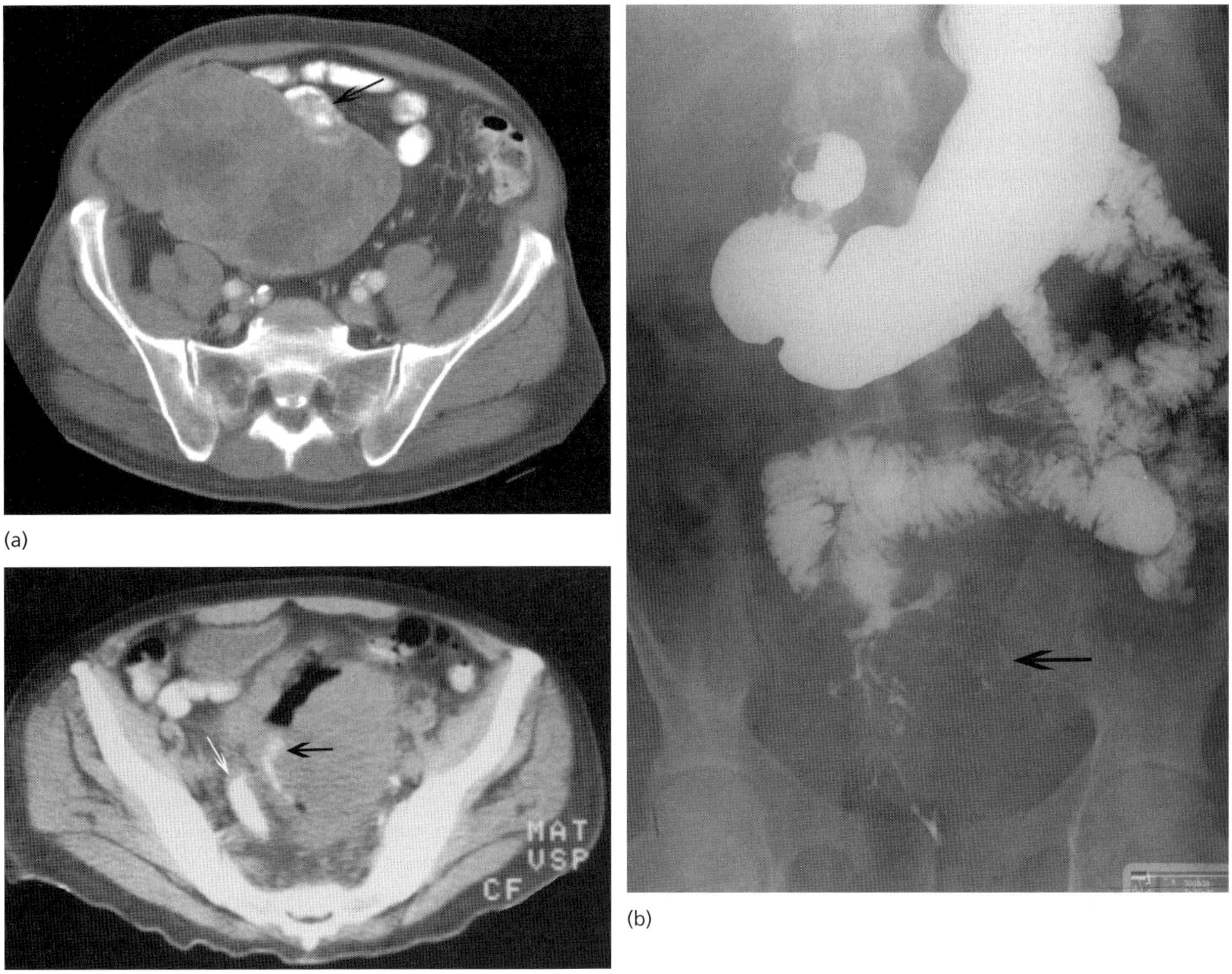

(a)

(b)

(c)

Fig. 8.9 Gastrointestinal stromal tumor (GIST). (a) Patient 1. Large heterogenous mass in the pelvis appears exophytic from the wall of an adjacent ileal loop (arrow). With exophytic GIST abutting many bowel loops preoperative imaging may fail to detect the tumor source precisely. (b) Patient 2. SBFT demonstrates irregular lumen of an ileum with extraluminal contrast (arrows) with no small bowel obstruction. (c) Patient 2. Large exophytic mass contains extraluminal barium (black arrow), which proves an origin of this tumor from the adjacent loop of ileum (white arrow).

Metastases to the small bowel

There are three pathways of secondary involvement of the SB.

1 Intraperitoneal spread: commonly from gastrointestinal and ovarian–uterine cancers. The areas most prone to involvement are the ileocecal valve and ileal loops in the cul-de-sac. Mesenteric metastases involve the mesenteric margin of the bowel. Desmoplastic reaction of these tumors commonly causes obstruction.

2 Hematogeneous dissemination. Lung cancer, breast cancer and melanoma have special affinity for SB involvement. Although SB metastasis in lung cancer is usually concomitant with overall progressive disease and is often clinically obscure, the situation may be different with melanoma (Fig. 8.10) and breast cancer. Metastases of these tumors can come to clinical attention as the only metastatic site years after the initial tumor has been removed.

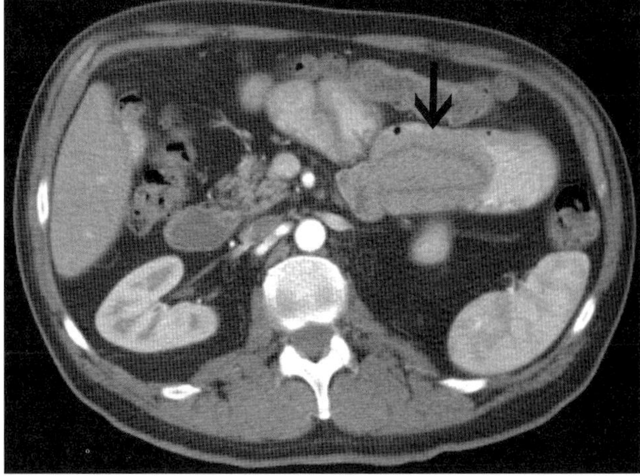

Fig. 8.10 Metastatic melanoma. Symptomatic jejunal mass with intussusception (arrow) was found in a patient with metastatic melanoma in the axilla.

Bender *et al.* (2001) report the polypoid pattern, equally distributed between the jejunum and ileum, to be the most common manifestation of metastatic melanoma to the SB. The target lesion was infrequently seen. SBFT (58% sensitivity) and conventional CT (66% sensitivity) seem to be unreliable in demonstrating melanoma metastases to the SB.

Swetter *et al.* (2002) report PET to be more sensitive and specific than CT for detection of melanoma metastasis. PET demonstrated 84% sensitivity and 97% specificity, whereas CT showed 58% sensitivity and 70% specificity for detection of melanoma metastases in total body imaging. In their study of 108 patients, they demonstrated that PET detected 86% of intra-abdominal metastases (including liver, pancreas, spleen, bowel, kidney, adrenal, and unspecified intra-abdominal metastases), whereas CT detected 72% overall. PET shows greater ability to detect soft tissue, SB, and lymph node metastasis that do not meet criteria designated as abnormal by CT.

3 Extension from an adjacent tumor either directly or via lymphatics. The most common primary tumor is colon cancer.

Treatment

Surgery

Ido Nachmany & Joseph M. Klausner

The only potential cure for small bowel adenocarcinoma is complete surgical resection. At operation, the resectability rate for cure is between 50% and 65%.

Discussion on the surgical treatment of small bowel tumors can be divided according to anatomy into tumors involving the duodenum, and those involving the rest of the small intestine, namely the jejuno-ileum. Lesions of the duodenum necessitate the comprehensive procedure of pancreaticoduodenectomy (Whipple's operation). The rest, including tumors of the distal duodenum, can be dealt with by relatively simple segmental resection, but since many patients are diagnosed with advanced disease, it is the decision making that most challenges the clinician and not the technical issues.

Adenocarcinomas, carcinoids and lymphomas should be resected with their regional lymph nodes within the mesentery. A 10-cm section of macroscopically normal bowel should be removed on both sides. GISTs on the other hand, tend to metastasize hematogenously and do not invade lymphatics. Therefore safe oncologic resection does not necessitate removal of the lymphatic basin.

The major challenge in surgical oncology of small bowel cancer is determining the place surgery should play in locally advanced disease, in patients with carcinomatosis and as a palliative mean, in the armamentarium of the multidisciplinary team.

This section will address the more complicated clinical issues encountered by the surgical oncologist regarding small bowel malignancies.

Surgery for periampullary duodenal polyps in FAP

The approach to periampullary lesions of the duodenum, in the context of familial adenomatous polyposis (FAP), is a complex one and demands multidisciplinary team work from the gastroenterologist, surgeon and oncologists.

The prevalence of periampullary duodenal adenocarcinoma is much higher in FAP patients compared to the general population (up to 200 to 300 times), but in absolute terms it is still low.

The increasing use of prophylactic proctocolectomy in FAP has caused a substantial reduction in the incidence of colorectal cancer, and proximal small bowel adenocarcinoma is one of the two leading causes of death (the other being desmoid tumors) in patients who have had their colon removed.

In 1989, Spigelman *et al.* described an endoscopic and histological classification system of five stages (0 to IV), for evaluation of the severity of duodenal adenomatosis. The Spigelman classification has since become the gold standard in studies of duodenal adenomatosis (Table 8.7).

In the largest prospective study of duodenal adenomatosis in FAP, Bülow *et al.* (2004) report on 368 patients. The prevalence of duodenal adenomatosis at first endoscopy was 65%. This is similar to values in the other major series in the literature. The cumulative incidence of adenomatosis development in the 128 patients without adenomas at study entry was 50% after 6 years and 68% after 8 years.

Combining the latter with the age distribution in patients with adenomas at study entry resulted in a 90% incidence of adenomatosis at age 70 years. Other authors report on similar incidence that may reach up to 100%.

Table 8.7 Spigelman classification of duodenal polyposis.

Number of points	1	2	3
Polyp number	1–4	5–20	>20
Polyp size (mm)	1–4	5–10	>10
Histology	Tubular	Tubulovillous	Villous
Dysplasia level	Mild	Moderate	Severe

Stages
Stage 0: 0 points
Stage I: 1–4 points
Stage II: 5–6 points
Stage III: 7–8 points
Stage IV: 9–12 points

The lifetime risk of Spigelman stage IV adenomatosis is variable in the literature, and is between 20 and 50% (Bjork *et al.* 2001; Bülow *et al.* 2004).

According to the literature reporting on treatment of advanced duodenal adenomas, recurrence is almost guaranteed unless the duodenum is removed. Polypectomy (endoscopic or surgical transduodenal) may be temporarily effective, but does not offer a permanent cure.

The results of pancreas-preserving duodenectomy or pancreaticoduodenectomy for benign or early malignant disease are good, with low recurrence and acceptable morbidity and mortality. The outcome of surgery for established cancer, on the other hand, is poor, with recurrence and death the usual outcome. Although the risk of duodenal/periampullary cancer is relatively low in patients with FAP, those with persistent high-grade dysplasia represent a high-risk group. Careful surveillance is needed, and conservative surgery or endoscopic therapy may be tried. If the severe dysplasia returns or persists, consideration must be given to duodenectomy.

Total pancreaticoduodenectomy (Whipple's operation), is presently used only in patients with carcinomas. A pancreas-sparing duodenectomy is a relatively new procedure. It is more demanding technically, but spares the pancreatic head and obviates the need for pancreaticojejunostomy, with its potential complications. It is recommended as a cancer prophylactic operation in patients with severe adenomatosis and in experienced hands, results in fewer complications and good quality of life (Sarmiento *et al.* 2002; Bülow *et al.* 2004).

Heated intraperitoneal chemotherapy (HIPC) for small bowel adenocarcinoma

In general, HIPC can be applied both in the context of curative attempt and as a palliative measure. Its curative value can be used in two scenarios: for the prevention of carcinomatosis in patients at high risk, and, combined with cytoreduction, for treatment of established peritoneal disease. The procedure can also be utilized on a palliative basis for the control of symptomatic malignant ascites.

Most studies on HIPC in gastrointestinal malignancies describe the effect and outcome in patients with colorectal or gastric cancer. Studies describing patients with small bowel adenocarcinoma are sparse, yet the same principles and indications learned from colorectal and gastric carcinoma should apply.

Many patients who have a free intraabdominal perforation of gastrointestinal cancer through the malignancy itself subsequently develop peritoneal seeding and may later suffer from peritoneal carcinomatosis. Patients with primary cancer adherent to adjacent organs or structures (T4 lesions) are also at great risk for peritoneal carcinomatosis. The same is true for patients with positive peritoneal cytology (Sugarbaker 2005).

The value of HIPC in the rare small bowel adenocarcinoma is hard to assess. Marchettini and colleagues report on six patients with carcinomatosis from small bowel adenocarcinoma. All were treated with an aggressive approach that utilized cytoreductive surgery plus perioperative intraperitoneal mitomycin C and 5-fluorouracil. Disease control in the abdomen and pelvis was achieved in four of these patients. Their median survival was 12 months, with one patient alive and well at 4.5 years (Marchinetti & Sugarbaker 2002).

Jacks *et al.* (2005) performed cytoreduction and HIPC with mitomycin C on six patients with carcinomatosis from small bowel primary tumors. Three of the six patients were still alive after a mean follow-up of 19.7 months. Three patients died of disease progression 29, 30, and 45 months after the procedure. Median survival after the operation was 30.1 months.

Therefore, although not evidence-based, cytoreduction and HIPC should be considered a serious option in patients with carcinomatosis from small bowel adenocarcinoma.

GIST

The mainstay of resectable GIST treatment was and is surgical. The surgical oncologist managing a GIST case must assess both the resectability of the tumor and the ability of the patient to withstand a major resection.

It is important to stress that although GISTs may present as a huge lesion, the 'pushing' nature of tumor growth may sometimes allow for the development of a safe plane of dissection. Unless the tumor is metastatic at presentation, the good surgical candidate should be given the chance of surgical exploration before the tumor is deemed unresectable. In this context, it is important to mention the part that imatinib may possibly play in the near future, as a neoadjuvant drug, given in an attempt to downstage a borderline case. In a retrospective study, Andtbacka *et al.* showed that patients with locally advanced primary, recurrent, or metastatic GISTs with a partial radiographic response to imatinib, had significantly higher complete resection rates than patients with progressive disease (Andtbacka *et al.* 2007).

Regarding a small bowel GIST, there may be a significant difference between tumors involving the jejunoileum and those of the duodenum. The most common surgical procedure performed in the jejunoileum is a segmental resection. Unlike adenocarcinoma or carcinoid tumor, that spread through lymphatics, GISTs metastasize hematogenously, obviating the need for removal of lymphatic drainage in the mesentery. The surgical goal is to remove the tumor completely in negative margins without 'breaking' the tumor. The fact that wide excisions with lymphatic resection need not be performed may be significant in the duodenum, allowing the surgeon to avoid a major procedure such as pancreaticoduodenectomy.

In the case of a large GIST, on the other hand, the surgeon and team must be prepared for a major procedure. He or she

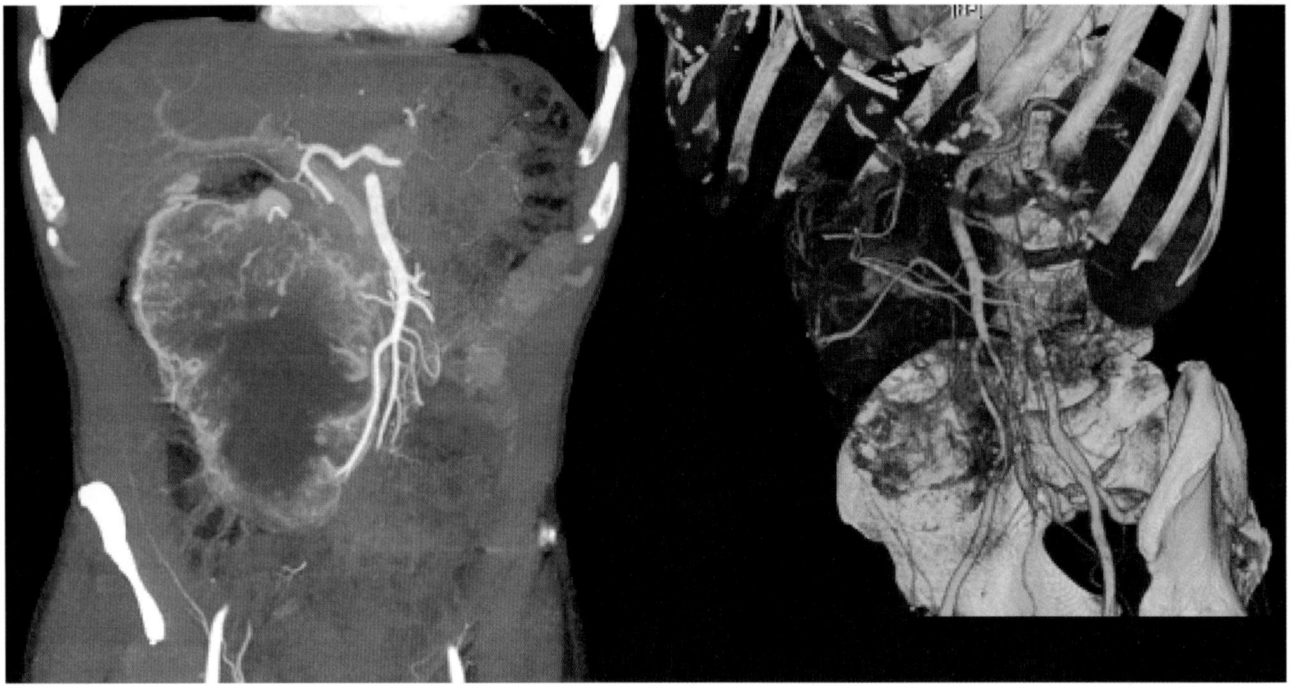

(a) (b)

Fig. 8.11 Huge duodenal GIST, as seen in CT angiography and a three-dimensional reconstruction. Note the 'heavy' vascularization (left) and the value of reconstruction in preoperative planning (right). (Courtesy of Dr Arye Blasher, Tel Aviv Sourasky Medical Center, Israel.)

must be familiar with the principles of adequate exposure and achievement of proximal and distal control over significant vascular structures, before trying to approach the tumor itself.

The surgeon preparing for such an adventure should use available imaging modalities to study the distorted anatomy to be expected when dealing with large GISTs (Fig. 8.11).

GISTs are highly vascularized and tend to rapture and bleed (see Fig. 8.11). This may be difficult to handle without preparation and may have significant impact on the oncologic outcome of the procedure.

Regarding all GISTs (gastric and small intestinal) complete excision is possible in approximately 85% of patients with primary, localized tumors. Negative microscopic margins are achieved in 70–95% of those completely resected.

Neuroendocrine tumors of the small intestine

Surgery is the most effective treatment for control of both local tumor effect and systemic endocrinopathy.

Resection can be performed either with curative intent or for palliation. In the case of palliative surgery, with incomplete removal of all the secreting tissue (liver metastases, lymph nodes), long-acting somatostatin analogs have proven efficacious in the management of the carcinoid syndrome.

A different issue is the surgical treatment of distant metastatic disease, most commonly in the liver, namely metastesectomy and liver transplantation.

Carcinoids of the jejunum and ileum

The usual procedure is a segmental resection. An important point to be remembered, especially in emergency operations for small bowel carcinoid (such as in bowel obstruction), is the association with other non-carcinoid neoplasms, which is evident in about 30% of patients. Also, there may be multiple lesions and liver metastases; therefore during such a procedure, one must thoroughly explore the abdomen, with significant emphasis on the colon.

Carcinoid syndrome, secondary to liver metastases, is reported to occur in up to 18% of patients with jejunoileal carcinoids but is rarely evident in carcinoids of the duodenum (Modlin *et al.* 2005).

If liver metastases are present at diagnosis, the primary tumor should nevertheless be resected to avoid later complications, which may include obstruction, bleeding, and perforation.

Duodenal neuroendocrine tumors

Most NE tumors are located in the second duodenum, around the papilla. There are different pathologic subtypes, including duodenal gastrinomas (about 65% of cases), somatostatinomas, non-functioning but hormone-producing tumors (such as serotonin, gastrin or calcitonin), poorly differentiated, predominantly ampullary NE carcinomas, and duodenal gangliocytic paragangliomas (Modlin *et al.* 2005).

The most common functional neuroendocrine tumor of the duodenum is gastrinoma, producing the Zollinger–Ellison syndrome (ZES). Since the vast majority of duodenal carcinoids are benign, gastrinomas serve as a prototype for other less common duodenal NE tumors. Pancreatic islet cell tumors, although usually considered together with gastrinomas, are naturally beyond the scope of this text.

Gastrinomas can occur sporadically or as part of multiple endocrine neoplasia type 1 (MEN1). The role surgery should play in MEN1 patients with ZES is probably limited to palliation only.

Sporadic ZES patients should undergo a surgical exploration in a curative attempt if they do not have diffuse liver metastases. There is no consensus as to the optimal extent of surgical treatment including the need for full-thickness duodenal resection and regional lymphadenectomy.

Duodenal gastrinomas are usually very small (less than 1 cm) and in many cases cannot be imaged preoperatively. Intraoperative localization is therefore very important.

During the operation, the search for neuroendocrine tumor is performed using palpation, intraoperative ultrasonography and an extended Kocher maneuver. Other options include intraoperative endoscopic transillumination of the duodenum and duodenotomy.

The most important maneuver in the exploration, when other techniques fail to locate the lesion, is the performance of wide longitudinal duodenotomy (Fig. 8.12).

Surgical treatment of hepatic metastases

Hepatic metastases from neuroendocrine tumors tend to progress slowly, but may become very symptomatic due to hormone secretion or pain. Although slow growing, these tumors confer a 5-year survival rate of no more then 20–40% and a median survival of 2–4 years, in the absence of aggressive surgical treatment.

Somatostatin analogs, that may be effective in symptom relief, do not have the same effect on tumor growth or prognosis. Thus, surgical therapy, which is possible in approximately 20% of these patients, remains one of the most effective treatments of metastatic NE tumors (Pascher *et al.* 2004).

Hepatic resection achieves symptom control and may also facilitate pharmacologic management in most patients but another significant benefit is survival extension, although recurrence is expected in the majority of patients.

Chen *et al.* (1998) compared 15 patients who underwent complete resection of liver metastases from neuroendocrine tumors with 23 patients with comparable tumor burden that were believed to be unresectable. The 5-year survival rate of patients who had complete resection was 73%, compared with 29% in the unresected group.

Sarmiento and colleagues describe 170 patients with metastatic NE tumors to the liver. Carcinoid was by far the most common (120 cases). Major hepatectomy was performed in 54% of patients. Operation controlled symptoms in 104 of 108 patients, but symptom recurrence rate at 5 years was 59%. Tumor recurred in 84% at 5 years and the overall survival was 61% and 35% at 5 and 10 years, respectively (Sarmiento *et al.* 2003).

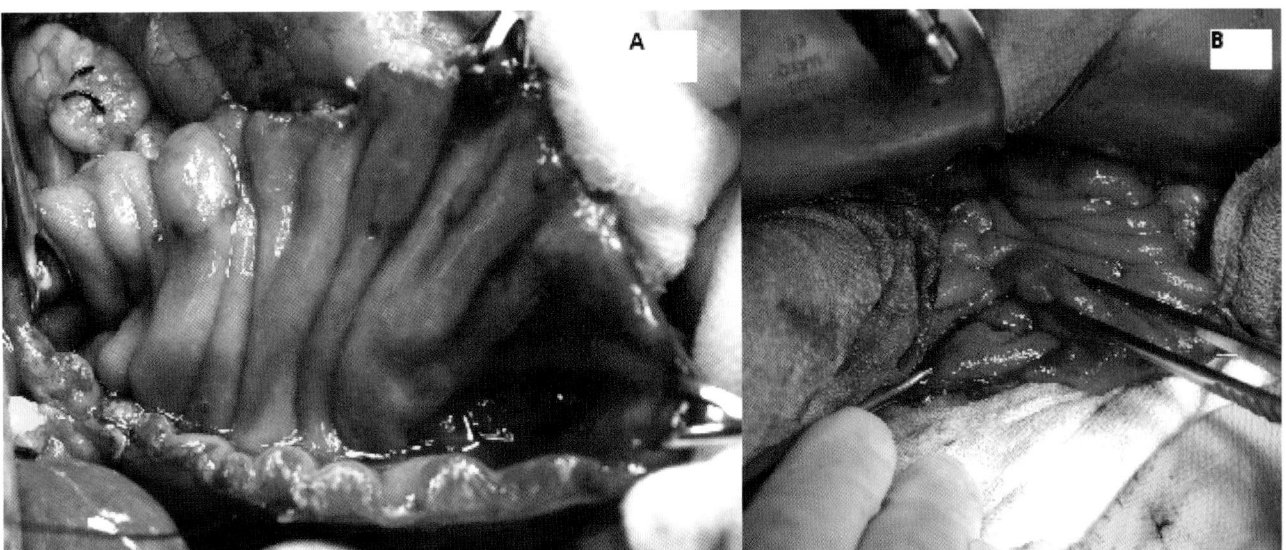

Fig. 8.12 Longitudinal duodenotomy (A) and localization of a small submucosal gastrinoma (B).

Before surgery, it is important to locate extrahepatic lesions. Perhaps the best use of indium^{111} pentetreotide is in the evaluation of disease beyond the liver, in the process of patient selection for surgery.

In a patient with a disease limited to the liver and a reasonable surgical risk, surgical outcome, morbidity and mortality justify operative intervention.

The main exception is the patient with carcinoid valvular disease. These patients are poor candidates for surgery and may develop a right-sided heart failure with an increase in the central venous pressure and massive hemorrhage during hepatectomy because of the difficulty in controlling backflow bleeding from hepatic veins. Correction of valvular disease should therefore be considered before liver resection.

Table 8.8 summarizes the single-center experience with surgical treatment of metastatic NE tumors.

Once the patient is planned for surgery, several steps need to be completed before the operation, to decrease the effect of specific endocrinopathies. For patients with symptoms related to carcinoid tumors, preoperative preparation with 150–500 μg of somatostatin decreases the chances of carcinoid crisis, which is manifested by hemodynamic instability. The use of this medication intraoperatively should be kept in mind because a carcinoid crisis can occur despite premedication (Modlin *et al.* 2005).

In conclusion, patients whose primary tumor can be controlled, who have no extrahepatic metastases or have limited and resectable extrahepatic disease, and who have a reasonable performance status are candidates for resection with curative intent (Sarmiento & Que 2003). This conclusion is not in doubt. The issue of palliative resection, on the other hand, is debatable. In selected cases, surgery probably offers a better palliation, allows a reduction of octreotide dose and even slightly improves survival compared with medical treatment. Since ablative procedures can usually control more than 90% of tumor load, a preoperative assessment that less than 90% of disease can be resected should be considered a contraindication to metastesectomy.

When surgical cytoreduction is impossible (or incomplete) due to the extent of disease, therapeutic options include one or a combination of the ablative techniques (hepatic artery ligation, chemoembolization, radiofrequency ablation and cryotherapy), medical treatment (with somatostatin analogs and chemotherapy), or liver transplantation.

Table 8.8 Single-center experience with surgical treatment of metastatic NE tumors. Adapted with permission from Pascher (2005).

Authors	Year	Number of patients	Perioperative mortality (%)	Symptom control (% patients)	Survival
McEntee *et al.*	1990	37	0	64	49% 1-year survival
Carty *et al.*	1992	17	0	–	79% 5-year survival
Soreide *et al.*	1992	75	2	–	70% 5-year survival
Que *et al.*	1995	74	1.6	90	74% 4-year survival
Dousset *et al.*	1996	17	5.9	88	46% 4-year survival
Ahlman *et al.*	1996	14	0	100	100% 5-year survival (R0)
Chen *et al.*	1998	15	0	–	73% 5-year survival
Chamberlain *et al.*	2000	34	6	Approximately 90	76% 5-year survival
Grazi *et al.*	2000	19	0	–	92% 4-year survival
Pascher *et al.*	2000	25	0	–	76% 5-year survival
Jaeck *et al.*	2001	13	0	–	91% 3-year survival
Nave *et al.*	2001	31	0	–	47% 5-year survival
Sarmiento *et al.*	2001	170	1.2	96	61% 5-year survival

Liver transplantation

The combination of the slow-growing nature of NE tumors and their relative resistance to chemotherapeutic agents led to the option of liver transplantation (OLT) in patients with isolated hepatic tumor burden beyond resectability. Unfortunately, the shortage of allografts, the complication rate and the cost of such a procedure has hampered this approach, and liver transplantation has not been common in clinical practice (no more than 200 cases were reported worldwide and most series include mixed patients with GI, pancreatic and pulmonary neuroendocrine tumors). Nonetheless, the oncologist should remember that the option of transplantation is still open in highly selected cases. The data is based on small and retrospective publications.

In a multicenter study from France, Le Treut reported a 5-year survival rate of 69% among 15 highly selected patients who underwent liver transplantation for metastatic carcinoid. Only 6 had the primary tumor in the small intestine. The authors concluded that OLT can achieve the control of hormonal symptoms and prolong survival in selected patients with liver metastasis of carcinoid tumours but not other NE tumors (Le Treut *et al.* 1997).

Rosenau *et al.* (2002) reported on 19 patients who underwent OLT for metastatic NE tumors. As in other papers on the subject, the study population was mixed and only 6 of the 19 had their primary tumor in the small intestine. Survival was found to be highly related to Ki67 and E-cadherin status in the metastases. After 7 years all five patients with low Ki67 and regular E-cadherin expression were alive, compared with none of the 12 with a high Ki67 or aberrant E-cadherin expression. The combination of Ki67 and E-cadherin had a specificity and sensitivity of 100% to predict survival 7 years after OLT ($p = 0.003$). The authors reported 1-, 5- and 10-year survival rates of 89, 80 and 50%, respectively.

van Vilsteren and colleagues, on the other hand, showed that the Ki67 proliferation index in 18 patients (most of them with pancreatic NE tumors) did not differentiate those with or without recurrence. The 1-year survival was 87% with an estimated 1-year recurrence-free rate of 77% (van Vilsteren *et al.* 2006).

There is no doubt about the value of liver surgery for almost all primary tumours and hepatic metastases, resectable radically with the aim of achieving a cure.

On the other hand, the role of orthotopic liver transplantation in the treatment of metastatic carcinoid tumors is not yet clear.

A strict selection of patients for transplantation must be the rule. The best selection criteria accepted today are the absence of extrahepatic metastases, young age (less than 50), low Ki67 index (less than 5%) and normal E-cadherin expression.

A survival of higher than 85% after the first year can be expected, but the long-term recurrence-free survival is probably no more then 25%.

Lymphoma

Non-Hodgkin's lymphomas (NHLs) may involve a variety of abdominal organs, including the liver, spleen, gastrointestinal tract, and retroperitoneum.

According to recent classifications of NHL (WHO and the REAL classification), lymphomas arising in the GI tract represent one of four subtypes:

- diffuse large B-cell lymphoma
- mucosal-associated lymphoid tissue (MALT)-associated lymphomas
- peripheral T-cell lymphoma
- Burkitt's lymphomas.

Chemotherapy is the primary therapeutic modality for most lymphomas. Lymphomas manifest a variable response to chemotherapy. The best overall cure rates with chemotherapy are seen with rapidly proliferating tumors, such as diffuse large-cell lymphomas. Slower-growing, indolent tumors, like mantle cell and follicular lymphomas, are frequently resistant to chemotherapy and in many cases chemotherapy will not change the outcome. Conversely, the most rapidly growing aggressive lymphomas, such as anaplastic lymphoma, also often demonstrate resistance to chemotherapy and, like the slow-growing indolent lymphomas, carry an overall lower cure rate. This phenomenon of variable responsiveness to chemotherapy based on rate of proliferation is a critical concept in the management of lymphoma. For the indolent localized lymphoma, surgical resection and local irradiation, alone or in combination, can play the primary role in treatment. On the other hand, chemotherapy remains the mainstay of therapy for the rapidly proliferating aggressive lymphomas, because these malignancies almost always extend beyond the local fields encompassed by surgery or radiation.

When isolated to the small intestine, the surgical treatment of segmental resection with adjuvant chemotherapy or radiation is the treatment of choice, but there is a paucity of data regarding the surgical treatment.

In an old retrospective study on 202 patients with abdominal lymphomas, Mentzer and colleagues report on 36 patients who underwent laparotomy before chemotherapy or radiation therapy. Twenty patients with localized disease demonstrated significantly better survival than those with extranodal and nodal involvement ($p < 0.05$). Four patients with local resection received no adjuvant therapy and were free of disease a median of 50 months after surgery (Mentzer *et al.* 1988).

Other treatments

Pascal Peeters, Eric Van Cutsem & Mario Dicato

Benign tumors

For adenomatous polyps located within the reach of upper

endoscopy, a simple endoscopic snare polypectomy is the treatment of choice. If technically not feasible, a surgical local excision is indicated. Complete resection is mandatory, since the villous adenomas in particular may harbour foci of malignancy in 25–45% of cases.

Endoscopic resection of periampullary sessile adenomas is often hampered by the risk of damaging the ampulla of Vater. Furthermore, after endoscopic resection in this region, local recurrences are seen in about half of patients. Close endoscopic follow-up is warranted.

Thus, due to the high rate of malignant degeneration, the propensity for local recurrence and the ampullary localization, the decision between endoscopic polypectomy and radical surgical approach (which means pancreaticoduodenectomy) remains difficult and should be individualized since it not only depends on the anatomic and histological features of the polyp, but also on the technical expertise of the endoscopist. Lesions in the first and second part of the duodenum should also be managed with pancreaticoduodenectomy if endoscopic resection is not feasible; lesions of the third and fourth portion of the duodenum can be treated with simple wedge resection. More distant polyps are surgically treated by segmental resection.

Since duodenal polyps can form part of the FAP syndrome, all patients with duodenal adenomas should undergo colonoscopy.

Lipomas should not be resected unless they are symptomatic. Benign leiomyomas should only be resected if they are symptomatic, if they cannot be differentiated from GISTs, or if there is doubt about their benign or malignant nature.

Neurofibromatas in patients with von Recklinghausen's disease are considered to be benign. Unless symptomatic, they should not be treated.

Hamartomatous polyps in Peutz–Jeghers syndrome (PJS) are generally not premalignant and they should only be resected when symptomatic (bleeding, invagination, obstruction), when the size exceeds 15 mm or when they have macroscopic or microscopic features suspicious for malignant degeneration (Wirtzfeld *et al.* 2001). Since polyps in PJS patients are abundant and there is a high lifetime risk of needing multiple interventions, appropriate surgical management consists of surgical enterectomy and polypectomy. If bowel resection is required, an absolute minimum length of bowel should be sacrificed in order to limit the risk for development of short bowel syndrome.

Appropriate surveillance of the proband and his or her first-degree relatives is warranted.

Adenocarcinoma

The type of surgery needed for treatment of small intestine adenocarcinomas depends upon localization. Pancreaticoduodenectomy is required for tumors located in the first and second and some of those located in the third portion of the duodenum. More distantly located adenocarcinomas can be treated by segmental resection, and tumors in the terminal part of the ileum need a right hemicolectomy. Wide surgical margins, with perioperative confirmation of the margin status by frozen section evaluation, and resection of the adherent mesentery and lymph nodes are standard requirements.

Until now, for duodenal adenocarcinomas no difference in survival has been shown after treatment with pancreaticoduodenectomy compared to local or segmental resection, which is associated with less morbidity and mortality. Thus, superficial duodenal tumors on the antimesenteric wall with an early stage confirmed by endoscopic ultrasound can also be treated by surgical local segmental excision, if technically feasible. On the other hand, the mortality associated with a Whipple procedure has reported to be improved dramatically when performed by an experienced surgeon, nowadays being only 1–3% (Dabaja *et al.* 2004).

There is not much information available on adjuvant chemotherapy for small bowel adenocarcinoma. There are no prospective randomized clinical trials on this topic, and in retrospective analyses no significant survival benefit could be demonstrated (Howe *et al.* 1999). Given the poor general prognosis it seems a logical approach to treat patients with adjuvant chemotherapy. However, as yet there is no evidence supporting this approach.

In metastatic disease, a palliative surgical resection of the primary tumor is frequently needed in order to prevent or treat complications as bowel obstruction or bleeding.

Palliative chemotherapeutic regimens are often based on 5-fluorouracil (5-FU) and cisplatin. Overall survival rates of 13–14 months are reported (Locher *et al.* 2005). Data on combination therapies with oxaliplatin and irinotecan, and on intraperitoneal hyperthermic chemotherapy are scarce.

Carcinoid tumors

Management of carcinoid tumors generally consists of resection of the tumor in localized disease, and control of carcinoid-related symptoms in the setting of unresectable or metastatic disease.

Localized disease

In comparison to other carcinoid localizations, small bowel carcinoids in particular tend to have a higher metastatic potential independent of their size (metastases in tumors even smaller than 1 cm). Therefore localized carcinoids should always be treated by wide en-bloc resection including the subjacent mesentery and lymph nodes. Regional lymph node metastasis is seen in up to 70% of small bowel carcinoids. Resection of the mesentery may be hampered by the presence of fibrosis and foreshortening.

Before surgery, a thorough examination of the entire gastrointestinal tract is indicated since all carcinoid tumors are associated with a significant risk of synchronous or metachronous non-carcinoid tumors (most likely adenocarcinomas) along the gastrointestinal tract, but also in the lung, the prostate, cervix and ovary. Of all carcinoid tumors, small intestinal carcinoids in particular tend to have the highest rate of association with synchronous or metachronous non-carcinoid tumors (29% for carcinoids of the small intestine versus 22% for all carcinoids taken together). One possible explanation for this observation is that these non-carcinoid tumors may result from prolonged exposure to growth factors secreted by the carcinoids (Modlin *et al.* 2003).

Advanced disease

Treatment of advanced disease is directed to control of carcinoid-related symptoms, for which different options are available including somatostatin analogs, interferon alpha, radiofrequency ablation, cryoablation, surgical resection, hepatic artery embolization or chemoembolization, radiolabeled therapies and systemic cytotoxic chemotherapy.

In cases of mild carcinoid syndrome, conventional measures are frequently sufficient. Alcohol intake should be limited since it typically induces flushing. Mild diarrhea and wheezing can be treated as in other patients. Diarrhea in patients with metastatic carcinoid tumors does not always occur as part of the carcinoid syndrome. It has to be differentiated from diarrhea resulting from wide segmental small bowel resection, or from removal of the ileocecal valve. These procedures can lead to bile acid loss and/or bacterial contamination of the terminal part of the small bowel with subsequent deconjugation of the bile acids. Specific treatment directed at these causes consists of cholestyramine and/or antibiotics. Diarrhea might also be an adverse effect of treatment with somatostatin analogs.

In the setting of moderate to severe carcinoid symptoms, treatment with the somatostatin analogs octreotide and lanreotide is considered as the gold standard. They are characterized by high affinity for somatostatin receptor 2, and to a lesser extent also receptor types 3 and 5. It is documented that tumors without somatostatin receptor 2 do not respond to treatment with somatostatin analogs (Arnold *et al.* 2000). The dose of octreotide needed to control symptoms varies from 50 μg up to 500 μg three times daily. In up to 75–85% of patients, symptoms are adequately controlled with acceptable toxicity. Biochemical responses (as defined as a more than 50% decrease in tumor markers) have been obtained in 30–75% of patients (Caplin *et al.* 1988; Öberg 1998, 1999; Rubin *et al.* 1999; Wymenga *et al.* 1999; Ducreux *et al.* 2000; Welin *et al.* 2004). Octreotide and lanreotide seem to be equally efficient in terms of symptom control and reduction in tumor cell markers for patients with the carcinoid syndrome (O'Toole *et al.* 2000). Furthermore, somatostatin analogs might have the potential of slowing tumor growth since objective radiographic tumor responses have been reported in a minority (3–10%) of patients (Öberg *et al.* 1998; Faiss *et al.* 1999; Ducreux *et al.* 2000; Aparicio *et al.* 2001; Öberg 2001; Leong & Pasieka 2002).

For patients with malignant midgut carcinoids, the median survival has been estimated at 36 months for somatostatin analog treatment (Öberg 2001). Potential side-effects include mild nausea, abdominal discomfort, bloating, loose stools and steatorrhea (presumably resulting from transient inhibition of pancreatic exocrine secretion and malabsorption of fat). The adverse effects start within hours of the first subcutaneous injection, are dose-dependent and usually tend to subside spontaneously within few weeks while continuing the treatment. There may be local pain and erythema at the injection site. Long-term treatment with somatostatin analogs induces the formation of gallstones or sludge in up to 50% of patients due to delayed postprandial gallbladder contractility and emptying. However, symptomatic gallstone disease is rare and only about 1% of patients require a cholecystectomy. More seldom, mild glucose intolerance occurs due to inhibition of insulin secretion (Öberg *et al.* 2004).

The optimum approach for using octreotide is to initiate therapy in the form of immediate-release subcutaneous injections to test for tolerability. The initial dose may range from 100 to 500 μg three times daily, with (if necessary) dose escalation every 3–4 days until achievement of maximum control of symptoms.

When treatment with octreotide or lanreotide is effective and well tolerated, it is advised to switch over to the long-acting formulas of both agents, which can be administered on a monthly basis because of their longer half-life. Octreotide is available as a long-acting release (LAR) formulation and administered by intramuscular injection at standard doses of 20 or 30 mg every 4 weeks; lanreotide initially as a prolonged release (PR) but recently as an autogel formulation, at standard doses of 60, 90 and 120 mg, also administered every 4 weeks. Pain at the injection site is a common complaint. It is shown that these depot forms are equally active as their original subcutaneous formulations (Rubin *et al.* 1999; Wymenga *et al.* 1999; Ducreux *et al.* 2000). The long-acting somatostatin analogs achieve a regression of carcinoid-related symptoms that is correlated to a biochemical response in 50–80% of patients. During the first 2 weeks after injection of octreotide LAR, supplemental subcutaneous octreotide is needed since the LAR formulations do not achieve therapeutic serum levels until that time. After that period, plateau serum levels of octreotide are maintained for almost 8 weeks. However, in individual patients, relapse of symptoms has been observed between 3 and 6 weeks after injection. Administration every 4 weeks has turned out to guarantee consistent elevated ocreotide serum concentrations providing pronounced suppression of the hormone releases (Arnold *et al.* 2000).

In some patients the carcinoid-related symptoms recur regularly in the week before the next injection. Options in this setting include addition of subcutaneous ocreotide during that period, but it is probably better to shorten the interval of the depot formulations to every 3 weeks instead of monthly intervals. Other patients symptoms are insufficiently controlled with the regular doses and they need dose escalations up to 60 mg of octreotide LAR each month (Öberg *et al.* 2004).

Treatment with interferon alpha has shown to control symptoms of hormonal hypersecretion in 40–50% of patients, to stabilize tumor growth in 20–40% of patients, and achieve an objective tumor regression in up to 15% of patients for a median duration of 32 months (Faiss *et al.* 1999; Öberg *et al.* 2004). Its mechanism of action is supposed to be multifactorial: triggering of the immune system and ability to stimulate natural killer cell function, a direct effect on the tumor cells by inducing apoptosis and differentiation, inhibiting the production of growth factor/receptors and other agents secreted by the tumor cells, and it is assumed that interferon alpha also exhibits an anti-angiogenic effect. It controls the release of tumor-derived hormonal products such as chromogranin A and serotonin reflected by a decrease in the urinary excretion of 5-HIAA. Interferon alpha seems to induce fibrosis within liver metastases, leading to a decrease in viable tumor cells which are replaced by fibroblasts and thus leading to less tumoral activity but without significant change in objective tumor size (Öberg 2000).

In patients resistant to somatostatin analogs, addition of interferon alpha has shown to be effective in controlling carcinoid-related symptoms, and to induce biochemical responses and objective tumor reduction (Frank *et al.* 1999; Öberg 2001). However, in a prospective randomized study no difference in antiproliferative effect could be demonstrated between patients treated with somatostatin analogs alone, with interferon alpha alone, or with the combination of both agents. The combination of both led to more side-effects and interruption of therapy (Faiss *et al.* 2003).

In comparison to treatment with somatostatin analogs, interferon alpha more frequently needs to be interrupted due to the adverse effects consisting of flu-like symptoms occurring in up to 90% of patients during the first 3–4 days after injection (which can be managed by paracetamol or aspirin), low-grade fever, anorexia and weight loss, chronic fatigue in about 50% of patients, and mental depression.

In the available clinical trials, the dose of interferon alpha varies from 3 to 9×10^6 units, administered subcutaneously three to seven times a week. Interferon alpha is somewhat myelosuppressive, causing anemia in 30% of patients and mild thrombocytopenia in up to 20%; leucopenia is mostly being the dose-limiting factor. Interferon alpha treatment needs to be individually titrated using a guideline index for leucocyte count not lower than 3.0×10^9/L. Mild hepatotoxicity is observed in 30% of patients, seldom leading to interruption of treatment, and autoimmune manifestations—mostly thyroid dysfunction—occur in up to 20% of patients (Öberg 2000).

During treatment with somatostatin analogs or interferon alpha, patients should be monitored using the biochemical parameters chromogranin A and urinary 5-HIAA combined with CT imaging every 3 months until stability is seen for two consecutive scans. From then, disease evaluation every 6 months seems to be sufficient (Öberg *et al.* 2004).

Until now, no chemotherapeutic regimen has shown to be of significant value. Many combinations have been tried, most of them including 5-fluorouracil, cisplatin, mitomycin C, streptozotocin, and doxorubicin, all with limited activity and associated with substantial side-effects. In comparison to the other digestive neuroendocrine tumors, response rates for carcinoids are substantially lower. In most studies, response rates vary between 15 and 25%, whereas response rates for other digestive neuroendocrine tumors may be as high as 40–60%. The response duration is often short lasting and no more than 3–4 months (Rougier & Mitry 2000). The combinations of streptozotocin and 5-fluorouracil and streptozotocin plus doxorubicin seem to be the most active (Sun *et al.* 2005). However, in approximately 50% of patients treated with streptozotocin and 5-FU or doxorubicin, grade 3 or 4 toxicities are seen. The main toxicities of this combinations include renal impairment, hepatotoxicity, nausea and vomiting, neutropenia and thrombocytopenia, and for the combination with doxorubicin, cardiac toxicity and alopecia. Given the minor activity and the substantial toxicity of cytotoxic chemotherapy combinations in carcinoid tumors, the benefit should counterbalance its toxicity and therefore patients should be carefully selected. The best criteria for initiating systemic chemotherapy seem to be: young patient age, highly proliferative and/or unresectable tumors, failure of chemoembolization, or tumor extension excluding locoregional treatment. In some cases a severe carcinoid syndrome that cannot be controlled by somatostatin analogs or other means can also be considered as a potential indication (Rougier & Mitry 2000). The proliferation index Ki-67 can be of use in the decision-making. The precise level of the proliferation index Ki-67 has not been determined but indices of more than 10% might support the use of systemic chemotherapy early in the treatment algorithm of an individual patient (Öberg 2001). Systemic chemotherapy is generally initiated after an observation period of many months—related to the slow rate of growth of carcinoids—but it should be started before impairment of the patient's general condition and major organ functions have developed.

More recent trials with newer agents as taxanes and gemcitabine failed to demonstrate significant anti-tumor activity (Kulke *et al.* 2004). Given the highly vascular nature of carcinoid tumors there could be a role for molecularly targeted therapies directed to the vascular endothelial growth factor (VEGF) such as bevacizumab and sunitinib. Preliminary results of small studies show the activity of these antiangiogenic agents, as well as from the mTOR (mammalian target of rapamycin) inhibitors, temsirolimus and everolimus (RAD001) (Yao 2007).

Preventive treatment with octreotide should be initiated preoperatively. It is often stated that there is a role for palliative surgery in patients with slow tumor growth and severe intractable hormonal symptoms in whom more than 90% of the metastatic load can be removed. A significant improvement in hormonal symptoms can be achieved with only minor complications in patients with extensive liver involvement and/or carcinoid syndrome by intervention with surgery and/or radiofrequency ablation (Ahlman *et al.* 2000; Gulec *et al.* 2002).

Radiofrequency ablation or cryoablation of liver metastases, and perctuaneous ethanol injections either alone or in combination with surgery, provide relief of symptoms in most patients if performed with curative intent. Data on these approaches are scarce.

The knowledge that liver metastases mainly get their blood supplied by the hepatic artery forms the rationale for hepatic artery embolization and hepatic artery chemoembolization (HACE). Normal liver tissue is relatively spared since it is supplied predominantly by the portal vein. It is assumed that embolization-induced ischemia sensitizes tumor cells to cytotoxic drugs, whose concentrations are increased by blood flow slowing down. The aims of HACE are the control of otherwise intractable hormone-related symptoms, the inhibition of tumor growth, and improving patients' survival. HACE mostly is carried out with the antineoplastic agents doxorubicin, cisplatin or streptozocin. In uncontrolled trials and retrospective analyses, a substantial improvement or relief of carcinoid symptoms is seen in 73–100% of patients. In concordance, a more than 50% decrease in the urinary excretion of the serotonin metabolite 5-HIAA is documented in 57–91% of patients undergoing HACE. Response, defined as radiographic regression of the lesions according to the WHO criteria, is reported in 33–80% of patients with a mean duration of 6–42 months (Moertel *et al.* 1994; Eriksson *et al.* 1998; Ruszniewski & Malka 2000). Patients with extensive liver involvement (more than 50%) may not benefit from this approach since it is shown that their outcome is very poor (Touzios *et al.* 2005). Liver embolizations performed relatively late in the clinical course appear to be as effective as procedures carried out earlier in the disease course (Eriksson *et al.* 1998). In comparison to simple embolization, chemoembolization is associated with more morbidity including leucocytosis, disturbed liver function tests, fever, nausea and abdominal pain. The rate of serious adverse events in most series is about 10%. Gallbladder perforation due to gallbladder ischemia, pancreatitis, liver abscess, vascular damage, hepatorenal syndrome and carcinoid crisis are seen in a minority of patients. In order to minimize these complications, several precautions can be undertaken such as prophylactic administration of octreotide, superselective catheterization with low risk of vascular damage, cholecystectomy at the time of initial surgery, and post-procedure hemodynamic monitoring and intravenous hydration. It is recommended that this type of procedure only be performed by an experienced interventional radiologist (Ahlman *et al.* 2000).

Given the morbidity, it is imperative to carefully select patients that might benefit from these procedures. Hepatic artery embolization or chemoembolization should be reserved for patients with unresectable liver metastases without extrahepatic spread, with progressive disease and/or severe carcinoid symptoms not responding to somatostatin analogs or interferon. Contraindications are tumor burden exceeding 50% of the liver volume, occlusion of the portal vein, and hyperbilirubinemia. However, some authors state that patients with extensive liver involvement can safely undergo this type of treatment using superselective catheters and treatment separated in time. When metastases are resectable, surgery remains the preferred approach (Ahlman *et al.* 2000; Ruszniewski & Malka 2000).

Another approach to tumor control consists of local irradiation by means of radiolabeled somatostatin analogs or metaiodobenzylguanidine (MIBG). The somatostatin analogs reach the tumor cells by binding to the somatostatin receptor while MIBG is stored in the neurosecretory granules. After binding to the somatostatin receptor, the radiolabeled somatostatin analog is internalized and translocated into the nucleus, which might be the explanation for the effectiveness of agents with a very short irradiation range such as indium-111 (Janson *et al.* 2000). The success of internalization of the radiolabeled somatostatin analogs depends on the types of somatostatin receptors expressed on the cellular membrane. Uptake of the somatostatin analogs in the tumoral tissue is seen to varying degrees; in some extent due to the peritumoral fibrosis, but possibly also due to a variable pattern of somatostatin receptors present on the cell membrane (Janson *et al.* 1997). Different agents are used: indium-111 octreotide, yttrium-90 octreotide, and lutetium-177 octreotate in patients with somatostatin receptor-positive tumors. In one series, 27% of patients with advanced neuroendocrine tumors achieved objective responses after treatment with lutetium-177 octreotate. In 82% of patients, at least a stabilization was noted, with a median time to tumor progression of more than 36 months. Severe grade 3 or 4 toxicity was very low. The likelihood of response was correlated with the intensity of uptake on pretreatment somatostatin receptor scintigraphy, and with limited disease comparing to more extensive metastatic disease (Kwekkeboom *et al.* 2005). Octreotide-based nuclear treatment is well tolerated; depression of bone marrow frequently is the dose-limiting factor.

As with SRS scans, therapy with the somatostatin analogs octreotide and lanreotide should be stopped before the administration of radiolabeled somatostatin analogs. Theoretically, occupation of the binding sites for somatostatin prevents the receptor sites from being occupied when the radionuclide combination is administered. It is recommended to stop a subcutaneous immediate release form 24 hours before radiotherapy, and to interrupt a depot formulation for at least 8 weeks (Öberg *et al.* 2004).

In a retrospective analysis, 15% of patients with metastatic carcinoids and positive diagnostic MIBG scintigraphy had objective radiographic responses and a significant decrease in the levels of 5-HIAA following treatment with Iodium-131 MIBG. An improvement in survival was not seen. Adverse effects of MIBG therapy include nausea, vomiting and hematologic toxicity (Safford *et al.* 2004).

Carcinoid crisis

Clinicians treating patients with advanced carcinoid tumors should be aware of the potential triggers of carcinoid crisis, and act in a preventive way by means of prophylactic administration of the somatostatin analog octreotide. In patients in whom symptoms are well controlled by a standard dose of a depot somatostatin analog, a supplementary bolus dose of 250–500 μg octreotide should be given subcutaneously within 1–2 hours before a procedure starts. For emergency surgery in therapy-naïve patients, a 500–1000-μg intravenous bolus of octreotide is recommended.

Once a carcinoid crisis has developed, an intravenous bolus of 500–1000 μg octreotide is given, with repetition at 5-min intervals until control of symptoms is achieved. Alternatively, following an intravenous bolus, continuous intravenous infusion of octreotide at a dose of 50–200 μg/h may be given (Öberg *et al.* 2004). Patients should be monitored and blood pressure should be corrected either by intravenous administration of antihypertensive agents or by colloids depending on the presence of hyper- or hypotension. When bronchodilating agents are needed, caution is needed not to worsen tachycardia.

Lymphoma

The majority of primary intestinal lymphomas are surgically treated at the time of diagnosis since in most cases no preoperative diagnosis can be made. A fresh resection specimen or biopsy should be sent to the pathologist in order to optimize histological interpretation.

The efficacy of *Helicobacter pylori* eradication as treatment for early-stage low-grade gastric extranodal marginal zone B-cell lymphoma of MALT type has repeatedly been demonstrated (Weber *et al.* 1994; Kulke & Mayer 1999; Roggero *et al.* 1995; Sackmann *et al.* 1997). Complete histological regression has been documented in 50–80% of patients. The anecdotal reports on the regression of intestinal MALT type lymphomas following eradication of *H. pylori* might also suggest a pathogenetic role for this organism (Nagashima *et al.* 1996).

The 'Western type' intestinal MALT lymphoma can be cured by surgery alone (resection of the affected segment of small bowel together with its subjacent mesentery) in the case of low-grade histology. After complete resection of a high-grade lymphoma (even if stage I) or in the presence of locoregional lymph node involvement, postoperative adjuvant chemotherapy is recommended by most authors because of the high relapse risk and the poor survival data following treatment with surgery alone (Coit 2001). Adjuvant radiation therapy is less recommended given the efficacy of the modern chemotherapeutic regimens and the important long-term side-effects of abdominal radiation therapy (Radaszkiewicz *et al.* 1992). Adjuvant combination chemotherapy has shown to improve disease-free and overall survival rates (Shih *et al.* 1994).

For patients with advanced disease (stages III and IV), combination chemotherapy is the treatment of choice, with CHOP being the preferred regimen. Palliative resection may be necessary to avoid or treat bleeding or perforation.

In Mediterranean lymphoma or immunoproliferative small intestinal disease (IPSID), remission can be induced by antibiotic treatment alone if diagnosis is made at an early stage when disease is limited to mucosa and/or submucosa. Antibiotic treatment is mostly directed against *Campylobacter jejuni* since most evidence points toward this organism as the culprit pathogenetic trigger in IPSID. Culture results of intestinal biopsy specimens in patients who had a dramatic response to treatment with antibiotics suggest the association between *C. jejuni* and IPSID (Lecuit *et al.* 2004). Ampicillin, tetracycline or metronidazole-based regimens are generally recommended.

However, after an initial treatment response, in the majority of patients IPSID will ultimately relapse and behave as an aggressive lymphoma necessitating combination chemotherapy and/or radiotherapy with nutritional support. Since the intestinal involvement is generally diffuse, surgery has a very little role.

Mantle cell lymphoma or lymphomatous polyposis can be treated by aggressive chemotherapy followed by autologous bone marrow transplantation but is considered to be incurable. Since its multifocal localization, surgery is only indicated in the setting of complications such as obstruction.

Sporadic Burkitt-like lymphomas are predominantly located in the ileocecal region. Aggressive chemotherapy is the mainstay of treatment and might be followed by autologous bone marrow transplantation. Complete surgical resection is usually performed in order to alleviate symptoms of mass effect and to avoid complications during chemotherapeutic treatment.

Enteropathy-associated T-cell lymphomas (EATLs) are almost always of high-grade histology, behave aggressively and are associated with poor prognosis. Five-year survival approximates 10%. Due to the likelihood of their causing ulceration and perforation, surgical intervention is frequently needed. Because of the late diagnosis of most EATLs and their underlying 'refractory' celiac disease with associated malnutrition, the frequent complications and their interventions, most patients are in a generally poor condition and are not able to tolerate multidrug chemotherapeutic regimens (Boot *et al.* 2004).

References

Ahlman H, Wängberg B, Jansson S *et al.* (2000) Interventional treatment of gastrointestinal neuroendocrine tumours. *Digestion* 62 (Suppl 1): 59–68.

Akahoshi K, Kubokawa M, Matsumoto M *et al.* (2006) Double-balloon endoscopy in the diagnosis and management of GI tract diseases: methodology, indications, safety, and clinical impact. *World J Gastroenterol* 12: 7654–59.

Andtbacka RH, Ng CS, Scaife CL *et al.* (2007) Surgical resection of gastrointestinal stromal tumors after treatment with imatinib. *Ann Surg Oncol* 14(1): 1–2.

Aparicio T, Ducreux M, Baudin E *et al.* (2001) Antitumour activity of somatostatin analogues in progressive metastatic neuroendocrine tumours. *Eur J Cancer* 37: 1014–9.

Arber N, Hibshoosh H, Yasui W *et al.* (1999) Abnormalities in the expression of cell cycle-related proteins in tumors of the small bowel. *Cancer Epidemiol Biomarkers Prev* 8(12): 1101–5.

Arber N, Sutter T, Miyake M *et al.* (1996) Increased expression of cyclin D1 and the Rb tumor suppressor gene in c-K-ras transformed rat enterocytes. *Oncogene* 12: 1903–8.

Arber N, Han EK, Sgambato A *et al.* (1997) A K-ras oncogene increases resistance to sulindac-induced apoptosis in rat enterocytes. *Gastroenterology* 113: 1892–900.

Arber N, Hibshoosh H, Yasui W *et al.* (1999) Abnormalities in the expression of cell cycle-related proteins in tumors of the small bowel. *Cancer Epidemiol Biomarkers Prev* 8(12): 1101–5.

Arber N, Shapira I, Ratan J *et al.* (2000) Activation of c-K-ras mutations in human gastrointestinal tumors. *Gastroenterology* 118: 1045–50.

Arbuna JCE. (1996) A factor responsible for resistance to cancer. *Curr Ther Res* 40: 745–9.

Arnold R, Simon B, Wied M. (2000) Treatment of neuroendocrine GEP tumours with somatostatin analogues. *Digestion* 62 (Suppl 1): 84–91.

Arslan H, Etlik O, Kayan M, Harman M, Tuncer Y, Temizoz O. (2005) Peroral CT enterography with lactulose solution: preliminary observations. *Am J Roentgenol* 185(5): 1173–9.

ASGE technology status evaluation report: wireless capsule endoscopy. (2006) *Gastrointest Endosc* 63: 539–45.

Bailey AA, Debinsky H, Appleyard M *et al.*(2004) Diagnosis and outcome of small bowel tumors found by capsule endoscopy: a three center Australian experience. *J Gastroenterol Hepatol* 19: S77.

Barkay O, Alon-Baron L, Shemesh E, Arber N. (2004) Endoscopically assisted wireless capsule endoscopy in a patient with familial adenomatous polyposis after total proctocolectomy and continent ileostomy. *Isr Med Assoc J* 6: 251–2.

Barshack I, Goldberg I, Chowers Y, Horowitz A, Kopolovic J. (2002) Different beta-catenin immunoexpression in carcinoid tumors of the appendix in comparison to other gastrointestinal carcinoid tumors. *Pathol Res Pract* 198: 531–6.

Begos DG *et al.* (1995) Metachronous small bowel adenocarcinoma in celiac sprue. *J Clin Gastroenterol* 20(3): 233–6.

Bender GN, Maglinte DD, McLarney JH, Rex D, Kelvin FM. (2001) Malignant melanoma: patterns of metastasis to the small bowel, reliability of imaging studies, and clinical relevance. *Am J Gastroenterol* 96(8): 2392–400.

Bessette JR, Maglinte DD, Kelvin FM, Chernish SM. (1989) Primary malignant tumors in the small bowel: a comparison of the small bowel enema and conventional follow-through examination. *Am J Roentgenol* 153: 741–4.

Bjork JA, Kerbrant H, Iselius L *et al.* (2001) Periampullary adenomas and adenocarcinomas in familial adenomatous polyposis: cumulative risks and APC gene mutations. *Gastroenterology* 121: 1127–35.

Blaker H, von Herbay A, Penzel R, Gross S, Otto HF. (2002) Genetics of adenocarcinomas of the small intestine: frequent deletions at chromosome 18q and mutations of the SMAD4 gene. *Oncogene* 21: 158–64.

Boot H, Aleman B, Mulder C, Zoetmulder F, Wobbes T. (2004) Malignant gastrointestinal lymphomas. In: J van Lanschot *et al.* eds. *Integrated Medical And Surgical Gastroenterology*, pp. 88–100. Bohn Stafleu Van Loghum, Houten, The Netherlands.

Bos JL. (1989) *ras* oncogenes in human cancer: a review. *Cancer Res* 49: 4682–9.

Bos JL, Fearon ER, Hamilton SR *et al.* (1987) Prevalence of ras gene mutations in human colorectal cancers. *Nature* 327: 293–7.

Boudiaf M, Jaff A, Soyer P, Bouhnik Y, Hamzi L, Rymer R. (2004) Small bowel diseases: prospective evaluation of multi-detector row helical CT enteroclysis in 107 consecutive patients. *Radiology* 233(2): 338–44.

Boyle W, Brenner D. (1995) Molecular and cellular biology of the small intestine. *Curr Opin Gastroenterol* 11: 121–7.

Bülow S, Björk J, Christensen IJ *et al.* (2004) Duodenal adenomatosis in familial adenomatous polyposis. *Gut* 53: 381–6.

Cai YC, Jiang Z, Vittimberga F *et al.* (1999) Expression of transforming growth factor-alpha and epidermal growth factor receptor in gastrointestinal stromal tumours. *Virchows Arch* 435: 112–5.

Caplin ME, Buscombe JR, Hilson AJ, Jones AL, Watkinson AF, Burroughs AK. (1998) Carcinoid tumour. *Lancet* 352: 799–805.

Catassi C, Bearzi I, Holmes GK. (2005) Association of celiac disease and intestinal lymphomas and other cancers. *Gastroenterology* 128 (4 Suppl 1): S79–86.

Chak A, Koehler MK, Sundaram SN, Cooper GS, Canto MI, Sivak MV. (1998) Diagnostic and therapeutic impact of push enteroscopy: analysis of factors associated with positive findings. *Gastrointest Endosc* 47: 18–22.

Chen CC, Neugut AI, Rotterdam H. (1994) Risk factors for adenocarcinomas and malignant carcinoids of the small intestine: preliminary findings. *Cancer Epidemiol Biomarkers Prev* 3(3): 205–7.

Chen H, Hardacre JM, Uzar A, Cameron JL, Choti MA. (1998) Isolated liver metastases from neuroendocrine tumors: does resection prolong survival? *J Am Coll Surg* 187: 88–92.

Cho RK, Vogelstein B. (1992) Genetic alterations in the adenoma-carcinoma sequence. *Cancer* 70: 1727–31.

Choi H, Charnsangavej C, de Castro Faria S *et al.* (2004) CT evaluation of the response of gastrointestinal stromal tumors after imatinib mesylate treatment: a quantitative analysis correlated with FDG PET findings. *Am J Roentgenol* 183(6): 1619–28.

Chompret A, Kannengiesser C, Barrois M *et al.* (2004) PDGFRA germline mutation in a family with multiple cases of gastrointestinal stromal tumor. *Gastroenterology* 126(1): 318–21.

Chow WH, Linet MS, McLaughlin JK *et al.* (1993) Risk factors for small intestine cancer. *Cancer Causes Control* 4(2): 163–9.

Chow JS, Chen CC, Ahsan H, Neugut AI (1996) A population-based study of the incidence of malignant small bowel tumours: SEER, 1973–1990. *Int J Epidemiol* 25(4): 722–8.

Coit DG. (2001) Cancer of the small intestine. In: VT DeVita *et al.* eds. *Cancer. Principles and Practice of Oncology*, 1204–16. Lippincott Williams & Wilkins, Philadelphia, USA.

Connacci-Sorrel ME, Ben Yedidia T, Shtutman M, Feinstein E, Einat P, Ben Ze'ev A. (2002) Nr-CAM is a target gene of the β-catenin/LEF-1 pathway in melanoma and colon cancer and its expression enhances motility and confers tumorigenesis. *Gene Dev* 16: 2058–72.

Dabaja BS, Suki D, Pro B, Bonnen M, Ajani J. (2004) Adenocarcinoma of the small bowel. *Cancer* 101: 518–26.

Dalla-Favera R, Martinotti S, Gallo RC, Erikson J, Croce CM. (1983) Translocation and rearrangements of the c-myc oncogene locus in human undifferentiated B-cell lymphomas. *Science* 219: 963–7.

Dansei R, McLellan CA, Myers CE. (1995)Specific labeling of isoprenylated proteins: application to study inhibitors of the post-translational farnesylation and gernaylgeranylation. *Biochem Biophys Res Commun* 206: 637–43.

Darke SG *et al.* (1973) Adenocarcinoma and Crohn's disease. A report of 2 cases and analysis of the literature. *Br J Surg* 60(3): 169–75.

De Giorgi U, Verweij J. (2005) Imatinib and gastrointestinal stromal tumors: Where do we go from here? *Mol Cancer Ther* 4: 495–501.

DeFranchis R, Rondonotti E, da Silva Aruajo Lopes LM. (2004) Small bowel malignancy. *Gastrointest Endosc Clin N Am* 14: 139–41.

DeMatteo RP *et al.* (2000) Two hundred gastrointestinal stromal tumors: recurrence patterns and prognostic factors for survival. *Ann Surg* 231(1): 51–8.

DiSario JA, Burt RW, Vargas H, McWhorter WP (1994) Small bowel cancer: epidemiological and clinical characteristics from a population-based registry. *Am J Gastroenterol* 89(5): 699–701.

Ducreux M, Ruszniewski P, Chayvialle JA *et al.* (2000) The antitumoral effect of the long-acting somatostatin analog lanreotide in neuroendocrine tumors. *Am J Gastroenterol* 95(11): 3276–81.

Eisen GM, Dominitz JA, Faigel DO. (2001) Enteroscopy. *Gastrointest Endosc* 53: 871–3.

Eliakim A. (2006) Video capsule endoscopy of the small bowel. *Curr Opin Gastroenterol* 22: 124–7.

Eriksson BK, Larsson EG, Skogseid BM, Löfberg AM, Lörelius LE, Öberg KE. (1998) Liver embolizations of patients with malignant neuroendocrine gastrointestinal tumors. *Cancer* 83: 2293–2301.

Faiss S, Räth U, Mansmann U *et al.* (1999) Ultra-high-dose lanreotide treatment in patients with metastatic neuroendocrine gastroenteropancreatic tumors. *Digestion* 60: 469–76.

Faiss S, Pape UF, Böhmig M *et al.* (2003) Prospective, randomized, multicenter trial on the antiproliferative effect of lanreotide, interferon alfa, and their combination for therapy of metastatic neuroendocrine gastroenteropancreatic tumors – the international lanreotide and interferon alfa study group. *J Clin Oncol* 21(14): 2689–96.

Feakins RM. (2005) The expression of p53 and bcl-2 in gastrointestinal stromal tumours is associated with anatomical site, and p53 expression is associated with grade and clinical outcome. *Histopathology* 46: 270–9.

Ferrucci PF, Zucca E. (2007) Primary gastric lymphoma pathogenesis and treatment: what has changed over the past 10 years? *Br J Haematol* 136(4): 521–38.

Frank M, Klose KJ, Wied M, Ishaque N, Schade-Brittinger C, Arnold R. (1999) Combination therapy with octreotide and α-interferon: effect on tumor growth in metastatic endocrine gastroenteropancreatic tumors. *Am J Gastroenterol* 94(5): 1381–7.

Gabos S, Berkel J, Band P, Robson D, Whittaker H (1993) Small bowel cancer in western Canada. *Int J Epidemiol* 22(2): 198–206.

Gayed I, Vu T, Iyer R *et al.* (2004) The role of 18F-FDG PET in staging and early prediction of response to therapy of recurrent gastrointestinal stromal tumors. *J Nucl Med* 45(1): 17–21.

Gerson LB. (2005) Double-balloon enteroscopy: the new gold standard for small bowel imaging? *Gastrointest Endosc* 62: 71–5.

Ghazizadeh M, Jin E, Shimizu H *et al.* (2005) Role of cdk4, p16INK4, and Rb expression in the prognosis of bronchioloalveolar carcinomas. *Respiration* 72: 68–73.

Giehl K. (2005) Oncogenic Ras in tumour progression and metastasis. *Biol Chem* 386: 193–205.

Ginzburg L, Schneider KM, Dreizin DH, Levinson C (1956) Carcinoma of the jejunum occurring in a case of regional enteritis. *Surgery* 39(2): 347–51.

Goldstein D, Tan BS, Rossleigh M, Haindl W, Walker B, Dixon J. (2005) Gastrointestinal stromal tumours: correlation of F-FDG gamma camera-based coincidence positron emission tomography with CT for the assessment of treatment response—an AGITG study. *Oncology* 69(4): 326–32.

Gortz B, Roth J, Krahenmann A *et al.* (1999) Mutations and allelic deletions of the MEN1 gene are associated with a subset of sporadic endocrine pancreatic and neuroendocrine tumors and not restricted to foregut neoplasms. *Am J Pathol* 154: 429–36.

Gourtsoyiannis N, Papanikolaou N, Grammatikakis J *et al.* (2001) MR enteroclysis protocol optimization: comparison between 3d FLASH with fat saturation after intravenous gadolinium injection and true FISP sequences. *Eur Radiol* 11: 908–13.

Gralnek IM. (2005) Obscure-overt gastrointestinal bleeding. *Gastroenterology* 128: 1424–30.

Greene FL, Page DL, Fleming ID *et al.* (2002) *AJCC Cancer Staging Manual*, 6th edn. Springer, New York.

Greenwald ES *et al.* (1962) Benign papillary adenoma of the ampullary region of the duodenum with intussusception. *Gastroenterology* 43: 344–50.

Gulec SA, Mountcastle TS, Frey D *et al.* (2002) Cytoreductive surgery in patients with advanced-stage carcinoid tumors. *Am Surg* 68: 667–72.

Hall M, Peters G. (1996) Genetics alterations of cyclins, cyclin-dependent kinases, and CDK inhibitors in human cancer. *Adv Cancer Res* 68: 67–108.

Hallak A, Arber N. (2003) Small bowel tumors—new insights of a rare disease. *Isr Med Assoc J* 5: 188–92.

Hara AK, Leighton JA, Sharma VK, Heigh RI, Fleischer DE. (2005) Imaging of small bowel disease: comparison of capsule endoscopy, standard endoscopy, barium examination, and CT. *RadioGraphics* 25: 697–711.

Harn SA, Seymour AB, Hoque ATMS *et al.* (1995) Allelotype of pancreatic adenocarcinomas using xenograft enrichment. *Cancer Res* 55: 4670–5.

Haselkorn T, Whittemore AS, Lilienfeld DE. (2005) *Incidence of small bowel cancer in the United States and worldwide: geographic, temporal, and racial differences. Cancer Causes Control* 16(7): 781–7.

Heiskanen I, Kellokumpu I, Jarvinen H. (1999) Management of duodenal adenomas in 98 patients with familial adenomatous polyposis. *Endoscopy* 31(6): 412–6.

Hemminki K, Li X. (2001) Incidence trends and risk factors of carcinoid tumors. A nationwide epidemiologic study from Sweden. *Cancer* 92: 2204–10.

Hermanek P. (1987) Adenoma/dysplasie-karzinom-sequence im dunndarm. *Z Gastroenterol* 25: 166–7.

Hessler PC, Braunstein E. (1978) Adenocarcinoma of the duodenum arising in a villous adenoma. *Gastrointest Radiol* 2(4): 355–7.

Hill MJ *et al.* (1971) Bacteria and aetiology of cancer of large bowel. *Lancet* 1(7690): 95–100.

Hong X, Choi H, Loyer EM, Benjamin RS, Trent JC, Charnsangavej C. (2006) Gastrointestinal stromal tumor: role of CT in diagnosis and in response evaluation and surveillance after treatment with imatinib. *Radiographics* 26(2): 481–95.

Horton KM, Fishman EK. (2004) Multidetector-row computed tomography and 3-dimensional computed tomography imaging of small bowel neoplasms: current concept in diagnosis. *J Comput Assist Tomogr* 28(1): 106–116.

Horton KM, Juluru K, Montogomery E, Fishman EK. (2004)Computed tomography imaging of gastrointestinal stromal tumors with pathology correlation. *J Comput Assist Tomogr* 28(6): 811–17.

Howe JR, Karnell LH, Menck HR, Scott-Conner C. (1999) Adenocarcinoma of the small bowel. Review of the national cancer database, 1985–1995. *Cancer* 86: 2693–706.

Hsu CM, Chiu CT, Su MY, Lin WP, Chen PC, Chen CH. (2007) The outcome assessment of double-balloon enteroscopy for diagnosing and managing patient with obscure gastrointestinal bleeding. *Dig Dis Sci* 52: 162–6.

Hunter T, Pines J. (1994) Cyclins and cancer. II: Cyclin D and CDK inhibitors come of age. *Cell* 79: 573–82.

Isaacson P, Wright DH. (1983) Malignant lymphoma of mucosa-associated lymphoid tissue. A distinctive type of B-cell lymphoma. *Cancer* 52(8): 1410–6.

Jacks SP, Hundley JC, Shen P, Russell GB, Levine EA. (2005) Cytoreductive surgery and intraperitoneal hyperthermic chemotherapy for peritoneal carcinomatosis from small bowel adenocarcinoma. *J Surg Oncol* 91(2): 112–7; discussion 118–9.

Jagelman DG, DeCosse JJ, Bussey HJ. (1988) Upper gastrointestinal cancer in familial adenomatous polyposis. *Lancet* 1(8595): 1149–51.

Jakobovitz G, Nass D, Demarco L *et al.* (1996) Carcinoid tumors frequently display genetic abnormalities involving chromosome 11. *J Clin Endocrinol Metab* 81: 3164–7.

Janson ET, Holmberg L, Stridsberg M *et al.* (1997) Carcinoid tumors: analysis of prognostic factors and survival in 301 patients from a referral center. *Ann Oncol* 8: 685–90.

Janson ET, Westlin JE, Öhrvall U, Öberg K, Lukinius A. (2000) Nuclear localization of 111In after intravenous injection of [^{111}In-DTPA-D-Phe^{1}]-octreotide in patients with neuroendocrine tumors. *J Nucl Med* 41: 1514–8.

Jemal A, Saegal R, Ward E *et al.* (2007) Cancer Statistics 2007. *CA Cancer J Clin* 57: 43–66.

Kaerlev L, Teglbjaerg PS, Sabroe S *et al.* (2000) Is there an association between alcohol intake or smoking and small bowel adenocarcinoma? Results from a European multi-center case–control study. *Cancer Causes Control* 11(9): 791–7.

Kaerlev L, Teglbjaerg PS, Sabroe S *et al.* (2001) Medical risk factors for small bowel adenocarcinoma with focus on Crohn disease: a European population-based case–control study. *Scand J Gastroenterol* 36(6): 641–6.

Kim SH, Roth KA, Moser AR, Gordon JI (1993) Transgenic mouse models that explore the multistep hypothesis of intestinal neoplasia. *J Cell Biol* 123(4): 877–93.

Kindblom LG, Remotti HE, Aldenborg F, Meis-Kindblom JM (1998) Gastrointestinal pacemaker cell tumor (GIPACT): gastrointestinal stromal tumors show phenotypic characteristics of the interstial cells of Cajal. *M J Pathol* 152: 1259–69.

Kleinerman RA *et al.* (1995) Second primary cancer after treatment for cervical cancer. An international cancer registries study. *Cancer* 76(3): 442–52.

Korman MU. (2002) Radiologic evaluation and staging of small intestine neoplasms. *Eur J Radiol* 42(3): 193–205.

Kovacs TO, Jensen DM. (2002) Recent advances in the endoscopic diagnosis and therapy of upper gastrointestinal, small intestinal and colonic bleeding. *Med Clin North Am* 86: 1319–56.

Kozuka S, Tsubone M, Yamaguchi A, Hachisuka K. (1981) Adenomatous residue in cancerous papilla of Vater. *Gut* 22: 1031–4.

Krugmann J, Dirnhofer S, Gschwendtner A *et al.* (2001) Primary gastrointestinal B-cell lymphoma. A clincopathological and immunohistochemical study of 61 cases with an evaluation of prognostic parameters. *Pathol Res Pract* 197: 385–93.

Kulke MH, Mayer RJ. (1999) Carcinoid tumors. *N Engl J Med* 340(11): 858–66.

Kulke MH, Kim H, Clark JW *et al.* (2004) A phase II trial of gemcitabine for metastatic neuroendocrine tumors. *Cancer* 101: 934–9.

Kumar R, Xiu Y, Potenta S *et al.* (2004) 18F-FDG PET for evaluation of the treatment response in patients with gastrointestinal tract lymphomas. *J Nucl Med* 45(11): 1796–803.

Kwekkeboom DJ, Teunissen JJ, Bakker WH *et al.* (2005) Radiolabeled somatostatin analog [^{177}Lu-DOTA^{0},Tyr^{3}] octreotate in patients with endocrine gastroenteropancreatic tumors. *J Clin Oncol* 23(12): 2754–62.

Lappas J, Heitkamp DE, Maglinte DD. (2003) Current status of CT enteroclysis. *Crit Rev Comput Tomogr* 44(3): 145–75.

Laqueur GL, Matsumoto H. (1966) Neoplasms in female Fischer rats following intraperitoneal injection of methylazoxy-methanol. *J Natl Cancer Inst*, 37(2): 217–32.

Lashner BA. (1992) Risk factors for small bowel cancer in Crohn's disease. *Dig Dis Sci* 37(8): 1179–84.

Le Treut YP, Delpero JR, Dousset B *et al.* (1997) Results of liver transplantation in the treatment of metastatic neuroendocrine tumors. A 31-case French multicentric report. *Ann Surg* 225: 355–64.

Lecuit M, Abachin E, Martin A *et al.* (2004) Immunoproliferative small intestinal disease associated with *Campylobacter jejuni*. *N Engl J Med* 350(3): 239–48.

Lee SK, Lee YC, Chung JB *et al.* (2004) Low grade gastric MALToma: Treatment strategies based on 10 year follow-up. *World J Gastroenterol* 10: 223–6.

Leong WL, Pasieka JL. (2002) Regression of metastatic carcinoid tumors with octreotide therapy: two case reports and a review of the literature. *J Surg Oncol* 79: 180–7.

Lewis B, Goldfarb N. (2003) Review article: the advent of capsule endoscopy—a not so-futuristic approach to obscure gastrointestinal bleeding. *Aliment Pharmacol Ther* 17: 1085–96.

Lewis B, Swain P. (2002) Capsule endoscopy in the evaluation of patients with suspected small intestinal bleeding: results of a pilot study. *Gastrointest Endosc* 56: 349–53.

Li H, Lochmuller H, Yong VW, Karpati G, Nalbantoglu J. (1997) Adenovirus-mediated wild-type p53 gene transfer and overexpression induces apoptosis of human glioma cells independent of endogenous p53 status. *J Neuropathol Exp Neurol* 56: 872–8.

Liberman E, Kraus S, Sagiv E, Dulkart O, Kazanov D, Arber N. (2007) The *APC* E1317Q and I1307K polymorphisms in non-colorectal cancers. *Biomed Pharmacother* 61: 566–9.

Lightdale C, Koepsell T, Sherlock P. (1982) Small intestine. In: Schottenfeld JFD Jr, ed. *Cancer Epidemiology and Prevention*, 1st edn, pp. 692–702. WB Saunders, Philadelphia.

Lipkin M, Higgins P. (1988) Biological markers of cell proliferation and differentiation in human gastrointestinal diseases. *Adv Cancer Res* 50: 1–24.

Locher C, Malka D, Boige V *et al.* (2005) Combination chemotherapy in advanced small bowel adenocarcinoma. *Oncology* 69: 290–4.

Lowenfels AB. (1973) Why are small bowel tumours so rare? *Lancet* 1(7793): 24–6.

Lowenfels AB. (1978) Does bile promote extra-colonic cancer? *Lancet* 2(8083): 239–41.

Lowenfels AB, Sonni A. (1977) Distribution of small bowel tumors. *Cancer Lett* 3(1–2): 83–6.

Maertens O, Prenen H, Debiec-Rychter M *et al.* (2006) Molecular pathogenesis of multiple gastrointestinal stromal tumors in NF1 patients. *Hum Mol Genet* 15: 1015–23.

Maggard MA, O'Connell JB, Ko CY. (2004) Updated population-based review of carcinoid tumors. *Ann Surg* 240(1): 117–22.

Manabe N, Tanaka S, Fukumoto A, Nakao M, Kamino D, Chayama K. (2006) Double-balloon enteroscopy in patients with GI bleeding of obscure origin. *Gastrointest Endosc* 64: 135–40.

Marchettini P, Sugarbaker PH. (2002)Mucinous adenocarcinoma of the small bowel with peritoneal seeding. *Eur J Surg Oncol* 28(1): 19–23.

Marmo R, Rotondano G, Piscopo R, Bianco MA, Cipolletta L. (2005) Meta-analysis: capsule enteroscopy vs. conventional modalities in diagnosis of small bowel diseases. *Aliment Pharmacol Ther* 22: 595–604.

Martin R. (1985) Malignant tumors of the small intestine. *Surg Clin North Am* 66: 779–785.

May A, Nachbar L, Ell C. (2005) Double-balloon enteroscopy (push-and-pull enteroscopy) of the small bowel: feasibility and diagnostic and therapeutic yield in patients with suspected small bowel disease. *Gastrointest Endosc* 62: 62–70.

Mentzer SJ, Osteen RT, Pappas TN, Rosenthal DS, Canellos GP, Wilson RE. (1988) Surgical therapy of localized abdominal non-Hodgkin's lymphomas. *Surgery* 103(6): 609–14.

Michelassi F *et al.* (1993) Adenocarcinoma complicating Crohn's disease. *Dis Colon Rectum* 36(7): 654–61.

Miettinen M, Fetsch JF, Sobin LH, Lasota J. (2006a) Gastrointestinal stromal tumors in patients with neurofibromatosis 1: a clinicopathologic and molecular genetic study of 45 cases. *Am J Surg Pathol* 30: 90–6.

Miettinen M, Lasota J. (2006b) Gastrointestinal stromal tumors of the jejunum and ileum: a clinicopathologic, immunohistochemical, and molecular genetic study of 906 cases before imatinib with long-term follow-up. *Am J Surg Pathol* 30(4): 477–89.

Mitomi H, Nakamura T, Ihara A *et al.* (2003) Frequent Ki-ras mutations and transforming growth factor-alpha expression in adenocarcinomas of the small intestine: report of 7 cases. *Dig Dis Sci* 48: 203–9.

Miyaki M, Kuroki T. (2003) Role of Smad4 (DPC4) inactivation in human cancer. *Biochem Biophys Res Commun* 306: 799–804.

Modlin IM, Lye KD, Kidd M. (2003) A 5-decade analysis of 13715 carcionoid tumors. *Cancer* 97: 934–59.

Modlin IM, Kidd M, Latich I, Zikusoka MN, Shapiro MD. (2005) Current status of gastrointestinal carcinoids. *Gastroenterology* 128: 1717–51.

Moertel CG, Johnson CM, McKusick MA *et al.* (1994) The management of patients with advanced carcinoid tumors and islet cell carcinomas. *Ann Intern Med* 120: 302–9.

Munkholm P *et al.* (1993) Intestinal cancer risk and mortality in patients with Crohn's disease. *Gastroenterology* 105(6): 1716–23.

Nagashima R, Takeda H, Maeda K, Ohno S, Takahashi T. (1996) Regression of duodenal mucosa associated lymphoid tissue lymphoma after eradication of *Helicobacter pylori*. *Gastroenterology* 111(6): 1674–8.

Neglia JP *et al.* (1995) The risk of cancer among patients with cystic fibrosis. Cystic Fibrosis and Cancer Study Group. *N Engl J Med* 332(8): 494–9.

Negri E *et al.* (1999) Risk factors for adenocarcinoma of the small intestine. *Int J Cancer* 82(2): 171–4.

Neugut AI, Santos J. (1993) The association between cancers of the small and large bowel. *Cancer Epidemiol Biomarkers Prev* 2(6): 551–3.

Neugut AI, Marvin MR, Rella VA, Chabot JA *et al.* (1997) An overview of adenocarcinoma of the small intestine. *Oncology (Williston Park)* 11(4): 529–36; discussion 545, 549–50.

Neugut AI, Jacobson JS, Suh S, Mukherjee R, Arber N *et al.* (1998) The epidemiology of cancer of the small bowel. *Cancer Epidemiol Biomarkers Prev* 7(3): 243–51.

Nishiyama K, Yao T, Yonemasu H, Yamaguchi K, Tanaka M, Tsuneyoshi M. (2002) Overexpression of p53 protein and point mutation of K-ras genes in primary carcinoma of the small intestine. *Oncol Rep* 9: 293–300.

Nugent KP, Spigelman AD, Williams CB, Talbot IC, Phillips RK *et al.* (1994) Surveillance of duodenal polyps in familial adenomatous polyposis: progress report. *J R Soc Med* 87(11): 704–6.

O'Toole D, Ducreux M, Bommelaer G *et al.* (2000) Treatment of carcinoid syndrome. A prospective crossover evaluation of lanreotide versus octreotide in terms of efficacy, patient acceptability, and tolerance. *Cancer* 88: 770–6.

Öberg K. (1998) Carcinoid tumors: current concepts in diagnosis and treatment. *Oncologist* 3: 339–45.

Öberg K. (1999) Neuroendocrine gastrointestinal tumors—a condensed overview of diagnosis and treatment. *Ann Oncol* 10 (Suppl 2): S3–S8.

Öberg K. (2000) Interferon in the management of neuroendocrine GEP-tumors. *Digestion* 62 (Suppl 1): 92–7.

Öberg K. (2001) Chemotherapy and biotherapy in the treatment of neuroendocrine tumours. *Ann Oncol* 12 (Suppl 2): S111–S114.

Öberg K, Kvols L, Caplin M *et al.* (2004) Consensus report on the use of somatostatin analogs for the management of neuroendocrine tumors of the gastroenteropancreatic system. *Ann Oncol* 15(6): 966–73.

Offerhaus GJA, Giardiello FM, Krush AJ *et al.* (1993) The risk of upper gastrointestinal cancer in familial adenomatous polyposis. *Gastroenterol* 102: 1980–2.

Orjollet-Lecoanet C, Menard Y, Martins A, Crombe-Ternamian A, Cotton F, Valette PJ. (2000) CT enteroclysis for detection of small bowel tumors. *J Radiol* 81(6): 618–27.

Papanikolaou N, Prassopoulos P, Grammatikakis I, Maris T, Gourtsoyiannis N. (2002) Technical challenges and clinical applications of magnetic resonance enteroclysis. *Magnetic Resonance Imaging in Bowel Imaging* 13(6): 397–408.

Parkin DMC, Whelan SL, Gao WT, Ferlay J. (1993) *Cancer Incidence in Five Continents*, 6th edn. IARC Scientific Publication #120. Oxford University Press, New York, NY.

Parsonnet J, Isaacson PG. (2004) Bacterial infection and MALT lymphoma. *N Engl J Med* 350(3): 213–5.

Pascher A, Klupp J, Neuhaus P. (2005) Transplantation in the management of metastatic endocrine tumors. *Best Pract Res Clin Gastroenterol* 19(4): 637–48.

Pennazio M. (2005) Small bowel endoscopy. *Endoscopy* 36: 32–41.

Perrone F, Tamborini E, Dagrada GP *et al.* (2005) 9p21 locus analysis in high-risk gastrointestinal stromal tumors characterized for c-kit and platelet-derived growth factor receptor alpha gene alterations. *Cancer* 104: 159–69.

Persson PG, Karlén P, Bernell O. (1994) Crohn's disease and cancer: a population-based cohort study. *Gastroenterology* 107(6): 1675–9.

Perzin HK, Bridge M. (1981)Adenomas of the small intestine: a clinicopathologic review of 51 cases and a study of their relationship to carcinoma. *Cancer* 48: 799–819.

Planck M, Ericson K, Piotrowska Z, Halvarsson B, Rambech E, Nilbert M. (2003) Microsatellite instability and expression of MLH1 and MSH2 in carcinomas of the small intestine. *Cancer* 97: 1551–7.

Potten CS. (1984) Clonogenic, stem and carcinogen-target cells in small intestine. *Scand J Gastroenterol Suppl* 104: 3–14.

Potten CS. (1992) The significance of spontaneous and induced apoptosis in the gastrointestinal tract of mice. *Cancer Metastasis Rev* 11(2): 179–95.

Radaszkiewicz T, Dragosics B, Bauer P. (1992) Gastrointestinal malignant lymphomas of the mucosa-associated lymphoid tissue: factors relevant to prognosis. *Gastroenterology* 102: 1628–38.

Rajesh A, Maglinte DD. (2006) Multislice CT enteroclysis: technique and clinical applications. *Clin Radiol* 61(1): 31–9.

Rashid A, Hamilton SR. (1997) Genetic alterations in sporadic and Crohn's-associated adenocarcinomas of the small intestine. *Gastroenterology* 113: 127–35.

Real MA, Fearon ER. (1996) Gene effects in colorectal tumorigenesis. In: Young GP, Rozen P, Levin B, eds. *Prevention and Early Detection of Colorectal Cancer,* pp 63–86. WB Saunders, London.

Reiber A, Aschoff A, Nussle K *et al.* (2000) MRI in the diagnosis of small bowel disease: use of positive and negative oral contrast media in combination with enteroclysis. *Eur Radiol* 10; 1377–82.

Ries L. (2006) *SEER Cancer Statistics Review, 1975–2003.* National Cancer Institute, Bethesda, MD.

Roggero E, Zucca E, Pinotti G *et al.* (1995) Eradication of *Helicobacter pylori* infection in primary low-grade gastric lymphoma of mucosa-associated lymphoid tissue. *Ann Intern Med* 122: 767–9.

Romano S, De Lutio E, Rollandi GA, Romano L, Grassi R, Maglinte DD. (2005) Multidetector computed tomography enteroclysis (MDCT-E) with neutral enteral and IV contrast enhancement in tumor detection. *Eur Radiol* 15(6): 1178–83.

Rosenau J, Bahr MJ, von Wasielewski R *et al.* (2002) Ki67, E-cadherin, and p53 as prognostic indicators of long-term outcome after liver transplantation for metastatic neuroendocrine tumours. *Transplantation* 73: 386–94.

Ross RK, Hartnett NM, Bernstein L, Henderson BE. (1991) Epidemiology of adenocarcinomas of the small intestine: is bile a small bowel carcinogen? *Br J Cancer* 63(1): 143–5.

Rougier P, Mitry E. (2000) Chemotherapy in the management of neuroendocrine malignant tumors. *Digestion* 62 (Suppl 1): 73–8.

Rubin J, Ajani J, Schirmer W *et al.* (1999) Octreotide acetate long-acting formulation versus open-label subcutaneous octreotide acetate in malignant carcinoid syndrome. *J Clin Oncol* 17(2): 600–6.

Rubin BP, Singer S, Tsao C *et al.* (2001) KIT activation is a ubiquitous feature of gastrointestinal stromal tumors. *Cancer Res* 61: 8118–21.

Ruszniewski P, Malka D. (2000) Hepatic arterial chemoembolization in the management of advanced digestive endocrine tumors. *Digestion* 62 (Suppl 1): 79–83.

Sackmann M, Morgner A, Rudolph B *et al.* (1997) Regression of gastric MALT lymphoma after eradication of *Helicobacter pylori* is predicted by endosonographic staging. *Gastroenterology* 113: 1087–90.

Safford SD, Coleman RE, Gockerman JP *et al.* (2004) Iodine-131 metaiodobenzylguanidine treatment for metastatic carcinoid. *Cancer* 101: 1987–93.

Salem PA, Estephan FF. (2005) Immunoproliferative small intestinal disease: current concepts. *Cancer J* 11(5): 374–82.

Samanic C, Gridley G, Chow WH *et al.* (2004) Obesity and cancer risk among white and black United States veterans. *Cancer Causes Control* 15(1): 35–43.

Sarmiento JM, Que FG. (2003)Hepatic surgery for metastases from neuroendocrine tumors. *Surg Oncol Clin N Am* 12(1): 231–42 [review].

Sarmiento JM, Thompson GB, Nagorney DM *et al.* (2002) Pancreas-sparing duodenectomy for duodenal polyposis. *Arch Surg* 137: 557–63.

Sarmiento JM, Heywood G, Rubin J *et al.* (2003) Surgical treatment of neuroendocrine metastases to the liver: a plea for resection to increase survival. *J Am Coll Surg* 197: 29–37.

Schottenfeld D, Islam SS. (1996) Cancers of the small intestine. In: D Schottenfeld, JF Fraumeni Jr, eds. *Cancer Epidemiology and Prevention,* 2nd edn, pp. 806–12. Oxford University Press, New York.

Schulman K, von Falkenhausen M, Krautmacher C *et al.* (2005) Feasibility and diagnostic utility of video capsule endoscopy for the detection of small bowel polyps in patients with hereditary polyposis syndromes. *Am J Gastroenterol* 100: 27–37.

Schulz S, Nyce JW. (1991) Inhibition of protein isoprenylation and p21 ras membrane association by dehydroepiandrosterone in human colonic adenocarcinoma cells in vitro. *Cancer Res* 51: 6563–7.

Seifert E, Schulte F, Stolte M. (1992) Adenoma and carcinoma of the duodenum and papilla of Vater: a clinicopathologic study. *Am J Gastroenterol* 87: 37–42.

Sellner F. (1990) Investigations on the significance of the adenoma-carcinoma sequence in the small bowel. *Cancer* 66: 702–15.

Semelka RC, John G, Kelekis NL, Burdeny DA, Ascher SM. (1996) Small bowel neoplastic disease: demonstration by MRI. *J Magn Reson Imaging* 6(6): 855–60.

Severson RK, Schenk M, Gurney JG, Weiss LK, Demers RY. (1996) Increasing incidence of adenocarcinomas and carcinoid tumors of the small intestine in adults. *Cancer Epidemiol Biomarkers Prev* 5(2): 81–4.

Sheldon CD, Assoufi BK, Hodson ME. (1993) A cohort study of cystic fibrosis and malignancy. *Br J Cancer* 68(5): 1025–8.

Shih L, Liaw S, Dunn P, Kuo T. (1994) Primary small intestinal lymphomas in Taiwan: immunoproliferative small intestinal disease and non-immunoproliferative small intestinal disease. *J Clin Oncol* 12 (7): 1375–82.

Sidransky D, Tokin T, Hamilton SR *et al.* (1992) Identification of Ras oncogene mutations in the stool of patients with curable colorectal tumors. *Science* 256: 102–5.

Spigelman AD, Williams CB, Talbot IC, Domizio P, Phillips RK. (1989) Upper gastrointestinal cancer in patients with familial adenomatous polyposis. *Lancet* 2(8666): 783–5.

Spigelman AD, Crofton-Sleigh C, Venitt S *et al.* (1990) Mutagenicity of bile and duodenal adenomas in familial adenomatous polyposis. *Br J Surg* 77: 878–81.

Spigelman AD, Talbot IC, Penna C. (1994) Evidence for adenoma-carcinoma sequence in the duodenum of patients with familial adenomatous polyposis. The Leeds Castle Polyposis Group (Upper Gastrointestinal Committee). *J Clin Pathol* 47(8): 709–10.

Stang A, Stegmaier C, Eisinger B *et al.* (1999) Descriptive epidemiology of small intestinal malignancies: the German Cancer Registry experience. *Br J Cancer* 80(9): 1440–4.

Sugarbaker PH. (2005) *Technical Handbook for the Integration of Cytoreductive Surgery and Perioperative Intraperitoneal Chemotherapy into the Surgical Management of Gastrointestinal and Gynecologic Malignancy.* December 5.

Sun W, Lipsitz S, Catalano P, Mailliard JA, Haller DG. (2005) Phase II/III study of doxorubicin with fluorouracil compared with streptozocin with fluorouracil or dacarbazine in the treatment of advanced carcinoid tumors: Eastern Cooperative Oncology Group Study E1281. *J Clin Oncol* 23(22): 4897–904.

Sun B, Rajan E, Cheng S *et al.* (2006) Diagnostic yield and therapeutic impact of double-balloon enteroscopy in a large cohort of patients with obscure gastrointestinal bleeding. *Am J Gastroenterol* 101: 2011–15.

Swetter SM, Carroll LA, Johnson DL, Segall GM. (2002) Positron emission tomography is superior to computed tomography for metastatic detection in melanoma patients. *Ann Surg Oncol* 9(7): 646–53.

Tarn C, Skorobogatko YV, Taguchi T, Eisenberg B, von Mehren M, Godwin AK. (2006) Therapeutic effect of imatinib in gastrointestinal stromal tumors: AKT signaling dependent and independent mechanisms. *Cancer Res* 66: 5477–86.

Touzios JG, Kiely JM, Pitt SC *et al.* (2005) Neuroendocrine hepatic metastases. Does aggressive management improve survival? *Ann Surg* 241: 776–85.

Tran T, Davila JA, El-Serag HB. (2005) The epidemiology of malignant gastrointestinal stromal tumors: an analysis of 1458 cases from 1992 to 2000. *Am J Gastroenterol* 100(1): 162–8.

Triester SL, Leighton JA, Leontiadis GI *et al.* (2005) A meta-analysis of the yield of capsule endoscopy compared to other diagnostic modalities in patients with obscure GI bleeding. *Am J Gastroenterol* 100: 2407–18.

Uppaputhangkule V, Maas LC, Gelzayd EA. (1976) Endoscopic diagnosis of villous adenoma of the duodenum. *Gastrointest Endosc* 23(2): 97–8.

van Vilsteren FG, Baskin-Bey ES, Nagorney DM *et al.* (2006) Liver transplantation for gastroenteropancreatic neuroendocrine cancers: defining selection criteria to improve survival. *Liver Transpl* 12(3): 448–56.

Verkarre V, Romana SP, Cellier C, Asnafi V, Mention JJ, Barbe U. (2003) Recurrent partial trisomy 1q22-q44 in clonal intraepithelial lymphocytes in refractory celiac sprue. *Gastroenterology* 125: 40–6.

Vogelstein B, Fearon ER, Hamilton SR *et al.* (1988) Genetic alterations during colorectal-tumor development. *N Engl J Med* 319: 525–32.

Vogelstein B, Kinzler KW. (1994)Colorectal cancer and the intersection between basic and clinical research. *Cold Spring Harbor Symp Quant Biol* 59: 517–21.

Wargovich MJ. (1996) Precancer markers and prediction of tumorigenesis. In: Young GP, Rozen P, Levin B, eds. *Prevention and Early Detection of Colorectal Cancer*, pp. 89–101. WB Saunders, London.

Wattenberg LW. (1966) Carcinogen-detoxifying mechanisms in the gastrointestinal tract. *Gastroenterology* 51(5): 932–5.

Weber DM, Dimopoulos MA, Anandu DP, Pugh WC, Steinbach G. (1994) Regression of gastric lymphoma of mucosa-associated lymphoid tissue with antibiotic therapy for *Helicobacter pylori*. *Gastroenterology* 107: 1835–8.

Weiss NS Yang CP. (1987) Incidence of histologic types of cancer of the small intestine. *J Natl Cancer Inst* 78(4): 653–6.

Welin SV, Tiensuu Janson E, Sundin A *et al.* (2004) High-dose treatment with a long-acting somatostatin analogue in patients with advanced midgut carcinoid tumours. *Eur J Endocrinol* 151: 107–12.

Wirtzfeld DA, Petrelli NJ, Rodriguez-Bigas MA. (2001) Hamartomatous polyposis syndromes: molecular genetics, neoplastic risk, and surveillance recommendations. *Ann Surg Oncol* 8: 319–27.

Wold PB, Fletcher JG, Johnson CD, Sandborn WJ. (2003) Assessment of small bowel Crohn disease: noninvasive peroral CT enterography compared with other imaging methods and endoscopy-feasibility study. *Radiology* 229: 275–81.

Wong RF, Tuteja AK, Haslem DS *et al.* (2006) Video capsule endoscopy compared with standard endoscopy for the evaluation of small bowel polyps in persons with familial adenomatous polyposis. *Gastrointest Endosc* 64: 530–7.

Wu AH, Yu MC, Mack TM. (1997) Smoking, alcohol use, dietary factors and risk of small intestinal adenocarcinoma. *Int J Cancer* 70(5): 512–7.

Wymenga AN, Eriksson B, Salmela PI *et al.* (1999) Efficacy and safety of prolonged-release lanreotide in patients with gastrointestinal neuroendocrine tumors and hormone-related symptoms. *J Clin Oncol* 17(4): 1111–17.

Yamamoto H, Sekine Y, Sato Y *et al.* (2001) Total enteroscopy with a nonsurgical steerable double-balloon method. *Gastrointest Endosc* 53: 216–20.

Yao JC. (2007) Neuroendocrine tumors. Molecular targeted therapy for carcinoid and islet-cell carcinoma. *Best Pract Res Clin Endocrinol Metab* 21: 163–72 [review].

Ye H, Gong L, Liu H *et al.* (2005) MALT lymphoma with t(14;18)(q32;q21)/IGH-MALT1 is characterized by strong cytoplasmic MALT1 and BCL10 expression. *J Pathol* 205: 293–301.

Zaman A, Sheppard B, Katon RM. (1999) Total peroral intraoperative enteroscopy for obscure GI bleeding using a dedicated push enteroscope: diagnostic yield and patient outcome. *Gastrointest Endosc* 50: 506–10.

Zhang LH, Zhang SZ, Hu HJ *et al.* (2005) Multi-detector CT enterography with iso-osmotic mannitol as oral contrast for detecting small bowel disease. *World J Gastroenterol* 11(15): 2324–9.

Zhu L, Kim K, Domenico DR, Appert HE, Howard JM. (1996) Adenocarcinoma of duodenum and ampulla of Vater: clinicopathology study and expression of p53, c-neu, TGF-alpha, CEA, and EMA. *J Surg Oncol* 61: 100–5.

Zonios D, Soula M, Archimandritis AJ *et al.* (2003) Cystlike hepatic metastases from gastrointestinal stromal tumors could be seen before any treatment. *AJR Am J Roentgenol* 181: 282.

9 Sarcoma and Gastrointestinal Stromal Tumors

Edited by Markku Miettinen

Introduction

Markku Miettinen

Gastrointestinal stromal tumor (GIST) is the designation for a specific type of mesenchymal tumor of the gastrointestinal (GI) tract that has a spectrum from benign to malignant. These tumors are driven by activating KIT and PDGFRA mutations, and they have a characteristic histologic spectrum including spindle or epithelioid morphology, and generally (~80%) express KIT receptor tyrosine kinase (CD117 in the nomenclature of leukocyte cluster of differentiation antigens). GIST has been known for almost a decade as an example of the first mesenchymal tumor with specific targeted treatment by tyrosine kinase inhibitors.

In previous literature, GISTs were classified as GI smooth muscle tumors and gastrointestinal autonomic nerve or nerve sheath tumors. Because GISTs are by far the most common mesenchymal tumors of the GI tract, they include a majority of tumors previously classified as other mesenchymal tumors of the GI tract, especially leiomyomas and leiomyosarcomas. Nevertheless, it should be noted that true smooth muscle tumors (benign and malignant) occur throughout the GI tract. Their frequency is low, except in the esophagus, where leiomyomas outnumber GISTs by a margin of 3 : 1, and in colon and rectum, where small polypoid leiomyomas of muscularis mucosae may be more common than GIST and the relative incidence of true leiomyosarcomas in the GI tract is the highest.

GISTs are believed to arise from interstitial cells of Cajal (ICC) or their multipotential precursors, KIT-positive spindle cells that are functional intermediaries between the autonomic nervous system and smooth muscle, and regulate autonomous nerve transmission and intestinal peristalsis. ICCs are located around myenteric plexus throughout the GI tract.

Gastrointestinal Oncology: A Critical Multidisciplinary Team Approach.
Edited by J. Jankowski, R. Sampliner, D. Kerr, and Y. Fong.

GISTs occur predominantly in older adults (median age 55–65 years), throughout the GI tract from distal esophagus to the rectum, and encompass a wide morphologic and clinicopathologic spectrum in all sites of their occurrence. They are very rare in children and relatively rare under the age of 40 years. The overall incidence of GIST has been estimated as 11–14 per million, and some series have shown a mild male predominance (55 : 45). The most common location is stomach (60%), followed by jejunum and ileum (30%), duodenum (5%), appendix and colon (1–2%), rectum (3–4%), and esophagus (<1%). Small numbers of GISTs have been reported as primary tumors in the omentum, mesentery and retroperitoneum, but most GISTs in these sites are metastatic, or perhaps secondarily separated from their GI tract origin. The frequency of malignant behavior varies by site, but is estimated as 20% for gastric and 40% for small intestinal GISTs.

Most GISTs (95%) are sporadic, but 5% occur in connection with three different syndromes: neurofibromatosis 1 (NF1), Carney triad and familial GIST with inheritable KIT or PDGFRA mutation. In NF1 patients, GISTs occur with a 100–200-fold frequency, compared with non-NF1 patients. In this context, the tumors typically occur in small intestine (including duodenum) and are often multiple. Although GISTs have a favorable clinical course in a majority of NF1 patients, some of these tumors are clinically malignant. The large studies on NF1 GISTs have not found GIST-specific KIT or PDGFRA mutations, suggesting that pathogenesis may differ from that of sporadic GISTs.

Carney triad includes three key manifestations: GIST, paraganglioma, and pulmonary chondroma (hamartoma); occurrence of two of these fulfils the set definition. In this syndrome, GISTs (almost xyz) always occur in the stomach and have epithelioid morphology. Most patients are females, and the GIST is usually diagnosed at a young age, sometimes in childhood. Some patients develop liver metastases, but the course of disease is typically protracted.

The histologic spectrum of GIST varies somewhat by primary site. In the stomach, approximately two-thirds are spindle cell tumors, and one-third has epithelioid morphology, with focal pleomorphism present in many tumors, especially those with epithelioid morphology; extensive pleomorphism is rare. Intestinal GISTs have a narrower morphologic spectrum; approximately 40–45% of tumors have distinctive extracellular collagen fibers.

Central to the diagnosis of GIST is detection of immunohistochemical positivity for KIT (CD117) that occurs in almost all GISTs. In most cases, there is strong membrane and cytoplasmic positivity. However, in some cases, especially in some PDGFRA mutant GISTs, KIT positivity can be weak or absent altogether. In KIT-negative GISTs, alternative markers such as protein kinase C theta and CD34 can be useful.

The frequency of malignant behavior varies by site, being lowest among gastric GISTs (20%), and approximately twice as high in intestinal GISTs (40%). Importantly, small intestinal GISTs behave more aggressively than gastric GISTs with similar tumor size and mitotic rate. The biologic background of this is unknown, although differences in gene expression profiles of gastric versus small intestinal GISTs have been noted.

Malignant GISTs typically metastasize anywhere to abdominal soft tissues and liver, often after an apparently complete excision. Abdominal metastases are the rule after incomplete resections. Rarely, metastases develop in bones (especially the axial skeleton) and peripheral soft tissues. However, lymph node and pulmonary metastases are exceptionally rare. In sarcomatous tumors with significantly elevated mitotic rates (>10 mitoses per 50 high-power fields, HPFs), metastases often develop 1–2 years after surgery, whereas less aggressive GISTs can develop metastases 5–20 years or more after surgery.

KIT or PDGFRA mutations occur in most GISTs. KIT exon 11 mutations (in frame deletions, point mutations, and duplications) occur in GISTs of all locations, whereas a characteristic duplication Ala502_Tyr503 is nearly specific for intestinal (versus gastric) tumors. In contrast, PDGFRA mutations are nearly specific for gastric GISTs. Mutation type influences therapy responsiveness, but fortunately only a minority of mutations (such as some KIT exon 17 mutants and PDGFRA exon 18 mutants) are imatinib resistant. Secondary KIT and PDGFRA mutations acquired during drug imatinib treatment cause drug resistance and this is a major problem limiting treatment success. Notably, pediatric GISTs and those occurring in NF1 patients do not have these mutations, suggesting a different pathogenesis.

Surgery is the main mode of treatment, and complete excision should be performed whenever possible. In the stomach, wedge resections are often sufficient, and especially smaller tumors are suitable for laparoscopic surgery. Intestinal GISTs usually require resections of an intestinal segment. It has not been determined whether preoperative use of imatinib would allow less radical surgery for sensitive sites, such as distal rectum.

Conventional sarcoma chemotherapy has generally been ineffective and radiation therapy impractical. New targeted treatment against oncogenic activation of KIT, PDGFRA (and other kinases) by specific tyrosine kinase inhibitors, such as imatinib mesylate, is now standard in metastatic and unresectable GISTs. In many cases, tumors develop resistance over 1–2 years. In such instances, other kinase inhibitors, such as sunitinib malate (inhibits KIT and some other tyrosine kinases), are used as rescue drugs. Use of these inhibitors as adjuvant treatment after complete excision or in neoadjuvant setting to improve tumor resectability or allow for more conservative surgical management is being investigated in clinical trials.

Pathology, prognosis and genetics of gastrointestinal stromal tumors (GISTs)

Markku Miettinen & Jerzy Lasota

Definition and terminology

Gastrointestinal stromal tumor (GIST) is the name for a specific, most common type of mesenchymal tumor in the gastrointestinal (GI) tract. This tumor is histogenetically related to interstitial cells of Cajal or their precursor, is immunohistochemically KIT (CD117) positive in >95% of cases, carries gain-of-function KIT or PDGFRA mutations, has a histologic spectrum including spindle cell, epithelioid and rarely pleomorphic variants, and varies in behavior from benign to malignant (Miettinen & Lasota 2006a).

In earlier times and in many centers until the late 1990s, GISTs were commonly classified as gastrointestinal smooth muscle tumors (leiomyomas, leiomyoblastomas, and leiomyosarcomas). Considering the rarity of true smooth muscle tumors in the stomach and small intestine, most tumors previously classified as smooth muscle tumors in these sites represent GISTs. Some GISTs were earlier believed to be nerve sheath tumors, and others were classified as non-specific sarcomas.

Gastrointestinal autonomic nerve tumor (GANT; originally named plexosarcoma) was described in the 1980s (Herrera *et al.* 1989). Although these tumors were then believed to be of neural derivation, they are now known to be histologically similar to GISTs, are immunohistochemically KIT-positive, and carry KIT mutations, thus justifying their reclassification as GISTs (Lee *et al.* 2001).

Based on the known relative frequencies of GIST and other mesenchymal tumors of the GI tract, a conversion table is provided here (Table 9.1). However, histologic review (and often KIT immunostaining) is necessary for accurate reclassification in individual cases.

Occurrence and epidemiology, and etiology of GIST

GISTs occur throughout the gastrointestinal tract from the

Table 9.1 Conversion guide from older terminology prior to application of KIT immunohistochemistry to the present terminology, in relation to GIST and other mesenchymal tumors of the gastrointestinal tract. Based on authors' experience in reclassification of large series of mesenchymal tumors at different sites. Based on Miettinen *et al.* (2000a,b, 2001, 2003, 2005a, 2006a).

Location	Diagnosis	Comment
Esophagus	Leiomyoma	Most are true leiomyomas and not GISTs
Esophagus	Leiomyosarcoma	Most are GISTs and very few are true leiomyosarcomas
Stomach	Leiomyoma	Most (>95%) are GISTs and only few are leiomyomas
Stomach	Leiomyoblastoma	Most are epithelioid GISTs
Stomach	Leiomyosarcoma	Almost all are GISTs and very few are true leiomyosarcomas
Small intestine	Leiomyoma	Most (>90%) are GISTs and very few are true leiomyomas
Small intestine	Leiomyosarcoma	Most are GISTs and few (5%) are true leiomyosarcomas
Colon and rectum	Leiomyoma	Mucosal lesions are true leiomyomas, and most mural ones are GISTs
Colon and rectum	Leiomyosarcoma	Most are GISTs, but up to 20% are true leiomyosarcomas
Stomach	Schwannoma or neurofibroma	One true Schwann cell tumor occurs in the stomach for every 50 GISTs
Small intestine	Schwannoma or neurofibroma	These tumors, especially in neurofibromatosis 1 patients, are mostly GISTs
Any location	Gastrointestinal autonomic nerve tumor (GANT)	These tumors are now classified as GISTs

mid esophagus to the anus. They are most common in the stomach (60%) and small intestine (30%), and are relatively rare in duodenum (5%), rectum (4%), and esophagus (<1%).

GISTs occur with a frequency of 11–19 per million according to population-based studies from Iceland, Norway and Sweden (Nilsson *et al.* 2005; Tryggvason *et al.* 2005; Steigen & Eide 2006). Assuming a similar incidence, this would translate into 3300–6220 new GISTs in the United States annually. The overall incidence could be even higher, considering the surprisingly high frequency of minimal incidental GISTs, reported in resections for gastroesophageal resections for carcinoma (14%) (Abraham *et al.* 2007). Of the GISTs annually detected in the United States, approximately 1000–1800 can be estimated to be clinically malignant. Intestinal GISTs are twice more often clinically malignant than gastric GISTs.

Worldwide incidence is not well studied. However, the apparent incidence of diagnosed cases depends on factors such as healthcare availability, number of endoscopic and surgical procedures that give an opportunity to detect incidental GIST, and on true variation in GIST population incidence. Median age at GIST diagnosis varies between 58 and 63 years, and only 10% are diagnosed before the age of 40 years. Presentation in childhood is very rare and essentially limited to second decade and gastric location; less than <1% of all GISTs are diagnosed before the age of 18 years, predominantly in girls. There is no clear sex difference in adult GISTs, except that malignant gastric and intestinal GISTs may be slightly more common in men (up to 55 : 45 male predominance).

Most GISTs are sporadic, but up to 5% are associated with tumor syndromes. Of these, neurofibromatosis 1 is the most common, and occurrence of multiple, usually indolent, small intestinal GISTs is typical. Carney triad (GIST, pulmonary chondroma, paraganglioma) and familial GIST syndrome are very rare.

The etiology of GIST, as for most other mesenchymal tumors, is poorly understood. It has not been delineated whether dietary carcinogenesis can play a role, especially in the genesis of gastric GISTs. Radiation does not seem to play a role, and in our experience, post-radiation sarcomas involving the intestine are uniformly non-GISTs.

Clinical presentation of GIST

Gastrointestinal bleeding is the most common symptomatic presentation. This results from ulcerated tumor, and occurs with benign and malignant GISTs at any site. Acute bleeding most commonly manifests as melena and rarely as hematemesis, and both can be a medical emergency requiring multiple blood transfusions. More commonly, the bleeding is insidious occult bleeding resulting in chronic anemia and associated symptoms that lead to the initial visit to the doctor. In earlier times, some patients had repeated episodes of acute bleeding or long-standing anemia before a GIST was eventually diagnosed; diagnostic delay was historically more common in small intestinal tumors.

Non-specific ulcer-like pain is a common complaint in gastric GISTs. Larger esophageal, intestinal and rectal GISTs can cause symptomatic obstruction: dysphagia, chronic or acute intestinal obstruction, and rectal obstruction. Intussusception is a rare complication of GIST. Larger cystic tumors may rupture into the abdominal cavity and cause an acute abdomen. Some patients with larger necrotic, possibly secondarily infected tumors, may have generalized infection-like symptoms such as fever, usually combined with abdominal pain.

Every third GIST is incidentally diagnosed in an asymptomatic patient during gastroscopy, abdominal surgery, radiologic tumor surveillance, or by palpation during pelvic or prostate examinations. In countries such as Japan, where gastroscopic screening for gastric carcinoma is widely practiced, small GISTs are often diagnosed as a byproduct generally promoting the detection of tumors at smaller size than elsewhere.

Patterns of metastasis

Malignant GISTs most commonly metastasize into abdominal soft tissues and liver. In the abdomen, the sites involved vary in a wide range depending of location of the primary tumor.

Metastases develop in sarcomatoid GISTs (with mitotic activity over 10–20 per 50 HPFs) in a high number of tumors, typically within 1–2 years from presentation, often even after apparently complete surgery. Tumors that have lower mitotic activity and that are relatively small (see prognostic section for details) metastasize less frequently; this may often be after a considerable delay that can be 10–20 years or more after surgery. This necessitates long-term follow-up for any GISTs, except minimal incidental tumors.

Common metastatic sites for gastric GISTs are the omentum and lesser omentum, peritoneal surfaces, around the colon, and the around spleen with secondary involvement of the exterior of these organs. Small intestinal and colonic GISTs often metastasize to mesenteries, peritoneal surfaces and the pelvic region where primary or metastatic intestinal GIST can simulate a gynecologic cancer.

Liver metastases are common for malignant GISTs of any origin, and the involvement varies from solitary or multiple nodules to diffuse involvement in advanced cases. Lung metastases are exceptionally rare in GISTs, in contrast to other types of soft tissue sarcomas. Also, histologically verifiable lymph node metastases are extremely rare.

Bone metastases occur rarely, and in our experience, the axial skeleton, pelvic bones and spine are most commonly involved. Peripheral soft tissue metastases are rare, with the exception of the abdominal wall. We have seen isolated cases of metastases into arm, axilla, posterior neck, distant sites of skin, parotid, and adrenal glands.

Diagnostic procedures

The location and size of the tumor and clinical circumstances dictate the strategy for sampling for morphologic diagnosis. Tumors that ulcerate gastrointestinal mucosa can often be reached via endoscopic biopsy, except when in the jejunum or ileum. Gastric tumors located beyond mucosa can be reached via ultrasound-guided endoscopic biopsy. CT-guided biopsy is used for larger abdominal tumors. Smaller tumors that are tentatively identified as GISTs are definitively diagnosed in the excision specimen. Saving multiple samples of frozen tissue in tumor bank should be considered whenever possible, because this will facilitate subsequent molecular genetic analysis.

Histologically GISTs can be relatively reliably identified by their characteristic morphologic features by an experienced pathologist, but the diagnosis should be confirmed by immunohistochemical demonstration of KIT and secondary immunohistochemical markers, such as CD34 and protein kinase C theta, and by GIST-specific KIT or PDGFRA mutations, whenever necessary. The pathology of GIST will be described below.

Histogenesis and pathogenesis of GIST

GISTs are immunophenotypically similar to interstitial cells of Cajal, the spindle cells present around the myenteric plexus and sometimes within the muscular layers of the GI tract. These cells express KIT and are KIT-dependent, and act as functional intermediaries between the autonomic nerve system and smooth muscle cells regulating the autonomic nervous system and gastrointestinal peristalsis (Maeda *et al.* 1992; Hirota *et al.* 1998; Kindblom *et al.* 1998). Based on these similarities, its is likely that GISTs arise from Cajal cells or related precursor cells.

Oncogenic activation of KIT or PFDGRA receptor tyrosine kinases via mutations that render constitutionally activated status to these signal proteins is believed to be the key pathogenetic event and best understood therapeutic target (Hirota & Isozaki 2006; Heinrich *et al.* 2003). Other as yet less well understood genetic changes seem to be necessary for tumor progression. The mutations will be described in detail below.

GIST of the esophagus

Esophageal GISTs are rare, comprising <1% of all GISTs; in this location, leiomyomas are three times more common, whereas true leiomyosarcomas are very rare. In the esophagus, GISTs occur nearly exclusively in the lower third, often close to the gastroesophageal junction. They typically cause dysphagia, but some form external masses bulging into the mediastinum and causing non-specific symptoms. Occasional tumors are found incidentally (Miettinen *et al.* 2000a).

Esophageal GISTs are usually >5 cm or have >5 mitoses per 50 HPFs, and most patients develop liver metastases. Long-term survivors are relatively few and include patients with small, mitotically inactive tumors. Histologically, esophageal GISTs generally resemble gastric GISTs, and most have spindle cell morphology, with the sarcomatous variants being most common. Due to the rarity of esophageal GISTs, prognostic factors are less developed than for other GISTs.

GIST of the stomach

This is a large, complex group that comprises approximately 60% of all GISTs. These tumors have a wide variation in clinical presentation, size, gross patterns, histology, KIT/PDGFRA mutation status, and prognosis. According to the largest series,

Table 9.2 Clinicopathologic characteristics of different histologic variants of gastric GISTs, including four spindle cell and four epithelioid variants. Based on data from Miettinen *et al.* (2005a).

Subtype	Typical histologic features	Usual range of mitotic rate	Metastatic rate
Spindle cell tumors			
Sclerosing	Paucicellular, collagen rich, often focally calcified	<5 per 50 HPFs	1.4%
Palisading vacuolated	Moderately cellular, nuclear palisading and perinuclear vacuoles prominent	<5 per 50 HPFs	2.2%
Hypercellular	Densely packed uniform spindle cells	5–10 per HPFs	14.6%
Sarcomatous	Densely cellular, cells often in fascicles separated by myxoid matrix	>20 per 50 HPFs	83.1%
Epithelioid tumors			
Sclerosing	Epithelioid cells in a collagenous stroma in a syncytial pattern	<5 per 50 HPFs	6.3%
Dyscohesive	Epithelioid cells with sharp cell borders, often separated by loose stroma	<5 per 50 HPFs	8.8%
Hypercellular	Densely cellular, with polygonal cells with sharp cell borders. No extracellular matrix	<5 per 10 HPFs	21.6%
Sarcomatous	Densely cellular, with polygonal cells with sharp cell borders. No extracellular matrix	>20/50 HPFs	64.3%

an average gastric GIST measures 6 cm, and has mitotic rate <5 per 50 HPFs. However, the tumor size can very from less than 1 mm to >40-cm tumors that can extend to the pelvis (Wong *et al.* 2003; Miettinen *et al.* 2005a). The great majority of pediatric GISTs are gastric, and all Carney triad GISTs are gastric, whereas GISTs in neurofibromatosis 1 patients rarely involve the stomach.

Any part of the stomach may be involved. Tumors with epithelioid morphology and pediatric gastric GISTs have a predilection for the antrum. Malignant behavior seems to be more common in GISTs involving the upper gastric body and gastroesophageal junction. Otherwise, clinicopathologic correlation of tumor location in various parts of the stomach is not well established.

Gastric GISTs of small size or focal gastric attachment are often treated by limited resections, especially wedge resections, and in the case of smaller tumors, increasingly by endoscopic or laparoscopic approach. Margins should be carefully evaluated to verify complete excision. Incomplete surgery may result in local gastric wall recurrences; these are often surgically curable.

Typical gross patterns include mural nodules producing luminally bulging dome-shaped elevations, external masses attached to gastric wall, sometimes with a pedicle, cystic external masses, and large, complex masses including intra- and extraluminal components. Posterior gastric wall tumors often fill the lesser omentum. Some tumors attach into the pancreas, spleen, transverse colon or left lobe of liver necessitating resections of these organs for attempted curative surgery. Large gastric GISTs sometimes clinically simulate primary tumors of neighboring organs. Omental and peritoneal dissemination correlates with malignant behavior. Lymph node involvement is extremely rare; extragastric tumor nodules around the stomach can almost never be verified as lymph nodes but rather represent peritoneal soft tissue metastases. Therefore, formal lymph node dissections are not necessary, but attention should be paid to extragastric peritoneal, omental or other tumor nodules.

Histologically gastric GISTs form a diverse group including spindle cell (60–70%), epithelioid (20–30%) and pleomorphic (<5%) variants. The main characteristics of these variants are shown in Table 9.2. These variants have a spectrum of different biologic potentials, with the sarcomatous spindled and epithelioid GISTs having a high metastatic rate. Spindle cell GISTs tend to have KIT mutations, whereas gastric epithelioid GISTs more often have PDGFRA mutations. The recognition of these variants helps to identify the full spectrum of GISTs, and it may also assist in determination of the biologic potential. Prognostic features are discussed in detail in a separate section.

Duodenal GISTs

Approximately 4–5% of all GISTs originate in the duodenum. GISTs can occur in any part of the duodenum, but are most common in the second part. Tumors involving the latter part can impinge on the pancreatic head and clinically simulate a pancreatic tumor. Clinicopathologic series have shown 35–50% tumor-related mortality in duodenal GISTs (Miettinen *et al.* 2003).

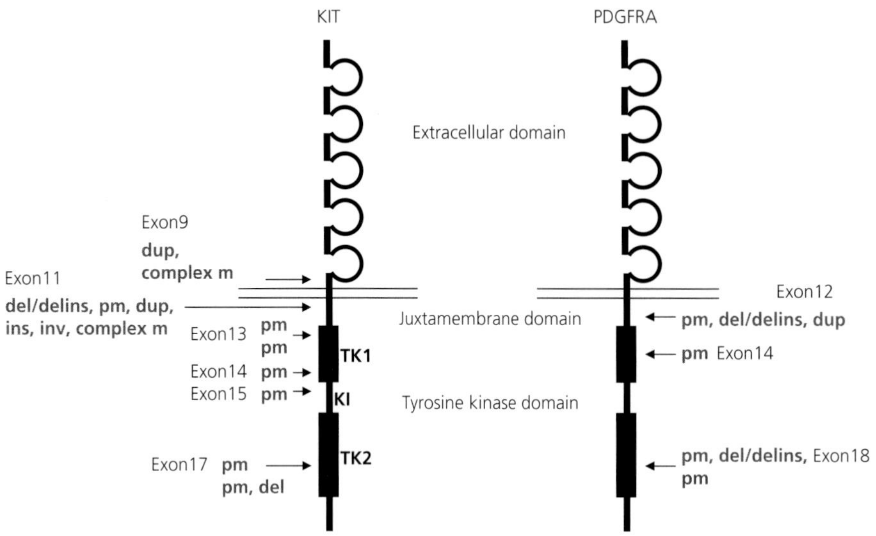

Fig. 9.1 Schematic structure of KIT and PDGFRA tyrosine kinase receptors and distribution of primary (grey) and secondary (red) mutations identified in different domains of these genes in GISTs. Abbreviations: TK1, first tyrosine kinse domain; TK2, second tyrosine kinase domain; KI, kinase insert; del, deletion; delins, deletion-insertion; dup, duplication; ins, insertion; inv, inversion; m, mutation; pm, point mutation.

Histologically duodenal GISTs are usually spindle cell tumors resembling small intestinal GISTs with half of the tumors containing skeinoid fibers. Hemangioma-like vascular proliferation is relatively common in duodenal GISTs and seems to be unique to this location. Epithelioid morphology is rare and represents malignant transformation rather than an independent type. Nearly all duodenal GISTs are KIT-positive.

The prognosis for small duodenal GISTs ≤2 cm with mitotic rate <5 per 50 HPFs is excellent, whereas metastases develop in patients with tumors of 2–5 cm with similarly low mitotic rate. Tumors that have >5 mitoses per 50 HPFs or that are >5 cm have a high tumor-related mortality.

Small intestinal GISTs

GISTs involving the jejunum or ileum comprise approximately 30% of all GISTs. Like other GISTs, they usually occur in older adults with a median age around 60 years; in this location occurrence in childhood is extremely rare. Small intestinal GISTs are more often malignant than gastric GISTs with overall 40–50% tumor-related mortality. The mortality is even higher with tumors >5 cm or with mitotic rate >5 per 50 HPFs. Location in the jejunum is more common than in the ileum by a factor of 1.6 : 1, but ileal tumors seem to be slightly more often clinically malignant (Miettinen *et al.* 2006a).

The tumors vary from diminutive nodules to complex masses >20–30 cm that extend into the abdomen. The common gross patterns include dumbbell-shaped lesions with internal and external components, solid outward bulging nodules, and large external cystic masses that can fistulate into lumen creating a diverticular appearance. These diverticula more likely represents a secondary structure formed by the tumor rather than origin from a structure such as Meckel's diverticulum, as sometimes suggested.

Small intestinal GISTs do not form distinctive histologic subtypes as gastric GISTs do, and most are spindle cell tumors. Nearly half contain distinctive, round, oval or elongated eosinophilic and PAS-positive aggregates of extracellular collagen fibers referred to as skeinoid fibers by their concentric lamellar ultrastructural appearance (Min 1992). These structures are more common in the non-malignant examples, and their presence has been found to be a statistically favorable prognostic feature. Collections of entangled cell processes surrounded by vague pseudorosettes are common. Despite their commonly malignant course, only a minority of small intestinal GISTs have histologically sarcomatous features with high mitotic activity, and pleomorphic forms are rare.

The epithelioid pattern in small intestinal GISTs (5%) is significantly linked with malignant tumors. It differs both morphologically and clinically from the gastric epithelioid GISTs and apparently represents morphologic tumor progression rather than a distinct subtype. Nearly all small intestinal GISTs are KIT positive (98%).

Pathology of GIST of colon and appendix

GISTs of the colon (excluding rectum) are rare, comprising no more than 1–2% of all GISTs. They occur throughout the colon but seem to be more common on the left side. They often present as large fungating masses >10 cm in diameter, and almost all are >5 cm. Overall tumor-related mortality is high, but prognosis generally correlates with tumor size and mitotic rate. Mitotically inactive tumors often contain skeinoid fibers, similar to small intestinal GISTs. Mitotically active tumors have variable morphology including spindle cell, epithelioid and pleomorphic patterns (Miettinen *et al.* 2000b).

Appendiceal GISTs are very rare, comprising less than 0.2% of all GISTs. Only handful of cases has been reported in adult patients. The reported tumors have been small <1 cm, KIT-positive, essentially incidental findings. Histologic features resemble those of small intestinal and colonic GISTs with low mitotic activity, and skeinoid fibers are common. Simple enucleation often leads to a recurrence (Miettinen & Sobin 2001).

Pathology of GISTs of rectum

GISTs of rectum comprise approximately 4% of all GISTs of defined localized origin. They vary from incidental minimal tumors to sarcomas. Larger tumors often present with rectal obstruction, bleeding or both. In particular, those rectal GISTs that involve the anterior rectum and extend to posterior aspect of the prostate can clinically simulate a prostate tumor (Miettinen *et al.* 2001; Hassan *et al.* 2006).

Histologically, rectal spindle cell GISTs can show spindle cell features somewhat similar to those seen in gastric GISTs, but perinuclear vacuolization is not prominent. Malignant examples can have a leiomyosarcoma-like fascicular pattern. Skeinoid fibers do not occur in rectal GISTs. Epithelioid morphology is rare.

Only tumors <2 cm with mitotic rate <5 per 50 HPFs seem to remain consistently free of metastases in follow-up studies; all other categories involve metastatic risk (see prognosis section and Table 9.5 below). Small, ≤2 cm, mitotically active (>5 per 50 HPFs) GISTs in the rectum have >50% of metastatic rate (Miettinen *et al.* 2001). Immunohistochemically GISTs of rectum are consistently KIT-positive and nearly always CD34-positive. However, they only rarely express smooth muscle actin, desmin and S100 protein.

Extragastrointestinal GISTs

GISTs have been reported outside of the tubular GI tract as apparent primary tumors. However, a great majority of GISTs in these locations are metastases from GI primaries. It is important to recognize GIST in this setting, and KIT immunostaining should therefore be performed on unclassified epithelioid and mesenchymal neoplasms in the abdomen, and also on suspected GIST metastases in peripheral tissues, so that the specific treatment can be made available to these patients (Miettinen *et al.* 1999; Reith *et al.* 2000; Yamamoto *et al.* 2004; Agaimy & Wunsch 2006).

The frequency of extragastrointestinal GISTs is low, no higher than 1% of all GISTs of defined origin. The more rigorous the definition for extragastrointestinal GISTs, and the better the investigation to rule out gastrointestinal origin, the fewer there are of such tumors. It is possible that some gastrointestinal GISTs have lost their primary connection to their GI tract origin and become secondarily attached as 'parasitic' masses to adjacent organs, omentum, mesenteries and retroperitoneum. Omental GISTs have histologic and prognostic features similar to gastric ones, whereas mesenteric GISTs closely mirror small intestinal GISTs.

We suspect that some reported GIST diagnoses outside of GI tract, especially those reported in the gallbladder and outside the abdomen, are based on overinterpretation of KIT immunostains in other mesenchymal tumors.

GISTs in children

Less than 1% of GISTs occur in children below 16 years; they are mostly in the second decade, in female patients and in the stomach, with a definite predilection to gastric antrum. Only isolated cases have been reported in the duodenum and intestines. Multinodularity and possible multifocality seem to be common in pediatric GISTs, predisposing patients to local recurrences and necessitating consideration of more radical surgery, with careful correlation of radiologic findings on tumor extent. The majority of pediatric GISTs (75%) have epithelioid morphology, and a few are associated with Carney triad in combination with pulmonary chondroma, paraganglioma or both. The prognosis of pediatric GISTs varies and seems to be somewhat unpredictable, with the correlation with mitotic rate, tumor size and prognosis being less distinct than in adult GISTs. No GIST-specific KIT or PDGFRA mutations have been found, suggesting that the pathogenesis of pediatric GISTs differs from that of adult GISTs (Prakash *et al.* 2005; Miettinen *et al.* 2005b).

GISTs in neurofibromatosis type 1 (NF1) patients

NF1 patients have a significant predilection to GISTs, and GISTs are the most common GI mesenchymal tumors in these patients outnumbering nerve sheath tumors. The NF1-associated GISTs typically occur in duodenum, jejunum and ileum and only rarely in the stomach or colon. They occur in slightly younger patients than sporadic GISTs, are often multiple, including minimal GIST precursors, and are accompanied by diffuse Cajal cell hyperplasia. The course is indolent in a majority of cases, although 10–15% of the patients have mitotically active and clinically malignant GIST, more often so in the duodenum. Morphologic features of NF1-associated GISTs are similar to those of sporadic intestinal GISTs and skeinoid fibers are common. NF1-associated GISTs have been negative for GIST-specific KIT and PDGFRA mutations (Kinoshita *et al.* 2004; Andersson *et al.* 2005; Miettinen *et al.* 2006b).

Carney triad

The combination of gastric GIST, pulmonary chondroma (hamartoma), and extra-adrenal paraganglioma constitute Carney triad; two of the three are required for the diagnosis, and the most common combination is GIST and pulmonary chondroma. The age of onset varies from 5–50 years, and there may be a long time span between the appearances of the different components. There is a strong female predominance (85%). There is no significant tendency to familial occurrence, and no genetic change specific to this syndrome has been identified to date (Carney 1999).

The GISTs in this syndrome preferentially occur in the antrum of the stomach and often have epithelioid morphology. The Carney triad-associated GISTs have many similarities with pediatric GISTs, including the fact that they do not seem to have GIST-specific KIT mutations. In the largest series reported by Carney, metastases developed in 28% of patients, most commonly to liver and abdomen, and only rarely outside the abdominal cavity. Despite metastases, many patients survive a long time with the disease.

Familial GISTs

At least 14 families have been reported worldwide with familial GIST syndrome, based on germline (inheritable) KIT (usually exon 11) or in one case, PDGFRA mutation. The syndrome is transmitted inan autosomal dominant pattern, and these patients typically develop multiple or sometimes diffuse GISTs, usually in middle age, and usually in the stomach or small intestine. Other signs of KIT activation can be present, including cutaneous hyperpigmentation, mastocytosis, and dysphagia (Table 9.3). Prognosis varies, and many patients live long with the disease. Experience with imatinib treatment in familial GIST is very limited (Antonescu 2006; Lasota & Miettinen 2006).

Two transgenic murine models with inheritable heterozygous KIT mutations, one representing a deletion of codon corresponding human Val559 and another substitution corresponding to human Lys641Glu, replicate human familial GIST syndrome (Sommer *et al.* 2003; Rubin *et al.* 2005).

Immunohistochemical markers

KIT (CD117) is expressed strongly in most GISTs and is detected by immunohistochemistry, usually using purified polyclonal antibodies. Detection of KIT in mast cells and Cajal cells and its absence in normal smooth muscle and fibroblasts serve as excellent internal controls to validate the sensitivity and specificity of KIT immunostaining. Because KIT is absent in most other tumors considered in the differential diagnosis of GIST, it is a useful immunohistochemical marker. However, melanoma, mastocytoma, Ewing sarcoma, and angiosarcoma are among non-GISTs that can be KIT-positive (Miettinen & Lasota 2005; Miettinen & Lasota 2006b).

Approximately 5% gastric GISTs and up to 2% of intestinal GISTs are KIT negative. Some gastric epithelioid GISTs express KIT focally or not at all; some of these tumors have PDGFRA mutations; however, most PDGFRA mutant GISTs express KIT. Regionally variable KIT expression or one appearing as perinuclear dots is seen in some GISTs. Currently, PDGFRA immunohistochemistry has not been standardized as a diagnostic marker for GIST (Lasota *et al.* 2004; Medeiros *et al.* 2004).

Protein kinase C theta is a protein kinase activated downstream in the KIT signaling pathway. This kinase is consistently present in GIST and generally absent in tumors to be considered in the differential diagnosis, and has also been suggested as a useful marker for GIST, especially for KIT-negative tumors; experience is rather limited (Blay *et al.* 2004; Duensing *et al.* 2004).

Table 9.3 Reported familial GISTs. Compilation adapted from Lasota and Miettinen (2006).

Location	Mutation	Dysphagia	Cutaneous hyperpigmentation	Mast cell tumors	Original reference
KIT-JM (exon 8)	Asp419del	Yes	No	Yes	Hartmann *et al.*
KIT-JM (exon 11)	Trp557Arg	No	No	No	Hirota *et al.*; O'Brien *et al.*
KIT-JM (exon 11)	Trp557Arg	No	Yes	No	Robson *et al.*
KIT-JM (exon 11)	Val559Ala	No	Yes	No	Maeyama *et al.*
KIT-JM (exon 11)	Val559Ala	No	Yes	Yes	Beghini *et al.*
KIT-JM (exon 11)	Val559Ala	No	Yes	No	Li *et al.*
KIT-JM (exon 11)	Val560del	No	Yes	No	Nishida *et al.*
KIT-JM (exon 11)	Gln575_Leu576dup	No	Yes	No	Carballo *et al.*
KIT-JM (exon 11)	Asp579del	No	No	No	Tarn *et al.*
KIT-JM (exon 11)	Asp579del	No	No	No	Lasota *et al.*
KIT-TK1 (exon 13)	Lys642 Glu	No	No	No	Isozaki *et al.*
KIT-TK2 (exon 17)	Asp820Tyr	Yes	No	No	Hirota *et al.*
KIT-TK2 (exon 17)	Asp820Tyr	Yes	No	No	O'Riain *et al.*
PDGFRA-TK2 (exon 18)	Asp846Tyr	No	No	No	Chompret *et al.*

Nestin, a type VI intermediate filament protein typical of neural and some other stem cells, is expressed in most GISTs, and also in GI schwannomas and melanomas (Sarlomo-Rikala *et al.* 2002).

CD34, the hematopoietic progenitor cell antigen, is expressed in 85–90% of gastric and rectal spindle cell GISTs and in 50% of gastric epithelioid GISTs and small intestinal GISTs in general. It can be a useful adjunct marker, although it is also expressed in some fibroblastic, lipomatous and vascular endothelial cell tumors (Miettinen & Lasota 2006b). Smooth muscle actin type of microfilament protein is expressed in 20% of gastric GISTs and 35% of small intestinal GISTs, often focal, sometimes extensively. However, positivity of desmin, the muscle type of intermediate filament protein, is detected in <5% of GISTs, usually in gastric examples, and generally focally. Variable expression of muscle cell markers probably reflects multipotentiality of Cajal cells, the ancestor cells of GIST. On the other hand, general lack of desmin helps to separate GIST from true smooth muscle tumors.

GISTs, especially the intestinal ones (10–20%), variably express S100 protein typical of nerve sheath and some other tumors. Neurofilament proteins (NF68) may also be present. The specific significance of these observations is currently unclear (Miettinen & Lasota 2006b).

KIT and PDGFRA mutations

Mutational activation of the closely related KIT or PDGFRA receptor tyrosine kinases is a central event in GIST pathogenesis and also has an implication for GIST diagnosis and tyrosine kinase inhibitor-based treatment. The mutations cause changes in the amino acid sequence of the KIT or PDGFRA proteins by substituting one amino acid for another, or by deleting or adding new amino acid residues. The mutant proteins are presumed to abnormally activate the KIT and PDGFRA signal transduction pathway, which under normal circumstances is activated by growth factor signals (stem cell factor for KIT and platelet-derived growth factors for PDGFRA). Because sensitivity to targeted kinase inhibitor treatment (especially for imatinib) depends on KIT or PDGFRA mutation type, mutation analysis is helpful in tailoring the therapy for individual patients. Also, detection of GIST-specific KIT or PDGFRA mutations is useful in verifying the diagnosis in cases that are negative for KIT expression. In GISTs, KIT and PDGFRA mutations are believed to be mutually exclusive and only one type of such mutation can be present in primary tumor and its recurrent or metastatic lesions. Approximately 75% of GISTs carry KIT and 10% PDGFRA mutations (Rubin *et al.* 2001; Corless *et al.* 2004; Lasota *et al.* 2004; Andersson *et al.* 2006; Hirota & Isozaki 2006; Lasota & Miettinen 2006). These mutations are usually heterozygous, but apparent hemizygous/homozygous mutations have been reported in a minority of cases (5%). Similar KIT and PDGFRA mutations were found in sporadic and familial GISTs. However GISTs in children, Carney triad, and NF1 patients lack KIT and PDGFRA mutations, implicating an alternative pathogenesis. The mutations detected in untreated tumors are referred to 'primary mutations' and those that are acquired in imatinib treated tumors are referred to 'secondary' mutations. Different types of primary and secondary KIT and PDGFRA mutations, their relative frequency, clinicopathologic correlation, and imatinib sensitivity are presented in Fig. 9.2 and Table 9.4.

KIT mutations

KIT exon 11 (juxtramembrane domain) is the most common site of mutations (90%). In order of decreasing frequency, these mutations represent deletions/deletion-insertions, missense (point) mutations, duplications, and in rare cases insertions. The majority of deletions cluster in the 5′ end of KIT exon 11; the most common deletion is Tryp557_Lys558del. Missense mutations affect exclusively codons Tryp557, Val559, Val560 and Leu576. Duplications occur in the 3′ end of KIT exon 11, usually in gastric tumors. Gastric GISTs with KIT exon 11 deletions show more aggressive behavior than tumors with missense mutations, whereas there seems to be no prognostic difference in small intestinal tumors. In general, KIT exon 11 mutant GISTs respond well to imatinib treatment (Rubin *et al.* 2001; Corless *et al.* 2004; Andersson *et al.* 2006; Hirota & Isozaki 2006; Lasota & Miettinen 2006).

Almost 100% of KIT exon 9 (extracellular domain) mutations represent two codon duplications Tyr502_Ala503dup. These mutations usually occur in intestinal as opposed to gastric GISTs. The behavior of tumors with such mutations is similar to small intestinal GISTs in general. KIT exon 9 mutant GISTs have a lesser response to imatinib treatment than tumors with KIT exon 11 mutations, and a higher imatinib dose has been suggested for these patients.

KIT exon 13 and 17 (first and second tyrosine kinase domain) missense mutations are rare. These mutations lead to single amino acid substitutions Lys642Glu and Asn822Lys or Asn-822His at the protein level. Data on prognosis are scant. However, some KIT exon 13 and 17 mutant GISTs have shown poor imatinib response. KIT exon 13, 14 (first tyrosine kinase domain) and 17 are common 'hot spots' for secondary mutations acquired during imatinib treatment and conferring secondary resistance (Antonescu *et al.* 2005; Chen *et al.* 2005; Debiec-Rychter *et al.* 2005; Wardelmann *et al.* 2005).

PDGFRA mutations

These mutations usually occur in gastric and rarely in duodenal GISTs, and some of these tumors have weak or no detectable KIT expression. A majority of PDGFRA mutant tumors have a favorable prognosis reflecting the prognosis of gastric GISTs. Most common (80%) are exon 18 (second tyrosine kinase domain) mutations, of which the one causing Asp842Val substitution is most frequent. However other mutations including deletions/deletion-insertions and insertions clustering in the

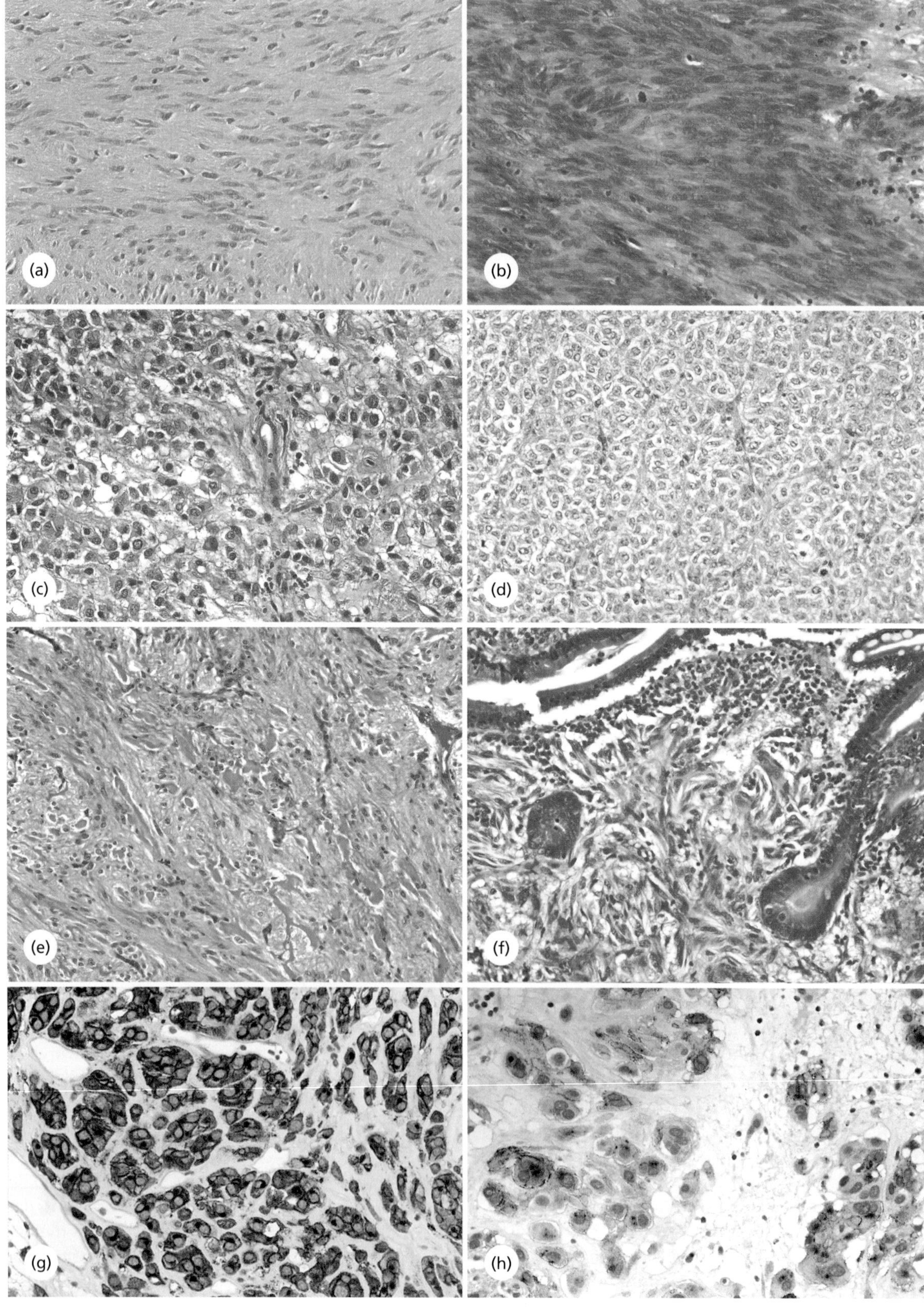
(a)
(b)
(c)
(d)
(e)
(f)
(g)
(h)

Fig. 9.2 Histologic spectrum of GIST and examples of immunohistochemical KIT positivity.
(a) Sclerosing spindle cell gastric GIST is paucicellular and mitotic activity is not detectable. (b) Sarcomatous spindle cell gastric GIST shows high nuclear density and nuclear atypia, and mitotic figures are present. (c) Epithelioid gastric GIST with low mitotic activity. (d) Epithelioid gastric GIST with high mitotic activity and sarcomatous features. (e) Small intestinal GIST with extracellular collagen globules (so-called skeinoid fibers). (f) Small intestinal GIST infiltrating between mucosal elements. This growth pattern, although rare, predicts malignant behavior. (g) Strong KIT positivity in a GIST is typically seen in the cytoplasm and often also as perinuclear dots. (h) Weaker but distinctive KIT positivity is often observed in gastric epithelioid GISTS.

Table 9.4 KIT and PDGFRA mutation types: frequency, common location, frequency, and imatinib response in primary sporadic GIST. Based on Lasota and Miettinen (2006) and Corless *et al.* (2005).

Gene	Domain	Mutation status	Common location and estimated overall frequency	Response to imatinib treatment and prognosis prior to imatibib
KIT	Extracellular (exon 9)	Duplication	Intestines 5% (10% of intestinal GISTs)	Incomplete response, might require a higher dosage (600–800 mg/day). Prognosis similar to that of intestinal GISTs in general.
	Juxtamembrane (exon 11)	Deletion Deletion-insertion Point mutation Duplication Insertion	Entire GI tract 65%	In general, responds well. Prognosis of different mutants varies. Gastric GISTs with deletions more malignant than those with point mutations.
	Tyrosine kinase 1 (TK1, exon 13)	Point mutation	Entire GI tract <2%	Response varies, poor in some cases. Clinicopathologic features not well-defined.
	Tyrosine kinase2 (TK2, exon 17)	Point mutation	Entire GI tract <2%	Response varies, poor in some cases. Predominantly seen in intestinal GISTs.
PDGFRA	JM (exon 12)	Point mutation Deletion Deletion-insertion Insertion	Stomach <2%	No clinical data on imatinib sensitivity; based on *in vitro* studies, expected to be sensitive.
	Tyrosine kinase 1 (TK1, exon 14)	Point mutation	Stomach <1%	No clinical data on imatinib sensitivity; based on *in vitro* studies, expected to be sensitive.
	Tyrosine kinase2 (TK2 exon 18)	Point mutation Deletion Deletion-insertion	Stomach 8–10%	Imatinib resistant *in vitro* and *in vivo*.
KIT	EC, JM, TK1, TK2	WT	Entire GI tract	Often poor response. Experience is limited.
PDGFRA	JM, TK1, TK2		10–15%	

vicinity of codon 842 and other than Asp842Val substitutions have been reported. PDGFRA exon 18-mutant GISTs are imatinib resistant. Moreover, acquired Asp842Val substitution causing secondary imatinib resistance was identified during a treatment.

PDGFRA exon 12 (juxtamembrane domain) mutations are relatively rare. These mutations form a heterogeneous group of missense mutations, deletions/deletion-insertions and duplications affecting codon 561 and its vicinity. The most frequent is point mutation leading toVal561Asp substitution at the protein level. PDGFRA exon 12-mutant GISTs are expected to be imatinib sensitive. PDGFRA exon 14 mutations (first tyrosine kinase domain) have been reported in a few cases. These mutations affect exclusively codon 659 and lead to Asn659Lys or Asn-659Tyr substitutions at the protein level. There are no specific clinical data on imatinib sensitivity of PDGFRA exon 14-mutant tumors (Heinrich *et al.* 2003; Corless *et al.* 2004; Lasota *et al.* 2004; Corless *et al.* 2005; Lasota & Miettinen 2006; Lasota *et al.* 2006).

Prognosis

The prognosis of GIST is highly variable, and best-documented prognostic markers are tumor size (maximum diameter) and mitotic activity (usually expressed per 50 HPFs equaling 5 mm^2). Additional but less documented prognostic markers are Ki67 (MIB1) labeling index and expression of p53. Approximately 20% of gastric GISTs and 40% of intestinal GISTs are clinically malignant (Miettinen & Lasota 2006b).

Table 9.5 summarizes the relationship of tumor size, mitotic rate and prognosis of GISTs of different sites. The tabularized data are based on the largest published site-specific clinicopathologic studies. In this table, GISTs are divided into eight groups based on these parameters. For rare sites some groups are merged because of the small number of cases.

As the table shows, GISTs of the stomach behave less aggressively than other GISTs with similar tumor size and mitosis parameters. For example, gastric GISTs >10 cm but with a low mitotic rate have a 12% metastatic rate, whereas small intestinal GISTs with similar parameters metastasize in 52% of cases. Similarly, the metastatic rate of gastric GISTs of 2–5 cm with mitotic rate >5 per 50 HPFs is 16%, whereas the metastatic rate for corresponding small intestinal GISTs is 73%.

Very small GISTs (<2 cm) with mitotic rate ≤5 mitoses per 50 HPFs seem to be indolent at any site, whereas tumors of 2–5 cm with similar mitotic rates have a very low (<2%) metastatic rate in the stomach but a somewhat higher metastatic rate in intestinal locations, varying from 4.3% to 8.5% at different sites. On the other hand, metastatic risk already exists in tumors <2 cm that have >5 mitoses per 50 HPFs, except for gastric tumors, based on Table 9.5. Relatively small tumors that unexpectedly metastasize often do so after considerable delay, sometimes 10–20 or more years after the primary surgery. We have seen patients whose GIST first metastasized over 40 years after primary surgery. Such tumor behavior necessitates long-term follow-up.

Irrespective of locations, GISTs >5 cm and with mitotic rate >5 per 50 HPFs have a high tumor-related mortality. with relatively short 1–2-year median survival times. Mitotic rates and sizes also predict survival times in patients who die of metastases. For example, patients with gastric GISTs who died of tumors with <5 mitoses per 50 HPFs have median survivals between 2–9 years, whereas the median survivals for patients with gastric GISTs >5 mitoses per 50 HPFs who die of tumor are 1–2.5 years in different tumor size categories. A similar but less clear tendency for longer survival time for patients with tumors of low mitotic rates exists for small intestinal GIST patients who died of tumor.

The expected prognosis in different size and mitosis rate-related categories may offer guidance for treatment and sur-

Table 9.5 Rates of metastases or tumor-related death in GISTs of stomach and small intestine by tumors grouped by mitotic rate and tumor size. Based on previously published long-term follow-up studies on 1055 gastric, 629 small intestinal, 144 duodenal, and 111 rectal GISTs (Miettinen *et al.* 2001, 2003, 2005a, 2006a).

Group	Tumor parameters		% of patients with progressive disease during long-term follow-up and characterization of risk for metastasis			
	Size	Mitotic rate	Gastric GISTs	Jejunal and ileal GISTs	Duodenal GISTs	Rectal GISTs
1	≤2 cm	≤5 per 50 HPFs	0 none	0 none	0 none	0 none
2	>2 ≤5 cm	≤5 per 50 HPFs	1.9 very low	4.3 low	8.3 low	8.5% low
3a	>5 ≤10 cm	≤5 per 50 HPFs	3.6 low	24 moderate		
3b	>10 cm	≤5 per 50 HPFs	12 moderate	52 high	34 high†	57* high†
4	≤2 cm	>5 per 50 HPFs	0*	50*	†	54 high
5	>2 ≤5 cm	>5 per 50 HPFs	16 moderate	73 high	50 high	52 high
6a	>5 ≤10 cm	>5 per 50 HPFs	55 high	85 high		
6b	>10 cm	>5 per 50 HPFs	86 high	90 high	86 high†	71 high†

* Denotes tumor categories with very small numbers of cases.

† Groups 3a and 3b or 6a and 6b are combined in duodenal and rectal GISTs because of small number of cases.

‡ No tumors of such category were included in the study.

Note that small intestinal and other intestinal GISTs show a markedly worse prognosis in many mitosis and size categories than gastric GISTs. Group refers to the grouping defined by a combination of size and mitotic rate, as used in the references.

HPFs, high power fields.

veillance strategies, and assist in determining the impact of adjuvant treatment. The data in Table 9.5 are based on the pre-imatinib era.

Proliferation markers such as Ki67 analogs and cyclins have been examined in GISTs. It is not clear whether they provide more accurate prognostic information than mitotic counts, although their use has been advocated by some. Standardized application is not possible, as no uniform cut-off values have been developed. As is the case with many other malignant tumors, sarcomatoid GISTs more often have nuclear p53 (TP53) positivity (Miettinen & Lasota 2006b). Loss of p16INK4A (cyclin-dependent kinase inhibitor subtype) has been found as an adverse prognostic factor.

References

Abraham SC, Krasinskas AM, Hofstetter WL, Swisher SG, Wu TT. (2007) 'Seedling' mesenchymal tumors (gastrointestinal stromal tumors and leiomyomas) are common incidental tumors of the esophagogastric region. *Am J Surg Pathol* 31(11): 1629–35.

Agaimy A, Wunsch PH. (2006) Gastrointestinal stromal tumours: a regular origin in the muscularis propria, but an extremely diverse gross presentation. A review of 200 to critically re-evaluate the concept of so-called extragastrointestinal stromal tumors. *Langenbecks Arch Surg* 391(4): 322–9.

Andersson J, Sihto H, Meis-Kindblom JM, Joensuu H, Nupponen N, Kindblom LG. (2005) NF1-associated gastrointestinal stromal tumors have unique clinical, phenotypic, and genotypic characteristics. *Am J Surg Pathol* 29(9): 1170–6.

Andersson J, Bumming P, Meis-Kindblom JM *et al.* (2006) Gastrointestinal stromal tumors with KIT exon 11 deletions are associated with poor prognosis. *Gastroenterology* 130: 1573–81.

Antonescu CR. (2006) Gastrointestinal stromal tumor (GIST). Pathogenesis, familial GIST and animal models. Review. *Semin Diagn Pathol* 23(2): 63–9.

Antonescu CR, Besmer P, Guo T *et al.* (2005) Acquired resistance to imatinib in gastrointestinal stromal tumor occurs through secondary gene mutation. *Clin Cancer Res* 11(11): 4182–90.

Blay P, Astudillo A, Buesa JM *et al.* (2004) Protein kinase C theta is highly expressed in gastrointestinal stromal tumors but not in other mesenchymal neoplasias. *Clin Cancer Res* 10(12 Pt 1): 4089–95.

Carney JA. (1999) Gastric stromal sarcoma, pulmonary chondroma, and extra-adrenal paraganglioma (Carney triad): Natural history, adrenocortical component, and possible familial occurrence. *Mayo Clin Proc* 74(6): 543–52.

Chen LL, Sabripour M, Andtbacka RH *et al.* (2005) Imatinib resistance in gastrointestinal stromal tumors. *Curr Oncol Rep* 7(4): 293–9.

Corless CL, Fletcher JA, Heinrich MC. (2004) Biology of gastrointestinal stromal tumors. *J Clin Oncol* 22(18): 3813–25.

Corless CL, Schroeder A, Griffith D *et al.* (2005) PDGFRA mutations in gastrointestinal stromal tumors: frequency, spectrum and in vitro sensitivity to imatinib. *J Clin Oncol* 23(23): 5357–64.

Debiec-Rychter M, Cools J, Dumez H *et al.* (2005) Mechanisms of resistence to imatinib mesylate in gastrointestinal stromal tumors and activity of the PKC412 inhibitor against imatinib-resistant mutants. *Gastroentereology* 128(2): 270–9.

Duensing A, Joseph NE, Medeiros F *et al.* (2004) Protein kinase C theta (PKCtheta) expression and constitutive activation in gastrointestinal stromal tumors (GISTs). *Cancer Res* 64(15): 5127–31.

Hassan I, You N, Dozois EJ *et al.* (2006) Clinical, pathologic, and immunohistochemical characteristics of gastrointestinal stromal tumors of the colon and rectum: Implications for surgical management and adjuvant therapies. *Dis Col Rectum* 49(5): 609–15.

Heinrich MC, Corless CL, Duensing A *et al.* (2003) PDGFRA activating mutations in gastrointestinal stromal tumors. *Science* 299(5607): 708–10.

Herrera GA, Cerezo L, Jones JE *et al.* (1989) Gastrointestinal autonomic nerve tumors. Plexosarcomas. *Arch Pathol Lab Med* 113(8): 846–53.

Hirota S, Isozaki K. (2006) Pathology of gastrointestinal stromal tumors. *Pathol Int* 56(1): 1–9.

Hirota S, Isozaki K, Moriyama Y *et al.* (1998) Gain-of-function mutations of c-kit in human gastrointestinal stromal tumors. *Science* 279(5350): 577–80.

Kindblom LG, Remotti HE, Aldenborg F, Meis- Kindblom JM. (1998) Gastrointestinal pacemaker cell tumor (GIPACT). Gastrointestinal stromal tumors show phenotypic characteristics of the interstitial cells of Cajal. *Am J Pathol* 153(5): 1259–69.

Kinoshita K, Hirota S, Isozaki K *et al.* (2004) Absence of c-kit gene mutations in gastrointestinal stromal tumours from neurofibromatosis type 1 patients. *J Pathol* 202(1): 80–5.

Lasota J, Miettinen M. (2006) KIT and PDGFRA mutations in gastrointestinal stromal tumors. *Semin Diagn Pathol* 23(2): 91–102.

Lasota J, Dansonka-Mieszkowska A, Sobin LH, Miettinen M. (2004) A great majority of GISTs with PDGFRA mutations represents gastric tumors of low or no malignant potential. *Lab Invest* 84(7): 874–83.

Lasota J, Stachura J, Miettinen M. (2006) GISTs with PDGFRA exon 14 mutations represent subset of clinically favorable gastric tumors with epithelioid morphology. *Lab Invest* 86(1): 94–100.

Lee JR, Joshi V, Griffin JW Jr, Lasota J, Miettinen M. (2001) Gastrointestinal autonomic nerve tumor: immunohistochemical and molecular identity with gastrointestinal stromal tumor. *Am J Surg Pathol* 25(8): 979–87.

Maeda H, Yamagata A, Nishikawa S *et al.* (1992) Requirement of c-kit for development of intestinal pacemaker system. *Development* 116(2): 369–75.

Medeiros F, Corless CL, Duensing A *et al.* (2004) KIT-negative gastrointestinal stromal tumors: proof of concept and therapeutic implications. *Am J Surg Pathol* 28(7): 889–94.

Miettinen M, Lasota J. (2005) KIT (CD117): a review on expression in normal and neoplastic tissues, and mutations and their clinicopathologic correlation. *Appl Immunohistochem* 13(3): 205–20.

Miettinen M, Lasota J. (2006a) Gastrointestinal stromal tumors: Review on morphology, molecular pathology, prognosis, and differential diagnosis. *Arch Pathol Lab Med* 130(10): 1466–78.

Miettinen M, Lasota J. (2006b) Pathology and prognosis of gastrointestinal stromal tumors. *Semin Diagn Pathol* 23(2): 70–83.

Miettinen M, Sobin LH. (2001) Gastrointestinal stromal tumors in the appendix. A clinicopathologic and immunohistochemical study of four cases. *Am J Surg Pathol* 25(11):1433–7.

Miettinen M, Monihan JM, Sarlomo-Rikala M *et al.* (1999) Gastrointestinal stromal tumors/smooth muscle tumors/GISTs in the omentum and mesentery—clinicopathologic and immunohistochemical study of 26 cases. *Am J Surg Pathol* 23(9): 1109–18.

Miettinen M, Sarlomo-Rikala M, Sobin LH, Lasota J. (2000a) Esophageal stromal tumors: a clinicopathologic, immunohistochemical, and molecular genetic study of 17 cases and comparison with esophageal leiomyomas and leiomyosarcomas. *Am J Surg Pathol* 24(2): 211–22.

Miettinen M, Sarlomo-Rikala M, Sobin LH, Lasota J. (2000b) Gastrointestinal stromal tumors and leiomyosarcomas in the colon. A clinicopathologic, immunohistochemical, and molecular genetic study of 44 cases. *Am J Surg Pathol* 24(10):1339–52.

Miettinen M, Furlong M, Sarlomo-Rikala M, Burke A, Sobin LH, Lasota J. (2001) Gastrointestinal stromal tumors, intramural leiomyomas, and leiomyosarcomas in the rectum and anus. A clinicopathologic, immunohistochemical, and molecular genetic study of 144 cases. *Am J Surg Pathol* 25(9):1121–33.

Miettinen M, Kopczynski J, Maklouf HR *et al.* (2003) Gastrointestinal stromal tumors, intramural leiomyomas, and leiomyosarcomas of the duodenum: a clinicopathologic, immunohistochemical, and molecular genetic study of 167 cases. *Am J Surg Pathol* 27(5): 625–41.

Miettinen M, Sobin LH, Lasota J. (2005a) Gastrointestinal stromal tumors of the stomach: A clinicopathologic, immunohistochemical, and molecular genetic studies of 1765 cases with long-term follow-up. *Am J Surg Pathol* 29(1): 52–68.

Miettinen M, Lasota J, Sobin LH. (2005b) Gastrointestinal stromal tumors of the stomach in children and young adults: a clinicopathologic, immunohistochemical, and molecular genetic study of 44 cases with long-term follow-up and review of the literature. *Am J Surg Pathol* 29(10): 1373–81.

Miettinen M, Makhlouf HR, Sobin LH, Lasota J. (2006a) Gastrointestinal stromal tumors (GISTs) of the jejunum and ileum – a clinicopathologic, immunohistochemical and molecular genetic study of 906 cases prior to imatinib with long-term follow-up. *Am J Surg Pathol* 30(4): 477–89.

Miettinen M, Fetsch JF, Sobin LH, Lasota J. (2006b) Gastrointestinal stromal tumors in patients with neurofibromatosis 1. A clinicopathologic study of 45 patients with long-term follow-up. *Am J Surg Pathol* 30(1): 90–6.

Min K-W. (1992) Small intestinal stromal tumors with skeinoid fibers. Clinicopathological, immunohistochemical, and ultrastructural investigations. *Am J Surg Pathol* 16(2): 145–55.

Nilsson B, Bumming P, Meis-Kindblom JM *et al.* (2005) Gastrointestinal stromal tumors: the incidence, prevalence, clinical course, and prognostication in the preimatinib mesylate era – a population-based study in western Sweden. *Cancer* 103(4): 821–9.

Prakash S, Sarran L, Socci N *et al.* (2005) Gastrointestinal stromal tumors in children and young adults: a clinicopathologic, molecular, and genomic study of 15 cases and review of the literature. *J Pediatr Hematol Oncol* 27(4): 179–87.

Reith JD, Goldblum JR, Lyles RH, Weiss SW. (2000) Extragastrointestinal (soft tissue) stromal tumors. An analysis of 48 cases with emphasis on histological predictors of outcome. *Mod Pathol* 13(5): 577–85.

Rubin BP, Singer S, Tsao C *et al.* (2001) KIT activation is a ubiquitous feature of gastrointestinal stromal tumors. *Cancer Res* 61(22): 8118–21.

Rubin BP, Antonescu CR, Scott-Browne JP *et al.* (2005) A knock-in mouse model of gastrointestinal stromal tumor harboring Kit K641E. *Cancer Res* 65(15): 6631–9.

Sarlomo-Rikala M, Tsujimura T, Lendahl U, Miettinen M. (2002) Patterns of nestin and other intermediate filament expression distinguish between gastrointestinal stromal tumors, leiomyomas and schwannomas. *APMIS* 110(6): 499–507.

Sommer G, Agosti V, Ehlers I *et al.* (2003) Gastrointestinal stromal tumors in a mouse model by targeted mutation of the Kit receptor tyrosine kinase. *Proc Natl Acad Sci USA* 100(11): 6706–11.

Steigen SE, Eide TJ. (2006) Trends in incidence and survival of mesenchymal neoplasms of the digestive tract within a defined population on northern Norway. *APMIS* 114(3): 192–200.

Tryggvason G, Gislason HG, Magnusson MK, Jonasson JG. (2005) Gastrointestinal stromal tumors in Iceland, 1990–2003: the Icelandic GIST study, a population-based incidence and pathologic risk stratification study. *Int J Cancer* 117(2): 289–93.

Wardelmann E, Thomas N, Merkelbach-Bruse *et al.* (2005) Acquired resistance to imatinib in gastrointestinal stromal tumours caused by multiple KIT mutations. *Lancet Oncol* 6(4): 249–51.

Wong NA, Young R, Malcomson RDG *et al.* (2003) Prognostic indicators for gastrointestinal stromal tumours: a clinicopathological and immunohistochemical study of 108 resected cases of the stomach. *Histopathology* 43(2): 118–26.

Yamamoto H, Oda Y, Kawaguchi K *et al.* (2004) c-kit and PDGFRA mutations in extragastrointestinal stromal tumor (gastrointestinal stromal tumor of the soft tissue). *Am J Surg Pathol* 28(4): 479–88.

Imaging and staging of gastrointestinal stromal tumors

Angela D. Levy

Introduction

Gastrointestinal stromal tumors have a diverse spectrum of imaging manifestations because they may develop at any location in the gastrointestinal tract and may be benign or malignant. Accordingly, GISTs may be small, incidentally discovered mural masses, or they may attain very large sizes, invade adjacent organs, and metastasize hematogenously. Since most GISTs involve the muscularis propria of the gastrointestinal tract wall, they share the unique feature of a well-defined mural mass on cross-sectional imaging studies, allowing them to be distinguished from epithelial neoplasms. An understanding of the imaging features of primary, metastatic, and recurrent GIST as well as the unique appearance of treated disease is important because GISTs can be effectively treated with KIT inhibitor therapy. In this section, the imaging features of primary, metastatic, and treated GIST and the role of imaging in the management of patients undergoing KIT-inhibitor therapy will be discussed.

Imaging features

Primary tumor

GISTs most commonly involve the muscularis propria of the gastrointestinal tract wall, forming an intramural mass. Since the muscularis propria is the outer muscular layer of the gastrointestinal wall, GISTs have a propensity for exophytic growth. The most common imaging appearance of GIST is a mass arising from the gastrointestinal wall and projecting into the

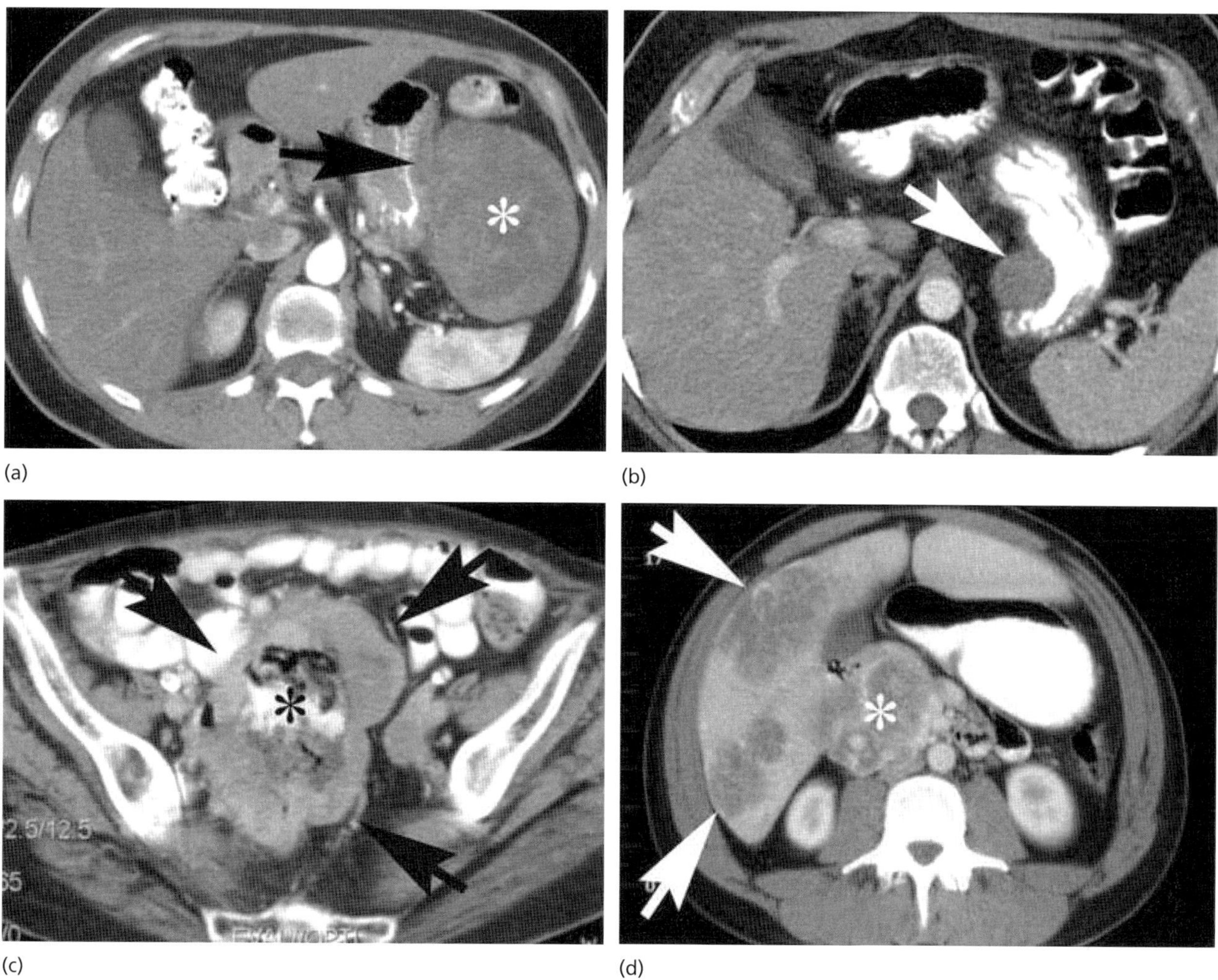

Fig. 9.3 CT findings of gastrointestinal stromal tumors. (a) CT shows a gastric GIST in a 57-year-old woman with a history of Conn syndrome who complained of upper abdominal fullness. There is a 9-cm well-defined mass (asterisk) with heterogeneous CT attenuation arising from the stomach and extending into the gastrosplenic ligament. The site of origin in the gastric wall shows focal mural thickening (arrow). (b) CT shows a gastric GIST in a 53-year-old man who complained of hematemesis. There is a 4-cm well-defined mass (arrow) in the gastric fundus near the gastroesophageal junction that is homogeneous in CT attenuation. (c) Small intestinal GIST in a 78-year-old woman who complained of lower abdominal pain and weight loss. There is a large cavitary mass (arrows) arising from the distal ileum. Gas, oral contrast, and fluid are present within the cavity (asterisk). (d) Duodenal GIST with liver metastasis in a 28-year-old man who complained of epigastric pain. CT scan shows a large, heterogeneous mass (asterisk) with peripheral enhancement in the second portion of the duodenum. Liver metastases (arrows) are present.

abdominal cavity (Fig. 9.3a) (Levy *et al.* 2003b). A focal area of mural thickening in the adjacent stomach or intestine can usually be identified to establish the origin of the mass (Fig. 9.3a). Less commonly, GISTs are intramural masses (Fig. 9.3b) or intraluminal polyps. In all morphologies, GISTs typically have smoothly marginated outer contours. As they enlarge, focal ulceration may occur on the mucosal surface overlying the tumor. Small GISTs are typically homogeneous on imaging studies. In contrast, large GISTs are more commonly heterogeneous on imaging studies because of degenerative, necrotic, and hemorrhagic regions within the tumor.

Sonography and endoscopy are commonly used as an initial imaging modality in a patient who complains of abdominal pain, nausea, or vomiting. As such, GISTs may be encountered on routine abdominal sonography or endoscopy. Once discovered, computed tomography (CT), magnetic resonance imaging (MRI), and positron emission tomography (PET) or PET/CT fusing imaging provide anatomic and functional imaging for staging. Intravenous contrast-enhanced CT and MRI show a peripheral enhancement pattern in the majority of GISTs, reflecting central tumor degeneration and necrosis (Fig. 9.3d) (Burkill *et al.* 2003; Levy *et al.* 2003b; Sandrasegaran *et al.* 2005). Less commonly, GISTs will have a homogenous pattern of contrast enhancement. Cavitation and fistula formation may occur in GISTs with extensive degenerative and necrotic changes. Cavitary GISTs may expand the caliber of the intestinal lumen, creating focally, irregularly marginated areas of luminal distension. Luminal contents, oral contrast agents, and gas may be identified within cavitary GISTs (Fig. 9.3c) (Levy *et al.* 2003b). Calcification is present in a minority of GISTs and the pattern of calcification may be coarse and chunky or finely stippled.

In the stomach, exophytic extension of the tumor beyond the stomach commonly occurs, particularly in malignant GISTs that attain large sizes. Extension into the gastrohepatic, gastrocolic, or gastrosplenic ligaments deviates the stomach and alters its contours. The gastric mucosa overlying the luminal surface of the tumor is often irregular, which reflects mucosal ulceration.

Small intestinal GISTs that extend into the small bowel mesentery may produce significant mass effect on adjacent organs or segments of intestine. It may be difficult on cross-sectional imaging studies to identify the small intestine as the origin of the tumor when extension into the small bowel mesentery occurs. In these cases, GISTs mimic primary and secondary tumors of the mesentery such as lymphoma, mesenteric fibromatosis, soft tissue sarcomas, and metastatic disease. Small bowel obstruction may occur from intussusception or luminal occlusion by the tumor. Hemorrhage from mucosal ulceration may produce significant bleeding such that angiography may be the initial radiologic exam performed in order to control bleeding through embolization of vessels. Angiographically, GISTs are characterized by twisted, irregular or ball-like vessels with neovascularity (Fang *et al.* 2004).

Focal, well-defined mural masses with or without mucosal ulceration are most characteristic of anorectal GISTs (Levy *et al.* 2003a). In the anorectal region, GISTs may extend into the ischiorectal fossa, perineum, or adjacent pelvic organs. Intraluminal polypoid masses are less common. Similar to gastric and small intestinal GISTs, the CT attenuation and intravenous contrast enhancement pattern is most commonly heterogeneous, reflecting intratumoral degeneration, necrosis, or hemorrhage.

MR imaging features of GISTs are variable. The degree of intratumoral degeneration, necrosis, and hemorrhage influences the signal intensity pattern. Solid portions of the tumor are typically low signal intensity on T1-weighted images, high signal intensity on T2-weighted images, and enhance after intravenous gadolinium administration. Areas of degeneration and necrosis do not show contrast enhancement. Hemorrhagic regions within the tumor will vary from high to low signal intensity on both T1 and T2-weighted images, depending on the age of the hemorrhage (Hasegawa *et al.* 1998; Levy *et al.* 2003b; Sandrasegaran *et al.* 2005).

Metastatic lesions

The liver and peritoneal cavity are the most common locations for GIST metastases. Rarely, GISTs may metastasize to the lung, bone, or pleura, or recur at the surgical site (Burkill *et al.* 2003). Lymphatic spread of tumor is so uncommon (Miettinen *et al.* 2005; Miettinen *et al.* 2006) that lymph node enlargement is not an imaging feature associated with GISTs. Hematogenous hepatic metastases are typically multifocal and low attenuation with respect to normal liver during the portal venous phase of intravenous contrast enhancement on CT (Fig. 9.3d). They may also have a heterogeneous pattern with central hypoattenuation or may be homogeneous (Burkill *et al.* 2003). Peritoneal metastases are focal mesenteric and omental soft tissue masses, nodules or focal confluent areas of increased attenuation within the mesentery and omentum. Peritoneal implants on visceral organs may occur.

Imaging during therapy

KIT-inhibitor therapy with imatinib mesylate (Gleevec, Glivec; Novartis AG, Basel, Switzerland) is the treatment of choice for patients with metastatic and recurrent GIST. The role of imatinib mesylate in adjuvant and neoadjuvant therapy is under investigation. Intravenous contrast-enhanced CT shows positive response to treatment with imatinib mesylate in primary and metastatic GIST as transformation of the lesion to a well-defined homogeneous, hypoattenuating cyst-like mass with disappearance of solid enhancing tumor (Fig. 9.4) (Chen *et al.* 2002; Warakaulle & Gleeson 2006). The cyst-like transformation of GIST following therapy has been attributed to myxoid degeneration with the development of myxohyaline stroma and a decreased density of tumor cells (Abdulkader *et al.* 2005). Treated lesions do not always decrease in size following therapy as traditionally seen in other solid tumors. Treated GIST may remain stable in size, decrease, or in some cases, paradoxically increase in size with imatinib mesylate therapy as the tumor becomes hypoattenuating and cyst-like in appearance on CT. Consequently, traditional tumor measurement protocols used to assess response to therapy that rely on dimensional measurements of the entire lesion do not apply to GIST treated with imatinib mesylate.

Disease progression in patients who previously had successful treatment with imatinib mesylate is the recurrence of solid, enhancing tumor nodules within the cyst-like lesions on CT. An overall increase in the size of the tumor and enhancement of previously hypoattenuating lesions is another indication of disease progression. The appearance of enhancing tumor nodules within a treated cyst-like lesion has been called the nodule within a mass pattern of recurrence (Shankar *et al.* 2005). In the majority of these cases, new focal FDG uptake on PET is seen, which confirms disease recurrence.

Staging

Although the roles of the various imaging modalities in staging and evaluating GIST response to therapy have not been established, evidence to date supports using both CT and PET imaging as complementary modalities. CT provides superior anatomic and spatial information to plan surgical intervention

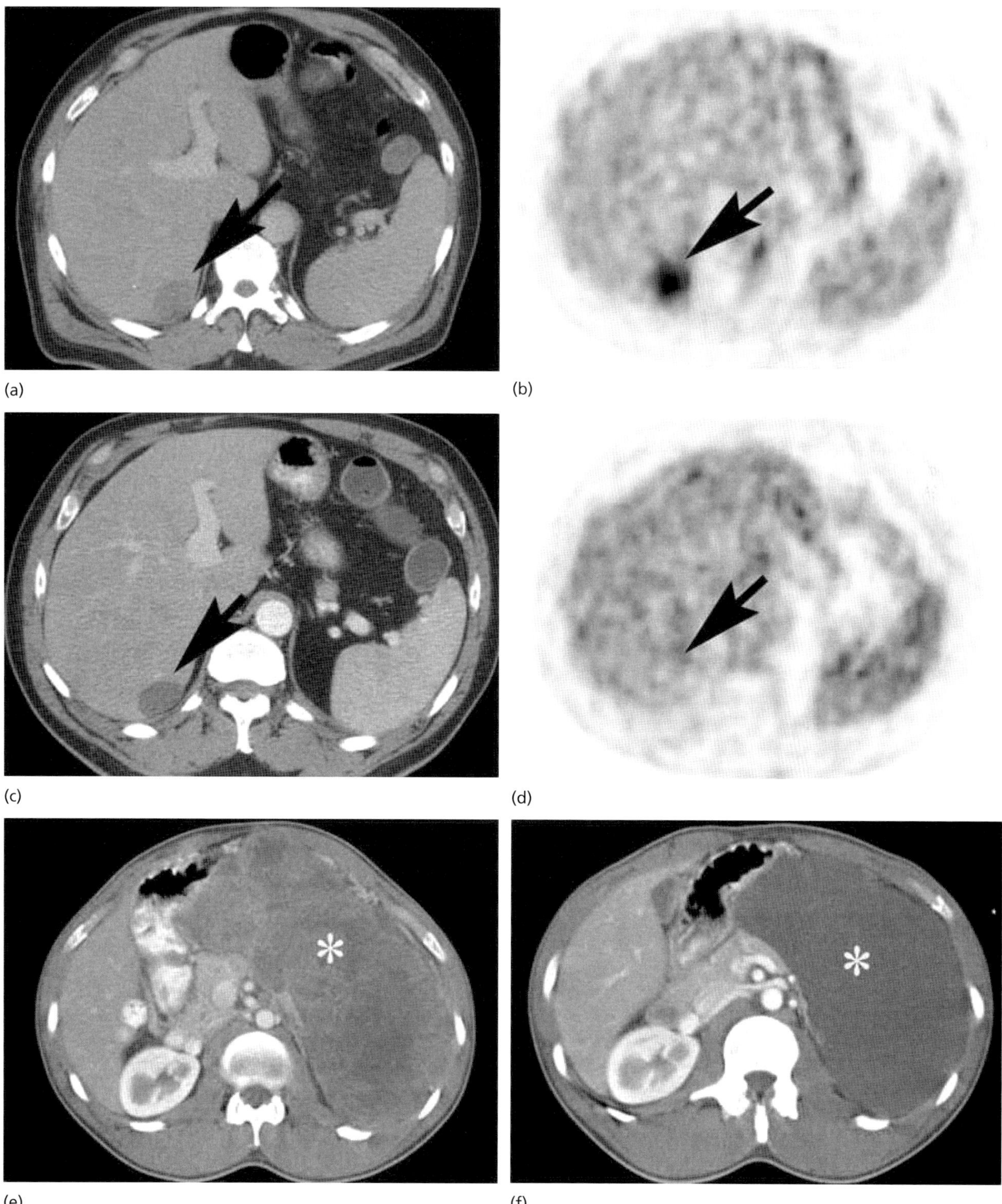

Fig. 9.4 Imaging of GIST treated with imatinib mesylate. (a–d) CT and PET-CT in a 52-year-old woman with liver metastasis from a small intestinal GIST shows a metastatic lesion in the right lobe of the liver on pretreatment CT (arrow in a) that is FDG avid on PET-CT (arrow in b). Following imatinib mesylate therapy, the liver lesion is better defined and more hypoattenuating (arrow in c) compared to the pretreatment scan and the lesion is no longer FDG avid on PET-CT (arrow in d). (e,f) CT scans in a 31-year-old man with a gastric GIST who received neoadjuvant therapy with imatinib mesylate. Pretherapy CT scan shows a large heterogeneously enhancing mass (asterisk in e) in the left upper abdomen. Post-therapy CT scan shows that the mass has become cyst-like and is homogenously hypoattenuating (asterisk in f).

and PET is essential to assess the degree of metabolic activity for evaluating response to treatment. For initial staging, reports suggest that CT and FDG-PET have comparable sensitivity and positive predictive value (Gayed *et al.* 2004; Goerres *et al.* 2005). Stroobants *et al.* have shown that FDG-PET obtained 8 days after the start of imatinib mesylate correctly predicted the therapy response and the PET showed a response before the anatomic changes were visible on CT (Stroobants *et al.* 2003). Goerres *et al.* suggest that a single post-treatment PET to identify the presence of FDG uptake is sufficient for the prediction of patient outcome and that a pretreatment scan is not needed to predict overall survival (Goerres *et al.* 2005). PET/CT imaging can be considered a reliable tool for assessment of GIST response and where available, should be used for initial staging and to follow tumor response in patients undergoing imatinib mesylate therapy (Antoch *et al.* 2004).

Conclusions

GISTs have a variable spectrum of imaging features at initial diagnosis and show unique imaging findings during imatinib mesylate therapy. CT and PET/CT are complementary imaging studies that should be used in the management of patients with GISTs.

References

Abdulkader I, Cameselle-Teijeiro J, Forteza J. (2005) Pathological changes related to imatinib treatment in a patient with a metastatic gastrointestinal stromal tumour. *Histopathology* 46: 470–2.

Antoch G, Kanja J, Bauer S *et al.* (2004) Comparison of PET, CT, and dual-modality PET/CT imaging for monitoring of imatinib (STI571) therapy in patients with gastrointestinal stromal tumors. *J Nucl Med* 45: 357–65.

Burkill GJ, Badran M, Al-Muderis O *et al.* (2003) Malignant gastrointestinal stromal tumor: distribution, imaging features, and pattern of metastatic spread. *Radiology* 226: 527–32.

Chen MY, Bechtold RE, Savage PD. (2002) Cystic changes in hepatic metastases from gastrointestinal stromal tumors (GISTs) treated with Gleevec (imatinib mesylate). *AJR Am J Roentgenol* 179: 1059–62.

Fang SH, Dong DJ, Zhang SZ, Jin M. (2004) Angiographic findings of gastrointestinal stromal tumor. *World J Gastroenterol* 10: 2905–7.

Gayed I, Vu T, Iyer R *et al.* (2004) The role of 18F-FDG PET in staging and early prediction of response to therapy of recurrent gastrointestinal stromal tumors. *J Nucl Med* 45: 17–21.

Goerres GW, Stupp R, Barghouth G *et al.* (2005) The value of PET, CT and in-line PET/CT in patients with gastrointestinal stromal tumours: long-term outcome of treatment with imatinib mesylate. *Eur J Nucl Med Mol Imaging* 32: 153–62.

Hasegawa S, Semelka RC, Noone TC *et al.* (1998) Gastric stromal sarcomas: correlation of MR imaging and histopathologic findings in nine patients. *Radiology* 208: 591–5.

Levy AD, Remotti HE, Thompson WM, Sobin LH, Miettinen M. (2003a) Anorectal gastrointestinal stromal tumors: CT and MR imaging features with clinical and pathologic correlation. *AJR Am J Roentgenol* 180: 1607–12.

Levy AD, Remotti HE, Thompson WM, Sobin LH, Miettinen M. (2003b) Gastrointestinal stromal tumors: radiologic features with pathologic correlation. *RadioGraphics* 23: 283–304, 456; quiz 532.

Miettinen M, Makhlouf H, Sobin LH, Lasota J. (2006) Gastrointestinal stromal tumors of the jejunum and ileum: a clinicopathologic, immunohistochemical, and molecular genetic study of 906 cases before imatinib with long-term follow-up. *Am J Surg Pathol* 30: 477–89.

Miettinen M, Sobin LH, Lasota J. (2005) Gastrointestinal stromal tumors of the stomach: a clinicopathologic, immunohistochemical, and molecular genetic study of 1765 cases with long-term follow-up. *Am J Surg Pathol* 29: 52–68.

Sandrasegaran K, Rajesh A, Rushing DA, Rydberg J, Akisik FM, Henley JD. (2005) Gastrointestinal stromal tumors: CT and MRI findings. *Eur Radiol* 15: 1407–14.

Shankar S, Vansonnenberg E, Desai J, Dipiro PJ, Van Den Abbeele A, Demetri GD. (2005) Gastrointestinal stromal tumor: new nodule-within-a-mass pattern of recurrence after partial response to imatinib mesylate. *Radiology* 235: 892–8.

Stroobants S, Goeminne J, Seegers M *et al.* (2003) 18FDG-positron emission tomography for the early prediction of response in advanced soft tissue sarcoma treated with imatinib mesylate (Glivec). *Eur J Cancer* 39: 2012–20.

Warakaulle DR, Gleeson F. (2006) MDCT appearance of gastrointestinal stromal tumors after therapy with imatinib mesylate. *AJR Am J Roentgenol* 186: 510–5.

Treatment

Heikki Joensuu & Ronald P. DeMatteo

Surgery

Primary localized GIST

Approximately 80% of patients presenting with GIST have primary localized disease without metastasis (Fig. 9.5). For them, complete surgical resection is the standard of care and offers the only chance of cure.

There are a number of notable surgical principles for treating primary GIST. GISTs are often fragile, especially when they are large or contain extensive intratumoral hemorrhage or necrosis. Consequently, biopsy carries a risk of inducing tumor dissemination or bleeding. In addition, preoperative biopsy may not be diagnostic if viable tumor is not sampled. If the radiologic or endoscopic findings are highly suggestive of the diagnosis, we do not routinely perform a preoperative biopsy when surgery is intended. During the operation, it is necessary that the surgeon be meticulous to avoid intraoperative tumor rupture, which is associated with a greater risk of intraperitoneal recurrence.

Typically, a wedge or segmental resection of the organ from which a GIST has arisen is sufficient. This is because GISTs grow exophytically from the gastrointestinal tract and do not usually spread within the bowel wall. Unlike gastrointestinal adenocar-

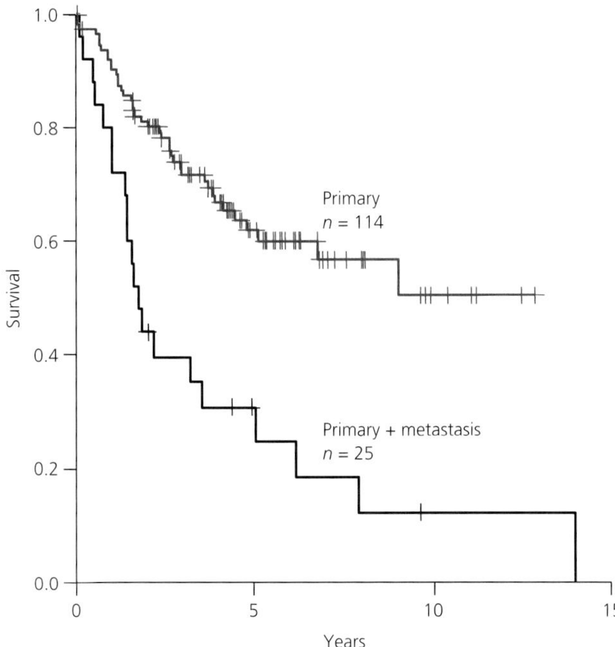

Fig. 9.5 Disease-specific survival depends on the stage of GIST at initial presentation. Unpublished data (DeMatteo) before the advent of imatinib.

cinomas, GISTs often just displace adjacent vital structures and do not invade them. Nevertheless, when tumor adherence to nearby structures does occur, partial resection of the involved organs in an en-bloc fashion may be necessary to achieve tumor clearance. The overall goal of surgery should be to achieve gross tumor clearance with negative microscopic margins whenever possible. There is no proof that wide margins (e.g. greater than 1 cm) provide additional benefit. The importance of negative microscopic margins on the resected organ is uncertain for GISTs larger than 10 cm in size, which may shed tumor cells into the peritoneum from anywhere along their surface. The management of a positive microscopic margin on final pathologic review depends on whether the surgeons thinks the margin is truly positive and whether the involved area could even be identified and removed at re-exploration. Surgical staplers can be used, although removal of the staples during pathologic processing from wedge resections of the stomach may confound examination of the true margin.

Laparoscopic resection can be performed by skilled surgeons and it is especially useful for small gastric GISTs. Unlike gastrointestinal adenocarcinomas, GISTs almost never metastasize to regional nodes and so lymphadenectomy is not performed routinely. The one notable exception to this is in pediatric patients, where GISTs tend to be multifocal and involve regional nodes. It is imperative that the surgeon performs a careful intraoperative evaluation for evidence or peritoneal or liver metastasis.

There are several institutional series documenting the outcome after resection of primary GIST (Table 9.6). There are

Table 9.6 Results of resection for primary localized GIST. Reproduced with permission from Gold JS, DeMatteo RP. (2006) Combined surgical and molecular therapy: The gastrointestinal stromal tumor model. *Ann Surg* 244: 176–84.

Author	Year	No. of patients	No. with completely resected primary localized disease	Median follow-up (months)	Number with recurrence (%)	5-year survival	Comments
DeMatteo	2000	200	80	24	32 (40%)	54% DSS	Tumor size prognostic variable of DSS
Wong	2003	108*	108	43		42% OS, 29% RFS	Mitotic index, Ki67 independent predictors of OS
Kim	2004	101	86	36	29 (34%)	78% OS	Tumor size, mitotic index, *KIT* mutation independent predictors of RFS
Martín	2005	162	162	42	42 (26%)	68% RFS	Tumor size, mitotic index, site of origin, cellularity, *KIT* amino acid 557-8 deletion independent predictors of RFS
Wu	2006	100†	85	33	44 (44%)	44% DFS	Mitotic index, cellularity, Ki67 independent predictors of DFS
Bümming	2006	259	221		38 (17%)		Tumor size, *KIT* exon 11 deletion, Ki67, independent predictors of recurrence

DSS, disease-specific survival; OS, overall survival; RFS, recurrence-free survival; DFS, disease-free survival; Ki67, graded assessment of immunohistochemical staining for the tumor proliferation marker Ki67.

* All tumors gastric in origin.

† All tumors small bowel in origin.

only a few large series, since the disease is uncommon. Most of the older data include patients with other intra-abdominal sarcomas (leiomyosarcoma in particular) because of the previous difficulties in the diagnosis and classification of GIST. Nevertheless, since most gastrointestinal tract sarcomas are in fact GISTs, the data are largely representative of GIST. We found that 80 (86%) of 93 patients who presented with a primary tumor and lacked metastasis were able to undergo complete surgical resection of their disease (DeMatteo *et al.* 2000). The 5-year disease-specific survival of the 80 patients was 54%.

There are no data regarding postoperative follow up of patients with completely resected GIST. In other words, there is no proof that earlier detection of recurrent GIST improves survival. Nevertheless, since there are now effective medical therapies for recurrent disease, it seems appropriate to perform routine radiologic surveillance for tumors that may recur. Because most recurrences happen within the first 3–5 years, the National Comprehensive Cancer Network (NCCN) and EORTC consensus guidelines advocate CT scans of the abdomen and pelvis with intravenous contrast every 3–6 months during the first 5 years after resection and yearly thereafter (Blay *et al.* 2004; Demetri *et al.* 2004).

Metastatic GIST

Before the imatinib era patients diagnosed with GIST metastases had a bleak outcome. The only exception were the rare patients who had slowly growing intra-abdominal metastases who may have survived for up to 20 years following the diagnosis (Miettinen *et al.* 2005; Nilsson *et al.* 2005). According to the United States National Cancer Institute (NCI) Surveillance, Epidemiology, and End Results (SEER) registry data the relative 5-year survival rate of GIST patients diagnosed in the United States in 1992 to 2000 was 45% (Tran *et al.* 2005). The 5-year survival rate ranged in the past from 40% to 65% after complete resection of localized primary tumor (DeMatteo *et al.* 2000), but nearly half of surgical patients develop postoperative recurrence or metastasis (Table 9.6). The median survival time of patients with metastatic or locally recurrent GIST was only 10–20 months before the imatinib era (DeMatteo *et al.* 2000).

GISTs frequently give rise to intra-abdominal and liver metastases. The intra-abdominal metastases are characteristically located on the peritoneal, omental, mesenteric, and other serosal surfaces. Metastases outside of the abdomen are relatively rare even in patients who have a large intra-abdominal tumor burden, but GIST metastases may occur in many organs systems such as the bone, soft tissues and very rarely in the brain. In the late stages of the disease GIST patients have a characteristic presentation with a greatly enlarged abdomen due to tumor burden (Fig. 9.6). Many of the intra-abdominal metastases probably result from tumor cell seeding from the primary tumor and subsequent implantation onto the intra-abdominal serosal surfaces, whereas liver metastases probably arise hematogeneously. GIST patients may sometimes have metastases in surgical scars and even in needle tracts reflecting the high tendency of GIST cells to seed and implant in soft tissues. Lymph node metastases are rare.

Once metastasis has occurred in GIST, the standard of care is tyrosine kinase inhibitor (TKI) therapy. Nevertheless, it is important to recognize the results of surgery alone for metastatic GIST to interpret the benefit of imatinib in the proper context and to consider the combined use of surgery and TKI therapy for metastatic disease, as will be discussed later. In highly selected patients, surgery achieved a 5-year survival of about 35% (Fig. 9.7) (Gold *et al.* 2006).

Complete surgical resection is possible in only a minority of patients with recurrent GIST isolated to the peritoneum. It is important to recognize that radiologic imaging usually underestimates the extent of peritoneal disease. Even when all peritoneal tumors can be removed, nearly all patients will develop additional peritoneal nodules. Eilber used a combination of peritoneal debulking and intraperitoneal mitoxantrone, a cytotoxic drug related to doxorubicin, in 19 patients with peritoneal GIST (Eilber *et al.* 2000). The 2-year actuarial survival was 33% compared to 0% in 8 patients who had surgery alone. Thus, the role of surgery is quite limited for peritoneal GIST. Intraperitoneal chemotherapy has been supplanted by TKI therapy.

Most patients with liver metastases from GIST have multiple, diffuse tumors and are therefore inoperable. In a series of 131 patients with liver metastases from GIST or intestinal leiomyosarcoma (some archival specimens could not be tested for KIT) treated at Memorial Sloan-Kettering Cancer Center, complete gross resection was possible in 34 patients (26%) (DeMatteo *et al.* 2001). The 1- and 3-year survival rates were 90% and 58%, respectively (Fig. 9.8). Nevertheless, as is the case after resection of peritoneal GIST, nearly all patients developed disease progression, with the liver being the most common site of relapse.

Chemotherapy

Treatment of advanced, inoperable GIST changed radically at the turn of the century, when imatinib mesylate was found to be effective first in a single patient (Joensuu *et al.* 2001) and later in prospective multicenter studies (Van Oosterom *et al.* 2001; Demetri *et al.* 2002). This discovery and subsequent introduction of other molecularly targeted agents (Demetri *et al.* 2006) have improved the outcome for patients diagnosed with advanced GIST.

Conventional chemotherapy

Attempts to treat malignant GISTs with conventional systemic chemotherapy have almost invariably been unsuccessful (reviewed in DeMatteo *et al.* 2002; Joensuu *et al.* 2002), though interpretation of many of the older chemotherapy series

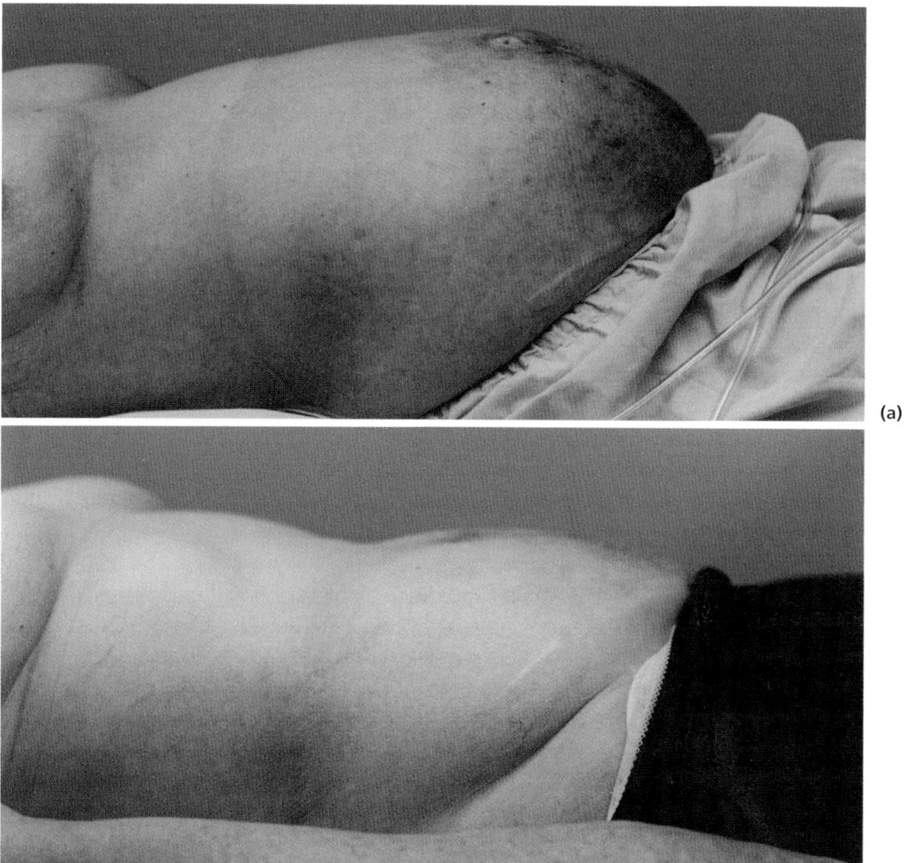

Fig. 9.6 Upper panel. Patient presenting with large intra-abdominal GIST tumors and a poor performance status (World Heath Organization performance status grade 4). Lower panel: Treatment result with imatinib. The abdomen is no longer extended and the performance status is normal (WHO 0). Produced with permission from Joensuu H. (2002) Tyrosine kinase inhibitors in the treatment of GIST. *Duodecim* 118: 2305–12.

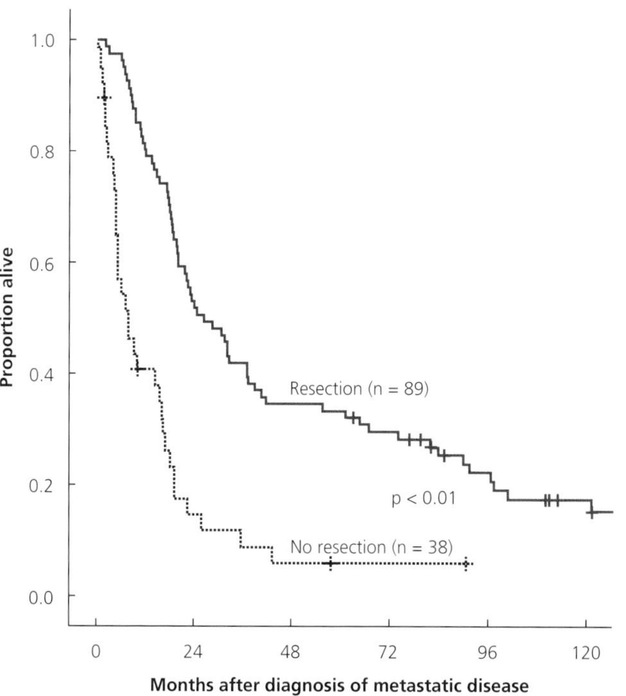

Fig. 9.7 Disease-specific survival in metastatic GIST based on whether surgical resection was performed. Based on data before the advent of imatinib. Reproduced with permission from Gold *et al.* (2007).

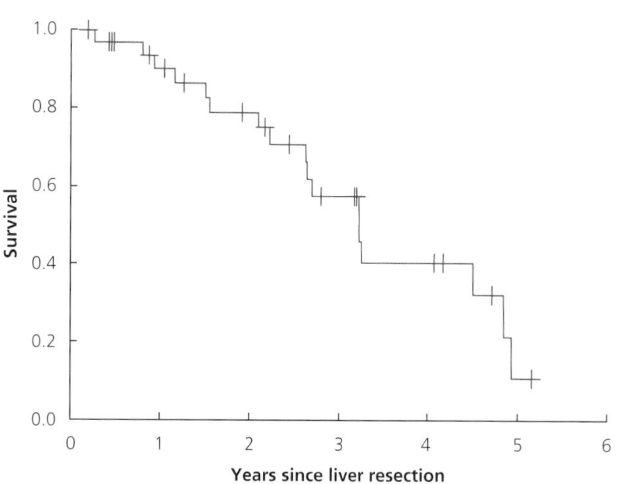

Fig. 9.8 Disease-specific survival after hepatectomy for liver metastases from GIST (n = 34). Reproduced with permission from DeMatteo *et al.* (2001).

reported before the year 2000 is often difficult since these series may consist of tumor types other than GIST. Response rates to combinations containing doxorubicin have generally been less than 10% in these series (Zalupski *et al.* 1991; Edmonson *et al.* 1999). In line with these findings, no responses were obtained in one study where gastrointestinal mesenchymal tumors were treated with ifosfamide and etoposide (Blair *et al.* 1994). Several of the more modern chemotherapy agents have not yet been evaluated in the treatment of GIST, but none of the 17 patients treated with temozolomide responded to treatment (Trent *et al.* 2003), and, similarly, no objective responses were found in a series of 28 GIST patients who were treated with ET743 (Blay *et al.* 2004).

Multidrug resistance has been associated with expression of proteins such as the P-glycoprotein, multidrug resistance protein (MDR1), and lung resistance protein (LRP). In one study consisting of 29 leiomyosarcomas and 26 GISTs, both P-glycoprotein and MDR1 were expressed in immunohistochemical stainings more often in GIST tissue samples than in samples consisting of leiomyosarcomas, whereas expression of lung resistance protein did not differ between these two types of sarcoma (Plaat *et al.* 2000). Most (85–100%) of GISTs express PKC-theta (Blay *et al.* 2004; Kim *et al.* 2006). This protein has been found to be associated with expression of multidrug resistance-associated protein (MRP) in acute myeloid leukemia (Beck *et al.* 1996) and MDR1 expression in the doxorubicin-resistant MCF-7 breast cancer cell line (Budworth *et al.* 1997). In sum, these findings are in line with the observed resistance of GISTs to many conventional chemotherapy agents in clinical series.

Systemic treatment with targeted agents

Imatinib mesylate

The standard first-line treatment of metastatic GIST is imatinib mesylate. Imatinib is an inhibitor of a few tyrosine kinases including the stem cell factor receptor (KIT), platelet-derived growth factor receptors (PDGFR-α and PDGFR-β), Abelson kinase (Abl), Breakpoint cluster region/Abelson oncogene (Bcr-Abl), Abl-related gene (ARG), and the macrophage colony-stimulating factor (M-CSF) receptor c-fms. It is administered orally at daily doses ranging from 300 mg to 800 mg. Imatinib binds to the ATP-binding pocket of the kinases competing with ATP in binding. An inactive conformation of the activation loop of the kinase (encoded by *KIT* exon 17) is needed for successful imatinib binding (Mol *et al.* 2004). The drug is eliminated predominantly via the bile in the form of metabolites, one of which (CGP 74588) shows comparable pharmacologic activity to the parent drug (Peng *et al.* 2005). The fecal to urinary excretion ratio is approximately 5:1. Imatinib is metabolized mainly by the cytochrome P450 (CYP) 3A4 or CYP3A5 as are many other drugs.

Approximately 50–70% of GIST patients achieve a partial response during imatinib treatment, and another 15–30% have stabilized disease (Verveij *et al.* 2004; Heinrich *et al.* 2005; Blanke *et al.* 2006). However, only few responses (5% or less) are radiologically or histologically complete. The median time to response is 3–4 months when response to imatinib is assessed using conventional response criteria that are based on tumor volume reduction. Patients may obtain subjective benefit within only a few days after starting imatinib, and diminished uptake of ^{18}F-fluorodeoxyglucose (FDG) in a PET scan may be found within a few hours or days after initiation of imatinib treatment (Joensuu & Dimitrijevic 2001). On the other hand, some GISTs shrink only slowly, and it may take up to 1 year to achieve tumor volume reduction justifying the definition of a partial remission. Imatinib therapy should be attempted even in cases where the patient's performance status is low (World Health Organization performance status 3 or 4), since even these patients may assume a normal lifestyle following initiation of imatinib mesylate.

Responding liver metastases characteristically become hypodense on CT or MR imaging following initiation of imatinib treatment. This is due to cell-rich tumor tissue being replaced by hyaline degeneration with only few surviving GIST cells (Joensuu *et al.* 2001). Hypodense GIST metastases are better delineated and more easily detected in a CT scan than the more dense untreated GIST lesions, which may result in visualization of a greater number of small liver lesions in a CT scan or MRI upon treatment (Fig. 9.9). This must not be misinterpreted as tumor progression (Linton *et al.* 2006). FDG-PET may be helpful in making a differential diagnosis between tumor progression and response in problematic cases. Decrease in metastatic lesion density usually heralds response and lesion volume reduction.

The median response duration of advanced GIST to imatinib treatment was 27 months in the US–Finland study (Blanke *et al.* 2006), and some patients with the longest follow-up times available to date have continued to respond over 6 years to imatinib. In the US–Finland study, patients who had stabilized disease (SD) achieved similar survival as those who had a partial response (PR) according to the South-West Oncology Group (SWOG) criteria suggesting that most of the responses judged as stabilized disease were in fact clinical responses to imatinib. Only 12% of the study participants had a GIST that was primarily resistant to imatinib. In the latest report of the study where the median follow-up time of the study participants was 52 months, the median survival time was 58 months and had not been reached in the subgroup of patients who had GIST with *KIT* exon 11 mutation (Blanke *et al.* 2006). These findings suggest that imatinib treatment prolongs survival approximately fourfold as compared to historical controls. This difference in outcome is considered so large that performing a randomized study where imatinib treatment is compared to a control arm of conventional chemotherapy is not likely to be conducted. Patients who have a small tumor burden at imatinib

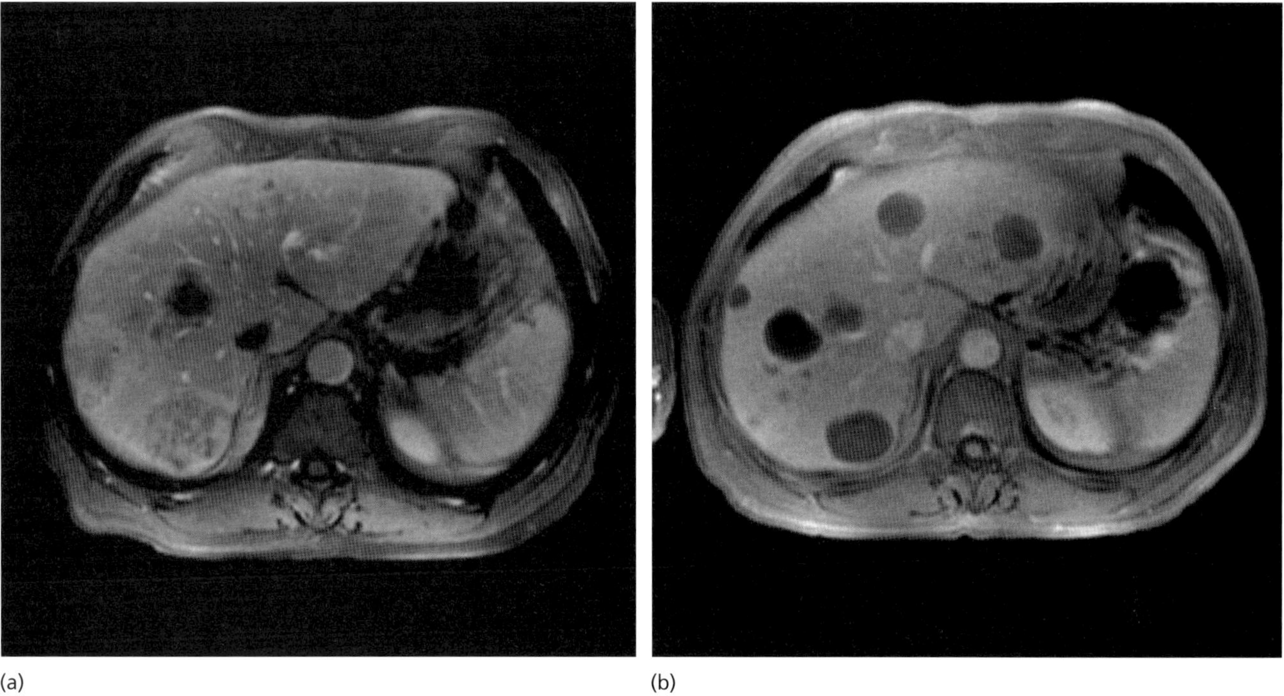

Fig. 9.9 GIST metastases in the liver. (a) Before initiation of imatinib. (b) The metastases have decreased in size and become hypointense following initiation of imatinib administration.

initiation survive longer than those who had a large burden, which lends support to early initiation of imatinib therapy for GIST patients who are diagnosed with metastatic disease.

The type of *KIT* or *PDGFRA* mutation and the gene exon where the *KIT* mutation is located predict for the likelihood of response to imatinib mesylate. GISTs with a *KIT* exon 11 mutation are generally the most responsive to imatinib therapy (Table 9.7). Patients with GIST with *KIT* exon 11 mutation achieve a partial remission in approximately 70–80% of cases with imatinib therapy, whereas approximately 40–50% of those who have GIST with exon 9 mutation achieve partial remission (Heinrich *et al.* 2003; Heinrich *et al.* 2005; Debiec-Rychter *et al.* 2006). The presence of *KIT* exon 11 mutation is also associated with a longer median time to imatinib failure as compared to exon 9 mutation (Heinrich *et al.* 2003; Debiec-Rychter *et al.* 2006). Patients who have no detectable mutation in either *KIT* or *PDGFRA* gene (who have 'wild-type GIST') respond less frequently to imatinib than patients whose GIST harbors mutation in *KIT* exon 11. In one series none of the patients with wild-type GIST responded to imatinib (Heinrich *et al.* 2003), whereas in two larger and more recent series 23% and 39% of the patients diagnosed with advanced wild-type GIST responded (Heinrich *et al.* 2005; Debiec-Rychter *et al.* 2006), suggesting that many of the patients who have wild-type GIST benefit from imatinib therapy.

Patients who have GIST with *KIT* exon 13 or 17 mutation, or *PDGFRA* mutation, may also respond to imatinib. The point

Table 9.7 Efficacy of imatinib in the treatment of advanced GIST.

	US-Finland B2222 n = 147	CALGB150105/ SWOG S0033 n = 746	EORTC/ISG/ AGITG 62005 n = 946
Response rate (CR+PR)			
All patients	68%	–	52%
Exon 11 mutation	87%	67%	68%
Exon 9 mutation	48%	40%	34%
Wild-type GIST	0%	39%	23%
Clinical benefit (CR, PR or SD)	84%	–	84%
Median duration of response	27 months	–	–
Median overall survival	58 months	–	–

mutation D816V (exon 17) that is common in systemic mastocytosis and that is resistant to imatinib is rare in GISTs that have not been exposed to imatinib. Metastatic GISTs that do not express the KIT protein (the 'KIT-negative GISTs', approximately 5% of GISTs) respond approximately as frequently to imatinib as those GISTs that express the KIT protein in immunohistochemistry. However, patients with KIT-positive advanced GIST appear to have somewhat more favorable survival than patients who have KIT-negative GIST when treated with imatinib (Blackstein *et al.* 2005). Based on these findings imatinib is considered as the first-line treatment for GIST patients who present with metastatic disease regardless of the location of the *KIT* or *PDGFRA* mutation and regardless of whether GIST expresses the KIT protein in immunohistochemistry or not. Patients who have a mutation that is known to be resistant to imatinib, such as the *PDGFRA* exon 18 D842V mutation, may be an exception to this principle (Corless *et al.* 2005). Similarly, pediatric patients who have wild-type GIST and patients diagnosed with the Carney triad may respond poorly to imatinib. A report consisting of three pediatric GIST patients suggests that sunitinib may be effective for pediatric GISTs that do not carry *KIT* or *PDGFR* mutation (Janeway *et al.* 2006).

The starting dose of imatinib mesylate is usually 400 mg once daily. Food has no relevant impact on the rate or extent of imatinib bioavailability (Peng *et al.* 2005), and because imatinib may cause local irritation, it is taken with food. Two large randomized trials (62005 and S0033) compared the imatinib dose of 400 mg administered twice daily (i.e. 800 mg/day) to 400 mg given once daily (Rankin *et al.* 2004; Verveij *et al.* 2004). Both trials had a cross-over design, allowing those patients who were allocated to the lower dose (400 mg daily) to cross over to the higher dose group (800 mg per day) at disease progression. In general, these two trials yielded similar results. The 800-mg dose was associated with a longer time to disease progression, which was statistically significant in the larger one of the trials (65002, Fig. 9.10). However, the response rates to imatinib were similar regardless of the dose administered, and in neither one of the trials the higher dose was associated with superior overall survival following cross-over. The 800-mg daily dose was associated with greater toxicity as compared with the 400-mg dose. In the US–Finland trial the study participants were randomly allocated to receive either 400 mg or 600 mg imatinib daily; in this study there was no difference in the time to disease progression or in survival between the allocation groups (Demetri *et al.* 2002; Blanke *et al.* 2006).

Based on these data, the 400-mg once daily dose may still be considered the standard starting dose of imatinib. According to one study (Judson *et al.* 2005) the frequency and severity of some imatinib-associated adverse effects decreases with time, suggesting that tissue exposure to imatinib might become somewhat less with prolonged imatinib administration. Since a higher dose than 400 mg per day may benefit some GIST patients, dose escalation beyond the 400-mg daily dose might be considered with prolonged imatinib administration. A retrospective analysis based on a limited number of patients suggests that patients with GIST with *KIT* exon 9 mutation may have a longer progression-free survival when 800 mg/day is administered as the starting dose as compared to the 400-mg once-daily dose (Debiec-Rychter *et al.* 2006). There was no difference in the duration of overall survival between the 400-mg and the 800-mg dose groups following dose escalation at the time of disease progression among patients whose GIST harbored *KIT* exon 9 mutation.

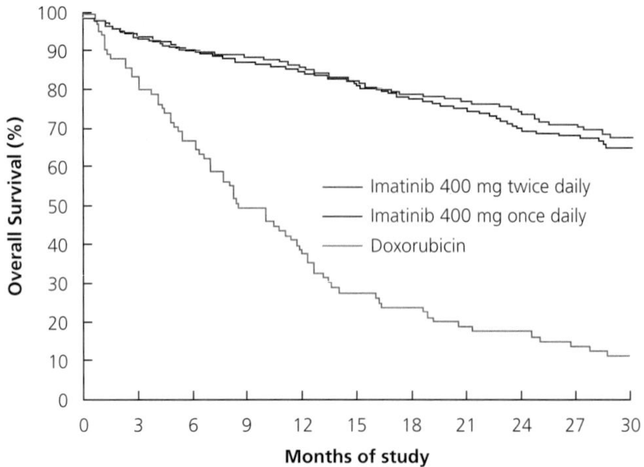

Fig. 9.10 Overall survival of GIST patients treated with either imatinib 400 mg once daily or with 400 mg twice daily in a randomized study. Survival of historical GIST patients treated with doxorubicin is shown for comparison. Reprinted from The Lancet Vol 364, Verweij J, Casali PG, Zalcberg J *et al.* Progression-free survival in gastrointestinal stromal tumours with high-dose imatinib: randomised trial, pp. 1127–1134. Copyright 2004, with permission from Elsevier.

Imatinib is recommended to be administered continuously without planned breaks in its administration. In a prospective multicenter trial (BFR14) 58 patients diagnosed with advanced GIST who were free from disease progression 12 months after starting imatinib treatment were randomly allocated either to continue imatinib therapy or to interrupt imatinib administration until disease progression (Le Cesne *et al.* 2005). Patients allocated to interrupt imatinib administration could start imatinib in case of progressive disease. Interruption of imatinib was associated with disease progression in 66% of the patients during a median observation time of 21 months, whereas only 15% of those who continued imatinib treatment progressed. The median time to disease progression was only 6 months following interruption of imatinib administration. There was no difference in overall survival between the two groups at the time of reporting of the trial, and most (79%) patients who progressed following imatinib administration interruption responded to imatinib reintroduction. Interruption of imatinib administration is unlikely to be beneficial, and continuous imatinib with no upper limit for administration duration is the current standard in the treatment of advanced GIST.

Since imatinib dose reductions are best avoided, it is important to know how to manage common adverse effects. Many adverse effects are mild to moderate in severity and may not require any specific therapy. The most frequent adverse effects of imatinib are periorbital or leg edema, occasional muscle cramps in fingers and feet, diarrhea, nausea/vomiting, fatigue, and skin rash. Grade 1 or 2 macrocytic anemia, neutropenia and elevation of serum transaminase levels are also common. Periorbital edema may respond to diuretics and muscle cramps to calcium or magnesium supplementation. Imatinib-related nausea may be alleviated when the daily imatinib dose is divided and administered twice daily. Imatinib therapy requires close surveillance, especially at the beginning of the treatment and when the patient is elderly or frail, and when multiple concomitant medications cannot be avoided. Generalized skin rash or edema, grade 3 or 4 cytopenias, and dyspnea (may herald interstitial lung disease) require prompt interruption of imatinib administration, and often lead to subsequent dose reduction. In one study the risk of imatinib-associated non-hematologic adverse effects (such as edema, nausea, diarrhea) was greater in females than in males, and in patients with advanced age or with a poor performance status (Glabbeke *et al.* 2006).

Tumor response to imatinib is usually monitored with CT or sometimes with MRI. Baseline imaging is recommended to be done within 2 weeks before initiation of imatinib administration, since some GISTs grow rapidly. No study has evaluated the optimal frequency of response evaluation examinations, which is currently unknown. In clinical practice the first follow-up CT is often carried out 1–2 months after initiation of imatinib, and the subsequent evaluations at approximately 3-month intervals. Metabolic imaging with FDG-PET may occasionally help in the clinical decision-making.

Combined surgery and TKI therapy for metastatic disease

TKI therapy is now the standard of care for nearly all patients with metastatic GIST. Since TKI therapy is not curative, the obvious question is whether surgery should be added to molecular therapy (Raut *et al.* 2006; DeMatteo *et al.* 2007). Combined therapy may prove to be curative or at least it may delay imatinib resistance, which occurs at a median of less than 2 years. We have put forward the hypothesis that the likelihood of resistance to imatinib is proportional to the amount of residual viable tumor after TKI therapy. Our general practice, therefore, is to treat patients with metastatic disease with imatinib for 3–6 months and then to consider surgery if all gross tumor can be removed. After surgery, patients should resume TKI therapy given the high risk of progression and the findings from the French study cited above in which imatinib was stopped in patients with metastatic GIST.

We performed surgery in 40 patients with metastatic GIST who were being treated with tyrosine kinase inhibitors. There were three groups of patients based on the status of their metastatic disease at the time of surgery: responsive disease, focal resistance, multifocal resistance. The median time of TKI therapy was 7, 21, and 26 months, respectively. Only 25% of the patients had a solitary tumor and the median size of the largest tumor was 9 cm. Operations involved the liver (43%), pancreas (13%), stomach/intestine (48%), and peritoneal tumors (68%). Gross tumor clearance was achieved in 85% of patients with responsive disease, but only 46% of those with focal resistance and 29% of those with multifocal resistance. There were no perioperative deaths. After a median follow-up of 15 months, progression-free survival was significantly different between the three groups (Fig. 9.11). In those with responsive disease, the 2-year progression-free survival was 61%. Meanwhile, patients with focal resistance had a median time to progression of 12 months and those with multifocal progression had a median time to postoperative progression of only 3 months. Obviously, these data and those from other centers are confounded by selection and lead time biases. Randomized trials of TKI therapy with or without surgery are now being designed. For now, patients with responsive metastatic disease or focal progression can be considered for surgical therapy. Patients with multifocal progression should be tried on other systemic therapies or clinical trials.

Treatment of imatinib-resistant GIST

Although primary resistance to imatinib is relatively rare, most GISTs acquire resistance to imatinib during prolonged therapy. Such GISTs often have a secondary *KIT* mutation that was not detectable before initiation of imatinib treatment. Interestingly, the second mutations often occur at those sites of the gene that encode the parts of the kinase that are involved with imatinib binding to the kinase. The acquired mutations are often found at the ATP/imatinib binding pocket (encoded by *KIT* exons 13 and 14), and approximately one half of the second mutations occur in *KIT* exon 17 that encodes the activation loop of the KIT kinase (Heinrich *et al.* 2006). These mutations interfere with imatinib binding. Mutations of exon 17 may cause the activation loop of the kinase to assume the active conformation, which prevents imatinib binding to the kinase, since imatinib only binds to the kinase when the activation loop assumes its inactive conformation (Schittenhelm *et al.* 2006). Other resistance mechanisms to imatinib may involve activation of other kinases and signaling routes, target gene amplification, increased imatinib metabolism, or development of drug resistance.

When GIST starts to progress during imatinib therapy progression may be either local or more generalized. In approximately 50% of all progressing GISTs only one (or a few) resistant tumor nodule emerges within or at the border of a pre-existing responding (hypodense) metastasis. This can be seen as a 'nodule within a mass' in a CT or MRI (Fig. 9.12). In one study (Desai *et al.* 2004), seven (78%) of nine such nodules harbored a new *KIT* mutation that was not detectable in a tissue sample resected prior to starting imatinib therapy. When the other known metastases continue to respond, surgical resection of the single growing nodule should be carefully considered, since

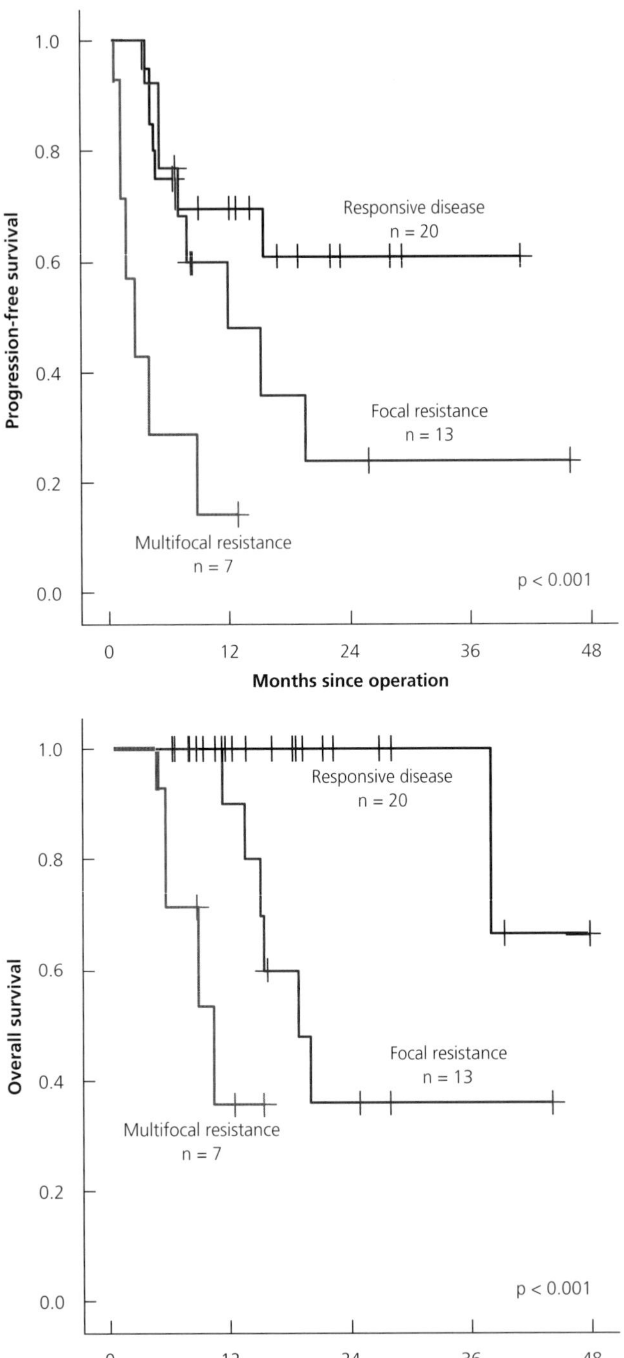

Fig. 9.11 Progression-free and overall survival after TKI therapy and resection of metastatic GIST. Reproduced with permission from DeMatteo RP, Maki RG, Singer SA, Gonen M, Brennan MF, Antonescu CR. (2007) Results of tyrosine kinase inhibitor therapy followed by surgical resection for metastatic gastrointestinal stromal tumor (GIST). *Ann Surg* (in press).

resection may lead to further disease control that may last for several months or a few years provided that imatinib administration is continued (Nishida *et al.* 2006). Radiofrequency ablation may be attempted when surgery is not feasible.

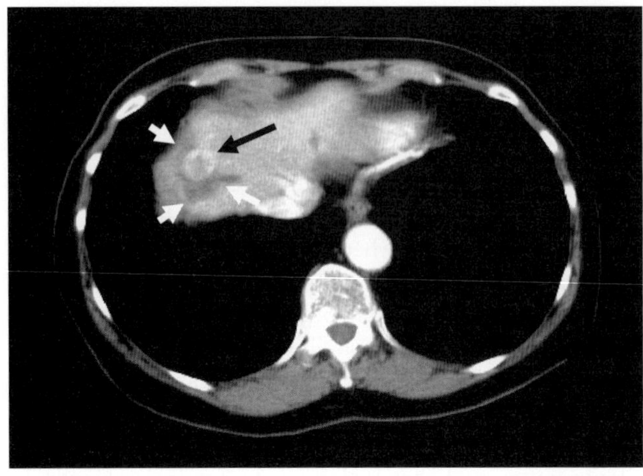

Fig. 9.12 Single growing liver metastasis in patient with GIST who responded to imatinib (nodule within a lesion). The black arrow points at the growing nodule, the white arrows at a hypodense lesion still responding to imatinib. Reprinted from The *Lancet* Vol 368, Joensuu H. Sunitinib for imatinib-resistant GIST, pp. 1303–4. Copyright 2006, with permission from Elsevier.

Compliance of imatinib administration needs to be assessed when GIST progresses during imatinib administration. Concomitant administration of enzyme-inducing antiepileptic drugs (EIAEDs) may also necessitate imatinib dose escalation. In one study EIAEDs reduced plasma exposure of imatinib by approximately 68% as compared with patients who did not use EIAEDs (Wen *et al.* 2006). Imatinib dose escalation up to 800 mg/day is recommended whenever feasible in patients who progress on a lower dose of imatinib. Approximately 5% of patients who progress on the standard dose of imatinib (400 mg/day) achieve a partial remission after imatinib dose escalation to 800 mg/day, and another 30% have stabilization of the disease (Rankin *et al.* 2004; Zalcberg *et al.* 2004). Patients who have disease progression and who progress despite imatinib dose escalation are candidates for a trial with other TKIs.

Sunitinib malate

Sunitinib malate is approved for clinical use in imatinib-resistant GIST and for patients who are intolerant to imatinib mesylate. Sunitinib is an oral multitargeted tyrosine kinase inhibitor with antiangiogenic and antitumor activity. It inhibits all three isoforms of the vascular endothelial cell growth factor receptor (VEGFR-1, -2, and -3), KIT, PDGFR-α, PDGFR-β, colony stimulating factor 1 receptor (CSF-1R), Fms-like tyrosine kinase-3 receptor (FLT-3), and the receptor encoded by the *ret* proto-oncogene (RET). In a prospective, randomized, placebo-controlled trial consisting of 312 patients whose GIST had either progressed during imatinib treatment or who were intolerant to imatinib the median time to tumor progression was 27.3 weeks for patients treated with sunitinib as compared to 6.4 weeks among those allocated to placebo (Demetri *et al.*

2006). The trial had a cross-over design allowing unblinding at the time of disease progression and administration of the active drug to those allocated to receive placebo. The objective response rate of sunitinib was relatively low in this trial (7%), but more patients (58%) treated with sunitinib had stable disease as compared with the placebo group (48%). Despite cross-over patients allocated to sunitinib had significantly longer overall survival.

In this trial imatinib therapy was interrupted before study entry. When only one or a few of GIST metastases begin to grow during imatinib treatment and treatment is discontinued, those metastases that were still controlled by imatinib may start to grow at an enhanced speed leading to 'tumor flare'. GIST patients may accumulate high blood concentrations of the stem cell factor (SCF) during imatinib treatment, which might speed up tumor growth upon imatinib discontinuation (Bono *et al.* 2004). Hypothetically, some patients assigned to placebo in the trial might thus have benefited from continued imatinib administration or gradual tapering down of the dose.

The most frequent adverse effects related to sunitinib are fatigue, diarrhea, hair and skin discoloration, nausea, leukopenia and thrombocytopenia (Demetri *et al.* 2006), but most adverse effects are mild (grade 1 or 2) in severity. Sunitinib may cause hypothyreosis in 4–50% of patients, and elevation of thyroid stimulating hormone (TSH) appears common in sunitinib-treated patients (Schoeffski 2006).

Ablation

Radiofrequency ablation

There are limited data regarding radiofrequency ablation (RFA) of liver metastases from GIST (Dileo *et al.* 2006). This technique uses radio waves to generate heat to kill a tumor. RFA can be performed percutaneously, via laparoscopy, or during laparotomy. Based on therapy of colorectal cancer metastatic to the liver and hepatocellular carcinoma, it is now clear that RFA is best used for tumors measuring less than 3 cm. Larger tumors have a high likelihood of subsequent tumor progression due to incomplete tumor kill. RFA is not recommended when a patient has more than 3–5 liver tumors. RFA is not as effective in tumors that lie next to major blood vessels and should be avoided when a tumor is situated near a major bile duct. RFA may be considered for a small, deep liver mass that is stable on imatinib therapy or for a liver tumor that shows early signs of progression (nodule within a mass) as described above.

Hepatic artery embolization

Hepatic artery embolization (HAE) is an effective palliative therapy for patients with liver metastases from GIST because the tumors tend to be hypervascular and derive most of their blood supply from the hepatic artery. The technique involves selectively occluding the major arterial branches supplying the tumors by injecting them with particles such as polyvinyl chloride. If there are diffuse metastases, then generally half of the liver is treated at one time. A post-embolization syndrome (abdominal pain, fever, and nausea) commonly occurs. HAE can be repeated several times. The benefit of adding a chemotherapeutic agent to the injected particles is unproven, especially since conventional agents are ineffective in GIST. HAE may be useful in patients with liver metastases who have pain or discomfort and is the treatment of choice in patients with acute hemorrhage from a liver metastasis. Although HAE may produce a dramatic reduction in tumor burden (Kobayashi *et al.* 2006; Maluccio *et al.* 2006) there is no conclusive evidence that it actually prolongs survival. It may be useful in patients with a single site of TKI resistance as an alternative to surgery.

Radiation therapy and palliative therapy

GISTs are often considered radiation therapy-resistant tumors (von Mehren 2006). This is unlike most other soft tissue sarcomas that are moderately radiation sensitive, and radiation sensitivity of GISTs has not been evaluated in prospective trials. At present, radiation therapy is considered to have little role in the primary treatment of GISTs, but it may sometimes be considered as palliative therapy of metastatic GISTs. It may be of benefit for rectal GIST. Radiation may have limited value at most other sites because of the risk of bowel toxicity.

Novel agents and adjuvant therapy

Continuation of imatinib despite disease progression might be beneficial when imatinib-sensitive and -resistant clones coexist in the same patient. In such cases imatinib therapy may be continued as long as there is evidence of continued benefit. Otherwise, sunitinib or newer agents should be tried.

Novel agents

Several other tyrosine kinase inhibitors that inhibit KIT and PDGFRs are currently being evaluated in the treatment of GIST. Like sunitinib, some of these agents inhibit also the VEGFRs and thus have anti-angiogenic function. The first results reported suggest that vatalanib (PTK787/ZK222584) that has a similar type tyrosine kinase inhibition spectrum as sunitinib, has activity against imatinib-resistant GIST (Joensuu *et al.* 2006).

Table 9.8 Novel agents being evaluated in the treatment of imatinib-resistant GIST.

Agent/combination	Comment
Single agents	
Dasatinib (BMS354825)	Abl, src, and KIT inhibitor
Vatalanib (PTK787)	VEGFR, KIT and PDGFR inhibitor
Nilotinib (AMN107)	KIT, PDGFRA and Bcr-Abl inhibitor
Everolimus (RAD001)	mTOR inhibitor
IPI-504	Hsp90 inhibitor
PKC412	KIT, PDGFRA, VEGFR and PKC inhibitor
AMG706	KIT, PDGFR, VEGFR and ret inhibitor
Sorafenib (BAY43–9006)	KIT, PDGFR, VEGFR, raf and ret
SDX-102	AMP synthesis inhibitor
Flavopiridol	Suppresses KIT mRNA expression
Combinations being evaluated	
Imatinib + nilotinib	
Imatinib +/– bevacizumab	
Imatinib + oblimersem sodium	

Table 9.9 'Consensus' assessment of the risk of recurrence in resectable GIST. Modified from Fletcher *et al.* (2002).

Risk category	Size	Mitotic count
Very low risk	<2 cm	<5/50 HPFs
Low risk	2–5 cm	<5/50 HPFs
Intermediate risk	<5 cm	6–10/50 HPFs
	5–10 cm	<5/50 HPFs
High risk	>10 cm	Any mitotic rate
	Any size	>10/50 HPFs
	>5 cm	>5/50 HPFs

HPF, high-power field.

Whereas imatinib and nilotinib (AMN107) require the activation loop of the kinase to be in the non-active conformation for KIT kinase binding, dasatinib (BMS354825) can bind to the kinase also when the activation loop assumes the active confirmation. This suggests that dasatinib might be active for some GISTs that harbor a *KIT* exon 17 mutation that renders the disease resistant to imatinib. Dasatinib also inhibits the src kinase, which is one of the downstream kinases that may be activated following KIT activation. Studies evaluating nilotinib and dasatinib in the treatment of imatinib-resistant GIST are being planned.

Activation of the KIT receptor tyrosine kinase often activates the PI3K-Akt-mammalian target of rapamycin (mTOR) pathway, and imatinib inhibits activity of this pathway (Rossi *et al.* 2006). These findings suggest that mTOR inhibitors might have activity in the treatment of GISTs. The first results from a clinical trial that evaluated an mTOR inhibitor everolimus suggest that this indeed may be the case (van Oosterom *et al.* 2005) and that other mTOR inhibitors might thus also have activity. Some novel agents that are currently being evaluated or planned to be evaluated in the treatment of GIST are listed in Table 9.8.

Adjuvant therapy

Since conventional chemotherapy is ineffective in GIST, the standard of care after complete resection of primary disease has been observation. Administration of adjuvant imatinib appears attractive following removal of GIST with a high risk for recurrence, but adjuvant use of imatinib is still considered experimental at present. The risk of GIST recurrence is often estimated using the proposed consensus approach for defining risk of aggressive behavior in GISTs, which is based on the tumor size and the mitotic count (Fletcher *et al.* 2002, Table 9.9). Tumor size and the mitotic count generally correlate well with outcome in most series on GIST patients. Somewhat different cut-off values may be optimal for gastric GISTs and for intestinal GISTs (Miettinen *et al.* 2005, 2006), and based on large cohorts of GIST patients with long follow-up Miettinen and Lasota have proposed a more detailed prognostic classification (Table 9.5). Other prognostic features such as the *KIT* mutation type might complement the consensus risk classification (Andersson *et al.* 2006). A variety of other prognostic factors have been identified, including aneuploidy, proliferative index, and percentage S-phase fraction. Despite these prognostic features, it is not possible to predict accurately the clinical behavior of any particular GIST. In fact, nearly all GISTs can exhibit malignant behavior and none, except perhaps the smallest tumors (1 cm or smaller in diameter), can be considered definitely benign.

Three randomized trials addressing the safety and efficacy of imatinib administered as adjuvant treatment are ongoing (Table 9.10). The North American trial carried out jointly by ACOSOG (American College of Surgical Oncology Group, trial Z9001), National Cancer Institute (NCI), Cancer and Leukemia Group-B (CALGB), Southwest Oncology Group (SWOG) and Eastern Cooperative Oncology Group (ECOG) and National Cancer Institute of Canada (NCI-C) compares 12 months of imatinib versus 12 months of placebo following macroscopically complete surgery of GISTs that are 3 cm or larger in diameter at the time of the diagnosis. The European Organization for Research and Treatment of Cancer (EORTC) adjuvant study allocates patients with an intermediate or high risk of recurrence according to the consensus criteria to either 24 months of imatinib or observation. The Scandinavian Sarcoma Group/German (AIO)

Table 9.10 Clinical trials testing adjuvant imatinib and surgery for primary GIST. Modified from van der Zwan S, DeMatteo RP. (2005) Gastrointestinal stromal tumor: 5 years later. *Cancer* 104: 1781–8.

Group/trial	Disease	Imatinib therapy	Eligibility	Dose	Accrual*
ACOSOG Z9000	Primary	Adjuvant	Any of the following: tumor ≥ 10 cm intraperitoneal tumor rupture/hemorrhage multifocal tumors (<5) Complete gross resection	400 mg/d × 12 months Open label	106/89†
ACOSOG Z9001	Primary	Adjuvant	Tumor ≥ 3cm Complete gross resection	400 mg/d vs placebo × 1 year Double blind	710/803
SSG XVIII/AIO	Primary ± mets	Adjuvant	Any of the following: tumor ≥ 10cm mitotic rate > 10 tumor > 5 cm and mitotic rate > 5 tumor rupture Complete gross resection	400 mg/d × 12 or 36 months Open label	240/280
EORTC 62024	Primary	Adjuvant	Any of the following: tumor > 5cm mitotic rate > 5 Complete resection	400 mg/d vs no treatment × 2 years Open label	400/750

* As of December 2006.

† Accrual completed.

ACOSOG, American College of Surgeons Oncology Group; SSG, Scandinavian Sarcoma Group; EORTC, European Organisation for the Research and Treatment of Cancer; mitotic rate, mitoses per 50 high-power fields; mets, metastases.

study randomly allocates patients with a high risk of recurrence according to the consensus criteria or with tumor rupture to receive imatinib for either 12 months or 36 months. The administered dose of imatinib is 400 mg daily in all three trials.

The American College of Surgeons Oncology Group (ACOSOG) is also conducting an intergroup phase II (Z9000) trial which met accrual in September 2003. There were 106 evaluable patients who underwent complete resection of a high-risk primary GIST (≥10 cm, intraperitoneal rupture or bleeding, or multifocal tumors) and were then treated for 1 year with imatinib 400 mg/day. The treatment was tolerated well (DeMatteo *et al.* 2005). There were no grade 4 or grade 5 toxicities. Overall, 83% of patients completed their prescribed therapy. Recurrence and survival data have not yet been released.

Patients who have tumor rupture into the abdominal cavity and those who have been rendered free from overt metastatic disease by surgery have a very high risk of tumor recurrence, and should probably be considered as candidates for imatinib therapy, although this practice has not been evaluated in clinical trials and the optimal duration of imatinib administration is unknown. Adjuvant radiation therapy and adjuvant conventional chemotherapy have no proven therapeutic value, and are not recommended.

A few small phase II trials currently evaluate primary systemic (neoadjuvant) treatment of large localized GISTs in an attempt to shrink the tumors and make them more amenable to organ-reserving surgery. In the ongoing trials imatinib is administered for 2–6 months before surgery. The optimal length of neoadjuvant TKI therapy has not been determined. Since most of the tumor shrinkage occurs within 6 months of therapy and the median time to imatinib mesylate resistance is less than 2 years, we have favored surgery within 6–9 months. Of course, the timing of surgery depends on the extent of the response and the surgeon should be consulted with each new CT scan. There may be other benefits besides increasing tumor resectability, such as decreasing intraoperative blood loss from these normally hypervascular tumors. Some of the trials also include adjuvant imatinib administration for 12–24 months following neoadjuvant therapy and surgery. As with adjuvant imatinib, neoadjuvant administration of imatinib is currently considered experimental. It may, however, benefit selected patients who otherwise might need to undergo extensive surgery such as total gastrectomy for gastric GIST or abdominoperineal resection for rectal GIST.

There are a few potential risks of neoadjuvant therapy. A needle biopsy needs to be taken to confirm the histologic diagnosis prior to initiating neoadjuvant treatment. The needle biopsy is preferentially taken at endoscopy to avoid intra-abdominal tumor cell seeding. Neoadjuvant administration of imatinib requires careful monitoring of the tumor size and

Table 9.11 Key principles in the management of GIST.

Clinical scenario	Management
Local disease (one tumor)	Complete surgical removal of the tumor with free (usually > 1 cm) margins. Avoid tumor rupture Adjuvant and neoadjuvant treatment with imatinib are being investigated in clinical trials and are considered experimental at present. Neoadjuvant imatinib may be considered for selected patients to achieve organ preservation. Adjuvant imatinib is recommended in case of tumor rupture Adjuvant radiation therapy or conventional chemotherapy have no proven value.
Recurrent/metastatic disease; first line therapy	Imatinib daily until treatment failure; the starting dose is usually 400 mg to 600 mg/day. Monitor blood cell counts, blood chemistry and treatment response (e.g. CT of the abdomen 1 month after starting imatinib, then at about 3-month intervals) Surgical resection of residual tumors of responding patients may be considered in selected cases, but the benefit is unproven. Removal of bleeding, infected or obstructing metastases may be necessary
GIST progresses during imatinib therapy	1) Check for compliance of taking imatinib. Patients who use enzyme-inducing drugs may need a higher dose than 400 mg/day. 2) Consider surgery for single growing metastases. Such metastases may harbor a new gene mutation that renders GIST resistant to imatinib. 3) Escalate imatinib dose up to 800 mg/day if feasible. 4) Sunitinib malate. 5) Participation in a clinical trial with novel agents. 6) Palliative surgery or radiation therapy in selected cases.

density during treatment, since not all GISTs respond to imatinib. Since 15% of patients have primary resistance to imatinib, the window to operate may be missed in a patient who has a marginally resectable GIST. For these patients, early (within a month) cross-sectional imaging is essential to determine whether they are responsive to therapy. Intraperitoneal hemorrhage does not occur often on TKI therapy but when it does it may lead to tumor dissemination.

The key principles of management of GIST are summarized in Table 9.11.

References

Andersson J, Bumming P, Meis-Kindblom JM *et al.* (2006) Gastrointestinal stromal tumors with KIT exon 11 deletions are associated with poor prognosis. *Gastroenterology* 130: 1573–81.

Beck J, Handgretinger R, Klingebiel T *et al.* (1996)Expression of PKC isozyme and MDR-associated genes in primary and relapsed state AML. *Leukemia* 10: 426–33.

Blackstein ME, Rankin C, Fletcher C *et al.* (2005) Clinical benefit of imatinib in patients with metastatic gastrointestinal stromal tumors (GIST) negative for the expression of CD117 in the S0033 trial. *Proc Am Soc Clin Oncol* 23: 818s (abstract).

Blair SC, Zalupski MM, Baker LH. (1994) Ifosfamide and etoposide in the treatment of advanced soft tissue sarcomas. *Am J Clin Oncol* 17: 480–4.

Blanke C, Demetri GD, Von Mehren M *et al.* (2006) Long-term follow-up of a phase II randomized trial in advanced gastrointestinal stromal tumor (GIST) patients treated with imatinib mesylate. *Proc Am Soc Clin Oncol* 24: 526s (abstract).

Blay JY, Bonvalot S, Casali P *et al.* (2005) Consensus meeting for the management of gastrointestinal stromal tumors. Report of the GIST Consensus Conference of 20–21 March 2004, under the auspices of ESMO. *Ann Oncol* 16: 566–78.

Blay JY, Le Cesne A, Verweij J *et al.* (2004) A phase II study of ET-743/trabectedin ('Yondelis') for patients with advanced gastrointestinal stromal tumours. *Eur J Cancer* 40: 1327–31.

Blay P, Astudillo A,Buesa JM *et al.* (2004) Protein kinase C theta is highly expressed in gastrointestinal stromal tumors but not in other mesenchymal neoplasias. *Clin Cancer Res* 10: 4089–95.

Bono P, Krause A, Blanke CD *et al.* (2004) Serum KIT, SCF and VEGF levels in gastrointestinal tumor patients treated with imatinib. *Blood* 103: 2929–35.

Budworth J, Gant TW, Gescher A. (1997) Co-ordinate loss of protein kinase C and multidrug resistance gene expression in revertant MCF-7/Adr breast carcinoma cells. *Br J Cancer* 75: 1330–5.

Bümming P, Ahlman H, Andersson J *et al.* (2006) Population-based study of the diagnosis and treatment of gastrointestinal stromal tumours. *Br J Surg* 93: 836–43.

Corless CL, Schroeder A, Griffith D *et al.* (2005) PDGFRA mutations in gastrointestinal stromal tumors: Frequency, spectrum and in vitro sensitivity to imatinib. *J Clin Oncol* 23: 5357–64.

Debiec-Rychter M, Sciot R, Le Cesne A *et al.* (2006) KIT mutations and dose selection for imatinib in patients with advanced gastrointestinal stromal tumours. *Eur J Cancer* 42: 1093–1103.

DeMatteo RP, Lewis JJ, Leung D *et al.* (2000)Two hundred gastrointestinal stromal tumors: Recurrence patterns and prognostic factors for survival. *Ann Surg* 231: 51–8.

DeMatteo RP, Shah A, Fong Y, Jarnagin WR, Blumgart LH, Brennan MF. (2001) Results of hepatic resection for sarcoma metastatic to liver. *Ann Surg* 234: 540–8.

DeMatteo RP, Heinrich MC, El-Rifai WM, Demetri G. (2002) Clinical management of gastrointestinal stromal tumors: Before and after STI-571. *Hum Pathol* 33: 466–77.

DeMatteo RP, Antonescu CR, Chadaram V *et al.* (2005) Adjuvant imatinib mesylate in patients with primary high risk gastrointestinal stromal tumor (GIST) following complete resection: Safety results from the U.S. Intergroup Phase II trial ACOSOG Z9000. *J Clin Oncol* 23: 9009.

DeMatteo RP, Maki RG, Singer SA, Gonen M, Brennan MF, Antonescu CR. (2007) Results of tyrosine kinase inhibitor therapy followed by surgical resection for metastatic gastrointestinal stromal tumor (GIST). *Ann Surg* (in press).

Demetri GD, von Mehren M, Blanke CD *et al.* (2002) Efficacy and safety of imatinib mesylate in advanced gastrointestinal stromal tumors. *N Engl J Med* 347: 472–80.

Demetri GD, Benjamin R, Blanke CD *et al.* (2004) Optimal management of patients with gastrointestinal stromal tumors (GIST): expansion and update of NCCN clinical practice guidelines. *J NCCN* 2 (Suppl 1): 1–26.

Demetri GD, van Oosterom AT, Garrett CR *et al.* (2006) Efficacy and safety of sunitinib in patients with advanced gastrointestinal stromal tumour following failure of imatinib mesylate due to resistance or intolerance. *Lancet* 368; 1329–38.

Desai J, Shankar S, Heinrich MC *et al.* (2004) Clonal evolution of resistance to imatinib in patients with gastrointestinal stromal tumor: Molecular and radiologic evaluation of new lesions. *Proc Am Soc Clin Oncol* 23: 197s (abstract).

Dileo P, Randhawa R, Vansonnenberg E *et al.* (2004) Safety and efficacy of percutaneous radio-frequency ablation (RFA) in patients with metastatic gastrointestinal stromal tumor (GIST) with clonal evolution of lesions refractory to imatinib mesylate. *J Clin Oncol* 22: 9024.

Edmonson J, Marks R, Buckner J *et al.* (1999)Contrast of response to D-MAP + sargramostin between patients with advanced malignant gastrointestinal stromal tumors and patients with other advanced leiomyosarcomas. *Proc Am Assoc Cancer Res* 18: 541s (abstract).

Eilber FC, Rosen G, Forscher C, Nelson SD, Dorey F, Eilber FR. (2000) Recurrent gastrointestinal stromal sarcomas. *Surg Oncol* 9: 71–5.

Fletcher CD, Berman JJ, Corless C *et al.* (2002) Diagnosis of gastrointestinal stromal tumors: A consensus approach. *Hum Pathol* 33: 459–65.

Glabbeke MV, Verweij J, Casali PG *et al.* (2006) Predicting toxicities for patients with advanced gastrointestinal stromal tumours treated with imatinib: A study of the European Organization for Research and Treatment of Cancer, the Italian Sarcoma Group, and the Australasian Gastro-Intestinal Trials Group (EORTV-ISG-AGITG). *Eur J Cancer* 42: 2277–85.

Gold JS, van der Zwan SM, Gonen M *et al.* (2007) Outcome of metastatic GIST in the era before tyrosine kinase inhibitors. *Ann Surg Oncol* 14: 134–42.

Heinrich MC, Corless CL, Demetri GD *et al.* (2003) Kinase mutations and imatinib response in patients with metastatic gastrointestinal stromal tumor. *J Clin Oncol* 21: 4342–9.

Heinrich MC, Corless CL, Demetri G *et al.* (2006)Molecular correlates of imatinib resistance in gastrointestinal stromal tumors. *J Clin Oncol* 24: 4764–74.

Heinrich MC, Shoemaker JS, Corless CL *et al.* (2005) Correlation of target genotype with clinical activity of imatinib mesylate in patients with metastatic GI stromal tumors (GISTs) expressing KIT. *Proc Am Soc Clin Oncol* 23: 3s (abstract).

Janeway KA, Matthews DC, Butrynski JE *et al.* (2006) Sunitinib treatment of pediatric metastatic GIST after failure of imatinib. *Proc Am Soc Clin Oncol* 24: 524s.

Joensuu H, De Braud F, Coco P *et al.* (2006)A phase II, open-label study of PTK787/ZK222584 in the treatment of metastatic gastrointestinal stromal tumors (GISTs) resistant to imatinib mesylate. *Proc Am Soc Clin Oncol* 24: 527s (abstract).

Joensuu H, Dimitrijevic S. (2001) Tyrosine kinase inhibitor imatinib (STI571) as anticancer agent in solid tumors. *Ann Med* 33: 451–55.

Joensuu H, Dimitrijevic S, Silberman S, Roberts PJ, Demetri GD. (2002) Management of gastrointestinal stromal tumours. *Lancet Oncol* 3: 655–64.

Joensuu H, Roberts P, Sarlomo-Rikala M *et al.* (2001) Effect of the tyrosine kinase inhibitor STI571 in a patient with metastatic gastrointestinal stromal tumor. *N Engl J Med* 344: 1052–6.

Judson I, Ma P, Peng B *et al.* (2005) Imatinib pharmacokinetics in patients with gastrointestinal stromal tumour: a retrospective population pharmacokinetic study over time. EORTC Soft Tissue and Bone Sarcoma Group. *Cancer Chemother Pharmacol* 55: 379–86.

Kim TW, Lee H, Kang Y-K *et al.* (2004) Prognostic significance of c-kit mutation in localized gastrointestinal stromal tumors. *Clin Cancer Res* 10: 3076–81.

Kim KM, Kang DW, Moon WS *et al.* (2005) Gastrointestinal stromal tumors in Koreans: its incidence and the clinical, pathologic and immunohistochemical findings. *J Korean Med Sci* 20: 977–84.

Kobayashi K, Gupta S, Trent JC *et al.* (2006) Hepatic artery chemoembolization for 110 gastrointestinal stromal tumors. *Cancer* 108: 2833–41.

Le Cesne A, Perol D, Ray-Coquard I, Bui B, Duffaud F, Rios M *et al.* (2005) Interruption of imatinib in GIST patients with advanced disease: updated results of the prospective French sarcoma group randomized phase III trial on survival and quality of life. *Proc Am Soc Clin Oncol* 23: 823s (abstract).

Linton KM, Taylor MB, Radford JA. (2006)Response evaluation in gastrointestinal stromal tumours treated with imatinib: misdiagnosis of disease progression on CT due to cystic change in liver metastases. *Br J Radiol* 79: e40–4.

Maluccio MA, Covey AM, Schubert J *et al.* (2006) Treatment of metastatic sarcoma to the liver with bland embolization. *Cancer* 107: 1617–23.

Martín J, Poveda A, Llombart-Bosch A *et al.* (2005) Deletions affecting codons 557–558 of the c-KIT gene indicate a poor prognosis in patients with completely resected gastrointestinal stromal tumors: a study by the Spanish Group for Sarcoma Research (GEIS). *J Clin Oncol* 23: 6190–8.

Miettinen M, Lasota J. (2006) Gastrointestinal stromal tumors: pathology and prognosis at different sites. *Semin Diagn Pathol* 23: 70–83.

Miettinen M, Makhlouf H, Sobin LH, Lasota J. (2006) Gastrointestinal stromal tumors of the jejunum and ileum: a clinicopathologic, immunohistochemical, and molecular genetic study of 906 cases before imatinib with long-term follow-up. *Am J Surg Pathol* 30(4): 477–89.

Miettinen M, Sobin LH, Lasota J. (2005) Gastrointestinal stromal tumors of the stomach: a clinicopathologic, immunohistochemical, and molecular genetic study of 1765 cases with long-term follow-up. *Am J Surg Pathol* 29: 52–68.

Mol CD, Dougan DR, Schneider TR *et al.* (2004) Structural basis for the autoinhibition and STI-571 inhibition of c-Kit tyrosine kinase. *J Biol Chem* 30: 31655–63.

Motegi A, Sakurai S, Nakayama H *et al.* (2005) PKC theta, a novel immunohistochemical marker for gastrointestinal stromal tumors (GIST), especially useful for identifying KIT-negative tumors. *Pathol Int* 55: 106–112.

Nilsson BP, Bumming P, Meis-Kindblom JM *et al.* (2005) Gastrointestinal stromal tumors: The incidence, prevalence, clinical course, and prognostication in the preimatinib mesylate era. *Cancer* 103: 821–9.

Nishida T, Hasegawa J, Nishitani A, Takahashi T, Kanda T, Hatakeyama K. (2006) Surgical interventions for focal progression of gastrointestinal stromal tumors under imatinib therapy. *Proc Am Soc Clin Oncol* 24: 531s (abstract 9548).

Peng B, Lloyd P, Schran H. (2005) Clinical pharmacokinetics of imatinib. *Clin Pharmacokinet* 44(9): 879–94.

Plaat BE, Hollema H, Molenaar WM *et al.* (2000) Soft tissue leiomyosarcomas and malignant gastrointestinal stromal tumors: differences in clinical outcome and expression of multidrug resistance proteins. *J Clin Oncol* 18: 3211–20.

Rankin C, Von Mehren M, Blanke C *et al.* (2004) Dose effect of imatinib in patients with metastatic GIST—Phase III Sarcoma Group Study S0033. *Proc Am Soc Clin Oncol* 23: 815 (abstract).

Raut CP, Posner M, Desai J *et al.* (2006) Surgical management of advanced gastrointestinal stromal tumors after treatment with targeted systemic therapy using kinase inhibitors. *J Clin Oncol* 24: 2325–31.

Rossi F, Ehlers I, Agosti V *et al.* (2006) Oncogenic Kit signalling and therapeutic intervention in a mouse model of gastrointestinal stromal tumor. *Proc Natl Acad Sci USA* 103: 12843–8.

Schittenhelm MM, Shiraga S, Schroeder A *et al.* (2006) Dasatinib (BMS-354825), a dual SRC/ABL kinase inhibitor, inhibits the kinase activity of wild-type, juxtamembrane, and activation loop mutant isoforms associated with human malignancies. *Cancer Res* 66: 473–81.

Schoeffski P, Wolter P, Himpe U *et al.* (2006) Sunitinib-related thyroid dysfunction: a single-center retrospective and prospective evaluation. *Proc Am Soc Clin Oncol* 24: 143s (abstract 3092).

Tran T, Davila JA, El-Serag HB. (2005) The epidemiology of malignant gastrointestinal stromal tumors: an analysis of 1458 cases from 1992 to 2000. *Am J Gastroenterol* 100: 162–8.

Trent JC, Beach J, Burgess MA *et al.* (2003) A two-arm phase II study of temozolomide in patients with advanced gastrointestinal stromal tumors and other soft tissue sarcomas. *Cancer* 98(12): 2693–9.

van Oosterom AT, Judson I, Verweij J *et al.* (2001) Safety and efficacy of imatinib (STI571) in metastatic gastrointestinal stromal tumours: a phase I study. *Lancet* 358: 1421–3.

van Oosterom A, Reichardt P, Blay J-Y *et al.* (2005) A phase I/II trial of oral mTOR-inhibitor everolimus and imatinib mesylate in patients with gastrointestinal stromal tumor (GIST) refractory to imatinib: Study update. *Proc Am Soc Clin Oncol* 23: 824s (abstract).

Verweij J, Casali PG, Zalcberg J *et al.* (2004) Progression-free survival in gastrointestinal stromal tumours with high-dose imatinib: randomised trial. *Lancet* 364: 1127–34.

Wen PY, Young WK, Lamborn KR *et al.* (2006) Phase I/II study of imatinib mesylate for recurrent malignant liomas: North American Brain Tumor Consortium Study 99–08. *Clin Cancer Res* 12: 4899–907.

von Mehren M. (2006) Imatinib-refractory gastrointestinal stromal tumors: the clinical problem and therapeutic strategies. *Curr Oncol Rep* 8: 192–7.

Wong NA, Young R, Malcomson RD *et al.* (2003) Prognostic indicators for gastrointestinal stromal tumours: a clinicopathological and immunohistochemical study of 108 resected cases of the stomach. *Histopathology* 43: 118–26.

Wu TJ, Lee LY, Yeh CN *et al.* (2006) Surgical treatment and prognostic analysis for gastrointestinal stromal tumors (GISTs) of the small intestine: before the era of imatinib mesylate. *BMC Gastroenterol* 6: 29.

Zalcberg JR, Verweij J, Casali PG *et al.* (2004) Outcome of patients with advanced gastrointestinal stromal tumors (GIST) crossing over to a daily imatinib dose of 800 mg after progression on 400 mg – an international, intergroup study of the EORTC, ISG and AGITG. *Proc Am Soc Clin Oncol* 23: 815 (abstract).

10 Rare Tumors of the Abdomen

Edited by Anil R. Prasad

Introduction

This chapter deals with the multidisciplinary team approach to rare mesenchymal tumors (<1 per 100,000 population) involving the gastrointestinal tract (GI) as well as certain rare epithelial neoplasms within the abdomen. Certain tumor-like lesions presenting as mass lesions within the abdominal cavity and involving the GI tract are also discussed. The mesenchymal neoplasms involving the GI tract discussed in this section are specific diagnostic entities such as neuromas, lymphangiomas, etc. These are divided into various sections based on their histogenesis such as smooth muscle tumors, tumors of adipose tissue, etc. There is a broad category of GI mesenchymal tumors which are difficult to categorize under any specific cell lineage and may have overlapping features of several other GI spindle cell tumors. These are classified as gastrointestinal stromal tumors or GISTs, which are discussed in Chapter 9.

The chapter is divided into eight parts, a part each for rare GI tumors of smooth muscle origin, vascular origin, adipose tissue origin, neural origin, myofibroblastic origin and mesothelial origin, and gastric lymphoma. Rare carcinomas and certain tumors and tumor-like lesions are discussed in the final part under the heading 'Rare miscellaneous tumors and tumor-like lesions.' This part also includes certain developmental cysts, rare but specific entities peculiar to certain regions of the GI tract, and the very rare GI tract rhabdomyosarcoma.

Smooth muscle and pericytic tumors

Mitual Amin, Malathy Kapali, Benjamin Paz, Sanjay Saluja & Tomislav Dragovich

Smooth muscle tumors of the gastrointestinal tract are relatively rare tumors and comprise 1% or less of all gastrointestinal neoplasms. Gastrointestinal stromal tumors and leiomyomas are the most common mesenchymal neoplasms and if these are excluded we are left with a handful of rare but fascinating entities.

Leiomyomatosis

Leiomyomatosis is an extremely rare condition of the GI tract where there is diffuse, contiguous and circumferential involvement of a localized segment of the GI tract by proliferation of smooth muscle cells. Because of this, this entity was also previously called giant muscular hypertrophy (Ferguson *et al.* 1969). This is differentiated clinically from multiple, multifocal leiomyomas that are composed of multiple discrete tumors. Leiomyomatosis is most commonly seen in the esophagus where it can be a cause of achalasia and can sometimes be associated with Alport's syndrome in familial cases (Lonsdale *et al.* 1992). An association of esophageal leiomyomatosis and anorectal leiomyomatosis has been reported in children (Azzie *et al.* 2003). There has been a recent case report of gallbladder leiomyomatosis and multifocal leiomyomas in liver, spleen, pancreas, intestinal tract and lung in an 8-year-old child with severe combined immunodeficiency in whom Epstein-Barr virus (EBV) was detected.

The lesion usually involves a portion of the esophagus and sometimes the proximal stomach. Gross examination shows confluent or non-confluent, diffuse nodularity causing marked diffuse thickening of the wall. Microscopic examination shows highly cellular smooth muscle proliferations that often surround blood vessels, and these do not show significant nuclear atypia or mitotic activity (Fig. 10.1).

Surgical resection in symptomatic cases is the treatment of choice.

Leiomyomatosis peritonealis disseminata

Leiomyomatosis peritonealis disseminata (LPD) is a rare entity

Gastrointestinal Oncology: A Critical Multidisciplinary Team Approach.
Edited by J. Jankowski, R. Sampliner, D. Kerr, and Y. Fong.
 ISBN: 978-1-4501-2783-7

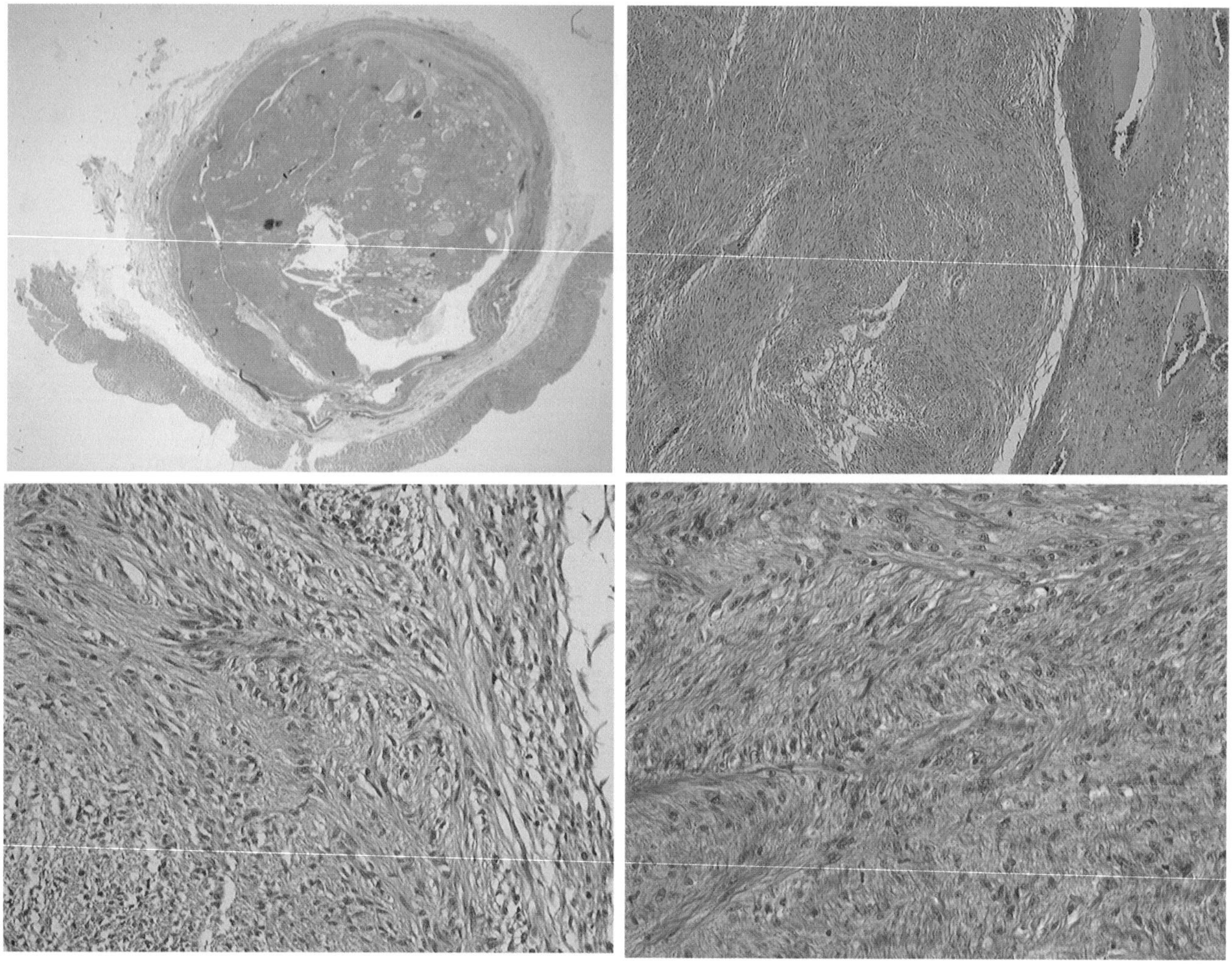

(a) (b) (c) (d)

Fig. 10.1 Leiomyoma colon. (a) A well circumscribed submucosal nodule within the wall of the colon. (b–d) Histopathology photomicrographs of the same lesion showing characteristic spindle cells with elongated cigar-shaped nuclei arranged in interlacing fascicles with nuclear palisading. Mitoses are rare.

characterized by multifocal nodules of varying sizes (a few mm to greater than 10 cm), composed of benign smooth muscle cells. This is a disease affecting women in the reproductive age group, although rare cases have been reported in postmenopausal women. This lesion is usually incidentally discovered during work-up of other medical complaints. It is a beingn entity despite its ominous appearance on CT; however malignant degeneration has been described in 10 cases. There are few reported descriptions of imaging findings in LPD because most of the described cases in the literature were incidentally detected at laparotomy. However ultrasonography and CT show multiple solid nodules with regular contours (Fig. 10.2). There is no ascites or other signs of malignancy. Imaging findings mimic peritoneal carcinomatosis which needs to be excluded by biopsy. The radiological differential diagnosis includes mesothelioma, desmoid tumors, tuberculosis, lymphoma and peritoneal metastases (Ruscelleda *et al.* 2006).

Grossly there are multiple nodules of varying sizes studding the peritoneal surfaces, especially that of the pelvic organs.

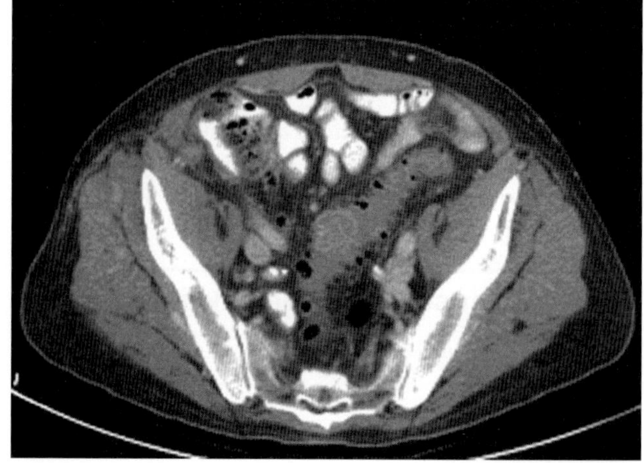

Fig. 10.2 Leiomyomatosis peritonealis disseminata. CT scan of the pelvis showing a large nodule embedded on the serosal surface of the sigmoid colon and another adjacent to the cecum. Peritoneal metastases could have a similar appearance on CT.

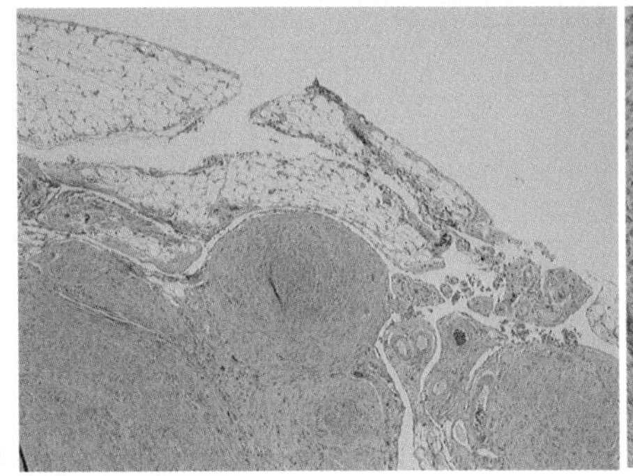
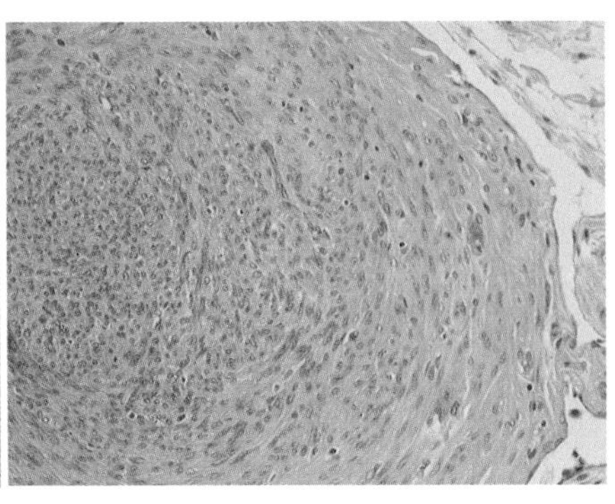

Fig. 10.3 Leiomyomatosis peritonealis disseminata. (a) Histopathology (H&E stain, ×40) shows multiple nodules studding the omentum. Photomicrograph (b) (H&E stain, ×100) highlights the nodular proliferation of smooth muscle cells, which lack cellular pleomorphism, mitotic activity or atypia.

Microscopically there are nodular proliferations of smooth muscle that in earlier phases are immediately subjacent to the peritoneal surface and in later phases may appear to grow in a permeative fashion. The cells usually show the characteristic morphology of smooth muscle cells and in some instances have a more fibroblastic or myofibroblastic appearance. There is lack of cytologic atypia, necrosis and mitotic activity (Fig. 10.3).

These lesions are usually positive for estrogen and progesterone receptors, suggesting an etiopathogenetic relationship (Shuterland & Wilson 1980). There is however also a discrete subset of cases without history of endogenous/exogenous estrogen exposure, negative for estrogen and progesterone receptors, without concomitant uterine leiomyomas, and cases occurring in postmenopausal women, that should be considered to have high malignant potential, and these associations seem to suggest a different pathway for tumorigenesis (Bekkers *et al.* 1999).

There are no established guidelines for therapy. Different drugs (gonadotrophin-releasing hormone agonists, megestrol acetate, danazol) have been considered in some cases with variable success. Surgical approach in symptomatic cases is indicated (Ghosh *et al.* 2000).

Hemangiopericytoma

Hemangiopericytomas are rare soft tissue tumors arising from pericytes surrounding small blood vessels. They occur in adults usually in the fifth and sixth decades, and can occur anywhere in the GI tract, the retroperitoneum and the mesentery. This lesion is found to occur in many different sites elsewhere in the body. These lesions appear to be closely linked with another similar histologic entity 'solidly fibrous tumor' that similarly occurs in almost any location in the body. Both lesions are associated with hypoglycemia and show positivity with CD34 immunostain.

The hallmark of hemangiopericytomas is their extreme hypervascularity, showing exuberant contrast enhancement. Foci of dystrophic calcification are often present. They are mildly hyperintense on T2 MRI images, hypointense on T1 images and show intense postgadolinium enhancement. Less commonly, they may contain some myxoid tissue that tends to be hyperintense on T2-weighted images. When malignant, the metastatic foci also show similar hypervascular features.

Hemangiopericytoma diagnosis rests on finding a lesion composed of bland spindle cells with a characteristic, elaborate branching pattern of small and large vessels, described as having a 'staghorn' or 'antler-like' configuration. CD34 immunoreactivity to tumors can range from focal to diffuse. Focal actin and desmin positivity also occur. The gross size varies from 1 cm to 23 cm, with an average size of 4–8 cm in diameter. They are generally well-circumscribed, and have a white-gray to red-brown cut surface that shows variable numbers of dilated vascular spaces with occasional areas of hemorrhage and cystic degeneration.

This is a difficult area both in making an accurate diagnosis and predicting the clinical behavior. This lesion is a difficult diagnostic entity as many lesions other than solitary fibrous tumor can be histologically similar, such as myopericytoma, infantile myofibromatosis, fibrous histiocytoma, synovial sarcoma, mesenchymal chondrosarcoma, juxtaglomerular cell tumor etc. Hemangiopericytoma is regarded by many as a diagnosis of exclusion (Gengler *et al.* 2006). The reported incidence of malignancy varies from 10% to 60% depending on diagnostic criteria and therapy.

Predicting the malignant potential of these neoplasms is difficult by usual histological methods. Mitotic activity, cellularity, hemorrhage and necrosis can be taken into account to predict for malignant potential. Tumors that are thought to be histologically benign may show metastasis after many years. In imaging studies, the presence of cystic areas of low attenuation consistent with necrosis, dystrophic calcifications, and invasion of the surrounding structures indicate that the tumor is probably malignant.

Complete surgical excision with adequate treatment is the method of choice with use of radiotherapy in an adjuvant setting.

Epstein–Barr virus-associated leiomyosarcoma

EBV has a known association with African Burkitt's lymphoma,

(a)

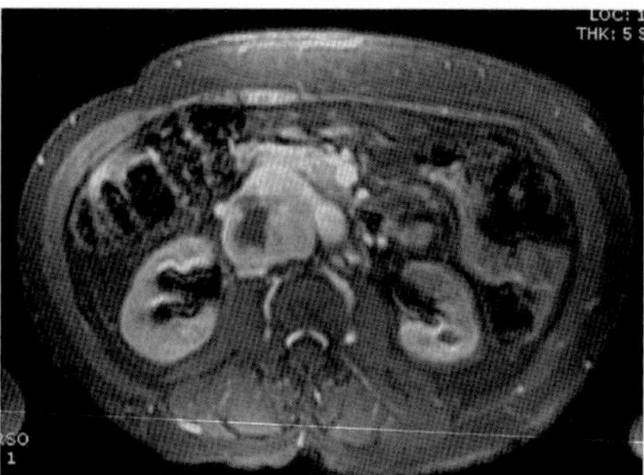

(b)

Fig. 10.4 Intra-abdominal leiyomyosarcoma. MRI images showing an inferior vena cava leiomyosarcoma. (a) A T2-weighted MRI with fat saturation showing a large lobulated neoplasm with a small amount of central fluid in the expected location of the inferior vena cava. (b) The same neoplasm after gadolinium administration showing solid enhancement. The lumen of the IVC has been displaced anteriorly. The neoplasm shows a predominantly extraluminal growth pattern.

nasopharyngeal carcinoma, Hodgkin's disease and B-cell lymphomas arising in immunodeficient patients (Hsu *et al.* 2000). Recently smooth muscle tumors have also been described to be associated with EBV in immunosuppressed patients. The causes of immunosuppression reported in these cases have been mostly those of acquired immunodeficiency syndrome (AIDS) or immunosuppression in organ transplant patients (Rogatsch *et al.* 2000). Evidence for EBV infection was found in leiomyosarcomas and leiomyomas from patients with HIV infection, but not in smooth muscle tumors from HIV-negative patients (McClain *et al.* 1995).

Grossly, the tumors are small, circumscribed and whorled, ranging in size from 1.5 to 3.2 cm. Microscopic examination shows cellular smooth muscle lesion with brisk mitotic activity. There may be infiltration of tumor by atypical lymphocytes. Differentiating benign from malignant cases may be difficult and there are no established guidelines due to the few numbers of cases reported in literature. The name 'EBV-associated smooth muscle tumor' has been suggested for these lesions rather than leiomyoma or leiomyosarcoma, as this appears to have a different etiopathogenetic mechanism and possibly different therapeutic implications as compared to non EBV-associated smooth muscle tumors (Shuterland & Wilson 1980).

Surgical removal and antiviral therapy combined with reduction of immunosuppression may play a critical role in successful long-term treatment. There is limited experience with chemotherapy, but some patients with EBV etiology have responded to antiviral therapy or withdrawal of immunosuppressive therapy.

Retroperitoneal leiomyosarcomas

These account for about 70% of all leiomyosarcomas and are more common in postmenopausal women. Very few leiomyosarcomas (non-GIST) originate in the abdominal cavity. They tend to have poor prognosis with a median survival ranging from 2 to 5 years, depending on the series (Ranchod *et al.* 1977; Rajani *et al.* 1999). Retroperitoneal and abdominal leiomyosarcomas are less amenable to radical surgery, due to anatomic considerations and their often advanced stage at presentation. T2-weighted MRI images show hyperintensity with solid enhancement (Fig. 10.4).

There is limited experience with chemotherapy, but some of the patients with EBV etiology have responded to antiviral therapy or withdrawal of immunosuppressive therapy.

In terms of systemic palliative chemotherapy for retroperitoneal/abdominal soft tissue sarcomas, agents such as antracyclines and ifosfamide that are commonly used for soft tissue sarcomas have demonstrated modest activity (Borden *et al.* 1987). A combination of ifosfamide with either doxorubicin or epirubicin yields a response rate approaching 25% in patients with metastatic disease (Frustaci *et al.* 1997). Other active chemotherapeutics are dacarbazine (DTIC), cisplatin and carboplatin. More recently a combination of gemcitabine and docetaxel 9 and temozolomide oral therapy have shown encouraging efficacy in leiomyosarcomas (Muro *et al.* 2001). However, the impact of palliative chemotherapy on patient survival is limited, failing to extend median survival beyond 12 months. For patients with slowly progressive disease, debulking and resection of metastases (particularly pulmonary metastases) should be considered. Younger patients with better performance status tend to derive greater benefit from the aggressive combination chemotherapy. Newer agents include marine-derived ecteinascidin 743 (Garcia-Carbonero *et al.* 2004) and novel drugs.

References

Azzie G, Bensoussan A, Spitz L. (2003) The association of anorectal leiomyomatosis and diffuse esophageal leiomyomatosis. *Pediatr Surg Int* 19(6): 424–6.

Bekkers RL, Willemsem WN, Schijf CP *et al.* (1999) Leiomyomatosis peritonealis disseminata: does malignant transformation occur? A literature review. *Gynecol Oncol* 75(1): 158–63.

Borden EC, Amato DA, Rosenbaum C *et al.* (1987) Randomized comparison of three adriamycin regiments for metastatic soft tissue sarcomas. *J Clin Oncol* 5: 840–50.

Ferguson TB, Woodbury JD, Roper CL, Burford TH. (1969) Giant muscular hypertrophy of the esophagus. *Ann Thorac Surg* 8: 209–18.

Frustaci S, Buonadonna A, Galligioni E *et al.* (1997) Increasing 4′-epidoxorubicin and fixed ifosfamide doses plus granulocytemacro-

phage colony-stimulating factor in advanced soft tissue sarcomas: a pilot study. *J Clin Oncol* 15: 1418–26.
Garcia-Carbonero R, Supko JG, Manola J *et al.* (2004) Phase II and pharmacokinetic study of ecteinascidin 743 in patients with progressive sarcomas of soft tissues refractory to chemotherapy. *J Clin Oncol* 22: 1480–90.
Gengler C, Guillou L. (2006) Solitary fibrous tumour and hemangiopericytoma: evolution of a concept. *Histopathology* 48: 63–74.
Ghosh K, Dorigo O, Bristow R, Berek J. (2000) Radical debulking of leiomyomatosis peritonealis disseminata from a colonic obstruction. A case report and review of literature. *J Am Coll Surg* 191: 212–15.
Hensley ML, Maki R, Venkatraman E *et al.* (2002) Gemcitabine and docetaxel in patients with unresectable leiomyosarcoma: results of a phase II trial. *J Clin Oncol* 20: 2824–31.
Hsu JL, Glaser SL. (2000) Epstein–Barr virus-associated malignancies: epidemiologic patterns and etiologic implications. *Crit Rev Oncol Hematol* 34(1): 27–53.
Lonsdale RN, Roberts PF, Vaughan R, Thiru S. (1992) Familial esophageal leiomyomatosis and nephropathy. *Histopathology* 20: 127–33.
McClain KL, Leach CT, Jenson HB *et al.* (1995) Association of Epstein–Barr virus with leiomyosarcomas in young people with AIDS. *N Engl J Med* 332: 12–18.
Muro XD, Pousa AL, Buesa JM *et al.* (2001) Temozolomide as a 6-week continuous oral schedule in advanced soft tissue sarcoma (STS): a phase II trial of the Spanish Group for Research on Sarcomas (GEIS) [abstract no. 1412]. *Proc Am Soc Clin Oncol* 20: 873.
Rajani P, Smith TA, Reith JD, Goldblum JR. (1999) Retroperitoneal leiomyosarcomas unassociated with the gastrointestinal tract: a clinicopathologic analysis of 17 cases. *Mod Pathol* 12: 12–28.
Ranchod M, Kempson RL. (1977) Smooth muscle tumors of the gastrointestinal tract and retroperitoneum. *Cancer* 39: 255–62.
Rogatsch H, Bonatti H, Menet A *et al.* (2000) Epstein-Barr virus-associated multicentric leiomyosarcoma in an adult patient after heart transplantation: case report and review of the literature. *Am J Surg Pathol* 24(4): 614–21.
Ruscelleda N, Eixarch E, Pages M *et al.* (2006) Leiomyomatosis peritonealis disseminata. *Eur Radiol* 16: 2879–82.
Shuterland JA, Wilson EA. (1980) Ultrastructure and steroid binding studies in leiomyomatosis peritonealis disseminata. *Am J Obstet Gynecol* 136: 992–96.

Vascular tumors

Mitual Amin, Malathy Kapali, Benjamin Paz, John Fetsch & Tomislav Dragovich

This section begins with a discussion of vascular tumors and tumor-like proliferations peculiar to specific sites in the GI tract followed by rare vascular lesions common to the entire GI tract.

Vascular lesions of the stomach

Gastric antral vascular ectasia

Gastric antral vascular ectasia (GAVE) or watermelon stomach is the most important vascular lesion of the stomach (Jabbari *et al.* 1984). It is an acquired vascular disease and the exact cause is unknown, but some cases are seen in association with mucosal trauma or mucosal prolapse through the pylorus. Patients present with upper GI bleeding and severe transfusion-dependent iron-deficiency anemia. As the name suggests the lesion typically occurs in the antrum but involvement of the proximal stomach has also been reported. The endoscopic findings are characteristic and consist of parallel red stripes at the crest of the mucosal folds in the antrum and thus resemble a watermelon. A biopsy of the reddened area shows an increase in the number of capillaries in the superficial lamina propria and the capillaries appears dilated. The dilated capillaries may contain fibrin thrombi and may be surrounded by eosinophilic homogenous material (fibrohyalinosis). Watermelon stomach should be considered in patients with acute or chronic upper GI bleeding and the diagnosis is usually based on the characteristic endoscopic appearance.

Vascular ectasia

Vascular ectasia can be seen in the stomach in association with portal hypertension (McCormack *et al.* 1985). It differs from GAVE in several respects. It involves the fundus and endoscopically these appear as flat red spots 2–5 mm in diameter. Histologically, it shows relatively mild degree of capillary dilatation, absence of fibrin thrombi and fibrohyalinosis. Vascular ectasia has also been reported following high-dose chemotherapy/hematopoetic stem cell transplantation. The vascular ectasia diffusely involves both the stomach and also the rest of the intestines (Schmidmaier *et al.* 2006).

Aneurysm of gastric vessels

Aneurysm of the gastric vessels known as Dieulafoys lesion (caliber persistence artery of the stomach) is an uncommon lesion thought to be of malformative rather than degenerative in origin. It is characterized by the presence of a single, unusually large and tortuous artery in the gastric submucosa, usually high in the lesser curvature. The vessel is normal histologically but is attached to the muscular mucosae. As the vessel compresses the mucosa there is gradual erosion of the overlying mucosa, which can eventually lead to perforation and bleeding from both the artery and the accompanying vein (Miko *et al.* 1988). Amyloid may deposit in the vessel wall. Unrecognized, the lesion has a high mortality rate (60%).

Other rare vascular lesions of the stomach include hemangiomas, lymphangiomas, and angiomatosis as part of the Osler–Weber–Rendu, Klippel–Trenaunay–Weber, and Maffucci's syndromes.

Glomus tumor

This benign tumor also known as glomangioma originates from

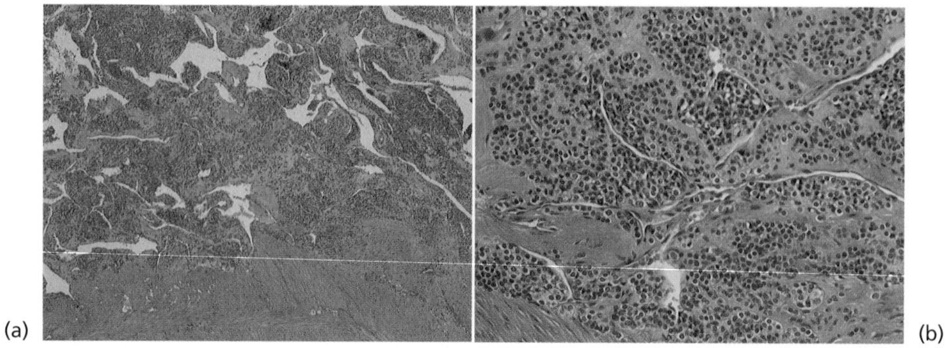

(a) (b)

Fig. 10.5 Glomus tumor (glomangioma) of the stomach. This submucosal lesion arose near the pyloric region along the greater curvature of the stomach. (a) Histopathology (H&E stain, ×40) photomicrograph depicting numerous vascular channels lined by endothelial cells. (b) High power (H&E stain, ×400) photomicrograph of the same which shows uniform small, round bland glomus cells surrounding the vascular channels.

neuromyoarterial glomus structures within the gut wall. In the GI tract most glomus tumors occur in the stomach. The tumor occurs predominantly in females and patients present with either bleeding or ulcer-like symptoms. The age range of patients is 38–89 years. The most common location within the stomach is the antral region. The tumors are usually submucosal in location and less than 3 cm. Grossly they appear as well-circumscribed intramural lesions. Histologically they are composed of proliferation of uniform round cells surrounding normal-appearing blood vessels (Fig. 10.5). Immunohistochemically they show positivity with myosin, actin and vimentin. Almost all tumors in the stomach behave in a benign fashion and surgical excision of the intramural nodule is the treatment of choice.

Vascular lesions of the colon

Intestinal vascular lesions can occur as isolated intestinal vascular abnormalities or in association with systemic syndromes.

Vascular ectasia of the right colon

This lesion is also known as angioma, angiodysplasia and arteriovenous malformation. It usually occurs in the elderly and is an important cause of recurrent low-grade lower gastrointestinal bleeding though some cases present with massive bleeding. The exact pathogenesis for these lesions is not known but they are thought to result from repeated partial obstruction to venous outflow caused by contraction of the muscularis propria. The lesion has been reported in association with aortic valvular stenosis and von Willebrand disease.

The lesions are small, multiple and usually confined to the cecum and ascending colon. They are easy to visualize by arterography but tend to collapse following colectomy. In resected specimens the best way to demonstrate them is to inject the fresh specimen vasculature with silicone rubber or other compounds followed by fixation and clearing of the specimen with methyl salicylate (Boley & Brandt 1986). The vascular ectasia usually appear as 1 mm–1 cm in diameter and have a coral-reef-like arrangement instead of the honeycomb pattern of normal vasculature.

Hemangiomas

Both capillary and cavernous hemangiomas may affect the intestinal tract. They can present as isolated lesions or in association with specific syndromes.

Capillary hemangiomas are more common in the small bowel, appendix and perianal skin than the colon. They are usually asymptomatic single, small lesions and histologically they are composed of closely packed capillaries (Camilleri *et al.* 1984).

Cavernous hemangiomas more commonly involve the mesentery and in the bowel involve the colon and rectum more than small bowel. When symptomatic they can present with rectal bleeding, mass lesion and anemia, or rarely with intussception. They are usually larger lesions than capillary hemangiomas and usually multiple. They consist of large blood-filled endothelial-lined sinuses with poorly defined borders on the CT scan. The presence of flebolith is highly suggestive of the diagnosis. Histologically they appear as sinus-like spaces filled with blood supported by scant connective tissue that contains smooth muscle.

The hemangiomas are thought to originate from embryonic sequestrations of mesodermal tissue. When patients present with hemangiomas it is important to rule out associated syndromes. The syndromes most commonly associated with hemangiomas are blue rubber bleb nevus syndrome and Klippel–Trenaunay syndrome. In Klippel–Trenaunay syndrome angiomas of the right leg with varices are associated with GI angiomas. There is soft tissue and bone hypertrophy in children with this syndrome.

In blue rubber bleb nevus syndrome, a rare congenital disorder, patients present with multifocal hemangiomas of the GI tract, skin and soft tissues (Fishman *et al.* 2005). Because of the large number of hemangiomas throughout the GI tract these lesions have to be treated more aggressively than the sporadic hemangiomas and an aggressive excisional approach is indicated. In other systemic syndromes like hereditary hemorrhagic telegenectasia, progressive systemic sclerosis and Turner syndrome the vascular abnormality affecting the GI tract is telangiectasia. Angiomatosis of the intestinal tract is seen in Osler–Rendu–Weber syndrome (hereditary hemorrhagic telangiectasia) along with telangiectasias of skin and mucous membranes.

Gastrointestinal vascular lesions are most effectively studied by angiography or endoscopy when accessible. Angiography demonstrates the extent of a vascular lesion and also identifies the presence of multiple lesions even if not clinically suspected. Hemangiomas are radiologically suspected when focal calcific densities (phleboliths) are detected within the intestinal wall. Massive hemorrhage as a major complication is noted in 25–50% of cases.

Phlebectasia

Phlebectasia or venous varicosity is most commonly seen in the lower esophagus in association with portal hypertension. It can occur in other sites like the rectosigmoid and small intestine. Phelebectasia can occasionally cause massive GI bleeding.

Angiosarcoma of the gastrointestinal tract

Angiosarcoma is very rare in the GI tract. There have been sporadic case reports of angiosarcomas affecting all sites within the GI tract with involvement of the stomach and small bowel being more common than the colon (Folpe *et al.* 2000). Angiosarcoma affecting the GI tract can be primary or metastatic. Colonic angiosarcoma was first reported by Steiner and Palmer in 1949 and according to the recent literature, there have been fewer than 20 cases reported so far. The tumor has been reported in association with prior history of radiation, Kaposi's sarcoma, and presence of foreign body (Izhak *et al.* 1992).

Clinically, they can present with abdominal pain, bleeding, and symptoms of intestinal obstruction. Grossly, they can present as blue-black nodules or masses with hemorrhagic appearance and the tumor is usually multifocal. Histologically, they are composed of atypical vascular channels showing infiltrative and destructive growth. The channels are lined with plump and layered endothelial cells (Fig. 10.6). The epithelioid variant of angiosarcoma is more common in the GI tract and the tumor has a sheet-like appearance with cleft-like spaces. Immunohistochemistry with vascular markers, cytokeratin and S-100 protein may help in the distinction between angiosarcoma, carcinoma, and melanoma (Dowed 1913).

Angiosarcomas of the GI tract are rapidly progressive. Though size of the tumor (smaller tumors have a better prognosis) and age of the patient (younger patients have more aggressive disease) are important, as a group they typically behave aggressively and metastasize early, with most cases being fatal within a few months of diagnosis. Surgical resection is the treatment of choice, though because of the infiltrative and multifocal nature complete excision may not be possible. Laparoscopic visualization may provide useful preoperative staging information before considering curative surgical resection. Patients often present with diffuse seeding of the liver, omentum and peritoneum with numerous nodules which appear red and hemorrhagic. With very few cases reported in the literature, the role of adjuvant treatment is not very clear. There have been reports of response to chemotherapy with drugs such as doxorubicin, DTIC, and paclitaxel (Fata *et al.* 1999).

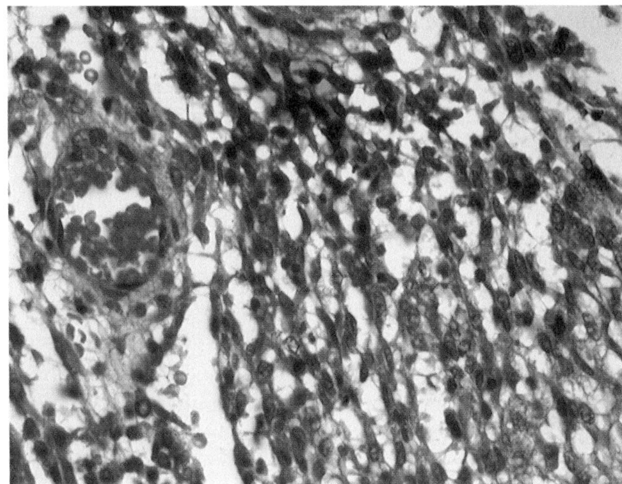
Fig. 10.6 Histopathology of angiosarcoma of the stomach. Light microscopy photomicrograph (H&E stain, ×40) of angiosarcoma composed of numerous irregular interanastomosing vascular channels. The channels are lined by atypical large hyperchromatic pleomorphic nuclei some of which show abnormal mitoses.

Because of the rarity of the lesion, a high index of suspicion, especially in patients with prior history of radiation is necessary to make the diagnosis. The distinction of this tumor from conventional carcinomas is important because of the extremely poor prognosis and the rapid course of the disease.

Kaposi's sarcoma

Kaposi's sarcoma, predominantly a cutaneous disease, can occasionally have visceral manifestations. GI involvement has been seen in 50% of homosexual men with cutaneous Kaposi's sarcoma and AIDS. But Kaposi's sarcoma of the GI tract outside the setting of AIDS is rare. Kaposi's sarcoma of the GI tract has also been reported in a patient post renal transplant. With the advances in antiretroviral therapy for AIDS the incidence of Kaposi's sarcoma in the HIV-positive population dropped from 40% in 1991 to less than 5% in 1999 (Biggar & Rabkin 1996).

Any part of the GI can be involved. The GI tract involvement can precede or be synchronous with the skin lesions or can occur without the skin lesions. The majority of cases are asymptomatic and when symptomatic (10% of cases) the presentation can mimic colitis with diarrhea, abdominal pain and protein-losing enteropathy.

Grossly, usually they present as multiple reddish-brown to purple submucosal/mucosal nodules, but can sometimes be a single lesion. Histologically, they resemble their cutaneous counterpart and are composed of malignant spindle cells with extravasation of red blood cells. The tumor cells infiltrate between as well as replace the epithelium. Immunohistochemically, Kaposi's sarcoma expresses CD34 and CD31 and is negative for S-100, desmin and muscle-specific actin which can help differentiate Kaposi's sarcoma from GIST and melanoma. A high index of suspicion, especially in a patient with AIDS, will usually help in arriving at the correct diagnosis.

Systemic therapy is indicated for the symptomatic, visceral disease. In addition, most patients benefit from highly active antiretroviral therapy (HAART). Active chemotherapy drugs include vicristine, etoposide and bleomycin. The current first-line therapeutic standards are liposomal anthracyclines (doxil, DaunoXome) (Stewart *et al.* 1998). Other biologic agents that have shown some activity include interferon-alpha and thalidomide.

Lymphangioma

Lymphangiomas are rare benign tumors of the lymphatics. Lymphangiomas may either be secondary to congenital malformations of the lymphatic system or represent acquired benign neoplasms. The majority of cases (90%) manifest before the age of 3 and both sexes are equally affected. They commonly affect the mesentery of the small and large bowel as well as retroperitoneal sites. The GI tract can be involved along with the adjacent involved mesentery or without mesenteric involvement. They are often seen in association with tumors at other sites.

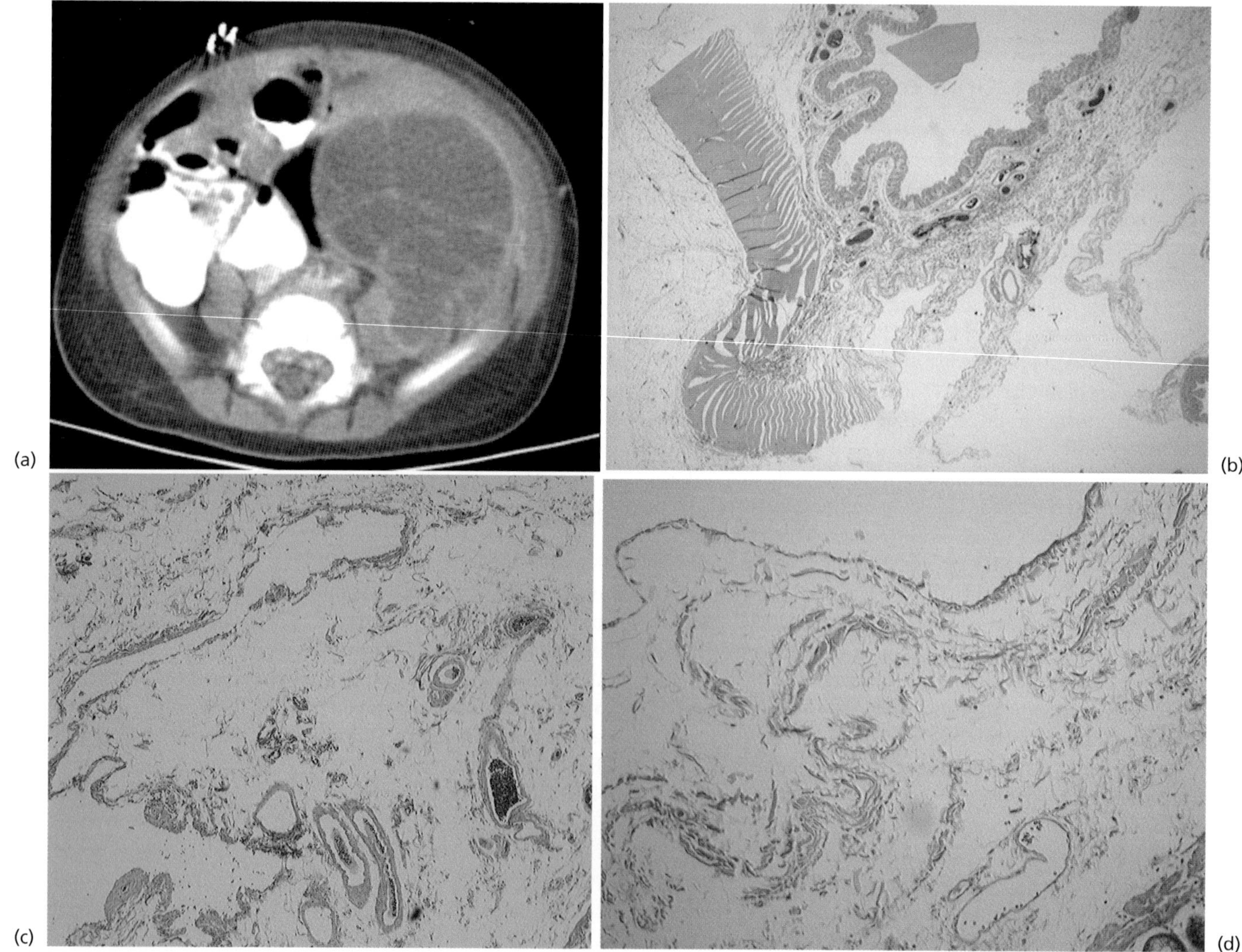

Fig. 10.7 Intra-abdominal lymphangioma. (a) A large intra-abdominal mass predominantly cystic with a thick capsule and multiple thick loculations with enhancing septations. The mass infiltrates the left psoas muscle. (b) Histopathology (H&E stain, ×20) shows a colonic segment involved by a large submucosal multicystic lymphangioma. Photomicrograph (c) (H&E stain, ×40) and photomicrograph (d) (H&E stain, ×100) depict the thin-walled cysts which contained clear yellowish fluid.

The exact etiology is still unclear but there are two schools of thought. One theory postulates that they arise from sequestrations of lymphatic tissue during embryonic development (Stewart *et al.* 1998). The other theory (by Godart) postulates that during development premature lymphatics appear as mesenchymal slits which coalesce and communicate with the venous system. Developmental failure to establish this communication may lead to lymphangiomas (Godart 1966). Both these theories might be possible since lymphangiomas do affect children more than adults and they preferentially occur at sites where lymphatic sacs occur. In contrast to children, development of lymphangiomas in adults is thought to be a phenomenon secondary to an inflammatory process or radiation therapy.

The clinical symptoms include abdominal pain, perforation, obstruction, or anemia. Typically they appear as large, thin-walled, multiloculated cysts on CT with barely visible cyst walls but vessels can be seen in between the cavities. On CT lymphangiomas have characteristically less attenuation than water due to the chylous content (Fig. 10.7a) (Hamrick-Turner *et al.* 1992). Grossly they are usually smooth, round to oval lesions, yellowish and translucent and easily compressible. Traditionally lymphangiomas are divided into three types: simple capillary, cavernous, and cystic lymphangiomas. All types are composed of dilated lymphatic channels lined with endothelial cells. The capillary type is composed of small thin-walled lymphatics, the cavernous type consists of larger lymphatics with advential coats and the cystic type consists of large macroscopic lymphatic spaces with collagen and smooth muscle (Fig. 10.7b–d). The differential diagnosis includes cavernous hemangiomas, cystic mesothelioma and microcystic adenomas in adult patients with lymphangiomas.

Lymphangiomas as a group are benign but may cause significant mortality because of their large size and critical location. Sometimes these tumors can transform into lympangiosarcoma after irradiation.

References

Appleman HD, Helwig EB. (1969) Glomus tumors of the stomach. *Cancer* 23: 203–13.

Biggar RJ, Rabkin CS. (1996) The epidemiology of AIDS-related neoplasms. *Hematol Oncol Clin North Am* 10: 997–1010.

Boley SJ, Brandt LJ. (1986) Vascular ectasias of the colon. *Dig Dis Sci* 31: 265–425.

Broion CJ, Falek VG, MacLean A. (2004) Angiosarcoma of the colon and rectum: report of a case and review of the literature. *Dis Colon Rectum* 47: 2202–07.

Camilleri M, Chadwick VS, Hodgson HJF. (1984) Vascular anomalies of the gastrointestinal tract. *Hepatogastroenterology* 31: 149–53.

Dowed CN. (1913) Hygroma cysticum coli. Its structure and etiology. *Ann Surg* 58: 102–32.

Fata F, O'Reilly E, Ilson D *et al.* (1999) Paclitaxel in the treatment of patients with angiosarcoma of the scalp or face. *Cancer* 86: 2034–7.

Fishman SJ, Smither CJ, Folkman J, Lund DP, Burrows PE, Mcullikan JB, Fox VL. (2005) Blue rubber bleb nevus syndrome: surgical eradication of gastrointestinal bleeding. *Ann Surg* 241(3): 523–8.

Folpe AL, Veikkala T, Valtola R, Weiss SW. (2000) Vascular endothelial growth factor receptor-3 (VEGFR-3): a marker of vascular tumors with presumed lymphatic differentiation, including Kaposi's sarcoma, kaposiform and Dobska-type hemangioendothaliomas, and a subset of angiosarcomas. *Mod Pathol* 13: 180–5.

Godart S. (1966) Embryological significance of lymphangiomas. *Arch Dis Child* 41: 204–6.

Hamrick-Turner JE, Chiechi MV, Abbit PL, Ros PR. (1992) Neoplastic and inflammatory processes of the peritoneum, omentum and mercentery: diagnosis with CT. *Radiographics* 12(6): 1051–68.

Izhak BD, Kerner H, Brenner B, Lichtig C. (1992) Angiosarcoma of the colon developing in a capsule of a foreign body. Report of a case with associated hemorrhagic diathesis. *Am J Clin Pathol* 97: 416–20.

Jabbari M, Cherry R, Lough JO, Daly DS, Kinnear DG, Goresky CA. (1984) Gastric antral vascular ectasia: the watermelon stomach. *Gastroenterology* 87: 1165–70.

McCormack TT, Sinr J, Eyre-Brook I *et al.* (1985) Gastric lesions in portal hypertension: inflammatory gastritis or competitive gastropathy. *Gut* 26: 1226–32.

Miko T, Thomazy VA. (1988) The caliber persistent artery of the stomach: a unifying approach to gastric aneurysm, Dieulafoy's lesion and submucosal arterial malformation. *Hem Pathol* 19: 914–21.

Schmidmaier R, Bittmann I, Gotzberger M, Straka C, Meinhardt G, Engler A. (2006) Vascular ectasia of the whole intestine as a cause of recurrent gastrointestinal bleeding after high dose chemotherapy. *Endoscopy* 38(9): 940–2.

Stewart S, Jablononski H, Goebel FD *et al.* (1998) Randomized comparative trial of pegylated liposomal doxorubicin versus bleomycin and vincristine in the treatment of AIDS-related Kaposi's sarcoma. *J Clin Oncol* 16: 683–91.

Adipose tissue tumors

John Fetsch, Anil R. Prasad, Sanjay Saluja & Benjamin Paz

There are several fatty lesions in the abdomen including lipomas, angiolipomas, myelolipomas, lipomatosis, liposarcoma, and lipomatous of the ileocecal valve. Most of these tumors are symptomatic especially when large (>2 cm) and they are found during routine imaging studies obtained for other clinical purposes. Most of the benign adipose tissue proliferations have unique characteristic CT findings that are usually diagnostic (Pereira *et al.* 2005). Knowledge of the clinical, anatomic, and imaging features is important in order to formulate an appropriate differential diagnosis and to guide patient care, often obviating the need for invasive diagnostic procedures.

Lipoma

Lipomas are rare in the GI tract and they comprise 6% of all GI tumors (Johnson *et al.* 1981). The colon is the most common

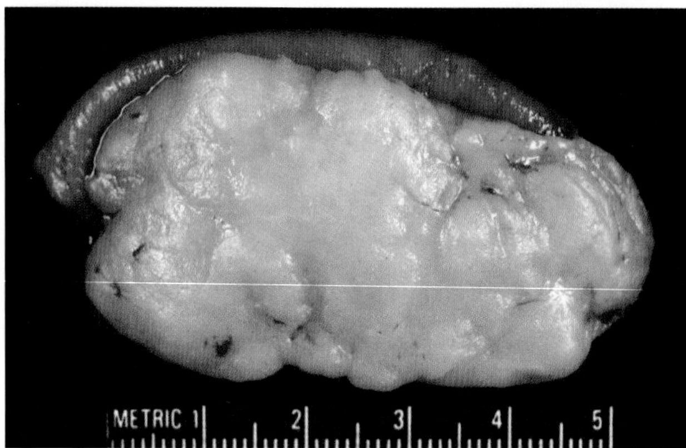

Fig. 10.8 Lipoma small intestine. Gross photograph depicting characteristic large lobulated encapsulated submucosal lesion, cut surface of which is bright yellow and greasy.

site affected followed by small bowel (ileum) with stomach being the least common. Lipomas can occur in any part of the stomach, except the cardiac and the pylorus and 75% occur in the antrum (Turkington 1965). Colon lipoma was initially described by Bauer in 1757 and nearly 90% are located on the right side. The lesion is more common among the elderly.

Gastric lipomas present with hemorrhage (most common), abdominal pain, pyloric obstruction or dyspepsia. Colon lipomas are usually asymptomatic. When symptomatic they can present with pain, diarrhea, rectal bleeding, constipation, or intussusception (usually seen with larger lesions). Predominantly fat-containing neoplasms are readily identified by CT as very low density masses. Their density measures less than 0 Hounsfield units, enabling a specific diagnosis of a fatty lesion by CT. However CT alone is not able to distinguish lipomas from liposarcomas.

Most gastrointestinal lipomas are submucosal in location with less than 10% being subserosal and they can be sessile or pedunculated (Fig. 10.8). They are usually less than 2 cm with an intact overlying mucosa. Grossly the tumors have smooth rounded configuration and uniform bright yellow parenchyma. Large lesions can have surface ulceration, due to a mechanical effect. Mesenteric lipomas are usually small and are incidental findings.

Histologically, the lipomas are well circumscribed and composed of mature adipocytes covered by attenuated mucosa. They do not usually extend into the mucosa or underlying muscle. Necrosis and hemorrhage can be seen in larger lesions. Atypical features similar to those seen in subcutaneous lipoma can be seen (atypical lipoma).

There is no reported malignant potential for lipomas and asymptomatic small lipomas do not need any surgical treatment. Surgery is currently indicated only when malignancy cannot be ruled out or the lipoma is symptomatic (Singh & Bawa 2004). The use of intraoperative frozen sections can avoid unnecessary resections.

Angiolipoma

These tumors grossly resemble lipomas; however, larger lesions may become hemorrhagic and present as acute abdomen. They contain a mixture of proliferating fat cells and capillaries. Complete surgical excision is curative.

Lipomatosis of the gastrointestinal tract

Multiple intestinal lipomas (lipomatosis) has been identified in 1–26% of collected series of patients (Comfort 1981) and has been described in the colon, small bowel, appendiceal epiploicae and pelvic connective tissue. In the small bowel, the ileum is the most common site of involvement with extension into the jejunum. Involvement of only jejunum or duodenum without ileal involvement is uncommon (Climie & Small 1981). Small intestinal lipomatosis has been reported to be associated with an increased incidence of diverticulosis of the affected area. Multiple lipomas commonly involve one segment of the intestine, though on occasions they can be diffuse.

In contrast to lipomas, lipomatosis are almost always symptomatic and present with abdominal pain, obstruction or intussuception. Grossly lipomatosis appear as distinctive usually submucosal fatty masses. They can have the appearance of multiple polyps in the colon for which the term lipomatosis polyposis has been used. Histologically they are composed of mature adipose tissue covered by attenuated mucosa. Focal ulceration can be present, especially when associated with intussception.

Lipomatosis is almost always symptomatic, patients present with weight loss and intestinal bleeding. Surgical resection of the affected areas appears to be the only practical option and is curative in all reported cases. There has been no reported incidence of malignant transformation.

Clinical and radiologic differential diagnosis of small bowel lipomatosis includes Peutz–Jeghers syndrome. However patient age and lack of cutaneous pigmentation can help differentiate the two entities. Although rare, lipomatosis should be considered in the differential diagnosis of patients presenting with multiple intraluminal masses.

Lipohyperplasia of ileocecal valve

This entity has also been described as lipoma or lipomatosis of the ileocecal valve. However, as the lesion is simply an increase in fatty tissue within the valve the term lipohyperplasia is more appropriate and distinguishes it from lipoma and lipomatosis which are true neoplastic proliferations of adipose tissue.

Lipohyperplasia of the ileocecal valve is fairly common. It consists of an excess of adipose tissue deposited circumferentially in the submucosa of the ileocecal valve. The exact cause for this disposition of fat is not known. It has been shown to be more common in obese individuals and it is postulated that mechanical propulsion of the mucosa and submucosa downstream into the lumen of the large bowel might create a sort of 'tissue vacuum' in the submucosal area that is filled by fat (Cabaud & Harris 1959). It is more common in females and in patients below 40 years of age. The lesion is usually asymptomatic and most often is an incidental finding in specimens resected for other conditions. It is often biopsied as it is easily recognized by the endoscopist. Rarely it can be symptomatic with subacute obstruction and is one cause of ileocecal valve syndrome. Right hemicolectomy has been performed as this lesion on occasions cannot be differentiated from carcinoma on radiographic examination.

Grossly there is enlargement, thickening and protrusion of the valve into the cecum. Histologically there is an excess of normal mature adipose tissue in the submucosa of the ileocecal valve. In contrast to lipoma which is focal accumulation of fat, in lipomatosis hyperplasia the fat accumulation is poorly circumscribed and non-encapsulated. The fat accumulation extends on both sides of the valve to involve the ileal and cecal surfaces. The overlying mucosa is usually intact, though on occasions the adipotic valve can become eroded with ulceration and bleeding. The underlying muscularis may become splayed superficially and intermingled with the adipose tissue.

Liposarcoma

Liposarcoma, one of the most common soft tissue sarcomas in adults, is exceedingly rare in the GI tract. Even though these tumors are usually found in the retroperitoneum, they can also arise from the omentum or bowel mesentery. There has been only a small number of cases reported from various sites within the GI tract.

Esophageal liposarcoma was first described by Mansour *et al.* in 1983 (Mansour *et al.* 1983) and so far at least 13 cases have been reported in the literature. Most liposarcomas (84.6%) of the esophagus are located in the upper esophagus. There is a slight male predominance (1.16 : 1) similar to that observed in soft tissue liposarcomas. The most common clinical symptoms include dysphagia, nausea, discomfort and foreign body sensation.

To our knowledge only eight cases of liposarcoma of the stomach have been reported in the literature. Men are more commonly affected than women and the age range of incidence is between 15 and 86 years. Most reported tumors are from the antrum and clinical symptoms are generally those of a space-occupying lesion of the stomach or abdominal cavity. The tumors can be submucosal (most common) or can be exophytic. Most tumors are well circumscribed, ranging in size from 5 to 30 cm.

Primary colonic liposarcoma was first described by Wood and Margenstein in 1989 (Wood & Morganstein 1989). This study was a case report of liposarcoma involving the ileocecal valve, cecum, and ascending colon. Following this there have been three reported cases of primary colonic liposarcoma. Two of these tumors involved the ascending colon and one the descending colon, and the right side of the colon seems to be more commonly affected. Of the reported cases, three out of four were in females (in contrast to that observed in soft tissue sarcomas) and the age ranged between 45 and 62 years.

Symptoms are non-specific and include weight loss, vomiting, abdominal pain, diarrhea, hematochesia and anemia. Extensive diffuse thickening of the intestinal wall is discovered on exploratory laporatomy (Fig. 10.9). The imaging profile of these neoplasms correlates well with their histologic subtypes. The well differentiated liposarcomas contain large amounts of macroscopic fat easily identified by CT. They may have foci of soft tissue attenuation within the neoplasm but these tend to be very small or minimal (Kim *et al.* 1996). The myxoid subtype shows low density content interspersed with foci of macroscopic fat. The fluid component of the myxoid neoplasms is also readily identified on MR as fluid signal on T2-weighted scans. However, following contrast enhancement, there is actual enhancement of this low-density material. The appearance of pleomorphic or round cell type is that of aggressive non-fatty soft tissue density masses making them indistinguishable from other non-fat-containing neoplasms (Fig. 10.10). It has been suggested that the greater the fat content within a liposarcoma, the lower the tumor grade histologically (Santhanam *et al.* 2006).

On gross examination most of these tumors were polypoid and intraluminal (Fig. 10.11). In the case reported by Chen the liposarcoma formed a dumbbell-shaped lesion with an intraluminal polypoid portion and a mesocolic component, and the

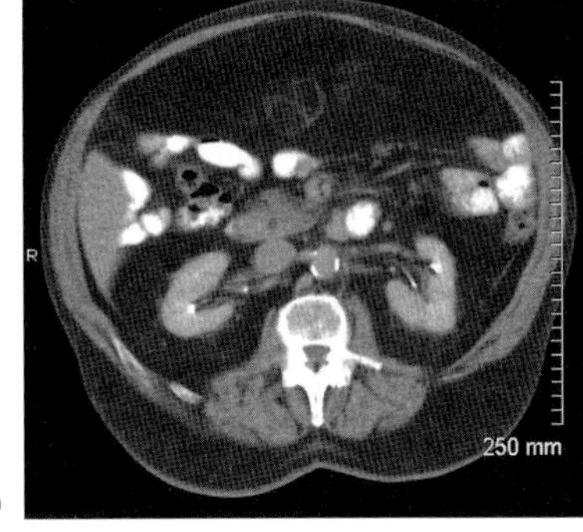

(a)

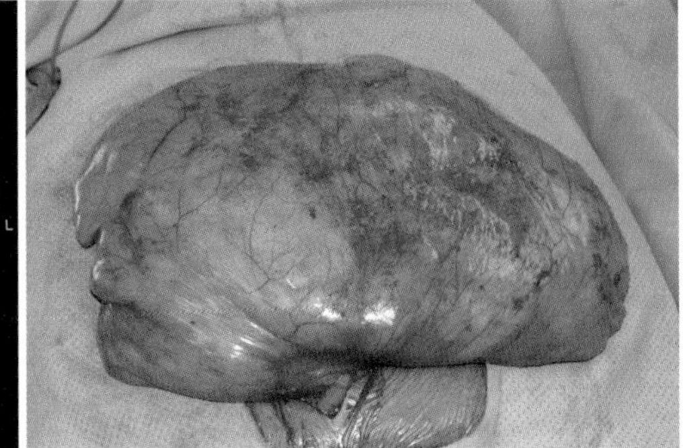
(b)

Fig. 10.9 Lipoma of sigmoid mesentery. (a) CT scan of the abdomen; the sigmoid mesentery vessels are well preserved without evidence of displacement or mass effect. (b) Surgical specimen of the same patient showing a large fatty tumor of the sigmoid mesentery.

(a) 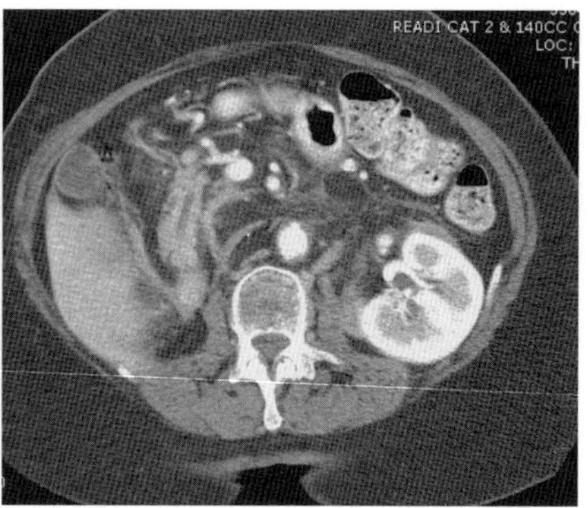 (b)

Fig. 10.10 Intraabdominal liposarcoma. (a) A 74-year-old female with a moderately differentiated reroperitoneal liposarcoma. There is a 3-cm round mass with ill-defined anterior margins (block arrow) immediately anterior to the inferior vena cava. The surrounding fat has a stranded appearance (dirty fat) especially in the left side of the retroperitoneum. (b) The same patient on a slice obtained a few cm higher than figure (a). The fat around the aorta shows significant amount of stranding and prominent vascular channels all consistent with a fatty neoplasm. Note how there are no distinct margins in this neoplasm.

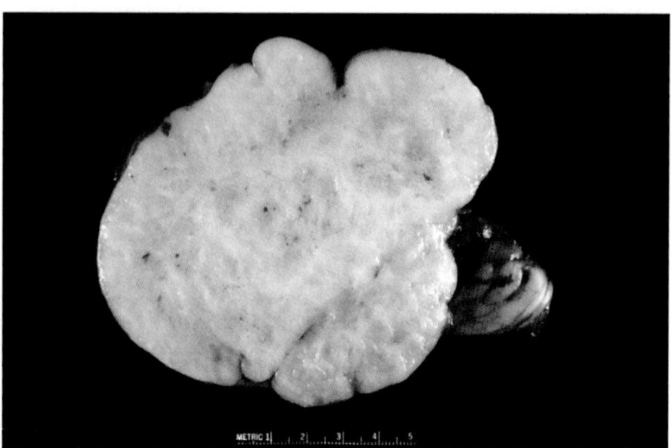

Fig. 10.11 Liposarcoma small intestine. Gross specimen photograph of liposarcoma involving the intestinal wall and partially obstructing the lumen. The lobular, greyish white yellow cut surface with focal areas of hemorrhage is fairly typical of these tumors.

case reported by Gutsu the tumor was located exclusively in the subserosa. Histologically, the diagnosis rests on the finding of lipoblasts in an adipocyte tumor. Liposarcomas are classified into five histologic subtypes: well-differentiated, myxoid, round cell, dedifferentiated, and pleomorphic. Except for the dedifferentiated type all other variants have been reported within the GI tract, with well-differentiated and myxoid being the most common. Immunohistochemically the tumor is positive for S-100 and vimentin and is negative for CD34. The differential diagnosis includes lipoma, GIST, and leiomyosarcoma.

The clinical outcome and prognosis are difficult to predict due to the small number of cases from the various sites within the GI tract. Surgical resection offers the only chance of cure and possible prolonged survival.

Fatty mass lesions in the mesentery are commonly fortuitously encountered during routine CT scanning of the abdomen, posing a diagnostic challenge. Many of these are benign and represent areas of lipodystrophy or fat necrosis but cannot reliably be distinguished from more malignant tumors such as liposarcomas by imaging features alone. These can be followed by CT serially to document stability. However in the more suspicious lesions, CT-guided biopsy or a surgical biopsy is necessary to obtain a tissue-specific diagnosis. If the biopsy results are equivocal, serial CT follow-up to assess the natural evolution is usually performed.

References

Cabaud PG, Harris LT. (1959) Lipomatosis of the ileocaecal valve. *Ann Surg* 150b: 1092–98.

Climie ARN, Small WR. (1981) Intestinal lipomatosis. *Arch Pathol Lab Med* 105: 40–42.

Comfort MW. (1981) Submucosa lipomata of the gastrointestinal tract. *Surg Gynecol Obstet* 52: 101–88.

Johnson DCI, DeHennara VA, Pizzi WF, Nealon TF. (1981)Gastric lipomas: A rare cause of massive upper gastrointestinal bleeding. *Am J Gastroenterol* 75: 299–301.

Kim T, Murakami T, O Hiromichi *et al.* (1996) CT and MR imaging of abdominal liposarcoma. *Am J Roentgenol* 166: 829–33.

Mansour KA, Fritis RC, Jacobs DM, Vellior F. (1983) Pedunculated liposarcoma of the esophagus: a first case report. *J Thorac Cardiovasc Surg* 86: 447.

Pereira JM, Sirlin CB, Pinto PS, Casola G. (2005) CT and MR imaging of antrahepatic fatty masses of the abdomen & pelvis: Techniques, diagnosis, differential diagnosis and pitfalls. *Radiographics* 25(1): 69–85.

Santhanam AN, Sillar RW, Roberts-Thomson IC. (2006) Gastrointestinal lipomas. *J Gastroenterol Hepatol* 21: 1628.

Singh R, Bawa AS. (2004) Lipoma of the stomach. *Indian J Surg* 66: 177–9.

Turkington RW. (1965) Gastric lipoma. Report of a case and review of the literature. *Am J Dig Dis* 10: 119–206.

Wood DI, Morganstein L. (1989) Liposarcoma of the ileocecal valve. A case report. *Mt Sinai J Med* 56: 62–4.

Neurogenic tumors

Anil R. Prasad, Markku Miettenen & Benjamin Paz

Primary neurogenic tumors of the GI tract and mesentery are rare. Most are of peripheral nerve sheath origin, i.e. neuromas, schwannomas and neurofibromas, while others arise from the sympathetic system, i.e. paraganglioma and ganglioneuromas.

Neuroma

Neuroma of the appendix is a fairly common entity and it is thought that most cases of so-called fibrous obliteration actually represent appendiceal neuromas. The frequency of neuroma increases with age and they can be single or multiple lesions. When single the tip of the appendix is usually affected, though any portion can be involved. When multiple the terms neuromatosis of the appendix, neuroganic appendicitis or neurogenic appendicopathy have been applied. Histologically they appear as a loose proliferation of spindle cells with entrapped fat, connective tissue and eosinophilic infiltrate. The spindle cells are positive for S-100 and neuron specific enolase. A small proportion of appendiceal neuromas have been associated with microcarcinoids. The lesion is favored to be a non-neoplastic neural proliferation induced by prior episodes of inflammation. Appendectomy is curative.

Neurofibromas

Gastrointestinal neurofibromas can be seen in the setting of von Recklinghausen's disease (which is more common) or as a solitary lesion. The prevalence of gastrointestinal involvement in von Recklinghausen's disease is around 11–25% and the small intestine is the most common gastrointestinal site of involvement (Pinsk *et al.* 2003). The colon and rectum are less commonly involved but even a solitary neurofibroma at this site should raise the possibility of von Recklinghausen's disease (Fig. 10.12). The neurofibroma of von Recklinghauren's disease presents most often with bleeding and sometimes with obstruction.

Schwannoma

Schwannomas are tumors that originate from the Schwann cells that form the nerve sheath. The stomach is the most common site affected within the GI tract, with involvement of esophagus and colon being rare. Schwannomas occur during middle to late adulthood and peak in the sixth decade of life. Grossly they are well circumscribed and submucosal with occasional cases having an intraluminal component (Fig. 10.13). Histologically they are composed of spindle cell proliferation with wavy or buckled nuclei. Cellularity varies within the tumor and they can have cellular Antoni A areas and hypocellular Antoni B areas in varied proportions. Nuclear atypia may be present but mitotic activity is usually low. In contrast to their peripheral counterparts, schwannomas of the gastrointestinal tract have a peripheral cuff of lymphocytes (Houy *et al.* 2006). Immunohistochemically they are positive for S-100 and negative for CD117 and muscle markers.

Schwannomas are most common among neurogenic tumors. They are usually round and well encapsulated with smooth margins. They do not infiltrate surrounding structures. There is mild to moderate enhancement following contrast administration. Their MRI features can be variable depending upon their cellular and fibrous content. Cellular components are hypointense to isointense on both T1- and T2-weighted images,

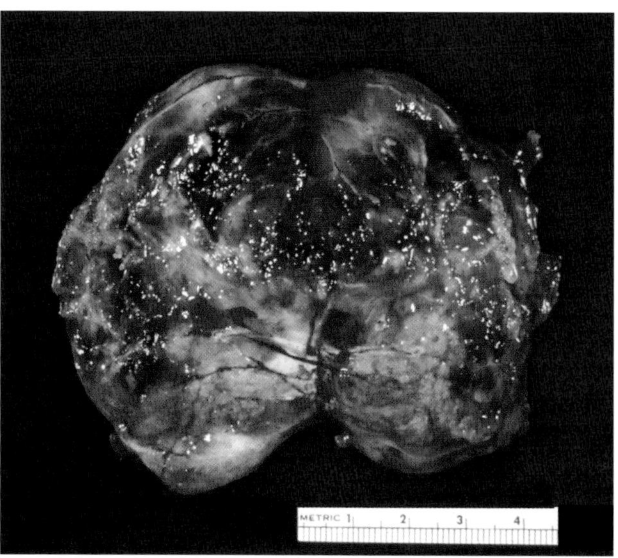

Fig. 10.13 Schwannoma involving small bowel. This well-encapsulated mass with a myxoid hemorrhagic cut surface was excised completely from the subserosal aspect of the small bowel.

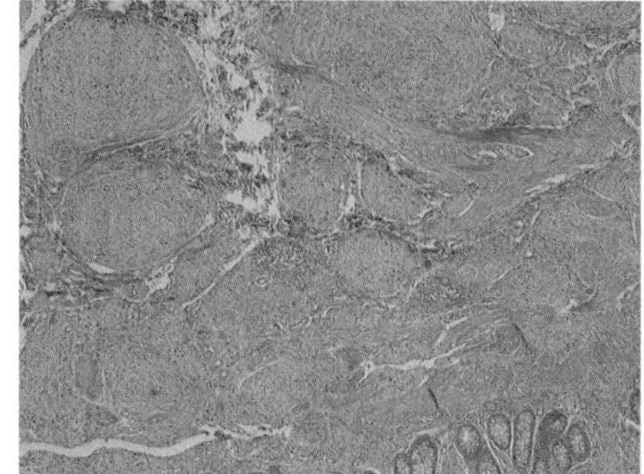
(a)

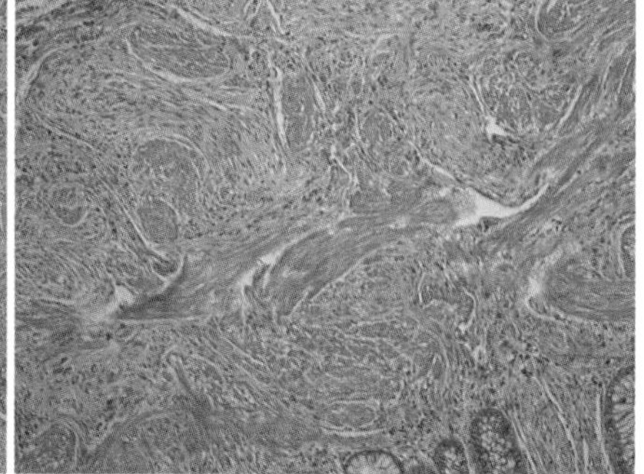
(b)

Fig. 10.12 Neurofibroma of the colon. Histopathology of a colon resection specimen in a patient with von Recklinghausen disease. Photomicrograph (a) (H&E stain, ×40) shows plexiform pattern of neurofibroma with expanded nerves forming nodules involving the colonic wall. Photomicrograph (b) (H&E stain, ×100) shows loose spindle cells and collagen bundles.

while predominantly fibrous lesions are markedly hypointense on both T1- and T2-weighted images. If myxoid tissue is present, the lesions tend to be hyperintense on T2-weighted images with delayed enhancement on the postgadolinium scans (Engleken & Ros 1997).

Granular cell tumors

Granular cell tumors (GCTs) are benign tumors of Schwann cell origin. They most often occur in the tongue or skin, with GI tract being a rare site of involvement. Within the GI tract, the distal esophagus is the most common site affected. They predominantly affect adults and are more common in females. They are usually single tumors discovered incidentally, though multiple tumor nodules can be seen throughout the GI tract. The lesions are usually submucosal in location and endoscopically they appear as yellowish-white submucosal nodules. Histologically they are composed of sheets of cells with abundant granular cytoplasm and bland nuclei. The granular cytoplasm is due to the accumulation of phagolysosomes. Immunohistochemically the cells are positive for S-100. In the esophagus the overlying squamous epithelium often shows pseudoepitheliomatous hyperplasia which can be mistaken for malignancy (David & Jakate 1999) if the underlying granular cell tumor has not been well sampled. Most GCT are benign, though malignant GCT has been reported.

Gangliocytic paraganglioma

The term gangliocytic paraganglioma was introduced by Kepes and Lacharean for a tumor composed of an admixture of Schwann cells, ganglion cells and nests of neuroendocrine cells that resembles paraganglioma. The second part of the duodenum at the level of the ampulla of Vater is the most common part affected (Burke & Helwig 1989). The lesion predominantly occurs in the fifth to sixth decades of life. Males are more commonly affected than females. CT scan usually shows an ill-defined solid enhancing mass (Fig. 10.14). Though the tumor contains endocrine cells they are non-functional and patients present with symptoms related to mass lesion or bleeding. Grossly they are non-encapsulated polypoid lesions (1–10 cm) with frequent ulceration of the overlying mucosa. Histologically (Fig. 10.15) they are composed of nested neuroendocrine cells (resembling paraganglioma) admixed with spindled Schwann cells and scattered ganglion cells. The tumors are considered to be benign and conservative management is recommended.

Ganglioneuromas

Ganglioneuromas (GNs) are benign neoplasms composed of nerve cells, ganglion cells and supporting cells. Colon and rectum are more commonly involved than stomach and small intestine. GN of the GI tract can occur as isolated polypoid ganglioneuromas, ganglioneuromatous polyposis, or diffuse ganglioneuromatosis. Isolated polypoid ganglioneuromas is the most common type and is usually not associated with NF or any syndromes. Ganglioneuromatous polyposis and diffuse ganglioneuromatosis arise in the setting of multiple endocrine neoplasia syndromes. Isolated polypoid ganglioneuromas present as single polypoid lesions whereas ganglioneuromatous polypo-

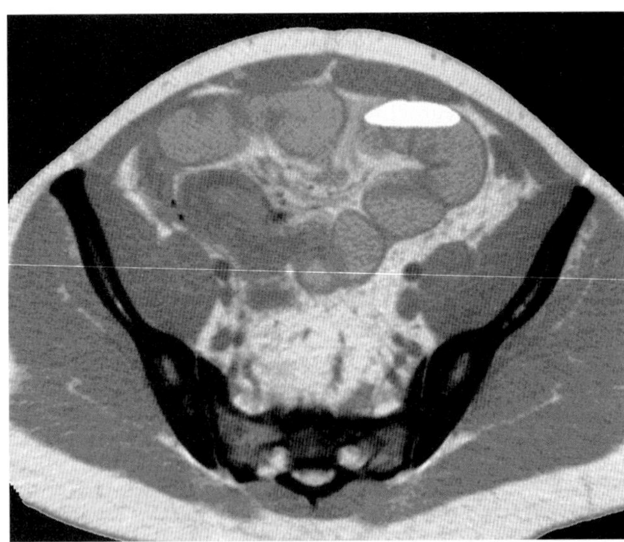

Fig. 10.14 Gangliocytic paraganglioma. CT scan shows a 33-year-old male with an ill-defined right lower quadrant solid mass with intense enhancement and foci of dystrophic calcification. The small bowel is obstructed. Histopathology showed a gangliocytic paraganglioma of the terminal ileum.

(a) 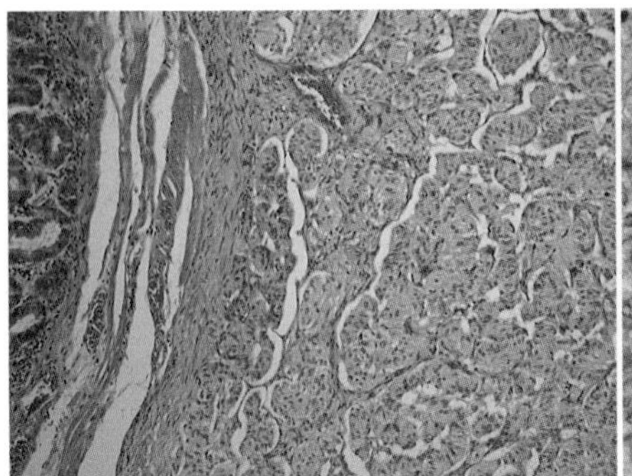

(b) 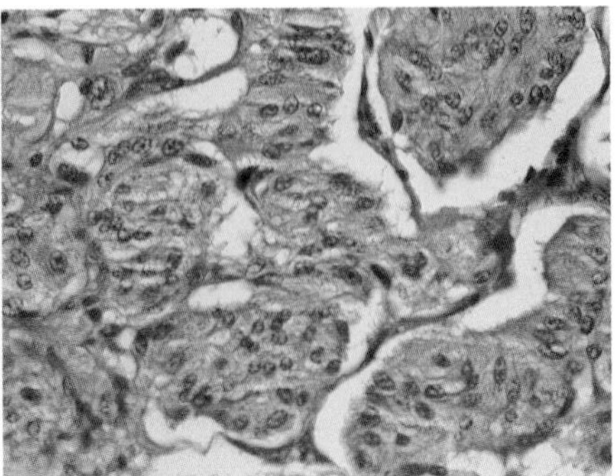

Fig. 10.15 Histopathology of gangliocytic paraganglioma. Photomicrograph (a) (H&E stain, ×100) shows typical spindle cells and round or polygonal epithelioid cells arranged in a 'zell ballen' pattern. (b) (H& E stain, ×200) shows the epithelioid cells surrounded by a capillary network. Abnormal mitoses are not present.

sis presents as multiple polyps (20 in number) as their name suggests. Histologically the tumor is composed of non-myelinated nerve fibres and varying proportions of ganglion cells.

Imaging features are not helpful in differentiating benign from malignant tumors. Features favoring the diagnosis of malignant lesion are presence of metastatic disease, irregular borders of the mass, internal heterogeneity and large size. Progressive enlargement and pain associated with the lesion are also suggestive of malignant transformation (Leslie & Cheung 1987; Levine *et al.* 1994). CT remains the mainstay of imaging. It is crucial for initial identification of the tumor, local and distant staging, planning biopsy, and follow-up after surgical removal.

References

Burke AP, Helwig EB. (1989) Gangliocytic paraganglioma. *Am J Clin Pathol* 92: 1–9.

David O, Jakate S. (1999) Multifocal granular cell tumor of the esophagus and proximal stomach with infiltrative pattern: a case report and review of literature. *Arch Pathol Lab Med* 123: 967–73.

Engleken JD, Ros PR. (1997) Retroperitoneal MR imaging. *Magn Reson Imaging Clin N Am* 5: 165–78.

Houy Y, Tan YS *et al.* (2006) Schwannoma of the gastrointestinal tract: a clinicopathological, immunohistochemical and ultrastructural study of 33 cases. *Histopathology* 48(5): 536–45.

Leslie MD, Cheung KY. (1987) Malignant transformation of neurofibromas at multiple sites in a case of neurofibromatosis. *Postgrad Med J* 63: 131–3.

Levine E, Huntrakoon M, Wetzel LH. (1994) Malignant nerve sheath neoplasms in neurofibromatosis: distinction from benign tumors by using imaging techniques. *AJR Am J Roentgenol* 163: 617–20.

Masson P. (1928) Carcinoids (argentaffian cell tumors) and nerve hyperplasia of the appendicular mucosa. *Am J Pathol* 4: 181–211.

Pinsk I, Dukhno O, Ovant A, Levy I. (2003) Gastrointestinal complications of von Recklinghausen's disease: two case reports and review of the literature. *Scand J Gastroenterol* 38(12): 1275–8.

Myofibroblastic and fibrous tumors

John Fetsch, Malathy Kapali, Benjamin Paz, Sanjay Saluja & Tomislav Dragovich

Mesenteric fibromatosis, sclerosing mesenteritis, inflammatory pseudotumor, and extrapleural solitary fibrous tumor constitute a loosely associated group of benign fibrous tumors and tumor like lesions of the mesentery (Levy *et al.* 2006). These lesions are rare but with a unique pathologic and biologic behavior. They are characterized by the presence of infiltrating fibrous tissue without malignant features. The clinical behavior of these lesions depends on their location, they usually present with abdominal distension, vague gastrointestinal or obstructive symptoms. These lesions are difficult to diagnose on imaging alone and needle biopsies can only rarely give a definitive diagnosis.

Intraabdominal or mesenteric fibromatosis (desmoid tumor)

Intraabdominal fibromatosis affecting the mesentery or reteroperitoneum has been referred to as fibrous dysplasia of the mesentery or desmoid. Mesenteric fibromatosis is considered the most frequent primary mesenteric tumor; it is a locally aggressive, but benign proliferative process. Intraabdominal fibromatosis arise with disproportionate frequency in patients with Gardner's syndrome (a variant of familial adenomatosis polyposis (FAP) (Enzinger & Weiss 1988).

Apart from APC gene mutations, other unknown genetic factors, hormones, and trauma (most desmoids that arise in association with FAP often appear after prophylactic colectomy) all play a role in their development and growth (Okuno 2006). Recent studies show that germline mutation distal to codon 1399 and a strong family history of desmoids are independent predictors for developing intra-abdominal fibromatosis.

The CT and MR imaging appearances of mesenteric fibromatosis are directly related to its underlying histologic characteristics and vascularity. Imaging is characterized by bowel displacement with associated bowel obstruction (Fig. 10.16). Desmoid tumors appear grossly as firm to hard well-circumscribed non-encapsulated masses. Cut surface appears a homogenous grey white (Fig. 10.17).

Fibromatosis is recognized by a uniform fibroplastic proliferation in the form of interlacing bundles of spindle cells. There is a tendency for the spindle cells to infiltrate the adipose tissue and outer muscular layer of the intestine. There is little associated inflammation (Fig. 10.18).

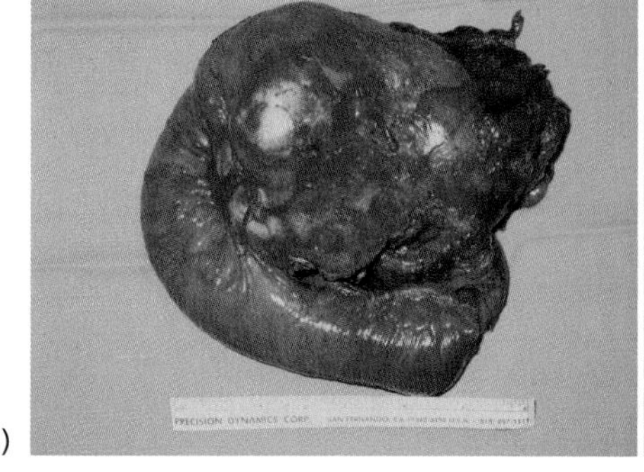
(a)

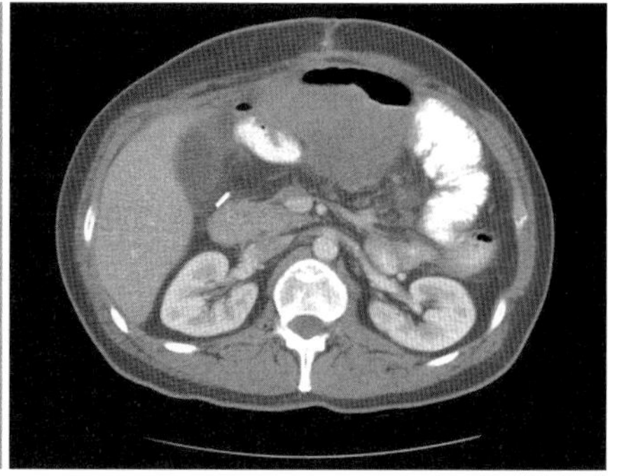
(b)

Fig. 10.16 (a) Intraoperative specimen picture of mesenteric fibromatosis; large ill-defined mass of the mesentery displacing the bowel wall and causing jejunal obstruction. (b) Mesenteric fibromatosis of the proximal jejunum forming a large mass with jejunal vessel involvement.

Fibromatosis can be misdiagnosed as GIST because it involves the bowel wall and is immunoreactive with CD34 and CD117 (c-kit) similar to GIST. However, in fibromatosis the reactivity with CD117 is only coarse cytoplasmic and is not present with some of the newer antibodies against this marker. Another distinguishing feature is the immunoreactivity of fibromatosis with beta-catenin in contrast to GIST, which is negative with this marker.

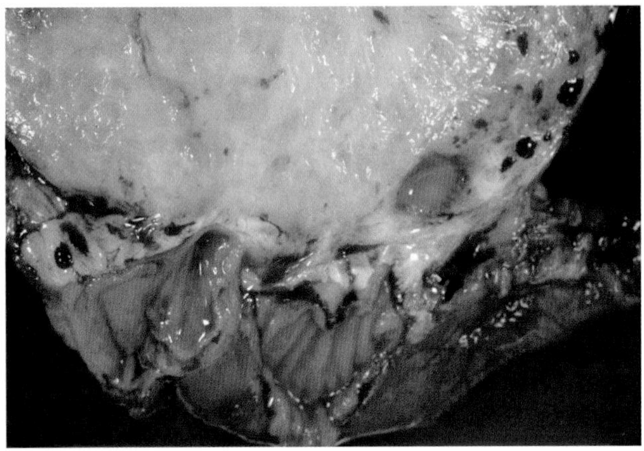

Fig. 10.17 Intraabdominal desmoid tumor. Gross specimen picture of a desmoid tumor involving the jejunal wall. Cut surface is grey white and has a characteristic fish flesh appearance. Mass is well circumscribed with partial infiltration into the intestinal wall.

The management of mesenteric fibromatosis is controversial. In sporadic cases the treatment of choice is resection and they frequently require the resection of the involved small and large bowel along with the mesenteric lesion. At surgery they often appear as a non-encapsulated fibrous mass with infiltrative margins. They may invade the bowel wall and they affect the mesenteric blood supply causing mucosal ulceration. In FAP a complete resection of the fibromatosis is often not possible without losing significant bowel function (Fig 10.19). In these cases, other non-surgical treatments should be considered including non-steroidal anti-inflammatory agents (sulindac), estrogen receptor antagonists, such as tamoxifen and teromifene, and chemotherapy with dactinomycin, vincristine, and cyclophosphamide. These treatments have been utilized, individually or in combinations, with variable degrees of success (Hansmann 2004). Though fibromatosis does not metastasize, it represents an important cause of death in patients with FAP due to its tendency for repeated recurrences.

Sclerosing mesenteritis

This is a rare idiopathic disorder that most commonly produces a stellate mass within the small bowel mesentery indistinguishable from metastatic disease. There are many synonyms in the literature for sclerosing mesenteritis: mesenteric panniculitis, retractile mesenteritis, mesenteric lipodystrophy, lipogranuloma of the mesentery, sclerosing lipogranulomatosis, primary

(a) 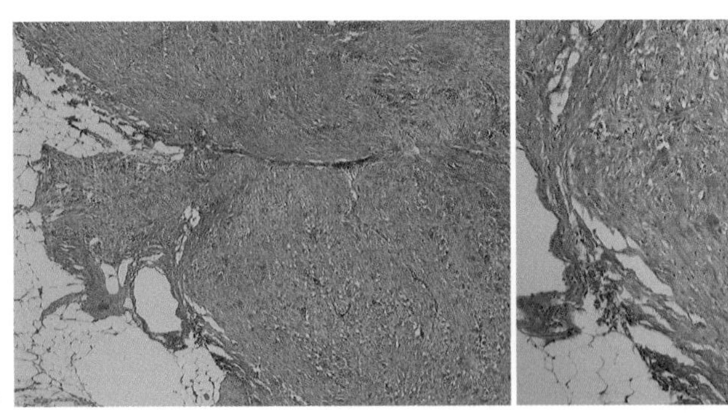 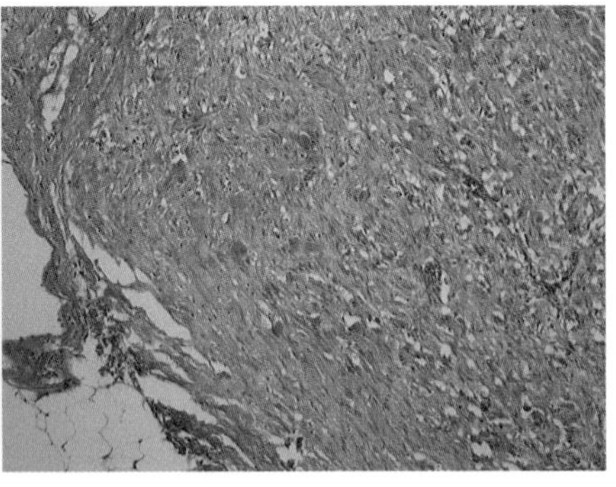 (b)

Fig. 10.18 Intraabdominal desmoid tumor (mesenteric fibromatosis). (a) Histopathology (H&E stain, ×40) shows a moderately cellular proliferation of spindle-shaped cells diffusely infiltrating the mesenteric adipose tissue. Photomicrograph (b) (H&E stain, ×100) shows extracellular collagen fibers separating individual cells with bland nuclei. Mitosis is occasional and necrosis is absent.

(a) 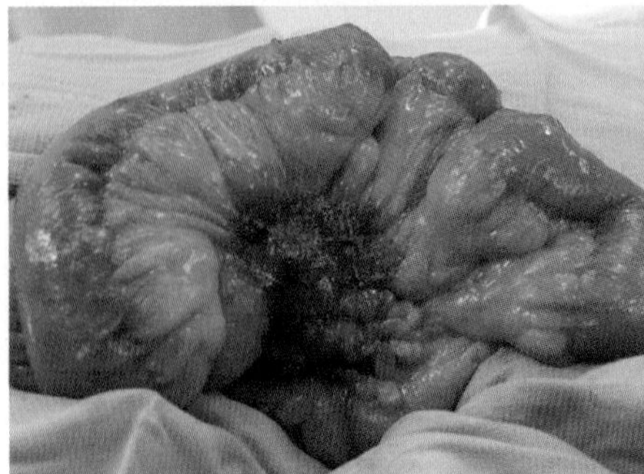 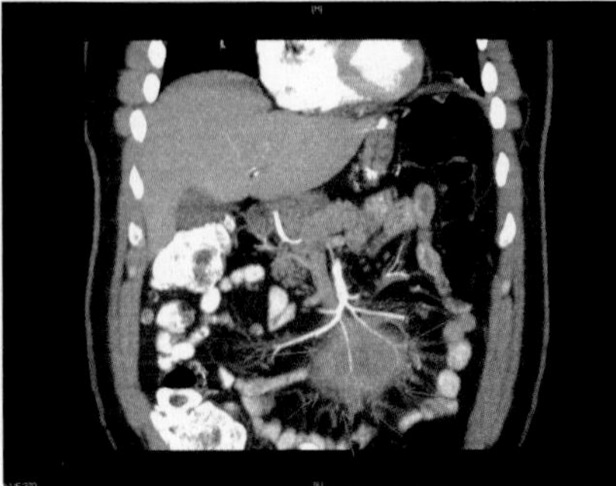 (b)

Fig. 10.19 (a) Gross picture of resected mesenteric desmoid tumor in a patient with Gardner's syndrome having multiple colonic polyps. The proximal jejunum is wrapped around the desmoid tumor. In this case the resection was possible since the main vessels were not involved.
(b) CT picture of same patient after 6 months of chemotherapy. Patient has necrosis of the desmoid tumor with jejunocolonic fistula. Notice the relation of the tumor to vessels. Besides a few jejunal branches there is no involvement of the inferior mesenteric artery or the distal jejunal branches.

liposclerosis of the mesentery, and multifocal subperitoneal sclerosis.

These lesions occur usually in older patients and they are more frequent in men (Kelly & Wei-Sek 1989). On histology (Fig. 10.20) they are difficult to distinguish from fibromatosis; one characteristic feature is that they never involve the intestinal wall. The clinical presentation is usually a palpable mass with gastrointestinal symptoms. On imaging, the CT frequently shows evidence of mesenteric shortening with angulation of the bowel and obstruction (Fig. 10.21). The most common differential diagnosis is with metastatic carcinoid. Somatostatin-receptor nuclear scintigram (with indium-111 pentetreotide) is often positive in carcinoid and negative in sclerosing mesenteritis. These lesions are frequently self-limited. Surgical resection is reserved for patients with complications. The use of immunosuppression and steroids is controversial.

Inflammatory myofibroblastic tumor

Inflammatory myofibroblastic tumor is extremely rare in the GI tract when compared to its pulmonary counterpart. This tumor in the past was more popularly known as plasma cell granuloma (Pettinato 1990) and inflammatory pseudotumor, and by various other names such as inflammatory myofibroblastic pseudotumor, extrapulmonary inflammatory pseudotumor, plasma cell pseudotumor, and inflammatory fibrosarcoma mainly due to the lack of understanding of the nature of the tumor. There have been isolated cases reported occurring in various parts of the GI tract and it can involve the peritoneum as well.

Inflammatory myofibroblastic tumor is more common in patients less than 20 years of age. They often present with intra-abdominal mass, fever, weight loss, polyclonal hypergammaglobulinemia and anemia, manifestations that often regress following removal of the mass (Day 1986).

On CT scans, inflammatory myofibroblastic tumor is a circumscribed, localized mass with heterogeneous attenuation. Involvement of adjacent bowel segments is rare.

Microscopically, it consists of myofibroblastic spindle cells arranged in a vaguely fascicular fashion admixed with rich inflammatory infiltrate composed predominantly of plasma cells and lymphocytes. Though most cases of inflammatory myofibroblastic tumor have a bland appearance and a favorable outcome following excision, there have been cases in which the myofibroblastic component has a more neoplastic appearance and a more aggressive clinical course including the development of metastasis (inflammatory fibrosarcoma). Because of this the more recent term inflammatory myofibroblastic tumor is preferred rather than plasma cell granuloma or inflammatory pseudotumor.

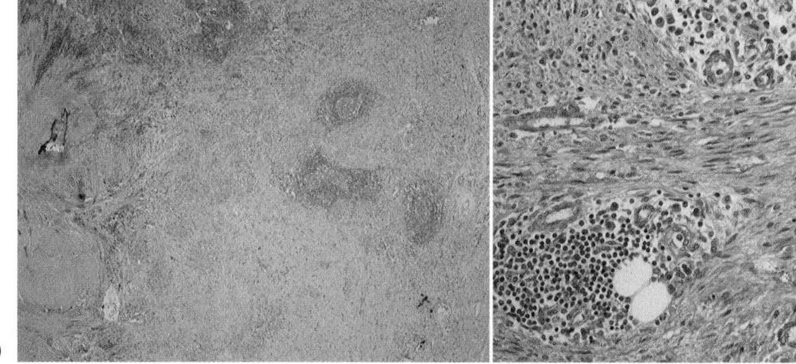
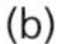

Fig. 10.20 Sclerosing mesenteritis. (a) Histopathology (H&E stain, ×40) shows a lesion composed of areas of fibrosis with collagen deposition; foci of calcifications may be seen occasionally as in this case. There is an intimate admixture of inflammatory cells with lymphoid aggregates. Photomicrograph (b) (H&E stain, ×100) shows a benign spindle cell proliferation along with a lymphoplasmacytic infiltrate with entrapped fat cells. (a) (b)

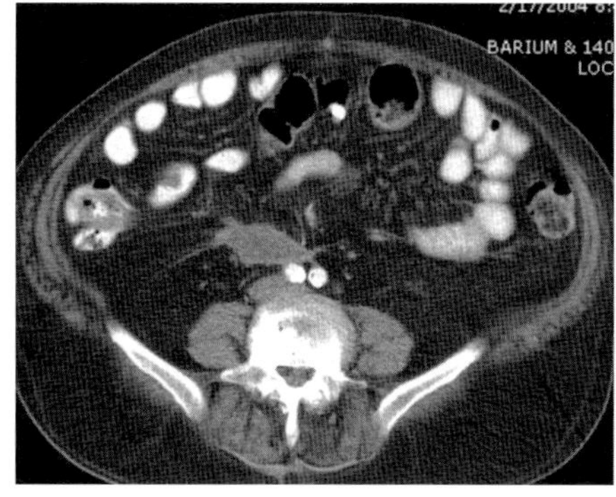

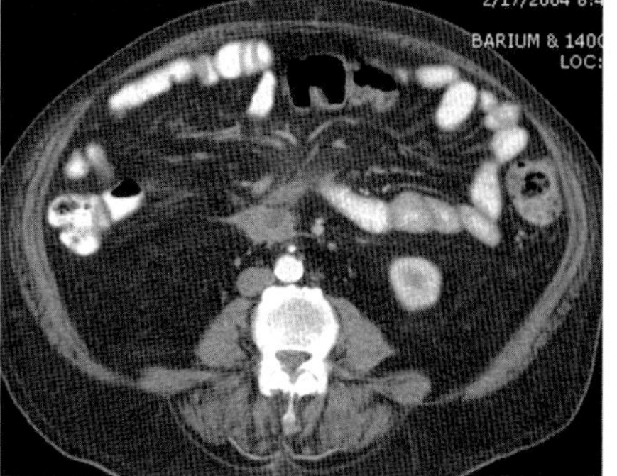

Fig. 10.21 (a,b) Sclerosing mesenteritis. A 62-year-old male with biopsy-proven sclerosing mesenteritis. The lesion presents as a spiculated mass with tethering at the edges. The traction can cause bowel obstruction. The lesion may shrink in size over time. (a) (b)

Extrapleural solitary fibrous tumor

This is a tumor of submesothelial origin that is identical to the solitary fibrous tumor of the pleura. When located in the mesentery or peritoneal cavity, this extrapleural solitary fibrous tumor has an imaging pattern that must be differentiated from metastatic disease, soft tissue sarcomas, and other benign and malignant neoplasms of the mesentery and peritoneum. On CT they appear as a well-circumscribed solitary solid and cystic mass. The diagnosis of benign fibrous tumors and tumor-like lesions of the mesentery should be considered during the preoperative evaluation of a mesenteric mass. They are spindle cell tumors on histology, with infrequent mitosis, and uncertain malignant potential. They are difficult to diagnose with a needle biopsy.

Malignant fibrous histiocytoma

The term malignant fibrous histiocytoma (MFH) was introduced by Weiss and Enzinger in 1978 for a group of tumors thought to arise from primitive mesenchymal cells that retain their histiocytic and fibrous potential. It commonly develops in the lower and upper extremities, reteroperitoneum and abdominal cavity, and has been reported in almost every site in the body . MFH affecting the GI tract is rare. Most cases have been reported in the colon. There have been isolated case reports of MFH affecting the esophagus, stomach and small bowel. Murata *et al.* (1993) reviewed 333 cases of MFH in the alimentary tract and half the cases occurred in the colon and rectum. Colonic MFH was initially described by Verma *et al.* in 1979 (Verma *et al.* 1979). Men are more commonly affected, with an average age of 55.7 years. Most colonic MFH occurred in the right side and most are large. Apart from presenting with symptoms related to GI tract these patients also present with fever, leucocytosis, and increased ESR. Histologically MFH is divided into four histologic types: storiform-pleomorphic, myxoid, giant cell type, and inflammatory type. The storiform-pleomorphic type is the most common type involving the colon. The prognosis of colonic MFH is poor. Surgical excision is usually the primary treatment modality in resectable lesions. Patients with metastatic and unresectable lesions (as most intra-abdominal lesions are) fare poorly and there is no evidence that chemotherapy given in the adjuvant or metastatic setting prolongs patient survival.

Fibrosarcoma

Fibrosarcomas are rare in the GI tract and histologically they resemble their peripheral counterparts with proliferation of spindle cells arranged in a herringbone pattern and intersecting fascicles. Most gastrointestinal cases reported in the literature have not had immunohistochemical studies performed. Surgical excision with good margins if possible is the treatment of choice.

References

Day DL, Sane S, Dehner LP. (1986) Inflammatory pseudotumor of the mesentery and small intestine. *Pediatr Radiol* 16: 210–15.

Enzinger FM, Weiss SW. (1988) *Soft Tissue Tumors.* CV Mosby, St. Louis.

Hansmann A, Adolph C, Vogel T, Unger A, Moeslein G. (2004) High-dose tamoxifen and sulindac as first-line treatment for desmoid tumors. *Cancer* 100(3): 612–20.

Hoehn JL, Hamilton GH, Beltaos E. (1980) Fibrosarcoma of the colon. *J Surg Oncol* 13: 223–26.

Kelly JK, Wei-Sek H. (1989) Idiopathic refractile (sclerosing) mesenteritis and its differential diagnosis. *Am J Surg Pathol* 13: 513–21.

Levy AD, Rimola J, Mehrotra AK, Sobin LH. (2006) From the archives of the AFIP: benign fibrous tumors and tumor like lesions of the mesentery: radiologic–pathologic correlation. *Radiographics* 26(1): 245–64.

Murata I, Makiyama K, Miyazaki K *et al.* (1993) A case of inflammatory malignant fibrous histiocytoma of the colon. *Gastroenterol Jpn* 28: 554–63.

Okuno S. (2006) The enigma of desmoid tumors. *Curr Treat Options Oncol* 7(6): 438–43.

Pettinato G, Manivel JC, De Rosa N, Dehner LP. (1990) Inflammatory myofibroblastic tumor (plasma cell granuloma). Clinicopathologic study of 20 cases with inmmunohistochemistry and ultrastructural observations. *Am J Clin Pathol* 94: 538–46.

Verma P, Chandra U, Bhatia PS. (1979) Malignant histiocytoma of the rectum: report of a case. *Dis Colon Rectum* 22: 179–82.

Mesothelial tumors

Anil R. Prasad, Malathy Kapali, Sanjay Saluja & Tomislav Dragovich

Mesothelial cysts (peritoneal inclusion cysts)

Mesothelial cysts can be unilocular or multilocular. These cysts predominantly occur in the peritoneal cavity of women of reproductive age though occasional cases have been reported in men (Michael *et al.* 1987).

The unilocular cysts form single or multiple small thin-walled translucent cysts that are either attached or lie free in the peritoneal cavity. Occasionally they involve the round ligament, simulating an inguinal hernia. Microscopically the cysts are lined by a single layer of flattened benign mesothelial cells. The unilocular mesothelial cysts are thought to be acquired cysts reactive in nature though some of these located in the mesocolon, retroperitoneum and splenic capsule may be developmental.

Multilocular peritoneal inclusion cysts (MPICs) have also been designated as cystic or multicystic benign mesothelioma, inflammatory cysts of the peritoneum or postoperative peritoneal cysts. There is often history of previous abdominal surgery, pelvic inflammatory disease or endometriosis (Roth 1973). MPICs are usually symptomatic with abdominal pain or palpable mass or both. Less often they are discovered incidentally at laparotomy or within hernial sac. Grossly, they appear as multilocular cysts 15–20 cm or more in diameter. They are usually attached to pelvic organs. The contents of the cyst can be serosanginous or bloody.

On histologic examination MPICs are lined by a single layer of flattened – cuboidal benign mesothelial cells. The lining cells can occasionally form small papillae and cribiform patterns. The septa between the cysts consist of loose fibrovascular sometimes abundant fibrous tissue.

Apart from the tendency for these lesions to recur (probably due to persistence of the original indicating factor) they behave in a benign fashion. Hence the term MPICs are preferred rather than benign cystic mesothelioma as there is no convincing evidence of a neoplastic nature.

Malignant mesotheliomas

Malignant peritoneal mesothelioma

Malignant peritoneal mesothelioma (MPM) is a relatively rare neoplasm of the abdominal and pelvic peritoneum strongly related to previous asbestos exposure. MPM represents approximately 15% of all mesotheliomas, but this figure varies in different studies from 3 to 50% (de Pangher Manzine 2005). Miller and Wynn in 1908 were the first to describe mesothelioma arising from the peritoneum. The DNA virus, Simian virus 40 (SV40), chronic inflammation, organic chemicals, irradiation, and genetic factors have been implicated as a cofactor in the causation of malignant mesothelioma. The overall annual incidence of malignant mesothelioma in the US is 15 cases per million habitants with the majority of cases presenting in the pleura, with only 200–400 cases of MPM per year (Lange 2004). In addition to the peritoneum it can affect other serosal cavities such as the pleura, the pericardium and the tunica vaginalis. It is more common in males than females, with a ratio of 5 : 1.

The clinical manifestations are usually non-specific and include increased abdominal girth, abdominal discomfort and weight loss. In some cases lympadenopathy due to metastatic disease can be the first manifestation of the disease. Ascites is present in the majority of cases. Thrombocytosis is present in up to 80% of patients; other frequent laboratory findings are anemia, hypoalbuminemia, and elevated erythrocyte sedimentation rate. Serum levels of mesothelin-related protein (SMRP), a soluble form of mesothelin, can be used as an adjuvant in the diagnosis of malignant mesothelioma. The SMRP level is elevated in 84% of patients with malignant mesothelioma and in less than 2% of patients with other pulmonary or pleural diseases. The elevation of SMRP may precede the clinical presentation of the disease by several years. Other serum markers frequently used but less specific are CA 15-3 and CA 125.

CT is the most useful imaging study (Fig 10.22a). There are three described CT manifestations. The 'dry painful' type is characterized by small multiple solid masses or one dominant abdominal mass localized in one quadrant of the abdomen. No ascites is seen. The second type is the 'wet' type, characterized predominantly by moderate to massive ascites associated with multiple small nodules studding the peritoneal surface. No dominant mass is seen. A third subtype shows mixed features of the above two types. In a lesion with a dominant nodule, CT-guided biopsy may be feasible to establish a diagnosis (Busch *et al.* 2002; Reuter *et al.* 1983). The solid nodules may show enhancement following contrast. The tumors may be present in any mesothelial surface either within the peritoneum or in the mesenteric folds. Mass effect on adjacent abdominal organs may be seen but the presence of visceral metastasis is infrequent. Pleural plaques are found in 20% of the patients. CT is crucial to surgical planning and staging. It can help identify organ involvement by the mass. The colon and liver are the two most involved abdominal organs, involved by local invasion. Colonic resection may be required at the time of debulking surgery. A recognized site for recurrence is the port for the trocar during laparoscopic surgery for initial diagnosis. Therefore the number of puncture sites should be limited (Hamrick-Turner *et al.* 1992). Positron emission tomography (PET) is useful in distinguishing between benign and malignant masses and establishing the extension of the tumor into the lymph nodes or other cavities.

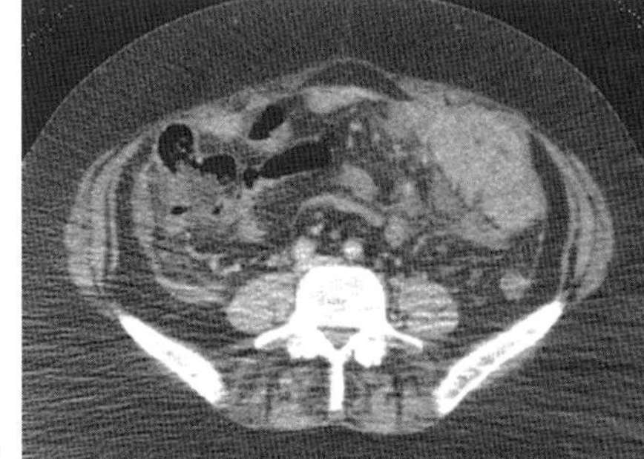
(a)

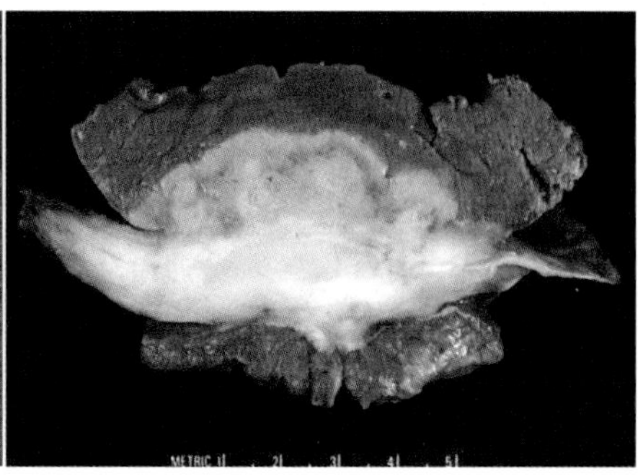
(b)

Fig. 10.22 Malignant mesothelioma of the peritoneum. (a) A large intensely enhancing aggressive-appearing mass in the anterior left abdominal cavity. There was some free intraperitoneal fluid on other slices (not shown). The lesion had completely infiltrated the omentum. (b) Gross specimen showing typical diffuse plaque-like lesion encasing the diaphragm involving liver and right parietal pleura and lower lobe of right lung.

Peritoneal cytology shows mesothelial cells and with the use of immunohistochemical markers it is possible to establish the diagnosis in 80% of cases. Occasionally peritoneal cytology is not diagnostic as it cannot differentiate between benign and malignant mesothelial cells. A diagnostic laparoscopy or laparotomy usually reveals the peritoneal and mesenteric implants. Robust biopsy samples may be obtained during this procedure to establish the definitive pathological diagnosis.

Grossly, visceral and parietal peritoneum can be diffusely thickened or extensively involved by multiple nodules or plaques. The adjacent viscera are often encased by tumor (Fig. 10.22b). Microscopically MPM can have a variety of appearances. The most common form is tubulopapillary with the tubules and papillae lined by atypical mesothelial cells (Fig. 10.23). In other instances they appear biphasic with mesothelial-like cells admixed with sarcomatoid spindle cells. The individual tumor cells retain some resemblance to mesothelial cells. They are fairly uniform with acidophilic or vacuolated cytoplasm. Nuclear atypicality varies from mild to moderate with variably prominent nucleoli. A rare morphologic variant of MPM occurs in an exclusive solid pattern of polygonal cells with abundant cytoplasm (decudoid MPMs). Though more common in young women it has been reported in both sexes and in association with asbestos exposure. In another rare variant 'lymphohistiocytic mesothelioma' the tumor contains prominent inflammatory infiltrate.

Well-differentiated papillary mesothelioma

Well-differentiated papillary mesotheliomas (WDPMs) are uncommon lesions, which show a great prediliction for women of reproductive age. Grossly, they appear as multiple gray white papillary or nodular lesions less than 2 cm in diameter. Microscopically, they are composed of fibrous papillae covered by a single layer of flattened to cuboidal mesothelial cells having bland nuclear features.

The overall prognosis of peritoneal mesothelioma is poor, with a median survival of 12 months at the time of diagnosis. The prognosis is worse in male patients and in patients with extensive disease and with poor performance status. Traditional chemotherapy combinations have shown poor responses (15–20%) in the treatment of malignant mesothelioma (O'Neal *et al.* 1989). Pemetrexed, a potent inhibitor of a number of proteins, including thymidylate synthase and dihydrofolate reductase, both of which are required for DNA synthesis, has shown effectiveness when combined with cisplatin in the treatment of pleural mesothelioma. A phase III multicenter study involving 448 patients treated with this combination showed an improvement of the median survival from 9 to 12 months (Reuter *et al.* 1983). The combination of gemcitabine and cisplatin showed objective responses of 33% and 48% in two studies with improvement in the quality of life and symptoms. Given the natural course and pattern of spread, important considerations have been given to the role of intraperitoneal chemotherapy. The most aggressive treatment protocols involve combination of cytoreductive surgery and intraperitoneal hyperthermic perfusion chemotherapy (IHPC). Some of the single-institution studies reported long-term survival in some patients, which justifies the further refinement of IHPC (Sugarbaker *et al.* 2006). Commonly used drugs for intraperitoneal administration are cisplatin (CDDP), mitomycin C (MMC) and doxorubicin. The rationale for using hyperthermic solution (40–42°C) is that hyperthermia generally increases sensitivity of cancer cells to chemotherapy. There is also evidence that hyperthermia increases formation of platinum–DNA adducts, thus resulting in an increased cell kill (Vaart *et al.* 1998). Some of the more recent series report increased survival with IHPC when compared to historical controls, and also excellent control of the ascites (Deraco *et al.* 2003). However, these results need to be interpreted with caution since most studies included patients with different histologies and were non-randomized trials, which introduce significant selection bias. In addition, this aggressive therapeutic approach requires a well-trained and skilled team which is currently available in very few medical institutions.

Though well-differentiated papillary mesothelioma for the most part behaves in an indolent fashion, recent studies have shown they it behave aggressively and hence should be treated as being potentially malignant.

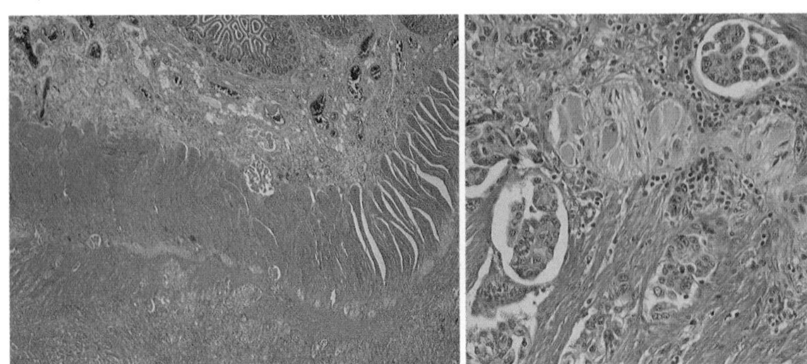

Fig. 10.23 Malignant peritoneal mesothelioma. Histopathology (H&E stain, ×20) of the tumor involving the serosal aspect as well as the muscle wall of the small intestine. Photomicrograph (b) shows tubulopapillary architecture of the tumor involving the bowel wall. Note normal intestinal wall myenteric nerve fibers with ganglion cells.

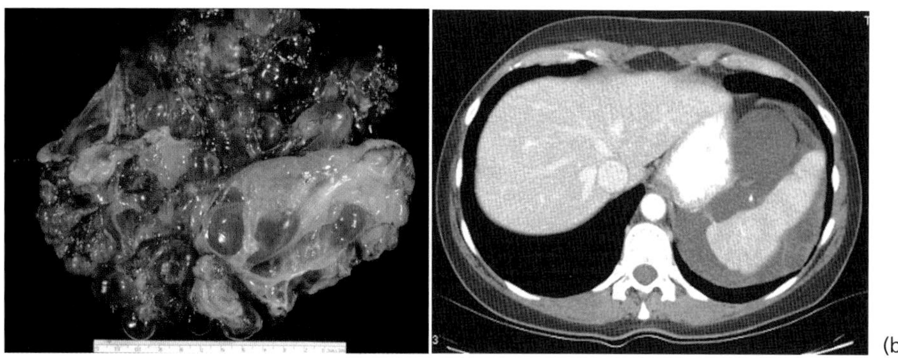

Fig. 10.24 Benign cystic mesothelioma of the peritoneum. (a) Gross specimen showing multiple serous fluid-filled cysts forming grape-like clusters. (b) A cystic multiloculated fluid collection with fine enhancing septations surrounding the spleen and extending into the gastrosplenic ligament. The lesion recurred locally despite multiple surgical excisions.

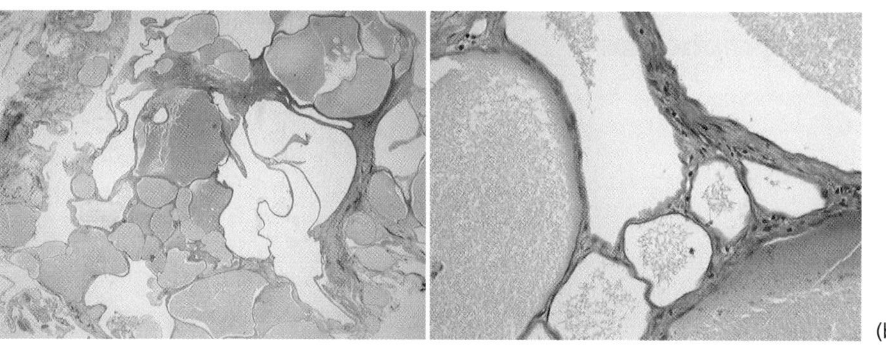

Fig. 10.25 Histopathology of benign cystic mesothelioma of the peritoneum. Photomicrograph (a) (H&E stain, ×20) shows a multicystic lesion containing pink serous fluid. (b) (H&E stain, ×200) shows the cyst lining composed of flattened benign mesothelial cells.

Cystic mesothelioma

This rare tumor is derived from the peritoneal mesothelium and is seen mostly in young and middle-aged females. The pelvic region is frequently involved. Cystic mesothelioma (CM) has a rare malignant potential, but recurs in 25–50% of cases. The lesion consists of multiple grapelike clusters (Fig. 10.24a) of single-lined mesothelial cysts separated by varying amounts of fibrous tissue (Fig. 10.25). The exact etiology of this disease is unknown but is presumed to be inflammatory with secondary mesothelial cell entrapment. Imaging is useful for initial diagnosis, preoperative planning, and postoperative follow-up of this lesion. Amongst the imaging modalities, CT scan is the most practical for routine issues. It reveals a thin-walled multicystic mass with several locules inside individual cysts containing water-density material. CT can also show the exact location of the cysts and their anatomic extension into planes between various intra-abdominal organs and sometimes even into the retroperitoneum (Fig. 10.24b). Ultrasound imaging typically shows the cyst and may be utilized if there is question as to whether the lesions are cystic or solid, but is limited as a modality in providing anatomic detail for surgical planning or follow-up. MRI is very sensitive to the fluid signal from the cyst contents but is of limited practical utility. For these reasons, CT is the most utilized modality (O'Neal *et al.* 1989).

The radiologic differential consists of other cystic lesions in the abdomen such as mesenteric/omental cysts, lymphangioma, pseudomyxoma peritonei, and cystic ovarian masses. Differentiation by CT alone between cystic mesothelioma and lymphangioma or pseudomyxoma peritonei may not be possible and histology is often necessary.

Occasionally, these tumors have an aggressive and recurrent behavior associated with significant abdominal distension and abdominal pain justifying a more radical tumor debulking and intraperitoneal chemotherapy (Sethna *et al.* 2003).

References

Busch JM, Kruskal JB, WUB. (2002) Best cases from the AFIP—malignant peritoneal mesothelioma. *Radiographics* 22: 1511–15.

de Pangher Manzine V. (2005) Malignant peritoneal mesothelioma. *Tumori* 91(1): 1–5.

Hamrick-Turner JE, Chiechi MV, Abbett PL, Ror PR. (1992) Neoplastic and inflammatory process of the peritoneum omentum and mesentery: diagnosis with CT. *Radiographics* 12: 1051–68.

Hanauske A-R. (2004) The role of Alimta in the treatment of malignant pleural mesothelioma: an overview of preclinical and clinical trials. *Lung Cancer* 45(Suppl 1): S121–4.

Lange JH. (2004) Re: 'Mesothelioma trends in the United States: an update based on surveillance, epidemiology and end results program data for 1973 through 2003'. *Am J Epidemiol* 160(8): 823.

Michael H, Stutton G, Rath LM (1987). Ovarian carcinoma with extracellular mucin production: reassessment of 'pseudomynoma ovarii et peritonei'. *Int J Gynecol Pathol* 6: 298–312.

O'Neal JD, Ross PR, Storm BL *et al.* (1989) Cystic mesothelioma of the peritoneum. *Radiology* 170: 333–7.

Reuter K, Raptapaulous V, Reele F *et al.* (1983) Diagnosis of peritoneal mesothelioma: computed tomography, sonography and fine needle aspiration biopsy. *AJR* 140: 1189–94.

Roth LM (1973). Endometriosis with perineural involvement. *Am J Clin Pathol* 59: 807–9.

Sethna K, Mohamed F, Marchettini P, Elias D, Sugarbaker PH. (2003) Peritoneal cystic mesothelioma. a case series. *Tumori* 89(1): 31–5.

Tomak S, Manegold C. (2004) Chemotherapy for malignant pleural mesothelioma: past results and recent developments. *Lung Cancer* 45(Suppl 1): S103–19.

Gastric lymphomas

Anil R. Prasad, Sanjay Saluja & Daniel O. Persky

Introduction

Primary gastric lymphomas represent about 5% of all gastric cancers, second in frequency after adenocarcinoma (Ferrucci & Zucca 2007). Lymphomas of the stomach are considered primary if the main bulk of disease is located at this site. They are non-Hodgkin's lymphomas (NHL), typically either diffuse large B-cell lymphomas (DLBCL) or extranodal marginal zone lymphomas of mucosa-associated lymphoid tissue (MZL). Follicular lymphomas and mantle cell lymphomas are less common in the stomach, the latter often presenting as multiple lymphomatous polyposis of the gastrointestinal tract. Primary Hodgkin's lymphoma is very rare in the gastrointestinal tract. DLBCL, an aggressive NHL subtype, represents about 60% of localized gastric lymphomas. A quarter of gastric DLBCL contains an MZL component, with DLBCL presumed to arise from MZL as a transformation. MZL is an indolent lymphoma that represents about 40% of gastric lymphomas. Follicular lymphoma, mantle cell lymphoma, and peripheral T-cell lymphomas account for less than 5% of primary gastric lymphoma incidence (Koch *et al.* 2005).

Clinical presentation

The symptoms of gastric lymphomas are non-specific, including dyspepsia, epigastric pain, nausea, anorexia, weight loss, and bleeding in up to 20–30% of patients at presentation. Diagnosis is usually via esophagogastroduodenoscopy (Fig. 10.26a), and should include a biopsy, preferably deep enough to include submucosa. DLBCLs sometimes present as significant submucosal nodules or masses and can be picked up by CT or PET scans (Fig.10.26b,c). Immunohistochemistry should be performed for B-cell markers and for *H. pylori.*

Gastric MZL is usually localized, with only 10–20% presenting at an advanced stage. It occurs predominantly in an older age group of patients with typical symptoms suggestive of gastritis or ulcer disease. The antrum is mainly affected, and the lymphoma is usually localized at diagnosis (stage IE or IIE). It rarely presents with systemic symptoms or bone marrow involvement, but may present with monoclonal gammopathy in up to a third of the patients. Overall, gastric MZL retains an excellent prognosis with an indolent course and an overall survival in excess of 80% at 10 years. Prognosis is more favorable than equivalent nodal disease.

Histopathology

The diagnosis of gastric lymphoma is not difficult when the lesion is high grade. Diagnostic problems in gastric lymphoma arise from distinguishing low-grade B-cell marginal zone lymphoma of mucosa-associated lymphoid tissue (MZL) from reactive lymphoid hyperplasia. In the past, many atypical lymphoid infiltrates within the gastric mucosa were interpreted as 'pseudolymphoma'. Isaacson and colleagues recognized that these lymphomas could be polymorphic, contain lymphoid

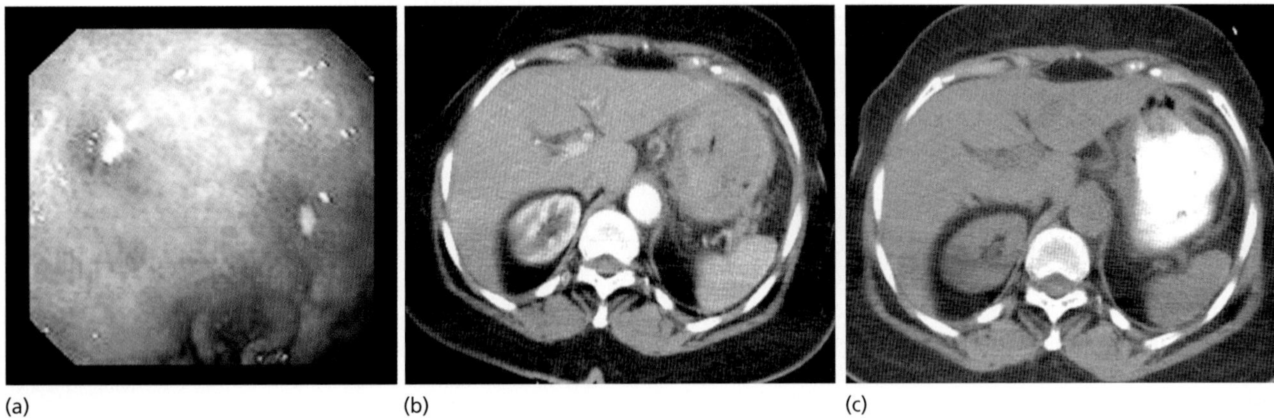

(a) (b) (c)

Fig. 10.26 (a) Endoscopic appearance of nodular mucosa of the stomach involved by MZL lymphoma. (b) Pretreatment CT shows diffusely thick-walled stomach involved by diffuse large B-cell lymphoma. (c) Post-treatment CT – note that the stomach walls are now normal in thickness.

follicles, and were diagnosable as lymphoma by demonstrating clonality by light chain restriction or gene rearrangement studies (Isaacson 1994; Isaacson *et al.* 1986). In fact, a retrospective review of cases that had previously been interpreted as pseudolymphoma of the stomach showed evidence of monoclonality in all (Isaacson *et al.* 1986).

MZL is characterized by a dense polymorphic lymphoid infiltrate, often accompanied by eosinophils and plasma cells. The lymphocytes resemble small, cleaved lymphocytes or monocytoid B-cells (Fig. 10.27a). These atypical lymphoid cells infiltrate the gastric epithelium to produce lymphoepithelial lesions, and ultimately destroy the epithelium (Fig. 10.27b). The diagnosis may be difficult purely on morphologic grounds and may require confirmatory ancillary studies that demonstrate clonality. The demonstration of light chain restriction by immunohistochemistry establishes the presence of a clonal proliferation. Characteristic immunophenotypic features of MZL extranodal lymphomas are as follows: CD20+, CD21+, CD35+ CD45+, bcl-2+, CD3–, CD5–, CD10–, and CD11c–.

Helicobacter pylori has been implicated in the etiology of MZL gastric lymphoma. The normal stomach does not contain lymphoid tissue. With *Helicobacter* infection, lymphoid tissue, including follicles with germinal centers, is recruited into the gastric mucosa and has been hypothesized to be the substrate on which gastric lymphoma may develop (Genta *et al.* 1993; Wotherspoon *et al.* 1993). Evidence of *Helicobacter* is present in over 90% of gastric MALT lymphoma cases and has been shown to precede the lymphoma (Parsonnet *et al.* 1994).

The stomach is commonly affected by diffuse large B-cell lymphomas which can be of germinal center or non-germinal center subtypes. DLBCL, germinal center subtypes are composed of diffuse infiltrates of large atypical lymphoid cells without lymphoepithelial lesions and plasma cells. Immunophenotypically they are CD20, CD79a, CD10, bcl-2, and bcl-6 positive, and negative for cytokeratin, CD3, and CD5 (Fig. 10.28). DLBCLs of non-germinal center subtype lack CD10, bcl-6 expression, but are positive for CD20, CD79a, CD45, and bcl-2.

Treatment

The majority of gastric MZL, particularly early-stage disease localized to the mucosa, is *H. pylori*-positive, and should be treated with antibiotic therapy. Several triple-therapy regimens exist, usually including antibiotics and a proton-pump inhibitor taken for 10–14 days. The regimens result in over 90% eradication of *H. pylori*, with approximately 60–80% complete remission (CR) rate in stage I disease (Fischbach *et al.* 2004; Nakamura *et al.* 2006). However, less than half of the patients maintain a molecular remission, making it unclear whether antibiotic therapy results in cure (Bertoni *et al.* 2002).

If the patient is still *H. pylori* positive on recheck esophagogastroduodenoscopy (EGD) at 3–6 months after treatment, triple therapy should be repeated. Submucosal invasion, translocation (11;18), and nuclear expression of bcl-10 predict for antibiotic resistance. In case of *H. pylori*-negative disease, an empiric course of triple therapy should still be considered as occasional responses have been seen (Nakamura *et al.* 2006; Raderer *et al.* 2006). If early-stage MZL is *H. pylori* negative or treatment resistant, 30 Gy of involved-field radiation therapy (IFRT) should be administered, as it resulted in disease-free survival of 77% and overall survival of 98% at 5 years in the largest retrospective series (Tsang *et al.* 2003). Radiation is preferred over surgery, which causes more morbidity and should be used very selectively (Koch *et al.* 2005).

If early-stage MZL recurs or is resistant to *H. pylori* treatment and to IFRT, it can be treated according to the same paradigm as advanced-stage disease. As with any indolent lymphoma in advanced stages, initial observation would be appropriate. Upon meeting criteria for treatment initiation (such as criteria used for follicular lymphoma; Brice *et al.* 1997), systemic therapy may be initiated. Four weekly doses of rituximab, a monoclonal antibody against CD20, resulted in 42–46% complete remission rate in studies of patients refractory to prior therapy, with longer duration of response in patients with fewer prior therapies (Martinelli *et al.* 2005). As a systemic treatment with fewest side effects, rituximab should be considered one of the first treatment options and may be used in combination regimens. Other treatment choices include oral daily chlorambucil or cyclophosphamide (75% CR, with about 50% still in CR at mean follow-up of 45 months) (Hammel *et al.* 1995), purine analogs such as fludarabine and cladribine (Zinzani *et al.* 2004), and combination chemotherapy such as CVP (cyclophosphamide, vincristine, and prednisone) or FM (fludarabine and mitoxantrone) (Zinzani *et al.* 2004). Anthracy-

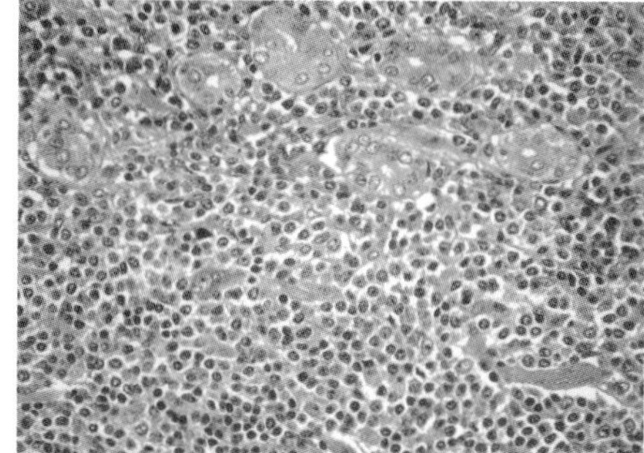
(a)

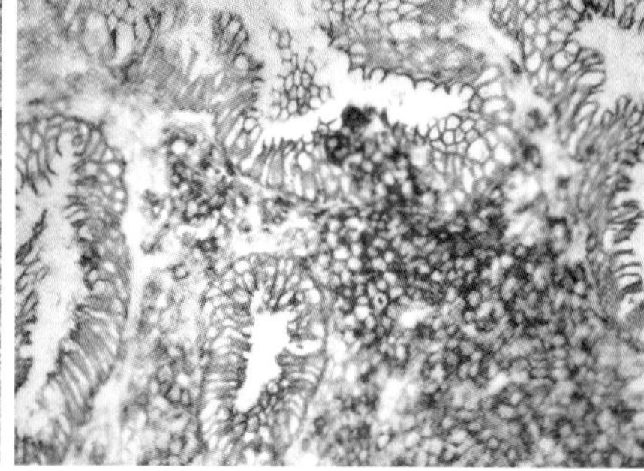
(b)

Fig. 10.27 (a) H&E photomicrograph (×100) shows diffuse small lymphocytic infiltrate involving gastric mucosa with lymphoepithelial lesions. (b) Cocktail CD20 (blue chromagen) and cytokeratin (brown chromagen) immunohistochemical stain, (×200), highlights the presence of lymphoepithelial lesions.

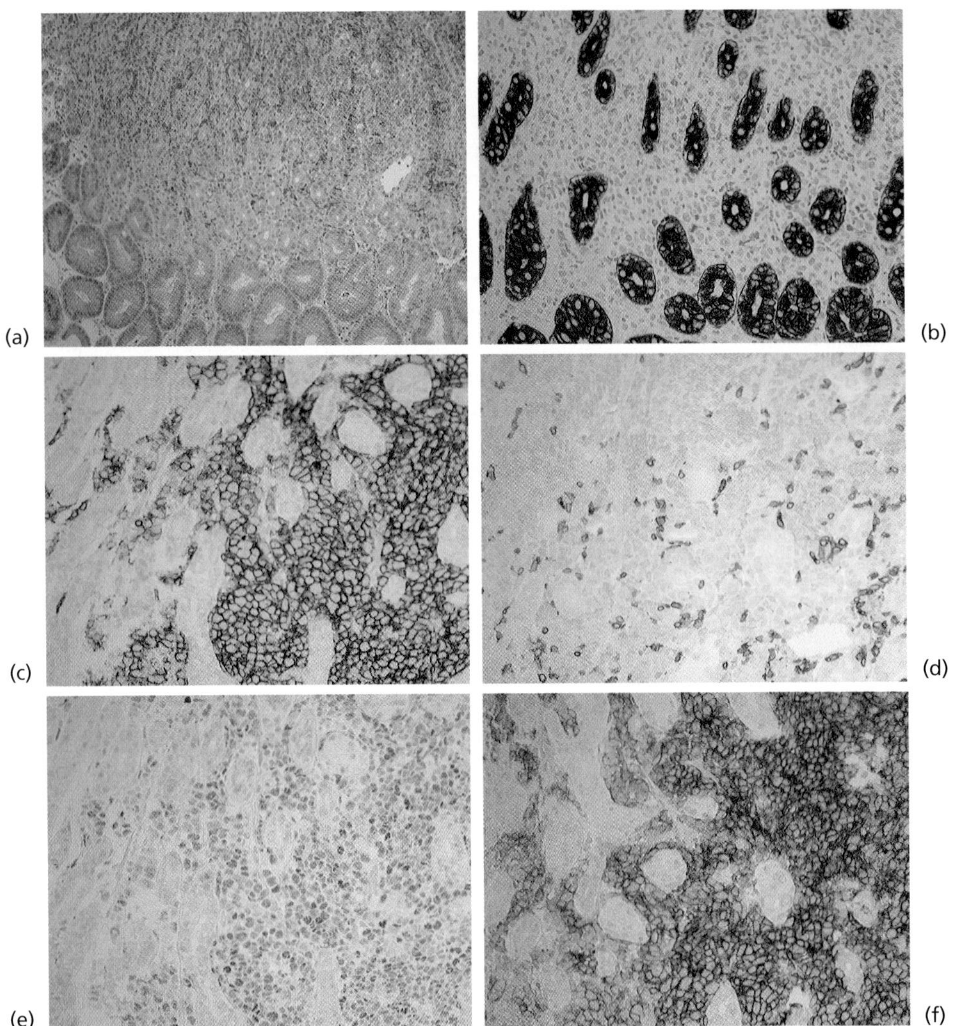

Fig. 10.28 (a) H&E photomicrograph (×200) shows diffuse large B-cell lymphoma, germinal cell subtype. Neoplastic lymphoid cells are (b) cytokeratin negative, native gastric glands stain positively. In contrast to the negative staining gastric glands, neoplastic lymphoid cells are (c) CD 20 positive, (d) CD 3 negative (e) CD 10 positive and (f) bcl-2 positive.

cline-containing regimens such as CHOP (cyclophosphamide, doxorubicin, vincristine, and prednisone) should be reserved for transformed or possibly bulky disease.

Gastric DLBCL is treated along the same paradigm as nodal DLBCL, particularly after a subgroup analysis of a large study showed that their survivals are similar (Salles *et al.* 1991). Early-stage gastric DLBCL is usually treated with 3–4 cycles of anthracycline-containing chemotherapy such as CHOP combined with rituximab, followed closely by 40 Gy of IFRT (Miller *et al.* 2004). Advanced-stage gastric DLBCL is treated with 6–8 cycles of CHOP combined with rituximab (Miller *et al.* 2004). The treatment of follicular lymphoma, mantle cell lymphoma, and peripheral T-cell lymphomas of the stomach is the same as that of the nodal disease.

References

Bertoni F, Conconi A, Capella C *et al.* (2002) Molecular follow-up in gastric mucosa-associated lymphoid tissue lymphomas: early analysis of the LY03 cooperative trial. *Blood* 99(7): 2541–4.

Brice P, Bastion Y, Lepage E *et al.* (1997) Comparison in low-tumor-burden follicular lymphomas between an initial no-treatment policy, prednimustine, or interferon alfa: a randomized study from the Groupe d'Etude des Lymphomes Folliculaires. Groupe d'Etude des Lymphomes de l'Adulte. *J Clin Oncol* 15(3): 1110–17.

Ferrucci PF, Zucca E. (2007) Primary gastric lymphoma pathogenesis and treatment: what has changed over the past 10 years? *Br J Haematol* 136(4): 521–38.

Fischbach W, Goebeler-Kolve ME, Dragosics B, Greiner A, Stolte M. (2004) Long term outcome of patients with gastric marginal zone B cell lymphoma of mucosa-associated lymphoid tissue (MALT) following exclusive *Helicobacter pylori* eradication therapy: experience from a large prospective series. *Gut* 53(1): 34–37.

Genta RM, Hamner HW, Graham DY. (1993) Gastric lymphoid follicles in *Helicobacter pylori* infection: frequency, distribution and response to triple therapy. *Hum Pathol* 24: 577–83.

Hammel P, Haioun C, Chaumette MT *et al.* (1995) Efficacy of single-agent chemotherapy in low-grade B-cell mucosa-associated lymphoid tissue lymphoma with prominent gastric expression. *J Clin Oncol* 13(10): 2524–9.

Isaacson P. (1994) Gastrointestinal lymphoma. *Hum Pathol* 25: 1020–9.

Isaacson PG, Spencer J, Finn T. (1986) Primary B-cell gastric lymphoma. *Hum Pathol* 17: 72–82.

Koch P, Probst A, Berdel WE *et al.* (2005) Treatment results in localized primary gastric lymphoma: data of patients registered within the German multicenter study (GIT NHL 02/96). *J Clin Oncol* 23(28): 7050–9.

Martinelli G, Laszlo D, Ferreri AJ *et al.* (2005) Clinical activity of rituximab in gastric marginal zone non-Hodgkin's lymphoma resistant to or not eligible for anti-Helicobacter pylori therapy. *J Clin Oncol* 23(9): 1979–83.

Miller TP, Unger JM, Spier C *et al.* (2004) Effect of adding rituximab to three cycles of CHOP plus involved-field radiotherapy for limited-stage aggressive diffuse B-cell lymphoma (SWOG-0014). *Blood* 104(11): 158a.

Nakamura S, Matsumoto T, Ye H *et al.* (2006) Helicobacter pylori-negative gastric mucosa-associated lymphoid tissue lymphoma: a clinicopathologic and molecular study with reference to antibiotic treatment. *Cancer* 107(12): 2770–8.

Parsonnet J, Hansen S, Rodriguez L *et al.* (1994) *Helicobacter pylori* infection and gastric lymphoma. *N Engl J Med* 330: 1267–71.

Raderer M, Streubel B, Wohrer S, Hafner M, Chott A. (2006) Successful antibiotic treatment of Helicobacter pylori negative gastric mucosa associated lymphoid tissue lymphomas. *Gut* 55(5): 616–18.

Salles G, Herbrecht R, Tilly H *et al.* (1991)Aggressive primary gastrointestinal lymphomas: review of 91 patients treated with the LNH-84 regimen. A study of the Groupe d'Etude des Lymphomes Agressifs. *Am J Med* 90(1): 77–84.

Tsang RW, Gospodarowicz MK, Pintilie M *et al.* (2003) Localized mucosa-associated lymphoid tissue lymphoma treated with radiation therapy has excellent clinical outcome. *J Clin Oncol* 21(22): 4157–64.

Wotherspoon AC, Doglioni C, Diss TC, Pan L *et al.* (1993) Regression of primary low-grade B-cell gastric lymphoma of mucosa-associated lymphoid tissue type after eradication of Helicobacter pylori. *Lancet* 342: 575–7.

Zinzani PL, Stefoni V, Musuraca G *et al.* (2004) Fludarabine-containing chemotherapy as frontline treatment of non-gastrointestinal mucosa-associated lymphoid tissue lymphoma. *Cancer* 100(10): 2190–4.

Rare miscellaneous tumors and tumor-like lesions

Anil R. Prasad, John Fetsch, Sanjay Saluja & Tomislav Dragovich

Fibrovascular polyp of the esophagus

This rare intraluminal tumor of the esophagus has been described by various names including angiofibrolipoma, myxoma, fibrolipoma, pedunculated lipoma, fibroma, and benign fibroepithelial polyp. Fibrovascular polyps of the esophagus are usually located in the upper one-third of the esophagus. Surprisingly, these tumors cause very little discomfort in spite of their large size. Occasionally they present with dysphagia, or regurgitation and rarely anemia. Regurgitation of the tumor has led to death in some patients due to laryngeal obstruction (Fries *et al.* 2003).

Fibrovascular polyp of the esophagus is usually seen in adult males. It characteristically causes a large polypoid intraluminal filling defect on barium swallow. It is often detected easily by endoscopy but tends to be missed sometimes as it is covered by an intact squamous mucosa.

Pathologically, the lesion is typically very large, pedunculated and covered by an intact smooth mucosal surface that can be focally ulcerated. Histologically, the tumor is composed of proliferating fibrous tissue (that often appears myxoid), adipose tissue and blood vessels in various proportions. This proliferation of fat, fibrous tissue and vessels expands and obliterates the lamina propria. Inflammation is minimal. The tumor is characteristically covered by a squamous mucosa that can be acanthotic.

Excision of fibrovascular polyp should be strongly considered in all cases. Due to the highly vascular nature of the tumor, caution is advised if one is considering removal through an endoscope.

Gastric xanthoma

Xanthomas are tumorous masses characterized by collections of foamy histiocytes, which accumulate free and esterified cholesterol, phospholipids and triglycerides. Xanthomas are associated with familial hyperlipidemias, acquired hyperlipidemic disorders and certain malignancies, but may arise without an underlying disorder. They are most commonly encountered in the subepithelial connective tissue of the skin and in tendons, but also occur in deep visceral organs. The entire gastrointestinal tract may be involved, but especially the stomach.

Gastric xanthoma is a well-recognized entity often encountered incidentally by endoscopists (Zafarni *et al.* 1980). It is asymptomatic and probably of little clinical significance. It appears to be more frequent, however, in patients with previous partial gastrectomy. It is more common in men (male: female ratio 3 : 2) and in the elderly, with a peak in the seventh decade of life. It is extremely rare in persons under 30 years. Typically, the lesions appear as yellow or white macules, slightly raised plaques or nodules. Occasional papillary configurations have been described. They vary between 0.5 and 3 mm in size. Very small lesions may be overlooked, and careful scrutiny of the stomach is required to detect them. This may partially explain the marked variability in the lesion's reported prevalence. They are multiple in more than two-thirds of reported cases, often located in the fundic region of the stomach.

Histologically, gastric xanthomas are characterized by the accumulation of foamy cells in the lamina propria. Very small lesions may be overlooked on H&E-stained sections. Chemical analysis has demonstrated these lesions to contain esterified cholesterol in all cases and triglycerides in 37% of cases. Stains for lipid are therefore always positive if performed on fresh-frozen tissue samples. Several morphologic features make gastric xanthoma prone to be initially misdiagnosed as early adenocarcinoma, particularly the signet-ring cell type (Drude *et al.* 1982). Unlike most signet-ring cell carcinomas, xanthomas are negative for mucicarmine, Alcian blue and PAS stains.

The cause of gastric xanthoma is not clear but they are often associated with chronic gastritis and are three times more common in stomachs with intestinal metaplasia. Intestinalized gastric mucosa is known to absorb fat, and this may play a role in the development of gastric xanthomas.

The natural history of gastric xanthoma is not well documented. Reduction in size and disappearance has been reported in many instances without intervention.

Adenoid cystic carcinoma of the esophagus

Adenoid cystic carcinomas constitute 0.75–5% of all esophageal carcinomas. These aggressive esophageal neoplasms that resemble their counterparts in salivary glands have a poor prognosis. They have a high rate of distant metastases at the time of diagnosis. Patients often present with progressive dysphagia and obstruction. Men are affected more frequently, with an average age of 65 years and a male : female ratio of 3 : 1.

Adenoid cystic carcinomas usually arise in the middle third of the esophagus (63%). Grossly, fungating or polypoid lesions occur most commonly. Similar to the histology of salivary gland tumors, there are two main cell types: duct-lining epithelial cells and myoepithelial cells. Microscopically, the tumor has expansile or infiltrating margins with tubular, cribriform, solid, or basaloid patterns. Hyalinized matrix is prominent. Esophageal tumors tend to show marked cellular pleomorphism and a higher mitotic index than those arising in salivary glands.

Wide surgical resection with negative margins is the standard primary therapy. Adjuvant radiation therapy is usually indicated for most tumors. Primary conventional radiotherapy has never been shown to provide sufficient local disease control. However, there are some data recently which suggest that neutron therapy, which involves larger particles of greater energy, can achieve reasonable local control (Prott *et al.* 1996). Adoptive immunotherapy in combination with chemoradiation therapy has shown promising results.

Developmental cysts

Based on morphology, developmental cysts are classified into epidermoid cysts, dermoid cysts, enteric or rectal duplication cysts, retrorectal cystic hamartomas, and cystic teratomas. Epidermoid and dermoid cysts are usually unilocular and are lined by stratified squamous epithelium. Dermal appendages are present in dermoid cysts, but not in epidermoid cysts. Duplication cysts are also unilocular and are lined by epithelium similar to epithelium of the gastrointestinal and respiratory tracts. The epithelium, often with villi, crypts, and glands, simulates the normal mucosa of the gut. The main distinctive feature is a well-formed muscular wall with two layers of muscle bundles containing nerve plexuses in between them. Anomalous lumen formation probably causes duplication cysts (Fig. 10.20). Some of these cysts communicate with the gut lumen. The rectal duplication cysts is recognized by the presence of a well-developed outer vascular layer recapitulating the muscularis propria of the bowel.

Developmental cysts in the retrorectal space are prone to infection and fistula and associated malignancy has been rarely reported. Therefore, total excision is recommended.

Retrorectal cystic hamartomas or tailgut cysts are rare congenital lesions that typically present as presacral masses (Hjermstad & Helwig 1988). They are usually multicystic or multilocated. The cysts are lined by a wide variety of epithelia which varies from cyst to cyst or even within the same cyst (Fig. 10.30): stratified squamous, transitional, stratified columnar, mucinous or ciliated columnar, ciliated pseudostratified columnar and gastric type (Prasad 2000). The cyst wall in most of the cases contain focal well-formed smooth muscle fibers. However, the muscle bundles are often disorganized and are present focally unlike the well-formed continuous two-layer muscle coat seen in duplication cysts. Theoretically, retrorectal cystic hamartomas can be classified as teratomas. They possess all three germ layers: ectoderm (squamous), endoderm (intestinal-type epithelium), and mesoderm (smooth muscle and fibrous tissue). However, the term teratoma should be reserved for cases with dermal appendages, neural elements, or other heterologous mesenchymal derivatives such as cartilage and bone.

Tailgut cysts or retrorectal cystic hamartomas are frequently clinically unrecognized and misdiagnosed. Malignant change as a rare complication has been occasionally documented (Hood *et al.* 1988; Prasad *et al.* 2000). These lesions require complete

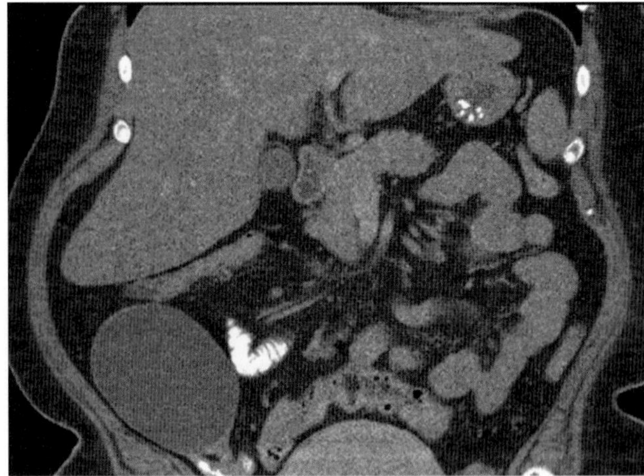

Fig. 10.29 Duplication cyst. A 34-year-old female presented with right lower quadrant abdominal pain. CT scan shows a 5-cm ovoid cyst adjacent to the cecum in the root of the mesentery. Findings are suggestive of a duplication cyst.

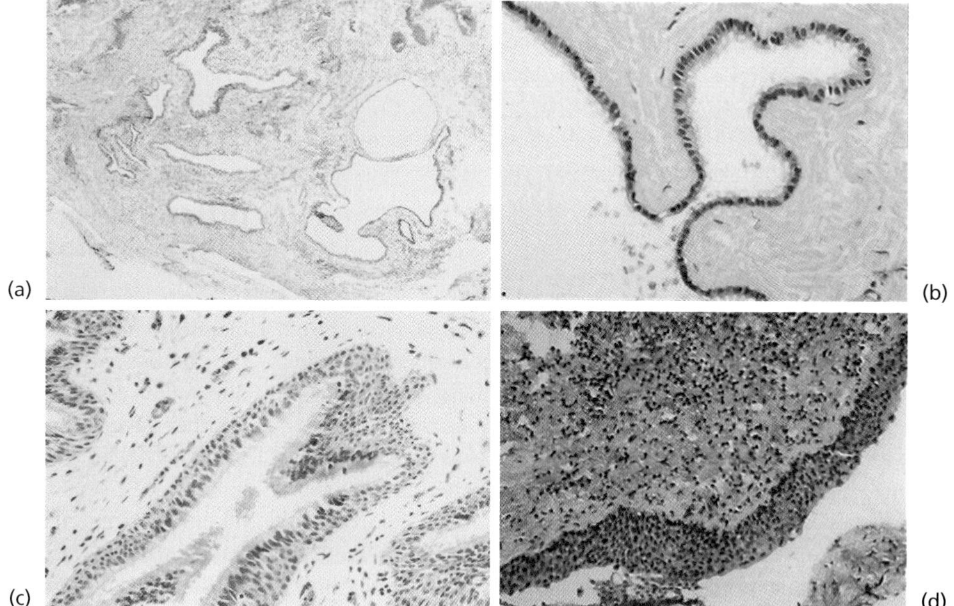

Fig. 10.30 Histopathology of retrorectal cystic hamartoma (tailgut cyst). (a) (H&E stain, ×20) shows a multicystic lesion composed of various cyst linings. (b–d) (H&E stain, ×100) show cuboidal epithelium, pseudostratified ciliated columnar epithelium, and transitional epithelium, respectively.

surgical excisions to prevent future recurrences and to preclude possible malignant transformation. The malignancies most commonly encountered in these lesions are neuroendocrine carcinomas and adenocarcinomas (Prasad *et al.* 2000) (Fig. 10.31).

Sacrococcygeal teratoma involving the retrorectal space must be distinguished from other developmental cysts. Sacrococcygeal teratomas typically occur in children, are multicystic, and contain elements of all three germ layers.

Malakoplakia of colon

Malakoplakia is a rare granulomatous disease that usually involves the urinary bladder (Long & Althausen 1989); however the colon is the commonest site of involvement after the urogenital tract. Patients with colonic malakoplakia range in age from 6 weeks to 88 years and have an equal sex distribution. This disease is seldom diagnosed clinically and is almost always detected upon pathological examination of resected tissue. The GI tract, especially the colon, is particularly affected in children (Chaudhry *et al.* 1979). Adults present with rectal bleeding, diarrhea, and abdominal pain. Patients with extensive disease experience intractable diarrhea, bowel obstruction, ulcers, fistulae, and even death. Children present with fever, failure to thrive, bloody diarrhea, and malnutrition. Endoscopically, gastrointestinal malakoplakia assumes three gross forms: unifocal lesions, widespread mucosal multinodular lesions, and large mass lesions.

Within the colon, the rectosigmoid and cecum are most commonly affected. Lesions may appear flat, yellowish-tan plaques or raised, tan-gray nodules. Overlying mucosa appears intact.

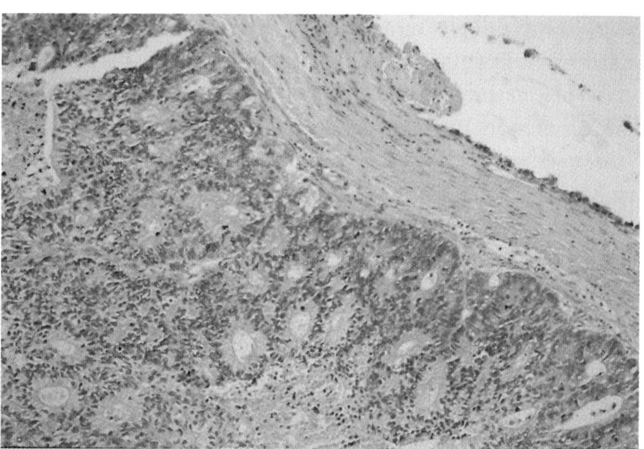

Fig. 10.31 Histopathology of adenocarcinoma arising in a retrorectal cystic hamartoma. The tumor (H&E stain, ×200) is a moderately differentiated tubular gland forming adenocarcinoma with necrosis arising within the wall of a retrorectal cystic hamartoma (tailgut cyst).

These lesions may mimic tumors and can appear polypoid or may even cause perforation and fistula formation. Histologic examination reveals the presence of numerous histiocytic granular cells with eosinophilic cytoplasm, called von Hansemann's cells. Ultrastructurally, the histiocytes contain giant polyphagolysosomes containing various forms of mineralized debris and partially digested bacteria. The presence of characteristic intracellular and extracellular Michaelis–Gutmann bodies clinches the diagnosis. Michaelis–Gutmann bodies vary in size from 2 to 6 mm and have a round, dense, or targetoid appearance due to the presence of concentric laminations. These stain blue with hematoxylin and are highlighted with the Von Kossa stain for calcium or with iron stains. Malakoplakia tends to be associated with adenomas and carcinomas; hence the tissues should be carefully evaluated for the presence of these neoplastic conditions (Chaudhry *et al.* 1979).

Surgical resection is usually curative in limited disease.

Rhabdomyosarcoma of the gastrointestinal tract

Rhabdomyosarcoma (RMSs) are highly aggressive soft tissue sarcomas differentiating toward smooth muscle. Most cases of rhabdomyosarcoma of the GI tract represent metastatic disease with primary involvement being rare. RMS has been reported affecting every part of the GI tract and most tumors in the upper GI tract have been isolated case reports. They can occur in children as well as adults. Reteroperitoneal RMS is limited mainly to infants and children. As with other sites, embryonal RMS is the predominant subtype encountered in the retroperitoneum. Apart from occurring as a separate entity rhabdomyomatous differentiation can form a component of other tumors like carcinosarcomas. The diagnosis of RMS is based on the identification of pleomorphic cells with marked nuclear atypia and strap cells with eosinophilic cytoplasm (Fig. 10.32). Cross striations are present and myoglobin positivity as evidence of striated muscle origin is seen.

Despite their aggressive behavior rhabdomyosarcomas are very responsive to cytotoxic therapy. The cure rate with multimodality treatment approaches 70%. The standard first-line induction chemotherapy regimen is vincristine–adriamycin–cisplatin (VAC) (Crist *et al.* 2001, 1995). Current investigational approaches focus on chemotherapy intensification and integration of newer drugs such as topoisomerase I inhibitors (Pappo *et al.* 2002). Other investigational drugs of interest include CpG oligopeptides (Weigel *et al.* 2003), tumor-specific peptide vaccines (Dagher *et al.* 2002) and pro-apoptotic peptides.

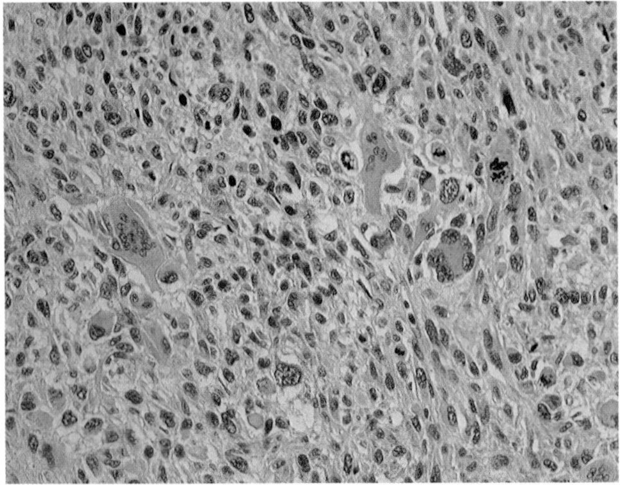

Fig. 10.32 Histopathology of rhabdomyosarcoma of the colon. Tumor is composed of bizarre, pleomorphic cells with abundant eosinophilic cytoplasm (strap cells) and multinucleate giant cells. Note the presence of numerous atypical mitotic figures (H&E stain, ×400).

Inflammatory fibroid polyp of the gastrointestinal tract

Inflammatory fibroid polyps are benign tumor masses that mainly occur in the small intestine (usually ileum) followed by the stomach and large intestine (Shimer & Helwig 1984). These uncommon lesions occur at all ages. Their cause is unknown, but they have been reported in pouches or the terminal ileum in patients with ulcerative colitis and Crohn's disease. These lesions have been described under various names such as eosinophilic granuloma, submucosal fibroma, hemangiopericytoma, inflammatory pseudotumor.

Clinical symptoms include episodic abdominal pain, vomiting, blood in the stool, diarrhea, constipation, abdominal distention, and weight loss. The vast majority of lesions are noted in the small intestine (mainly in the ileum); however, they can occur less commonly in the colon. The lesions are polypoid and mainly submucosal, and range in size from 1.5 to 13 cm (average, 3.0–4.0 cm). Occasionally these polyps may infiltrate into the muscularis propria and serosa. On cut surface they tend to be tan-gray and the overlying mucosa is usually focally eroded or ulcerated. Microscopic examination reveals a 'fibrocytic'-like lesion in a loose vascular stroma along with an inflammatory infiltrate. The stroma appears loose and myxoid, especially around vessels. The stroma is composed of stellate and spindle-shaped fibroblasts with indistinct basophilic cytoplasm (Fig. 10.33). Eosinophils, lmphocytes, plasma cells, macrophages, and mast cells are noted. Eosinophils are frequent and may form dense aggregates. It is notoriously difficult to diagnose inflammatory fibroid polyps in small endoscopic biopsies, as all one usually sees is ulcerated epithelium with what appears like granulation tissue underneath.

This lesion must be distinguished from malignant mesenchymal tumors as sometimes brisk mitosis is present within these benign polyps and an infiltrative pattern with dissection between the muscle fibers is also seen. Immunohistochemistry shows a heterogenous lesion derived from myofibroblasts, histiocytes or fibroblasts.

Inflammatory fibroid polyps are benign, and surgical resection is curative.

Small cell carcinoma of the colon

Small cell carcinoma (SCC) is a rare large intestinal tumor that is more prevalent in Japan than in the US. Patients range in age from 38 to 74 years, with a mean of 65 years. SCC mainly arises in the right colon. Patients are usually asymptomatic or may complain of crampy abdominal pain, malaise, weight loss, fever,

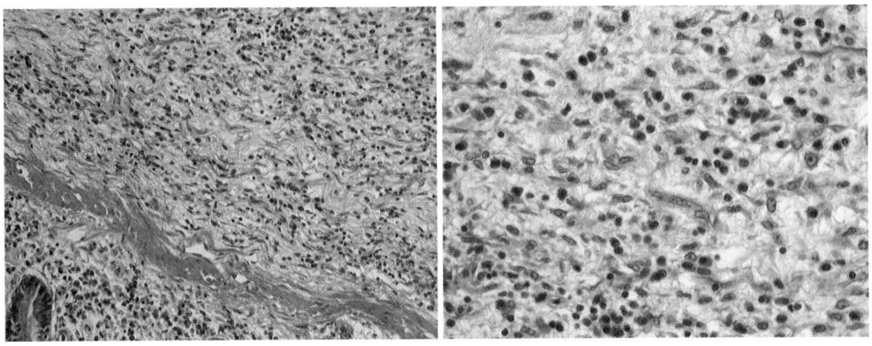

(a) (b)

Fig. 10.33 (a,b) Histopathology of inflammatory fibroid polyp of the stomach. The lesion is composed of slender stellate to spindled cells with features of fibroblasts admixed with numerous eosinophils and macrophages (a, H&E stain, ×40; b, H&E stain, ×200).

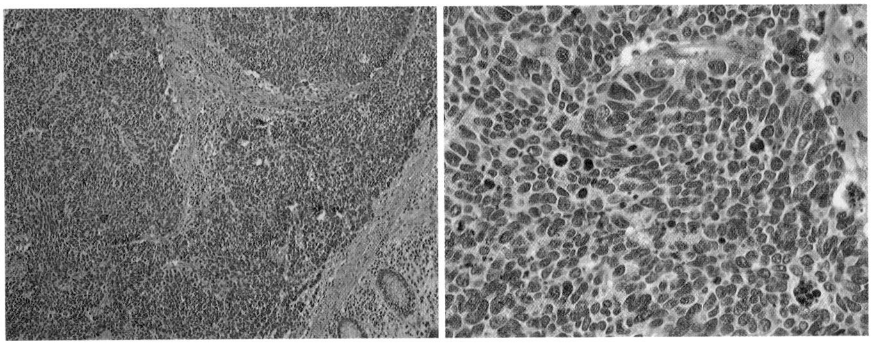

(a) (b)

Fig. 10.34 Histopathology of small cell carcinoma of the colon. (a) (H&E stain, ×40) A small blue cell tumor involving the colon. (b) (H&E stain, ×200) Typical small cell carcinoma cells with fine nuclear granular 'salt & pepper' chromatin, abundant mitoses and apoptotic figures. Nuclear moulding is present.

diarrhea, and rectal bleeding. At the time of surgery almost all patients have metastases in the regional lymph nodes and the liver. Seventy-one per cent of tumors metastasize to the liver; 64% of patients are dead at 5 months. Even after aggressive treatment, patients die between 3 and 12 months following diagnosis. CT scan shows submucosal thickening or intraluminal polypoid masses.

The tumors are usually bulky and polypoid. Histologically, colorectal SCC resembles small cell carcinomas of the lung and appear undifferentiated (Fig. 10.34) and show features of neuroendocrine differentiation. The tumor contains sheets and nests of densely packed, small, oval-, spindle-, or fusiform-shaped anaplastic cells with dark hyperchromatic nuclei, coarse chromatin, and scant cytoplasm. The cells may also be intermediate or larger in size similar to that seen in lung. Nuclei are hyperchromatic and approximately twice the diameter of mature lymphocytes. Tumors are mitotically very active with focal necrosis and vascular invasion present in most cases. The lesions may infiltrate transmurally, with limited involvement of the lamina propria, or they may be predominantly intramucosal, with only focal submucosal invasion. Cytokeratin stains may show punctate perinuclear cytoplasmic reactivity. Immunostaining with antibodies to chromogranin and synaptophysin are strongly positive.

Small cell carcinomas have a poor prognosis and tend to disseminate rapidly, a finding consistent with their high frequency of lymphatic and blood vessel involvement. Patients tend to die within less than a year of diagnosis. Median survival is 3.1 months. Many patients have metastatic disease at the time of presentation. Survival directly relates to depth of invasion. Lesions invading the underlying submucosa or muscle have a 5-year survival rate of up to 90%, whereas those invading into soft tissue have a 5-year survival rate of 33%, and those with nodal metastases a 5-year survival rate of 28.6–38%.

Despite rare reports of long-term survivors, surgery alone is inadequate therapy, even for apparently localized disease. Adjuvant radiotherapy (RT) for incompletely resected disease and systemic chemotherapy are widely recommended, although the effectiveness of a combined modality approach has not been established.

The selection of chemotherapy regimens, either as an adjuvant after surgery or for the treatment of metastatic disease, is based on individual experience. For patients with limited-stage disease combination chemotherapy with a platinum-based regimen, in conjunction with concurrent RT is recommended. Chemotherapy with the platinum-based regimen is usually administered with radiation beginning with cycle 1 or 2 of chemotherapy. The combination of cisplatin plus etoposide is preferable since it is compatible with concurrent RT. The usual dose of RT is either 45 Gy in 1.5-Gy twice daily fractions; an alternative regimen for which there are less data is 54–61 Gy in 1.8-Gy daily fractions (Brenner *et al.* 2004).

In the case of extensive-stage disease combination chemotherapy with a platinum-based regimen is recommended. A two-drug combination of etoposide plus either carboplatin or cisplatin is suggested. Regimens substituting irinotecan, topotecan, or epirubicin for etoposide are reasonable alternatives. The use of maintenance chemotherapy, three- or four-drug combinations, and alternating or sequential non-cross-resistant regimens have not been shown to offer substantial benefits compared to a two-drug combination; thus, these approaches are not routinely utilized (Brenner *et al.* 2004).

Desmoplastic small round cell tumor

Desmoplastic small round cell tumor (DSRCT) is an aggressive tumor of multiphenotype differentiation which typically affects the abdominal or pelvic cavity of adolescents and young adults. The tumor is more common in males. CT appearance is that of multiple rounded peritoneal masses with or without ascites. Grossly the tumor presents as single or multiple nodules within the abdominal cavity and or pelvic region and can extend to involve the serosal surfaces of the gastrointestinal organs. Histologically the tumor is composed of small round monotonous cells with a high nuclear cytoplasmic ratio. The cells are arranged in islands separated by abundant desmoplastic stroma. The tumor cells coexpress epithelial, mesenchymal, myogenic and neural markers, with a very characteristic perinuclear dot-like staining pattern with vimentin and desmin. Cytogenetically they have a unique and specific translocation at (11:22) (p13;q12) and the EWS-WT1 fusion transcript can be detected in formalin-fixed paraffin embedded tissue by RT-PCR. Nodal or visceral metastases are present in at least 50% of patients at the time of diagnosis (Dagher *et al.* 2002). The most aggressive therapeutic approaches adopted by some institutions involves treatment with systemic chemotherapy consisting of seven courses of multiagent chemotherapy (cyclophosphamide, doxorubicin, vincristine, ifosfamide, and etoposide) followed by aggressive tumor debulking and total abdominal radiation (La Quaglia & Brennan 2000; Lal *et al.* 2005). These patients had a 44% 3-year survival, with better survival among those patients that received multiagent chemotherapy and had a complete debulking surgery.

Choriocarcinoma of the colon

Pure primary choriocarcinomas of the colon are rare. These tumors are otherwise indistinguishable from gestational and gonadal tumors. The tumors arise in both sexes with a mean age of 55–57 years. The metastases show both mixed and pure patterns, although a pure choriocarcinomatous overgrowth is more common. Metastases involve the lymph nodes, lungs, liver, pancreas, and intraabdominal organs due to direct or transperitoneal spread. Histologically, transitions occur from the trophoblastic areas to the more classical colonic glandular phenotype. The trophoblastic cells which are large polyhedral cells with abundant eosinophilic cytoplasm (Fig. 10.35) in the tumor produce human chorionic gonadotropin (hCG), sometimes causing Leydig cell hyperplasia and gynecomastia in males. Women present with abnormal uterine bleeding due to endometrial hyperplasia, secretory changes in the breast, and a decidual reaction of the endometrium. The adenocarcinomatous component of this tumor is usually negative for hCG but positive for cytokeratin and carcinoembryonic antigen (CEA), by immunohistochemistry. Treatment is composed of initial surgical resection with adequate margins followed by multiagent chemotherapy composed of methotrexate and actinomycin D. Radiotherapy (4000 Gy) has been tried concomitantly in some cases (Motzer *et al.* 1996).

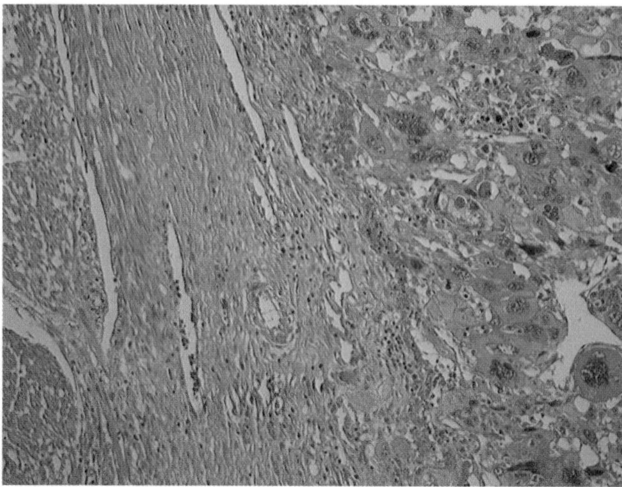

Fig. 10.35 Histopathology of primary choriocarcinoma of the colon. The tumor (H&E stain, ×100) is composed of a dimorphic population of large polyhedral cytotrophoblastic cells with abundant cytoplasm and multinucleated syncytiotrophoblasts similar to that seen in tumors arising from the placenta. lymphoid cells are (b) cytokeratin negative, native gastric glands stain positively. In contrast to the negative staining gastric glands, neoplastic lymphoid cells are (c) CD 20 positive, (d) CD 3 negative (e) CD 10 positive and (f) bcl-2 positive.

References

Brenner B, Shah MA, Gonen M *et al.* (2004) Small cell carcinoma of the gastrointestinal tract, a retrospective study of 64 cases. *Br J Cancer* 90: 1720–26.

Chaudhry AP, Saigal KP, Intengan M *et al.* (1979) Malakoplakia of the large intestine found incidentally at necropsy: Light and electron microscopic features. *Dis Colon Rectum* 22: 73–6.

Crist WM, Anderson JR, Meza JL *et al.* (2001) Intergroup Rhabdomyosarcoma Study-IV: results for patients with nonmetastatic disease. *J Clin Oncol* 19: 3091–102.

Crist WM, Gehan EA, Ragab AH *et al.* (1995) The Third Intergroup Rhabdomyosarcoma Study. *J Clin Oncol* 13: 610–30.

Dagher R, Long LM, Read EJ *et al.* (2002) Pilot trial of tumor-specific peptide vaccination and continuous infusion interleukin-2 in patients with recurrent Ewing sarcoma and alveolar rhabdomyosarcoma: an inter-institute NIH study. *Med Pediatr Oncol* 38: 158–164.

Drude RB, Balart LA, Herrington JP *et al.* (1982) Gastric xanthoma: Histological similarity to signet ring cell carcinoma. *J Clin Gastroenterol* 4: 217–21.

Fries MR, Galindo RL, Flint PW *et al.* (2003) Giant fibrovascular polyp of the esophagus. A lesion causing upper airway obstruction and syncope. *Arch Pathol Lab Med* 127(4): 485–7.

Hjermstad BM, Helwig EB. (1988) Tailgut cysts. Report of 33 cases. *Am J Clin Pathol* 89: 139–47.

Hood DL, Petras RE, Grundfest-Broniatowski S, Jagelman DG. (1988) Retrorectal cystic hamartoma: report of five cases with carcinoid tumor arising in two. *Am J Clin Pathol* 89: 433–6.

La Quaglia MP, Brennan MF. (2000) The clinical approach to desmoplastic small round cell tumor. *Surg Oncol* 9: 77–81.

Lal DR, Su W, Wolden SL, Loh KC, Modak S, La Quaglia MP. (2005) Results of multimodal treatment for desmoplastic small round cell tumors. *J Pediatr Surg* 40: 251–5.

Long JP, Althausen AF. (1989) Malakoplakia: A 25-year experience with a review of the literature. *J Urol* 141: 1320–6.

Motzer RJ, Mazumdar M, Bosl GJ *et al.* (1996) High-dose carboplatin, etoposide, and cyclophosphamide for patients with refractory germ cell tumors: Treatment results and prognostic factors for survival and toxicity. *J Clin Oncol* 14: 1098–1105.

Pappo AS, Lyden E, Breitfeld PP *et al.* (2002) Irinotecan (CPT-11) is active against pediatric rhabdomyosarcoma (RMS): a phase II window trial from the Soft Tissue Sarcoma Committee (STS) of the Children's Oncology Group (COG). *Proc Am Soc Clin Oncol* 21: 393a.

Prasad AR, Amin MB, Randolph TL, Lee CS, Ma CK. (2000) Retrorectal cystic hamartoma: report of 5 cases with malignancy arising in two. *Arch Pathol Lab Med* 124(5): 725–9.

Prott FJ, Haverkamp U, Willich N *et al.* (1996) Ten years of fast neutron therapy in Munster. *Bull Cancer Radiother* 83: 115S–121S.

Shimer GR, Helwig EB. (1984) Inflammatory fibroid polyps of the intestine. *Am J Clin Pathol* 81: 708–714.

Weigel BJ, Rodeberg DA, Krieg AM *et al.* (2003) CpG oligodeoxynucleotides potentiate the antitumor effects of chemotherapy or tumor resection in an orthotopic murine model of rhabdomyosarcoma. *Clin Cancer Res* 9: 3105–14.

Zafarni ES, Bitoun A, Paillard A *et al.* (1980) Gastric xanthelesma: endoscopic and pathologic study of 10 cases. *Gastroenterol Clin Biol* 4(3): 194–9.

2 Colorectal Cancer

Edited by David Kerr

11 Epidemiology and prevention of colorectal cancer

Paul Moayyedi

Introduction

Colorectal cancer (CRC) is the second most common cancer in the Western world, the third commonest cancer worldwide with over one million cases annually, and is also the fourth commonest cause of death worldwide (GLOBOCAN 2002) (Fig. 11.1). The main causes of the three cancers ahead of CRC in the global 'league tables' have all been elucidated, and these cancers may be largely preventable. Lung cancer could be prevented by cessation of smoking, gastric cancer by eradication of *Helicobacter pylori,* and hepatocellular carcinoma by immunization against hepatitis B. CRC is therefore the most common cause of cancer death for which the causes are largely unknown. Epidemiology has been instrumental in determining the etiologic factors in lung, stomach and liver cancer and may also be helpful in our understanding of the causes of CRC. It has been argued that whilst the cause of CRC is uncertain we understand that most cancers are derived from adenomatous polyps so we can largely prevent this disease by removing these precancerous lesions (Walsh & Terdiman 2003). The epidemiologic evidence will be reviewed to determine whether there is strong evidence to support the concept that CRC incidence could be reduced by public health measures, chemoprevention or endoscopic screening to remove polyps.

Geographical variation and time trends in colorectal cancer

There is an over 50-fold variation in incidence of CRC, with Congo having the lowest age-standardized rate (ASR) of 1.0 and the Czech Republic having the highest at 58.5 per 100,000 in men, with similar relative differences in women. There is a stark contrast between developed and developing countries with the incidence of CRC being higher in the former (ASR 40.0 vs 10.2 per 100,000) (Fig. 11.2) (GLOBOCAN 2002). This variability could be due to environmental or genetic factors but studies suggest that the environment plays the larger role. Migrants moving from lower- to higher-risk regions take on a CRC incidence similar to their new country within the first generation (McMichael *et al.* 1980; Monroe *et al.* 2003; Flood *et al.* 2000; Stirbu *et al.* 2006; Yavari *et al.* 2006). Indeed Japanese born in the USA have higher rates of CRC than both US whites and those born in Japan (Flood *et al.* 2000), and in some areas such as Hawaii and Los Angeles the incidence rates are amongst the highest in the world (Parkin 2004).

CRC has remained stable or declined slightly in developed countries in recent years (Fig. 11.3). In some developing countries such as those in Africa and central Asia the incidence of CRC has been relatively low and remained stable over time. In many Eastern Europe and south east Asian countries, however, there has been a dramatic increase in CRC rates (Sung *et al.* 2005) over the last three decades (Fig. 11.3). The marked rise in CRC rates in these countries suggest that environmental factors are playing a key role. The putative environment factors are likely to be related to affluence given the geographic distribution of CRC and the populations which are noting the most rapid rise in CRC rates are usually those experiencing rapid economic growth. What is it about an affluent lifestyle that leads to an increased risk of CRC? If this can be elucidated then preventative strategies can potentially be developed.

Modifiable risk factors for colorectal cancer

The incidence of CRC increases with age, with only 5% of cases in those under the age of 40 years in the US (Reis *et al.* 1998–2002). There is a steady increase in CRC incidence with age which plateaus in the sixth decade (Reis *et al.* 1998–2002). There may also be a shift in the site of CRC from distal to more proximal with age (Cooper *et al.* 1995). CRC is also more common in men and this is true of all countries and races although gender differences are modest compared with many other common cancers such as lung, liver and stomach. Worldwide the age-standardized incidence rate is 10.2 for men and

Gastrointestinal Oncology: A Critical Multidisciplinary Team Approach.
Edited by J. Jankowski, R. Sampliner, D. Kerr, and Y. Fong.
 ISBN: 978-1-4501-2783-7

7.6 per 100,000 for women. As women tend to live longer the crude rates and absolute number of cases of CRC are very similar between the sexes. There is also a well-known increased risk of CRC in those with a positive family history. Studies suggest a two to threefold increase in risk in those with first-degree relatives that have colon cancer (Johns & Houlston 2001; Andrieu *et al.* 2004). Patients with ulcerative colitis and possibly

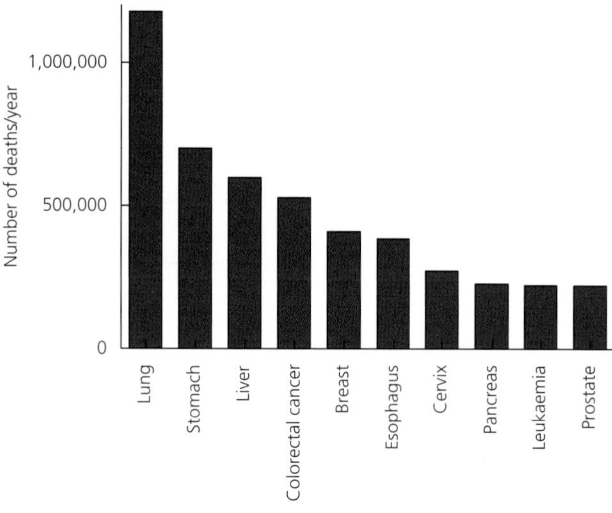

Fig. 11.1 The top ten causes of cancer death worldwide (GLOBOCAN 2002).

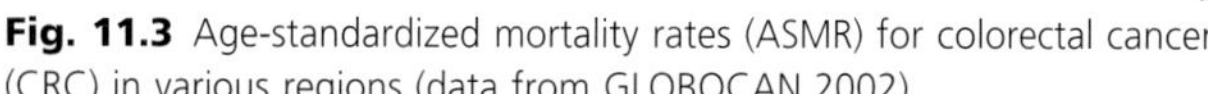

Fig. 11.3 Age-standardized mortality rates (ASMR) for colorectal cancer (CRC) in various regions (data from GLOBOCAN 2002).

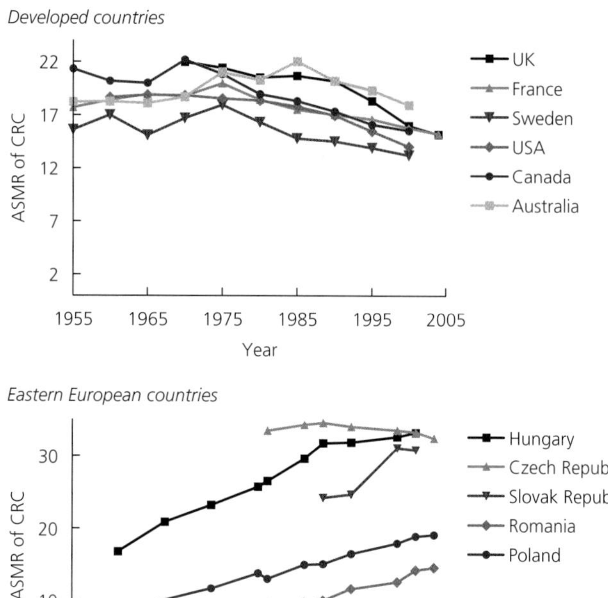

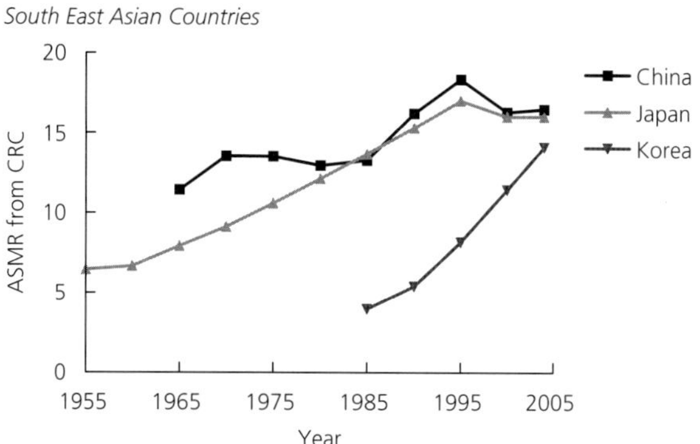

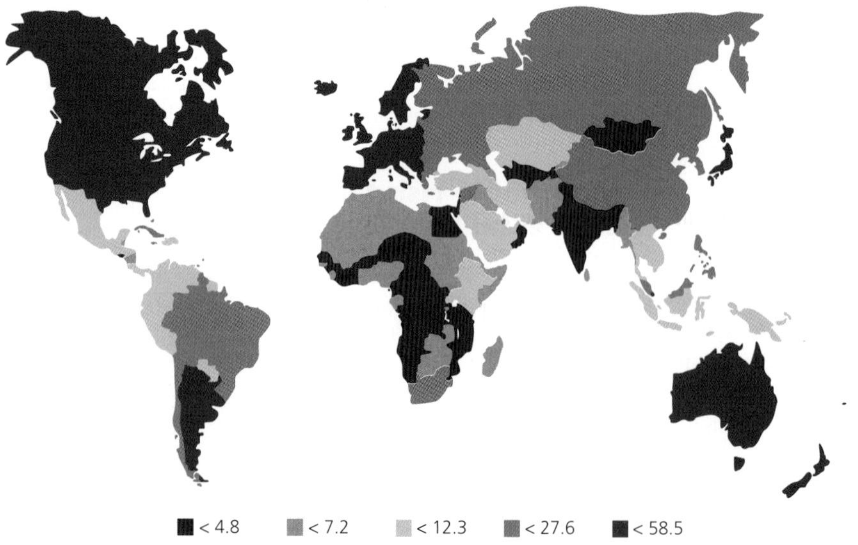

Fig. 11.2 Geographical distribution of age standardized CRC rates in men (GLOBOCAN 2002).

large bowel Crohn's disease also have an increased risk of CRC (Jess *et al.* 2006). These factors, however, are not modifiable and are not related to affluence. Prevention programs would be helped by data on potentially modifiable risk factors such as obesity, diet, physical activity and to a lesser extent socioeconomic status.

Body mass index

Rates of obesity are increasing dramatically in most Western nations (Anonymous 2006) and this is a major concern given the association between body mass index (BMI) and age- and sex-adjusted mortality (McTigue *et al.* 2006). Obesity is associated with an increased risk of a variety of diseases such as diabetes mellitus, gallstones and ischemic heart disease as well as some cancers (Wyatt *et al.* 2006). In particular, there is a consistent association between BMI and risk of CRC. A systematic review (Bergstrom *et al.* 2001) identified 19 papers (12 cohort and 7 case–control studies) that evaluated the association between BMI and CRC with 15 reporting a statistically significant positive relationship. Overall there was a 1.03 (95% confidence interval (CI) 1.02–1.04) relative risk (RR) of CRC for every unit increase in BMI. The proportion of CRC attributable to excess weight was estimated at 11% which translates to 21,000 CRC cases annually in Europe (Bergstrom *et al.* 2001). Most studies attempted to adjust for confounders such as socioeconomic status, age, diet and physical activity but few papers adjusted for all of these factors and it is possible that some of the association between BMI and CRC is due to residual confounding. A similar association exists between waist to hip ratio and CRC risk (Pischon *et al.* 2006). Indeed this study suggested that abdominal obesity was a more important risk factor for CRC than BMI alone (Pischon *et al.* 2006). These epidemiologic data therefore suggest that encouraging the population not to gain weight is a good public health strategy that may prevent CRC as well as many other diseases.

Dietary fiber

The observation that CRC was uncommon in Africa where the intake of dietary fiber is high has led some to suggest that roughage may be protective (Burkitt 1969). A systematic review of 13 case–control studies (Howe *et al.* 1992) would support this hypothesis with a consistent reduction in CRC risk in the highest fiber intake quintile compared with the lowest (odds ratio [OR] 0.53; 95% CI 0.47–0.61) and this was supported by a further review of the literature (Trock *et al.* 1990). Large cohort studies have been less consistent. The European Prospective Investigation in Cancer and Nutrition study suggested that dietary fiber was protective (Bingham *et al.* 2003), whilst the Nurses Health Study and the Health Professionals Follow-up Study found no association between fiber intake and CRC risk (Michels *et al.* 2005). A major problem with epidemiologic studies on dietary fiber is the difficulty in discriminating between the fiber and non-fiber effect of vegetable intake. This can be overcome by randomized controlled trials (RCTs) of fiber supplements versus placebo. A systematic review (Asano & McLeod 2002) identified five studies involving 3641 patients undergoing polyp surveillance. Dietary fiber did not reduce the incidence of colonic adenomas (RR 1.08; 95% CI 0.94–1.23) and there was an increased risk of CRC (RR 2.71; 95% CI 1.07–6.86). The increased risk of CRC with fiber intake may be a chance finding as the absolute number of cancers in this review was small but these data certainly do not support the hypothesis that fiber is protective.

Meat consumption

Ecologic data from 27 countries showed a strong correlation between CRC incidence and average per capita meat consumption (Ognjanovic *et al.* 2006). This is supported by case–control and cohort studies, and the World Health Organization concluded that the consumption of red meat is likely to be associated with CRC (Scheppach *et al.* 1999). This decision is consistent with systematic reviews that report an increased risk of CRC in those in the highest red and processed meat categories compared with the lowest (Norat *et al.* 2001; Sandhu *et al.* 2001). High red meat intake is also associated with colonic adenomatous polyps (Yoon *et al.* 2000). The main concern is that the association was not consistent across all studies. An updated systematic review (Larsson & Wolk 2006), however, found no heterogeneity between studies and a consistent albeit modest effect of both red and processed meat and risk of CRC. The overall RR for CRC from 15 prospective studies (involving 7367 CRC cases) was 1.28 (95% CI 1.15–1.42) for the highest versus the lowest red meat intake category. There were 14 studies (involving 7903 CRC cases) that evaluated processed meat intake and CRC risk and found a similar association to red meat (RR 1.20; 95% CI 1.11–1.31). For both red and processed meat the relative risk did not change when only studies that adjusted for BMI, physical activity, and other dietary intake were included. There was also a dose–response relationship between the amount of red or processed meat eaten and the risk of CRC with an approximately 10% excess relative risk for every 30 g of meat eaten (Norat *et al.* 2001; Larsson & Wolk 2006). Conversely there is an inverse association between fish intake and CRC risk (Kimura *et al.* 2007; Norat *et al.* 2005).

There is strong epidemiologic evidence to support the hypothesis that a diet rich in red and processed meats may increase the risk of CRC. There have been several biologic explanations for this apparent association. Red meat contains higher amounts of heme iron which can damage colonic mucosa and stimulate proliferation (Cross *et al.* 2003). Furthermore, heme iron supplementation has increased fecal excretion of N-nitroso compounds which are potent carcinogens (Cross *et al.* 2003; Lee *et al.* 2004; Cross & Sinha 2004). Cooked meat also contains heterocyclic amines and polycylic aromatic hydrocarbons which are also carcinogenic (Lee *et al.* 2004). The extent to which these compounds increase cancer risk may depend on genetically determined activation of metabolic enzymes (Ognjanovic *et al.* 2006). Whatever the explanation for the association it would seem sensible to advise less red and processed meat consumption and possibly encourage more fish in the diet.

Fruit and vegetable intake

Fruit and vegetables are an important source of antioxidants and fiber and have been reported to reduce the risk of a variety of cancers. The impact on CRC is less clear with both positive (Terry *et al.* 2001a) and negative studies (Voorrips *et al.* 2000). A systematic review (Riboli & Norat 2003) identified 28 case–control and 12 cohort studies evaluating vegetable and/or fruit intake and CRC risk. Overall the case–control studies reported a reduction in CRC risk for both fruit and vegetables but there was no statistically significant association in cohort studies. The polyp prevention trial (Schatzkin *et al.* 2000) also failed to show any impact of high vegetable and fruit intake on colonic polyp recurrence despite subjective and objective evidence that those randomized to dietary intervention had adhered to their diet (Lanza *et al.* 2001). A diet high in vegetable and fruit may have other health benefits but is unlikely to have a major impact on CRC rates.

Dairy products

Milk and other dairy products are a rich source of calcium and vitamin D which animal studies suggest may protect against CRC (Lamprecht & Lipkin 2001). Fermented dairy products also promote lactobacilli which may protect against the effects of mutagens (Norat & Riboli 2003). Conversely, the saturated fat content of milk may increase CRC risk (Norat & Riboli 2003). A pooled analysis (Cho *et al.* 2004a) of 10 cohort studies involving over 530,000 subjects with 6–10 years of follow-up suggested milk intake was associated with a decreased risk of CRC (RR of CRC in highest compared with the lowest category of intake 0.85; 95% CI 0.78–0.94) particularly in the distal colon. A systematic review (Norat & Riboli 2003) also found that dairy products were consistently associated with a reduced CRC risk in cohort studies. The same review (Norat & Riboli 2003) found the evidence from case–control studies was divergent. There were 11 case–control studies, with three finding a statistically significant increased risk and three a statistically significant decreased risk of CRC in those taking high quantities of dairy products. Overall there was no statistically significant effect of dairy products on CRC risk when results from case–control studies were synthesized. The conflicting nature of epidemiologic evidence and the divergent theoretical effects on carcinogenesis suggest there is currently insufficient evidence to promote dairy product consumption as a public health measure to prevent CRC.

Alcohol, smoking and coffee consumption

Alcohol is associated with a variety of cancers including the oral cavity, pharynx, larynx and esophagus (Boffetta *et al.* 2006). Alcohol may have a general effect on increasing the risk of neoplasia due to direct genotoxic effects, production of reactive oxygen species and interference with folate metabolism (Boffetta & Hashibe 2006). A review of 16 cohort studies (Moskal *et al.* 2007) found that there was an increased risk of CRC in those in the highest compared to the lowest alcohol intake category. There was also a dose–response relationship with a 15% increase in risk of CRC with each 100 g per week of alcohol consumed (Moskal *et al.* 2007). There does not appear to be any difference in risk according to the type of alcohol consumed (Cho *et al.* 2004b).

Smoking tobacco produces a variety of genotoxic agents such as heterocyclic amines, nitrosamines and polynuclear aromatic hydrocarbons. It is therefore not surprising that cigarette smoking is associated with an increased incidence of a variety of cancers including lung, stomach, bladder and pancreas (Giovannucci 2001). Smoking is also associated with colorectal adenomas with a two- to threefold increase in risk after 20–40 pack years (Giovannucci 2001). Epidemiologic data on smoking and CRC have been less consistent (Giovannucci 2001), but large cohort studies have generally suggested there is a positive association (Terry *et al.* 2001b; Mizoue *et al.* 2006). The evidence in isolation would not be sufficient to mandate public health measures to curb smoking to prevent CRC. There is, however, overwhelming evidence that advising smoking cessation will prolong life because of the impact on other diseases.

A systematic review (Giovannucci 1998) suggested that high coffee consumption was associated with a reduced risk of CRC in 12 case–control studies. The author was cautious in interpreting these data as the result could be due to confounding and bias. For example, individuals at high risk of CRC may avoid coffee. Furthermore the five cohort studies in the same review (Giovannucci 1998) did not suggest an association between coffee intake and CRC overall. Subsequent cohort studies (Terry *et al.* 2001c) have generally been negative, suggesting modulating coffee consumption is unlikely to have any major impact on CRC incidence.

Physical activity

A sedentary lifestyle increases the risk of a number of chronic diseases including cancer and is associated with reduced survival (Warburton *et al.* 2006). The reasons for this are unclear but exercise has effects on the immune function, hormones and prostaglandin synthesis (Quadrilatero & Hoffman-Goetz 2003). Physical activity may influence these to protect against CRC as may the effects of exercise on gut transit time (Quadrilatero & Hoffman-Goetz 2003). Variation in CRC rates in US states is correlated with indices of a sedentary lifestyle (Lai *et al.* 2006). A systematic review of 19 cohort studies (Samad *et al.* 2005) found that increased physical activity consistently reduced the risk of CRC. Twenty-eight case–control studies also reported an association between physical activity and a reduction in CRC risk (Samad *et al.* 2005). Overall the highest category of physical activity had a 20–25% reduction in CRC compared with the lowest category. There was usually a dose–response relationship between the amount of physical activity and CRC risk. These findings have been confirmed in subsequent cohort studies (Friedenreich *et al.* 2006; Isomura *et al.* 2006; Johnsen *et al.* 2006; Larsson *et al.* 2006; Mai *et al.* 2007). The effect is seen in both men and women and in numerous countries. The association could be due to confounding factors, the most obvious of which is obesity. Many studies have controlled for BMI as well as dietary and other confounding factors in the analyses and this has not reduced the association (Samad *et al.* 2005; Isomura *et al.* 2006; Friedenreich *et al.* 2006; Johnsen *et al.* 2006; Larsson *et al.* 2006; Mai *et al.* 2007). There is therefore strong epidemiologic evidence that physical activity protects against CRC and given the other health benefits of exercise this should be encouraged.

Socioeconomic status

It is arguable whether socioeconomic status is a 'modifiable' risk factor, but it is important to consider it as this is an indicator of how affluence may impact on CRC risk. A systematic review (Palmer & Schneider 2005) identified that there was a surprising paucity of data on socioeconomic status and CRC incidence. There was a rich literature on ethnicity, socioeconomic status and screening uptake, but fewer data pertaining to other aspects of CRC (Palmer & Schneider 2005). Low socioeconomic status is associated with a lower uptake of screening (Singh *et al.* 2004), later stage of disease at diagnosis and lower survival (Parikh-Patel *et al.* 2006). Two cohort studies have shown that there is a significant increase in CRC incidence in the highest versus lowest social class groups (van Loon *et al.* 1995; Weiderpass & Pukkala 2006). This observation is supported by one case–control study (Tavani *et al.*1999). Two studies suggest that higher education status is also associated with increased CRC risk (Tavani *et al.*1999; Shipp *et al.* 2005). These data are consistent with the geographical and time trend data that suggest CRC may be the price society pays for increasing affluence.

Chemoprevention to reduce colorectal cancer incidence

There are a number of dietary and other lifestyle factors that may decrease or increase the risk of CRC. This would suggest that appropriate public health programs may reduce CRC in the population although these measures are often difficult to adhere to and therefore meet with limited success. Taking a tablet to prevent cancer is much easier than dietary modification and therefore may meet with higher compliance. The efficacy of these strategies can be tested by RCTs more readily than lifestyle measures. There is therefore the potential for the efficacy of these strategies to be more precisely defined. Chemoprevention has mainly focused on dietary supplements but other approaches could be considered including modulating gut flora and inhibiting cyclo-oxygenase pathways.

Antioxidant vitamins

Cell injury through oxidative stress can cause gene mutation and carcinogenesis. Epidemiologic evidence suggests a diet rich in antioxidants may protect against CRC, although the data are conflicting. This could be due to the difficulties in accurately assessing dietary intake, and antioxidant vitamin supplements such as vitamins A, C and E may be a more effective approach to ensuring CRC prevention. A systematic review (Bjelakovic *et al.* 2006) of eight RCTs found that β-carotene, and vitamins A, C and E either alone or in combination was not effective in reducing the development of colorectal adenomas. There was also no significant effect of these antioxidants in preventing CRC in a systematic review of four RCTs involving over 76,000 participants with 2–12 years' follow-up (Bjelakovic *et al.* 2004a,b). The use of antioxidant supplements is further questioned by a systematic review (Bjelakovic *et al.* 2007) that suggested that in 47 low-bias RCTs involving almost 181,000 participants there was a small but statistically significant increase in all-cause mortality. These data suggest antioxidant vitamin supplements should not be used in CRC prevention.

Folate

Dietary folate may prevent carcinogenesis through maintaining DNA synthesis and methylation. Conversely, folate deficiency causes an increased frequency of chromosomal breaks and gene mutations (Blount *et al.* 1997). Folate supplementation therefore has the potential to reduce the risk of CRC particularly in those that have a deficiency of this vitamin. Reviews of the literature (Giovannucci 2002; Sanjoaquin *et al.* 2005) have suggested that there is a 25% reduction in CRC risk in those in the highest category of dietary folate compared with the lowest in both case–control and cohort studies (Sanjoaquin *et al.* 2005). These results are consistent, with little heterogeneity between studies, but are difficult to interpret as folate intake is strongly correlated with other vitamin and fiber consumption and the protective effect may be due to confounding from these other dietary factors. Analyses attempt to adjust for these confounders but as it is difficult to precisely estimate nutrient intake the possibility of residual confounding persists. Indeed the three cohort and three case–control studies (Sanjoaquin *et al.* 2005) that evaluated the impact of folate supplements on CRC risk found no association between these variables. There have been no RCTs evaluating the effect of folate supplements on CRC although one trial found no statistically significant effect on colorectal adenoma recurrence after 2 years (Paspatis & Karamanolis 1994).

Calcium and vitamin D

Observational studies have generally found that increased calcium (Norat & Riboli 2003) and vitamin D (Gorham *et al.* 2005) intake are associated with a reduced risk of CRC. They may act by binding bile acid salts and inhibiting the proliferation of colonic epithelial cells (Lamprecht & Lipkin 2003). Systematic reviews of RCTs that evaluated the effect of calcium in secondary prevention of colorectal adenomas (Shaukat *et al.* 2005; Weingarten *et al.* 2005) have suggested there is a 20% reduction in recurrent polyps in those given supplements compared with placebo. There was also a statistically non-significant trend to reduced CRC incidence. Calcium and vitamin D therefore looked to be promising chemoprevention agents until the results of an RCT from the US Women's Health Initiative (Wactawski-Wende *et al.* 2006) that looked primarily at the role of these supplements in preventing hip fracture: 36,282 postmenopausal women aged 50–79 years were randomized to receive 1 g of elemental calcium (as calcium carbonate) plus 400 IU of vitamin D_3 or matching placebo, and followed up for 7 years. Colorectal cancer was a planned secondary analysis. There were 322 cases of colorectal cancer, with 168 in the supplement group and 154 in the control group (hazard ratio 1.08; 95% CI 0.86–1.34).

Selenium

The trace element selenium has had increasing attention as a possible cancer chemoprevention agent. The main dietary sources of selenium are meat and grain. It is an antioxidant as well as being required for a variety of selenoproteins, many of which have unknown functions. Ecologic data suggest that those living in regions of low selenium consumption have the highest rates of CRC (Schrauzer *et al.* 1977). Cohort studies (Fernandez-Banares *et al.* 2002; Jacobs *et al.* 2004; Peters *et al.* 2006) have also suggested that the incidence of colorectal adenomas is reduced in those with highest serum selenium levels although this is not a universal finding (Wallace *et al.* 2003). One RCT (Hofstad *et al.* 1998) of a combination of -carotene, vitamin C, vitamin E, calcium and selenium or placebo did not show any impact of this supplement cocktail on colorectal adenoma recurrence after 2 years. Two cohort studies (Knekt *et al.* 1988; van den Brandt *et al.* 1993) of over 157,000 participants followed up over 3–10 years failed to show any association between low selenium levels and subsequent CRC risk. On the other hand, there is intriguing RCT evidence that suggests selenium supplementation may protect against CRC. The National Prevention of Cancer Trial (Duffield-Lillico *et al.* 2002) was originally designed to evaluate the efficacy of selenium supplementation in preventing non-melanoma skin cancer. There was no effect of selenium on skin cancer in the 1250 participants randomized to selenium 200 μg or placebo followed up for a mean of 7.4 years. The trial did note there was an overall reduction in cancer mortality in the group treated with selenium and this seemed to be due to reduced rates of prostate, lung and colorectal cancers in the treatment group. There was a 54% reduction in CRC in those given selenium (Duffield-Lillico *et al.* 2002), although this was of marginal statistical significance (hazard ratio 0.46; 95% CI 0.21–1.02, $p = 0.057$). This is an interesting secondary analysis which has prompted a large RCT involving over 32,000 men in the US, Canada and Puerto Rico followed up for 12 years (Lippman *et al.* 2005). The primary aim of the SELECT trial is to evaluate the efficacy of selenium and/or vitamin E in preventing prostate cancer but CRC incidence is a predefined secondary endpoint. The results of this trial are awaited with interest.

Modulating gut flora

The discovery that *Helicobacter pylori* infection is associated with gastric cancer (Moayyedi & Hunt 2004) had stimulated interest in microbes as a cause for cancer in other sites. CRC is an obvious candidate as there are up to 10^{12} bacterial cells per gram of feces and there is some evidence that microbes have an important role in carcinogenesis (Hope *et al.* 2005). There are a number of mice models where colon cancer can be induced, and germ-free mice have a lower incidence of tumor formation compared with conventionally reared animals (Engle *et al.* 2002). Colonic flora can produce metabolites that are potent mutagens and the interaction with diet is particularly important in this regard. There is also epidemiologic evidence that some bacterial species are associated with colorectal cancer. Case–control studies have suggested adherent strains, and intracellular *Escherichia coli* are common in patients with CRC but rare in healthy controls (Swidsinski *et al.* 1998; Martin *et al.* 2004). Sulfate-producing bacteria have also been implicated in neoplasia as these produce hydrogen sulfide which damages the colonic epithelial barrier (Deplancke *et al.* 2003). Hydrogen sulfide levels are higher in CRC cases compared to healthy controls (McGarr *et al.* 2005). It may be possible to modulate gut flora in a way that could promote the health of colonic epithelium and reduce the risk of CRC (Rafter 2003; Geier *et al.* 2006). As yet we know little of the biodiversity within the gut lumen so at this stage this remains a hypothetical approach. The only RCT evaluating probiotics in preventing CRC in high-risk individuals was negative (Ishikawa *et al.* 2005). This remains an avenue worthy of further laboratory study and once there is a better understanding of host–microbe interactions this could be the subject of clinical studies.

Non-steroidal anti-inflammatory drugs

Non-steroidal anti-inflammatory drugs (NSAIDs) have come under increasing scrutiny as possible chemoprevention agents for esophageal (Jankowski & Moayyedi 2004), stomach (Wang *et al.* 2003), and colorectal cancer (Rostom *et al.* 2007). A systematic review identified three cohort studies evaluating non-aspirin NSAIDs and found a 40% relative risk reduction in CRC incidence which was statistically significant (95% CI 23–52%) (Rostom *et al.* 2007). The benefits of aspirin chemoprevention is being tested on polyp growth as a secondary outcome in the ASPECT trial. There was a similar finding in the nine case–control studies reporting on CRC incidence and NSAID use (Rostom *et al.* 2007). These studies reported that longer duration of use (over 2–5 years) was associated with greater benefit. This systematic review also found one RCT evaluating non-aspirin NSAIDs and three RCTs evaluating cyclo-oxygenase 2 inhibitors (COX-2) in preventing recurrence of colorectal adenomas. Cox-2 inhibitors were associated with a statistically significant 44% reduction in advanced colorectal adenomas (Rostom *et al.* 2007). There were no RCTs evaluating the impact of non-aspirin NSAIDS or COX-2 inhibitors on CRC incidence. Whilst these agents may have a protective effect on CRC the gastrointestinal toxicity of non-aspirin NSAIDs and the cardiotoxicity of COX-2 inhibitors suggest the risk–benefit ratio will not be favorable as a chemoprevention strategy for the general population.

A systematic review also evaluated the effectiveness of aspirin in preventing CRC (Dube *et al.* 2007). Two cohort studies and five case–control studies found a 10–30% relative risk reduction in colorectal adenoma recurrence (Dube *et al.* 2007) which was statistically significant. There was also one small RCT which showed a trend towards a reduction in adenoma incidence but this did not reach statistical significance (Dube *et al.* 2007). There were six cohort and seven case–control studies that suggested a 20–30% relative risk reduction in CRC incidence in those taking aspirin, particularly if this had been for more than 5 years (Dube *et al.* 2007). Two RCTs involving almost 62,000 participants followed up for 5–10 years (the Physicians Health Study and the Women's Health Study) however failed to show an impact of aspirin on CRC incidence (RR 1.02; 95% CI 0.84–1.25) (Dube *et al.* 2007). A small beneficial effect of aspirin cannot be excluded by these trials and it is possible that longer duration of aspirin therapy may confer benefit. Nevertheless current RCT data would not support the use of aspirin to prevent CRC.

Screening flexible sigmoidoscopy and colonoscopy to prevent colorectal cancer

There is increasing awareness of colorectal screening as a strategy to prevent CRC mortality (Cram *et al.* 2003). The three most common approaches are fecal occult blood (FOB) testing, flexible sigmoidoscopy, and colonoscopy (Winawer *et al.* 2003a). FOB testing has the most evidence of efficacy, with four RCTs with up to 18 years follow-up (Hewitson *et al.* 2007). FOB is associated with a 16% reduction in CRC mortality but most studies do not report any decrease in CRC incidence (Hewitson *et al.* 2007). The likely impact of FOB on CRC mortality is therefore to detect the disease early. One trial did report a reduced incidence of CRC in the FOB test groups (Mandel *et al.* 2000), but this study had the highest rate of colonoscopy which may explain this outlying result.

Flexible sigmoidoscopy has the advantage of being more sensitive than FOB for diagnosing CRC distal to the splenic flexure. This represents approximately 60% of all CRC and this strategy will also identify and remove left-sided polyps. This approach should therefore prevent colorectal cancer as well as detect disease early. Colonoscopy views the whole colon, which is an important consideration as approximately 40% of all colorectal cancer is in the proximal colon and not detectable by flexible sigmoidoscopy (Lieberman *et al.* 2000). Most CRC is believed to be derived from polyps and these can be removed throughout the colon at colonoscopy so this approach has the greatest potential to prevent colorectal adenocarcinoma.

The main driver of the interest in flexible sigmoidoscopy and colonoscopy screening is the hypothesis that most CRC is derived from adenomatous polyps. It is very difficult to conduct an exhaustive literature search around this issue as many papers date before the scope of electronic databases. My impression is, however, that in the 1940s to 1960s opinion was equally divided as to whether adenomatous polyps were precancerous or not. There were statements in prominent medical journals such as 'there is increasing evidence that they [colorectal adenomas] may have no more sinister significance than benign polyps of the nose' (Anonymous 1962) and 'The belief . . . that adenomatous polyps of the colon often become malignant has very little factual support' (Castleman & Krickstein 1962) that questioned the importance of polyps. In the 1970s Basil Morson (Morson 1974) and others eloquently outlined the adenoma–carcinoma hypothesis of colorectal carcinogenesis, and clinicians stopped questioning whether colorectal adenomas had malignant potential. The reason for the cessation of debate is not clear but certainly does not relate to the emergence of high-quality epidemiologic evidence supporting the hypothesis. I can find four studies (Colvert & Brown 1948; Achord & Galambos 1970; Stryker *et al.* 1987; Murakami *et al.* 1990) that have looked at the natural history of colorectal adenomas over time. Participants have been followed up for a mean of 2.5–7 years with an annual incidence rate of 0–1.5% (Table 11.1). Overall the incidence of CRC does appear to be higher than would be expected from the general population, although only two studies compared the CRC rates with a control group (Morson 1974). These

Table 11.1 Studies evaluating the natural history of unresected colorectal polyps.

Author	No. of subjects	Mean follow-up (years)	% with colorectal cancer
Colvert & Brown 1948	43	7	6.9%
Achord & Galambos 1970	67	2.5	0%
Stryker *et al.* 1987	226	5.7	9%
Murakami *et al.* 1990	305	6.3	2.6%

studies (Colvert & Brown 1948; Murakami *et al.* 1990) compared CRC rates in those that did and did not have large colorectal polyps resected. There was an increase in the risk of CRC in those with polyps left *in situ* but this did not reach statistical significance in either study (Table 11.2). The relative risk increase was modest and the population-attributable risk (not given in the papers but calculated from them) was only 30–50%. Furthermore, the reason why some patients had polyps resected and others did not was not clearly outlined and the results may be due to confounding factors. This is supported by the observation that the risk of gastric cancer was also increased in those that did not have colorectal polypectomy compared to those that did (Murakami *et al.* 1990). There are studies that assessed the incidence of CRC in those undergoing polyp surveillance with colonoscopy compared to the general population and the literature has been well summarized (Winawer *et al.* 2006). These studies have shown very heterogeneous results, with some (Winawer *et al.* 1993b; Citarda *et al.* 2001) reporting CRC significantly reduced in those undergoing polyp surveillance and others (Robertson *et al.* 2005; Jorgensen *et al.* 1995) showing CRC incidences very similar to the general population (Fig. 11.4).

Table 11.2 Studies comparing colorectal cancer in patients with colorectal polyps that did and did not have polypectomy.

Author	Relative risk	95% CI	Population-attributable risk
Colvert & Brown 1948	2.72	0.64–11.34	30%
Murakami *et al.* 1990			
CRC	3.56	0.59–21.9	46%
Gastric cancer	2.01	0.50–8.82	25%

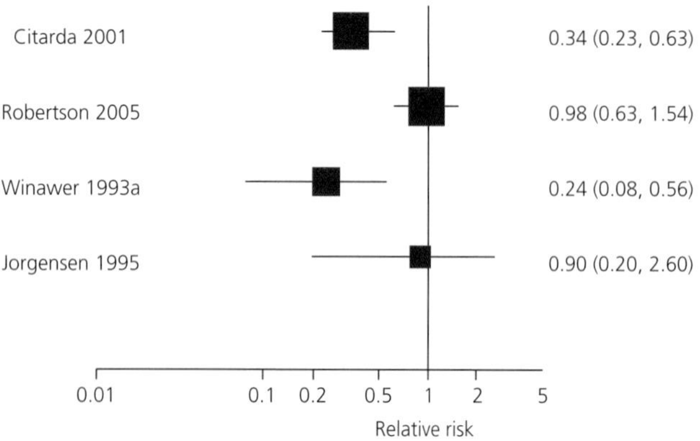

Fig. 11.4 A Forest plot of the relative risk of colorectal cancer compared with normal controls in patients undergoing polypectomy and colonscopic surveillance.

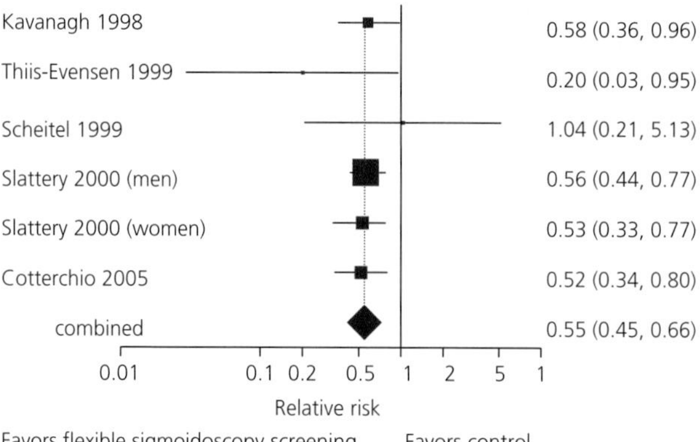

Fig. 11.5 A Forest plot of observational studies evaluating the association between CRC incidence and having flexible sigmoidoscopy screening. This is not a systematic review but data synthesized for ease of presentation as there was little heterogeneity between studies (Cochran Q = 2.08, df = 5; p = 0.84; I^2 = 0%, 95% CI 0–61%) and most gave similar results.

Epidemiologic data supporting the adenoma carcinoma hypothesis are hardly overwhelming but the belief is so well ingrained in clinical practice that it would be unethical to leave large adenomas untreated. It is therefore inappropriate to study this further and instead we should concentrate on whether flexible sigmoidoscopy or colonoscopy screening reduce CRC mortality compared with an alternative strategy (such as FOB screening or no screening). There have been no recent systematic reviews on the efficacy of colonoscopy and flexible sigmoidoscopy in reducing colorectal cancer incidence and mortality. Three RCTs have evaluated flexible sigmoidoscopy against no screening in 358,724 subjects. All RCTs suggest CRC is detected at an earlier stage (UK FSSTI 2002; Weissfeld *et al.* 2005; Segnan *et al.* 2005), but there are currently no data on CRC incidence or mortality. There are also two cohort studies (Kavanagh *et al.* 1998; Thiis-Evensen *et al.* 1999) with 25,543 subjects and three case–control studies (Scheitel *et al.* 1999; Slattery *et al.* 2000; Cotterchio *et al.* 2005) with 5605 subjects evaluating flexible sigmoidoscopy with no screening. This is not a systematic review but all studies gave similar results and pooling the results suggests overall flexible sigmoidoscopy is associated with a reduced CRC incidence (RR 0.55; 95% CI 0.45–0.66) (Fig. 11.5). There are no published RCTs that evaluate the efficacy of colonoscopy screening, and only one case–control study evaluating 2915 subjects (Cotterchio *et al.* 2005). There was no statistically significant difference between colonoscopy and no screening (RR 0.69; 95% CI 0.44–1.07) although this study was underpowered.

Conclusions

CRC is a global health problem, particularly in rapidly developing nations and developed countries. Epidemiologic studies suggest public health programs that reduce obesity, encourage physical activity and discourage excessive meat consumption could dramatically decrease CRC incidence (Platz *et al.* 2000). RCTs evaluating chemoprevention of specific dietary supplements have been largely disappointing. Selenium still deserves attention as does aspirin or possibly NSAID derivatives that avoid gastrointestinal and cardiovascular harms. The main strategy adopted in some countries is to screen the population over a certain age threshold for colorectal polyps with either flexible sigmoidoscopy or colonoscopy. This theoretically could have the greatest impact on CRC incidence although data are far from conclusive and it is a sad indictment of the international academic community and funding organizations that there are no adequately powered randomized studies on colonoscopy screening.

References

Achord JL. Galambos JT. (1970) The natural history of adenomatous rectal polyps. *South Med J* 63: 1464.

Andrieu N, Launoy G, Guillois R, Ory-Paoletti C, Gignoux M. (2004) Estimation of the familial relative risk of cancer by site from a French population based family study on colorectal cancer (CCREF study). *Gut* 53: 1322–8.

Anonymous. (1962) *JAMA* editorial: Rectal polyps and cancer. *JAMA* 181: 134.

Anonymous. (2006) Curbing the obesity epidemic. *Lancet* 367: 1549.

Asano T, McLeod RS. (2002) Dietary fibre for the prevention of colorectal adenomas and carcinomas. *Cochrane Database* Syst Rev (2): CD003430.

Bergstrom A, Pisani P, Tenet V, Wolk A, Adami HO. (2001) Overweight as an avoidable cause of cancer in Europe. *Int J Cancer* 91: 421–30.

Bingham SA, Day NE, Luben R *et al.* (2003) European Prospective Investigation into Cancer and Nutrition. Dietary fibre in food and protection against colorectal cancer in the European Prospective Investigation into Cancer and Nutrition (EPIC): an observational study. *Lancet* 361: 1496–501.

Bjelakovic G, Nikolova D, Simonetti RG, Gluud C. (2004a) Antioxidant supplements for preventing gastrointestinal cancers. *Cochrane Database Syst Rev* (4): CD004183.

Bjelakovic G, Nikolova D, Simonetti RG, Gluud C. (2004b) Antioxidant supplements for prevention of gastrointestinal cancers: a systematic review and meta-analysis. *Lancet* 364: 1219–28.

Bjelakovic G, Nagorni A, Nikolova D, Simonetti RG, Bjelakovic M, Gluud C. (2006) Meta-analysis: antioxidant supplements for primary and secondary prevention of colorectal adenoma. *Aliment Pharmacol Ther* 24: 281–91.

Bjelakovic G, Nikolova D, Gluud LL, Simonetti RG, Gluud C. (2007) Mortality in randomized trials of antioxidant supplements for primary and secondary prevention: systematic review and meta-analysis. *JAMA* 297: 842–57.

Blount BC, Mack MM, Wehr CM *et al.* (1997) Folate deficiency causes uracil misincorporation into human DNA and chromosome breakage: implications for cancer and neuronal damage. *Proc Nat Acad Sci USA* 94: 3290–5.

Boffetta P, Hashibe M. (2000) Alcohol and cancer. *Lancet Oncol* 7: 149–56.

Boffetta P, Hashibe M, La Vecchia C, Zatonski W, Rehm J. (2006) The burden of cancer attributable to alcohol drinking. *Int J Cancer* 119: 884–7.

Burkitt DP. (1969) Related disease–related cause? *Lancet* ii: 1229–31.

Castleman B, Krickstein HI. (1963) Polyps of the colon. *Surg Gynae Obs* 116: 752–3.

Cho E, Smith-Warner SA, Spiegelman D *et al.* (2004a) Dairy foods, calcium, and colorectal cancer: a pooled analysis of 10 cohort studies. *J Natl Cancer Inst* 96: 1015–22.

Cho E, Smith-Warner SA, Ritz J *et al.* (2004b) Alcohol intake and colorectal cancer: a pooled analysis of 8 cohort studies. *Ann Intern Med* 140: 603–13.

Citarda F, Tomaselli G, Capocaccia R, Barcherini S, Crespi M. Italian Multicentre Study Group. (2001) Efficacy in standard clinical practice of colonoscopic polypectomy in reducing colorectal cancer incidence. *Gut* 48: 812–5.

Colvert JR, Brown CH. (1948) Rectal polyps: diagnosis, 5 year follow-up, and relation to carcinoma of the rectum. *Am J Med Sci* 215: 24–32.

Cooper GS, Yuan Z, Landefeld CS *et al.* (1995) A national population-based study of incidence of colorectal cancer and age: implications for screening older Americans. *Cancer* 75: 775–81.

Cotterchio M, Manno M, Klar N, McLaughlin J, Gallinger S. (2005) Colorectal screening is associated with reduced colorectal cancer risk: a case-control study within the population-based Ontario Familial Colorectal Cancer Registry. *Cancer Causes Control* 16: 865–75.

Cram P, Fendrick AM, Inadomi J, Cowen ME, Carpenter D, Vijan S. (2003) The impact of a celebrity promotional campaign on the use of colon cancer screening: the Katie Couric effect. *Arch Intern Med* 163: 1601–5.

Cross AJ, Sinha R. (2004) Meat-related mutagens/carcinogens in the etiology of colorectal cancer. *Environ Mol Mutagen* 44: 44–55.

Cross AJ, Pollock JR, Bingham SA. (2003) Haem, not protein or inorganic iron, is responsible for endogenous intestinal N-nitrosation arising from red meat. *Cancer Res* 63: 2358–60.

Deplancke B, Finster K, Graham WV, Collier CT, Thurmond JE, Gaskins HR. (2003) Gastrointestinal and microbial responses to sulfate-supplemented drinking water in mice. *Exp Biol Med* 228: 424–33.

Dube C, Rostom A, Lewin G *et al.* (2007) U.S. Preventive Services Task Force. The use of aspirin for primary prevention of colorectal cancer: a systematic review prepared for the U.S. Preventive Services Task Force. *Ann Intern Med* 146: 365–75.

Duffield-Lillico AJ, Reid ME, Turnbull BW *et al.* (2002) Baseline characteristics and the effect of selenium supplementation on cancer incidence in a randomized clinical trial: a summary report of the Nutritional Prevention of Cancer Trial. *Cancer Epidemiol Biomarkers Prev* 11: 630–9.

Engle SJ, Ormsby I, Pawlowski S *et al.* (2002) Elimination of colon cancer in germ-free transforming growth factor beta 1-deficient mice. *Cancer Research* 62: 6362–6.

Fernandez-Banares F, Cabre E, Esteve M *et al.* (2002) Serum selenium and risk of large size colorectal adenomas in a geographical area with a low selenium status. *Am J Gastroenterol* 97: 2103–8.

Flood DM, Weiss NS, Cook LS, Emerson JC, Schwartz SM, Potter JD. (2000) Colorectal cancer incidence in Asian migrants to the United States and their descendants. *Cancer Causes Control* 11: 403–11.

Friedenreich C, Norat T, Steindorf K *et al.* (2006) Physical activity and risk of colon and rectal cancers: the European prospective investigation into cancer and nutrition. *Cancer Epidemiol Biomarkers Prev* 15: 2398–407.

Geier MS, Butler RN, Howarth GS. (2006) Probiotics, prebiotics and synbiotics: a role in chemoprevention for colorectal cancer? *Cancer Biol Ther* 5: 1265–9.

Giovannucci E. (1998) Meta-analysis of coffee consumption and risk of colorectal cancer. *Am J Epidemiol* 147: 1043–52.

Giovannucci E. (2001) An updated review of the epidemiological evidence that cigarette smoking increases risk of colorectal cancer. *Cancer Epidemiol Biomarkers Prev* 10: 725–31.

Giovannucci E. (2002) Epidemiologic studies of folate and colorectal neoplasia: a review. *J Nutr* 132(8 Suppl): 2350S–2355S.

GLOBOCAN. (2002) International Agency for Research on Cancer. http://www-dep.iarc.fr/ [accessed May 15, 2007]

Gorham ED, Garland CF, Garland FC *et al.* (2005) Vitamin D and prevention of colorectal cancer. *J Steroid Biochem Mol Biol* 97: 179–94.

Hofstad B, Almendingen K, Vatn M *et al.* (1998) Growth and recurrence of colorectal polyps: a double-blind 3-year intervention with calcium and antioxidants. *Digestion* 59: 148–56.

Hope ME, Hold GL, Kain R, El-Omar EM. (2005) Sporadic colorectal cancer—role of the commensal microbiota. *FEMS Microbiol Lett* 244: 1–7.

Howe GR, Benito E, Castelleto R *et al.* (1992) Dietary intake of fiber and decreased risk of cancers of the colon and rectum: evidence from the combined analysis of 13 case-control studies. *J Natl Cancer Inst* 84: 1887–96.

Hewitson P, Glasziou P, Irwig L, Towler B, Watson E. (2007) Screening for colorectal cancer using the faecal occult blood test, Hemoccult. *Cochrane Database Syst Rev* 1 CD001216. DOI: 10.1002/14651858.CD001216.pub2.

Ishikawa H, Akedo I, Otani T *et al.* (2005) Randomized trial of dietary fiber and *Lactobacillus casei* administration for prevention of colorectal tumors. *Int J Cancer* 116: 762–7.

Isomura K, Kono S, Moore MA *et al.* (2006) Physical activity and colorectal cancer: the Fukuoka Colorectal Cancer Study. *Cancer* Sci 97: 1099–104.

Jacobs ET, Jiang R, Alberts DS *et al.* (2004) Selenium and colorectal adenoma: results of a pooled analysis. *J Natl Cancer Inst* 96: 1669–75.

Jankowski J, Moayyedi P. (2004) Cost effectiveness of aspirin chemoprevention for Barrett's esophagus. *J Natl Cancer Inst* 96: 885–7.

Jess T, Loftus EV Jr, Velayos FS *et al.* (2006) Risk of intestinal cancer in inflammatory bowel disease: a population-based study from olmsted county, Minnesota. *Gastroenterology* 130: 1039–46.

Johns LE, Houlston RS. (2001) A systematic review and meta-analysis of familial colorectal cancer risk. *Am J Gastroenterol* 96: 2992–3003.

Johnsen NF, Christensen J, Thomsen BL *et al.* (2006) Physical activity and risk of colon cancer in a cohort of Danish middle-aged men and women. *Eur J Epidemiol* 21: 877–84.

Jorgensen OD, Kronborg O, Fenger C. (1995) A randomized surveillance study of patients with pedunculated and small sessile tubular and tubulovillous adenomas. The Funen Adenoma Follow-up Study. *Scand J Gastroenterol* 30: 686–92.

Kavanagh AM, Giovannucci EL, Fuchs CS, Colditz GA. (1998) Screening endoscopy and risk of colorectal cancer in United States men. *Cancer Causes Control* 9: 455–62.

Kimura Y, Kono S, Toyomura K *et al.* (2007) Meat, fish and fat intake in relation to subsite-specific risk of colorectal cancer: The Fukuoka Colorectal Cancer Study. *Cancer* Sci 98: 590–7.

Knekt P, Aromaa A, Maatela J *et al.* (1988) Serum vitamin E, serum selenium and the risk of gastrointestinal cancer. *Int J Cancer* 42: 846–50.

Lai SM, Zhang KB, Uhler RJ, Harrison JN, Clutter GG, Williams MA. (2006) Geographic variation in the incidence of colorectal cancer in the United States, 1998–2001. *Cancer* 107 (5 Suppl): 1172–80.

Lamprecht SA, Lipkin M. (2001) Cellular mechanisms of calcium and vitamin D in the inhibition of colorectal carcinogenesis. *Ann NY Acad Sci* 952: 73–87.

Lamprecht SA, Lipkin M. (2003) Chemoprevention of colon cancer by calcium, vitamin D and folate: molecular mechanisms. *Nat Rev Cancer* 3: 601–14.

Lanza E, Schatzkin A, Daston C *et al.* (2001) PPT Study Group. Implementation of a 4-y, high-fiber, high-fruit-and-vegetable, low-fat dietary intervention: results of dietary changes in the Polyp Prevention Trial. Am J Clin Nutr 74: 387–401.

Larsson SC, Wolk A. (2006) Meat consumption and risk of colorectal cancer: a meta-analysis of prospective studies. *Int J Cancer* 119: 2657–64.

Larsson SC, Rutegard J, Bergkvist L, Wolk A. (2006) Physical activity, obesity, and risk of colon and rectal cancer in a cohort of Swedish men. *Eur J* Cancer 42: 2590–7.

Lee DH, Anderson KE, Harnack LJ, Folsom AR, Jacobs DR Jr. (2004) Heme iron, zinc, alcohol consumption, and colon cancer: Iowa Women's Health Study. *J Natl Cancer Inst* 96: 403–7.

Lieberman DA, Weiss DG, Bond JH, Ahnen DJ, Garewal H, Chejfec G. (2000) Use of colonoscopy to screen asymptomatic adults for colorectal cancer. Veterans Affairs Cooperative Study Group 380. *N Engl J Med* 343: 162–8.

Lippman SM, Goodman PJ, Klein EA *et al.* (2005) Designing the Selenium and Vitamin E Cancer Prevention Trial (SELECT). *J Natl Cancer Inst* 97: 94–102.

Mandel JS, Church TR, Bond JH *et al.* (2000) The effect of fecal occult-blood screening on the incidence of colorectal cancer. *N Engl J Med* 343: 1603–7.

Mai PL, Sullivan-Halley J, Ursin G *et al.* (2007) Physical activity and colon cancer risk among women in the California Teachers Study. *Cancer Epidemiol Biomarkers Prev* 16: 517–25.

Martin HM, Campbell BJ, Hart CA *et al.* (2004) Enhanced *Escherichia coli* adherence and invasion in Crohn's disease and colon cancer. *Gastroenterology* 127: 80–93.

McGarr SE, Ridlon JM, Hylemon PB. (2005) Diet, anaerobic bacterial metabolism, and colon cancer: a review of the literature. *J Clin Gastroenterol* 39: 98–109.

McMichael AJ, McCall MG, Hartshorne JM, Woodings TL. (1980) Patterns of gastro-intestinal cancer in European migrants to Australia: the role of dietary change. *Int J Cancer* 25: 431–7.

McTigue K, Larson JC, Valoski A *et al.* (2006) Mortality and cardiac and vascular outcomes in extremely obese women. *JAMA* 296: 79–86.

Michels KB, Fuchs CS, Giovannucci E *et al.* (2005) Fiber intake and incidence of colorectal cancer among 76,947 women and 47,279 men. *Cancer Epidemiol Biomarkers Prev* 14: 842–9.

Mizoue T, Inoue M, Tanaka K *et al.* (2006) Research Group for the Development, Evaluation of Cancer Prevention Strategies in Japan. Tobacco smoking and colorectal cancer risk: an evaluation based on a systematic review of epidemiologic evidence among the Japanese population. *Jpn J Clin Oncol* 36: 25–39.

Moayyedi P, Hunt R. (2004) *Helicobacter pylori* public health implications. *Helicobacter* 9 (Suppl 1): 67–72.

Monroe KR, Hankin JH, Pike MC *et al.* (2003) Correlation of dietary intake and colorectal cancer incidence among Mexican-American migrants: the multiethnic cohort study. *Nutr* Cancer 45: 133–47.

Moskal A, Norat T, Ferrari P, Riboli E. (2007) Alcohol intake and colorectal cancer risk: a dose–response meta-analysis of published cohort studies. *Int J Cancer* 120: 664–71.

Morson B. (1974) The polyp–cancer sequence in the large bowel. *Proc Roy Soc Med* 67: 451–7.

Murakami R, Tsukuma H, Kanamori S *et al.* (1990) Natural history of colorectal polyps and the effect of polypectomy on occurrence of subsequent cancer. *Int J Cancer* 46: 159–64.

Norat T, Riboli E. (2003) Dairy products and colorectal cancer. A review of possible mechanisms and epidemiological evidence. *Eur J Clin Nutr* 57: 1–17.

Norat T, Lukanova A, Ferrari P, Riboli E. (2002) Meat consumption and colorectal cancer risk: dose-response meta-analysis of epidemiological studies. *Int J Cancer* 98: 241–56.

Norat T, Bingham S, Ferrari P *et al.* (2005) Meat, fish, and colorectal cancer risk: the European Prospective Investigation into cancer and nutrition. *J Natl Cancer Inst* 97: 906–16.

Ognjanovic S, Yamamoto J, Maskarinec G, Le Marchand L. (2006) NAT2, meat consumption and colorectal cancer incidence: an ecological study among 27 countries. *Cancer Causes Control* 17: 1175–82.

Palmer RC, Schneider EC. (2005) Social disparities across the continuum of colorectal cancer: a systematic review. *Cancer Causes Control* 16: 55–61.

Parikh-Patel A, Bates JH, Campleman S. (2006) Colorectal cancer stage at diagnosis by socioeconomic and urban/rural status in California, 1988–2000. *Cancer* 107(5 Suppl): 1189–95.

Parkin DM. (2004) International variation. *Oncogene* 23: 6329–40.

Paspatis GA, Karamanolis DG. (1994) Folate supplementation and adenomatous colonic polyps. *Dis Colon Rectum* 37: 1340–1.

Peters U, Chatterjee N, Church TR *et al.* (2006) High serum selenium and reduced risk of advanced colorectal adenoma in a colorectal cancer early detection program. *Cancer Epidemiol Biomarkers Prev* 15: 315–20.

Pischon T, Lahmann PH, Boeing H *et al.* (2006) Body size and risk of colon and rectal cancer in the European Prospective Investigation Into Cancer and Nutrition (EPIC). *J Natl Cancer Inst* 98: 920–31.

Platz EA, Willett WC, Colditz GA, Rimm EB, Spiegelman D, Giovannucci E. (2000) Proportion of colon cancer risk that might be preventable in a cohort of middle-aged US men. *Cancer Causes Control* 11: 579–88.

Quadrilatero J, Hoffman-Goetz L. (2003) Physical activity and colon cancer. A systematic review of potential mechanisms. *J Sports Med Phys Fitness* 43: 121–38.

Rafter J. (2003)Probiotics and colon cancer. *Best Pract Res Clin Gastroenterol* 17: 849–59.

Reis LAG, Eisner MR, Kosary CL *et al.* (1998–2002) Age distribution of incidence cases by site, 1998–2002. SEER Cancer Statistics Review 1975–2002. National Cancer Institute, Bethesda, USA 2007.

Riboli E, Norat T. (2003) Epidemiologic evidence of the protective effect of fruit and vegetables on cancer risk. *Am J Clin Nutr* 78(3 Suppl): 559S–569S.

Robertson DJ, Greenberg ER, Beach M *et al.* (2005) Colorectal cancer in patients under close colonoscopic surveillance. *Gastroenterology* 129: 34–41.

Rostom A, Dube C, Lewin G *et al.* (2007) U.S. Preventive Services Task Force. Nonsteroidal anti-inflammatory drugs and cyclooxygenase-2 inhibitors for primary prevention of colorectal cancer: a systematic review prepared for the U.S. Preventive Services Task Force. *Ann Intern Med* 146: 376–89.

Samad AK, Taylor RS, Marshall T, Chapman MA. (2005) A meta-analysis of the association of physical activity with reduced risk of colorectal cancer. *Colorectal Dis* 7: 204–13.

Sandhu MS, White IR, McPherson K. (2001) Systematic review of the prospective cohort studies on meat consumption and colorectal cancer risk: a meta-analytical approach. *Cancer Epidemiol Biomarkers Prev* 10: 439–46.

Sanjoaquin MA, Allen N, Couto E, Roddam AW, Key TJ. (2005) Folate intake and colorectal cancer risk: a meta-analytical approach. *Int J Cancer* 113: 825–8.

Schatzkin A, Lanza E, Corle D *et al.* (2000)Lack of effect of a low-fat, high-fiber diet on the recurrence of colorectal adenomas. Polyp Prevention Trial Study Group. *N Engl J Med* 342: 1149–55.

Scheppach W, Bingham S, Boutron-Ruault MC *et al.* (1999) WHO consensus statement on the role of nutrition in colorectal cancer. *Eur J Cancer Prev* 8: 57–62.

Scheitel SM, Ahlquist DA, Wollan PC, Hagen PT, Silverstein MD. (1999) Colorectal cancer screening: a community case-control study of proctosigmoidoscopy, barium enema radiography, and fecal occult blood test efficacy. *Mayo Clin Proc* 74: 1207–13.

Schrauzer GN, White DA, Schneider CJ. (1977) Cancer mortality correlation studies. IV: associations with dietary intakes and blood levels of certain trace elements, notably Se-antagonists. *Bioinorg Chem* 7: 35–56.

Segnan N, Senore C, Andreoni B *et al.* (2005) SCORE2 Working Group–Italy. Randomized trial of different screening strategies for colorectal cancer: patient response and detection rates. *J Natl Cancer Inst* 97: 347–57.

Shaukat A, Scouras N, Schunemann HJ. (2005) Role of supplemental calcium in the recurrence of colorectal adenomas: a metaanalysis of randomized controlled trials. *Am J Gastroenterol* 100: 390–4.

Shipp MP, Desmond R, Accortt N, Wilson RJ, Fouad M, Eloubeidi MA. (2005) Population-based study of the geographic variation in colon cancer incidence in Alabama: relationship to socioeconomic status indicators and physician density. *South Med J* 98: 1076–82.

Singh SM, Paszat LF, Li C, He J, Vinden C, Rabeneck L. (2004) Association of socioeconomic status and receipt of colorectal cancer investigations: a population-based retrospective cohort study. *CMAJ* 171: 461–5.

Slattery ML, Edwards SL, Ma KN, Friedman GD. (2000) Colon cancer screening, lifestyle, and risk of colon cancer. *Cancer Causes Control* 11: 555–63.

Stirbu I, Kunst AE, Vlems FA *et al.* (2006) Cancer mortality rates among first and second generation migrants in the Netherlands: Convergence toward the rates of the native Dutch population. *Int J Cancer* 119: 2665–72.

Stryker SJ, Wolff BG, Culp CE, Libbe SD, Ilstrup DM, MacCarty RL. (1987) Natural history of untreated colonic polyps. *Gastroenterology* 93: 1009–13.

Sung JJ, Lau JY, Goh KL, Leung WK. (2005) Asia Pacific Working Group on Colorectal Cancer. Increasing incidence of colorectal cancer in Asia: implications for screening. *Lancet Oncol* 6: 871–6.

Swidsinski A, Khilkin M, Kerjaschki D *et al.* (1998) Association between intraepithelial *Escherichia coli* and colorectal cancer. *Gastroenterology* 115: 281–6.

Tavani A, Fioretti F, Franceschi S *et al.* (1999) Education, socioeconomic status and risk of cancer of the colon and rectum. *Int J Epidemiol* 28: 380–5.

Terry P, Giovannucci E, Michels KB *et al.* (2001a) Fruit, vegetables, dietary fiber, and risk of colorectal cancer. *J Natl Cancer Inst* 93: 525–33.

Terry P, Ekbom A, Lichtenstein P, Feychting M, Wolk A. (2001b) Long-term tobacco smoking and colorectal cancer in a prospective cohort study. *Int J Cancer* 91: 585–7.

Terry P, Bergkvist L, Holmberg L, Wolk A. (2001c) Coffee consumption and risk of colorectal cancer in a population based prospective cohort of Swedish women. *Gut* 49: 87–90.

Thiis-Evensen E, Hoff GS, Sauar J, Langmark F, Majak BM, Vatn MH. (1999) Population-based surveillance by colonoscopy: effect on the incidence of colorectal cancer. Telemark Polyp Study I. *Scand J Gastroenterol* 34: 414–20.

Trock B, Lanza E, Greenwald P. (1990) Dietary fiber, vegetables, and colon cancer: critical review and meta-analyses of the epidemiologic evidence. *J Natl Cancer Inst* 82: 650–61.

UK FSSTI. (2002) Single flexible sigmoidoscopy screening to prevent colorectal cancer. *Lancet* 359: 1291–1300.

van den Brandt PA, Goldbohm RA, van't Veer P *et al.* (1993) A prospective cohort study on toenail selenium levels and risk of gastrointestinal cancer. *J Natl Cancer Inst* 85: 224–9.

van Loon AJ, van den Brandt PA, Golbohm RA. (1995) Socioeconomic status and colon cancer incidence: a prospective cohort study. *Br J* Cancer 71: 882–7.

Voorrips LE, Goldbohm RA, van Poppel G, Sturmans F, Hermus RJ, van den Brandt PA. (2000) Vegetable and fruit consumption and risks of colon and rectal cancer in a prospective cohort study: The Netherlands Cohort Study on Diet and Cancer. *Am J Epidemiol* 152: 1081–92.

Wactawski-Wende J, Kotchen JM, Anderson GL, Assaf AR, Brunner RL, O'Sullivan MJ *et al.* (2006) Calcium plus vitamin D supplementation and the risk of colorectal cancer. *N Engl J Med* 354: 684–96.

Wallace K, Byers T, Morris JS *et al.* (2003) Prediagnostic serum selenium concentration and the risk of recurrent colorectal adenoma: a nested case–control study. *Cancer Epidemiol Biomarkers Prev* 12: 464–7.

Walsh JM, Terdiman JP. (2003) Colorectal cancer screening: scientific review. *JAMA* 289: 1288–96.

Wang WH, Huang JQ, Zheng GF, Lam SK, Karlberg J, Wong BC. (2003) Non-steroidal anti-inflammatory drug use and the risk of gastric cancer: a systematic review and meta-analysis. *J Natl Cancer Inst* 95: 1784–91.

Warburton DE, Nicol CW, Bredin SS. (2006) Health benefits of physical activity: the evidence. *CMAJ* 174: 801–9.

Weiderpass E, Pukkala E. (2006) Time trends in socioeconomic differences in incidence rates of cancers of gastro-intestinal tract in Finland. *BMC Gastroenterol* 6: 41.

Weingarten MA, Zalmanovici A, Yaphe J. (2005) Dietary calcium supplementation for preventing colorectal cancer and adenomatous polyps. *Cochrane Database Syst Rev* (3):CD003548.

Weissfeld JL, Schoen RE, Pinsky PF *et al.* (2005) PLCO Project Team. Flexible sigmoidoscopy in the PLCO cancer screening trial: results from the baseline screening examination of a randomized trial. *J Natl Cancer Inst* 97: 989–97.

Winawer SJ, Zauber AG, Ho MN *et al.* (1993a) Prevention of colorectal cancer by colonoscopic polypectomy. The National Polyp Study Workgroup. *N Engl J Med* 329: 1977–81.

Winawer S, Fletcher R, Rex D *et al.* (2003b) Gastrointestinal Consortium Panel. Colorectal cancer screening and surveillance: clinical guidelines and rationale-Update based on new evidence. *Gastroenterology* 124: 544–60.

Winawer SJ, Zauber AG, Fletcher RH *et al.* (2006) US Multi-Society Task Force on Colorectal Cancer. American Cancer Society. Guidelines for colonoscopy surveillance after polypectomy: a consensus update by the US Multi-Society Task Force on Colorectal Cancer and the American Cancer Society. *Gastroenterology* 130: 1872–85.

Wyatt SB, Winters KP, Dubbert PM. (2006) Overweight and obesity: prevalence, consequences, and causes of a growing public health problem. *Am J Med Sci* 331: 166–74.

Yavari P, Hislop TG, Bajdik C *et al.* (2006) Comparison of cancer incidence in Iran and Iranian immigrants to British Columbia, Canada. *Asian Pac J Cancer Prev* 7: 86–90.

Yoon H, Benamouzig R, Little J, Francois-Collange M, Tome D. (2000) Systematic review of epidemiological studies on meat, dairy products and egg consumption and risk of colorectal adenomas. *Eur J* Cancer *Prev* 9: 151–64.

12 The Molecular Pathology of Sporadic and Hereditary Colorectal Cancer

Massimo Pignatelli, Nahida Banu & Zsombor Melegh

Colorectal cancer is the second most common cancer in the Western world, the third most common cancer worldwide and the fourth commonest cause of death worldwide. The past decade has witnessed a considerable growth in the understanding and management of colorectal cancer, and although there has been a decrease in mortality, it is still the second highest cause of cancer death (Lieberman & Atkin 2004). It causes some 5,500,000 deaths annually worldwide and is thus a major health problem (Gupta *et al.* 2002). Colorectal cancer is mainly sporadic and is generally observed in the elderly, with about 95% of the cases occurring in individuals over the age of 50 (Kinzler & Vogelstein 1996). A person over the age of 50 has approximately a 5% chance of developing colorectal cancer and a 2.5% chance of dying from it (Trujillo *et al.* 1994). It occurs at an earlier age in individuals with the hereditary forms of colorectal cancer such as familial adenomatous polyposis (FAP) or hereditary non-polyposis colorectal cancer (HNPCC) which account for about 5% of colorectal cancers (Kinzler & Vogelstein 1996; Maughan & Quirke 2002). Here we will review the molecular pathways that are involved in the development of sporadic and hereditary colorectal cancer.

Chromosomal instability in colorectal cancer

Colorectal cancers, whether sporadic or hereditary, are caused by genetic alterations. There are at least two different pathogenic pathways for colorectal cancer: the chromosomal instability pathway and the microsatellite instability pathway. Chromosomal instability is found in about 80% of colorectal cancer and it allows fast and 'efficient' accumulation of cancerous mutations. It involves inactivation of tumor suppressor genes by deletion or mutation, activation of proto-oncogenes by mutation, and dysregulated expression of diverse molecules. Chromosomal unstable or instability (CIN) tumors develop losses or gains of whole chromosome at a rate that is 10–100 times higher than that of normal cells. Investigators have discovered alterations that could lead to CIN. The first described were mutational inactivation of a human homolog of the yeast BUB1 gene (Cahill *et al.* 1998). More recently loss of function of APC was implicated in appearance of CIN. Familial adenomatous polyposis, a major inherited syndrome, is an example of the CIN pathway (Tejpar & Cutsem 2002).

Gastrointestinal Oncology: A Critical Multidisciplinary Team Approach.
Edited by J. Jankowski, R. Sampliner, D. Kerr, and Y. Fong.

Familial adenomatous polyposis

Familial adenomatous polyposis is a rare autosomal dominant disease with almost 100% penetrance (Strate & Syngal 2005). The disease is maintained in the population at a frequency of about 1 in 8000 (Bodmer 1996), is characterized by a large number of colorectal adenomas (Fig. 12.1) (more than 100), and accounts for approximately 1% of all colorectal cancer.

Genetics

The identification of an interstitial deletion on chromosome 5q21 in a patient with Gardner's syndrome, followed by linkage analysis, led to the positional cloning of the *adenomatous polyposis coli* (APC) gene in 1991 (Groden *et al.* 1991). Familial adenomatous polyposis is caused by germline mutations of this tumor suppressor gene APC. APC is a large gene, encompassing 15 exons with an open reading frame of 8538 base pairs. It encodes a protein of 2843 amino acids with a molecular weight of 310 kDa (Lal & Gallinger 2000). More than 800 different germline mutations in the APC gene have been published and the most (> 90%) are nonsense mutations and frameshift mutations that lead to premature stop codons. The resulting protein is truncated and presumably non-functional (Strate & Syngal 2005). Most of these germline mutations are clustered at the 5' end of exon 15, otherwise referred to as the mutation cluster region (Galiatsatos & Foulkes 2006).

Genotype–phenotype correlation in FAP

It is not the mutation itself that is of relevance, but its localization within the gene, since it defines the length of the mutant

APC protein. The FAP phenotype (age of onset, type and number of intestinal polyps and extracolonic tumors) correlates somewhat with the type and location of APC mutations (Lal & Gallinger 2000). Generally, mutations in the central region of the gene (codons 1290–1400) give a profuse polyposis phenotype with thousands of intestinal polyps (Lipton & Tomlinson 2006). A deletion of 5 base pairs at codon 1309 is the most frequent mutation (18% of all FAP patients). This leads a severe phenotype, with an onset of disease 10 years earlier than in patients with mutations between codons 168 and 1580 (except codon 1309). Another frequent mutation is a deletion of 5 bp at codon 1061 (12%) of all FAP patients. Patients with mutations proximal to codon 168 or distal to codon 1580 are diagnosed predominantly at an older age (more than 50 years) and display attenuated phenotype. Approximately 80% of FAP patients present with congenital hypertrophies of the retinal pigment epithelium (CHRPE). CHRPE is associated with mutations in the central portion of the APC gene (codon 463–1387). Mandibular osteomas and desmoid tumors are more prevalent in patients with mutation after codon 1400 (Lipton & Tomlinson 2006). The localization of the APC germline mutation may be of clinical value in the surgical management of colorectal polyposis, since mutations between codon 1250 and 1500 are associated with an increased risk of cancer in the rectal stump after subtotal colectomy (Schulmann *et al.* 2002).

Despite the above genotype–phenotype correlations, various reports suggest that the location of the mutation along the APC gene is not the sole determinant of phenotype, and the other genetic and environmental factors may play a role. For example, a modifier locus (Mom-1) has been shown to regulate polyp number in multiple intestinal neoplasia (Min) mice (Lal & Gallinger 2000).

Tumor progression/APC β-catenin pathway

An important function of the APC gene is the prevention of accumulation of β-catenins, as essential component of the adherens junctions, where it provides the link between E-cadherin and β-catenin, and binds actin and actin-associated proteins (Fodde 2002). β-catenin also represents a very important component of the Wnt/wingless signal transduction pathway. In the absence of Wnt signalling, a cytoplasmic degradation complex (consisting of APC, axin, GSK-3β and β-catenin) leads to the phosphorylation of both β-catenin and axin by GSK-3β. This promotes ubiquitination of β-catenin and its degradation by the proteosomes. Thus at the steady state in the absence of Wnt signalling, β-catenin is rapidly degradated in the cytoplasm. In colorectal cancer there is dysregulation of the Wnt/APC/β-catenin signalling pathway (Fig. 12.1). Wnt signalling reduces the phosphorylation and degradation of β-catenin, leading to its accumulation in the nucleus. In the nucleus β-catenin binds to TCF/LEF transcription factors and activates the target genes such as c-myc and cyclin D1 (Tejpar & Van Cutsem 2002).

Furthermore, APC stabilizes microtubules, thus promoting chromosomal stability. Inactivation of APC can lead to defects in mitotic spindles and chromosomal missegregation, with the resulting aneuploidy leading to cancer (Galiatsatos & Foulkes 2006).

Clinicopathologic presentation

The majority of patients with FAP develop hundreds to thousands of colorectal polyps. Polyp development starts in the distal colorectum at an average age of 15 years, and most patients become symptomatic by the age of 25–30 years. The number and size of these polyps increases with time, ultimately reaching 100 to 5000 in number (Strate & Syngal 2005). Usually there is a positive family history; however, up to 25% of FAP patients do not have a family history, suggesting spontaneous germline mutations in these patients.

Individual colon adenomas in patients with FAP are endoscopically and histologically identical to sporadic adenomatous polyps. The size of polyps is usually <1 cm, they may be

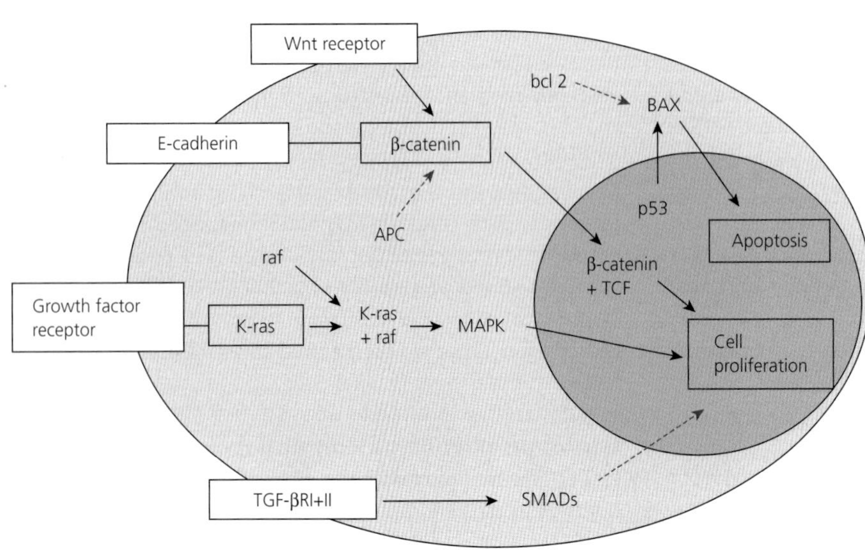

Fig. 12.1 Overview of effector pathways in colorectal carcinogenesis. Black arrows show a positive, red arrows a negative control. Wnt, Wingless pathway; APC, adenomatous polyposis coli; MAPK, mitogen-activated protein kinase; SMAD, mothers against decapentaplegic homolog; TCF, T-cell factor; TGF-β, transforming growth factor-β; BAX, bcl-2-associated X protein.

pedunculated or sessile, with tubular, tubulovillous or villous histology (Lal & Gallinger 2000) (Fig. 12.2). These adenomatous polyps can progressively develop into invasive cancer (Figs 12.3 & 12.4), but they do not have an increased malignant potential in comparison to sporadic polyps. However, nearly in all patients with untreated FAP there is malignant transformation in at least one of these polyps by the fifth decade due to the vast number and early onset of polyps (Strate & Syngal 2005;

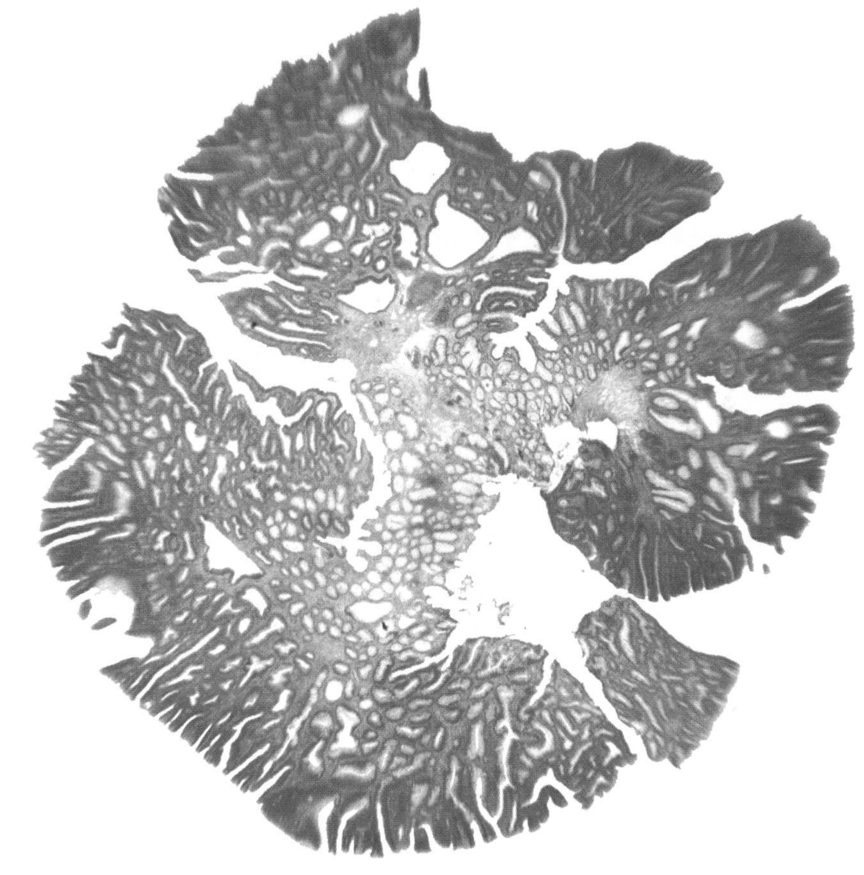

(a)

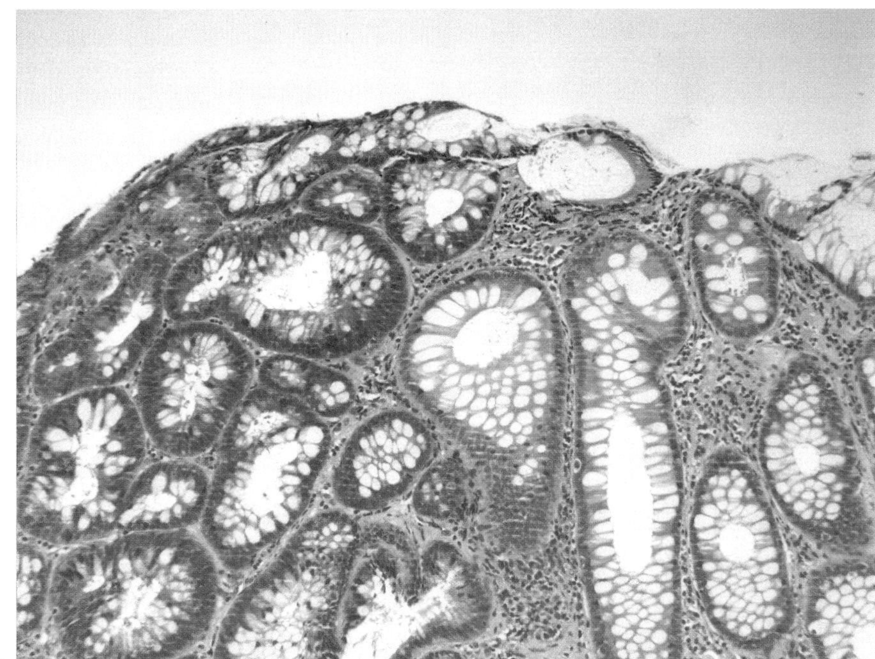

(b)

Fig. 12.2 (a) Tubulovillous adenoma, hematoxylin eosin staining, low magnification. (b) Tubular adenoma, hematoxylin eosin staining, high magnification. Low-grade dysplasia is evident in the adenomatous crypts (left) in a background of normal epithelium (right). *Continued on p. 308.*

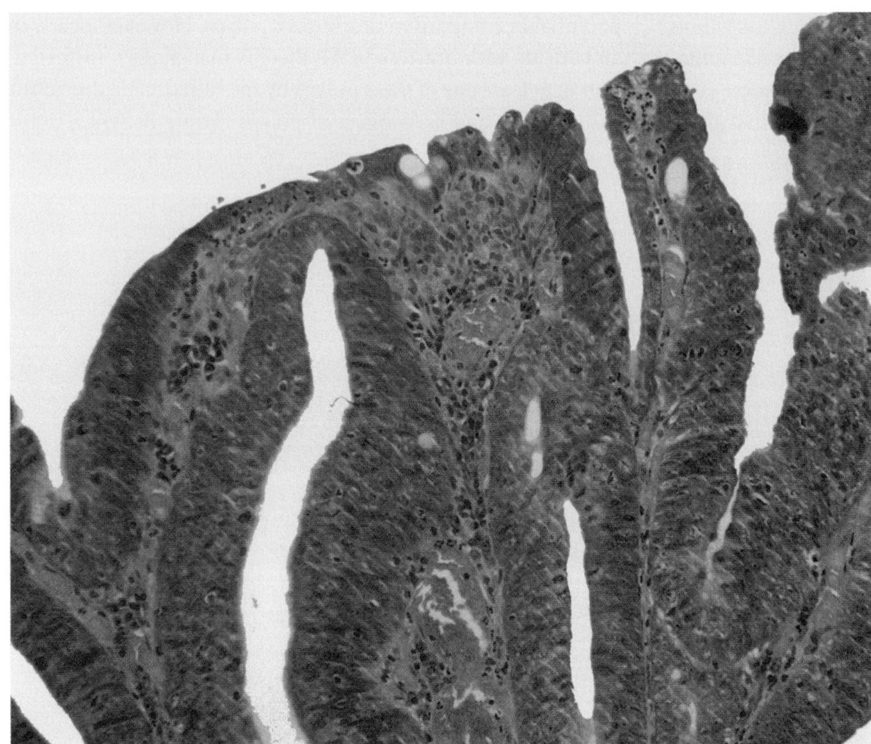

Fig. 12.2 *Continued* (c) Villous adenoma, hematoxylin eosin staining, high magnification. This adenoma shows a villous architecture and high-grade dysplasia.

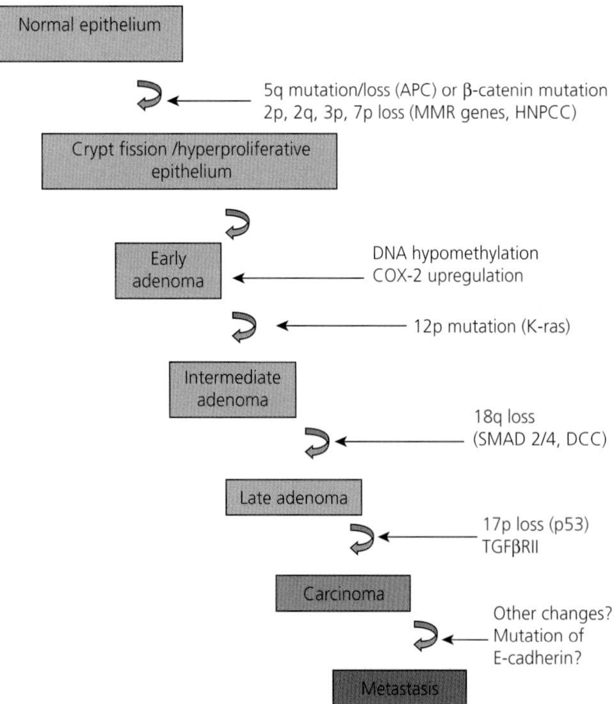

Fig. 12.3 A schematic representation of colorectal tumor development (adapted from Janne & Mayer 2000). Colon cancers result from a series of pathologic changes that transform normal colonic epithelium into adenoma and finally into invasive carcinoma.

Lipton & Tomlinson 2006). The anatomic distribution of colorectal cancers in FAP is similar to the distribution in sporadic cancers (i.e. a preponderance of left-sided and rectal tumors) (Lal & Gallinger 2000). About 70% of patients with FAP who underwent proctocolectomy develop polyps in the upper gastrointestinal tract, often flat adenomas of the duodenum. Roughly 30–40% of FAP patients develop fundic gland polyposis and 5–10% develop gastric adenomas. The risk of gastric cancer is not increased, whereas duodenal cancer and ampullary cancer are the major cause of death in colectomized patients with FAP. Malignancies outside the gastrointestinal tract also occur at an increased frequency in patients with FAP. These lesions include papillary carcinoma of thyroid, hepatoblastoma, adrenal hyperplasia and carcinoma and various central nervous system tumors (Strate & Syngal 2005).

Familial adenomatous polyposis variants

There are three variants of FAP syndrome: Gardner syndrome, Turcot syndrome and attenuated familial adenomatous polyposis (AAPC). In addition, biallelic mutations in the MYH gene may account for up to 30% of families with multiple adenomas who do not exhibit an autosomal dominant pattern of inheritance or a germline mutation in the APC gene (Strate & Syngal 2005).

Gardner syndrome includes manifestations of FAP and the development of benign extracolonic tumors including desmoid

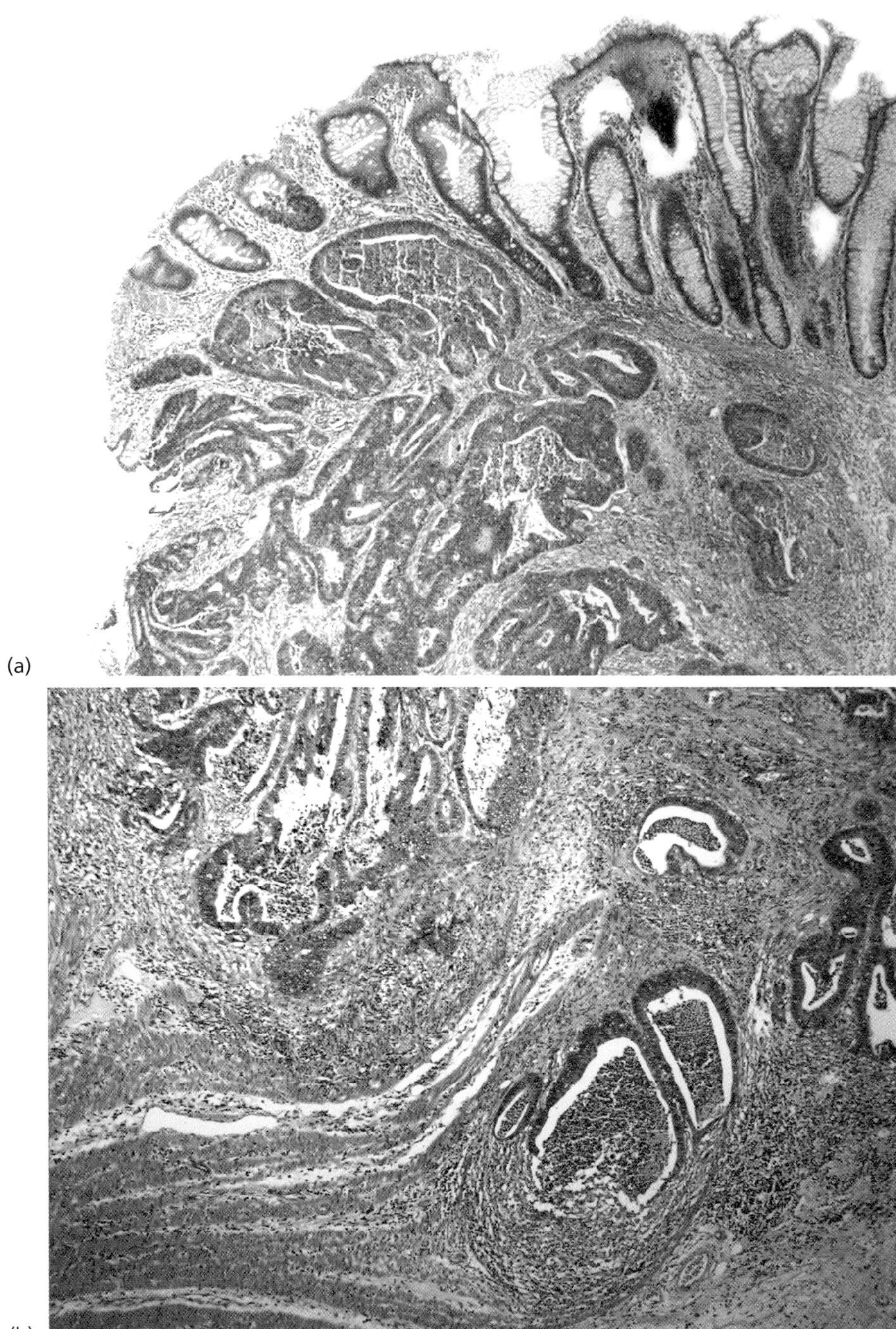

Fig. 12.4 (a) Invasive adenocarcinoma, hematoxylin eosin staining, low magnification. The tumor is infiltrating the bowel wall (left). Residual normal epithelium is also seen in the background (upper right). (b) Invasive adenocarcinoma, hematoxylin eosin staining, high magnification. The tumor is infiltrating between the muscle fibers of the muscular layer of the bowel wall.

tumors, soft tissue tumors, osteomas, epidermoid cysts and dental abnormalities. Desmoids are benign tumors of the connective tissues that can lead to life-threatening complications through their sheer size and impingement on vital structures. They occur in 5–10% of FAP patients, most often in the mesentery or abdominal wall following surgical trauma (Strate & Syngal 2005; Lipton & Tomlinson 2006).

The combination of polyposis and CNS tumors is defined as Turcot's syndrome. The CNS tumors include medulloblastomas, astrocytomas and ependymomas.

The existence of an attenuated form of FAP had been suggested in 1990 by Leppert who showed linkage to 5q in a large family with an attenuated polyposis phenotype (Leppert *et al.* 1987). Approximately 10% of FAP patients present with an attenuated phenotype (AAPC) characterized by milder course of disease, a late onset of colorectal adenomatosis and carcinoma, and a more limited expression of the extracolonic features (Knudsen *et al.* 2003). These patients have fewer than 100 polyps and the predominant development of right-sided colon adenomas, which are often of the flat adenoma type. AAPC is mostly diagnosed between the age of 50 and 55 years, on average 15 years later than classical FAP. The risk of colon malignancy, although very high, is not 100% (Strate & Syngal 2005). The mutations in families with attenuated FAP are located in the proximal or distal parts of the APC gene (Schulmann *et al.* 2002).

Sporadic colorectal cancer with chromosomal instability

Colorectal cancers not associated with hereditary cancer syndromes are defined as sporadic. The lifetime risk of developing sporadic colorectal cancer after age 50 is approximately 5% for average-risk individuals. In addition to genetic predisposition, environmental factors including a diet low in fiber, vegetables and folate but high in fat, red meat and alcohol, sedentary occupation, and cigarette smoking are believed to be associated with an increased colorectal cancer risk.

Genetics

Genomic destabilization is an early step in sporadic tumor development. Stoler and colleagues state that this supports a model in which genomic instability is a cause rather than an effect of colorectal carcinogenesis (Stoler *et al.* 1999). Inactivation of the APC gene is the first molecular event in sporadic colorectal cancer (Fig. 12.5). Somatic APC mutations are identified in approximately 60–80% of sporadic colorectal cancers and adenomas (Narayan & Roy 2003). Nakamura and his colleagues identified in somatic APC mutations a 'mutation cluster region' (MCR) of the gene, which accounted for about 60% of all somatic mutations (Bodmer 2006). Within the MCR there are two hot spots for somatic mutations at codons 1309 and 1450. APC mutation within the MCR results in a truncated APC protein that lacks all of the axin binding sites and all but one or two of its 20-amino acid β-catenin binding sites (Fearnhead *et al.* 2001). About 50% of sporadic tumors with intact APC are reported to show mutations of β-catenin itself, resulting in the accumulation of β-catenin (Takayama *et al.* 2006). P53 mutations have been identified in 40–50% of sporadic colorectal cancers. P53 mutation occurs at the time of transition from adenoma to cancer. Most mutations occur in highly conserved areas of exon 5 to 8 and the majority are missense mutations (GC to AT). The frequency of p53 mutation is higher in distal colon and rectal cancers than in proximal colon cancers. Patients with cancers involving a p53 mutation have a worse outcome and shorter survival time than patients without p53 mutations. K-ras mutation has been found in 15–68% of sporadic colorectal adenomas and in 40–65% of cancers. The majority of k-ras mutations occur as an activating point mutation in codons 12, 13 and 64. Mutated k-ras protein activates a variety of effector pathways including raf/MAPK, Jun N-terminal kinase (JNK) and phosphatidylinositol-3 kinase (PI3-K), which leads to constitutive growth promotion. Some of the downstream gene targets of k-ras include the cyclin D1, DNA methyltransferase, and vascular endothelial growth factors (Takayama *et al.* 2006). Allelic losses on chromosome 18q have been identified in approximately 70% of primary colorectal cancers, particularly in advanced colorectal cancers, with metastasis (Fearon & Vogelstein 1990). Point mutations of the DCC gene have been identified in approximately 6% of sporadic colorectal cancers (Cho *et al.* 1994).

Recently the candidacy of this gene has been called into question. Mice heterozygous for DCC have been reported to lack the tumor predisposition phenotype. SMAD4/2, a tumor suppressor gene has been reported on 18q, and SMAD4 has been causally associated with progression of cancers (Takayama *et al.* 2006).

Microsatellite instability in colorectal cancer

In contrast to the chromosomal instability pathway, there is a distinct group of colorectal cancers that do not show large chromosomal abnormalities. These usually diploid tumors have a

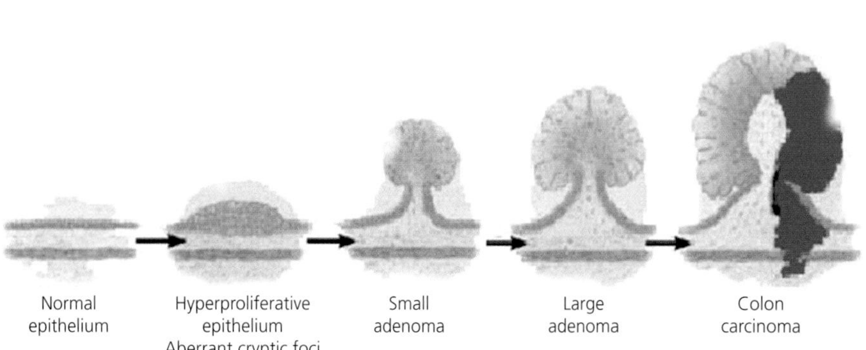

Fig. 12.5 A genetic model for colorectal tumorigenesis (adapted from Fearon & Vogelstein 1990). Tumorigenesis proceeds through a series of genetic alterations involving oncogenes and tumor suppressor genes. Somatic mutations in at least four or five genes of a cell are required for malignant transformation. The accumulation of these changes rather than their order in respect to each other seems most important. Tumors continue to progress once carcinomas have formed and the accumulated loss of suppressor genes on additional chromosomes correlates with the ability of the carcinomas to metastasize and cause death.

different background of the genetic instability, in which the abnormalities are at the nucleotide level. The propensity for deletion or gain of short DNA sequences in these tumors has been termed microsatellite instability.

Microsatellite instability

Microsatellites are short sequences in the genomic DNA comprising repetition of one to four nucleotides. These mono/di/tri/tetranucleotides can be repeated ten to hundred times in the sequence. The most common microsatellite in human is the repetition of citosine–adenine dinucleotide (i.e. CACACACACA). Due to the repetitive nature of these sequences they are liable to changes during DNA replication. Under normal conditions these mistakes are corrected by DNA repair enzymes during cell replication. These enzymes and the process of DNA repair are highly conserved throughout the philogenesis. If the repair process is damaged the microsatellite sequences can lose or gain nucleotides and this phenomenon is termed microsatellite instability (MSI). As a consequence, alteration of the length of the microsatellites is a marker of an underlying DNA repair malfunction.

The detection of microsatellite instability is possible with current diagnostic processes only if there are numerous cells bearing the same abnormality, i.e. the cells are part of a clonal process. Clonal proliferation is a characteristic of neoplastic processes, which consequently means that a microsatellite instability detected by current diagnostic methods is indicative of a clonal neoplastic process (Soreide *et al.* 2006).

Loss or gain of nucleotides in coding microsatellites or in other coding sequences changes the amino acid sequence of the coded protein by means of frame shift mutation. In frame shift mutation deletion or insertion of a single nucleotide shifts the reading frame of the DNA polymerase and in turn changes the amino acid sequence of the gene product. Frame shift mutations in microsatellites or in other sequences can cause loss of function in genes which play important roles in the life cycle of the cells. Ultimately, loss of function of DNA repair proteins results in genomic instability which promotes mutations in other genes and facilitates malignant transformation.

Human non-polyposis colorectal cancer

It became clear in the mid 1990s that the human non polyposis colorectal cancer (HNPCC) or Lynch syndrome that was originallly described by Warthin in 1913 and further characterized by Lynch in the mid 1960s (Lynch *et al.* 1998), is associated with MSI (Peltomaki *et al.* 1993; Thibodeau *et al.* 1993). HNPCC is responsible for up to 6% of colorectal cancers (Aaltonen *et al.* 1998) and hence it is the most common form of hereditary colorectal cancer syndromes. The syndrome is characterized by increased risk of carcinogenesis in the gastrointestinal tract, endometrium, and ovary, and rarely in the urogenital tract, hepatobiliary tract and pancreas (Aarnio *et al.* 1999). The lifetime 5–6% risk of developing colorectal cancer that is seen in the normal population is increased to 70–80% in HNPCC (Aarnio 1999; Chung & Rustgi 2003). Lifetime risk of endometrial cancer is increased by a similar magnitude (around 60%), while the lifetime risk of other cancers is only moderately increased (by between 2 and 13%).

Similarly to FAP, HNPCC shows an autosomal dominant inheritance, but the underlying cause is germline mutation of DNA repair genes. The most commonly mutated genes are human MutL homologue 1 (hMLH1) found on chromosome 3p and human MutS homologue 2 (hMSH2) located to chromosome 2p. The name 'Mut' originates from the work on *E. coli* that showed that inactivation of these genes gave rise to hypermutable strains. Other, less commonly involved genes in HNPCC are human MutS homologue (hMSH6), and human postmeiotic segregation increased 2 (hPMS2) and 1 (hPMS1). The later two were first described in the *Saccharomyces cerevisiae* genome.

Tumor progression in HNPCC

It seems that the genetic pathway leading to tumor genesis in HNPCC considerably overlaps with CIN, but there are differences in the involvement of the different genes. Tumors of the HNPCC pathway also show mutations of APC, p53 and K-ras genes (Huang *et al.* 1996), but the incidence of p53 and K-ras mutation is less frequent than in CIN (Samowitz *et al.* 2001b). In addition, there are certain genes with important roles in the regulation of the cell growth that have coding microsatellite sequences, such as transforming growth factor β1 receptor II (TGF-βRII) (Parsons *et al.* 1995), retinoblasstoma-protein-interacting zinc fingers (RIZ) (Piao *et al.* 2000), T-cell factor 4 (TF4) (Duval *et al.* 1999), bcl-2-associated X protein (BAX) (Ouyang *et al.* 1998), and insulin-like growth factor II receptor (IGFRIIR) (Souza *et al.* 1996). Among these, the tumorigenic role of TGF-βRII and BAX mutations is the best characterized (Fig. 12.1). Mutation of TGF-βRII is the most common among the above-mentioned genes, occuring in about 90% of MSI-associated cancers. Change of function of this receptor leads to dysregulation of the SMAD protein pathway that has an important role in transcription regulation. The BAX gene is affected in about 33% of MSI-associated cancers, and the mutation of this gene leads to disruption of the function of B-cell CLL/lymphoma 2 (bcl-2) mediated apoptosis pathway.

Microstatellites are also found in the coding sequences of DNA repair genes such as hMSH6, hMSH2 and hMSH3, but the importance of this is not yet fully understood (Yamamoto *et al.* 1998).

Clinicopathologic features

Cancers in HNPCC tend to localize to the right side of the colon, proximal to the splenic flexure (Lynch *et al.* 1993). They appear about 20 years earlier than sporadic colorectal cancers; the mean age at diagnosis is about 44 years. There is an increased risk of multiplicity of colorectal cancers that can be either synchronous (multiple colorectal cancers at or within 6 months after surgical resection for colorectal cancer) or metachronous (colorectal cancer occurring more than 6 months after resection for colorectal cancer) (Lynch & de la Chapelle 1999).

Histologically, a characteristic feature is the presence of tumor-infiltrating lymphocytes and a Crohn's disease-like peritumoral lymphocytic reaction. On immunohistochemical analysis it has been demonstrated that the tumor-infiltrating lymphocytes are CD8+ T cells, while the peritumoral lymphoctes are B cells surrounded by T cells. This prominent imflamatory response is found to be associated with the improved survival seen in HNPCC (Samowitz *et al.* 2001a). These cancers are also more commonly poorly differentiated or show a mucinous phenotype (Jass 2000). The inflammatory reaction is not always prominent in these tumors, but usually still seen in the non-mucinous areas of a mucinous carcinoma.

Patients do not usually present with the large number of adenomas as seen in AFP, yet the adenomas tend to be slightly more frequent than in the age-matched normal population. However, these adenomas do not show a predilection to the right side of the colon and are evenly distributed throughout the large bowel. In addition, they show more prominent villous architecture and high-grade dysplasia, histologic features that are associated with increased cancer risk (Jass 1994).

HNPCC variants

Muir–Torre syndrome is characterized by an association of internal malignancies and uncommon sebaceous skin tumors (Schwartz & Torre 1995). The striking similarity of the internal cancers to those seen in HNPCC led to the assumption that Muir–Torre is a rare variant of HNPCC. Investigation of DNA repair genes located the mutation to hMSH2 but in exceptional cases it can be seen in hMLH1 (Kolodner *et al.* 1994).

Turcot syndrome, an association of colorectal and of brain tumors, can be caused not just by FAP mutation but also by microsatellite instability (Hamilton *et al.* 1995). In the latter case the brain tumor is usually a glioma that can arise in childhood but is also seen in adults. The underlying mutation is found in hMLH1, hMSH2 and also hPMS2. Association of hPMS2 with Turcot syndrome is of special interest, since the few cases of hPMS2 mutation described in the literature were nearly exclusively identified in families showing features of Turcot syndrome.

Similar to FAP, an attenuated phenotype of HNPCC is also seen in certain families, where there is a reduced penetrance and late onset of cancer (Lucci-Gordisco *et al.* 2003).

In exceptional cases patients can carry homozygous germline mutations of DNA repair genes (Hamilton 1995; Lucci-Gordisco 2003). These patients present with a phenotype which shows a striking similarity to those seen in neurofibromatosis type 1 (café-au-lait spots, dermal neurofibromas, axillary freckling) as well as development of leukemia or lymphoma. Unfortunately mutation of the neurofibromatosis 1 gene is yet to be investigated in these cases and hence it is not clear whether a secondary mutation of neurofibromatosis 1 gene is behind these changes.

Genetic testing for HNPCC

In order to capture individuals with HNPCC the so-called Amsterdam criteria were established in 1990, primarily for research purposes (Vasen *et al.* 1991) (Table 12.1). These criteria were based on the patient's age and presence of colorectal malignancies in the patient's relatives. As it became clear that the syndrome can also have extracolonic manifestations, these criteria were revised to incorporate extracolonic malignancies (Vasen *et al.* 1999). Several modifications of the Amsterdam criteria have been also proposed, but these were not intended

Table 12.1 Amsterdam criteria.

The Amsterdam criteria (1990)

At least three relatives with colorectal cancer plus all the following:
- one affected patient is a first-degree relative of the other two
- two or more successive generations affected
- at least one affected relative diagnosed with colorectal cancer at age <50 years
- familial adenomatous coli excluded
- tumors verified by pathologic examination

Amsterdam II criteria (1997)

There should be at least three relatives with an HNPCC-associated cancer.
- One affected patient is a first-degree relative of the other two
- Two or more successive generations affected
- At least one affected relative diagnosed with colorectal cancer at age < 50 years
- Familial adenomatous coli excluded
- Tumors verified by pathologic examination

Modified Amsterdam criteria

Only one of these criteria need to be met.
- In very small families a patient can be considered to have HNPCC with colorectal cancer even if only two first-degree relatives had colorectal cancer, if at least two generations had the cancer and at least one case of colorectal cancer was diagnosed at age < 50 years
- In families where two first-degree relatives are affected by colorectal cancer, the presence of a third relative with an unusual early-onset neoplasm or endometrial cancer is sufficient for the diagnosis of HNPCC

Young age at onset criterion

If an individual is diagnosed at age <40 years and does not have a family history that fulfils the Amsterdam or modified Amsterdam criteria they are still considered to have HNPCC

HNPCC variant criterion

If an individual has a family history that suggests HNPCC but does not fulfil the Amsterdam or modified Amsterdam criteria or young age of onset criterion, they are considered to have HNPCC variant for diagnostic purposes (Benatti et al. 1993; Bellacosa et al. 1996).

The Bethesda criteria (Rodriguez-Bigas et al. 1997) and their modified version (Umar et al. 2004) were introduced to recognize patients and families who would benefit from genetic testing (Table 12.2). These criteria take further clinicopathologic features into account, such as undifferentiated phenotype, right-sided predominance and multiplicity of colorectal cancer.

Further testing for mutations in microsatellites is recommended in those individuals who correspond to any of the Bethesda criteria (Burt & Neklason 2005; Kaz & Brentnall 2006). This PCR-based method requires samples from both normal and tumor tissue. Those tumors that show mutation in at least 40% of the examined microsatellites are termed microsatellite instability high (MSI-H), those with less than 40% microsatellite instability low (MSI-L), and those with no mutation microsatellite stable (MSS) tumors (Boland et al. 1998). Since usually five microsatellites are used for testing, in practice this means that a tumor is called MSI-H if at least two out of five markers show mutation. The most commonly used microsatellite markers are Bat 25 and Bat 26, which contain mononucleotide repeats, and D5S346, DS123 and D17S250, which contain dinucleotide repeats.

Table 12.2 Bethesda guidelines for identification of patients with colorectal tumors who should undergo genetic testing for microsatellite instability.

Bethesda Guidelines (1997)

Only one of these criteria needs to be met.

- Individuals with cancer in families meeting the Amsterdam criteria
- Individuals with two HNPCC-related cancers, including synchronous and metachronous colorectal cancers or associated extracolonic cancers
- Individuals with colorectal cancer and a first-degree relative with colorectal cancer or HNPCC-related extracolonic cancer or a colorectal adenoma, one of the cancers diagnosed at age <45 years, and the adenoma diagnosed at age <40 years
- Individuals with colorectal cancer or endometrial cancer diagnosed at age <45 years
- Individuals with right-sided colorectal cancer with an undifferentiated pattern on histopathology diagnosed at age <45 years
- Individuals with signet-ring cell-type colorectal cancer diagnosed at age <45 years
- Individuals with adenomas diagnosed at age <40 years

Revised Bethesda (2004)

Only one of these criteria needs to be met.

- Colorectal cancer diagnosed in individual at age <50 years
- Presence of synchronous, metachronous colorectal, or other HNPCC-associated tumors, regardless of age
- Colorectal cancer with the MSI-H histology at age < 60 years
- Colorectal cancer in one or more first-degree relatives with colorectal cancer or other HNPCC-related tumor, with one of the cancers being diagnosed at age <50 years (this includes adenoma which must be diagnosed at age <40 years)
- Colorectal cancer diagnosed in two or more first- or second-degree relatives with colorectal cancer or other HNPCC-related tumors, regardless of age

As we will see, microsatellite instability can be also seen in about 15%% of sporadic colorectal cancers, and therefore an MSI-H tumor itself is not diagnostic for HNPCC. Hence further mutational analysis of hMLH1and hMSH2 is also recommended in MSI-H tumors.

Loss of expression of DNA mismatch repair genes can also be detected by immunohistochemistry, but this method has lower sensitivity and specificity than the PCR-based methods (Shia et al. 2003).

Sporadic MSI-associated colorectal cancer

Only about 6% of colorectal cancers are associated with either HNPCC or APC. The vast majority of the remaining tumors are sporadic. Most of these sporadic colorectal cancers follow the CIN pathway, but about 15% of them show a different pathway and these are associated with deficient mismatch repair. In contrast to HNPCC, these sporadic MSI-H-associated colorectal cancers carry no germline mutation of DNA repair genes, the underlying mechanism is usually epigenetic silencing of the genes. Epigenetic changes affect the gene function by methylation of cytosine residues of citosine- and guanine-rich 0.5–2-kb regions, so-called CpG islands (the ‘p’ stands for the phosphodiester bond between the two nucleotides) in promoter sequences. As a consequence, there is no transcription of the gene, hence the gene is ‘silenced’. Methylation in MSI-H-associated colorectal cancer most commonly occurs at the promoter region of hMLH1 (Kane 1997).

CpG island methylation phenotype

Methylation of the genome on one hand is considered as a normal aging process, in as much it shows an increased frequency with progressive age. It is also more commonly found in females. As a consequence, MSI-H-associated sporadic colorectal cancer is more frequent in elderly females (Malkhosyan et al. 2000). On the other hand it is possible that in some instances there is a predisposition to increased genomic methylation. Colorectal tumor development against a background of increased genomic methylation is designated CpG island methylation phenotype (CIMP). CIMP is characterized by promoter methylation of multiple genes that are methylated in cancer but not in normal tissue (Toyota et al. 1999). This type of methylation is termed Type C in contrast to age-related Type A methylation. Some authors consider CIMP merely one extreme within the normal distribution of methylation events (Yamashita 2003; Anacleto 2005), while others suggest that this is a third pathway of tumor genesis in addition to the MSI and the CIN pathways (Ogino 2006; Weisenberger et al. 2006). Unfortunately, it is still not clearly defined what degree of methylation would make a certain tumor belong to the CIMP group. Furthermore, the fact that high level of methylation is also seen in MSI-H tumors suggests that the group of MSI-H and CIMP-associated tumors hugely overlap. However, excess level of b-raf mutation is uniformly seen in CIMP-associated MSI-H and MSS colorectal cancers (Samowitz et al. 2005; Ogino et al. 2006). This leads to a further assumption, namely that hMLH1 methylation in MSI-H sporadic cancers is merely a consequence of a broader epigenetic control defect that is seen in CIMP (Weisenberger 2006), while the same epigenetic control defect does not affect hMLH1 in other MSS-associated CIMP cases.

Clinicopathologic features

Although they show much similarity, sporadic MSI-H-associated cancer should not be simply considered as a sporadic counterpart of HNPCC, as they differ not just in their genetic background but also in clinical and pathologic features. As we have seen, sporadic MSI-H-associated colorectal cancers tend to be more common among females and are seen in older individuals, usually above 65 years of age. They also have a greater tendency to develop in the proximal colon than it is seen in HNPCC (Jass 2004). Histologically they are very similar to the colorectal cancers seen in HNPCC, but are also more commonly heterogeneous with areas of different degrees of differentiation (Jass et al. 2002) or contain a mucinous component (Jass 2004). There is also increasing evidence that while HNPCC develops from traditional colorectal adenomas (Iino et al. 2000), most if not all sporadic MSI-H colorectal cancers arise from serrated polyps.

Tumor progression in MSI-associated sporadic colorectal tumors/serrated pathway

The recently characterized and still evolving group of serrated polyps comprises classic hyperplastic polyps and serrated adenomas, all of which show a serrated architecture of the crypts. There are three morphologically distinct groups of hyperplastic polyps; these are termed goblet cell rich, microvesicular and mucin poor (Snover et al. 2005). The originally described serrated adenoma (Longacre & Fenoglio-Preiser 1990), which showed features of both traditional adenomas and hyperplastic polyps is now retermed as traditional serrated adenoma. Sessile serrrated adenomas show architectural atypia with no overt cytologic dysplasia (Torlakovic & Snover 1996). Mixed polyps are also seen, usually showing features of tubular adenoma and sessile serrated adenoma in the same polyp (Snover et al. 2005).

Among these, similar molecular features have been described in microvesicular hyperplastic polyps and sessile serrated adenomas. These tumors show high frequency of b-raf mutation and microsatellite instability (Kambara et al. 2004), while k-ras mutation rate was found to be very low (Wynter et al. 2004). B-raf is a part of the mitogen activating protein (map) kinase activating cascade, which regulates various cellular activities, such as gene expression, mitosis, differentiation, and cell survival/apoptosis. B-raf mutation is also common in sporadic MSI-H-associated colorectal cancers, while k-ras mutation is infrequent in these tumors (Koinuma et al. 2004). The fact that among these three entities the frequency of b-raf mutation and MSI is the lowest in microvesicuar hyperplastic polyps and highest in MSI-H-associated sporadic cancer led to the assumption that MSI-associated sporadic cancer is an endpoint of a microvesicular hyperplastic polyp–sessile serrated adenoma–carcinoma sequence (O'Brien et al. 2006; Spring et al. 2006). This theory has been also supported on morphologic grounds, namely that serrated lesions are seen adjacent to an MSI-associated carcinoma (Makinen et al. 2001; Jass 2004).

As we have seen before, the map kinase cascade is also affected in the CIN-associated tumorigenesis in the form of k-ras mutation. This fact emphasizes the important role of dysregulation of the map kinase cascade in colorectal carcinogenesis and also shows that the same cascade can be affected at different points in the two tumorigenetic pathways. It is also important to underline that either k-ras or b-raf mutation alone is enough for the disruption of the cascade; therefore mutation of the two genes is usually not seen in the same tumor (Ogino et al. 2006).

Conclusion

Our evolving knowledge of its pathology and elucidation of the genetic background of colorectal cancer showed that it is a heterogeneous disease with different pathways involved in cancer development. Identification of specific stepwise mutations is a potential tool to predict prognosis or response to therapy in an individual and also provides a basis to develop novel strategies based on molecular targeting.

Identification of a germline mutation in a hereditary syndrome can confirm risk, and consequently a reduced mortality and morbidity can be achieved in affected individuals and families. Germline APC mutations carry a 99% risk of CRC by 40 years of age. Therefore it is important that physicians be familiar not just with appropriate cancer screening and surgical prophylactic methods, but also with the biologic background of familial cancer syndromes.

References

Aaltonen LA, Salovaara R, Kristo P *et al.* (1998) Incidence of hereditary nonpolyposis colorectal cancer and the feasibility of molecular screening for the disease. *N Engl J Med* 338(21): 1481–7.

Aarnio M, Sankila R, Pukkala E *et al.* (1999) Cancer risk in mutation carriers of DNA-mismatch-repair genes. *Int J Cancer* 81(2): 214–8.

Bellacosa A, Genuardi M, Anti M, Viel A, Ponz de Leon M. (1996) Hereditary nonpolyposis colorectal cancer: review of clinical, molecular genetics, and counseling aspects. *Am J Med Genet* 62(4): 353–64.

Benatti P, Sassatelli R, Roncucci L *et al.* (1993) Tumour spectrum in hereditary non-polyposis colorectal cancer (HNPCC) and in families with 'suspected HNPCC'. A population-based study in northern Italy. Colorectal Cancer Study Group. *Int J Cancer* 54(3): 371–7.

Bodmer WF. (2006) Cancer genetics: colorectal cancer as a model. *J Hum Genet* 51(5): 391–6.

Boland CR, Thibodeau SN, Hamilton SR *et al.* (1998) A National Cancer Institute Workshop on Microsatellite Instability for cancer detection and familial predisposition: development of international criteria for the determination of microsatellite instability in colorectal cancer. *Cancer Res* 58(22): 5248–57.

Burt R, Neklason DW. (2005) Genetic testing for inherited colon cancer. *Gastroenterology* 128(6): 1696–716.

Cahill DP, Lengauer C, Yu J *et al.* (1998) Mutations of mitotic checkpoint genes in human cancers. *Nature* 392(6673): 300–3.

Cho KR, Oliner JD, Simons JW *et al.* (1994) The DCC gene: structural analysis and mutations in colorectal carcinomas. *Genomics* 19(3): 525–3.

Chung DC, Rustgi AK. (2003) The hereditary nonpolyposis colorectal cancer syndrome: genetics and clinical implications. *Ann Intern Med* 138(7): 560–70.

Duval A, Gayet J, Zhou XP, Iacopetta B, Thomas G, Hamelin R. (1999) Frequent frameshift mutations of the TCF-4 gene in colorectal cancers with microsatellite instability. *Cancer Res* 1;59(17): 4213–5.

Fearnhead NS, Britton MP, Bodmer WF. (2001) The ABC of APC. *Hum Mol Genet* 10(7): 721–33.

Fearon ER, Vogelstein B. (1990) A genetic model for colorectal tumorigenesis. *Cell* 61(5): 759–67.

Fodde R. (2002) The APC gene in colorectal cancer. *Eur J Cancer* 38(7): 867–71.

Galiatsatos P, Foulkes WD. (2006) Familial adenomatous polyposis. *Am J Gastroenterol* 101(2): 385–98.

Groden J, Thliveris A. Groden J *et al.* (1991) Identification and characterization of the familial adenomatous polyposis coli gene. *Cell* 66(3): 589–600.

Gupta RA, DuBois RN, Wallace MC. (2002) New avenues for the prevention of colorectal cancer: targeting cyclo-oxygenase-2 activity. *Best Pract Res Clin Gastroenterol* 16: 945–56.

Hamilton SR, Liu B, Parsons RE *et al.* (1995) The molecular basis of Turcot's syndrome. *N Engl J Med* 332(13): 839–47.

Huang J, Papadopoulos N, McKinley AJ *et al.* (1996) APC mutations in colorectal tumors with mismatch repair deficiency. *Proc Natl Acad Sci USA* 93(17): 9049–54.

Iino H, Simms L, Young J *et al.* (2000) DNA microsatellite instability and mismatch repair protein loss in adenomas presenting in hereditary non-polyposis colorectal cancer. *Gut* 47(1): 37–42.

Janne PA, Mayer RJ. (2000) Chemoprevention of colorectal cancer. *N Engl J Med* 342: 1960–8.

Jass JR. (2000) Pathology of hereditary nonpolyposis colorectal cancer. *Ann NY Acad Sci* 910: 62–73.

Jass JR. (2004) HNPCC and sporadic MSI-H colorectal cancer: a review of the morphologic similarities and differences. *Fam Cancer* 3(2): 93–100.

Jass JR, Stewart SM, Stewart J, Lane MR. (1994) Hereditary non-polyposis colorectal cancer–morphologies, genes and mutations. *Mutat Res* 310(1): 125–33.

Jass JR, Walsh MD, Barker M, Simms LA, Young J, Leggett BA. (2002) Distinction between familial and sporadic forms of colorectal cancer showing DNA microsatellite instability. *Eur J Cancer* 38(7): 858–66.

Kambara T, Simms LA, Whitehall VL *et al.* (2004) BRAF mutation is associated with DNA methylation in serrated polyps and cancers of the colorectum. *Gut* 53(8): 1137–44.

Kaz AM, Brentnall TA. (2006) Genetic testing for colon cancer. *Nat Clin Pract Gastroenterol Hepatol* 3(12): 670–9.

Kinzler KW, Vogelstein B. (1996) Lessons from hereditary colorectal cancer. *Cell* 87, 159–70.

Knudsen AL, Bisgaard ML, Bulow S. (2003) Attenuated familial adenomatous polyposis (AFAP). A review of the literature. *Fam Cancer* 2(1): 43–55.

Koinuma K, Shitoh K, Miyakura Y *et al.* (2004) Mutations of BRAF are associated with extensive hMLH1 promoter methylation in sporadic colorectal carcinomas. *Int J Cancer* 108(2): 237–42.

Kolodner RD, Hall NR, Lipford J *et al.* (1995) Structure of the human MSH2 locus and analysis of two Muir-Torre kindreds for msh2 mutations. *Genomics* 24(3): 516–26. Erratum in *Genomics* (1995) 28(3): 613.

Lal G, Gallinger S. (2000) Familial adenomatous polyposis. *Semin Surg Oncol* 18(4): 314–23.

Leppert M, Dobbs M, Scambler P *et al.* (1987) The gene for familial polyposis coli maps to the long arm of chromosome 5. *Science* 238(4832): 1411–3.

Lieberman DA, Atkin W. (2004) Review article: balancing the ideal versus the practical considerations of colorectal cancer prevention and screening. *Aliment Pharmacol Ther* 19 Suppl 1: 71–6.

Lipton L, Tomlinson I. (2006) The genetics of FAP and FAP-like syndromes. *Fam Cancer* 5: 221–6.

Longacre TA, Fenoglio-Preiser CM. (1990) Mixed hyperplastic adenomatous polyps/serrated adenomas. A distinct form of colorectal neoplasia. *Am J Surg Pathol* 14(6): 524–37.

Lucci-Cordisco E, Zito I, Gensini F, Genuardi M. (2003) Hereditary nonpolyposis colorectal cancer and related conditions. *Am J Med Genet A* 122(4): 325–34.

Lynch HT, Smyrk TC, Watson P *et al.* (1993) Genetics, natural history, tumor spectrum, and pathology of hereditary nonpolyposis colorectal cancer: an updated review. *Gastroenterology* 104(5): 1535–49.

Lynch HT, Smyrk T, Lynch JF. (1998) Molecular genetics and clinical-pathology features of hereditary nonpolyposis colorectal carcinoma (Lynch syndrome): historical journey from pedigree anecdote to molecular genetic confirmation. *Oncology* 55(2): 103–8.

Lynch HT, de la Chapelle A. (1999) Genetic susceptibility to non-polyposis colorectal cancer. *J Med Genet* 36(11): 801–18.

Makinen MJ, George SM, Jernvall P, Makela J, Vihko P, Karttunen TJ. (2001) Colorectal carcinoma associated with serrated adenoma—prevalence, histological features, and prognosis. *J Pathol* 193(3): 286–94.

Malkhosyan SR, Yamamoto H, Piao Z, Perucho M. (2000) Late onset and high incidence of colon cancer of the mutator phenotype with hypermethylated hMLH1 gene in women. *Gastroenterology* 119(2): 598.

Maughan NJ, Quirke P. (2002) Pathology—a molecular prognostic approach. *Br Med Bull* 64: 59–74.

Narayan S, Roy D. (2003) Role of APC and DNA mismatch repair genes in the development of colorectal cancers. *Mol Cancer* 12(2): 41.

O'Brien MJ, Yang S, Mack C *et al.* (2006) Comparison of microsatellite instability, CpG island methylation phenotype, BRAF and KRAS status in serrated polyps and traditional adenomas indicates separate pathways to distinct colorectal carcinoma end points. *Am J Surg Pathol* 30(12): 1491–501.

Ogino S, Cantor M, Kawasaki T *et al.* (2006) CpG island methylator phenotype (CIMP) of colorectal cancer is best characterised by quantitative DNA methylation analysis and prospective cohort studies. *Gut* 55(7): 1000–6.

Ouyang H, Furukawa T, Abe T, Kato Y, Horii A. (1998) The BAX gene, the promoter of apoptosis, is mutated in genetically unstable cancers of the colorectum, stomach, and endometrium. *Clin Cancer Res* 4(4): 1071–4.

Parsons R, Myeroff LL, Liu B *et al.* (1995) Microsatellite instability and mutations of the transforming growth factor beta type II receptor gene in colorectal cancer. *Cancer Res* 55(23): 5548–50.

Peltomaki P, Lothe RA, Aaltonen LA *et al.* (1993) Microsatellite instability is associated with tumors that characterize the hereditary non-polyposis colorectal carcinoma syndrome. *Cancer Res* 53(24): 5853–5.

Piao Z, Fang W, Malkhosyan S *et al.* (2000) Frequent frameshift mutations of RIZ in sporadic gastrointestinal and endometrial carcinomas with microsatellite instability. *Cancer Res* 60(17): 4701–4.

Rodriguez-Bigas MA, Boland CR, Hamilton SR *et al.* (1997) A National Cancer Institute Workshop on Hereditary Nonpolyposis Colorectal Cancer Syndrome: meeting highlights and Bethesda guidelines. *J Natl Cancer Inst* 89(23): 1758–62.

Samowitz WS, Curtin K, Ma KN *et al.* (2001a) Microsatellite instability in sporadic colon cancer is associated with an improved prognosis at the population level. *Cancer Epidemiol Biomarkers Prev* 10(9): 917–23.

Samowitz WS, Holden JA, Curtin K *et al.* (2001b) Inverse relationship between microsatellite instability and K-ras and p53 gene alterations in colon cancer. *Am J Pathol* 158(4): 1517–24.

Samowitz WS, Albertsen H, Herrick J *et al.* (2005) Evaluation of a large, population-based sample supports a CpG island methylator phenotype in colon cancer. *Gastroenterology* 129(3): 837–45.

Schulmann K, Reiser M, Schmiegel W. (2002) Colonic cancer and polyps. *Best Pract Res Clin Gastroenterol* 16(1): 91–114.

Schwartz RA, Torre DP. (1995) The Muir-Torre syndrome: a 25-year retrospect. *J Am Acad Dermatol* 33(1): 90–104.

Shia J, Ellis NA, Paty PB *et al.* (2003) Value of histopathology in predicting microsatellite instability in hereditary nonpolyposis colorectal cancer and sporadic colorectal cancer. *Am J Surg Pathol* 27(11): 1407–17.

Snover DC, Jass JR, Fenoglio-Preiser C, Batts KP. (2005) Serrated polyps of the large intestine: a morphologic and molecular review of an evolving concept. *Am J Clin Pathol* 124(3): 380–91.

Soreide K, Janssen EA, Soiland H, Korner H, Baak JP. (2006) Microsatellite instability in colorectal cancer. *Br J Surg* 93(4): 395–406.

Souza RF, Appel R, Yin J *et al.* (1996) Microsatellite instability in the insulin-like growth factor II receptor gene in gastrointestinal tumours. *Nat Genet* 14(3): 255–7. Erratum in *Nat Genet* (1996) 14(4): 488.

Spring KJ, Zhao ZZ, Karamatic R *et al.* (2006) High prevalence of sessile serrated adenomas with BRAF mutations: a prospective study of patients undergoing colonoscopy. *Gastroenterology.*131(5): 1400–7.

Stoler DL, Chen N, Basik M *et al.* (1999) The onset and extent of genomic instability in sporadic colorectal tumor progression. *Proc Natl Acad Sci USA* 96(26): 15121–6.

Strate LL, Syngal S. (2005) Hereditary colorectal cancer syndromes. *Cancer Causes Control* 16(3): 201–13.

Takayama T, Miyanishi K, Hayashi T, Sato Y, Niitsu Y. (2006) Colorectal cancer: genetics of development and metastasis. *J Gastroenterol* 41(3): 185–92.

Tejpar S, Van Cutsem E. (2002) Molecular and genetic defects in colorectal tumorigenesis. *Best Pract Res Clin Gastroenterol* 16(2): 171–85.

Thibodeau SN, Bren G, Schaid D. (1993) Microsatellite instability in cancer of the proximal colon. *Science* 260(5109): 816–9.

Torlakovic E, Snover DC. (1996) Serrated adenomatous polyposis in humans. *Gastroenterology* 110(3): 748–55.

Toyota M, Ahuja N, Ohe-Toyota M, Herman JG, Baylin SB, Issa JP. (1999) CpG island methylator phenotype in colorectal cancer. *Proc Natl Acad Sci USA* 96(15): 8681–6.

Trujillo MA, Garewal HS, Sampliner RE. (1994) Nonsteroidal antiinflammatory agents in chemoprevention of colorectal cancer. At what cost? *Dig Dis Sci* 39, 2260–6.

Umar A, Boland CR, Terdiman JP *et al.* (2004) Revised Bethesda Guidelines for hereditary nonpolyposis colorectal cancer (Lynch syndrome) and microsatellite instability. *J Natl Cancer Inst* 96(4): 261–8.

Vasen HF, Mecklin JP, Khan PM, Lynch HT. (1991) The International Collaborative Group on Hereditary Non-Polyposis Colorectal Cancer (ICG-HNPCC). *Dis Colon Rectum* 34(5): 424–5.

Vasen HF, Watson P, Mecklin JP, Lynch HT. (1999) New clinical criteria for hereditary nonpolyposis colorectal cancer (HNPCC, Lynch syndrome) proposed by the International Collaborative group on HNPCC. *Gastroenterology* 116(6): 1453–6.

Weisenberger DJ, Siegmund KD, Campan M *et al.* (2006) CpG island methylator phenotype underlies sporadic microsatellite instability and is tightly associated with BRAF mutation in colorectal cancer. *Nat Genet* 38(7): 787–93.

Wynter CV, Walsh MD, Higuchi T, Leggett BA, Young J, Jass JR. (2004) Methylation patterns define two types of hyperplastic polyp associated with colorectal cancer. *Gut* 53(4): 573–80.

Yamamoto H, Sawai H, Weber TK, Rodriguez-Bigas MA, Perucho M. (1998) Somatic frameshift mutations in DNA mismatch repair and proapoptosis genes in hereditary nonpolyposis colorectal cancer. *Cancer Res* 58(5): 997–1003.

13 Screening for Colorectal Cancer

Robert J.C. Steele

Introduction

Colorectal cancer is the second most common cancer in the Western world, the third most common worldwide, and the fourth commonest cause of death worldwide. In the United Kingdom there are approximately 30,000 cases and 20,000 result in deaths each year (Cancer Research Campaign 1992). Currently, overall 5-year survival is less than 50% and this is largely due to the fact that the majority of symptomatic patients present with relatively advanced disease (Black *et al.* 1993). The most effective way of improving prognosis is early detection but available evidence would suggest that using the symptomatic route to achieve this would not be particularly fruitful (Ahmed *et al.* 2005). The only reliable method of consistently detecting early disease is by screening and in this chapter the following areas are covered: the principles of screening for colorectal cancer, the evidence relating to currently available screening modalities, the disbenefits of screening, the economics of screening, and novel approaches.

The principles of screening for colorectal cancer

Screening involves testing individuals in order to diagnose the disease at an early stage of its development thereby improving the outcomes of treatment. There is, however, some confusion regarding the purpose of colorectal screening and the philosophy varies markedly according the healthcare system. If the main aim is to reduce the burden of disease on a population then it is essential to have a test which is economically affordable, acceptable and above all safe. If on the other hand the purpose is to inform an individual about their disease status then the emphasis must be on sensitivity and specificity of the test. In this chapter we shall be dealing largely with population screening, although case finding on demand has an important role to play in many countries and may indeed explain the reduction in the incidence of colorectal cancer that has been seen in the United States (Winawer *et al.* 2006).

Currently accepted criteria for an effective screening program are attributed to Wilson and Jungner (Wilson & Jungner 1968). The benefits of screening are seemingly obvious, but screening is associated with inbuilt biases that result in screen-detected disease being associated with a better prognosis than symptomatic disease regardless of whether or not the screening process has actually affected the outcome.

These biases are volunteer bias, length bias and lead-time bias. Volunteer bias results from the fact that invitations to be screened are more likely to be accepted by those who are health conscious than those who are not. Thus people who accept invitations to be screened are likely to have a better outcome from the disease process for reasons other than early detection; for example they are less likely to smoke and more likely to take exercise. Length bias occurs because intermittent screening tests tend to pick up indolent disease that is more likely to have a good prognosis than aggressive disease which is more likely to be symptomatic and present between screening intervals. Lead-time bias is a product of early diagnosis itself; early diagnosis inevitably leads to an apparently improved duration of survival by shifting the point of diagnosis forward in time so that screening appears to prolong survival without having a real effect on the time course of the disease. To allow for these biases, population-based randomized trials are necessary. In these trials the group randomized to screening must be analysed as a whole, *including* those who develop interval cancers (cancers that present with symptoms after a negative screening test) and those who do not participate in the screening process. This group must then be compared with a randomly selected control group that is not offered screening and only if a significant improvement in disease-specific mortality is observed in the test group can the screening process be deemed beneficial.

According to the criteria of Wilson and Jungner, there is little doubt that colorectal cancer is a suitable candidate for screening. It is certainly an important health problem in the Western world, and the second most common cause of cancer death in the United Kingdom (Cancer Research Campaign 1992). The

Gastrointestinal Oncology: A Critical Multidisciplinary Team Approach.
Edited by J. Jankowski, R. Sampliner, D. Kerr, and Y. Fong.

treatment for colorectal cancer is evidence based (SIGN 2003), and the natural history is reasonably well understood; the evidence for the adenoma–carcinoma sequence is strong and it is generally accepted that the majority of invasive cancers arise from pre-existing benign adenomatous polyps (Leslie *et al.* 2002). Thus if screening detects significant adenomas there is an opportunity to reduce the incidence of colorectal cancer. It is also well documented that the prognosis for colorectal cancer is highly dependent on stage at diagnosis. However, the most important evidence supporting screening for colorectal cancer comes from population-based randomized trials.

Fecal occult blood test (FOBT) screening

The technology for testing feces for blood has been available for many years but it is only relatively recently that tests specific for human hemoglobin have become available and all the published population-based screening trials employ the indirect guaiac test. The guaiac test reacts to heme in its free form or bound to protein such as globin, myoglobin and some cytochromes by virtue of its peroxidase activity and is not capable of detecting the degradation products of heme (Young *et al.* 1996). As a dietary component heme enters the gastrointestinal tract as myoglobin or hemoglobin and when it reaches the colon the heme is modified by microflora and loses its peroxidase activity. Thus although guaiac tests can detect dietary heme this is relatively unusual. For the same reason guaiac tests are much more sensitive for distal bleeding lesions than for proximal lesions.

The clinical sensitivity of guaiac in a screening context is quite difficult to estimate but when the test is unrehydrated studies of interval cancer rates suggest that it will only pick up around 50% of cancers in a population accepting screening. This low sensitivity is presumably due to the fact that cancers bleed intermittently. Specificity (proportion of subjects without the disease with a negative test) is around 98% but, although this appears to be high, because the majority of the population do not have colorectal cancer this leads to a fairly high false-positive rate. False-positive results are caused by a combination of factors including bleeding from benign lesions and dietary components containing hemoglobin, myoglobin or peroxidase.

Reyhdration of the guaiac test increases its sensitivity by lysing red cells and exposing more heme. However, although this will detect more cancers it will also detect blood from relatively trivial lesions and this has an adverse effect on specificity. It has been suggested that specificity can be improved by appropriate dietary restriction but a recent meta-analysis suggests that this approach is ineffective (Pignone *et al.* 2001).

In terms of FOBT technology by far the most exciting development has been the fecal immunological occult blood tests (FITs). These are specific for human hemoglobin or its early degradation forms, and are based on a number of methods including reverse passive hemagglutination (using erythrocytes coated in antihuman hemoglobin that agglutinate in the presence of human hemoglobin) and immunochromatography. Until recently the commercially available versions of these tests have been set at high analytic sensitivities which means that although the clinical sensitivity is high the specificity is very low and the false-positive rate is high. However, tests are now available which can be set to a wide range of analytic sensitivities (Janssens 2005). It is clear that a test with high analytic sensitivity has a high clinical sensitivity for colorectal cancer but any increase in sensitivity is counterbalanced by a decrease in specificity. Thus by using a FIT with variable analytic sensitivity it is possible to set a detection limit that will result in a given positivity rate for a screening population. This approach has been employed by workers in Australia and will be discussed later in this section.

All the population-based trials of FOBT screening to date have employed the guaiac-based Haemoccult II test. These trials were carried out in United States, England, Denmark, France, and Sweden, and the results are considered below. The American study, which was carried out in Minnesota, involved randomizing volunteers to an observation group, a group offered biennial screening and a group offered annual screening using rehydrated Haemoccult II without dietary restriction. Colonoscopy was used to investigate all with a positive test and it was found that colorectal cancer mortality dropped by 21% in the biennial group and by 33% in the annual group after a follow-up period of 18 years (Mandel *et al.* 1993). The use of the rehydrated test resulted in a 10% positivity, and in the group offered annual screening 38% underwent colonoscopy at least once. For population screening therefore, the positivity rate was rather higher than most countries could cope with and the implications of this study for a non-volunteer population is not entirely clear. It is, however, important to note that after 18 years of follow-up in the Minnesota study the incidence of colorectal cancer in the groups offered screening dropped significantly below that in the control group (Mandel *et al.* 2000). This has not been seen in any of the other trials of faecal occult blood test screening but given the high colonoscopy rate in the Minnesota study it is likely that this reduction in incidence was related to colonoscopic polypectomy.

The English study was carried out in Nottingham (Hardcastle *et al.* 1996). Here approximately 150,000 subjects were randomized by household into an observation group and into a group offered screening. The screening group, aged between 50 and 74, was offered non-rehydrated Haemoccult II testing on a 2-yearly basis. For most of the study dietary restriction was not specified but if a weakly positive test was returned a retest with dietary restriction was offered. This approach resulted in a much lower rate of test positivity than in the Minnesota study with a 2% investigation rate following the first (prevalence) round and a 1.2% investigation rate in the subsequent (incidence) rounds. Thus, over five screening rounds, colonoscopy was only performed in 4% of the population offered screening.

Uptake was variable from one round to another, but overall 60% of the group that was offered screening completed at least one evaluable test. The cancers that were detected by screening were likely to be highly favorable with 57% being diagnosed at Dukes Stage A. However, there were a large number of interval cancers and in fact about 50% of the cancers diagnosed amongst those who had accepted at least one screening invitation were not actually detected by screening. This means that, in the Nottingham study at least, the Haemoccult II test was only about 50% sensitive in a screening context. Despite the relatively low uptake and sensitivity, however, when the group offered screening was compared to the control group a statistically significant 15% reduction in death rate from colorectal cancer was seen after a median of 7.8 years of follow-up. At a median of 11 years of follow-up this reduction in mortality was still seen, albeit reduced to 13% (Scholefield *et al.* 2002).

Another important issue is the effect of a screening program on the presentation of symptomatic disease and the Nottingham study sheds some light on this. It was observed that in the control group (i.e. those who were not offered screening) the proportion of patients presenting with Dukes Stage A rectal cancer increased from 9% in the first half of the recruitment period to 28% in the second half (Robinson *et al.* 1993). Thus it would appear that the screening program had an effect even on those who were not invited for screening and although the reasons for this are not clear it may be related to increased awareness of rectal bleeding as a significant symptom, amongst both general practitioners and the general population itself. A related topic is that of the emergency presentation of colorectal cancer, and during the Nottingham study there were significantly fewer emergency admissions in the group offered screening when compared to the control group (Scholefield *et al.* 1998). This indicates that a policy of screening leads to a reduction in the numbers of patients presenting as emergencies with possible consequences for reduced operative mortality and improved long-term outcome.

The Danish randomized control trial carried out in Funen differed from the Nottingham study in that dietary restriction was utilized at the first invitation. In other respects the design of the Funen and Nottingham trials was very similar. In the Danish study 61,933 men and women were randomized into an observation group or a group that was offered screening by means of the Haemocult II test (Kronborg *et al.* 1996; Jorgensen *et al.* 2002). The acceptance rate for the first screening round was 67%, with more than 90% accepting repeated screening invitations. Surprisingly, however, the overall positivity rate was only 1% following the first round and dropped to 0.8% in the second round. However the positivity rate increased with subsequent rounds and by the fifth screening round it had reached 1.8%. At diagnosis the stage of screen-detected cancer was favorable with 48% being diagnosed at Dukes Stage A and only 8% had distinct metastases. Interval cancers made up about 30% of all cancers diagnosed in the group offered screening. Thus the performance the Danish screening strategy was very similar to that seen in Nottingham and indeed the mortality reduction after five rounds was 18%.

In Burgundy, France a rather different approach was taken (Faivre *et al.* 2004). Rather than carrying out a randomized trial on an individual basis small geographic areas were allocated to screening or no screening. Again, this employed testing with the non-rehydrated Haemoccult II test, and a total of 91,199 individuals between the ages of 50 and 74 were offered screening without dietary restriction. The positivity rate was 1.2 in the first round but in subsequent rounds it was slightly higher at 1.4 on average. Uptake in the first round was 52.8% and remained fairly constant in subsequent rounds. Again, very much in keeping with Nottingham and Denmark, the disease-specific mortality reduction was 16%.

In the Swedish city of Goteborg all those born between 1918 and 1931 were randomized into a group offered Haemoccult II screening or into an observation group (Kewenter *et al.* 1994). Initial uptake was 63%, dropping to 60% in subsequent screening rounds. In the first round the positivity rate was 4.4% and as with all other screening studies screen-detected cancers were diagnosed at a generally favorable stage. Unfortunately mortality data were never obtained for this study.

Of these five studies, four studies were randomized, four were truly population based and four have reported mortality data. Using information from all five studies a meta-analysis has indicated that offering screening to a population should bring about a reduction in colorectal cancer mortality of 16% and that this should go up to 23% when adjusted for uptake (Towler *et al.* 1998). Thus, although the FOBT is fairly insensitive and uptake is relatively poor, the statistically significant effects seen at the randomized trials demonstrate beyond doubt that early detection of colorectal cancer by screening is beneficial even if the guaiac test is not ideal.

In the United Kingdom the National Screening Committee recommended to the United Kingdom Government Health Departments that a demonstration pilot of colorectal cancer screening using guaiac FOBT should be performed in order to find out whether or not the results of the randomized trials could be reproduced within the country's National Health Service (Steele *et al.* 2001). This was put into effect in two areas in the United Kingdom, one in England and one in Scotland. In total, 478,250 subjects were invited to take part over a 2-period with a view to simulate the first round of a biennial screening program. This process demonstrated that the short-term outcomes of the screening programs could be reproduced with an uptake of 56.8% and a positivity rate of 1.9%. It was also encouraging to find that 48% of all cancers detected by screening were Dukes Stage A and only 1% of patients identified by screening had distant metastases at the time of diagnosis (Steele 2004). Independent evaluators compared the results of this demonstration pilot with the results found in the MRC (Nottingham) randomized study, and the conclusions indicated that a British National Screening Program based on guaiac FOBT should bring about a clinically significant reduction in death rates from colorectal cancer (DoH 2003). As a result the United Kingdom Health Departments are currently rolling out a National Screening Program.

Until recently, most of the research on fecal occult blood test screening has employed the guaiac test but there is an increasing body of evidence relating to the use of immunologic fecal occult blood testing or faecal immunological testing (FIT) (Janssens 2005). Within the context of the United Kingdom Screening Pilot it has been shown that the use of an analytically highly sensitive FIT in those with a weakly positive guaiac test can reliably identify those without significant neoplastic disease (Fraser *et al.* 2006). Until recently, the high analytic sensitivities of the commercially available FIT tests have made them rather unattractive as first-line population screening tools owing to the high false-positive rate. However it is now possible to set the analytic sensitivity of a number of FIT tests to produce a positivity rate that is acceptable to a community's needs. This approach has been taken in Australia and extensive evaluation of a variable cut-off FIT test has demonstrated that a positivity rate of about 8% will detect nearly all cancers. This does, however, result in a fairly high false-positive rate with approximately 75% of colonoscopies showing no neoplastic disease (G. Young, personal communication).

Flexible sigmoidoscopy

As approximately three-quarters of all colorectal cancers are in the rectum or sigmoid colon it seems reasonable to use flexible sigmoidoscopy with a 60-cm instrument as a screening tool, particularly as the finding of a significant distal adenoma may act as an index of proximal disease. Based on these premises it has been proposed that a single flexible sigmoidoscopy at about the age of 60 years with removal of all adenomas at the time of examination and performing colonoscopy for those with high-risk adenomas or cancers would be an effective screening modality for colorectal cancer (Atkin *et al.* 2001). In addition, this strategy might be expected to reduce the incidence of colorectal cancer by removal of adenomas.

This approach is currently being studied by two multicenter randomized controlled trials, one being carried out in Italy (Segnan *et al.* 2002) and the other in the United Kingdom (UK Flexible Sigmoidoscopy Screening Trial Investigators 2002). In the British arm of the trial subjects aged between 60 and 64 from 14 centers were asked by questionnaire whether or not they would attend for flexible sigmoidoscopy screening if they were invited. This questionnaire was sent to 354,262 people and 55% responded positively. Of these, 170,432 people were randomized using a 2:1 ratio of controls to invitees. The process then involved a flexible sigmoidoscopy with the removal of all polyps, going on to colonoscopy for those with high-risk adenomas (three or more adenomas, a villous or severely dysplasia adenoma, or an adenoma greater than 1 cm) or cancer. Overall 57,254 people were invited for screening and 71% attended. This study is, therefore, essentially a volunteer study and the population uptake rate can be estimated at little more than 30%.

The results to date, however, are extremely promising. Adenomas were found by flexible sigmoidoscopy in 12%, and cancer in 0.3%. Subsequent colonoscopy revealed proximal adenomas in 18.8% and cancer in 0.4%. Of all the cancers found by this screening protocol 62% were Dukes Stage A. The Italian study (SCORE) produced very similar results. Overall 236,568 individuals aged between 55 and 64 were approached but only 23.9% replied that they would undergo a screening if invited. Disappointingly, of the 17,148 invited for screening only 58% attended. The stage of cancer at diagnosis was also extremely favorable, with 54% having Dukes Stage A cancers.

In the United States a randomized trial of flexible sigmoidoscopy as part of a study looking at prostate, lung, colorectal and ovarian cancer screening has been carried out (Schoen *et al.* 2003). So far there are no data on uptake or pathology yield but it has been found that repeat flexible sigmoidoscopy at 3 years after initial examination revealed significant adenomas or cancers in the distal colon. This raises the question of whether or not repeated flexible sigmoidoscopy would be preferable to the once-only approach.

Currently, evidence suggests that flexible sigmoidoscopy is an extremely effective screening tool although as yet there is no clear evidence relating to mortality reduction or reduction in colorectal cancer incidence. In addition, it is not yet clear what the uptake of flexible sigmoidoscopy in an unselected population is likely to be, although there are ongoing pilot studies to resolve this issue (W. Atkin, personal communication).

Colonoscopy

Colonoscopy itself would, on the surface, appear to be the ideal screening tool as it has a specificity of 100% and a very high sensitivity. That sensitivity is not 100% is evidenced by a study in which back-to-back colonoscopies clearly demonstrated that adenomas and occasionally carcinoma can be missed even by the most experienced colonoscopist (Rex *et al.* 1997). Furthermore, a recent study has compared colonoscopy with high-quality CT colography which suggests that the sensitivity of colonoscopy for adenomas may only be in the region of 90% (Pickhardt *et al.* 2003). Nevertheless colonoscopy is widely used for opportunistic screening throughout the developed world and there is a good circumstantial evidence that colonoscopy is associated with reduction of colorectal cancer mortality and incidence by means of endoscopic polypectomy (Winawer *et al.* 1993).

However, the use of colonoscopy as a population screening tool remains highly controversial. There are no appropriate randomized trials although there are two studies from which some conclusions can be drawn. The first was conducted amongst US military veterans and consisted of a study of 4,411 veterans dying of colorectal cancer between 1992 and 1998 (Muller & Sonnenberg 1995). The control group was recruited from living and dead patients without colorectal cancer matched by age, sex and race to each of the cases dying of colorectal cancer. This revealed that colonoscopy appeared to reduce mortality from colorectal cancer with an odds ratio of 0.41 (95% CI 0.33–0.50). However, the indications for colonoscopy in the study group were varied and included some investigations for symptoms and the results cannot be fully extrapolated into a population screening context. The second study was again carried out amongst veterans and involved using colonoscopy in asymptomatic individuals aged 50–75 years as a screening modality for colorectal neoplasia (Lieberman *et al.* 2000). There were 17,732 potential subjects and of these 3121 underwent total colonoscopy. The majority (97%) were male and the mean age was 63 years. A significant adenoma (>1 cm in diameter) was found in 7.9%, and cancer in 1%. Thus it would appear that if colonoscopy was used for population screening in men between the ages of 50 and 75 years uptake would only be in the region of 20% and the cancer detection rate would only be 1%. If these figures are an accurate reflection of performance of colonoscopy as a population screening tool then it is clearly far from ideal. If, however, a society is prepared in terms of both uptake and financial cost to use colonoscopy as a screening tool there is very good evidence that a single examination at around the age of 60 would be highly effective given that an individual with a 'clean' colon at this age is highly unlikely to develop and die of colorectal cancer within their remaining lifetime (Brenner *et al.* 2006).

Radiology

There is no good evidence relating to the use of barium enema as a screening modality but there is increasing interest in the use of CT colography in this context. There are a number of studies purporting to examine this technology as a screening tool, although there are no population-based data. It does seem, however, that CT colography can be highly sensitive and specific as evidenced by the results of a study carried out in Bethesda, Maryland. Here 1233 asymptomatic individuals around the age of 60 underwent both colonoscopy and CT colography on the same day (Pickhardt *et al.* 2003). A final colonoscopy with the hindsight of the results of the two previous investigations was used as the reference standard. On this basis, sensitivity of CT colography was 93.8% for adenomas of >1 cm in diameter compared with the sensitivity of 87.5% for colonoscopy. The specificity of CT colography for these lesions was 96%. Thus it would appear that in the right hands CT colography is highly sensitive and specific and given adequate uptake could be used as a population screening tool.

Comparative studies

The comparative studies of different screening technologies carried out to date have all compared FOBT and flexible sigmoidoscopy. In Nottingham, a randomized study comparing FOBT along with flexible sigmoidoscopy plus FOBT showed that the yield of adenomas and cancers was four times greater in those undergoing the combined approach, but while uptake of FOBT was 50%, in those who were offered both tests only 20% agreed to have flexible sigmoidoscopy (Berry *et al.* 1997). In a Swedish study FOBT alone was compared with flexible sigmoidoscopy alone and here uptake of FOBT was approximately 60% and for flexible sigmoidoscopy 50% (Brevinge *et al.* 1997). Overall the yield of neoplasia in the group offered flexible sigmoidoscopy was three times that in the group offered FOBT, suggesting that in the Swedish population flexible sigmoidoscopy may be more effective as a screening tool despite the lower uptake. This was, however, a small study and the results should be interpreted with caution. In Norway the Norwegian Colorectal Cancer Prevention (NORCCAP) Study randomized 20,780 individuals aged between 50 and 64 to flexible sigmoidoscopy or a combination of flexible sigmoidoscopy and FOBT (Gondal *et al.* 2003). Here the yield of neoplastic pathology in the two groups was identical. It was concluded that very little benefit accrued from adding FOBT to a flexible sigmoidoscopy.

These three studies appear to indicate that while the uptake of flexible sigmoidoscopy tends to be lower than that for FOBT, the sensitivity of the endoscopic examination is significantly superior. However, it must be remembered that these studies are comparing a single episode of FOBT with a single flexible sigmoidoscopy and in the randomized studies of FOBT repeated biennial or annual tests were employed. In a Danish study comparing once-only flexible sigmoidoscopy with FOBT against FOBT alone over 16 years found that after four rounds of FOBT screening the diagnostic yield of this approach was at least as high as a single flexible sigmoidoscopy (Rasmussen *et al.* 2003). Thus, the debate surrounding flexible sigmoidoscopy compared with a FOBT screening program based on regular testing has not yet been resolved and clearly merits a formal randomized controlled trial comparing the two strategies.

Disbenefits of screening

Although performing a faecal occult blood test is without hazard and flexible sigmoidoscopy is a safe investigation, subsequent colonoscopy has the potential to cause morbidity and even mortality. In addition to this, false-negative FOBT results are inevitable owing to relatively low sensitivity of this investigation and there is concern that a negative result may falsely reassure an individual to such an extent that they may ignore symptoms and delay the diagnosis of colorectal cancer ('the certificate of health effect'). Both of these issues have been studied by the Nottingham Group who have looked at investigation- and treatment-related mortality and the stage at presentation of interval cancers (Robinson *et al.* 1999). No colonoscopy-related deaths were noted and the mortality after surgery for screen-detected cancers was less than 2%. The 0% mortality rate from colonoscopy was mirrored in the recent UK pilot (Steele 2004) and probably represents the effect of close auditing within these studies. As far as the certificate of health effect is concerned, the Nottingham Group found that the stage distribution of interval cancers was similar to that of all cancers in the control group and the survival after diagnosis of an interval cancer was significantly better than for the cancers in the control group (Robinson *et al.* 1999). These findings indicate that an appreciable certificate of health effect did not occur within the Nottingham Study.

Concerns have been raised that all-cause mortality does not appear to be affected by colorectal cancer screening and that, in the Nottingham Study, it was in fact found to be increased in the group offered screening (Black *et al.* 2002). It must be appreciated, however, that colorectal cancer only accounts for approximately 2% of all deaths and a 15% reduction in disease-specific mortality would only be expected to reduce overall mortality by 0.3%. To demonstrate such an effect it would require a randomized trial that would be too big to be feasible. It must also be emphasized that the finding of increased all-cause mortality was statistically non-significant and thus may have been a chance observation.

The effect of screening on psychological morbidity must also not be forgotten. In the randomized study of FOBT screening carried out in Sweden a questionnaire study indicated that 4.7% participants experienced worry as a result of receiving the invitation letter and that this increased to 15% after the reporting of a positive test (Lindholm *et al.* 1997). However, this worry rapidly decayed after the screening process was over and at 1 year 96% of participants indicated that they were pleased to have had the opportunity to be screened. A similar study was carried out within the Nottingham trial; psychiatric morbidity was detected in those with a positive test result, but in those with false/positive tests it returned almost to normal the day after the colonoscopy and remained at low levels after 1 month (Parker *et al.* 2002). It therefore appears that screening does cause anxiety but it tends to be short lived.

Finally, there is the issue of whether or not to investigate patients with false-positive FOBT results. Despite the fact that upper gastrointestinal bleeding is relatively unlikely to cause a positive guaiac test, concern remains that significant upper gastrointestinal pathology may be missed if no further investigations are carried out after a negative colonoscopy. To address this issue the Nottingham Group studied a cohort of 283 FOBT-positive cases in whom no adenomas or carcinomas had been found on colonoscopy (Thomas & Hardcastle 1990). Five per cent of this group had undergone upper gastrointestinal endoscopy because of symptoms and one was found to have a gastric cancer. The others who were asymptomatic were followed up for a median period of 5 years and only one who continued to have symptoms after a previous partial gastrectomy was eventually diagnosed as having gastric cancer. Thus it would appear that individuals who have no upper gastrointestinal symptoms do not require upper gastrointestinal endoscopy after a negative colonoscopy. This has been confirmed by a study carried out in Aberdeen as part of the UK demonstration pilot in which a cohort of patients underwent upper gastrointestinal endoscopy after a negative colonoscopy. In this instance no significant neoplastic pathology was found in the upper gastrointestinal tract (NAG Mowat, personal communication).

Economics of screening

Before any society embarks on a screening program it is important to have information on cost effectiveness. Unfortunately there are no data available from the randomized controlled trials, and all estimates of the cost effectiveness of colorectal cancer screening come from health economic models. In a relatively recent study 25 papers examining the cost effectiveness of colorectal cancer screening were identified, although eight had to be rejected as they calculated cost per cancer detected rather than cost per life year saved (Steele *et al.* 2004). In the remaining papers 5-yearly sigmoidoscopy, 10-yearly colonoscopy or a combination of these approaches were addressed. Unfortunately, there was no reliable information on biennial FOB testing or 'once-off' sigmoidoscopy. Using specific statistical techniques, known as Monte Carlo simulations of a Markov model, yearly FOB testing, 5-yearly sigmoidoscopy and 10-yearly colonoscopy were compared with one another. This suggested that FOB screening costs 8900 Euros per life year saved compared with 8000 Euros per life year saved by sigmoidoscopy and 28,500 Euros for colonoscopy. Given the quality of data, however, there was a great deal of uncertainty surrounding these figures and when this uncertainty was taken into account it appeared that it is 95% certain that annual FOB testing is cost effective providing society is willing to pay 30,000 Euro per life year saved whereas for colonoscopy the same figure was 90,000 Euros per life year saved. Although sigmoidoscopy appeared to be cheaper than FOB testing, when uncertainty was brought in to the picture there was less than 80% certainty that sigmoidoscopy is more cost effective than annual FOB test screening even at an infinite willingness to pay per life year saved. This seemingly anomalous result is due to the lack of mortality data in any studies of flexible sigmoidoscopy and this will certainly be addressed by the MRC study. The main conclusion of these findings is that FOBT is highly likely to be cost effective at a reasonable cost whereas this is extremely unlikely with colonoscopy.

Novel approaches to screening

A number of proteins found in stool have been studied, including transferrin (Miyoshi *et al.* 1992), albumen (Saitoh *et al.* 1995), and alpha-1 antitrypsin (Moran *et al.* 1995), but none of these have proven to be sufficiently sensitive and specific to act as screening tools. There has also been interest in the calcium binding protein calprotectin that is found in neutrophils, but although a fecal calprotectin test has been shown to be more sensitive for cancers and adenomas than FOBT specificity appears to be highly variable owing to the fact that levels are raised by inflammatory conditions (Tibble *et al.* 2001). Another interesting approach is stool cytology aided by immunohistochemical detection of the MCM2 protein which is found to be ubiquitously expressed by neoplastic epithelium (Davies *et al.* 2002). It is likely, however, that even with immunohistochemical aid stool cytology would be too labor intensive to form the basis of a colorectal screening program.

A great deal is now known about the different types of genetic mutations that are associated with colorectal cancer. This has led to the development of tests that can detect these genetic mutations in DNA that is extracted from stool samples (Mak *et al.* 2004). DNA extraction is now quite feasible and it is then reasonably straightforward to amplify mutations using a polymerase chain reaction. However, because of the heterogeneity of genetic mutations in both cancers and adenomas, to develop a test that will be reasonably sensitive it is essential to look at a panel of different mutations in the different genes. The genes most commonly studied are *Kras*, *APC* and *p53*, and the mononucleotide BAT26 has been used as a marker of microsatellite instability (Ahlquist *et al.* 2000). It is also possible to use DNA non-specifically, in the sense that long DNA is likely to be shed from tumors, whereas cells shed from the colonic epithelium undergoing apoptosis give rise to short segments of DNA.

Using this technology a number of groups have demonstrated high sensitivity for colorectal cancer and adenomas and a recent study has compared the effectiveness of detecting mutations in stool with the FOBT (Imperiale *et al.* 2004). Even more recently, a custom-built chip looking at 28 different mutations in four separate cancer-associated genes has been developed but as yet has to undergo clinical trials (FitzGerald *et al.* 2005).

This approach to screening is very exciting but is still at a very early stage. Currently in most countries it would be seen as too expensive for a population screening tool but if it proves to be of real value in terms of sensitivity and specificity there is potential for bringing down costs by means of automation.

Conclusions

There is now extremely good evidence that early detection of colorectal cancer by screening reduces colorectal cancer mortality and less good but reasonably convincing evidence that detection of adenomas may reduce the incidence of colorectal cancer. Currently the only modality that has been shown to reduce mortality in a population sense is FOB testing but it is highly likely that, given adequate uptake, flexible sigmoidoscopy will also be a useful tool. Colonoscopy is clearly effective, but can only really be used on an individual basis as both uptake and costs are likely to prohibit its widespread use in population screening. Currently research is focusing on developing new sensitive and specific tests that will be both safe and acceptable to the population and on examining methods for increasing uptake. The bowel cancer screening programmes in the UK and USA will, in the near future, determine whether longevity occurs in addition to decreased cancer rates.

References

Ahlquist DA, Skoletsky JE, Boynton KA *et al.* (2000) Colorectal cancer screening by detection of altered DNA in stool: feasibility of a multitarget assay panel. *Gastroenterology* 119: 1219–27.

Ahmed S, Leslie A, Thaha M, Carey FA, Steele RJC. (2005) Lower gastrointestinal symptoms do not discriminate for colorectal neoplasia in a faecal occult blood scree-positive population. *Br J Surg* 92: 478–81.

Atkin WS, Edwards R, Wardle J *et al.* (2001) Design of a multicentre randomised trial to evaluate flexible sigmoidoscopy in colorectal cancer screening. *J Med Screen* 8: 137–44.

Berry DP, Clarke P, Hardcastle JD, Vellacott KD. (1997) Randomized trial of the addition of flexible sigmoidoscopy to faecal occult blood testing for colorectal neoplasia population screening. *Br J Surg* 84: 1274–6.

Black RJ, Sharp L, Kendrick SW. (1993) *Trends in Cancer Survival in Scotland 1968–1990.* ISD Publication, Edinburgh.

Black WC, Haggstrom DA, Welch HG. (2002) All-cause mortality in randomised trials of cancer screening. *JNCI* 94: 167–73.

Brenner H, Chang-Claude J, Seiler CM, Shurmenr T, Hoffmeister M. (2006) Does a negative screening colonoscopy ever need to be repeated? *Gut* 55: 1145–50.

Brevinge H, Lindholm E, Buntzen S, Kewenter J. (1997) Screening for colorectal neoplasia with faecal occult blood testing compared with flexible sigmoidoscopy directly in a 55 years' old population. *Int J Colorectal Dis* 12: 291–5.

Cancer Research Campaign. (1992) *Cancer in the European Community.* Factsheet 5.2 1992.

Davies RJ, Freeman A, Morris LS, Bingham S, Dilworth S, Scott I *et al.* (2002) Analysis of minichromosome maintenance proteins as a novel method for detection of colorectal cancer in stool. *Lancet* 359: 1917–19.

DoH. (2003) *Evaluation of the UK colorectal screening pilot. A report for the UK Department of Heal*th. http://www.cancerscreening.nhs.uk/colorectal/finalreport.pdf Department of Health, June 2003.

Faivre J, Dancourt V, Lejeune C *et al.* (2004) Reduction in colorectal cancer mortality by fecal occult blood screening in a French controlled study. *Gastroenterology* 126: 1674–80.

FitzGerald SP, Lamont JV, McConnell RI, Benchikhel O *et al.* (2005) Development of a high-throughput automated analyser using biochip array technology. *Clin Chem* 51: 1165–76.

Fraser CG, Matthew CM, Mowat NAG, Wilson JA, Carey FA, Steele RJC. (2006) Immunochemical testing of individuals positive for guaiac faecal occult blood test in a screening programme for colorectal cancer: an observational study. *Lancet Oncol* 7: 127–31.

Gondal G, Grotmol T, Hofstad B, Bretthauer M, Eide TJ, Hoff G. (2003) The Norwegian Colorectal Cancer Prevention (NORCCAP) screening study: baseline findings and implementations for clinical work-up in age groups 50–64 years. *Scand J Gastroenterol* 38: 635–42.

Hardcastle JD, Chamberlain JO, Robinson MHE, Moss SM, Amar SS, Balfour TW *et al.* (1996) Randomised controlled trial of faecal occult blood screening for colorectal cancer. *Lancet* 348: 1472–7.

Imperiale TF, Ransohoff DF, Itzkowitz SH, Turnbull BA, Ross ME. (2004) Fecal DNA versus fecal occult blood for colorectal-cancer screening in an average-risk population. *N Engl J Med* 351: 2704–14.

Janssens JF. (2005) Faecal occult blood test as a screening test for colorectal cancer. *Acta Gastroenterol Belg* 68: 244–6.

Jorgensen OD, Krongborg O, Fenger C. (2002) A randomised study of screening for colorectal cancer using faecal occult blood testing: results after 13 years and seven biennial screening rounds. *Gut* 50: 29–32.

Kewenter J, Brevinge H, Engaras B, Haglin E, Ahren C. (1994) Results of screening, rescreening, and follow-up in a prospect randomized study for detection of colorectal cancer by fecal occult blood testing. Results for 68,308 subjects. *Scand J Gastroenterol* 29: 468–73.

Kronborg O, Fenger C, Olsen J, Jorgensen OD, Sondergaard O. (1996) Randomised study of screening for colorectal cancer with faecal occult blood test. *Lancet* 348: 1467–71.

Leslie A, Carey FA, Pratt NR, Steele RJC. (2002) The colorectal adenoma–carcinoma sequence. *Br J Surg* 89: 845–60.

Lieberman DA, Weiss DG, Bond JH, Ahnen DJ, Garewal H, Chejfec G. (2000) Use of colonoscopy to screen asymptomatic adults for colorectal cancer. Veterans Affairs Cooperative Study Group 380. *N Engl J Med* 343: 162–8.

Lindholm E, Berglund B, Kewenter J, Halind E. (1997) Worry associated with screening for colorectal carcinomas. *Scand J Gastroenterol* 32: 238–45.

Mak T, Lalloo F, Evans DGR, Hill J. (2004) Molecular stool screening for colorectal cancer. *Br J Surg* 91: 790–800.

Mandel JS, Bond JH, Church JR *et al.* (1993) Reducing mortality from colorectal cancer by screening for faecal occult blood. *N Engl J Med* 328: 1365–71.

Mandel JS, Church TR, Bond JH *et al.* (2000) The effect of fecal occult-blood screening on the incidence of colorectal cancer. *N Engl J Med* 343: 1603–7.

Miyoshi H, Ohshiba s, Asada S, Hirata I, Uchida K. (1992) Immunological determination of fecal haemoglobin and transferrin levels: a comparison with other fecal occult blood tests. *Am J Gastroenterol* 87: 67–73.

Moran A, Robinson M, Lawson N, Stanley J, Jones AF, Hardcastle JD. (1995) Fecal alpha 1-antitrypsin detection of colorectal neoplasia. An evaluation using HemoQuant. *Dig Dis Sci* 40: 2522–5.

Muller AD, Sonnenberg A. (1995) Protection by endoscopy against death from colorectal cancer. A case-control study among Veterans. *Arch Intern Med* 155: 1741–8.

Parker MA, Robinson MH, Scholefield JH, Hardcastle JD. (2002) Psychiatric morbidity and screening for colorectal cancer. *J Med Screen* 9: 7–10.

Pickhardt PJ, Choi JR, Hwang I *et al.* (2003) Computed tomographic virtual colonoscopy to screen for colorectal neoplasia in asymptomatic adults. *N Engl J Med* 349: 2191–200.

Pignone M, Campbell MK, Carr C, Phillips C. (2001) Meta-analysis of dietary restriction during faecal occult blood testing. *Eff Clin Pract* 4: 150–6.

Rasmussen M, Fenger C, Kronborg O. (2003) Diagnostic yield in a biennial Haemoccult-II screening programme compared to a once-only screening with flexible sigmoidoscopy and Haemoccult-II. *Scand J Gastroenterol* 38: 114–8.

Rex DK, Cutler CS, Lemmel GT *et al.* (1997) Colonoscopic miss rates of adenomas determined by back-to-back colonoscopies. *Gastroenterology* 112: 24–28.

Robinson MHE, Thomas WM, Hardcastle JD, Chamberlain J, Mangham CM. (1993) Change towards earlier stage at presentation of colorectal cancer. *Br J Surg* 80: 1610–12.

Robinson MHE, Hardcastle JD, Moss SM *et al.* (1999) The risks of screening: data from the Nottingham randomised controlled trial of faecal occult blood screening for colorectal cancer. *Gut* 45: 588–92.

Saitoh O, Matsumoto H, Sugimori K, Sugi K, Nakagawa K, Miyoshi H *et al.* (1995) Intestinal protein loss and bleeding assessed by fecal hemoglobin, transferrin, albumin and alpha-1-antitrypsin levels in patients with colorectal diseases. *Digestion* 56: 67–75.

Schoen RE, Pinsky PF, Weissfeld JL *et al.* (2003) Results of repeat sigmoidoscopy 3 years after a negative examination. *JAMA* 290: 41–8.

Scholefield JH, Robinson MH, Mangham CM, Hardcastle JD. (1998) Screening for colorectal cancer reduces emergency admissions. *Eur J Surg Oncol* 24: 47–50.

Scholefield JH, Moss S, Sufi F, Mangham CM, Hardcastle JD. (2002) Effect of faecal occult blood screening on mortality from colorectal cancer: results from a randomised controlled trial. *Gut* 50: 840–4.

Segnan N, Senore C, Andreoni B *et al.* SCORE working group. (2002) Baseline findings of the Italian multicenter randomized controlled trial of 'once-only sigmoidoscopy' – SCORE. *J Natl Cancer Inst* 94:1763–72.

SIGN (Scottish Intercollegiate Guidelines Network). (2003) *Guidelines on the Management of Colorectal Cancer*. SIGN, Edinburgh.

Steele RJC, Parker R, Patnick J *et al.* (2001) A demonstration pilot for colorectal cancer screening in the United Kingdom: a new concept in the introduction of health care strategies. *J Med Screen* 8: 197–202.

Steele RJC for the UK Colorectal Cancer Screening Pilot Group. (2004) Results of the first round of a demonstration pilot of screening for colorectal cancer in the United Kingdom. *BMJ* 329: 133–5.

Steele RJC, Gnauck R, Hrcka R *et al.* (2004) ESGE/UEGF Colorectal Cancer – Public Awareness Campaign The Public/Professional Interface Workshop, Oslo, Norway, June 20–22, 2003. Methods and Economic Considerations: Group 1 Report. *Endoscopy* 36: 349–53.

Thomas WM, Hardcastle JD. (1990) Role of upper gastrointestinal investigations in a screening study for colorectal neoplasia. *Gut* 31: 1294–97.

Tibble J, Sigthorsson G, Foster R, Sherwood R, Fagerhol M, Bjarnason I. (2001) Faecal calprotectin and faecal occult blood tests in the diagnosis of colorectal carcinoma and adenoma. *Gut* 49: 402–8.

Towler B, Irwig L, Glasziou P, Kewenter J, Weller D, Silagy C. (1998) A systematic review of the effects of screening for colorectal cancer using the faecal occult blood test, Hemoccult. *BMJ* 317: 559–65.

UK Flexible Sigmoidoscopy Screening Trial Investigators. (2002) Single flexible sigmoidoscopy screening to prevent colorectal cancer: baseline findings of a UK multicentre randomized trial. *Lancet* 359: 1291–1300.

Winawer SJ, Zauber AG, Ho MN *et al.* (1993) Prevention of colorectal cancer by colonoscopic polypectomy. The National Polyp Study Working Group. *N Engl J Med* 329: 1977–81.

Winawer SJ, Zauber AG, Fletcher AG *et al.* (2006) Guidelines for colonoscopy surveillance after polypectomy: a consensus update by the US Multi-Society Task Force on colorectal cancer and the American Cancer Society. *Gastroenterology* 130: 1872–85.

Wilson JM, Jungner F. (1968) Principles and practice of screening for disease. Public Health Papers No. 34. WHO, Geneva.

Young GP, Macrae FA, St John DJB. (1996) Clinical methods for early detection: basis, use and evaluation. In: Young GP, Rozen P, Levin B, eds. *Prevention and Early Detection of Colorectal Cancer*, pp. 241–70. WB Saunders, Philadelphia.

14 Cancer of the Colon and Rectum

Edited by Rachel S. Midgley

Diagnosis

Clinical presentation

Omar Khan, Rachel S Midgley & Andrew Weaver

Introduction

The aim of this section of the book is to exemplify the importance of the multidisciplinary team in looking after patients with colorectal cancer, from the pathologists and the radiologists who provide diagnosis and prognostication, the surgeons who provide the mainstay of therapy, the oncologists who administer chemotherapy and radiotherapy to decrease recurrence rates and to palliate, and finally to the specialist nurses who provide the central integral role of coordinating the patient pathway, counselling patients and providing advice and support about stoma care.

Patients with colorectal cancer can present with a myriad of symptoms and signs and to a wide variety of health professionals, including GPs, A&E doctors, hospital specialists and practice nurses. It is important therefore that anyone who might come into contact with such patients should be able to recognise the common presentation patterns.

By studying the case presentations given below you will become familiar with these patterns and you will learn what investigations should be performed and how they should be interpreted. A number of questions will be posed at the end of each case. You may not be able to answer these until you have read the rest of this chapter about the MDT approach to colorectal cancer. However once you have read these sections you should be able to answer all of the questions fully. If you are still struggling, in the final section you will find complete explanations.

Gastrointestinal Oncology: A Critical Multidisciplinary Team Approach. Edited by J. Jankowski, R. Sampliner, D. Kerr, and Y. Fong.

Case 1

A 62 year old man presents with a 3-month history of tiredness and right iliac fossa pain. On examination he appears pale and has some tenderness in the right iliac fossa associated with a firm mass. Investigations reveal a hypochromic microcytic anemia consistent with iron deficiency. His blood biochemistry and liver function tests are within normal limits. Colonoscopy reveals a cecal mass with no other abnormalities in the colon or rectum; biopsy confirms adencocarcinoma. A computed tomography (CT) scan demonstrates no evidence of distant metastases.

He undergoes a right hemicolectomy. Histologic analysis reveals a Duke's C, T3N2MX stage IIIC poorly differentiated adencocarcinoma of the colon. He is enrolled onto the QUASAR 2 trial and is randomized to receive adjuvant capecitabine and bevacizumab.

Questions

1 Was it appropriate for this patient to be offered chemotherapy after his surgery?
2 What is the evidence for 5-FU-based chemotherapy?
3 What is the QUASAR 2 trial?

Case 2

A 68-year-old woman presents with a 1-month history of rectal bleeding, tenesmus and altered bowel habit. On examination she has a firm midrectal tumor felt on digital rectal examination. Investigations reveal a normal full blood count. Her blood biochemistry and liver function tests are within normal limits. Rectal biopsy confirms poorly differentiated carcinoma. CT scan reveals no distant metastases. Magnetic resonance imaging (MRI) of the pelvis reveals a T3N1MX midrectal tumor with a threatened mesorectal margin.

She undergoes preoperative chemoradiotherapy. MRI scanning after treatment reveals significant reduction of the tumor mass with no significant change in morphology of the lymph nodes.

She subsequently has a low anterior resection and coloanal anastomosis. Histology reveals a ypT2N0M0 tumor. Excision margins are clear of tumor.

She has adjuvant chemotherapy with 5-FU and folinic acid.

Questions

1 Should this patient have been offered radiotherapy alone before surgery?
2 What is the evidence for combined chemoradiotherapy in downstaging rectal tumors?

Case 3

A 43-year-old woman presents with a 4-month history of weight loss, loss of appetite and right upper quadrant pain. On examination she is cachectic and not clinically jaundiced. She has firm, non-tender hepatomegaly of 4 cm below the costal margin with an irregular edge. Investigations reveal a mild normocytic, normochromic anemia. Blood biochemistry is normal but her AST and ALT are abnormally elevated. Serum albumin, bilirubin and clotting are all normal. CEA is grossly elevated at 4500. CT scan reveals multiple liver metastases in both lobes of the liver as well as small-volume pulmonary metastases. There is an area of abnormality in the sigmoid colon. Sigmoidoscopy reveals a non-obstructing mass in the sigmoid colon and biopsy confirms adencocarcinoma.

She is commenced on palliative chemotherapy with oxaliplatin and modified de Gramont chemotherapy. She has a rapid improvement in symptoms and a concurrent fall in CEA. CT scan after 6 cycles of chemotherapy reveals a good partial response in the liver and pulmonary lesions. She develops worsening peripheral neuropathy after 9 cycles of treatment and chemotherapy is stopped.

Ten months later she presents with weight loss and a return of her right upper quadrant pain. CEA is elevated at 1050 and CT scan confirms disease progression in the liver. She is commenced on irinotecan and modified de Gramont chemotherapy and has clinical benefit. Six months after completion of chemotherapy she presents with jaundice, weight loss and a distended abdomen. Clinical examination reveals gross hepatomegaly and ascites. Liver function tests reveal a very high bilirubin and low albumin. Ultrasound of the abdomen confirms ascites which is drained for symptomatic relief. She is not considered fit enough for palliative chemotherapy and further management is palliative.

Questions

1 What extra benefit does oxaliplatin give when added to 5-FU in the treatment of advanced colorectal cancer?
2 What is the evidence for the use of monoclonal antibodies in this setting?

Case 4

A 52-year-old man presents with change in bowel habit and mild left-sided abdominal discomfort. Clinical examination reveals fullness in the left iliac fossa. Flexible sigmoidoscopy reveals a mass in the sigmoid colon with impending obstruction. Staging investigations demonstrate no distant metastases. He undergoes a sigmoid colectomy and makes a good postoperative recovery.

Histology reveals a Duke's C, T3N1M0 stage IIIB moderately differentiated adencocarcinoma of the sigmoid colon. He received eight cycles of adjuvant chemotherapy with capecitabine.

One year later, a routine follow-up CT scan demonstrates one large liver metastasis in the right lobe of the liver. He is asymptomatic and liver function is normal. CEA is elevated at 96. A PET scan demonstrates no evidence of extrahepatic disease. His case is discussed at the multidisciplinary meeting and he is offered downsizing chemotherapy with oxaliplatin and modified de Gramont chemotherapy. He receives four cycles and has a fall in CEA to 34. CT scan demonstrates significant reduction in size of the liver metastasis in the right lobe. He has four more cycles of chemotherapy but develops neutropenic sepsis after the eighth cycle.

Chemotherapy is stopped and a further CT scan shows further reduction in the size of the right lobe metastasis. He undergoes liver resection. He has a good postoperative recovery. Fourteen months later he has a routine CT scan and this shows another isolated liver metastasis now in the left lobe of the liver, which is considered inoperable.

He undergoes radiofrequency ablation of his tumor. He is currently under follow-up and remains fit and well with no evidence of recurrent disease.

Questions

1 What criteria are accepted as defining absolute unresectability of liver metastases?
2 Name three features that may define adverse prognosis in patients undergoing hepatic resection?
3 What is the evidence for radiofrequency ablation in these situations?

Have you been able to answer fully all of the questions above? If so, then perhaps you do not need to read the rest of this chapter! However, if you feel that there are gaps in your knowledge, read on through the following sections and you will soon have the confidence to answer the questions with ease.

Histopathology

Daniel Royston & Bryan Warren

Introduction

Patients and clinicians expect and deserve a consistent and

informed approach to the reporting of colorectal cancer specimens by pathologists (Shepherd & Quirke 1997). In turn, pathologists can provide valuable audit data on the accuracy of preoperative radiologic staging and the quality of the surgical resection margin. Systematic review of all original colorectal pathology reports, macroscopic images/descriptions and slides also acts to audit the quality and consistency of reporting within the pathology department. Pathologists are therefore well placed to help establish and maintain high standards of clinical care for colorectal cancer patients as part of the MDT.

This section addresses a number of issues relating to the pathologic assessment and reporting of colorectal adenocarcinoma. It considers areas of diagnostic difficulty and sources of potentially confused communication between pathologists and other members of the MDT. The specimens examined by the pathologist will be considered separately, starting from the initial assessment of diagnostic biopsies and progressing through local excisions to resections. This approach broadly corresponds to the order in which surgical specimens are examined as patients progress along the colorectal cancer care pathway.

Biopsy diagnosis of large bowel adenocarcinoma

Frequently, the pathologist is required to interpret biopsies taken from a polypoid, ulcerated or flat lesion which is endoscopically suspicious of malignancy. The aim is to confirm the diagnosis of malignancy, classify the type of malignancy (including primary versus secondary) and assess the tumor grade. Less frequently, biopsies taken from sites other than the colon and rectum may contain deposits of colorectal adenocarcinoma. In such cases the pathologist is strongly aided by detailed clinical information, including appropriate radiologic imaging, and may require the use of special immunohistochemical stains. Depending upon the biopsy appearance, a report of metastatic adenocarcinoma may be suggestive of primary colorectal malignancy.

Endoscopic biopsy confirmation of colorectal adenocarcinoma depends upon the identification of unequivocal evidence of invasion by tumor cells through the muscularis mucosae into the submucosa. A desmoplastic stromal reaction may provide a clue to the diagnosis. Unfortunately, tumor biopsies are often entirely composed of superficial fragments of 'dysplastic' epithelium with no relation to the muscularis mucosae. Occasionally, they contain only necrotic tissue. In such cases, despite possibly overwhelming clinical and radiologic evidence of an invasive tumor, the pathologist is unable to independently verify the diagnosis of malignancy. Small biopsies from invasive tumors may also fail to accurately represent the true tumor grade, while areas of ulceration and associated inflammation from superficial parts of the tumor may lead to the mistaken interpretation of a poorly differentiated tumor.

In cases where biopsies are composed of adenoma, the degree of dysplasia and the architectural pattern of the lesion (tubular, tubulovillous, villous or serrated) should be recorded. Clearly, any features suggestive of possible underlying malignancy such as stromal sclerosis should also be highlighted. A repeat biopsy in such cases is usually necessary.

Local excision specimens

In some circumstances, a biopsy diagnosis of adenocarcinoma may be followed by planned local excision. Lesions may be removed by endoscopic polypectomy or, in the case of low rectal tumors, Parks' per anal excision or transanal endoscopic microsurgery (TEM).

Polypectomy

It is generally accepted that the majority of large bowel adenocarcinomas arise from pre-existing adenomas. Careful assessment and reporting of these premalignant lesions requires a standardized approach to cut-up and the use of consistent terminology amongst pathologists, gastroenterologists and colorectal surgeons. This is particularly important if inappropriate over- or undertreatment of patients is to be avoided, as has been reported in the literature (Rex *et al.* 2005).

There is considerable international debate about the correct terminology to be used when categorizing the dysplastic features of adenomas, in particular the use of the terms 'high-grade dysplasia', 'carcinoma *in situ*' and 'intramucosal adenocarcinoma'. In the United Kingdom, three grades of dysplasia are recognized (mild, moderate and severe), based upon the tissue architecture, nuclear changes and cytoplasmic differentiation of adenomas. The terms carcinoma *in situ* and intramucosal carcinoma are not used in the United Kingdom. By definition, invasive adenocarcinoma requires the presence of malignant crypts within the submucosa. This is often difficult to assess, even with multiple step sections, and care must be taken to avoid the misinterpretation of benign glands or artefactually misplaced dysplastic crypts within the submucosa. Lack of stromal sclerosis may be helpful in misplaced crypts which are accompanied by their lamina propria.

In cases of definite adenocarcinoma which have developed within an adenomatous polyp, the pathologic description should include: (i) the proximity of the tumor to the endoscopic resection margin; (ii) the degree of tumor differentiation; and (iii) the presence or absence of lymphovascular invasion by tumor cells. Haggitt *et al.* (1985) described a classification system for early adenocarcinoma confined to the submucosa of pedunculated polyps (Fig. 14.1a). Level 0 represents non-invasive carcinoma (not used in the United Kingdom) with levels 1–3 representing increasing submucosal invasion within the polyp, and level 4 signifying invasion beyond the polyp stalk but above the muscularis propria. Completely excised, well or moderately differentiated carcinomas with no evidence of lymphovascular invasion that correspond to levels 0–3 require no further treatment. Any tumor involving level 4,

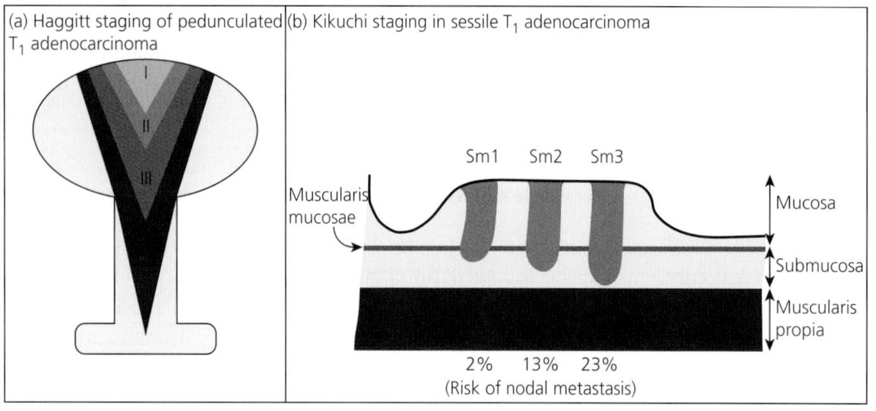

Fig. 14.1 Substaging of T1 cancer. (a) Haggitt staging of pedunculated T1 adenocarcinoma. (b) Kikuchi staging in sessile T1 adenocarcinoma.

however, should prompt surgical resection. Although initially applied to pedunculated and sessile polyps, this classification is most readily applied to pedunculated lesions. The classification of sessile T1 adenocarcinomas is briefly discussed below in relation to local rectal excision specimens.

Local rectal excision

In selected patients, local excision of early rectal cancer may be an alternative to the more radical anterior and abdominoperineal resection procedures. Traditionally used for patients considered unfit for major abdominal surgery, local resection is now being considered as a potentially curative procedure for patients with early-stage rectal cancer. Several local excision techniques have been developed, including Parks' per anal excision and transanal endoscopic microsurgery (TEM). Each procedure removes a full-thickness piece of rectal wall without regional lymph node sampling. Dukes staging is therefore not possible with these local excision specimens.

Pathologic assessment relies upon the fresh specimen being carefully pinned out on to cork board to prevent distortion and curling during formalin fixation. Following careful macroscopic examination, with particular attention being paid to the mucosal margin, the tumor should be thoroughly sampled and examined microscopically at multiple levels. Of particular importance is the total tumor size, degree of differentiation, presence of ulceration and lymphovascular invasion (Nastro *et al.* 2005). It has been suggested that high-grade or mucinous tumors showing evidence of budding, lymphovascular invasion or ulceration are not appropriate for local excision. Kikuchi *et al.* (1995) suggested a classification system for the horizontal and vertical invasion of submucosa in these large and often flat lesions (Fig. 14.1b). The vertical component divides the submucosa into upper, middle and lower thirds. 'Sm1' describes infiltration by tumor into the upper third of the submucosa, 'Sm2' describes infiltration into the middle third, and 'Sm3' describes infiltration into the lower third of the submucosal layer. The incidence of lymph node metastasis in Sm1, Sm2 and Sm3 lesions is 3%, 13% and 23% respectively.

Resection specimens

Colorectal resection specimens require careful handling and assessment if key prognostic data are to be determined reliably and accurately. The critical role of a skilled surgical technique and its effect on patient outcome (morbidity and mortality) is well established for anterior resection (AR) and abdominoperineal resection (APER) procedures. Increasingly, audit of the adequacy of the surgical technique is regarded as a valuable source of feedback to colorectal surgeons.

The fresh colorectal specimen should be photographed and carefully examined. In rectal specimens, particular attention should be given to the macroscopic assessment of the mesorectum (Fig. 14.2a). Ideally, the mesorectal 'fat package' should be intact, with only minor irregularities of a smooth mesorectal fascia. No defect deeper than 5 mm should be seen and there should be no coning towards the distal margin of the specimen. A three-tier scoring system has been proposed, namely: *complete* (as described above); *nearly complete*; and *incomplete* (Nagtegaal *et al.* 2002). This important information should be clearly recorded in the final macroscopic report and audited. For APER specimens, two scores should be provided, one for the mesorectum above the level of the anterior reflection of the peritoneum, and a second for the region below.

Having externally examined the fresh specimen, the resection should be opened anteriorly from the proximal end until one reaches the peritoneal reflection or just above the tumor with care taken not to open the tumor. The formalin-fixed mesorectal excision margin should be inked prior to serial slicing of the tumor. The transverse tumor slices should be carefully ordered and photographed with particular attention given to the inked circumferential margin of excision (CRM). This method of CRM assessment has the combined benefit of allowing careful tumor measurements and provides audit data for comparison with preoperative CT or MRI imaging. The tumor should be thoroughly sampled, with particular attention given to areas of close macroscopic mesorectal and circumferential margin involvement. Areas suspicious of peritonealized surface involvement should also be sampled. Traditionally associated with

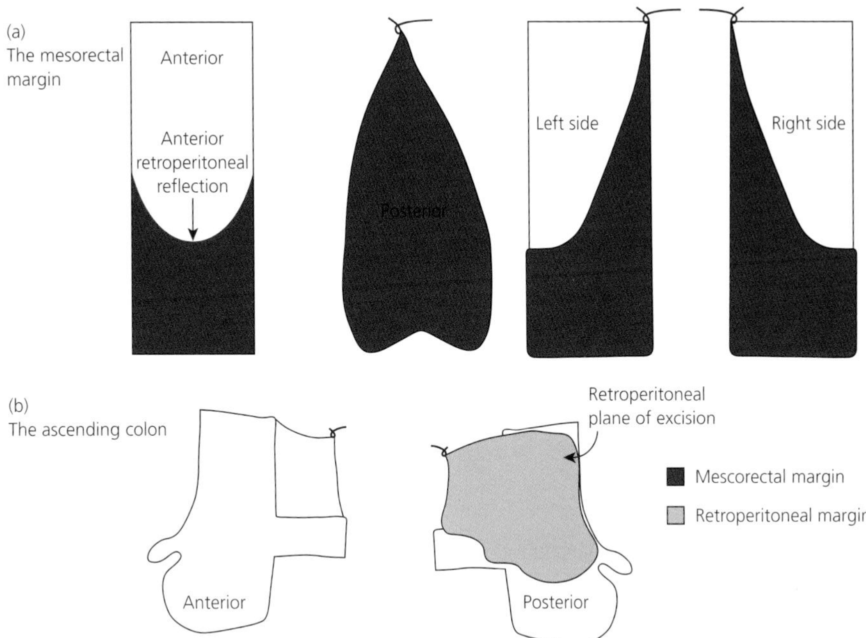

Fig. 14.2 Margins in rectal and colonic cancer resections. (a) The mesorectal margin. (b) The ascending colon.

rectal resection specimens, the prognostic significance of retroperitoneal surgical margin involvement in distal cecal and proximal ascending colon carcinomas has also been highlighted (Bateman *et al.* 2005) (Fig. 14.2b). Finally, the lymph nodes should be exhaustively sampled along with any suspicious dilated extramural vascular channels.

In addition to detailed macroscopic description, the pathology report should include information relating to the tumor type and differentiation, extent of local tumor invasion (pT), character of invasive margin (pushing versus infiltrative), presence of peritumoral lymphocytic infiltrate, nodal involvement (including apical node for Dukes staging), presence of extramural vascular invasion and any other abnormalities present in the specimen. Amongst these features, the degree of tumor differentiation, extent of local spread, character of invasive margin, peritumoral lymphocytic infiltrate and lymph node involvement are of independent prognostic significance. A guide to the pathologic reporting of these cases has been published by the Royal College of Pathologists as the 'Minimum Dataset for Colorectal Cancer Histopathology Reports'. Regular audit of resection specimen reports should ensure that all of the relevant data is consistently and accurately recorded in the final report.

Preoperative chemoradiotherapy-related changes in surgical specimens

It has long been established that postoperative (adjuvant) chemoradiotherapy is of benefit to patients with locally advanced rectal tumors and/or lymph node involvement. More recently however, preoperative (neoadjuvant) chemoradiotherapy is increasingly recommended for the downsizing of advanced rectal tumors and for internal sphincter preservation. It is also claimed to be associated with improved patient outcomes. The response of tumors to preoperative chemoradiotherapy is highly variable and likely reflects differences in tumor volume, treatment regimes (short-course versus long-course therapy) and tumor biology.

When dealing with a rectal cancer specimen following preoperative chemotherapy and/or radiotherapy, the pathologist is faced with a number of new histologic features in the tumor and normal tissues. Tumors may show evidence of extensive regression with widespread necrosis and stromal fibrosis, although the extent to which this is due to neoadjuvant therapy is often uncertain. Alterations in the appearance of the advancing front of tumor cells and a reduced lymphocytic response is also frequently seen. In some circumstances, the tumor may be entirely absent from the specimen despite extensive sampling. All the scarred area is processed as large blocks and cut at three levels. Alternatively, small foci of residual tumor cells may appear isolated within the rectal wall. Lymph nodes, critical for accurate pathologic staging, may be small and difficult to find and display features of necrosis. Clearly, these changes will reduce the amount of useful prognostic data obtained from the pathologic examination of the specimen. In addition to these tumor-related features, changes within the 'normal' bowel may require the distinction of chemoradiotherapy-induced inflammatory features from inflammatory bowel diseases.

In order to allow meaningful comparisons of resected rectal tumors and to establish the prognostic value of histologic chemoradiotherapeutic changes, a tumor regression grade (TRG) has been proposed based upon a similar model applied to esophageal carcinomas (Mandard *et al.* 1994). The Mandard grading system ranges from TRG 1 (no residual cancer cells) to TRG 5 (no regression) with intermediate grades reflecting the relative proportions of tumor cells and fibrosis. This grading system has proven difficult to reproduce and Wheeler *et al.* (2004) have suggested a simpler three-tier grading system (TRG 1–3). Some studies using such grading systems have claimed independent prognostic significance, although this remains controversial. It is clear, however, that pathologists should be encouraged to document the tumor regression grade of tumors in all patients receiving preoperative long-course chemoradiotherapy.

Summary

This section has discussed the important aspects of the pathologic reporting of colorectal cancer specimens that are relevant to the MDT. Specimen data enabling systematic audit of preoperative radiologic staging should be made readily available. In addition, careful macroscopic examination of resection specimens to determine the quality of surgical excision should be included in the main report and be the subject of regular audit. Finally, review of all colorectal cancer pathology reports, slides and macroscopic images should act to audit the quality of reporting within the pathology department.

References

Bateman AC, Carr NJ, Warren BF. (2005) The retroperitoneal surface in distal caecal and proximal ascending colon carcinoma: the Cinderella surgical margin? *J Clin Pathol* 58(4): 426–8.

Haggitt RC *et al.* (1985) Prognostic factors in colorectal carcinomas arising in adenomas: implications for lesions removed by endoscopic polypectomy. *Gastroenterology* 89(2): 328–36.

Kikuchi R *et al.* (1995) Management of early invasive colorectal cancer. Risk of recurrence and clinical guidelines. *Dis Colon Rectum* 38(12): 1286–95.

Mandard AM *et al.* (1994) Pathologic assessment of tumor regression after preoperative chemoradiotherapy of esophageal carcinoma. Clinicopathologic correlations. *Cancer* 73(11): 2680–6.

Nagtegaal ID *et al.* (2002) Macroscopic evaluation of rectal cancer resection specimen: clinical significance of the pathologist in quality control. *J Clin Oncol* 20(7): 1729–34.

Nastro P *et al.* (2005) Local excision of rectal cancer: review of literature. *Dig Surg* 22(1–2): 6–15.

Rex DK, Ulbright TM, Cummings OW. (2005) Coming to terms with pathologists over colon polyps with cancer or high-grade dysplasia. *J Clin Gastroenterol* 39(1): 1–3.

Shepherd NA, Quirke P. (1997) Colorectal cancer reporting: are we failing the patient? *J Clin Pathol* 50(4): 266–7.

Wheeler JM *et al.* (2004) Preoperative chemoradiotherapy and total mesorectal excision surgery for locally advanced rectal cancer: correlation with rectal cancer regression grade. *Dis Colon Rectum* 47(12): 2025–31.

Imaging and staging

Margaret Betts

The treatment of colonic cancer is almost invariably surgical, whether with curative intent or to control local symptoms. Although there is currently no universally accepted preoperative strategy for patients with colon cancer, there are a number of objectives for preoperative imaging. There should be an attempt to accurately stage the tumor in accordance with the TNM classification, with an emphasis on the extent of local invasion or extension into adjacent structures. Imaging should detect complications such as perforation or bowel obstruction. It should allow the identification of potentially difficult surgical cases, such as those complicated by perforation or tumor invasion. As part of the staging process the presence and extent of local and distant nodal disease and metastatic disease should be noted.

Colonic cancer

Appearances of the primary tumor

Computed tomography (CT) of the chest, abdomen and pelvis is the primary imaging staging investigation. The appearance of the primary tumor is usually either as a soft tissue mass or bowel wall thickening that may be associated with luminal narrowing. The mass will typically enhance in a similar fashion to the bowel wall, though large lesions may undergo central necrosis.

CT is able to demonstrate both the colon and its surrounding tissues. This allows the assessment of the extent of local spread. Extracolonic spread is seen as a mass or soft tissue infiltration of the pericolonic fat. In the ascending and descending colon, posterior extracolonic spread is likely to represent T3 disease. However, CT is unable to resolve the peritoneal covering of the colon. Since involvement of the peritoneum represents T4 disease, CT is often unable to differentiate advanced T3 from T4 disease. The involvement of adjacent organs is suggested by loss of the fat planes between the tumor, or by direct tumor invasion.

Bowel obstruction, perforation and fistulation are the commonest complications from colonic cancer, all of which can be readily identified on CT.

Lymph node involvement

CT is reliable in the detection of enlarged nodes with the pelvis and abdomen. With a cut-off of 10 mm short axis, CT is specific although not sensitive. Pathologically enlarged nodes may not contain tumor and smaller nodes may have microscopic tumor involvement. The patterns of lymphatic spread are highly dependent on the primary tumor site so, for example, right colon cancers have lymphatic spread along the small bowel mesentery and sigmoid tumors spread initially along the inferior mesenteric vessels. Retroperitoneal, pelvic or inguinal lymph node enlargement constitutes metastatic disease in colonic cancer.

Rectal cancer

The introduction of total mesorectal excision (TME) as a surgical technique and preoperative downsizing chemoreadiotherapy have markedly improved both local recurrence rates and survival for rectal cancers, to the extent that survival is similar to that of colonic cancers. The role of imaging is to provide detailed staging, including an assessment of the tumor in relation to the circumferential resection margin (CRM) and the presence or absence of poor prognostic factors. This will then allow discussion on the suitability and planning of optimal surgery or neoadjuvant pre operative treatment.

Involvement of the circumferential resection margin by tumor is associated with a high recurrence rate regardless of the local stage of the tumor (Adam *et al.* 1994). The extent of tumor penetration through the mesorectum has been shown to be an independent predictor of outcome, with spread beyond 5 mm having a significantly worse outcome (Cawthorn *et al.* 1990). Other predictors of poor prognosis include extramural vascular invasion, involvement of the peritoneum by tumor, and nodal status (Talbot *et al.* 1980; Gunderson *et al.* 2004).

Imaging modalities that are available are endorectal ultrasound, CT and magnetic resonance imaging (MRI). Enodrectal ultrasound will display the different layers of the wall of the rectum and allow the distinction between T1 and T2 tumors, though its accuracy for the more common tumors that penetrate the bowel wall is lower (Garcia-Aguilar *et al.* 2002). It cannot assess tumors that pass deep into the mesorectum or predict a clear CRM, and is limited in its ability to detect nodal involvement. Both CT and MRI can obtain high-resolution images through the pelvis that allow assessment of the tumors, lymph nodes and CRM. However, MRI has a number of advantages. The mesorectal fascia is consistently demonstrated and hence tumor extending to the CRM may be identified. The contrast resolution of MRI allows distinguishing of tumor from perirectal fibrosis, desmoplastic response or vascular cuffing. The outer layer (muscularis propria) is seen as a distinct layer and the true distance of extramural spread from the outer muscle can be measured on images obtained perpendicular to the rectal wall. Studies have consistently shown that MRI is most useful for the assessment of lateral tumor spread (Brown *et al.* 1999; Blomqvist *et al.* 1999; Beets-Tan *et al.* 2001). Thus high-resolution MRI is the mainstay of local staging of rectal cancer, with CT reserved for the staging of distant disease.

Appearances of the primary tumor

The rectal wall cannot be fully resolved by MRI. The mucosal layer of the bowel wall appears as a fine, low signal intensity line with the thicker, higher signal intensity submucosal layer beneath. The muscularis propria is seen as a low-intensity outer layer that may occasionally be depicted as two distinct layers—the inner circular layer and the outer longitudinal layer. The outer layer has an irregular corrugated appearance and numerous surface interruptions caused by vessels entering the rectal wall. The perirectal fat displays high signal intensity surrounding of the muscularis propria. Vessels are depicted as signal voids within this. The mesorectal fascia is seen as a fine, low signal layer enveloping the perirectal fat and rectum (Brown *et al.* 1999).

Tumors typically appear as intermediate signal lesions on MRI, i.e. higher signal than muscle but lower signal than fat or the rectal submucosa. Thus a T1 tumor will appear as low signal in the higher signal submucosa layer, which does not extend into the muscularis propria. T2 tumors appear as intermediate signal within the low signal outer muscle layer. The tumor does not extend beyond the outer rectal muscle into the perirectal fat. The MRI diagnosis of T3 disease is based on the presence of tumor signal extending into the perirectal fat with a rounded or nodular advancing margin and in continuity with the intramural portion of the tumor.

The muscularis propria often has an irregular corrugated appearance in the absence of tumor and interruptions of this outer layer may occur normally due to penetrating blood vessels. Thus irregularity or disruption of the low signal muscularis propria itself is not sufficient to diagnose T3 disease. Spiculation within the mesorectal fat adjacent to the tumor is not necessarily a manifestation of extramural tumor spread. The tumor often may elicit a desmoplastic response or cause perivascular cuffing of the penetrating vessels. Non-malignant spiculation is distinguished from tumor on MRI as it returns lower signal intensity and forms fine strands in the perirectal fat. MRI cannot differentiate between T2 and early T3 tumors but this differentiation is not clinically important as the outcome of patients with minimal T3 tumors is good with surgery alone (Brown *et al.* 2003a). Tumor extension into adjacent organs, pelvic sidewall or peritoneal reflection represents T4 disease.

Circumferential resection margin

The circumferential resection margin at TME is the mesorectal fascia. This is identified as a thin low signal intensity linear structure encompassing the mesorectum (Fig 14.3). The mesorectum itself is the fatty tissue containing blood vessels and lymphatics that surrounds the rectum. Once identified, the presence of tumor close to the mesorectal fascia may imply a threatened margin. The tumor may directly spread to the CRM or may be present within lymph nodes or as tumor islands. MRI is extremely accurate in predicting CRM involvement if the tumor is within 1 mm of the mesorectal fascia (Blomqvist *et al.* 1999; MERCURY 2006).

In the upper rectum, the anterior wall is covered by peritoneum, rather than mesorectum. Identification of the peritoneal

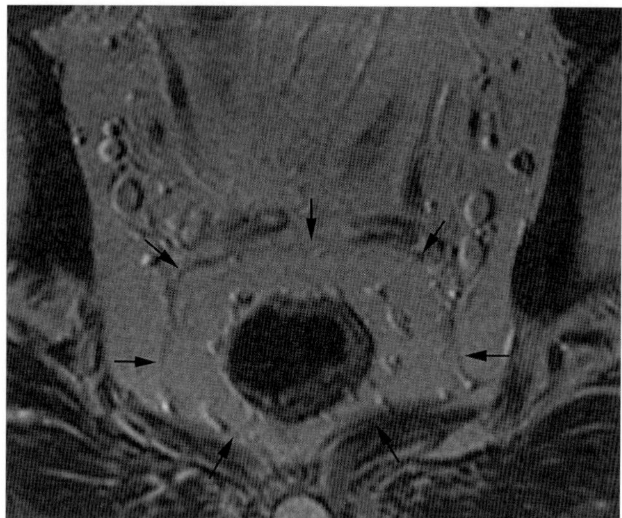

Fig. 14.3 High-resolution T2-weighted MR image obtained in a patient with a stage T2 rectal adenocarcinoma shows the mesorectal fascia as a low signal intensity layer (arrows) enveloping the high signal intensity mesorectal fat.

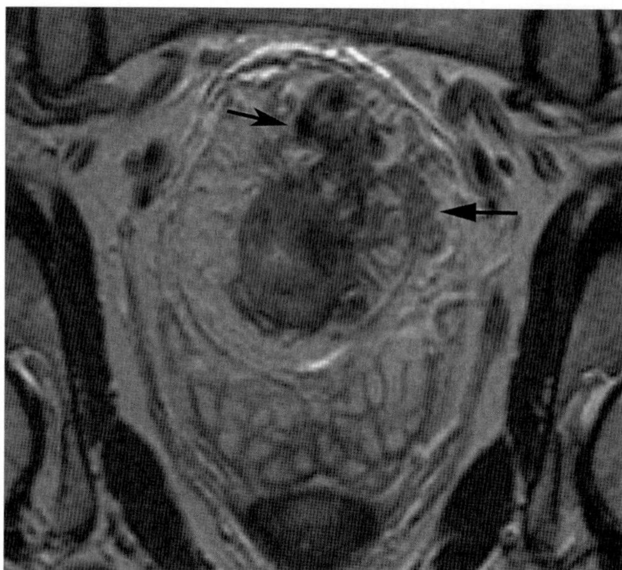

Fig. 14.4 High resolution T2-weighted MR image shows extramural vascular invasion (curved arrowhead) and involvement of the mesorectal fascia by tumor (arrow).

reflection is important as peritoneal involvement by tumor represents T4 disease. Although the peritoneal reflection is a variable structure, it may be readily identified on the sagittal images as a low signal intensity structure passing over the bladder, which passes posteriorly to its point of attachment to the rectum.

Vascular invasion

In addition to direct extension, tumor may invade along blood vessel and lymphatics. On thin-section MRI, extramural venous invasion by tumor can be readily identified and is demonstrated as serpiginous or tubular extension of tumor beyond the muscle coat and when this is identified this has a high positive predictive value when compared with histopathologic assessment of extramural venous spread (Brown 2005) (Fig 14.4).

Nodal involvement

As with colonic cancer, CT can only use size as a criterion for nodal involvement by tumor and as such suffers the same limitations. However, with the contrast resolution provided by MRI other criteria have been developed. There have been a wide variety of suggested cut-off values for lymph node size ranging from 3 to 10mm, with variable sensitivities and specificities. Other criteria based on the morphology of the node have been developed. An irregular or indistinct border has consistently been shown to be a specific marker of likely lymph node positivity. Similarly, an irregular or heterogeneous signal from within the node also correlates with likely nodal positivity (Kim *et al.* 2004). Preservation of the chemical-shift artefact around lymph nodes seems to correlate with being reactive or uninvolved. These criteria are independent of nodal size. When combined, these criteria can increase the sensitivity and specificity of nodal staging to 90% (Brown 2005). However, there remains the limitation for imaging in the detection of micrometastases (tumor deposits around 1–2mm) within individual nodes.

Local nodes are located within the mesorectal fat. As with colonic cancer, the second group of nodes is related to the arterial blood supply. However, the rectum receives supply both from the inferior mesenteric artery, via its hemorrhoidal vessels and the internal iliac artery, via branches of the pudendal artery. Thus it is possible for nodal metastases to occur outside the mesorectum along the internal iliac chain with lateral spread to the pelvic sidewall or retroperitoneally.

Metastatic disease

The imaging of rectal and colonic metastatic disease is similar, as is the patterns of spread. The liver is the predominant site of metastatic disease; 10–15% of patients have metastases at diagnosis and 70% of patients that die do so from their liver disease. The presence of metastatic disease at presentation is an indicator of poor prognosis. The development of metastatic disease after surgery may be suitable for treatment with either a survival benefit or curative intent. Imaging of metastases in these different contexts will be different.

Metastatic disease at presentation

The staging CT is the primary imaging modality for the detection of metastatic disease and at best will detect 90% of lesions greater than 1 cm (Kuszyk *et al.* 1996). Optimal detection of metastases requires intravenous contrast and scanning in the portal venous phase of enhancement. With this imaging strategy, liver metastases usually appear as masses of decreased attenuation compared to the liver parenchyma, though with an absolute attenuation above that of water. Cystic lesions in the liver may be due to mucinous tumor metastases making differentiation from simple cysts more difficult. Imaging by either ultrasound or MRI may be helpful.

Other sites of metastatic disease are lung, lymph nodes such as retroperitoneal, inguinal or thoracic sites, and less commonly bone. Staging CT is able to demonstrate these with an acceptable sensitivity. As with small liver lesions, sub-centimeter lung parenchymal nodules cannot be accurately characterized and again may need follow-up imaging.

Metastatic disease after tumor resection

Metastatic disease occurring some time after resection of the primary tumor may be suspected due to symptoms or a rise in serum chorioembryonic antigen (CEA), or detected on follow-up imaging. The liver is the commonest site of metastatic disease. The role of imaging in this instance is slightly different from that at disease presentation. For liver disease, there may be the option of either surgical resection or radiofrequency ablation and a comprehensive assessment of all potential lesions is required.

Magnetic resonance imaging at 1.5-tesla field strength and with i.v. contrast (gadolinium)-enhanced sequences is superior to contrast-enhanced CT for the detection of lesions above and below 1 cm in diameter. On a per patient basis, it does not perform as well as PET/CT. However, for colorectal cancer, it is not sufficient to simply diagnose the presence of metastatic disease within the liver. If the potential treatment is surgical resection then it is necessary to detect all lesions and also to characterize their location. In this regard, the per lesion performance of MRI is significantly better than PET/CT (Bipat *et al.* 2005; Sahani *et al.* 2005). It is therefore the imaging modality of choice for the assessment of metastatic disease of the liver.

PET/CT

Although PET/CT is a sensitive modality for the detection of the primary tumor it does not have any advantage over other imaging modalities. Similarly, its performance for nodal staging is not much superior to CT alone; the intense uptake of trace by the primary tumor seems to obscure uptake in adjacent local nodes (Furukawa *et al.* 2006). Therefore there does not seem to be a role in the initial staging investigations.

In patients with hepatic metastases, although MRI is the investigation of choice for the characterization of the liver lesions, PET/CT is used to exclude disease elsewhere. It may detect extrahepatic metastatic disease in up to 29% of patients considered for surgery, hence altering the decision-making (Khan *et al.* 2006).

The detection and assessment of locally recurrent rectal disease is problematical with conventional imaging. Despite the convenience of CT, it has a low specificity in this regard and follow-up imaging is usually required with a consequent delay in treatment. MRI may perform better, with the differentiation of local recurrence from scar tissue but again there are limitations with respect to tumor size and overall specificity. However, PET/CT has been shown to more accurately demonstrate locally recurrent disease (Votrubova *et al.* 2006).

Imaging guiding the MDT discussion

The radiologic findings for individual patients are often the starting point for the MDT discussion. Whilst the histopathologic stage of the surgical specimen remains the gold standard, the radiologic stage is increasingly used for decisions on preoperative therapy. For colonic cancer it is known that T4 stage, N2 stage (four or more malignant nodes), extramural venous invasion, and either an emergency clinical or a radiologic complicated presentation are all independent indicators of poor prognosis. The image interpretation should pay particular attention to this. Obviously, the presence at diagnosis of extensive metastatic disease will also predict poor prognosis to the extent that non-surgical therapy may be deemed more appropriate; again imaging will direct this discussion. It may be anticipated with the increasing interest in laparoscopic surgery for colonic tumors that imaging will have a role in the selection of suitable cases and predicting potential problems, which may result in conversion to open surgery.

For rectal tumors, there is a clear role for preoperative therapy and imaging has a key role in the selection of patients. Central to this is the identification of the circumferential resection margin and prediction as to its involvement. Patients with extensive local disease on imaging can be identified and selected for neoadjuvant therapy that may downstage the tumor and improve surgical outcome and survival. Conversely in patients with favorable localized tumors then optimal surgery is the initial treatment and decisions on adjuvant treatment can be based on the histologic stage.

The discussion with regard to metastatic disease is more complicated and the evidence less secure. A more aggressive approach to liver metastases is being adopted. The primary role of imaging is to confirm the presence and distribution of disease to allow an assessment of surgical suitability. The absence of disease elsewhere is confirmed by the imaging investigation. If surgery is not an option, then alterative strategies such as radiofrequency ablation or high-intensity focused ultrasound may be considered. The accurate anatomic location of disease within the liver is key to this discussion.

Conclusion

In conclusion, the role of the radiologist in the colorectal cancer MDT is paramount, from the initial staging of the primary to guide resection, the determination of the presence of metastatic disease to guide the oncologist, and the characterization of that metastatic disease to guide the liver surgeons or the interventional radiologists with respect to the rationale for metastatic resection or ablative therapies.

References

Adam IJ, Mohamdee MO, Martin IG, Scott N, Finan PJ, Johnston D *et al.* (1994) Role of circumferential margin involvement in the local recurrence of rectal cancer. *Lancet* 344: 707–11.

Beets-Tan RG, Beets GL, Vliegen RF *et al.* (2001) Accuracy of magnetic resonance imaging in prediction of tumour-free resection margin in rectal cancer surgery. *Lancet* 357: 497–504.

Bipat S, van Leeuwen MS, Comans EF *et al.* (2005) Colorectal liver metastases: CT, MR imaging, and PET for diagnosis—meta-analysis, *Radiology* 237: 123–31.

Blomqvist L, Rubio C, Holm T, Machado M, Hindmarsh T. (1999) Rectal adenocarcinoma: assessment of tumour involvement of the lateral resection margin by MRI of resected specimen. *Br J Radiol* 72: 18–23.

Brown G, Richards CJ, Newcombe RG *et al.* (1999) Rectal carcinoma: thin-section MR imaging for staging in 28 patients. *Radiology* 211: 215–22.

Brown G, Radcliffe AG, Newcombe RG, Dallimore NS, Bourne MW, Williams GT. (2003a) Preoperative assessment of prognostic factors in rectal cancer using high-resolution magnetic resonance imaging. *Br J Surg* 90: 355–64.

Brown G, Richards CJ, Bourne MW *et al.* (2003b) Morphologic predictors of lymph node status in rectal cancer with use of high-spatial-resolution MR imaging with histopathologic comparison. *Radiology* 227: 371–7.

Brown G. (2005) Thin section MRI in multidisciplinary pre-operative decision making for patients with rectal cancer. *Br J Radiol* 78: S117–27.

Cawthorn SJ, Parums DV, Gibbs NMA *et al.* (1990) Extent of mesorectal spread and involvement of lateral resection margin as prognostic factors after surgery for rectal cancer. *Lancet* 335: 1055–9.

Furukawa H, Ikuma H, Seki A *et al.*(2006) Positron emission tomography scanning is not superior to whole body multidetector helical computed tomography in the preoperative staging of colorectal cancer. *Gut* 55: 1007–11.

Garcia-Aguilar J, Polack J, Lee SH *et al.* (2002) Accuracy of endorectal ultrasonography in preoperative staging of rectal tumors. *Dis Colon Rectum* 45: 10–15.

Gunderson LL, Sargent DJ, Tepper JE *et al.* (2004) Impact of T and N stage and treatment on survival and relapse in adjuvant rectal cancer: a pooled analysis. *J Clin Oncol* 22: 1785–96.

Khan S, Tan YM, John A *et al.* (2006) An audit of fusion CT-PET in the management of colorectal liver metastases. *Eur J Surg Oncol* 32: 564–7.

Kim JH, Beets GL, Kim MJ, Kessels AG, Beets-Tan RG. (2004) High-resolution MR imaging for nodal staging in rectal cancer: are there any criteria in addition to the size? *Eur J Radiol* 52(1): 78–83.

Kuszyk BS, Bluemke DA, Urban BA *et al.* (1996) Portal-phase contrast-enhanced helical CT for the detection of malignant hepatic tumors: sensitivity based on comparison with intraoperative and pathologic findings, *Am J Roentgenol* 66: 91–5.

MERCURY Study Group. (2006) Diagnostic accuracy of preoperative magnetic resonance imaging in predicting curative resection of rectal cancer: prospective observational study. *BMJ* 333: 779–82.

Sahani DV, Kalva SP, Fischman AJ *et al.* (2005) Detection of liver metastases from adenocarcinoma of the colon and pancreas: comparison of mangafodipir trisodium-enhanced liver MRI and whole-body FDG PET. *Am J Roentgenol* 185: 239–46.

Talbot IC, Ritchie S, Leighton MH, Hughes AO, Bussey HJ, Morson BC. (1980) The clinical significance of invasion of veins by rectal cancer. *Br J Surg* 67: 439–42.

Votrubova J, Belohlavek O, Jaruskova M *et al.* (2006) The role of FDG-PET/CT in the detection of recurrent colorectal cancer, *Eur J Nucl Med Mol Imaging* 33: 779–84.

Treatment

Overview of therapy modalities

Rachel S. Midgley

So we have now diagnosed our colorectal cancer patient with the help of the histopathologist, we have staged the patient with respect to local infiltration and distant metastatic spread with the aid of the radiologist, and the patient is being presented at the colorectal MDT meeting. What do we do next?

What we do largely depends on the evidence presented by the professionals above. However the mainstay of treatment with bowel cancer is usually surgery to remove the cancer. The ease with which this is done without any prior treatment will usually depend on the local extent and the site of the tumor. Tumors in the rectum are harder to access and are more likely to have impinged upon surrounding structures. Further up in the colon there is more space for the tumor to grow and surgery is easier, frequently nowadays being performed through laporoscopic incisions.

There are occasions when we cannot, or choose not, to do immediate surgery. For example, a T3/T4 low tumor in the rectum is likely to leave a positive R1 resection margin or necessitate an operation that will result in impotence or incontinence unless it is downsized by chemoradiotherapy.

Or, the patient may have very little in the way of symptoms from the primary tumor but may have a heavy burden of disease in the liver. Under these circumstances it may be more appropriate for the patient to be referred directly to the oncologist for palliative chemotherapy. If this does happen, there must be very rapid referral pathways set up for immediate access to surgery should the patient develop obstruction or perforation.

When the patient has had his or her primary removed, again their case should be brought back to the MDT for further clinical decision-making. Frequently at this point they will be referred for consideration of adjuvant chemotherapy to reduce the chances of recurrence of their cancer in the future.

The patient may have secondary disease in the liver or the lung that is potentially operable and then they should be referred through to the appropriate specialist MDT to be considered for surgery or ablative therapy. Often these specialist MDTs will only be available at tertiary referral centers, but these should be made easily accessible to patients being treated at cancer units.

If a patient with metastatic disease has explored all standard chemotherapy regimens and is still of good performance status and is highly motivated, then consideration should be given for their referral to a center that runs phase I trials. Many of the agents that are being explored in phase I trials in colorectal cancer at the present time are discussed later in this chapter.

So, in summary, there is a complex myriad of potential treatments open to patients with colorectal cancer (see Figs 14.5 & 14.6). Make sure that your MDT has the necessary skills and knowledge to keep all avenues of treatment open to your patients by reading the following sections.

Surgery

Baljit Singh & Chris Cunningham

The surgical plan in the majority of colorectal cancer cases discussed at a multidisciplinary meeting is logical and uncontroversial. The surgical approach is based on radical excision aimed at removing the primary cancer, draining lymphatics and any involved adjacent structures. However, there are important instances where the surgical plan is less certain and the subtleties of management are determined by expert assessment of histology and radiologic imaging. These are considered with patient factors including symptoms, fitness, life expectancy and, of course, personal wishes. This chapter aims to provide an evidence-based approach for surgical decision-making in these difficult cases. In addition it will present some of the recent advances to be embraced by the MDT.

Early colorectal cancer

Early cancer is increasingly diagnosed and treated endoscopically, and a large population of patients now exists where

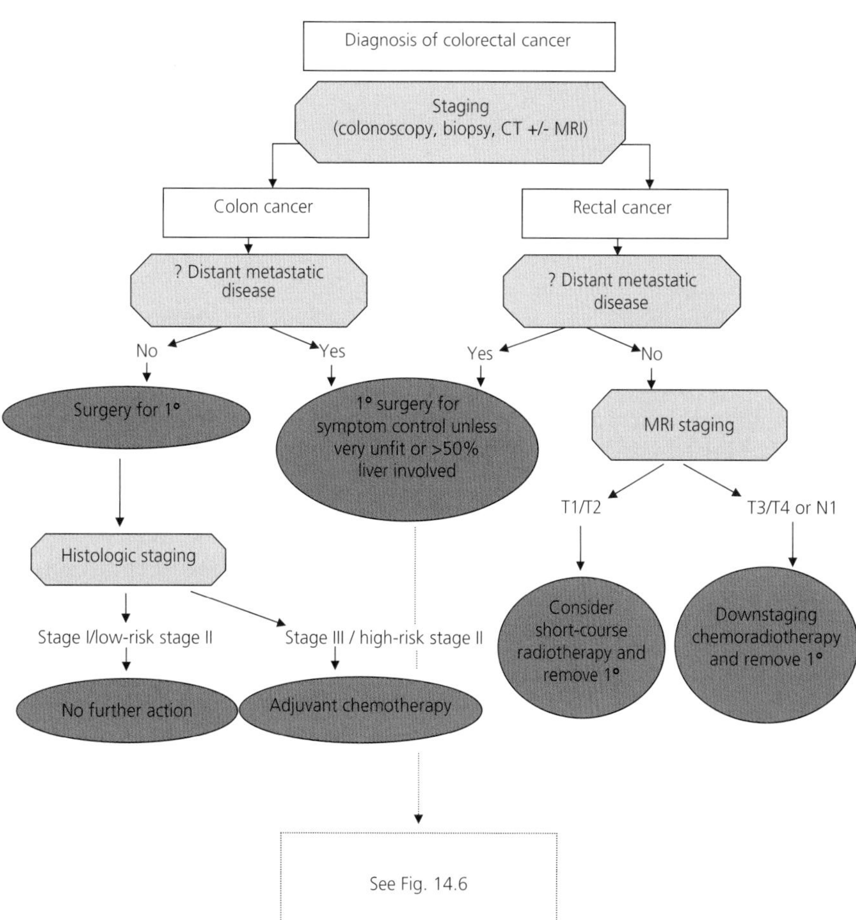

Fig. 14.5 The colorectal cancer treatment pathway for primary colorectal cancer.

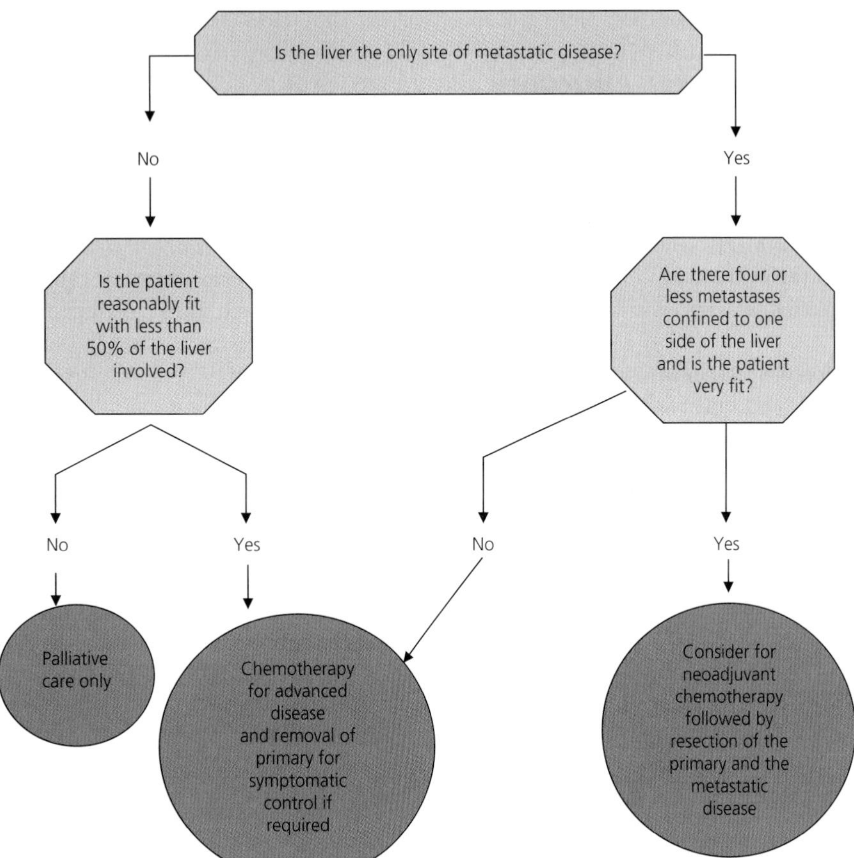

Fig. 14.6 The colorectal cancer treatment pathway when distant metastatic disease is present at diagnosis.

traditional radical excision is abandoned in favor of local excision. This has many advantages but inevitably will compromise the oncologic treatment of some patients. A key role of the MDT is to determine the balance of benefits of local excision for individual patients: protecting those for whom oncologic compromise is too great by use of local excision alone, and at the same time ensuring that those with early cancer are not unnecessarily 'overtreated' by major surgery.

Many cancers arising within polyps are removed completely by snare polypectomy or the more advanced technique of endoscopic mucosal resection. The need for further surgery is dictated by depth of invasion and the presence of adverse features including poor differentiation, tumor budding, lymphovascular invasion and suspicion of resection margin involvement (Bretagnol *et al.* 2007). These factors predict the likelihood of lymph node involvement and local recurrence in the bowel wall. Pedunculated malignant polyps are commonly assessed according to Haggitt classification of stalk invasion, whereas in sessile polyps the Kikuchi classification of submucosa invasion is employed. Figure 14.1 summarizes Haggitt and Kikuchi classifications and risk of lymph node involvement. T1 cancers which penetrate the lower third of the submucosa (Kikuchi SM3) or base of polyp stalk (Haggitt level IV) have a reported risk of lymph node metastases of up to 25%, and in all but the most frail patients this would support further treatment with radical surgical resection. In contrast, early T1 lesions (Kikuchi SM1, or Haggitt I/II) have a less than 5% incidence of involved lymph nodes and the benefits of radical surgery may only be realized in patients where the risks of surgery are minimal.

In early rectal cancer the therapeutic options are increased with per anal excision by either conventional approaches or the use of transanal endoscopic microsurgery (TEM). TEM facilitates the precise removal of rectal lesions with full thickness of the muscularis propria under direct vision with sophisticated instrumentation. The technique is safe and well tolerated by patients. Major complications such as bleeding, abscess formation and intraperitoneal perforation are reported, but occur in less than 4% of cases. This technique can provide adequate local excision of advanced T1 and even T2 tumors, but the critical determinant for most patients is the likelihood of lymph node involvement which, for the most part, is determined by histologic assessment. Preoperative staging by rectal MRI and particularly endorectal ultrasound is important in determining suitability for local excision by assessing depth of invasion and the presence of suspicious mesorectal lymph nodes.

Initial results from TEM databases were disappointing, suggesting local recurrence rates of 6–20% for T1 lesions and 20–59% for T3 lesions (Bach *et al.* 2006) which compare badly with the expected results from total mesorectal excision. However, these results include many patients where oncologic compromise was accepted. In contrast to many surgical techniques, the introduction of TEM has been characterized by rigorous data collection and this has allowed a robust prediction of prognostic factors following excision. Analysis of the national UK TEM database has shown that local recurrence correlated with age, tumor area and pT stage (Bach *et al.* 2006). In an optimum setting with a well-differentiated T1 cancer of less than 2 cm in size with no vascular invasion, the recurrence rate was less than 2%. In those with unfavorable histologic factors early recourse to salvage surgery is effective and does not compromise long-term survival.

It is intriguing to consider the use of TEM resection coupled with adjuvant or even neoadjuvant treatment as a means of dealing with nodal disease and thereby extending the proportion of rectal tumors where local excision may be acceptable. The evolving complexities of managing early rectal cancer support the recent directive from UK Cancer Networks that decision-making in these cancers should be concentrated in regional centers of interest.

Total mesorectal excision

Total mesorectal excision for rectal cancer exemplifies the principles which should be applied to all colorectal cancers, i.e. the precise anatomic dissection of the affected bowel with its mesentery enclosed within an intact fascial plane. This can be technically demanding, but meticulous technique has lead to a radical improvement in local control of rectal cancer and reduced complications such as pelvic nerve injury (Fig. 14.7). The widespread adoption of TME has been associated with a reduction in recurrent rectal cancer to 10% or less in most institutions with adequately trained surgeons compared to historical rates of 30% (Visser *et al.* 2006). It is good routine practice for postoperative MDT discussion to include an assessment of quality of mesorectal dissection. A poor grade of mesorectal excision has been shown to correlate with recurrence (Maslekar *et al.* 2007).

Adam *et al.* have shown that local recurrence correlates with an involved circumferential resection margin (CRM) (Adam *et al.* 1994). An involved or threatened CRM should be identified on preoperative MRI and will indicate the need for neoadjuvant treatment. However, a threatened CRM is not the only risk factor for tumor recurrence. Chan *et al.* found that anterior rectal tumors had a significantly higher recurrence rate and poorer 5-year survival compared to rectal tumors in other positions (Chan *et al.* 2006). Furthermore, Lee *et al.* reported that outcome was worse for anterior rectal tumors in males compared to females (Lee *et al.* 2005). Patient habitus is an important factor in rectal dissection which Salerno *et al.* have explored with MRI modelling which can be helpful in predicting the technical difficulty of TME (Salerno *et al.* 2006).

Extended resections for anterior rectal cancer

Low rectal cancers

Whilst TME has become the established surgical technique for rectal dissection there is still controversy surrounding the management of very low rectal cancers where local recurrence following abdominoperineal (APR) resection ranges from 4 to

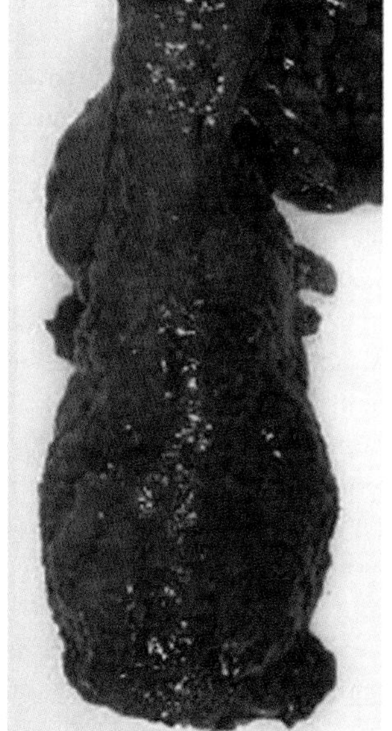

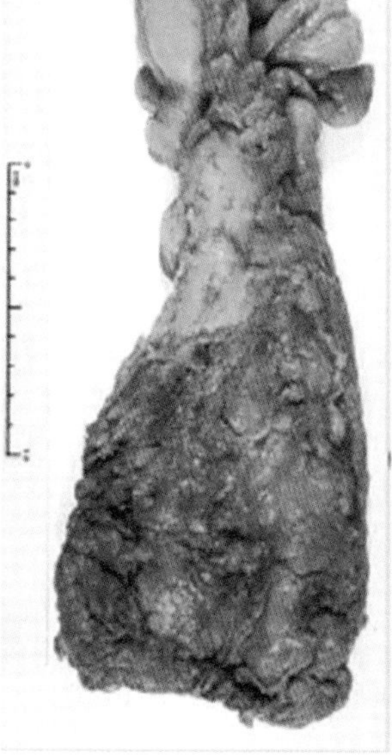

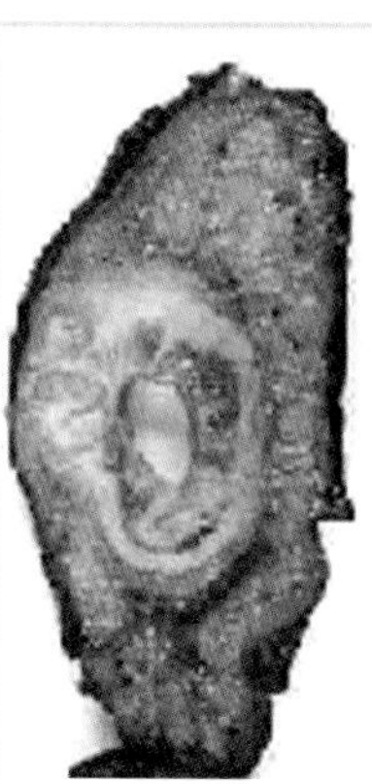

Fig. 14.7 A total mesorectal excision resection specimen.

33%. Marr *et al.* found that the volume of tissue outside the muscularis propria at abdominoperineal resection was significantly less than at anterior resection (Marr *et al.* 2005). Consequently, for a similar T stage a low rectal cancer is closer to the CRM compared to a mid- or high rectal tumor. The anatomic explanation rests with the fact that the mesorectum tapers or 'cones in' distally and this, at least in part, accounts for the higher rate of CRM involvement in APR. Adequate oncologic clearance for a low rectal cancer demands cylindrical excision outside of the mesorectal fascia where it is adherent to the pelvic floor. Miles' original description of APR detailed an abdominal mobilization of the rectum to the levator muscle and a perineal excision including removal of the coccyx and division of the lateral attachment of the levator muscle. Thus, it appears we are returning to the original description. Experience from Scandinavia would suggest that the perineal procedure is optimized with the patient placed in the prone position and closure of the large defect is facilitated by a myocutaneous flap reconstruction. In addition, selective en bloc partial resection of the prostate or vagina may be important in improving local control of anterior rectal cancers after neoadjuvant treatment.

Neoadjuvant chemoradiation for rectal cancer: timing of surgery and use of pretreatment defunctioning stoma

Details of short-course radiotherapy and neoadjuvant chemoradiation are presented elsewhere. However, two areas of surgical management in relation to neoadjuvant chemoradiation are discussed: timing of surgery and use of pretreatment ileostomy. Francois *et al.* looked at patients who underwent preoperative radiotherapy for rectal cancer and subsequent surgery at an interval of either 2 weeks or 6–8 weeks following downsizing (Francois *et al.* 2005). The longer interval was associated with a better rate of clinical and pathologic response as well as a higher rate of sphincter-saving surgery. Similarly, Moore *et al.* found a better pathologic response rate at day 44 or greater compared to a time point before this (Moore *et al.* 2004). However it is unclear from the literature whether delaying surgery beyond this allows for improved response. Several modalities have been employed to assess response to neoadjuvant therapy and specifically to identify those with a complete clinical response in whom surgery may be avoided. These can predict rectal cancer regression to some extent but cannot reliably identify complete pathologic response. Habr-Gama *et al.* explored non-operative management of the 28% of patients determined to have a complete clinical response by clinical examination, ultrasound, CT scan and biopsy. These patients were followed by regular clinical assessment with early recourse to resection if disease progression was identified. The 5-year overall and disease-free survival favored the observational group (100% and 92% respectively) compared to the operative group (88% and 83% respectively). The authors propose that major surgery and its associated morbidity can be avoided in patients demonstrating a complete clinical response if structured intensive surveillance is maintained (Habr-Gama 2006). Rigorous examination of this non-operative approach to patients with complete clinical response appears reasonable and may be helped by advances in radiologic assessment such as PET-CT.

In the UK around 14% of rectal cancer patients undergo stoma formation before treatment. For most this is driven by the need to control intolerable rectal symptoms such as incipient obstruction or tenesmus. However, many institutions employ defunctioning stoma as a routine in the belief that chemoradiation is better tolerated with reduced likelihood of breaks in therapy through side-effects. This is against a background understanding that all of these patients would have a protective stoma fashioned at the time of resection. The literature tends to support the use of a defunctioning ileostomy rather than colostomy but there is a lack of evidence on the routine use of defunctioning stoma. Practices in the UK vary widely and only prospective randomized controlled trials (RCTs) are likely to influence surgical practice towards uniformity.

Laparoscopic surgery

In 2000, the UK National Institute for Health and Clinical Excellence (NICE) expressed concerns over minimally invasive surgery in colorectal cancer based on fears that laparoscopic resection may compromise the oncologic aspects of colorectal resections with port-site metastases and less radical resections. However, a meta-analysis of 12 RCTs in North America, UK and mainland Europe has shown equivalence in oncologic outcomes with advantages in terms of quicker postoperative recovery (Reza *et al.* 2006). Laparoscopic procedures generally take longer and use more consumables than open equivalents. However, cost analysis is complex and when reduced hospital stay, earlier return to normal function and potential longer term benefits are considered, the overall cost impact may well be neutral. In 2006, NICE reviewed the position and advocated the use of laparoscopic surgery for cancer resections in suitable patients with appropriately trained surgical teams. With these apparent advantages it is incumbent on MDTs to ensure that suitable patients are not disadvantaged by lack of access to these techniques.

While laparoscopic surgery for colon and upper rectal cancer has obvious advantages, the situation in cancer of the lower rectum is less reassuring. Despite the conclusion of a Cochrane Review (Breukink *et al.* 2006) supporting laparoscopic TME there are worrying reports from high-volume centers with expertise in this surgery suggesting an unacceptable increase in anastomotic leaks and pelvic autonomic nerve injury. It is likely that these will be reduced as training and instrumentation improve, but for the moment laparoscopic mesorectal excision should be approached with caution and in the authors' opinion should not be undertaken outside of specialist centers.

Lacy *et al.* report a survival advantage in patients with stage II disease undergoing laparoscopically assisted compared to open resection. This may be a real phenomenon and it is interesting to speculate that reduced immunologic assault or perhaps earlier progression to adjuvant chemotherapy may contribute in the laparoscopic group (Lacy *et al.* 2002). This is an exciting period in colorectal surgery as laparoscopic techniques and expertise evolve. To date, many trials have been of poor quality and often involving surgeons with modest experience. Laparoscopic surgery will not provide an alternative to open resections in all cases but with time there will be a defined population which will benefit from rapid recovery, cost saving and perhaps even oncologic advantage.

Management of primary colorectal cancer with liver metastases

Twenty per cent of colorectal cancer patients present with synchronous liver metastases. Standard teaching is that the primary lesion should be removed and hepatic resection performed after a delay of months. This dogma has been challenged, however, with comparable mortalities for combined hepatic resection and delayed hepatic resection. However Tanaka *et al.* noted synchronous resection involving four or more liver metastases had a poorer outcome than delayed hepatic resection (Tanaka *et al.* 2004). A response in the primary tumor is seen in 50–75% of patients receiving oxaliplatin-based treatment. Early palliative chemotherapy has been associated with prolongation of survival and improved quality of life.

Patients with extensive or inoperable metastatic liver disease should avoid surgery unless the bowel primary cancer is causing significant symptoms. In most cases anemia can be controlled with iron supplements and mild obstructive symptoms helped by osmotic laxatives. Indications for intervention are usually obstructive symptoms, intractable anemia or the presence of rectal symptoms such as tenesmus, bleeding and mucous discharge. Rectal cancers can be adequately palliated by transanal resection with a urologic-type resectoscope or laser ablation. In patients who present with colonic obstruction an alternative to emergency surgery is the insertion of a self-expanding metallic stent (SEMS) (Fig. 14.8). This is an attractive option, especially for left-sided tumors. If SEMS insertion fails or the tumor is inaccessible then resection can be considered.

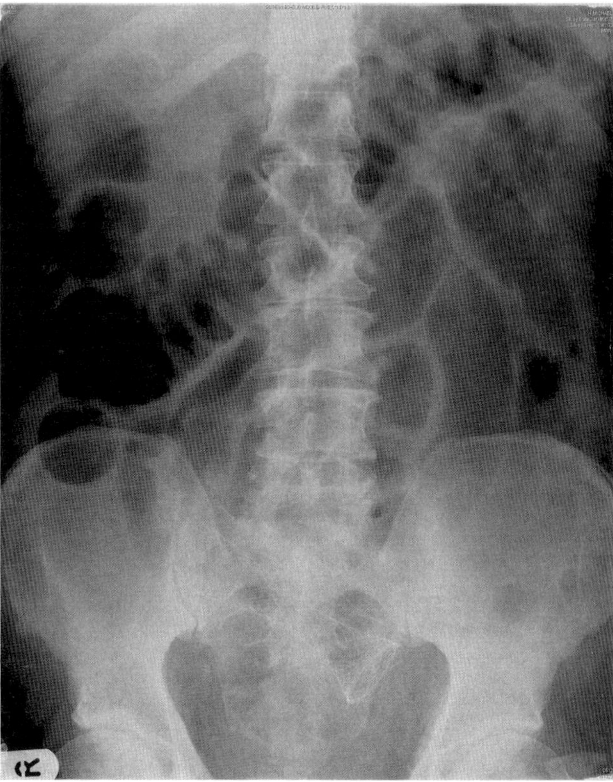

Fig. 14.8 A self-expanding metallic stent used to alleviate acute colonic obstruction.

Management of multivisceral involvement

The management of advanced colorectal cancer which involves multiple organs is challenging. Organ involvement commonly includes the urinary tract (bladder, kidney and ureter), large or small bowel involvement and (male or female) genital organs. Detailed and thorough preoperative assessment of the tumor is essential in planning a surgical strategy and involvement of other surgical specialities such as plastic surgeons, urologists and gynecologists. However imaging cannot always discriminate between inflammatory changes and tumor invasion of surrounding structures. Histologic tumor involvement correlates with a reduction in survival (Gall *et al.* 1987). Therefore, tumors suspected of local invasion must be removed en bloc. Multivisceral surgery is associated with considerable morbidity ranging from 11 to 50% with the commonest being infective complications. The 5-year survival rate following curative multivisceral resection ranges from 49 to 77% (Gall *et al.* 1987).

Recurrent cancer

It is essential to accurately preoperatively stage patients with recurrent cancer before considering surgical excision. PET-CT is valuable in this setting, identifying patients with metastases elsewhere which render resection futile. It can affect management in up to 37% of patients with recurrent cancer.

Isolated intra-abdominal recurrence of colonic cancer can be treated with resection after accurate staging to exclude disease elsewhere. Isolated pelvic recurrence after rectal cancer surgery may be amenable to resection after assessment in a rigorous multidisciplinary environment. Pelvic recurrence may occur centrally, usually associated with anastomosis or laterally on the pelvic side wall or sacrum. Mortality has been reported as 1.4% with a morbidity of 35%.

Acute presentation of colonic tumors

Large bowel obstruction can be the initial presentation of a colonic tumor in the emergency setting. Whilst surgery is feasible, the risk of stoma formation is higher compared to the elective setting. An alternative strategy is to utilize a SEMS to alleviate acute left-sided obstruction. This technique can be used as a 'bridge to surgery' and following resolution of the acute obstruction allows for adequate staging of the cancer prior to definitive surgery. A review of 1198 cases with large bowel obstruction treated with SEM found the risks of perforation (3.8%), migration (11.8%) and reobstruction (7.3%) (Sebastian *et al.* 2004).

There are few studies which have compared the results of stenting versus emergency surgery in patients with left-sided obstruction. Ng *et al.* compared case-matched patients presenting with left-sided obstruction that either underwent emergency surgery or stent insertion and delayed surgery (Ng *et al.* 2006). A primary anastomosis was performed in 95% who had initial stent insertion compared to 75% who underwent emergency surgery. Furthermore, stent insertion and delayed surgery was associated with a shorter hospital stay. This optimism is tempered by reports of a recent randomized trial of SEMS versus surgery in patients with incurable cancer resection which was abandoned due to unacceptable delayed perforation associated with stenting (van Hooft *et al.* 2006).

If resection is undesirable then a defunctioning proximal stoma can be valuable, particularly in distal colorectal cancers. Stoma formation can usually be achieved by minimally invasive techniques.

Conclusion

Colorectal cancer for many years was treated surgically without due scrutiny. In recent years the MDT has supported assessment and decision-making in colorectal cancer care encouraging the dissemination of best practice. This is seen is several key areas. The adoption of TME alone has reduced pelvic recurrence of rectal cancer by more than 50% and this has been augmented by improvements in neoadjuvant therapies. The development of new techniques in local excision such as TEM offers cure in patients who would previously have required major surgery. More recently the use of laparoscopic resection, as supported by NICE, has allowed the same high standards of surgical resection to be undertaken in a minimally invasive way offering tangible benefits to patients. This is an exciting time in the surgical management of colorectal cancer and inevitably increased choice is associated with increased complexity in decision-making. A robust MDT approach is vital is encouraging education and training and most importantly providing optimum treatment for all patients with colorectal cancer.

References

Adam IJ, Mohamdee MO, Martin IG *et al.* (1994) Role of circumferential margin involvement in the local recurrence of rectal cancer. *Lancet* 344: 707–11.

Bach S, Mortensen N. (2006) Analysis of national database for TEM resected rectal cancer. *Colorectal Dis* 8(9): 815.

Bretagnol F, Rullier E, George B, Warren BF, Mortensen NJ. (2007) Local therapy for rectal cancer: still controversial? *Dis Colon Rectum* 50(4): 523–33.

Breukink S, Pierie J, Wiggers T. (2006) Laparoscopic versus open total mesorectal excision for rectal cancer. *Cochrane Database Syst Rev* 2006(4): CD005200.

Chan CL, Bokey EL, Chapuis PH, Renwick AA, Dent OF. (2006) Local recurrence after curative resection for rectal cancer is associated with anterior position of the tumour. *Br J Surg* 93(1): 105–12.

Francois Y, Nemoz CJ, Baulieux J *et al.* (1999) Influence of the interval between preoperative radiation therapy and surgery on downstaging and on the rate of sphincter-sparing surgery for rectal cancer: the Lyon R90–01 randomized trial. *J Clin Oncol* 17(8): 2396.

Gall FP, Tonak J, Altendorf A. (1987) Multivisceral resections in colorectal cancer. *Dis Colon Rectum* 30(5): 337–41.

Habr-Gama A. (2006) Assessment and management of the complete clinical response of rectal cancer to chemoradiotherapy. *Colorectal Dis* 8 Suppl 3: 21–4.

Lacy AM, Garcia-Valdecasas JC, Delgado S *et al.* (2002) Laparoscopy-assisted colectomy versus open colectomy for treatment of non-metastatic colon cancer: a randomized trial. *Lancet* 29: 2224–9.

Lee SH, Hernandez de Anda E, Finne CO, Madoff RD, Garcia-Aguilar J. (2005) The effect of circumferential tumor location in clinical outcomes of rectal cancer patients treated with total mesorectal excision. *Dis Colon Rectum* 48(12): 2249–57.

Marr R, Birbeck K, Garvican J *et al.* (2005) The modern abdominoperineal excision: the next challenge after total mesorectal excision. *Ann Surg* 242(1): 74–82.

Maslekar S, Sharma A, Macdonald A, Gunn J, Monson JR, Hartley JE. (2007) Mesorectal grades predict recurrences after curative resection for rectal cancer. *Dis Colon Rectum* 50(2): 168–75.

Moore HG, Gittleman AE, Minsky BD *et al.* (2004) Rate of pathologic complete response with increased interval between preoperative combined modality therapy and rectal cancer resection. *Dis Colon Rectum* 47(3): 279–86.

Ng KC, Law WL, Lee YM, Choi HK, Seto CL, Ho JW. (2006) Self-expanding metallic stent as a bridge to surgery versus emergency resection for obstructing left-sided colorectal cancer: a case-matched study. *J Gastrointest Surg* 10(6): 798–803.

Reza MM, Blasco JA, Andradas E, Cantero R, Mayol J. (2006) Systematic review of laparoscopic versus open surgery for colorectal cancer. *Br J Surg* 93(8): 921–8.

Salerno G, Daniels IR, Brown G, Heald RJ, Moran BJ. (2006) Magnetic resonance imaging pelvimetry in 186 patients with rectal cancer confirms an overlap in pelvic size between males and females. *Colorectal Dis* 8(9): 772–6.

Sebastian S, Johnston S, Geoghegan T, Torreggiani W, Buckley M. (2004) Pooled analysis of the efficacy and safety of self-expanding metal stenting in malignant colorectal obstruction. *Am J Gastroenterol* 99(10): 2051–7.

Tanaka K, Shimada H, Matsuo K *et al.* (2004) Outcome after simultaneous colorectal and hepatic resection for colorectal cancer with synchronous metastases. *Surgery* 136(3): 650–9.

van Hooft JE, Fockens P, Marinelli AW, Bossuyt PM, Bemelman WA. (2006) Premature closure of the Dutch Stent-in I study. *Lancet* 368(9547): 1573–4.

Visser O, Bakx R, Zoetmulder FA *et al.* (2006) The influence of total mesorectal excision on local recurrence and survival in rectal cancer patients: A population-based study in greater Amsterdam. *J Surg Oncol* 95(6): 447–54.

Chemotherapy

Ami Sabharwal & David Kerr

Introduction

The last 20 years have seen significant advances in the use of chemotherapy in the treatment of colorectal cancer patients. Increased understanding of the pharmacology of 5-fluorouracil (5-FU) and the discovery of modulators of its activity e.g. leucovorin (LV) resulted in some initial improvements in treatment. However, over the past 5 years, the discovery of a number of new cytotoxic drugs (e.g. oxaliplatin and irinotecan) and monoclonal antibodies (e.g. bevacizimab and cetuximab), which have proven efficacy in large bowel cancer, has significantly improved patient outcome and prognosis. Systemic chemotherapy now has a clear role as an adjunct to surgery to improve survival in stage III and certain 'high-risk' stage II colorectal cancer patients. Appropriate chemotherapy in the metastatic setting will also prolong survival and improve quality of life. The evolution of chemotherapy use as well as current practice in the adjuvant and metastatic setting will now be discussed.

Adjuvant chemotherapy

Almost half of patients who have undergone potentially curative resection for colon cancer will relapse and die of metastatic disease because of the presence of clinically occult micrometastases. The aim of postoperative adjuvant chemotherapy is to eradicate these micrometastases in patients with high-risk disease, therefore reducing the risk of recurrence and increasing the probability of cure.

Leucovorin-modulated 5-FU

A number of trials of adjuvant 5-FU/LV have been undertaken in patients with resected stage II/III colon cancer, demonstrating an improvement in survival compared to resection alone (IMPACT 1995; O'Connell *et al.* 1997; Zaniboni *et al.* 1998). In subgroup analysis, this benefit was almost entirely limited to node-positive (Stage III) patients. The relative reduction in rates of mortality were 21% (95% confidence interval [CI] 14–47%, $p = 0.24$) in the stage II patients, versus 28% (95% CI 34–46%, $p = 0.03$) in the stage III patients. Reduction in event-free recurrence rates was 24% (95% CI 10–48%, $p < 0.155$) in stage II patients compared with 39% (95% CI 19–54%, $p < 0.001$) for stage III patients (Zaniboni *et al.* 1998) and therefore adjuvant chemotherapy with 5-FU/LV was adopted as the standard of care for resected stage III colon patients in the early 1990s. Further randomized studies from Europe and the USA subsequently defined the optimal 5-FU/LV-based regimen. To summarize, these show that 5-FU/low-dose LV (20 mg/m^2) is equivalent to 5-FU/high-dose LV (200–500 mg/m^2); there is no significant difference between the two most commonly used bolus 5-FU/LV regimens (Mayo regimen for six cycles and Roswell Park regimen for three to four cycles); 5-FU/LV given for 6 months is equivalent to 12 months of treatment; continuous infusional 5-FU (de Gramont) is comparable to bolus 5-FU, but continuous infusional 5-FU has a more favorable toxicity profile (Benson 2005). The modified de Gramont regimen is the preferred infusional 5-FU/LV regimen commonly used in the UK.

Oral fluoropyrimidines

The orally active fluropyrimidine prodrug capecitabine is converted to 5-FU in the presence of thymidine phosphorylase (TP). It offers increased patient convenience with theoretically increased therapeutic ratio as TP is present at consistently higher levels in tumor compared to normal tissue, therefore potentially enhancing selectivity for tumor cells and sparing normal tissue. The X-ACT study randomized patients with resected stage III colon cancer to capecitabine monotherapy or bolus 5-FU/LV (Mayo regimen). With median follow-up of 3.8 years, it demonstrated capecitabine had therapeutic equivalence to 5-FU/LV in terms of disease-free survival (DFS) (64.2 vs 60.6%; $p = 0.05$) and a trend towards increased overall survival (OS) (81.3 vs 77.6%; $p = 0.07$). The incidence of adverse effects was also lower in patients treated with capecitabine than those treated with 5-FU/LV, with the exception of hand–foot syndrome (Gramont 2005). Capecitabine is now widely used for the adjuvant therapy of stage III colon cancer.

Combination treatment

Oxaliplatin-based regimens

The MOSAIC trial was the first RCT to show benefit for adding oxaliplatin to 5-FU/LV in patients with completely resected stage II/III colon cancer. Patients were randomized to 6 months of short-term infusional 5-FU/LV (De Gramont regimen) or the same regimen of 5-FU/LV with oxaliplatin (FOLFOX4). With a median follow-up of 48.6 months, 4-year DFS was significantly higher with FOLFOX4 (24% reduction in relative risk of relapse with FOLFOX4 compared to 5-FU/LV; $p = 0.0008$); OS however was similar in both groups (84.3 vs 82.7% for

FOLFOX4 and 5-FU/LV respectively). The main toxicity seen with FOLFOX4 regimen was peripheral neuropathy (92%), which was severe (grade 3) in 12.4%; 3.4% of patients had persistent grade 2/3 symptoms 4 years after completion of treatment (Chau & Cunningham 2006). This is important as absolute survival benefits are small in some groups of patients so a 1 in 30 risk of significant chronic neuropathy needs to be taken into careful consideration.

Improved DFS with the addition of oxaliplatin to bolus 5-FU/LV was also reported in NSABP trial C-07, which randomly assigned patients with stage II/III resected colon cancer to three cycles of 5-FU/LV (Roswell Park regimen) with or without oxaliplatin (Chau & Cunningham 2006). Therefore, although mature data are not yet available for OS, an oxaliplatin-containing regimen may be considered as one option postoperatively for stage III colon cancer patients.

Irinotecan-based treatment

In contrast, three RCTs have failed to show benefit from adding irinotecan to bolus or continuous infusional 5-FU/LV. Therefore irinotecan is not recommended routinely in the adjuvant setting (Chau & Cunningham 2006).

Targeted therapy

A number of ongoing phase III trials are investigating the role of cetuximab and bevacizumab in the adjuvant setting (PETACC-8, AVANT, QUASAR-2, NCCTG-N0147, and E5202). The NSABP C-08 trial comparing infusional 5-FU/LV and oxaliplatin with and without bevacizumab in patients with resected stage II/III colon cancer has closed and results are awaited.

Stage II colon cancer and any stage rectal cancer

In contrast to the clear benefit for adjuvant chemotherapy in patients with node-positive (stage III) disease, its role in resected stage II colon cancer and in any stage rectal cancer is more controversial. Many early trials including a mixture of patients with stage II and III colon cancer failed to demonstrate a significant survival benefit in patients with stage II disease from 5-FU-based adjuvant chemotherapy. However many of these were insufficiently powered to detect small differences in outcome in this subgroup. Three meta-analyses were therefore conducted to evaluate the benefit of adjuvant chemotherapy in patients with stage II resected colon cancer, none of which demonstrated a survival advantage (Midgley & Kerr 2005; Chau & Cunningham 2006).

The QUASAR 1 study was the first trial that was specifically designed and appropriately powered to try to address the issues of stage II colon and any stage rectal cancer. This study randomly assigned 3239 patients (92% stage II) to 5-FU-based therapy or observation following resection of colon (71%) or rectal cancer. With a median follow-up of 4.2 years, taking all patients into consideration, adjuvant chemotherapy was associated with a significantly lower risk of disease recurrence (relative risk 0.78, 95% CI 0.67–0.91; $p=0.001$) and reduced risk of death (HR 0.83, 95% CI 0.71–0.97; $p=0.02$). In analysis of the stage II patients alone ($n=2{,}948$) of which over 70% were 'good-risk' stage II patients, there was a 3–4% absolute improvement in overall survival ($p=0.04$) (Midgley & Kerr 2005). Despite these findings from the QUASAR 1 trial, current guidelines recommend against the routine administration of 5-FU-based chemotherapy in resected stage II colon cancer. Instead therapy is generally considered for certain poor prognosis subsets of patients including those with poorly differentiated histology, lymphovascular or perineural invasion, T4 lesions and/or bowel perforation at presentation.

Other modes of therapy in the adjuvant setting

Regionally delivered adjuvant chemotherapy

The liver is the main site of recurrence in approximately half of patients undergoing potentially curative resection of colon cancer. This has lead to exploration of regional therapy directed at the liver with the use of prophylactic portal vein infusion therapy or hepatic intra-arterial infusion of 5-FU, following resection of localized colon cancer. Several trials have failed to show any benefit to this approach and therefore adjuvant regional therapy is not currently recommended in any setting.

Metastatic colorectal cancer therapy

Approximately one-third of patients with colon or rectal cancer will present with metastatic disease, which cannot be cured by surgery, except for a small subset with liver-isolated disease. For all other patients with metastatic disease, treatment is palliative and likely to involve systemic chemotherapy, possibly with additional local measures such as surgery or radiotherapy.

First-line chemotherapy treatment

5-FU/LV

5-FU was the standard of care for the treatment of patients with metastatic colorectal cancer for 40 years. To summarize the outcomes of the studies conducted over this period defining the optimal 5-FU/LV schedule of treatment: 5-FU administered as a continuous infusion resulted in a higher response rate than bolus 5-FU (Mayo protocol) (22 vs 14%; $p=0.002$), but with similar median survival times (12.1 vs 11.3 months; $p=0.04$); continuous infusional 5-FU had a more favorable toxicity profile than bolus 5-FU with fewer hematologic and gastrointestinal side-effects; 5-FU/LV had a twofold higher response rate (21 vs 11%; $p=0.0001$) and a significant increase in OS compared to 5-FU alone (11.7 vs 10.5 months; HR 0.90; $p=0.004$) (Venook 2005). Therefore patients with metastatic colorectal cancer were mainly being treated with 5-FU/LV using a short-term infusional schedule (de Gramont or modified de Gramont) until the introduction of doublet cytotoxic therapy (see later) and subsequently monoclonal antibodies. For patients not medically fit enough for aggressive combination therapy, infusional 5-FU/LV may still be considered a reasonable treatment option.

Capecitabine has been shown to have similar efficacy to bolus 5-FU in two large phase III trials for first-line treatment of metastatic colorectal cancer (Varadhachary & Hoff 2005). Both studies compared capecitabine to the Mayo 5-FU/LV regimen; the study reported by Van Cutsem *et al.* demonstrated similar response rates (19 vs 15%), time to tumor progression (TTP) (5.2 vs 4.7 months; p = 0.65), and median OS (13.2 vs 12.1 months; p = 0.33). It is therefore an alternative to 5-FU/LV in patients who cannot be considered for more aggressive combination therapy.

Irinotecan-based therapy

Second-line irinotecan monotherapy has been shown in two phase III trials to have a survival advantage compared to treatment with infusional 5-FU/LV or best supportive care (BSC) in 5-FU-refactory patients. One-year survival rates were 36.2% with irinotecan and BSC vs 13.8% with BSC alone (p = 0.0001); and 45% with irinotecan vs 32% with 5-FU/LV (p = 0.035) (Rougier & Lepere 2005). Subsequently, three pivotal phase III trials demonstrated a survival benefit for combined irinotecan and 5-FU/LV (bolus and infusional regimens) compared to 5-FU/LV alone as first-line treatment for metastatic colorectal cancer (Venook 2005). In one of these studies, Douillard *et al.* randomized 385 patients to infusional 5-FU/LV with irinotecan or weekly infusional 5-FU/LV and irinotecan vs infusional 5-FU/LV alone, and demonstrated a better response rate (34.8% vs 21.9%; p < 0.005) and a statistically significant improvement in OS (17.4 vs 14.1 months; p = 0.031) with combination chemotherapy compared with 5-FU/LV alone. Combination treatment with 5-FU/LV and irinotecan was therefore established as possible first-line treatment for metastatic colorectal cancer.

Oxaliplatin-based combination therapy

Single-agent oxaliplatin therapy has fairly low response rates and is therefore not considered an appropriate choice for first-line therapy. However, oxaliplatin synergises with 5-FU/LV and at least two studies have demonstrated significantly longer progression-free survival (PFS) but similar OS with FOLFOX4 or FUFOX (weekly oxaliplatin with weekly infusional 5-FU/LV) compared to 5-FU/LV alone (Venook 2005). These results are similar to those of 5-FU/LV and irinotecan combination treatment. The failure to show a significant difference in OS is likely to be due to patient crossover in these studies with patients receiving salvage treatment with oxaliplatin and/or irinotecan. The Intergroup N9741 study compared bolus 5-FU/LV and irinotecan and FOLFOX inpatients with untreated colorectal cancer (Goldberg *et al.* 2006) and demonstrated significantly better outcome for patients treated with FOLFOX (OS 19.0 vs 16.3 months; p = 0.026). On the basis of these results, oxaliplatin-based regimens were approved for first-line treatment of patients with advanced colorectal cancer.

Other combination therapies

Irinotecan and capecitabine (XELIRI) in combination therapy has been shown to be efficacious in early phase studies (Venook 2005) but toxicity, principally gastrointestinal, has necessitated alterations in dose and administration schedules.

A number of RCTs have been conducted to explore whether capecitabine and oxaliplatin (XELOX) provides similar efficacy and tolerability as other fluropyrimidine/oxaliplatin combinations (Hochster *et al.* 2005; Sastre *et al.* 2005). Early data from these studies suggest that XELOX has similar antitumor efficacy to oxaliplatin/5-FU/LV combinations but may be associated with more toxicity, especially diarrhea. The recently presented phase III XELOX-1/NO16966 study randomized over 2000 patients in a 2×2 factorial trial to XELOX vs FOLFOX with bevacizumab or placebo (see later) in metastatic colorectal cancer (Hochster *et al.* 2005). This study demonstrated that XELOX was non-inferior to FOLFOX in terms of PFS (HR 1.05, 97.5% CI 0.94–1.18). Mature survival data from this study are awaited.

Sequential combination treatments; benefits of second-line therapy

The relative benefits of first-line irinotecan vs oxaliplatin-based combination therapy are difficult to assess.

Treatment of patients who progress after first-line chemotherapy is guided by treatment given, patient response, duration of response, and type and severity of toxicity. Patients who have been treated with an oxaliplatin-based regimen, as occurs in the majority of cases, may be treated with an irinotecan-based regimen and vice versa. The GERCOR V308 study (Rougier & Lepere 2005) randomized patients with metastatic colorectal cancer to FOLFIRI followed by FOLFOX6 (oxaliplatin and modified de Gramont regimen) or the reverse sequence to determine optimal drug sequencing. This study showed first-line FOLFOX6 followed by second-line FOLFIRI resulted in a similar survival time to that produced by the reverse sequence (20.6 vs 21.5 months; p = 0.99). However a significant percentage of patients (30%) did not receive second-line treatment. Although both first-line treatments achieved similar RRs (FOLFIRI 56% vs FOLFOX6 54%; p = 0.26), second-line FOLFIRI achieved a significantly lower RR than FOLFOX6 (4 vs 15%; p = 0.05). A second phase III study found that FOLFOX4 was far superior in response rate (9.6%) to oxaliplatin (1.1%) and to 5-FU/LV alone (0.7%) in patients with recurrent/progressive disease following primary irinotecan-based treatment (Rougier & Lepere 2005). The choice of the second-line therapy may be determined by the relative toxicity profiles and the acceptability for the individual patient.

Targeted therapy

Bevacizumab

Bevacizumab, the antivascular endothelial growth factor (VEGF) receptor antibody, has been shown to have activity in combination with 5-FU/LV and both alone and in combination with irinotecan or oxaliplatin. It significantly improves survival time when used in combination with IFL (infusional 5-FU/LV and irinotecan) compared with IFL alone (20 vs 15.6 months; p = 0.001) as first-line treatment in the metastatic setting. The addition of bevacizumab to IFL also significantly improved RR, duration of response and PFS times. Toxicities accredited to bevacizumab with this regimen included mild hypertension managed with standard antihypertensives, and gastrointestinal events including bowel perforation (Venook 2005). The phase II AVIRI study treated patients with first-line FOLFIRI and bevacizumab (Sobrero *et al.* 2006). Estimated 6-month PFS with combination treatment was 82% and the regimen was well tolerated (Sobrero *et al.* 2006). Combination therapy with 5-FU/LV and bevacizumab has also produced favorable results in first-line treatment and should therefore be considered in patients who are not considered able to tolerate oxaliplatin- or irinotecan-based combination treatment (Venook 2005).

The phase III XELOX-1/NO16966 study (see above) demonstrated that patients treated with XELOX and bevacizumab/FOLFOX and bevacizumab had a superior PFS compared to those treated with XELOX and placebo/FOLFOX and placebo (HR 0.83, 97.5% CI 0.72–0.95; p = 0.0023) (Cassidy *et al.* 2006). In subgroup analysis, the addition of bevacizumab to XELOX (9.3 months vs 7.4 months; HR 0.77; p = 0.0026) and FOLFOX (9.4 months vs 8.6 months; HR 0.89; p = 0.1871) prolonged PFS compared with respective placebo arms; however, suprisingly, it did not show statistical significance with the FOLFOX regimen. Second-line treatment with bevacizumab in combination with FOLFOX4 has been shown to improve survival from early phase III data (12.5 vs 10.7 months; p = 0.0024). More mature data and the results of other ongoing studies are awaited.

Cetuximab

A number of phase II studies have evaluated the role of cetuximab, an epidermal growth factor receptor (EGFR) antibody, with irinotecan or oxaliplatin with or without 5-FU/LV or capecitabine or as a single agent. In a pivotal study, irinotecan and cetuximab combination treatment in 329 patients with irinotecan-refractory colorectal cancer demonstrated RRs of 22.9% compared to 10.8% for cetuximab monotherapy (Venook 2005), with TTP of 4.1 months vs 1.5 months (p < 0.001) and median OS of 8.6 vs 6.9 months (p = 0.48). Side-effects of cetuximab included hypersensitivity, fatigue and acne-like rash.

A number of studies have been conducted in the first-line setting in metastatic colorectal cancer. The CALGB group randomized patients to either FOLFOX or FOLFIRI, with or without cetuximab in chemonaive patients (Venook *et al.* 2006). This study showed no difference in RR between FOLFOX and FOLFIRI, but did show a significantly higher RRs for the chemotherapy regimens containing antibody (49 vs 33%; p = 0.014) (Venook *et al.* 2006).

Duration of treatment

The optimal duration for treatment in responding patients is controversial as to whether to discontinue treatment after one to two cycles beyond best response, or continue treatment until progressive disease. This issue has been addressed by at least two studies, neither of which demonstrated a survival advantage with continuous treatment (Maughan *et al.* 2003; Lal *et al.* 2004). More recently, the OPTIMOX1 study randomized patients with previously untreated metastatic colorectal cancer between FOLFOX continuously until progression or a simplified 5-FU/LV regimen with high-dose oxaliplatin (FOLFOX7) for six cycles. Patients in the latter arm then continued on maintenance treatment without oxaliplatin for 12 cycles followed by reintroduction of FOLFOX7 (Tournigand *et al.* 2006). This study found no statistical difference in median PFS (9.0 vs 8.7 months [continuous vs intermittent]; HR = 1.06; 95% CI 0.89–1.2; p = 0.47) or OS (19.3 vs 21.2 months [continuous vs intermittent]; HR = 0.93; 95% CI 0.72–1.11; p = 0.49). The OPTIMOX2, a randomized phase II study, subsequently compared intermittent FOLFOX7 with maintenance 5-FU/LV (the second arm of the OPTIMOX1 study) with six cycles of FOLFOX7 alone (Maindrault-Goebel *et al.* 2006). This study reported found an improvement in median PFS in the maintenance arm (36 vs 28 weeks; p = 0.01); however, this small advantage of disease control must be balanced in the quality of life of almost 6 months of chemotherapy-free time in the intermittent treatment arm. Current treatment policy in our center is therefore generally to treat to one to two cycles beyond best response and to encourage 'drug holidays'.

Conclusion

There have been significant advances in the treatment of colorectal cancer in both the adjuvant and metastatic settings resulting in improvements in patient survival and quality of life over the past two decades. Combination chemotherapy has a well-defined role in the adjuvant setting for stage III colon cancer. It is also beneficial for patients with resected stage II disease, with a similar proportional reduction in recurrence and death but smaller absolute benefits. In metastatic colorectal cancer, the development of newer agents has shifted treatment from mono- to combination chemotherapy, although the most appropriate setting, doses, combination and sequences for each of these agents/regimens still needs to be determined (Fig. 14.9).

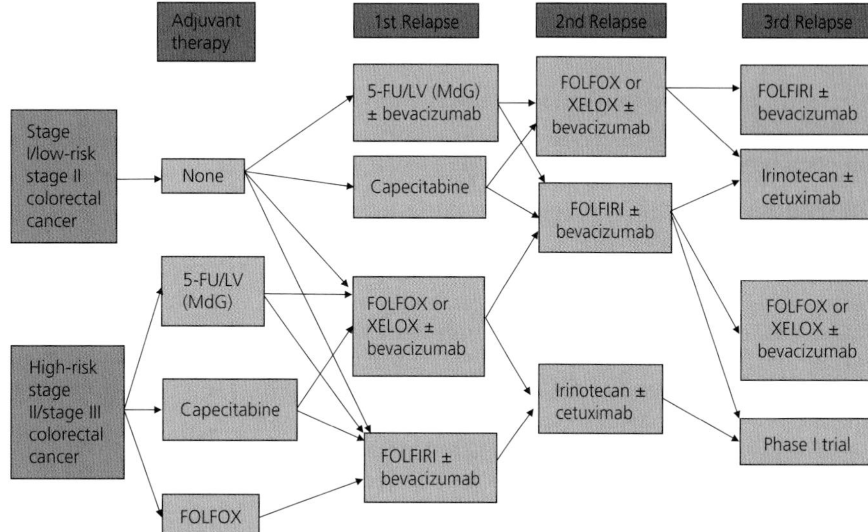

Fig. 14.9 Chemotherapy treatment sequence. 5-FU/LV (MdG), 5-fluorouracil and leucovorin (modified de Gramont regimen); FOLFOX, oxaliplatin and 5-FU/LV; XELOX, oxaliplatin and capecitabine; FOLFIRI, irinotecan and 5-FU/LV.

Ongoing properly powered clinical trials will continue to define the role of emerging biologic agents.

Glossary

X-ACT: Xeloda in adjuvant colon cancer therapy

MOSAIC: Multicentre international study of oxaliplatin/5-flurouracil/leucovorin in the adjuvant treatment of colon cancer

NSABP: National Surgical Adjuvant Breast and Bowel Project

QUASAR: quick and simple and reliable

References

Benson AB III. (2005) Adjuvant chemotherapy of stage III colon cancer. *Semin Oncol* 32: S74–77.

Cassidy J, Clarke S, Diaz Rubio E *et al.* (2006) First efficacy and safety results from XELOX-1/NO16966, a randomised 2x2 factorial phase III trial of XELOX vs FOLFOX4 + bevacizumab or placebo in first-line metastatic colorectal cancer (MCRC). *ESMO: Ann Oncol* Abstract no. LBA3.

Chau I, Cunningham D. (2006) Adjuvant therapy in colon cancer—what, when and how? *Ann Oncol* 17(9): 1347–59.

Goldberg RM, Sargent DJ, Morton RF *et al.* (2006) Randomized controlled trial of reduced-dose bolus fluorouracil plus leucovorin and irinotecan or infused fluorouracil plus leucovorin and oxaliplatin in patients with previously untreated metastatic colorectal cancer: a North American Intergroup Trial. *J Clin Oncol* 24: 3347–53.

Gramont A. (2005) Adjuvant therapy of stage II and III colon cancer. *Semin Oncol*32: 11–14.

Hochster HS, Welles L, Hart L *et al.* (2006) Safety and efficacy of bevacizumab (Bev) when added to oxaliplatin/fluoropyrimidine (O/F) regimens as first-line treatment of metastatic colorectal cancer (mCRC): TREE 1 & 2 Studies. *ASCO Annual Meeting Proceedings J Clin Oncol*: Abstract no. 3515.

IMPACT. (1995) Efficacy of adjuvant fluorouracil and folinic acid in colon cancer. International Multicentre Pooled Analysis of Colon Cancer Trials (IMPACT) investigators. *Lancet* 345: 939–44.

Lal R, Dickson J, Cunningham D *et al.* (2004) A randomized trial comparing defined-duration with continuous irinotecan until disease progression in fluoropyrimidine and thymidylate synthase inhibitor-resistant advanced colorectal cancer. *J Clin Oncol* 22: 3023–31.

Maindrault-Goebel F, Lledo G, Chibaudel B *et al.* (2006) OPTIMOX2, a large randomized phase II study of maintenance therapy or chemotherapy-free intervals (CFI) after FOLFOX in patients with metastatic colorectal cancer (MRC). A GERCOR study. *J Clin Oncol* 24, no. 18S, Abstract no. 3504.

Maughan TS, James RD, Kerr DJ *et al.* (2003) Comparison of intermittent and continuous palliative chemotherapy for advanced colorectal cancer: a multicentre randomised trial. *Lancet* 361: 457–64.

Midgley R, Kerr DJ. (2005) Adjuvant chemotherapy for stage II colorectal cancer: the time is right! *Nat Clin Pract Oncol* 2: 364–9.

O'Connell MJ, Mailliard JA, Kahn MJ *et al.* (1997) Controlled trial of fluorouracil and low-dose leucovorin given for 6 months as postoperative adjuvant therapy for colon cancer. *J Clin Oncol* 15: 246–50.

Rougier P, Lepere C. (2005) Second-line treatment of patients with metastatic colorectal cancer. *Semin Oncol* 32: S48–54.

Sastre J, Massuti B, Tabernero JM *et al.* (2005) Preliminary results of a randomized phase III trial of the TTD Group comparing capecitabine and oxaliplatin (CapeOx) vs oxaliplatin and 5-fluorouracil in continuous infusion (5-FU CI) as first line treatment in advanced or metastatic colorectal cancer (CRC). *ASCO Annual Meeting Proceedings J Clin Oncol*: Abstract no. 3524.

Sobrero A, Ackland S, Carrion RP *et al.* (2006) Efficacy and safety of bevacizumab in combination with irinotecan and infusional 5-FU as first-line treatment for patients with metastatic colorectal cancer. *ASCO Annual Meeting Proceedings J Clin Oncol*: Abstract no. 3544.

Tournigand C, Cervantes A, Figer A *et al.* (2006) OPTIMOX1: a randomized study of FOLFOX4 or FOLFOX7 with oxaliplatin in a stop-and-go fashion in advanced colorectal cancer—a GERCOR study. *J Clin Oncol* 24: 394–400.

Varadhachary GR, Hoff PM. (2005) Front-line therapy for advanced colorectal cancer: emphasis on chemotherapy. *Semin Oncol* 32: S40–2.

Venook A. (2005) Critical evaluation of current treatments in metastatic colorectal cancer. *Oncologist* 10: 250–61.

Venook A, Niedzwiecki D, Hollis D *et al.* (2006) Phase III study of irinotecan/5FU/LV (FOLFIRI) or oxaliplatin/5FU/LV (FOLFOX) ± cetuximab for patients (pts) with untreated metastatic adenocarcinoma of the colon or rectum (MCRC): CALGB 80203 preliminary results. *ASCO Annual Meeting Proceedings J Clin Oncol*: Abstract no. 3509.

Zaniboni A, Labianca R, Marsoni S *et al.* (1998) GIVIO-SITAC 01: A randomized trial of adjuvant 5-fluorouracil and folinic acid administered to patients with colon carcinoma—long term results and evaluation of the indicators of health-related quality of life. Gruppo Italiano Valutazione Interventi in Oncologia. Studio Italiano Terapia Adiuvante Colon. *Cancer* 82: 2135–44.

Radiotherapy

Robert Glynne-Jones

Introduction

Better preoperative imaging, innovations in surgical technique, more accurate histopathologic reporting, clearer indications for radiotherapy, more accurate planning techniques and greater precision of its delivery have improved the treatment of rectal cancer. However, adjuvant radiotherapy remains a controversial issue. Radiotherapy has many aims: to reduce the risk of local recurrence; to improve the likelihood of achieving a curative surgery with a pathologically complete resection margin as defined by a clear circumferential margin greater than 1 mm; to facilitate sphincter-sparing procedures; as a definitive treatment in the elderly and frail; and finally as a means of palliation.

Reducing local recurrence

Approximately one-third of patients will present with locally advanced cancers (T3/T4), which have a high risk of local recurrence and poor survival (50–65% at 5 years). Local failure is especially high for cancers below the peritoneal reflection where the serosa is lacking, and in the lower rectum even after potentially curative surgery, so radiotherapy is frequently recommended. The rectum is a fixed structure within the pelvis and hence easy to target. Thus both preoperative and postoperative radiotherapy have an important role, and can reduce recurrence rates about threefold.

Three systematic reviews/meta-analyses examine the role of radiotherapy in resectable rectal cancer (Camma *et al.* 2000; Colorectal Cancer Collaborative Group 2001; Munro & Bentley 2002). The Colorectal Cancer Collaborative Group meta-analysis (Colorectal Cancer Collaborative Group 2001) identified 22 RCTs, which compared both preoperative radiotherapy (14 trials, a total of 6350 patients) and postoperative radiotherapy (8 trials, a total of 2157 patients) versus surgery alone. This meta-analysis concluded that for preoperative radiotherapy a biologically equivalent dose (BED) of >30 Gy is more effective in reducing local relapse. The use of inadequate dose schedules, crude planning techniques and unnecessarily large treatment fields in these historical studies may have contributed to a higher mortality compared to surgery alone (Anonymous 1997).

Pre- versus postoperative radiotherapy

Randomized trials have confirmed better local control, lower toxicity (both acute and late) and better compliance if preoperative radiotherapy or CRT is administered rather than postoperative (Frykholm *et al.* 1993; Sauer *et al.* 2004), with a dose–response effect favoring preoperative radiotherapy (Glimelius *et al.* 1997). Local recurrence in the German AIO/CRO/ARO study was 6% with preoperative CRT and 13% in the postoperative CRT arm (Sauer *et al.* 2004). However, there was no difference in the rate of distant metastases (36% versus 38% respectively at 5 years), or disease-free or overall survival.

Facilitating sphincter-sparing procedures

The low position of some rectal cancers (3–6 cm from the anal verge), and bulky anterior tumors in obese men with a narrow pelvis may make it technically demanding to achieve sphincter-sparing surgery (SPSS). Long-course preoperative radiotherapy or chemoradiation followed by a planned delay prior to surgery may result in shrinkage back from the distal margin, and enable SPSS. Subset analysis of randomized trials suggests preoperative chemoradiation offers a 10% (Roh *et al.* 2001) or even a 20% (Sauer *et al.* 2004) higher chance overall in achieving SPSS. Yet a randomized trial testing SCPRT against preoperative chemoradiation with the endpoint of SPSS failed to show any difference. Surgeons did not change their initial decision (Bujko *et al.* 2004). The validity of this approach remains unproven (Bujko *et al.* 2006), and data on late function of the sphincter mechanism following CRT remain elusive.

Radiotherapy as definitive treatment

The use of radiotherapy as a definitive treatment is based on observational series of endocavitary, local contact therapy or brachytherapy either alone or in combination with external-beam radiotherapy in selected patients with early cancers (Papillon 1982). Higher total doses to the pelvis with external-beam radiotherapy alone are limited by the tolerance

Table 14.1 Trial design: preoperative radiotherapy versus surgery alone or selective postoperative radiation/chemoradiation.

Trial	Duration of trial	Patient nos	Randomization	Nos	TME	Primary endpoint	Local recurrence	Metastases	Overall survival	Dease-free survival	PCR	Pathology CRM/R1
Resectable rectal cancer												
Swedish Rectal Cancer Trial (1997)	1987–1997 10 years	1168	25 Gy/5#	553			63/553 = 11%	23%	58%	Not stated	0%	57/553 10%
			vs									
			Surgery alone	557	No	OS	150/157 = 27% at 5 years	24%	48%		0%	63/557 11% (not CRM)
Dutch Trial CKVO 95-04 (2001)	1996–2001 5 years	1861	25 Gy/5#	897			2.4%	14.8%	82%	Not stated	0%	16%
			vs									vs
			Surgery alone	908	Yes	OS	8.2% at 2 years	16.8% at 2 yrs	81.8% at 2 years		0%	18% (CRM)
CRO7 (Abstract only Sebag-Montefiore 2006)	1995–2005 10 years	1350	25 Gy/5#	674	Yes	Local recurrence	5%	?	81%	80%	0%	13% (CRM) overall)
			vs				vs		vs	vs		
			Selective postoperative CTRT	676			11% at 3 years	?	79% at 3 years	75% at 3 years	0%	
Borderline resectable rectal cancer (fixed and tethered)												
MRC2 (1996)	1981–1996 14 years	279	40 Gy	139	No	OS	50/139 = 48%	49/139	34% at 5 yrs	Improved with RT	0%	Not stated
			vs									
			Surgery alone	140			65/140 = 57%	67/140	29% at 5 yrs		0%	

Duration, start of trial to publication; TME, total mesorectal excision; PCR, pathologic complete response rate; R0, curative resection or CRM < 1 mm if documented; OS, overall survival; DFS, disease-free survival; SPS, sphincter-sparing surgery.

Table 14.2 Trial design: preoperative radiotherapy versus preoperative chemoradiation.

Trial	Duration of trial	Patient nos	Randomization	Nos	TME	Primary endpoint	Local recurrence	Metastases	Overall survival	Disease-free survival	PCR	Pathology CRM
Resectable rectal cancer												
EORTC (Boulis-Wassif 1984)	1972–1984 12 years	247	34.5 Gy vs	121	No	OS	15%	30% overall	59%	72%	2.5%	Not Quirke
			5-FU + 34.5 Gy	126	No		15% at 5 years		46% at 5 years	68% at 3 years	5%	
EORTC 22921 (Bosset 2006)	1992–1994 12 years	1011	45 Gy25# / vs	506	No	OS	17.1% vs	34.4% overall	64.8% vs	54.4% vs	5%	Not Quirke
			FUFA + 45 GY	505	No		8.7% at 5 years		65.8% at 5 years	56.1% at 5 years	14%	
FFCD 9203 (Gerard 2006)	1993–2005 12 years	762	45 Gy25# / vs	367	No	OS	16.5% vs	No data	67.9% vs	No data	3.6%	Not Quirke
			FUFA + 45 GY	375	No		8.1% at 5 years		67.4% at 5 years		11.4%	
POLISH TRIAL (Bujko et al. 2004, 2006)	1999–2004 5 years	316	25 Gy /5# vs	155	?YES	SPS	11% vs	No data	67.2% vs	58.4% vs	1%	13%
			FUFA + 50 Gy	157	?YES		16.5% at 5 years		66.2% at 4 years	55.6% at 4 years	16%	4% (CRM)
Trans-Tasman Radiation Oncology Group TROG	2001–2006 5 years	310	25 Gy /5# vs 50.4 Gy + PVI 5 FU	No data	?YES	Local recurrence	No data	No data	No data	No data	No data	Not Quirke No data
Unresectable rectal cancer												
Frykholm (2001)	1988–2001 13 years	70	46 Gy /23 fractions 5 FU/MTX + Split 40 Gy	27 29	No No	Curative resection	12/27 = 17% 5/29 = 44%	Not stated	18% 29% (NS)	Not stated	1/27 (4%) 3/29 (12%)	36% 26% Not Quirke

Table 14.3 Trial design: preoperative chemoradiation versus postoperative chemoradiation.

Trial	Duration of trial	Patient nos	Randomization	Nos	TME	Primary endpoint	Local recurrence	Metastases	Overall survival	Disease-free survival	PCR	Pathology CRM
Resectable rectal cancer												
INTO 147 (No data)	5 years	53	Preop 50.4 Gy+ FUFA Vs Postop 50.4 Gy + FUFA	No data	No	OS	No data Closed early →					
NSABP RO3 (Abstracts only Hyams 1997, Roh 2004, Roh 2005)	1993–2003 10 years	267	Preop 45 Gy + FUFA Vs Postop 45 Gy + FUFA	130 137	No	OS	5% vs 9% at 5 years	Not stated	74% vs 66% at 5 years	64% vs 53% at 5 years	16% 0%	No data
CAA/ARO/AIO-94 (Sauer 2004)	1995–2004 9 years	823	Preop 50.4 Gy + 5-FU Vs	405	? YES in later years	OS	6%	36%	76%	68%	8%	2%
			Postop 50.4 Gy + 5-FU	394			13% at 5 years	38%	74% at 5 yrs	66% at 5 yrs	0%	3% Not Quirke

of structures such as bladder and small bowel. Doses of 100 Gy or more can be delivered to a small volume with high rates of local control without risk of unacceptable late complications (Gerard *et al.* 2003). The curative use of radiotherapy as a sole modality of treatment has been confined to specialists with considerable expertise.

Short-course preoperative radiotherapy (SCPRT)

A short hypofractionated accelerated preoperative radiation schedule of 25 Gy in 5 fractions with surgery performed within a few days of completion of radiation reduces local recurrence. The Swedish rectal cancer trial (Anonymous 1997) originally demonstrated not only a significant reduction in local recurrence but also a 10% absolute improvement in survival, which led to the widespread adoption of SCPRT in Europe. Further trials examined SCPRT when added to total mesorectal excision (TME) surgery (Kapiteijn *et al.* 2001). If a negative circumferential resection margin (>2 mm) is achieved, local recurrence is less than 10% at 2 years (Nagtegaal *et al.* 2002).

Preliminary results of the CR07 trial (Sebag-Montefiore *et al.* 2006), suggests SCPRT and TME significantly impacts on both local recurrence and 3-year disease-free survival compared to surgery alone. The difference in favor of the preoperative arm was noted for all tumor locations, all pathologic stages, and good, average or poor-quality surgery. A previous study from Manchester (Marsh *et al.* 1994) showed an improvement in local control from preoperative pelvic radiotherapy using a lower dose of 20 Gy in four fractions when compared to immediate surgery. Recent audit data appear to confirm the effectiveness of this approach.

However, SCPRT represents a blanket approach, preceding the use of high-quality MRI to select high-risk patients.

Rendering borderline/unresectable tumors resectable

Radiotherapy is also used to shrink the primary tumor, and enable a curative (R0) resection of an unresectable cancer. SCPRT is therefore unsuitable for this purpose as surgery is recommended within 5 days to avoid added morbidity and excess mortality and downstaging will not occur.

A single small phase III trial (Frykholm *et al.* 2001) in unresectable rectal cancer has compared radiation alone with CRT, demonstrating improved resectability and local control with the use of CRT. Local recurrence-free survival at 5 years was 35% versus 66% ($p = 0.03$) and 5-year survival was 18% versus 29% (non-significant) for radiotherapy versus CRT respectively. A recent abstract also supports the use of 5-FU-based CRT in this setting (Braendengen *et al.* 2005).

Recent studies in resectable T3/T4 rectal cancers (Bosset *et al.* 2006; Gerard *et al.* 2006) have shown an advantage in reducing the rates of local recurrence for preoperative chemoradiation (CRT) with 45 Gy and 5-FU-based chemotherapy over radiation alone. Surgery is undertaken 4–12 weeks following CRT to allow the patient to recover, and enable tumor shrinkage. The presence of tumor cells within 1 mm of the radial or circumferential resection margin (CRM) is associated with a high risk of local recurrence and poor survival (Quirke *et al.* 1986; Wibe *et al.* 2002; Nagtegaal *et al.* 2005), particularly in the lower rectum (Nagtegaal *et al.* 2005). This finding reflects both the extent of the tumor beyond the muscularis propria, invasion into the intersphincteric space, and the quality of surgical resection. MRI offers an opportunity to predict accurately whether the surgical resection margin will be clear or involved by tumor (Mercury 2006), and select which patients may benefit from preoperative CRT.

Postoperative chemoradiation

Postoperative adjuvant chem-radiotherapy is the North American standard of care (NIH 1990; Krook *et al.* 1991; O'Connell *et al.* 1994). Clinicians are able to use information gained at laparotomy, and the histopathologic specimen, to define suitability for treatment, field size and dose intensity. Postoperative radiotherapy has been tested in numerous RCTs that use surgery alone as a control arm. A recent overview demonstrated a statistically significant reduction in local recurrence when postoperative radiation was given (Colorectal Cancer Collaborative Group 2001). Only one individual trial (MRC Rectal Cancer Working Party 1996) demonstrated a statistically significant reduction in local recurrence, but most of the trials were small and underpowered to detect modest improvements. A further seven trials have tested the role of chemoradiation postoperatively, of which three have a surgery-alone arm and three have a chemotherapy-alone arm. In addition, the risks of toxicity, particularly from small bowel trapped within the sacral bay following surgery, and from adhesions in the pelvis, remain considerable.

Acute toxicity of radiotherapy

Acute toxicity comprises mainly gastrointestinal effects. The level of grade 3/4 toxicity is acceptable in the preoperative setting, and toxic deaths are rare. Hence compliance to preoperative radiation is in the range of 90–95% (Sauer *et al.* 2004; Bosset *et al.* 2006; Sebag-Montefiore *et al.* 2006) compared to 50–70% in the postoperative setting.

Surgical morbidity

There are concerns that preoperative SCPRT and CRT increase the risk of infections and poor wound healing in the sacral cavity and in the perineum following AP excision of the rectum, or an anastomotic leak if an anterior resection is performed. A significantly higher leak rate was observed after preoperative radiotherapy in the Swedish Rectal Cancer Trial (Anonymous

1997). However, in both the Dutch TME study (Kapiteijn *et al.* 2001) and the German AIO study (Sauer *et al.* 2004) the clinical anastomotic leak rate was not statistically different whether the patient had received preoperative radiotherapy or surgery alone.

Late effects

Pelvic radiotherapy is associated with significant risks of radiation damage to the urinary and gastrointestinal tract—from minor side-effects to serious and life-threatening complications, and a major impact on quality of life. About 5–10% of patients will experience grade 3 or 4 late morbidity (Dahlberg *et al.* 1998; Tepper *et al.* 2002). Small bowel tolerance is the main dose-limiting factor, and the volume of the small bowel in the radiation field is crucial (Letschert *et al.* 1994). Effects on sexual function, urinary incontinence (Pollack *et al.* 2006), bowel function (Peeters *et al.* 2005), including a doubling of bowel frequency, and an increase in incontinence, have been documented after SCPRT (Dahlberg *et al.* 1998).

These complications depend on technique, the radiation field, shielding, the overall treatment time, the fraction size, and total dose. Mature results of the Swedish Rectal Cancer Trial confirm an increase in hospital admissions for a variety of gastrointestinal problems after RT, particularly bowel obstruction (after approximately 8 years) and abdominal pain (Birgisson *et al.* 2006). There are other unexplained late cardiac effects (Pollack *et al.* 2006). Finally there is an increased risk of a second malignancy after preoperative radiotherapy (Birgisson *et al.* 2006). As follow-up in the majority of studies is generally short, there is likely to be a major underestimate of the real risks of late effects.

Radiotherapy planning

In the past, standardized radiation fields have been based on patterns of locoregional relapse (Gunderson *et al.* 1974), which predate the widespread use of TME and Quirke-style pathology. The conventional reference points for two standardized fields for upper and low rectum have been the bony landmarks within the pelvis (particularly the sacrum). Currently these fields would be considered excessively large. Recent more relevant data for patterns of relapse following TME and modern pathologic reporting techniques are available (Syk *et al.* 2006). With this evidence and current anatomical knowledge of nodes at risk from MRI, individualized treatment volumes with three-dimensional planning are recommended (Roels *et al.* 2006). Accurate target definition, and obtaining the best functional outcome from the combination of surgery and radiotherapy, requires collaboration between radiologists, surgeons, and radiation oncologists.

Radiotherapy should encompass the gross tumor volume (GTV); that is, all gross sites of disease (primary and nodal) according to the MRI with a 1-cm margin. The clinical target volume (CTV) should also include the mesorectum at all levels and the relevant locoregional lymph node groups. The external anal margin can be visualized on MRI, and marked for CT planning with a ball bearing. Alignment tattoos are used as external reference points. The radiotherapy dose is prescribed to the intersection point ensuring the 95% isodose covers the target volume. All fields are treated daily, five times a week.

References

Anonymous. (1997) Improved survival with preoperative radiotherapy in resectable rectal cancer. Swedish rectal cancer trial. *N Engl J Med* 336: 980–7.

Birgisson H, Pahlman L, Glimelius B. (2006) Adverse effects of preoperative radiation therapy for rectal cancer: long-term follow-up of the Swedish rectal Cancer Trial. *J Clin Oncol* 23: 8697–8705.

Bosset JF, Collette L, Calais G *et al.* (2006) Chemotherapy with preoperative radiotherapy in rectal cancer. *N Engl J Med* 355: 1114–23.

Braendengen M, Tveit KM, Berglund A *et al.* (2005) A randomised phase III study (LARCS) comparing preoperative radiotherapy alone with chemoradiotherapy in non-resectable rectal cancer. *Eur J Cancer* Suppl 3(2): 172 abstr 612.

Bujko K, Nowacki MP, Nasierowska-Guttmejer A *et al.* (2004) Sphincter preservation following preoperative radiotherapy for rectal cancer: report of a randomized trial comparing short-term radiotherapy vs conventionally fractionated radiochemotherapy. *Radiother Oncol* 72: 15–24.

Bujko K, Kepka L, Michalski W, Nowacki MP. (2006) Does rectal cancer shrinkage induced by preoperative radio(chemo)therapy increase the likelihood of anterior resection? A systematic review of randomised trials. *Radiother Oncol* 80: 4–12.

Camma C, Giunta M, Fiorica F, Pagliaro L, Craxi A, Cottone M. (2000) Preoperative radiotherapy for resectable rectal cancer: A meta-analysis. *JAMA* 284: 1008–15.

Colorectal Cancer Collaborative Group. (2001) Adjuvant radiotherapy for rectal cancer: a systematic overview of 8507 patients from randomised trials. *Lancet* 358: 1291–304.

Dahlberg M, Glimerlius B, Graff W *et al.* (1998) Preoperative radiation affects functional results after surgery for rectal cancer: results from a randomised study. *Dis Colon Rectum* 41: 543–9.

Frykholm GJ, Glimelius B, Pahlman L. (1993) Preoperative or postoperative irradiation in adenocarcinoma of the rectum: Final results of a randomised trial and an evaluation of late secondary effects. *Dis Colon Rectum* 36: 564–72.

Frykholm GJ, Pahlman L, Glimelius B. (2001) Combined chemo- and radiotherapy vs radiotherapy alone in the treatment of primary nonresectable cancer of the rectum. *Int J Radiat Oncol Biol Phys* 50: 433–40.

Gerard JP, Romestaing P, Baulieux J *et al.* (2003) Local curative treatment of rectal cancer by radiotherapy alone. *Colorectal Dis* 5: 442–4.

Gerard JP, Conroy T, Bonnetain F *et al.* (2006) Preoperative radiotherapy with or without concurrent fluorouracil and leucovorin in T3-T4 rectal cancers: results of FFCD 9203. *J Clin Oncol* 24: 4620–5.

Glimelius B, Isaacson U, Jung B *et al.* (1997) Radiotherapy in addition to radical surgery in rectal cancer: evidence for a dose–response effect favouring preoperative treatment. *Int J Radiat Oncol Biol Phys* 37: 281–7.

Kapitejn E, Marijnen CA, Nagtegaal ID *et al.* (2001) Preoperative radiotherapy combined with total mesorectal excision for resectable rectal cancer. *N Engl J Med* 345: 639–46.

Krook JE, Moertel CG, Gunderson LL *et al.* (1991) Effective surgical adjuvant therapy for high-risk rectal carcinoma. *N Engl J Med* 324: 709–15.

Letschert JGJ, Lebesque JV, Aleman VMP. (1994) The volume effect in radiation related late small bowel complications: results of a clinical study of the EORTC Radiotherapy Co-operative Group in patients treated for rectal carcinoma. *Radiother Oncol* 32: 116–23.

Marsh PJ, James RD, Schofield PF. (1994) Adjuvant preoperative radiotherapy for locally advanced rectal carcinoma. Results of a prospective randomised trial. *Dis Colon Rectum* 37: 1205–14.

MERCURY Study Group. (2006) Diagnostic accuracy of preoperative magnetic resonance imaging in predicting curative resection of rectal cancer; prospective observational study. *BMJ* 333: 779.

MRC Rectal Cancer Working Party. (1996) Randomised trial of surgery alone versus radiotherapy followed by surgery for potentially operable locally advanced rectal cancer. *Lancet* 348: 1605–10.

Munro AJ, Bentley AHM. (2002) Adjuvant radiotherapy in operable rectal cancer: a systematic review. *Sem Colon Rectal Surg* 13: 31–42.

Nagtegaal ID, Marijnen CA, Kranenbarg EK *et al.* (2002) Circumferential margin involvement is still an important predictor of local recurrence in rectal cancer: not 1 millimetre but 2 millimetres is the limit. *Am J Surg Pathol* 26: 350–7.

Nagetgaal ID, Van de Velde CJ, Marijnen CA *et al.* (2005) Low rectal cancer: a call for a change of approach in abdominoperineal resection. *J Clin Oncol* 23: 9257–64.

National Institutes of Health Consensus Conference. (1990)Adjuvant therapy for patients with colon and rectal cancer. *JAMA* 264: 1444–50.

O'Connell MJ, Martenson JA, Weiand HS *et al.* (1994) Improving adjuvant therapy for rectal cancer by combining protracted infusional fluorouracil with radiation therapy after curative surgery. *N Engl J Med* 331: 502–7.

Papillon J. (1982) *Rectal and Anal Cancers: Conservative Treatment by Irradiation: an Alternative to Radical Surgery*. Springer-Verlag, New York.

Peeters K, van de Velde C *et al.* (2005) Impact of short-term preoperative radiotherapy on health-related quality of life and sexual functions in primary rectal cancer; report of a multicenter randomised trial. *J Clin Oncol* 23: 1847–58.

Pollack J, Holm T, Cedermark B *et al.* (2006) Late effects of short-course preoperative radiotherapy in rectal cancer. *Br J Surg* 93(12): 1519–25.

Quirke P, Durdey P, Dixon MF, Williams NS. (1986) Local recurrence of rectal adenocarcinoma due to inadequate surgical resection: histopathological study of lateral tumor spread and surgical excision. *Lancet* ii: 996–9.

Roels S, Duthoy W, Haustermans K *et al.* (2006) Definition and delineation of the clinical target volume for rectal cancer. *Int J Radiat Oncol Biol Phys* 65(4): 1129–42.

Roh M, Petrelli N, Wieand H *et al.* (2001) Phase III randomised trial of preoperative versus postoperative mutimodality therapy in patients with carcinoma of the rectum (NSABP R-03). *J Clin Oncol Proc ASCO* 20: abstract 123.

Sauer R. Becker H. Hohenberger W *et al.* (2004) German Rectal Cancer Study Group. Preoperative versus postoperative chemoradiotherapy for rectal cancer. *N Engl J Med* 351: 1731–40.

Sebag-Montefiore D, Steele R, Quirke P *et al.* (2006) Routine short course preop radiotherapy or selective post-op chemoradiotherapy for resectable rectal cancer? Preliminary results of MRC CR07 randomised trial. *J Clin Oncol* 24: 185 abstract 3511.

Syk E, Torkzad, Blomqvist L *et al.* (2006) Radiological findings do not support lateral residual tumour as a major cause of local recurrence of rectal cancer. *Br J Surg* 93(1): 113–9.

Tepper JE, O'Connell, Nieddzwiecki D *et al.* (2002) Adjuvant therapy in rectal cancer: analysis of stage, sex and local control – final report of Intergroup 0114. *J Clin Oncol* 20: 1744–50.

Wibe A, Rendedal PR, Svensson E, Norstein J, Eide TJ, Myrvold HE, Soreide O. (2002) Prognostic significance of the circumferential resection margin following total mesorectal excision for rectal cancer. *Br J Surg* 89(3): 327–34.

Surgery for liver metastases

Zahir Soonawalla

Introduction

Hepatic metastases occur in at least 50% of patients with colorectal cancer, and the liver is the only identifiable site of spread in about 40% of these cases. As the venous drainage of the colon and upper rectum drains directly into the liver, it has reasonably been presumed that the liver may be the only affected site of metastasis, and that resection of liver metastases may potentially cure the disease. Despite the lack of randomized trials supporting this concept, liver resection has become well established as a potentially curative treatment. The long-term cure rates that have been achieved following hepatic metastatectomy are not encountered in comparable patients who do not have surgical treatment, and clearly demonstrate the usefulness of such an approach. Historical series show that patients with untreated liver metastases from colorectal cancer almost never survived 5 years, whereas patients who underwent liver resection could expect a 30–40% chance of 5-year survival (Cummings *et al.* 2007). With the improvements in staging and multimodality therapies that have recently transformed the management of colorectal liver metastases, 5-year survival in excess of 50% is expected (Choti *et al.* 2002).

The morbidity and mortality associated with liver surgery is nowadays very acceptable, with many major centers reporting 1–3% mortality for resection of colorectal liver metastases. As liver surgery has become safer, and as the scope for these procedures has expanded, the majority of patients with liver-only metastases can feasibly be treated with liver-directed surgical and/or ablative therapies. This makes the task of an MDT all the more difficult, as it must decide not only whether a procedure may be feasible, but which subset of patients is likely to benefit from it. There is also considerable scope to combine various modalities, so that many patients will be treated by at least two, if not all, of the main therapeutic options (systemic chemotherapy, liver resection, and ablation). The MDT will often need to deliberate on which of these options to use, and in what order. As the armamentarium of available therapeutic options grows, so does the complexity of the decisions facing an MDT. This is compounded by the lack of robust evidence in the literature on which to base decisions.

Principles of liver resection

Is the disease technically resectable?

The first decision that faces a liver team is whether the liver metastases are technically resectable. One must be able to resect all the involved liver with clear resection margins, leaving behind sufficient liver parenchyma to support synthetic function, and ensuring adequate vascular inflow and outflow to this tissue. This decision is very important, as postoperative liver failure is a major cause of mortality. This decision is based on careful assessment of the cross-sectional imaging, and can be assisted by three-dimensional reformatting and computerized volumetric measurements.

About 20% of normal healthy vascularized liver volume is usually sufficient to provide adequate liver synthetic function and prevent serious liver failure. This is dependent on the liver parenchyma being healthy, and conditions that are known to affect the function of the remnant liver, such as hepatic steatosis, need to be taken into consideration. There is also the potential to jeopardize the vascular supply or venous drainage of part of the remnant, thereby reducing the volume of functional liver tissue. This is particularly relevant to the venous drainage of the parts of the liver supplied by the middle hepatic vein. There is considerable variability between different liver surgeons as to what is deemed resectable, and this is covered in more detail later in this section.

What techniques can make surgery possible in borderline cases?

Various preoperative and operative maneuvers have been described to enable one to resect disease that may seem technically unresectable.

Preoperative portal vein embolization

A unilateral portal vein, usually the right portal branch, can be embolized by percutaneous intervention from the same or opposite hemiliver (Kokudo & Makuuchi 2004). This results in compensatory hypertrophy of the opposite hemiliver, taking 3–5 weeks to achieve measurable increase in volume. It is also possible to selectively embolize the branch to segment IV at the same time, and this will result in more impressive hypertrophy of the left lateral segments, without stimulation of tumor growth in segment IV. Portal vein embolization may be useful for disease that is amenable to resection by extended right hepatectomy in patients with a small left lateral segment (residual liver mass less than 20–25% of total normal liver volume or less than 0.4–0.5 g/kg body weight). It is erroneous to measure the residual liver mass as a proportion of the total liver volume, particularly in cases with bulky tumor burden; the absolute residual liver volume is a more relevant measure in such cases.

There is considerable variation in the use of portal venous embolization across liver centers. Some units use this technique frequently, and would recommend it for the majority of patients undergoing extended right hepatectomy. Others rarely resort to it, and report equally good outcomes. Patients may then be subject to a higher incidence of postoperative liver dysfunction, but, in the absence of postoperative complications, this is transient and recovers spontaneously. Therefore the decision to use preoperative portal vein embolization depends on local expertise and surgical practices. However, it is important that a patient is not deemed unresectable due to a small left lateral remnant, without consideration being given to this technique.

Vascular reconstruction

The experience gained with liver transplantation has made liver surgeons more aware of the importance of venous drainage of the remaining parenchyma (Lang *et al.* 2005). It has also increased surgical experience of vascular reconstruction as a method of achieving better venous drainage and thereby improving the function of the residual liver. When tumor involves the portal inflow to or the venous outflow from the residual liver parenchyma, it may be possible to resect the disease and perform vascular reconstruction. Though long-term outcomes do not appear to be as good, such procedures are still recommended in the absence of any other potentially curative option (Aoki *et al.* 2004). Vascular reconstruction may also be necessary for tumors that involve the inferior vena cava. It is worth noting that occasionally all three hepatic veins can be sacrificed, if a large accessory right hepatic vein can be preserved. During such resections, one may need to resort to total vascular exclusion of the liver, or other similar technical steps to reduce bleeding.

Staged resections

Patients with extensive bilateral disease that would be unsafe to resect at one operation can be treated by sequential resections. The first operation removes the side of the liver that carries the bulk of the disease. When the patient has recovered from this operation, the residual liver has usually hypertrophied sufficiently to permit a second resection to remove the residual disease. Chemotherapy is advised after the first resection, to reduce the impact of growth factors on residual tumor in the remnant liver.

In the experience of the Paul Brousse Hospital, France, 5% of their patients who underwent liver resection required a staged resection (Adam *et al.* 2000). Of their 16 patients who were planned for two-stage procedures, three developed distant metastases after the first hepatectomy. They found that the second operation had a higher morbidity and mortality, and the overall mortality from this approach was 15%. The 3-year survival for the 13 patients who underwent staged resections was 35%. This strategy, though successful, clearly has considerable risks. It would be useful to compare this to a strategy of resection combined with ablation, which is likely to have a higher risk of local recurrence, but be safer. In view of the higher morbidity and mortality of staged resections, it seems prudent to reserve this strategy for patients who are not suitable for combined resection with operative ablation, or who then go on to develop local recurrence at the site of ablation.

Resection combined with ablation

Patients with bilateral deposits in the liver that are deemed inoperable or at very high risk for complete resection may be treated by a combination of resection and ablation. These patients may also be suitable for staged resections, and there are presently no guidelines to select patients for one or other therapy. The favored form of operative ablation at present is radiofrequency ablation. Experience with this technique suggests that complete ablation of a lesion may be more successfully achieved during open surgery than by percutaneous means. The most common scenario where this technique would be indicated is where the bulk of the disease is on one side, and can only be resected by hemihepatectomy/extended hepatectomy, and there is a small (<5-cm) deposit in the remnant whose location precludes minor non-anatomical excision.

At present there is insufficient evidence in the literature to be able to compare the merits of this technique with other options, such as staged resections. It is also unclear from the literature whether patients who undergo surgery with ablation, and then fail due to local recurrence at the site of ablation, have a good chance of being salvaged by a second resection. However, the M D Anderson experience does suggest that there is a higher rate of local recurrence following ablation (9%) when compared to excision of metastases (2%) (Abdalla *et al.* 2004). Surgical excision of all metastases at one operation still remains the treatment of choice, when it can be performed safely.

The decision for liver resection

Does the patient's overall prognosis justify resection of the metastases?

The more contentious issue that the MDT needs to address is the selection of patients who are likely, or unlikely, to benefit from liver surgery. Certain contraindications to liver resection are uncontroversial: the presence of extrahepatic disease (though localized extrahepatic disease, such as an isolated lung metastasis, has been resected with significant success), and the inability to completely excise the metastases (debulking surgery has no proven survival benefit). However, a proportion of patients will have potentially resectable liver metastases but a poor overall prognosis, and the decision to resect metastases in such patients becomes difficult to justify. Various retrospective prognostic variables that influence outcomes after resection of colorectal liver metastases have been identified, and it is reasonable to use these variables to gauge the utility of liver surgery for individual cases (Mann *et al.* 2004). Patients with a poor prognosis are often offered neoadjuvant chemotherapy rather than liver surgery, despite having potentially resectable liver metastases. Some patients will have progressive disease despite chemotherapy, and may no longer be amenable to liver resection. However, Adam *et al.* show that patients whose disease progresses on chemotherapy do very poorly after liver resection, and operating on them at an earlier stage is not likely to have provided any benefit (Adam *et al.* 2004a). In this manner, the response of the disease to chemotherapy can be used as an additional prognostic variable to select patients for liver surgery.

Can the metastases be downstaged and made resectable?

There is convincing evidence that patients with inoperable bulky liver metastases can be successfully downstaged with chemotherapy. Adam *et al.* show that 12.5% of their patients with inoperable liver metastases became operable following neoadjuvant combination chemotherapy (Adam *et al.* 2004b). When there is a good response to chemotherapy, tumor deposits occasionally disappear, and it can then be difficult to decide whether and how to treat these patients. In view of the fact that these patients are never cured by chemotherapy, one should presume that there would be residual cancer at the previously identified sites of metastases. The author therefore believes that, in general, surgery for such patients should be planned with a view to treating all the previously affected sites of disease.

Restaging patients who have received neoadjuvant chemotherapy is difficult and often inaccurate. Cross-sectional imaging is more difficult to interpret, and tumor deposits may not be sufficiently metabolically active to be detected on PET scanning. PET scans done soon after chemotherapy are likely to be falsely negative, and though activity seems to recover if the scan is performed several weeks after completion of chemotherapy, it is still not as accurate as when performed before the start of chemotherapy. Treatment decisions at that stage often need to be based on the cross-sectional images of the liver obtained prior to chemotherapy. Therefore it is strongly recommended that the liver disease is accurately imaged and discussed within an MDT prior to neoadjuvant therapy.

PET scanning can be used to gauge the metabolic response of the tumor to chemotherapy, and may eventually be shown to be a good early predictor of chemosensitivity (Findlay *et al.* 1996). It may then be possible to predict response to chemotherapy soon after starting treatment. This would help prevent patients from receiving unhelpful courses of chemotherapy. It may also be useful for patients with borderline resectable disease, who would be at risk of progressing to an unresectable stage if the chemoresistant nature of their disease is not identified at an early stage.

Controversies in liver resection

What number of metastases can be excised with a reasonable prospect of cure?

The number of metastases in the liver has been shown to be a prognostic variable that affects survival after liver metastatectomy. Traditionally liver resection was not recommended for patients who had more than three metastases or who had bilobar disease. However, there has been sufficient evidence to refute this outdated tenet, and all liver units would agree that good long-term outcomes can be achieved with resection of more advanced disease (Pawlik *et al.* 2006). Though the absolute number of lesions present no longer determines whether one deems the disease inoperable, this is certainly one variable that should be considered; the literature suggests that patients with eight or more metastases have a very poor outcome after metastatectomy (Malik *et al.* 2007). It is also suggested that the volume of affected liver parenchyma appears to be a more significant determinant of outcome than the number of affected sites, and this is another variable that one must weigh in assessing the chance of cure (Ercolani *et al.* 2002).

Is staging laparoscopy useful?

Laparoscopy has been used as a method of identifying patients with unresectable disease, and thereby avoiding a large abdominal incision. The technique has been hampered by a significant failure rate due to adhesions from previous surgery. Jarnagin, however, has reported successful laparoscopy in over 90% of patients, and was able to identify more than half the patients who had unresectable disease (Jarnagin *et al.* 2001). Grobmyer, from the same group, confirmed in a follow-up study that laparoscopy identified 41% of the 24% of patients who had unresectable disease (Grobmyer *et al.* 2004). They also advocate that laparoscopy can be avoided in patients with a good prognostic score, and is valuable in patients with a poor prognostic score. The majority of liver units do not offer this procedure routinely, largely because it is cumbersome to perform due to previous surgery. Recent developments in imaging, surgical techniques, and the use of surgery with ablation have reduced the number of patients who are found to be untreatable at operation. Many centers nowadays report low rates of unresectability consistently below 10%, and do not feel that routine laparoscopy can be justified.

What margin of resection is sufficient?

There is no doubt that surgically involved margins are associated with worse outcomes, and every effort should be made during surgery to obtain clear margins. The traditional teaching was for liver surgeons to maintain a minimum resection margin of at least 1 cm. However, evidence suggests that a smaller margin is adequate and is associated with low rates of local recurrence and equal long-term outcomes. Lodge *et al.* show that any margin more than 1 mm is sufficient to obtain tumor clearance, and patients should not be deemed unresectable because a 1-cm margin would not be possible to achieve (Hamady *et al.* 2006). The technique of parenchymal transection used during liver surgery, whether by ultrasonic dissection, waterjet or coagulation, destroys a wide area of liver parenchyma and the true resection margin is likely to be considerably greater than the pathologic margin.

Should neoadjuvant chemotherapy be used in patients with resectable liver metastases?

There is insufficient evidence to help us decide whether patients with resectable liver metastases would do better with neoadjuvant chemotherapy followed by surgery, when compared to proceeding with liver resection and then providing adjuvant chemotherapy. Proceeding directly with surgery has the advantages of avoiding delays and treating patients with chemoresistant disease. The administration of neoadjuvant chemotherapy can help select out patients who are likely to do poorly with surgery, and avoid unnecessary operations. The administration of chemotherapy may cause hepatic steatosis or veno-occlusive reaction in the liver; this has the potential to make liver surgery more difficult, with increased blood loss and impaired function of the residual parenchyma. This effect is more pronounced when patients have received long courses of chemotherapy. It is therefore best to minimize neoadjuvant chemotherapy to six cycles, and to have a window of at least 4 weeks between completion of chemotherapy and surgery.

The present trend is to use a variety of prognostic scoring systems, and to give neoadjuvant chemotherapy to patients whose outcome is gauged to be poor. There is little robust evidence to support this practice, but it is logical and presently appears to be appropriate.

What is the optimal timing of liver surgery for patients with synchronous metastases?

There is considerable evidence to show that synchronous colorectal and liver resections can be performed safely and with reasonable outcomes. Martin and colleagues show that these resections are safe, have a reduced overall complication rate as compared to two staged operations, and also have equivalent long-term survival benefits (Martin *et al.* 2003). However there is no direct comparison of synchronous versus staged resections of colorectal cancers and their synchronous metastases that shows which is superior. The obvious advantage of synchronous resection is to clear all the disease at one operation, thereby avoiding the risk of progression and further metastases. This becomes particularly relevant when the patient develops a complication from the first operation, and takes several months to recover. The main downside of synchronous resection is that a number of patients with poor prognostic disease will undergo unnecessary surgery.

Liver surgeons often prefer a separate upper abdominal incision, and exposure of the liver and the rectum may be difficult to obtain with common access. Initial resection of the primary tumor provides prognostic information that may be valuable and may preclude liver surgery. It also allows the use of neoadjuvant chemotherapy, and this further helps to select out patients with poor prognosis from undergoing unnecessary surgery. Whether the benefits gained from delaying resection of the secondaries are greater than the downsides of delaying their removal remains unknown.

Staged resections are performed in the majority of the Western world. The logistic problems of arranging synchronous surgery, when two separate teams perform the operations, will continue to be a major factor against synchronous resection of a colorectal cancer and its liver metastases.

How should we manage patients with rectal cancer and synchronous liver metastases?

Primary rectal cancers with synchronous liver metastases are particularly problematic. The rectal primary requires more complex preoperative staging investigations, and is often treated with neoadjuvant chemoradiotherapy. These factors result in considerable delay before treatment can be considered to control the liver metastases. It seems inappropriate to focus one's therapy for several months on the primary tumor, when the patient is very likely to die from systemic disease rather than local recurrence. It is important to consider the benefits of aggressive chemotherapy that has the potential to control the systemic disease, while providing a good response at the primary site. Such a strategy has been shown to work, and may obviate the need for radiotherapy in some cases (Mentha *et al.* 2006). It is particularly important in patients with small primary tumors and bulky liver metastases. Liver resection can be considered before removal of the primary, if the liver disease is felt to be at greater threat of progressing to an incurable stage.

Is repeat liver resection safe and effective?

The majority of patients will develop recurrent metastases after liver resection, and about one-third of them will have liver-only disease. There are several reports attesting to the safety of repeat hepatic resection for this group of patients, and it is now established as part of the armamentarium. A meta-analysis of 21 studies including 3741 patients found that repeat liver surgery was safe and obtained equivalent long-term outcomes to the first liver resection (Antoniou *et al.* 2007). Third and fourth hepatectomies have also been performed with favorable outcomes; the Paul Brousse Hospital, France, report that of 115 patients with liver-only recurrences after second hepatectomy, they proceeded with surgery in 68 (59%), and were able to resect the disease in 60 of 68 cases (88%) (Adam *et al.* 2003). They conclude that third hepatectomy is safe and provides an additional survival benefit similar to that of first and second liver resections.

It is more difficult to select patients suitable for repeat surgery, particularly if there is more than one deposit or when the disease-free interval after the previous hepatic resection is short. It is also more difficult to plan the operation, and many of these procedures will be non-anatomic excisions.

Conclusions

Liver surgery, when possible, remains the mainstay of treatment for patients with hepatic metastases from colorectal cancer. The management of these patients has become increasingly complex, as the available therapeutic options have increased. The use of various combinations of chemotherapy, surgery and ablative methods allows us to treat patients who, in the past, would have been deemed unresectable. The complexity and range of decisions that an MDT faces accentuates the importance of a multidisciplinary environment in the care of these patients. The lack of robust evidence in the literature also highlights the need for evaluating these therapies in a scientific fashion within trials.

References

Abdalla EK, Vauthey JN, Ellis LM *et al.* (2004) Recurrence and outcomes following hepatic resection, radiofrequency ablation, and combined resection/ablation for colorectal liver metastases. *Ann Surg* 239(6): 818–25.

Adam R, Laurent A, Azoulay D, Castaing D, Bismuth H. (2000) Two-stage hepatectomy: A planned strategy to treat irresectable liver tumors. *Ann Surg* 232(6): 777–85.

Adam R, Pascal G, Azoulay D, Tanaka K, Castaing D, Bismuth H. (2003) Liver resection for colorectal metastases: the third hepatectomy. *Ann Surg* 238(6): 871–83.

Adam R, Pascal G, Castaing D *et al.* (2004a) Tumor progression while on chemotherapy: a contraindication to liver resection for multiple colorectal metastases? *Ann Surg* 240(6): 1052–61.

Adam R, Delvart V, Pascal G *et al.* (2004b) Rescue surgery for unresectable colorectal liver metastases downstaged by chemotherapy: a model to predict long-term survival. *Ann Surg* 240(4): 644–57.

Antoniou A, Lovegrove RE, Tilney HS *et al.* (2007) Meta-analysis of clinical outcome after first and second liver resection for colorectal metastases. *Surgery* 141(1): 9–18.

Aoki T, Sugawara Y, Imamura H *et al.* (2004) Hepatic resection with reconstruction of the inferior vena cava or hepatic venous confluence for metastatic liver tumor from colorectal cancer. *J Am Coll Surg* 198(3): 366–72.

Choti MA, Sitzmann JV, Tiburi MF *et al.* (2002) Trends in long-term survival following liver resection for hepatic colorectal metastases. *Ann Surg* 235(6): 759–66.

Cummings LC, Payes JD, Cooper GS. (2007) Survival after hepatic resection in metastatic colorectal cancer: a population-based study. *Cancer* 109(4): 718–26.

Ercolani G, Grazi GL, Ravaioli M *et al.* Liver resection for multiple colorectal metastases: influence of parenchymal involvement and total tumor volume, versus number or location, on long-term survival. *Arch Surg* (2002) 137(10): 1187–92.

Findlay M, Young H, Cunningham D *et al.* (1996) Noninvasive monitoring of tumor metabolism using fluorodeoxyglucose and positron emission tomography in colorectal cancer liver metastases: correlation with tumor response to fluorouracil. *J Clin Oncol* 14(3): 700–8.

Grobmyer SR, Fong Y, D'Angelica M, Dematteo RP, Blumgart LH, Jarnagin WR. (2004) Diagnostic laparoscopy prior to planned hepatic resection for colorectal metastases. *Arch Surg* 139(12): 1326–30.

Hamady ZZ, Cameron IC, Wyatt J, Prasad RK, Toogood GJ, Lodge JP. (2006) Resection margin in patients undergoing hepatectomy for colorectal liver metastasis: a critical appraisal of the 1cm rule. *Eur J Surg Oncol* 32(5): 557–63.

Jarnagin WR, Conlon K, Bodniewicz J *et al.* (2001) A clinical scoring system predicts the yield of diagnostic laparoscopy in patients with potentially resectable hepatic colorectal metastases. *Cancer* 91(6): 1121–8.

Kokudo N, Makuuchi M. (2004) Current role of portal vein embolization/hepatic artery chemoembolization. *Surg Clin North Am* 84(2): 643–57.

Lang H, Radtke A, Hindennach M *et al.* (2005) Impact of virtual tumor resection and computer-assisted risk analysis on operation planning and intraoperative strategy in major hepatic resection. *Arch Surg* 140(7): 629–38.

Malik HZ, Hamady ZZ, Adair R *et al.* (2007) Prognostic influence of multiple hepatic metastases from colorectal cancer. *Eur J Surg Oncol* 33(4): 468–73.

Mann CD, Metcalfe MS, Leopardi LN, Maddern GJ. (2004) The clinical risk score: emerging as a reliable preoperative prognostic index in hepatectomy for colorectal metastases. *Arch Surg* 139(11): 1168–72.

Martin R, Paty P, Fong Y *et al.* (2003) Simultaneous liver and colorectal resections are safe for synchronous colorectal liver metastasis. *J Am Coll Surg* 197(2): 233–41.

Mentha G, Majno PE, Andres A, Rubbia-Brandt L, Morel P, Roth AD. (2006) Neoadjuvant chemotherapy and resection of advanced synchronous liver metastases before treatment of the colorectal primary. *Br J Surg* 93(7): 872–8.

Pawlik TM, Abdalla EK, Ellis LM, Vauthey JN, Curley SA. (2006) Debunking dogma: surgery for four or more colorectal liver metastases is justified. *J Gastrointest Surg* 10(2): 240–8.

Ablative treatments

Fergus Gleeson

Introduction

It has long been accepted that it is possible to locally ablate tumor within the liver, initially using percutaneous ethanol injection for hepatocellular carcinoma, and then more recently using thermal mechanisms delivered via a variety of different technologies as the method of ablation. Radiofrequency ablation (RFA), cryoablation, laser ablation, high-intensity focused ultrasound (HIFU), and microwave therapy have all been used as means of causing tumor cell death and ablating focal areas of disease within the liver. Ablative therapy may be used as the sole means of treatment or in combination with resection or may be used after a reduction in volume of tumor has been achieved following either chemotherapy or chemoembolization.

The different techniques have various advantages and disadvantages compared to each other. There are a number of limitations when compared to surgical resection, and there are recognized risks associated with each technique. One of the major difficulties using ablative techniques when compared to resection is the difficulty in determining that complete ablation of all disease has been achieved, and careful follow-up to detect local disease relapse is necessary. At present the most readily available and frequently used technique is radiofrequency ablation (Fig. 14.10), but newer techniques such as HIFU are the subject of intense research interest, offering potentially decreased morbidity and mortality, and the ability to monitor ablation in real time. This section will briefly review the most commonly used methods of ablation, the morbidity and mortality of the procedures, choice of lesions for ablation and the methods of assessing whether the ablation has been successful.

Types of ablative therapy

Radiofrequency ablation

The use of RFA to ablate liver lesions was initially reported in 1990 (McGahan *et al.* 1990; Rossi *et al.* 1990). Since that time the number of articles published on the technique has steadily increased, and it is now possible to comment on which lesions are most amenable to ablation, with new developments aimed at increasing both the number of lesions that may be targeted and the volumes of ablation that may be achieved (Lucey 2006). RFA is the technique of inducing coagulation and hence cell death using an electromagnetic energy source, most commonly using frequencies in the 375–500 kHz range. One of the difficulties experienced when performing RFA is the local effect of heating, resulting in charring of the adjacent tissue preventing consistent heat delivery and reducing the volume of tissue that can be ablated. Much of the variety in the different RFA techniques is centered on attempts to enable consistent heat delivery to as large a volume as possible. At present most devices use a single monopolar 'active' electrode dissipating the current generated into return grounding pads with ablation occurring adjacent to the electrode. This differs from bipolar devices which have two 'active' electrodes with contiguous coagulation, i.e. ablation occurring between the electrodes. There are also many different types of electrode available with which to deliver the thermal energy. The different types aim to either increase the volume of tissue ablated, or to deliver a very consistent thermal dose enabling a reproducible ablation to be performed. The electrodes may be single or, if a large area is to be ablated,

(a)

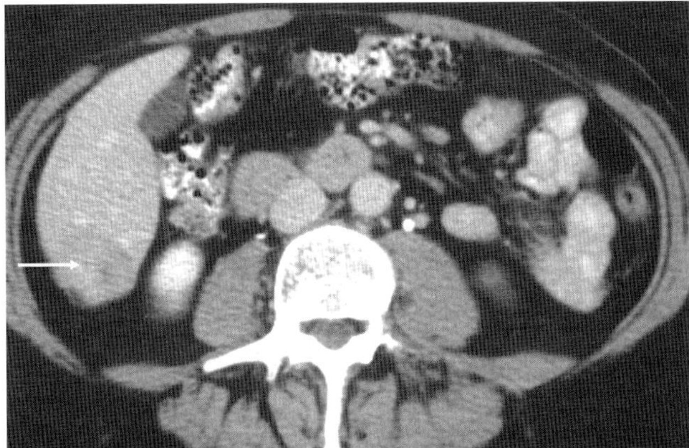

(b)

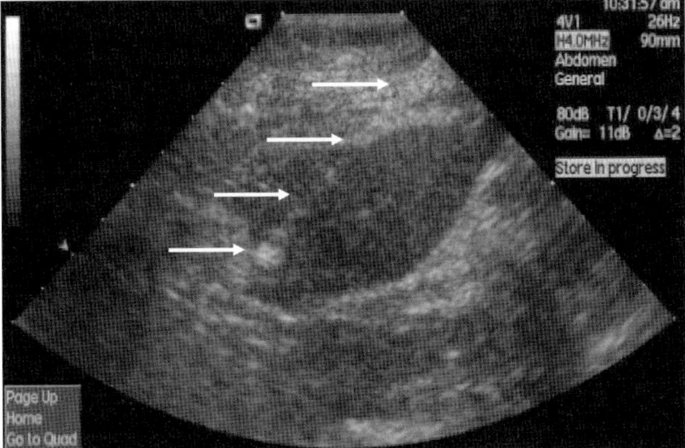

(c)

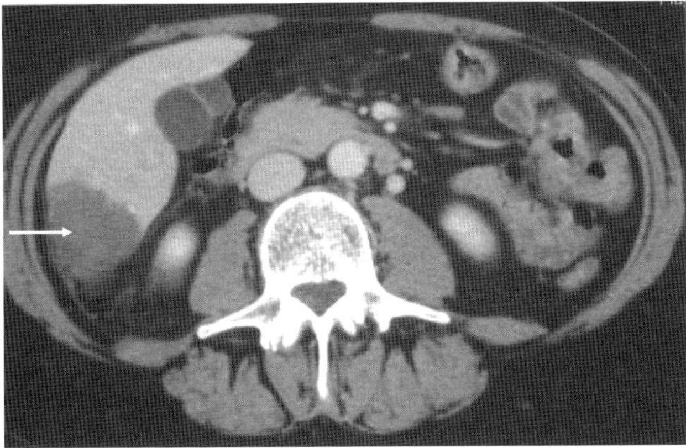

Fig. 14.10 (a) Contrast-enhanced CT scan demonstrating a hepatic metastasis (arrowed) suitable for RFA. (b) Ultrasound image demonstrating the RFA probe *in situ* (arrowed). (c) Contrast-enhanced CT scan performed the day after RFA demonstrating successful ablation of the metastasis.

greater than 3 cm in diameter, then either multiple electrodes or an umbrella array, consisting of multiple electrode tines expanding out from a single centrally positioned electrode may be used. Some devices have mechanisms that allow water to flow either along an internal lumen not in contact with the patient to keep the electrode at a consistent temperature, or to flow from small apertures at the tip potentially allowing heat to be transmitted a greater distance from the tip.

Cryoablation

This is the destruction of tissue by applying low-temperature freezing. In hepatic ablative therapy, cryoablation is performed by placing a closed cryoprobe in the target area. The cold temperatures are predominantly achieved using argon gas or either gas or liquid nitrogen. It has been used sparingly as a method of liver ablative therapy, due to the need in the past to use large delivery probes, and concerns over hemorrhage (Onik *et al.* 1993) and reports of liver cracking (Selfert & Morris 1999). Newer probes that are smaller and more accurately monitor the temperature at the site of ablation may allow it to be more extensively investigated and used (Shock *et al.* 2005).

Laser ablation

Laser ablation has in the past been referred to as laser interstitial tumor therapy, laser coagulation therapy and laser interstitial photocoagulation. This technique was first described in 1983 and destroys tumor cells by direct heating using a low-power laser light energy delivered via thin optical fibers (Vogl *et al.* 2001). It causes minimal damage to surrounding tissues, and its success is critically dependent on accurate placement of the optic fibers and monitoring of the effects of treatment. It may be performed using either ultrasound or magnetic resonance imaging, and although not as commonly used as RFA or HIFU the published reports suggest it to be an effective means of producing tumor ablation.

Microwave ablation

As microwave ablation does not rely on tissue conduction of heat and electricity it is not limited by charring. This allows temperatures greater than 100°C to be reached, allowing a large ablation zone to be achieved in a relative fast treatment time, and this may allow ablation of areas adjacent to vessels that are difficult to treat successfully using techniques such as RFA (Wright *et al.* 2005). Additionally, work is now ongoing to develop microwave ablation units that can deliver more power, enabling larger tumor volumes to be ablated more quickly, although this may result in a reduction in the ability to carefully target the area to be ablated (Hines-Pealta *et al.* 2006).

High-intensity focused ultrasound

HIFU (Kennedy *et al.* 2003) relies on the effect of a focused ultrasound beam of sufficient energy causing a local rise in the tissue on which it is aimed resulting in tissue necrosis. As it uses the same principles as conventional diagnostic ultrasound, the unfocused ultrasound beam is able to pass harmlessly through tissue until it reaches the target or focused area and because of this has the obvious attraction of not needing interventional needle placement to deliver energy at the site of ablation. It has the advantage of being able to be tightly focused, but has the disadvantage of only being able to deliver ablative energy to a small volume, and is consequently slower as a means of ablation than alternative techniques. It cannot be used of course if the lesion cannot be visualized using ultrasound, and this also limits its utility.

Morbidity and mortality

Aside from the expected risks associated with percutaneous image-guided needle placement (not of concern if the ablative technique is HIFU, or if the procedure is performed at laparotomy), injuries reported secondary to ablative therapy are predominantly due to inadvertent thermal damage of structures adjacent to the target area. Complications reported from liver ablative therapy include bowel perforation, biliary perforation and stricture formation, diaphragmatic injury, abscess formation and sepsis, and hemorrhage (Lucey 2006). Attempts to minimize these risks include meticulous attention to detail for needle placement, choosing access routes that avoid structures that cannot be safely traversed, and performing the procedure laparoscopically or at laparotomy if necessary. Other techniques may also be used to move away structures adjacent to the target area at risk from thermal injury. The most commonly used technique is the infusion of 5% dextrose in water into the peritoneal space as a method of protecting the body wall and bowel (Lucey 2006). Large bowel is at greatest risk when lesions adjacent to the caudal hepatic capsular surface are ablated (Fig. 14.11).

The risk of postablation hemorrhage when withdrawing the needle, and needle-track seeding are reduced by withdrawing the needle whilst hot (Lucey 2006).

Lesion suitability for ablation

Intuitively, both small lesions and limited numbers of lesions correlate with procedure success, although each case referred for ablation needs to be considered on its own merit (Goldberg *et al.* 2005). The surgical gold standard for resection is to achieve where possible a margin of 1 cm between the tumor and the resection edge, with a lesser margin associated with an increase in local recurrence. A tumor-free margin of 1 cm is also desirable when using ablative therapy but is frequently not attainable due to lesion position. There are also two difficulties experienced by ablative therapy not encountered surgically: the effect of adjacent vessels on heat production within the lesion, and the size of lesions that may be ablated. The edge of lesions adjacent to vessels may not achieve a sufficient rise in temperature to produce necrosis, as large vessels greater than 4 mm in diameter act as heat sumps, drawing heat away from the tumor. Single needle ablations are limited by the volume of tumor/liver that can be heated sufficient to achieve cell death, with non-needle ablative therapies such as HIFU similarly limited by their inability to heat large volumes. A reasonable assumption is that lesions above 4 cm in diameter have a reduced likelihood of being successfully ablated, with a rapid fall-off in successful ablations above 5 cm. Similarly, an increase in the number of lesions requiring ablation results in a decrease in the likelihood of successful treatment, with more than four lesions reducing the likelihood of complete tumor ablation.

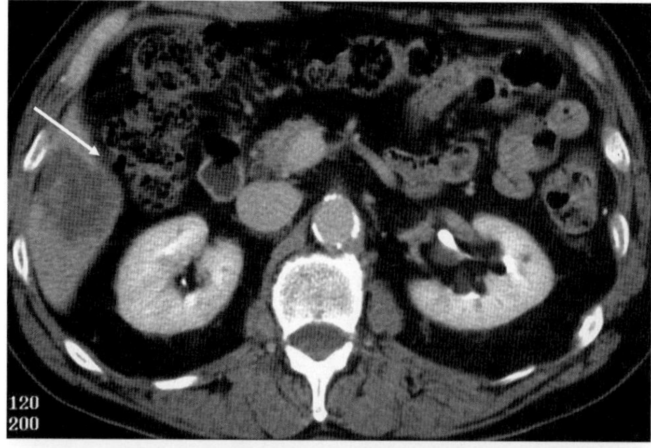

(a)

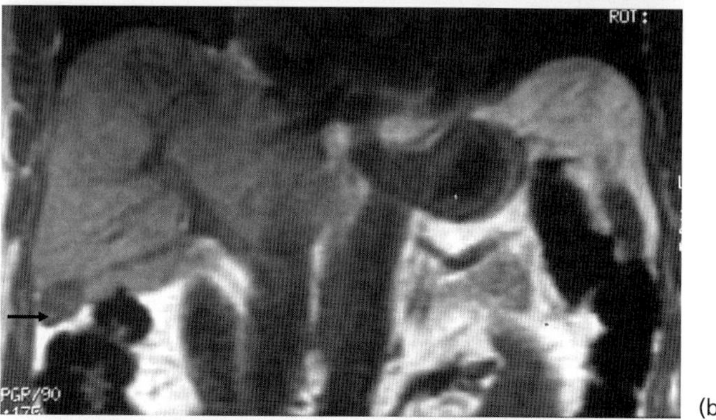

(b)

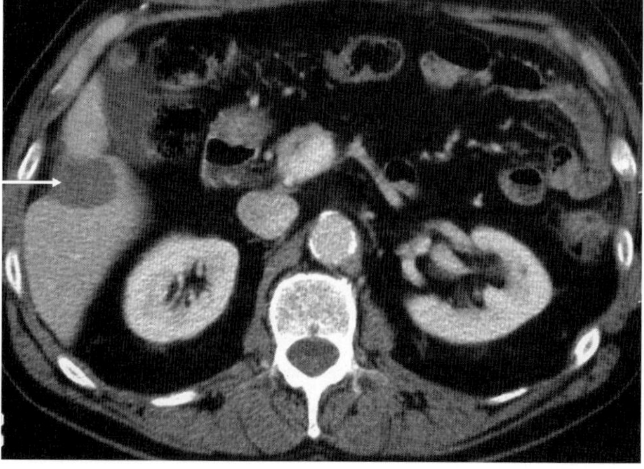

(c)

Fig. 14.11 (a) Contrast-enhanced CT scan demonstrating a hepatic metastasis adjacent to colon (arrowed). (b) A coronal T1-weighted MRI scan showing the proximity of the metastasis (arrowed) to the adjacent colon. The metastasis was subsequently ablated using RFA laparoscopically. (c) Contrast-enhanced CT scan showing the characteristic reduction in size of the metastasis 6 months post ablation.

Assessment of ablation

The success of surgical resection for metastatic disease can be readily determined by histologic assessment of the resected specimen and analysisof the resection margins, as described earlier. This is in contradistinction to ablative therapy, when direct assessment of the area ablated is not possible (Goldberg *et al.* 2005). Attempts to confirm that all the tumor has been ablated is one of the areas currently under intense research. If it is immediately possible post ablation to identify a small area that has not been completely ablated it is possible to repeat the procedure in this area. The use of MRI both to allow accurate lesion targeting when placing the ablative needles (MRI-safe needles are now commonplace), and to assess whether the procedure has been successful is now increasing. Alternative techniques such as the use of microbubble-performed ultrasound may also help in determining whether a repeat procedure is necessary. Careful and regular follow-up scanning, most commonly contrast-enhanced CT, is obviously critical in identifying local disease recurrence and new disease within the liver or in other organs such as the lungs.

References

Goldberg SN, Grassi CJ, Cardella JF *et al.* (2005) Image-guided tumor ablation: standardisation of terminology and reporting criteria. *Radiology* 235: 728–39.

Hines-Pealta AU, Pirani N, Clegg P *et al.* (2006) Microwave ablation: results with a 2.45-GHz applicator in ex vivo bovine and in vivo porcine liver. *Radiology* 239: 94–102.

Kennedy JE, ter Haar GR, Cranston D. (2003) High intensity focused ultrasound: surgery of the future? *Br J Radiol* 76: 590–9.

Lucey BC. (2006) Radiofrequency ablation. *Am J Roentgenol* 186: S237–S333.

McGahan JP, Browning PD, Brock JM, Tesluk H. (1990) Hepatic ablation using radiofrequency electrocautery. *Invest Radiol* 25: 267–70.

Onik GM, Atkinson D, Zemel R, Weaver ML. (1993) Cryosurgery of liver cancer. *Semin Surg Oncol* 9: 309–17.

Rossi S, Fornari F, Pathies C, Buscarini L. (1990) Thermal lesions induced by 480-kHz localised current field in guinea pig and pig liver. *Tumori* 76: 54–7.

Selfert JK, Morris DL. (1999) World survey on the complications of hepatic and prostate cryotherapy. *World J Surg* 23: 109–13.

Shock SA, Laeseke PF, Sampson LA *et al.* (2005) Hepatic hemorrhage caused by percutaneous tumour ablation: radiofrequency ablation versus cryoablation in a porcine model. *Radiology* 236: 125–31.

Vogl TJ, Eichler K, Straub R *et al.* (2001) Laser-induced thermotherapy of malignant liver tumours: general principles, equipment, procedure side-effects, complications and results. *Eur J Ultrasound* 13: 117–27.

Wright AS, Sampson LA, Warner TF, Mahvi DM, Lee FT. (2005) Radiofrequency versus microwave ablation in a hepatic porcine model. *Radiology* 236: 132–9.

Novel therapies

Carlos Escriu, Mark Middleton & Rachel S. Midgley

Introduction

Recent advances in basic molecular biology, pharmacology, genetics, epigenetics and immunology have opened the door to new treatments by targeting specific molecular abnormalities in cancer cells.

The aim of these therapies is:

- to directly target the growth mechanisms of cancer cells
- to improve the efficacy and restore sensitivity to current cytotoxic and radiologic therapies
- to potentiate or create a new immune response against cancer cells.

Molecular abnormalities can have also a use in cancer staging and prediction of response to treatment. Although some of these therapies have already a niche within current treatment guidelines, most of them are still under investigation and their future role is uncertain.

In colorectal cancer treatment, novel therapies have made an important impact through endothelial growth factor receptor (EGFR) and vascular endothelial growth factor (VEGF) pathways.

EGFR belongs to the ErbB family of receptors. All of them have a ligand-binding domain, a transmembrane segment, and an intracellular protein tyrosine kinase domain with a regulatory carboxyl terminal segment. Their physiologic homodimer activation can be triggered through the ligand-binding domain or by interacting with other activated homodimers from the same family. The formation of heterodimeric complexes triggers phosphorylation cascades that involve PI3/Akt and RAS/MAPK pathways (Figs 14.12 & 14.13). The EGFR ligands are epidermal growth factor (EGF) and tumor growth factor (TGF) α.

EGFR, also called ErbB1 or HER1, is abnormally expressed in 70–80% of colorectal cancers, and is involved in apoptosis inhibition, metastasis and cell differentiation (Zhang *et al.* 2006). The tyrosine kinase domain can be activated in cancer cells through ligand-independent mechanisms such as urokinase plasminogen receptor or G-protein-coupled receptors. EGFR is present in normal tissues such as the skin and the loop of Henle, both sites of special relevance when considering the side-effects of EGFR blockers: rash and hypomagnesemia.

VEGF is a cytokine with four major isoforms of identical biologic activity but different ability to bind heparin and extracellular matrix. It is suggested that those VEGF isoforms have tissue-specific expression patterns. In the normal cell, VEGF is upregulated by hypoxia. VEGF interacts with four cell surface tyrosine kinase receptors with similar domain structure to EGFR:

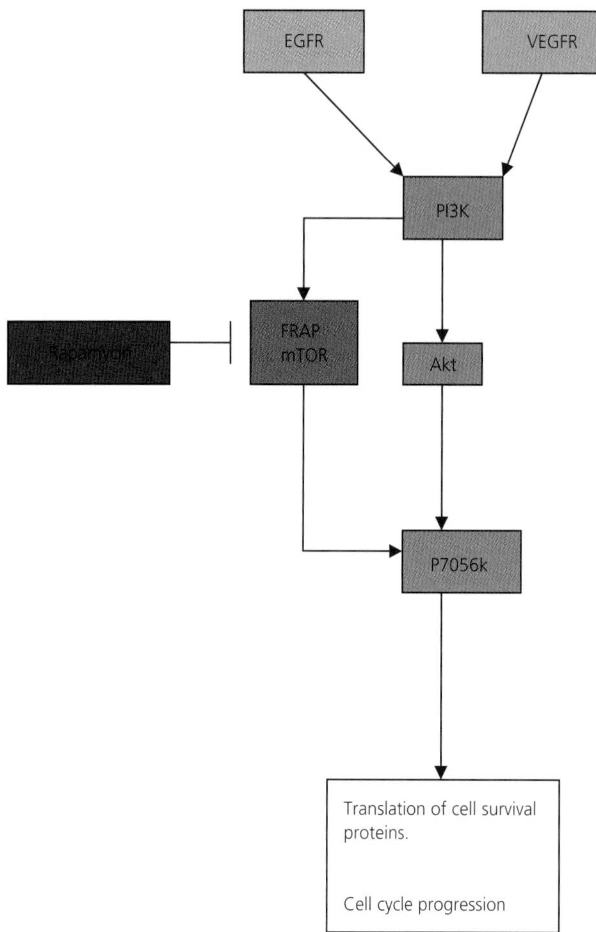

Fig. 14.12 PI3K/Akt pathway.

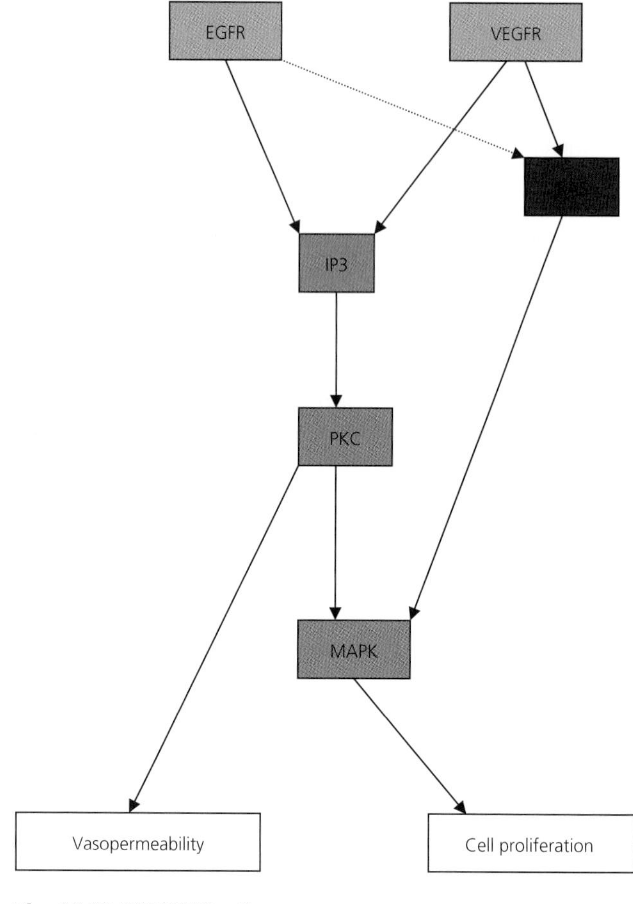

Fig. 14.13 RAS/MAPK pathway.

- VEGFR-1 and VEGFR-2, selectively expressed on vascular endothelial cells
- VEGFR-3, expressed in lymphatic and vascular endothelium
- neuropilin receptor, expressed in vascular endothelium and neurons.

VEGF/VEGFR binding triggers phosphorylation cascades down the PI3/Akt and RAS/MAPK pathways.

In physiologic conditions, VEGF enhances microvascular permeability, causes vasodilatation, stimulates cell migration and growth, upregulates antiapoptotic proteins, stimulates proliferation, and induces enzymes necessary for the degradation of the basement membrane. Accordingly, in cancer cells, VEGF is involved in the metastasis and angiogenesis processes. The side-effects of its blockade are hypertension (opposite to vasodilatation), a tendency to bleed due to decreased renewal capacity of endothelial cells, and an increase of thrombotic events, due to tissue factor activation secondary to exposure of subendothelial collagen (Kilickap *et al.* 2003).

Both receptors' signalling pathways interact so that EGFR expression upregulates VEGF signalling, and VEGF upregulation contributes to resistance to EGFR inhibition.

The effects of other growth factors and cytokines like HER-2, insulin-like growth factor receptor (IGF-IR), hepatocyte growth factor, platelet-derived growth factors (PDGFs), prostaglandins and prostaglandin-endoperoxide synthase (COX) interact with both EGFR and VEGF pathways.

Novel therapies

There are several strategies to inhibit VEGF and EGFR:

- monoclonal antibodies, either blocking the EFGR ligand (e.g. cetuximab and panitumumab), or neutralizing VEGF or VEGFR (e.g. bevacizumab)
- low molecular weight molecules, like tyrosine kinase inhibitors.

Monoclonal antibodies (mAbs)

mAbs are given intravenously and work by blocking with different degrees of reversibility the targeted receptors (Table 14.4).

They also have an indirect action mediated by the immune system through immunoglobulin-mediated mechanisms. The elimination of cancer cells is achieved through:

Table 14.5 Simplified classification of EGFR inhibitors rash.

Grade 1	Grade 2	Grade 3	Grade 4
Rash: desquamation			
Asymptomatic rash	<50% of body surface	>50% of body surface	Exfoliative, ulcerative or bullous erythroderma
Rash: acne/acneiform			
Intervention not indicated	Intervention indicated	. Pain, disfigurement, ulceration or desquamation	–

Table 14.4 mAbs and targeted receptors.

EGFR inhibitors	VEGF inhibitors
Cetuximab Panitumumab Matuzumab Nimotuzumab	Bevacizumab

1 *cellular toxicity mechanisms*: complement-dependent cytotoxicity (CDC) and antibody-dependent cellular cytotoxicity (ADCC) and

2 *humoral toxicity mechanisms*: complement-dependent cell-mediated cytotoxicity (CDCC), through tumor cell opsonization (Imai & Takaoka 2006).

Antibodies targeting similar extracellular epitopes have shown different phosphorylation activity downstream as well as different clinical activity (Meira *et al.* 2007).

Cetuximab

Cetuximab is a chimeric IgG1 monoclonal antibody that binds to EGFR with high specificity and with a higher affinity than either EGF or TGFα.

Preclinical data showed an optimal biologic dose of 200–400 mg/m^2/week determined by antibody clearance. On patient biopsies that dose of cetuximab was proven to be sufficient to block EGFR (Mendelsohn & Baselga 2003). Doses of up to 500 mg/m^2/week have been well tolerated in clinical trials. New studies are investigating the pharmacodinamics and pharmacokinetics of a 2-weekly schedule (Cervantes *et al.* 2007).

In phase I and II trials cetuximab monotherapy achieved response rates (RR) of approximately 22.5% and median duration response (MDR) of 6.2 months (Mendelsohn & Baselga 2003).

The side-effects of cetuximab are skin rash, fatigue, diarrhea, hypomagnesemia and anaphylactoid or anaphylactic reactions (2%). Non-neutralizing human antibodies against chimeric antibodies were found in 4% of patients, but were not related to allergic reactions and had no pharmacokinetic effect on weekly cetuximab infusions. When combined with other chemotherapies diarrhea and neutropenia appear to be more severe, although as frequent as in the chemotherapy arms (Mendelsohn & Baselga 2003).

The dose-dependent acneiform skin rash appears within the first 3 weeks of cetuximab treatment and is self-limiting, although it can require treatment dose modification (see Table 14.5). Microscopically the rash appears as a neutrophilic folliculitis and perifolicullitis. It is confined to seborrheic areas (face, neck, retroauricular areas, shoulders, upper trunk [V shaped] and scalp). Palms and soles are spared. It may evolve into pustules that may dry out in yellow crusts. This rash may be accompanied by pruritus and its treatment is based on antihistamines and topical antibiotic cream.

As well as the acneiform rash, patients can present telangiectasia or more importantly, dry skin over weeks, resembling the xerosis in atopic eczema. That is why as soon as the pustules have dried, hydrating cream must be applied. Xerosis is worse in old age, previous cytotoxic therapy, and background of eczema. Its distribution is in the same areas as the acneiform rash. It may develop into chronic asteatotic eczema and can involve the mucosa, causing vaginal dryness or aphthous ulcers of the mouth and nose.

At a later time, between 4 and 8 weeks, 10–15% of patients present with paronychia that can evolve into pyogenic granuloma of the nail fold and/or secondary infection with *Staphylococcus aureus*. Hair changes like trichomegaly, patchy hair loss and hyperthricosis have been reported.

Postinflammatory hyperpigmentation can be a long-term sequela and early treatment of the acneiform rash, as well as suncream protection, are advised (Sagaent *et al.* 2005).

In the BOND study acneiform rash appeared in 88.9% of the patients, but only grade 3–4 in 5.2% of patients treated with cetuximab monotherapy and 9.4% in those patients who received combination treatment (Cunningham *et al.* 2004).

Retrospectively, patients with rash had better outcomes. In that respect, the EVEREST study (Tejpar *et al.* 2006) assessed the need for dose escalation until grade 2–3 rash in 166 irinotecan-refractory patients. The patients who were on dose escalation to rash had a RR of 30%, whereas those who presented the rash on normal doses had a RR of 22%, and those with no rash a RR of 13%. However, the results did not reach statistic significance and the question of dosing to rash remains open.

Most trials have selected patients to receive cetuximab only if they are EGFR positive on immunohistochemistry. It is advocated that PCR quantification (qPCR) or FISH might be better techniques for patient selection (Arteaga 2003; Imai & Takaoka 2006).

Cetuximab has been shown to restore sensitivity to cytotoxic therapy in the second-line setting. The BOND study (Cunningham *et al.* 2004) was a multicenter phase III trial in 329 stage IV colorectal cancer patients who had progressed within 3 months of irinotecan-based treatment.

Patients were randomized to receive an initial dose of 400 mg/m^2 of cetuximab followed by 250 mg/m^2 monotherapy (111 patients) or cetuximab plus irinotecan (218 patients). 56 patients who presented with disease progression on cetuximab were crossed over to have irinotecan with the antibody.

RR were 10.8% in the cetuximab arm and 22.9% in the cetuximab plus irinotecan arm. In patients who progressed during or within 1 month of irinotecan chemotherapy the RR was 14.1% in the monotherapy arm and 25.2% in the combination therapy. The MDR was 4.2 months in the cetuximab arm and 5.7 months in the cetuximab plus irinotecan arm.

In the first-line treatment of metastatic colorectal cancer, cetuximab seems to have shown high response rate in combination with FOLFOX (Rubio *et al.* 2005) and XELOX (Borner *et al.* 2006) in several phase II trials, according to preliminary data. When cetuximab plus FOLFOX-4 was given to 48 EGFR-positive patients until progressive disease or unacceptable toxicity, the overall confirmed response rate was 72% (9% complete responses and 63% partial responses); 23% had stable disease. Acne-like rash was only observed in 30.2% of patients.

Antibody combined with a VEGF inhibitor was analysed in the BOND 2 study (Lenz *et al.* 2007). That was a phase II trial on irinotecan-refractory and bevacizumab-naïve patients. The RR of cetuximab, bevacizumab and irinotecan versus cetuximab and bevacizumab was 38% and 23% respectively. The toxicity profile of antibody combination was similar to that of a single antibody administration.

The current indication of cetuximab is for EGFR-positive irinotecan-refractory metastatic colorectal cancers (mCRCs). Current studies are assessing its possible role on EGFR-negative mCRC and non-irinotecan-refractory mCRC.

Panitumumab

Panitumumab is a G2 MAb against the EGFR extracellular ligand-binding domain which has been shown to be effective as a treatment of colorectal cancer. As it is a fully human MAb it virtually eliminates the risk of immunogenic reaction. Panitumumab causes skin rash in 100% of patients after at least three doses of 2.5 mg/kg/week (Cohenuram & Saif 2007). It is administered with no loading dose or premedication.

Its advantage over cetuximab is the longer half-life and a substantially lower inhibitory concentration (50%), needing less frequent doses and allowing the patient to have a better quality of life by reducing hospital visits. It can be administered in different schedules ranging between 1 and 3 weekly doses, although in phase III trials it has been given at 6 mg/kg every 2 weeks.

As a single agent in chemoresistant disease after irinotecan and/or oxaliplatin it has shown a 46% reduction in the risk of tumor progression and a partial response rate of 8%, with an MDR of 7.9 months in a phase II trial with 148 patients (Gibson *et al.* 2006). Disease response has also been recorded on immunohistochemistry-defined EGFR-negative patients treated with panitumumab.

Although generally well tolerated, panitumumab's side-effects are diarrhea, fatigue, hypomagnesemia and skin rash. The latter persisted, usually without worsening, through the entire treatment period, and was also predictive of outcome. This typical skin rash from EGFR inhibitors is present in 90% of patients, and of grade 3–4 in 14% of patients.

A large phase III trial compared panitumumab monotherapy versus best supportive care (BSC) in 463 pretreated patients with metastatic colorectal cancer. The overall RR was 36% in the antibody arm and 10% in those patients who had BSC, with an MDR of 17 weeks. The progression-free survival was 18% and 5% respectively at 6 months, a difference maintained at 8 months (10% vs 4%).

No significant difference was found in overall survival, although 75% of patients on BSC crossed over to panitumumab, from which 9% achieved partial response and 32% stable disease (Peeters *et al.* 2006).

In view of those results, panitumumab is expected to be approved soon in the USA as second-line monotherapy treatment for mCRC patients. Ongoing studies are analysing the role of panitumumab in the first-line setting in combination with VEGF inhibitors and several chemotherapeutic regimes.

Bevacizumab

Bevacizumab is a recombinant humanized version of a murine antihuman VEGF G1 monoclonal antibody. In addition to its direct antiangiogenic effects, bevacizumab may also improve the delivery of chemotherapy by altering tumor vasculature and decreasing the elevated interstitial pressure in tumors, according to several studies comparing drug penetration in animal tissues with different vasculature changes induced by VEGFR2 blockade (Tong 2004). A common dosage schedule is 5 mg/kg every 2 weeks in 8-week cycles.

High-dose (10 mg/kg) bevacizumab was assessed in a phase III trial in the second-line setting, alone and in combination with FOLFOX4, and compared with a third arm of FOLFOX4 alone. The RR of bevacizumab alone was 3.3%, 8.6% for the FOLFOX4-alone arm, and 22.7% for the combination arm. The median PFS was 2.7 months for the antibody-alone arm, 4.7 months for the FOLFOX4 arm, and 7.3 months for the combination arm. The median duration of survival was 10.2 months, 10.8 months, and 12.9 months respectively (Giantonio *et al.* 2007).

The side-effects of bevacizumab are:

- grade 3 or 4 hemorrhage in 5% of the patients (4% in the gastrointestinal tract)
- venous thrombosis (5.9%)

- hypertension (4%) and supraventricular arrhythmia
- grade 4 arterial thromboembolitic events (<1%)
- bowel perforation, likely to be multifactorial (previous adjuvant radiotherapy, recent sigmoidoscopy or colonoscopy and primary tumor tract), which is rare but obviously severe, and warrants stopping bevacizumab treatment.

So far, patients with known proteinuria, deranged liver function, active or recent cardiovascular disease or cerebrovascular accident, recent major surgery, bleeding diathesis, coagulopathy or full-dose anticoagulation have been excluded from bevacizumab trials.

In the second-line setting, a phase II multicenter trial assessed the use of bevacizumab plus 5-FU/LV in patients with advanced refractory mCRC. Of the first 100 assessable patients, 4 had partial response and 50 stable disease. Four patients were not adequately assessed. The second phase of the trial opened then as a compassionate access so that the total patient number went up to 339, from which the median PFS was 3.7 months and the overall survival 9.1 months.

The frequency and severity of the side-effects previously described were obtained from this last group of patients (Chen *et al.* 2006).

In the first line, a phase III trial with 813 patients with mCRC compared 5-FU plus bevacizumab versus 5-FU plus placebo. The RRs were 44.8% and 34.8% respectively. The median duration of response was 10.4 months in the antibody arm, and 7.1 months in the placebo arm. Grade 3 hypertension appeared in 11% of patients treated with bevacizumab and in 2.3% of patients treated with placebo. The median duration of survival was 20.3 months and 15.6 months, respectively. The 1- year survival rate was 74.3% in the 5-FU/bevacizumab group and 63.4% in the 5-FU/placebo group (Hurwitz *et al.* 2004).

Bevacizumab has now been approved by the FDA in combination with chemotherapy in first and second treatment lines for metastatic colorectal cancer.

Preliminary data are available now on a phase II study of FOLFOX, bevacizumab and erlotinib (a tyrosine kinase inhibitor) as a first-line treatment for 35 mCRC patients. The main side-effects were rash, neuropathy and diarrhea; 51% withdrew due to adverse events, and 26% withdrew consent due to toxicity.

From the information available the RR was 34%, but PFS calculation was not possible (Meyerhardt *et al.* 2007).

Tyrosine kinase inhibitors (TKIs)

These small-molecule agents are administered orally and behave as ATP mimetics, competing for the binding site of the tyrosine kinase with ATP (Table 14.6). They have better tissue penetration, tumor retention and blood clearance, but their plasma concentrations tend to vary at a given dose between patients. Overall, small-molecule agents are less expensive and more convenient to administer than mAbs (Imai & Takaoka 2006).

Table 14.6 Tyrosine kinase inhibitors and targeted receptors.

EGFR inhibitor	VEGF inhibitor	EGFR and VEGF inhibitor
Gefitinib (ZD1839)	Sunitinib (SUO11248)	Sorefanib (BAY43–9006)
Erlotinib (OSI-774)	Vatalanib (PTK787/ZK222584)	
Lapatinib (ZD1839)	Recentin (AZD2171)	

Different molecules have been tested to block EGFR and VEGFR tyrosine kinases. Gefitinib (Iressa) and erlotinib (Tarceva) selectively inhibit EGFR. Sorefanib (Nexavar) inhibits Raf serine kinase, VEGFR, EGFR and PDGFR. Sunitinib malate (Sutent) is also multitargeted to inhibit VEGFR, PDGFR, KIT and FLT3. Lapatinib (Tykerb) reversibly and specifically inhibits both EGFR and ErbB2.

Erlotinib

Erlotinib is a small-molecule quinazolinamine that reversibly inhibits EGFR tyrosine kinase. It is continuously administered orally at 150 mg/day in 28-day cycles. Its most common side-effects are in keeping with EGFR blockade: rash, fatigue and diarrhea, although gastrointestinal toxicity is more common (up to 60% of patients) (Fownsley *et al.* 2006).

Monotherapy in solid tumors including refractory colorectal cancer has shown RRs of 8%, although results have been variable (Tabernero 2007). In a phase II study of single-agent erlotinib administered to 31 evaluable patients with mCRC, 39% had stable disease with a median time to progression of 123 days (4.1 months) (Meyerhardt 2006).

Another phase II study of erlotinib in 38 patients with unresectable or metastatic hepatocellular cancer (88% EGFR positive) showed 32% PFS at 6 months, disease control in 59% of patients with a median time to relapse of 3.8 months, and a median overall survival of 13 months. Dose reductions were mainly toxicity related (26%) and 34% had grade 3 toxicities: skin rash (13%), diarrhea (8%) and fatigue (8%).

A similar study on advanced biliary cancer patients with 42 patients (81% EGFR positive), also in the second-line setting, showed 17% PFS at 6 months, with three partial responses, all of which had skin rash. Disease control was achieved in 50% of patients with a median duration of 5.1 months (Fownsley *et al.* 2006).

No pharmacodynamic interactions have been found in combination with FOLFOX chemotherapy. Preliminary results from phase I and II studies of erlotinib combination with FOLFOX or XELOX in the second-line setting suggest beneficial effects in patients with esophageal or gastroesophageal junction cancer (RR up to 15%), but no activity in gastric cancer patients (Tabernero 2007).

Erlotinib is currently approved in several countries as a second-line treatment for metastatic non-small cell lung cancer, and in the first line with gemcitabine for pancreatic cancer.

Gefitinib

Gefitinib is a low molecular weight molecule anilinoquinazoline that reversibly inhibits EGFR tyrosine kinase. Monotherapy has failed to show clinical activity (objective clinical response) in two phase II trials in metastatic colorectal cancer patients (Rothenberg *et al.* 2005; Mackenzie *et al.* 2007).

In combination with FOLFOX it has shown beneficial effects in two other phase II trials, with RR of 74% and median time to progression of 9.5 months in the first-line setting, and RR of 23% and median time to progression of 5.2 months in the second-line setting (Fisher *et al.* 2004; Zampino *et al.* 2005).

Similar to erlotinib, gefitinib monotherapy has proven of value in esophageal and gastroesophageal junction cancer but not in gastric cancer (Tabernero 2007).

Vatalanib

Vatalanib is a small molecule that potently inhibits the VEGF-R2 intracellular tyrosine kinase as well as kinases of other VEGF receptors, platelet-derived growth factor and basic fibroblast growth factor. Theoretically that is an advantage over bevacizumab, which only inhibits the commonest receptor VEGF-A.

In phase I trials, vatalanib proved to be well tolerated, and although variability of the drug action was not defined in phase II studies, they were followed by two phase III trials: CONFIRM-1 and CONFIRM-2. Both assessed the combination of oxaliplatin and 5-FU with or without vatalanib, the first in the first-line setting, and the second in the second-line setting (Hecht *et al.* 2005). No significant benefit in PFS was demonstrated in any of them.

It is hypothesized that those results might be due to insufficient duration of receptor inhibition, insufficient dose in a proportion of the patients, or to adverse effects from inhibition of kinases other than VEGF-R2 (O'Dwyer 2006). More detailed analyses of tumor samples will be needed in further trials to find the answer.

In general terms, ongoing research is looking at the mechanisms that make mAbs more effective, the rationale for their different activity, why TKIs, unlike mAbs, do not seem to overcome chemoresistance or potentate the effects of radiotherapy, and overall, what is the best combination of mAbs and/or TKIs for each treatment line.

Other novel therapies

There are many other strategies to target cancer cells. The most obvious is to target molecules down the phosphorylation cascade that fuels the abnormal behaviour of cancer cells. We can distinguish those drugs according to the two phosphorylation cascades previously mentioned (Figs 14.12 & 14.13).

IP3/MAPK pathway

There are several drugs targeted to the same pathway at different levels. *MAPK/ERK kinase (MEK) inhibitors* (like AZD 6244) have proven initially disappointing, although the recent finding of exquisitely sensitive cell lines with B-raf mutations have increased the expectation of finding a role for them after genetic-based colorectal patient selection.

PI3K/Akt pathway

Small interfering RNA (siRNA) molecules suppress expression of target genes. Studies in animal models with siRNA targeted to PI3K pathway components showed hopeful results. It is thought that a combination of siRNA might potentiate the effect of standard chemotherapy.

Rapamycin is known to block mTOR and thus the PI3K pathway. However, despite full inhibition of S6, it causes Akt phosphorylation *in vitro*. In different cell lines, coadministration of erlotinib showed encouraging results in blocking rapamycin-stimulated Akt activity (Buck 2006; Nozawa 2007).

Other pathways like COX2, FAK and NO that are related to those two pathways are also being investigated.

New advances in cancer epigenetics are also providing interesting potential therapeutic targets. Epigenetics is the study of non-DNA sequence heritable information through potentially reversible promoter sequence and/or histone methylation or hypomethylation (Laird 2005). There are two main therapeutic groups.

1 DNA methyltransferase (DNMT) inhibitors, such as 5-aza-2′-deoxycytidine (5-aza-CdR), clinically referred to as *decitabine*, which can induce cytosine methylation and chromatin remodeling. It has a short half-life and cell divisions are required for its action. Myelosuppression is a major side-effect, although substantial improvement was found at low (5–2 mg/m^2/day) prolonged administration. *Zebularine* has a longer half-life. Another drug in this group is *MG98*, a phosphorothioate antisense oligodeoxynucleotide, a specific inhibitor of DNA methyltransferase mRNA. Phase II trials are ongoing.

2 Histone deacetylase (HDAC) inhibitors like *Trichostatin A* (TSA), which leads to hyperacetylation of histones and upregulation of cell cycle inhibitors, are effective even in non-proliferating tumor cells *in vitro*. Phase I and II trials are now under way for solid tumors (Miyamoto & Ushijima 2005).

Many other novel therapies are being investigated and their role is also uncertain (Morabito *et al.* 2006).

Individualizing therapy: prognostication and prediction

The present anatomic staging system is most useful in therapeutic decisions that involve local treatment.

New biologic targets can already help in diagnosing colorectal cancer by identifying tissue-specific molecular profiles, differentiating it from ovarian cancer in abdominal metastatic disease with an unknown primary. They can also help defining prediction of response to targeted treatments and can have a prognostic value.

Different strategies have been established to identify molecular abnormalities that could be used as markers with a possible role in screening, diagnosis, prognosis and treatment response prediction and monitoring (Ludwig & Weinstein 2005).

DNA techniques

DNA techniques identify changes within the DNA like silent nucleotide polymorphisms, chromosomal aberrations, changes in DNA copy number, microsatellite instability and promoter activation (methylation) status.

It has been reported that 70% of patients with CRC have lost part of chromosome 17q or 18q or both. 17q contains p53, which is mutated in 40–60% of CRC patients. When p53 was assessed by immunohistochemistry and polymerase chain reaction (PCR) single-stranded conformational polymorphism (SSCP), it did not prove to be an independent prognostic factor in early CRC; whereas its role as a predictive marker of response to 5-FU remains controversial.

On the other hand, loss of 18q or lack of its protein expression has proved to correlate with poor prognosis. Retention of both 18q alleles also correlated with better outcome after adjuvant 5-FU-based chemotherapy in stage III CRC. DPC4 and JV18–1 might have also prognostic significance.

Microsatellite instability (MSI) is present in 50–75% of sporadic colon cancers. The MSI-high (MSI-H) phenotype improves survival in stage II and III CRC by 22%. Moreover, MSI has proved to increase recurrence-free survival, and adjuvant chemotherapy does not seem to benefit these patients. MSI-H phenotype has also been associated with transforming growth factor beta (TGFβ) RII mutation (61% of stage III CRC), whose presence increases 5-year survival following adjuvant 5-FU by 28%.

Oncogene K-ras mutation is also present in 30% of CRC patients. More than 80% of cases of K-ras mutations are located in codons 12 and 13. K-ras mutation is associated with recurrence and poorer long-term survival, whereas valine mutation on codon 12 suggests more aggressive biologic behaviour.

In relation with prediction to response to oxaliplatin, ERCC1 is a protein involved in the cleavage of damaged DNA, and ERCC1 gene expression levels have shown significant independent correlation with overall survival after 5-FU/oxaliplatin therapy in refractory mCRC patients.

The XPD gene (also known as ERCC2) might also have a role in platinum drug resistance (Allen & Johnston 2005).

RNA-based techniques

RNA-based techniques like microarray techniques, involve converting RNA to cDNA with a reverse transcriptase and then performing PCR, so that gene profile expression can be established. Overexpressed and underexpressed transcripts can be correlated with prognosis and treatment response.

From a study of 204 CRC patients with minimum follow-up of 5 years gene profile expression was defined using oligonucleotide printed microarrays and Affymetrix arrays. When correlated they achieved prediction rates of 77% and 84% respectively. Despite the different technologies, both retained their prognostic power (Lin *et al.* 2007). The greatest challenge of this technique is to define the most predictive gene expression combination for each stage of disease. Current microarray research in CRC is still in the early stages.

Protein markers

Protein markers like cell receptors have been investigated in more depth, and it is known that EGFR and VEGF are poor prognostic markers. In a pivotal trial with 813 patients, VEGF and thrombospondin-2 expression, and microvessel density were not suggestive to predict response to bevacizumab treatment in patients with colorectal cancer (Jubb *et al.* 2006). EGFR expression is not a good predictor of EGFR inhibition response.

There are currently no markers to efficiently predict the benefit from EGFR-targeted therapy. That might be down to the immunohistochemical detection methods used, the different expression patterns within the same tumor, or the receptor functional state. In that respect, specific EGFR mutations and the measurement of downstream molecules like MAPK, PI3K, Akt, p27 and Stat3 could give a clue as to how functional the receptor is, and how likely the cancer is to overcome its inhibition by growth stimulation through other pathways.

Other protein markers are tumor antigens like carcinoembrionic antigen (CEA), phosphorylation states, carbohydrate determinants, and released peptides. Of those, only CEA is recommended preoperatively as a prognostic marker and postoperatively to monitor response of metastatic disease to systemic therapy (Locker *et al.* 2006). One recent development is evidence that topoisomerase 1 may be both a predictive and prognostic biomarker for CRC outcomes.

Functional molecular imaging

Functional molecular imaging is also gaining importance in prognostication. MRI, PET or optical imaging can be used to identify function and molecular expression distribution in different cancers.

Recent international guidelines describe the need for further studies on most of the mentioned techniques before they can be recommended in standard practice (Locker *et al.* 2006).

There is, therefore, not only a need to obtain more information on action mechanisms that would fully explain the clinical effects of novel therapies, but also a need to identify treatment response markers to establish what treatment is necessary (individualizing therapy), and a need to develop further prognostication techniques to determine when and if each treatment should be given.

References

Allen WL, Johnston PG. (2005) Role of genomic markers in colorectal cancer treatment. *J Clin Oncol* 23: 4545–52.

Borner M. *et al.* (2006) The impact of cetuximab on the capecitabine plus oxaliplatin (XELOX) combination in first-line treatment of metastatic colorectal cancer (MCC): A randomized phase II trial of the Swiss Group for Clinical Cancer Research (SAKK). *J Clin Oncol ASCO Annual Meeting Proceedings* 24, no. 18S: 3551.

Buck E. (2006) Rapamycin synergizes with EGFR inhibitor erlotinib in NSCLC, pancreatic, colon and breast tumors. *Mol Cancer Ther* 5(11): 2676–84.

Carlos L, Arteaga EGF. (2003) Receptor as a therapeutic target: patient selection and mechanisms of resistance to receptor-targeted drugs. *J Clin Oncol* 21: 289S–291S.

Cervantes A *et al.* (2007) *Optimal dose of cetuximab administered every 2 weeks: A phase I safety, pharmacokinetics (PK) and pharmacodynamics (PD) study of weekly and 2 weekly schedules in patients with metastatic colorectal cancer.* Abstract LB-352 presented at the AACR 2007.

Chen HX *et al.* (2006) Phase II multicenter trial of bevacizumab plus fluorouracil and leucovorin in patients with advanced refractory colorectal cancer: An NCI treatment referral center trial TRC-0301. *J Clin Oncol* 24: 3354–60.

Chung Y *et al.* (2005) Cetuximab shows activity in colorectal cancer patients with tumors that do not express the epidermal growth factor receptor by immunohistochemistry. *J Clin Oncol* 23: 1803–10.

Cohenuram M, Saif MW. (2007) Panitumumab the first fully human monoclonal antibody: from the bench to the clinic. *Anticancer Drugs* 18(1): 7–15.

Cunningham D *et al.* (2004) 'Cetuximab monotherapy and cetuximab plus irinotecan in irinotecan-refractory metastatic colorectal cancer. *N Engl J Med* 351: 337–45.

Ferrara N, Davis-Smyth T. (1997) The biology of vascular endothelial growth factor. *Endocrin Rev* 18(1): 4–25.

Fisher GA *et al.* (2004) A phase II study of gefitinib in combination with FOLFOX-4 (IFOX) in patients with metastatic colorectal cancer. *J Clin Oncol* 22: 248s.

Fownsley CA *et al.* (2006) Phase II study of erlotinib (OSI-774) in patients with metastatic colorectal cancer. *Br J Cancer* 94(8): 1136–43.

Giantonio BJ *et al.* (2007) Bevacizumab in combination with oxaliplatin, fluorouracil, and leucovorin (FOLFOX-4) for previously treated metastatic colorectal cancer: results from the Eastern Cooperative Oncology Group Study E3200. *J Clin Oncol* 25(12): 1539–44.

Gibson TN *et al.* (2006) Randomized phase III trial results of panitumumab, a fully human anti-epidermal growth factor receptor monoclonal antibody, in metastatic colorectal cancer. *Clin Colorectal Cancer* 6(1): 29–31.

Goffin JR, Talavera JR. (2006) Overstated conclusions of a Poole analysis of bevacizumab in colon cancer. *J Clin Oncol* 24(3): 528–9.

Hecht JR *et al.* (2005)A randomized, double-blind, placebo-controlled, phase III study in patients with metastatic adenocarcinoma of the colon or rectum receiving first-line chemotherapy with oxaliplatin/5-fluorouracil/leucovorin and PTK787/zk 222584 or placebo (CONFIRM-1). Presented at the 2005 Annual Meeting of the American Society of Clinical Oncology, Orlando, FL, May 13–17.

Hicklin DJ, Ellis LM. (2005) Role of the vascular endothelial growth factor pathway in tumor growth and angiogenesis. *J Clin Oncol* 23(5): 1011–27.

Hurwitz H *et al.* (2004) Bevacizumab plus irinotecan, fluorouracil, and leucovorin for metastatic colorectal cancer. *New Engl J Med* 350: 2335–42.

Imai K, Takaoka A. (2006) Comparing antibody and small-molecule therapies for cancer. *Nat Rev Cancer* 6: 714–27.

Jubb M *et al.* (2006) Impact of vascular endothelial growth factor-A expression, thrombospondin-2 expression, and microvessel density on the treatment effect of bevacizumab in metastatic colorectal cancer. *J Clin Oncol* 24(2): 217–27.

Kabbinavar F *et al.* (2005) Combined analysis of efficacy: the addition of bevacizumab to fluorouracil/leucovorin improves survival for patients with metastatic colorectal cancer. *J Clin Oncol* 23(16): 3706–12.

Kilickap S *et al.*(2003) Bevacizumab, bleeding, thrombosis, and warfarin. *J Clin Oncol* 21(18): 3542.

Laird PW. (2005) Cancer epigenetics. *Hum Mol Genet* 14, Review Issue 1: R65–R76.

Lenz H *et al.* (2007) Pharmacogenomic analysis of a randomized phase II trial (BOND 2) of cetuximab/bevacizumab/irinotecan (CBI) versus cetuximab/bevacizumab (CB) in irinotecan-refractory colorectal cancer. *ASCO* abstract no. 401.

Lin YH *et al.* (2007) Multiple gene expression classifiers from different array platforms predict poor prognosis of colorectal cancer. *Clin Cancer Res* 13(2 Pt 1): 498–507.

Locker GY *et al.* (2006) ASCO 2006 update of recommendations for the use of tumor markers in gastrointestinal cancer. *J Clin Oncol* 24(33): 5313–27.

Ludwig JA, Weinstein JN. (2005) Biomarkers in cancer staging, prognosis and treatment selection. *Nat Rev Cancer* 5, 845–56.

Mackenzie MJ *et al.* (2005) A phase II trial of ZD1839 (Iressa) 750mg per day, an oral epidermal growth factor receptor-tyrosine kinase inhibitor, in paitents with metastatic colorectal cancer. *Invest New Drugs* 23: 165–70.

Meira DD *et al.* (2007) Differences in activity between matuzumab and cetuximab in A431 cells may rely on MAPK cascade inhibition. Abstract #336 presented at the American Association for Cancer Research (AACR) 2007.

Mendelsohn J, Baselga J. (2003) Status of epidermal growth factor receptor antagonists in the biology and treatment of cancer. *J Clin Oncol* 21(14): 2787–99.

Meyerhardt JA. (2006) Phase II study of capecitabine, oxaliplatin, and erlotinib in previously treated patients with metastatic colorectal cancer. *J Clin Oncol* 24(12): 1892–7.

Meyerhardt J *et al.* (2007) Phase II study of FOLFOX, bevacizumab and erlotinib as first-line therapy for patients with metastatic colorectal cancer. *Ann Oncol* 18(7): 1185–9.

Miyamoto K, Ushijima T. (2005) Diagnostic and therapeutic application of epigenetics. *Jpn J Clin Oncol* 35(6): 293–301.

Morabito A *et al.* (2006) Tyrosine kinase inhibitors of vascular endothelial growth factor receptors in clinical trials: current status and future directions. *Oncologist* 11(7): 753–64.

Nozawa H. (2007) Phosphorylation of ribosomal p70S6 kinase and rapamycin sensitivity in human colorectal cancer. *Cancer Lett* 251(1): 105–13.

O'Dwyer PJ. (2006) The present and future of angiogenesis-directed treatments of colorectal cancer. *Oncologist* 11(9): 992–8.

Peeters M *et al.* (2006) A Phase III, multicentre, randomized controlled trial of panitumumab plus best supportive care (BSC) vs BSC alone in patients with metastatic colorectal cancer. *Proc Am Assoc Cancer Res* 47:A CP-1, abstr.

Rothenberg ML *et al.* (2005) Randomized phase II trial of the clinical and biological effects of two dose levels of gefitinib in patients with recurrent colorectal adenocarcinoma. *J Clin Oncol* 23: 9265–74.

Rubio D *et al.* (2005) Cetuximab in combination with oxaliplatin/5-fluorouracil (5-FU)/folinic acid (FA) (FOLFOX-4) in the first-line treatment of patients with epidermal growth factor receptor (EGFR)-expressing metastatic colorectal cancer: An international phase II study. *J Clin Oncol ASCO Annual Meeting Proceedings* Vol 23, no. 16S: 3535.

Sagaent S *et al.* (2005) Clinical signs, pathophysiology and management of skin toxicity during therapy with EGFR inhibitors. *Ann Oncol* 16(9): 1425–33.

Tabernero J. (2007) The role of VEGF and EGFR inhibition: implications for combining anti-VEGF and anti-EGFR agents. *Mol Cancer Res* 5: 203–20.

Tejpar *et al.* (2006) Dose-escalation study using up to twice the standard dose of cetuximab in patients with metastatic colorectal cancer (mCRC) with no or slight skin reactions on cetuximab standard dose treatment (EVEREST study): Preliminary data. *J Clin Oncol ASCO Annual Meeting Proceedings* Vol 24, No 18S: 3554.

Tong RT. (2004) Vascular normalization by VEGFR2 blockade induces a pressure gradient across the vasculature and improves drug penetration in tumors. *Cancer Res* 64: 3731–6.

Zampino MG *et al.* (2005) First-line Gefitinib combined with simplified FOLFOX-6 in patients with epidermal growth factor receptor-positive advanced colorectal cancer. *J Clin Oncol* 23: 285s.

Zhang W *et al.* (2006) Novel approaches to treatment of advanced colorectal cancer with anti-EGFR monoclonal antibodies. *Ann Med* 38(8): 545–51.

Stomas

Ann MacArthur & Julia Liddi

This section begins by looking at the role of the clinical nurse specialist, before focusing on stoma formation in relation to colorectal cancer and some of the potential physiologic complications that may occur. Stoma formation can have an immense impact on a patient's quality of life and it is vital that these patients have access to a clinical nurse specialist with stoma care expertise.

What is the role of the colorectal clinical nurse specialist?

The role of the clinical nurse specialist has many facets, incorporating competencies such as clinical practice, patient pathway coordination, management, consultation, education and research/audit (Marshall & Luffingham 1998). The hospital-based clinical nurse specialist in colorectal cancer can be dual-trained in stoma care as well as oncology; alternatively, the oncology clinical nurse specialist will work closely alongside specialist stoma care nurses in order to provide a high standard of holistic care to patients with colorectal cancer. Specialist nurse teams can vary depending on the size and location of hospitals and the needs of the local population.

Clinical nurse specialists have a pivotal role in the care of individuals with colorectal cancer and their families, providing information and support from diagnosis, throughout treatment and during follow-up or palliative care. NICE guidance from 2004 states that patients should be able to contact a clinical nurse specialist from the time of their diagnosis and that this should ensure continuity of care and practical help in dealing with the effects of colorectal cancer. The nurse specialist works as an autonomous practitioner with a caseload of patients, being an expert resource with a sound knowledge base and it is imperative that the care delivered is research-based and of a high standard.

To ensure a smooth pathway through various disciplines the nurse specialist liaises with other members of the MDT, acting as the patient's advocate when treatment decisions are being made. They also communicate frequently with primary care teams, particularly in the light of recent government guidelines such as the 2-week wait system. The recommendation that patients with certain symptoms are investigated promptly and within 2 weeks of referral from their GP puts the nurse specialist at the center of the patient care pathway, coordinating further referrals to appropriate specialities and informing GPs of relevant diagnoses.

Education and sharing of expertise are paramount in the role of the clinical nurse specialist. The teaching of patients, their families and generalist colleagues on all aspects of stoma care and colorectal cancer is pivotal to providing optimal overall care. In addition, the empowering and motivation of ward nurses, clinic staff and primary care teams that the nurse specialist can engender allows the building of good working relationships and a more cohesive network of professionals.

In order to provide up-to-date care, the clinical nurse specialist should be actively involved in the auditing of services and setting of standards and protocols. It is very important that the results of audit are incorporated into standard practice, and the clinical nurse specialist can facilitate this by acting as a change agent and adapting practice appropriately (Rose *et al.* 2006).

All you need to know about stomas

A major part of the role of the clinical nurse specialist in colorectal cancer involves caring for patients with stomas. The number of patients requiring a permanent stoma has decreased with advances in surgical management. Restorative resections, conserving the anal sphincter, are performed whenever possible, even in the case of low rectal tumors. However, as a result, there has been a rise in the number of temporary stomas, most commonly the loop ileostomy.

A loop stoma is generally formed for diversion or palliation. An end stoma is generally formed in association with a Hartman's procedure or an abdominoperineal excision of rectum. There are two main types of fecal stoma: A colostomy is most commonly formed in the sigmoid colon. The stoma should be red, moist and fairly flush to the skin. The output is generally formed stool and patients usually wear a 'closed' appliance, which they change, on average, twice daily. An ileostomy is most commonly formed in the terminal ileum. The stoma should be red, moist and spouted. The output varies from liquid to porridge-like consistency and is extremely corrosive to skin, as it contains proteolytic enzymes. A 'drainable' appliance is worn, enabling the patient to empty it several times during the day. On average 500–700 mL of effluent is passed daily (Cushiere *et al.* 1995). As a rough guide, this equates to the patient emptying the bag approximately four or five times daily.

Stoma complications

High stoma output

High stoma output is most commonly seen in patients with an ileostomy and can cause rapid depletion of water and sodium and a subsequent state of dehydration. High output needs to be dealt with promptly and effectively; if not the outcome can be renal failure and ultimately death (Cottam 2003). The most important facet of treatment is restoration of fluid and electrolyte balance. In general, intravenous methods are required, but sometimes oral supplementation may suffice. Antidiarrheal medication should be commenced. These are most effective taken 30–60 minutes before meals, which will facilitate absorption before the gut is stimulated by the presence of food. Encourage foods low in soluble fiber and high in starch, which will avoid intestinal irritability and facilitate sodium and water absorption such as rice, mashed potatoes, bread and bananas. Foods that contain gelatine help to firm stoma output.

Isotonic fluids should be encouraged in place of hypotonic. An accurate fluid balance should be monitored on a daily basis, as should the patient's serum sodium, normal values being 134–145 mol/L. A high-output appliance may be used, which can be attached to a drainage system. This will keep the patient comfortable and avoid overfilling and possible leakage from their usual appliance and also facilitate accurate monitoring of their output.

Parastomal herniae

Most parastomal hernias occur within 2 years of stoma formation and the incidence rate varies depending on the type of stoma (Carne *et al.* 2003). The risk factors for developing a hernia include age, obesity, previous hernia repair and possibly smoking (McGrath *et al.* 2006). Potential complications related to parastomal hernia include mechanical bowel obstruction, bowel incarceration, perforation, appliance leakage and subsequent peristomal skin soreness. The hernia presents as a complete or partial bulge around the immediate peristomal area. This may reduce when the patient is lying and increase when sitting/standing (Fig. 14.14).

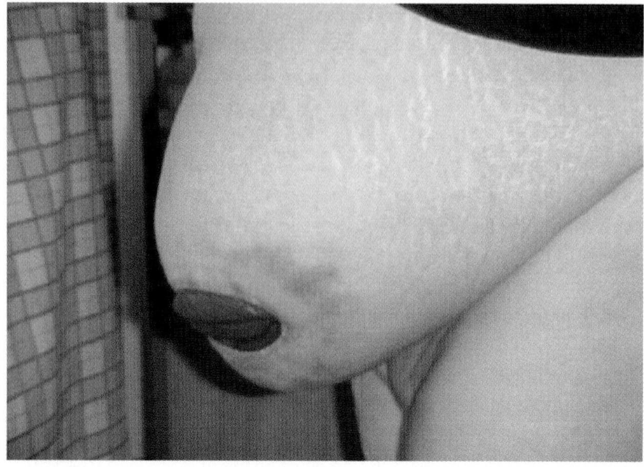

Fig. 14.14 A parastomal hernia.

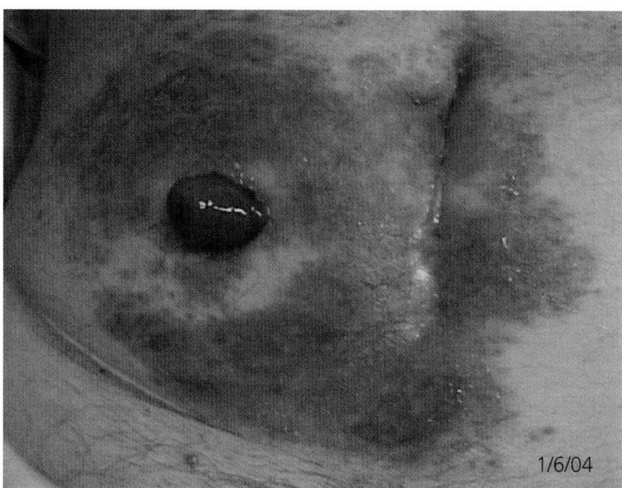

Fig. 14.15 Peristomal skin soreness.

In some cases when the hernia is only minimal with no complications, the hernia may be managed conservatively. A surgical support garment can reduce the effect of weak abdominal muscles and provide support. These are specifically designed for stoma patients and aim not to compromise stoma function. However, when the hernia causes complications, surgical intervention may be necessary.

Peristomal skin soreness

Sore skin, particularly from stoma effluent, is the most common cause of peristomal skin problems and affects up to two-thirds of all stoma patients at some time (Fig. 14.15) (Lyon & Smith 2001). Identifying risk factors for the occurrence of peristomal skin complications can help optimize assessment and management approaches. Treatment can be based upon etiology; for example chemical injury (irritant contact dermatitis), mechanical injury (pressure/shearing, stripping, mucocutaneous separation), infection (*Candida*, folliculitis), and disease-related lesions (varices, pyoderma gangrenosum, malignancy). It is extremely important to first elicit the cause for the skin soreness in order to implement the effective treatment. Careful assessment by the clinical nurse specialist before treatment is recommended cannot be overemphasized. Treatments will generally include topical application of specialist stoma skin preparations (e.g. seals, pastes, powders, skin barriers) to help promote a healing environment.

Stoma retraction

Retraction occurs when the stoma is drawn or pulled back below skin level; this may be partial or complete. Approximately 25% of patients will develop retraction (Arumugam *et al.* 2003). Retraction can occur early in the postoperative phase or as a later complication. Postoperative stoma retraction results secondary to poor surgical stoma construction. This may be because of insufficient stomal length, tension on the mesentery, inadequate fixation of the bowel to the peritoneum, or secondary to abdominal anomalies such as thickened abdominal wall due to edema, abdominal distension or obesity. Retraction as a later complication may be the result of weight gain.

The aim of managing a retracted stoma is to maintain a secure leak-free seal between the appliance and skin. There are specifically designed convex appliances and stoma accessories available to deal with this, which should only be used after careful assessment by the clinical nurse specialist.

Stoma prolapse

Stoma prolapse can happen at any time and is more prevalent with loop stomas. Prolapse etiology may involve difficulties with stoma construction; for example, creating an excessively large opening in the abdominal wall for an edematous bowel, which will be larger than necessary as the edema subsides, or inadequate fixation of the bowel to the abdominal wall. A larger appliance will be necessary to accommodate the stoma, which may also be edematous. The patient needs to observe the stoma for signs of ischemia and obstruction and to report any changes in colour or bowel function.

Some prolapses can be manually reduced and gently manipulated back into the body. This is done by the patient lying down to decrease intra-abdominal pressure and continuously applying a gentle pressure to the stoma. If the stoma is edematous, applying a cold compress or sugar/salt application (osmotic therapy) for 30 minutes before reduction reduces the edema, allowing the stoma to be gently manipulated back in (Fligelstone *et al.* 1997). A stoma shield may be worn over the appliance with the aim of keeping the prolapse in. If the patient cannot tolerate the prolapse, or if further complications develop, surgical repair may be undertaken.

Summary

Stoma complications can occur at any time and it is vital that the advice of clinical nurse specialists is sought. With their specialist knowledge and expertise, they can help to greatly improve the patient's quality of life.

References

Arumugam P, Bevan L, Macdonald L *et al.* (2003) A prospective audit of stomas—analysis of risk factors and complications and their management. *Colorectal Dis* 5(1): 49–52.

Carne PW, Robertson GM, Frizelle FA. (2003) Parastomal hernia. *Br J Surg* 90(7): 784–93.

Cottam J. (2003) The high output ileostomy following rectal resection: Why it happens and how it should be managed. *Gastrointest Nurs* 1(7): 19–23.

Cuschiere A, Giles GR, Moosa AR. (1995) *Essential Surgical Practice*, 3rd edn. Butterworth Heinemann, Oxford.

Fligelstone L *et al.* (1997). Osmotic therapy for acute irreducible stoma prolapse. *Br J Surg* 84(3): 390.

Lyon C, Smith A. (2001) *Abdominal Stomas and their Skin Disorders. An Atlas of Diagnosis and Management.* Martin Dunitz, London.

Marshall Z, Luffingham N. (1998) Does the specialist nurse enhance or deskill the general nurse? *Br J Nursing* 7(11).

McGrath A, Porrett T, Heyman B. (2006) Parastomal hernia: and exploration of the risk factors and the implications. *Br J Nursing* 15(6): 317–21.

National Institute for Health and Clinical Excellence (NICE). (2004) *Healthcare services for bowel (colorectal) cancer.* Understanding NICE guidance – information for the public. National Institute for Health and Clinical Excellence, London.

Rose SB, All AC, Gresham D. Role preservation of the clinical nurse specialist practitioner. *Internet J Adv Nursing Pract* ISSN: 1523–6064.

Answers to case scenarios

Omar Khan, Rachel S. Midgley & Andrew Weaver

We hope that you have now read and absorbed all of the sections in this chapter. You should now be able to answer all of the questions that we posed in the first section. If you are still struggling, please read through the responses given below, which will act as a revision summary for you.

Case 1: adjuvant chemotherapy

The rationale for use of adjuvant chemotherapy in colon cancer is to eradicate clinically occult micrometastatic disease that is present at the time of surgery. It is recommended that all patients with stage III disease (nodal disease present) should be offered adjuvant chemotherapy to reduce the risk of recurrence and improve overall survival. The benefit of chemotherapy in patients with resected stage II cancer is less clear.

Early regimes consisting of 5-FU monotherapy did not show improved 5- year survival (Buyse *et al.* 1990). The discovery of 5-FU activity modulators such as folinic acid (FA) and levamisole (an antihelminthic with immunomodulatory properties) as well as reports of benefits seen with combination regimes containing 5-FU led to a reappraisal of the role of 5-FU in the adjuvant setting in colon cancer. In 1990, an NIH consensus conference established adjuvant 5-FU-containing chemotherapy (either with FA or levamisole) as the standard of care for resected stage III colon cancer (NIH 1990).

The use of levamisole has now declined as studies have shown that in combination with 5-FU, it is inferior to FA (Wolmark *et al.* 1999). In addition, weekly bolus 5-FU and higher-dose FA is thought to be less toxic than a 5-day bolus regime with low-dose FA (Mayo regime). There is no significant difference in effectiveness and the optimum duration of treatment with this regime seems to be 6 months (Haller *et al.* 2005).

The orally active fluoropyrimidines, capecitabine and uracil tegafur (UFT), are much more convenient for the patient and less labor-intensive for units delivering chemotherapy. Capecitabine is absorbed through the intestinal wall and converted to 5-FU in enzymatic reactions including thymidine phosphorylase. This enzyme is present in higher levels in tumor and there is theoretically better selectivity for tumor cells. Trials have confirmed that 6 months of capecitabine monotherapy is at least as effective as 5-FU/FA with less toxicity other than hand–foot syndrome (Twelves *et al.* 2005). Similar results have been seen with UFT (Lembersky *et al.* 2006).

More recently, oxaliplatin and irinotecan have been studied in the adjuvant setting. Benefit from adding oxaliplatin to 5-FU/FA adjuvant chemotherapy was first demonstrated in the MOSAIC trial (Andre *et al.* 2004). This trial randomized 2246 patients with completely resected stage II (40%) or III (60%) to 6 months of the following regimes.

1 Short-term infusional 5-FU/FA administered according to the de Gramont regime (LV 200 mg/m^2 as a 2-hour infusion, followed by bolus 5-FU 400 mg/m^2 and then a 22-hour infusion of 5-FU 600 mg/m^2 on two consecutive days).

2 The same regime with oxaliplatin (85 mg/m^2 day 1 every 14 days) – FOLFOX4.

After a median follow-up of 38 months, 3-year disease-free survival (DFS) was significantly higher with FOLFOX (78% vs 73%). In patients with stage II disease there was no significant difference. Overall survival (OS) benefit has also not been seen so far. Toxicity was greater with FOLFOX but not considered to be prohibitive to its use. The FOLFOX regime has been approved for use in the adjuvant treatment of stage III colon cancer in the USA and more recently in the UK. Studies of irinotecan-containing regimes have not so far shown any benefit on DFS with greater toxicity and therefore their use in the adjuvant setting cannot be recommended.

In resected stage II colon cancer the benefits of adjuvant chemotherapy are less clear. Most trials have shown either a trend towards improved DFS and OS or no benefit. The American Society of Clinical Oncology (ASCO) guidelines for adjuvant therapy in colorectal cancer issued in 2004 recommended against routine administration of 5-FU-based chemotherapy in stage II disease (Benson *et al.* 2004). Adjuvant therapy may have a role in patients with poor prognosis risk factors such as T4 lesions, perforation, poorly differentiated histology, inadequately sampled lymph nodes, and vascular or lymphatic invasion. There is also controversy over which regime to use. Although the FOLFOX regime in the MOSAIC trial was shown to be superior to 5-FU/FA and the trial included stage II patients, it was not adequately powered to compare the efficacy of chemotherapy separately. Current practice is to offer 5-FU/FA or capecitabine monotherapy to the majority of patients but offer high-risk, young patients the FOLFOX regime.

There is interest in novel targeted agents based on their effectiveness in the metastatic setting. A number of trials are ongoing exploring their role in the adjuvant setting including the QUASAR II trial (capecitabine alone or in combination with bevacizumab).

Case 2: preoperative therapy in rectal cancer

Most patients with rectal cancer have deeply invasive cancers requiring extensive surgery. Tumors of the upper and middle third of the rectum can usually be managed by undertaking an anterior resection, coloanal anastomosis and preservation of the anal sphincter. Preservation of the pelvic autonomic nerves using the technique of total mesorectal excision can reduce the risk of sexual and urinary dysfunction. Tumors of the distal rectum are considerably more challenging in terms of local tumor control and preservation of the anal sphincter. Abdominoperineal resection (APR) is the standard operation for tumors with a distal edge up to 6 cm from the anal verge. The disadvantages of APR are the need for a permanent colostomy and damage to pelvic nerves leading to a high incidence of urinary and sexual dysfunction.

Preoperative radiotherapy and combined chemotherapy and radiotherapy are utilized to 'downstage' or 'downsize' larger (T3 or T4) tumors of the distal rectum in an attempt to avoid APR and enable a sphincter-sparing procedure or to increase the chance of obtaining clear resection margins (i.e. an R0 resection). Preoperative treatment is also increasingly used for proximal rectal tumors that are large, locally invasive or clinically node positive.

Accurate staging is essential for all patients being considered for sphincter-sparing procedures. Endoscopic rectal ultrasound and MRI scanning are considered to have greater accuracy than CT scanning. CT scanning is performed to detect distant metastatic disease.

A landmark Swedish study published in 1997 demonstrated a survival benefit and improved local control for a short course of high-dose radiotherapy (25 Gy in five fractions) used preoperatively in patients with rectal cancer (SRCT 1997). Longer term toxicity of gastrointestinal disorders such as bowel obstruction and abdominal pain was significantly greater in patients who had received radiotherapy compared with those not receiving radiotherapy. Two meta-analyses have shown reduction in local recurrence with preoperative radiotherapy but overall survival was improved in only one of the analyses (Camma *et al.* 2000; CCCG 2001).

A randomized trial comparing radiotherapy alone (45 Gy over 5 weeks) against concomitant 5-FU and folinic acid given in the first and final week of treatment in patients with T3/4 rectal cancer has demonstrated improved pathologic complete remission (pCR) in the combined treatment arm (Gerard *et al.* 2005). There was also a significantly lower local recurrence rate but overall survival was similar.

Similar results were seen in a trial that utilized the same chemotherapy and radiotherapy regime but also randomized patients to receive adjuvant chemotherapy using 5-FU and folinic acid or no adjuvant treatment (Bosset *et al.* 2005). The impact of chemotherapy was to reduce local recurrence but no impact on overall survival was seen. There is no conclusive evidence that postoperative chemotherapy with 5-FU/FA improves outcomes in patients who have had preoperative chemoradiotherapy but there was a trend towards improved PFS in the group of patients who had received adjuvant chemotherapy.

A German study investigated the effects of preoperative compared to postoperative chemoradiotherapy (50.4 Gy in 28 daily fractions with concurrent infusional 5-FU in the first and last week of treatment) (Sauer *et al.* 2004). There was a lower pelvic relapse rate and increased likelihood of undergoing a sphincter-sparing operation in patients who received preoperative treatment. Disease-free and overall survival rates were similar. The fear that preoperative treatment may lead to greater operative morbidity was not borne out in this trial. The role of oral fluoropyrimidines as a replacement for intravenous 5-FU is under investigation.

Case 3

Most patients with colorectal cancer present with apparently resectable localized disease but about half develop disseminated advanced disease and ultimately most will die from it. In such cases, providing the patient is fit enough, most are offered palliative chemotherapy. There is also occasionally a role for palliative surgery and radiotherapy. The main aims of these palliative treatments are to improve symptoms, quality of life and survival.

Over the last 5 years a number of new chemotherapeutic agents have become available that have significantly altered the management of advanced colorectal cancer. The key component of treatment remains 5-FU. Newer agents include the topoisomerase I inhibitor irinotecan, the third-generation platinum compound oxaliplatin, and the oral fluoropyrimidines capecitabine and uracil tegafur (UFT). In addition, two humanized monoclonal antibodies that target vascular endothelial growth factor (bevacizumab) and the epidermal growth factor receptor (cetuximab) have become available.

Systemic chemotherapy has been shown to improve median OS and PFS even though 5-year survival rates have not changed significantly. 5-FU combined with the biomodulator folinic acid (FA) increases the response rate (RR) compared to 5-FU alone (21 vs 11%) and confers a small but significant survival advantage (11.7 vs 10.5 months) (Thirion *et al.* 2004). Continuous infusional 5-FU also has superior efficacy and less toxicity than bolus treatment (Meta-analysis Group in Cancer 1998a,b).

Capecitabine and UFT offer the convenience of oral delivery as well as response rates similar to those seen with 5-FU/FA. Capecitabine has been shown to have a higher RR and similar median time to progression (TTP) and OS to 5-FU/FA (Van Cutsem *et al.* 2004). It has also been shown to have lower overall toxicity.

Two pivotal phase III trials have demonstrated a survival benefit for irinotecan in combination with 5-FU/FA (Douillard *et al.* 2000; Saltz *et al.* 2000). A European trial investigated infusional 5-FU/FA regimens and a US trial investigated a bolus 5-FU/FA regimen. The addition of irinotecan conferred a significant clinical benefit in terms of RR, PFS and OS compared to 5-FU/FA alone. There was greater toxicity in the regimens involving bolus 5-FU/FA and irinotecan, especially grade 3/4 neutropenia and diarrhea. Excessive mortality was also noted with this combination, with most patients dying from a similar combination of dehydration, neutropenia and sepsis (Sargent *et al.* 2001).

Two pivotal phase III trials demonstrated an improvement in RR and median PFS but not OS using oxaliplatin in combination with 5-FU/FA compared to 5-FU/FA alone (de Gramont *et al.* 2000; Giacchetti *et al.* 2000). Dose-limiting toxicities include neurotoxicity and neutropenia. A late-onset cumulative sensory neuropathy can occur which usually improves rapidly once the drug is stopped.

Oxaliplatin combined with infusional 5-FU/FA (FOLFOX) was compared to irinotecan combined with bolus 5-FU/FA (IFL) in patients with previously untreated metastatic colorectal cancer (Goldberg *et al.* 2004). The results suggest that FOLFOX is the superior regimen but it is known that bolus 5-FU is not as efficacious as infusional 5-FU so criticisms have been levelled at the validity of this comparison.

In a crossover study patients were randomized to receive either FOLFOX or irinotecan and infusional 5-FU/FA (FOLFIRI) until disease progression or unacceptable toxicity and then switched to the other regime (Tournigrand *et al.* 2004). Median overall survival was similar in both arms; 21.5 months in arm A (FOLFIRI followed by FOLFOX) and 20.6 months in arm B (FOLFOX followed by FOLFIRI). More patients in arm B had their metastatic disease rendered operable. One of the most important observations was in both arms the median overall survival was greater than 20 months.

A pivotal study in which patients who had progressed during or immediately after irinotecan-based therapy and then were randomized to receive either irinotecan plus cetuximab or cetuximab alone, demonstrated improved RR and TTP for the combination therapy arm (Cunningham *et al.* 2004). This has led to its approval in Europe and the US for use in combination with irinotecan as second-line therapy in colorectal cancer patients in whom prior irinotecan treatment has failed.

Bevacizumab has been investigated in combination with irinotecan/bolus 5-FU/FA in a placebo-controlled trial (Hurwitz *et al.* 2004). There was improved overall survival, RR and PFS. First-line use with oxaliplatin has been investigated in the TREE-1 and TREE-2 trials. The TREE-1 study compared FOLFOX, oxaliplatin/bolus 5-FU/FA, and capecitabine and oxaliplatin (CAPOX). TREE-2 was initiated once bevacizumab was approved and the addition of bevacizumab has shown improvement in RR and median TTP in all arms of the study (Hochster *et al.* 2006).

Case 4

Hepatic metastatic disease from colorectal cancer is common and in about one-third of patients with metastatic disease, the liver is the only site of disease. In such cases, regional treatment can be considered as an alternative to systemic chemotherapy. The options include surgical resection, local tumor ablation, regional hepatic intra-arterial chemotherapy or chemoembolization.

The only potentially curative option for patients with isolated liver metastases is surgical resection. After resection, mean 5- year relapse-free survival is about 33% (Registry of Hepatic Metastases 1988). However, less than a fifth of patients with isolated liver metastases are amenable to resection.

There is no consensus on optimal patient selection. Most liver surgeons would agree that the following criteria define absolute unresectability:

- extrahepatic disease
- surgically unfit patient
- involvement of >50% or four segments of the liver.

There should also be no radiologic evidence of main portal vein, major bile duct and hepatic artery involvement. It is also essential that there is adequate post-resection hepatic functional reserve.

There are a number of adverse prognostic factors in patients who undergo resection for liver metastases:

- initially node-positive colorectal cancer
- disease-free interval of less than 12 months
- more than one liver metastasis
- any metastasis greater than 5 cm in size
- a carcinoembryonic antigen (CEA) level greater than 200.
- positive resection margin.

PET is increasingly used to identify occult extrahepatic disease as well as defining the extent of liver metastases. In an analysis of six trials, sensitivity and specificity of PET scans were significantly better for hepatic and extrahepatic disease when compared to CT scans (Wiering *et al.* 2005). Interpretation of PET scans in patients scanned soon after chemotherapy can be difficult due to decreased cellular metabolic activity of the tumor. Restaging PET scans should be interpreted with caution if performed soon after chemotherapy.

In patients who may be initially deemed unresectable, 'down-staging' chemotherapy is routinely offered to increase the chance of the tumor becoming resectable. Between 12 and 22% of patients initially deemed unresectable become resectable and 5-year survival rates average 30–35%. The chemotherapy regimes used most frequently are oxaliplatin or irinotecan based, usually with 5-FU and folinic acid.

There is some concern that chemotherapy with these agents may cause hepatotoxicity. There has been an increased incidence of non-alcoholic steatohepatitis (NASH) and sinusoidal dilatation with irinotecan and oxaliplatin respectively. Patients with NASH have significantly higher 90-day mortality than those without (Vauthey *et al.* 2006).

In patients who are not surgical candidates, options include systemic chemotherapy, regional tumor ablation and regional chemotherapy via the hepatic artery.

Lesions that are amenable to surgical resection also lend themselves to ablative treatments. Radiofrequency ablation (RFA) produces localized tumor destruction by heating the soft tissues in the vicinity of the RFA electrode. Local recurrence rates after RFA of colorectal cancer liver metastases range from 0 to 39% with surgical approaches having lower rates of recurrence than percutaneous ones (Decadt & Siriwardena 2004).

Long-term outcomes are difficult to assess as most published trials have limited follow-up. A prospective trial in which 135 patients underwent laparoscopic RFA demonstrated a median survival of 29 months (Berber *et al.* 2005). Patients with lower pretreatment CEA levels, tumor size less than 5 cm and fewer than three tumors had significantly better survival. Data on the use of post RFA chemotherapy were not provided by the authors and it is likely that some of the prolonged survival was due to salvage chemotherapy.

While there are no prospective comparisons between RFA and open resection of liver metastases from colorectal cancer, a small retrospective analysis showed that median survival for patients treated by RFA was 37 months versus 41 months for those treated by resection (Oshowo *et al.* 2003).

RFA has low morbidity and mortality. A recent meta-analysis of 95 published series reported a complication rate of 8.9% (Mulier *et al.* 2002). There is a risk of portal vein thrombosis, damage to the biliary tree, perforation of adjacent organs, liver abscess and hemorrhage.

Liver macrometastases derive most of their blood supply from the hepatic arterial circulation and normal hepatocytes are supplied primarily by the portal system. Hepatic intra-arterial chemotherapy (HIAC), administered via a hepatic artery catheter, enables the delivery of cytotoxic agents to the tumor with relative sparing of normal liver tissue. A much greater concentration of drug can be achieved, and due to first-pass metabolism, the actual systemic effects can be minimized.

Early phase III trials demonstrated only a trend towards improved survival; there was considerable toxicity from the agent used (floxuridine) as well as surgical complications including catheter dislodgement and gastrointestinal misperfusion (Hohn *et al.* 1986). There have been improvements in the technique of pump placement as well as increased use of less hepatotoxic drugs such as mitomycin and mitoxantrone (Link *et al.* 2001). Recently, a number of early phase trials have reported some success using intrahepatic arterial oxaliplatin and irinotecan.

References

Andre T, Boni C, Mounedji-Boudiaf L *et al.* (2004) Oxaliplatin, fluorouracil, and leucovorin as adjuvant treatment for colon cancer. *N Engl J Med* 350: 2343–51.

Benson A III, Schrag D, Somerfield M *et al.* (2004) American Society of Clinical Oncology recommendations on adjuvant chemotherapy for stage II colon cancer. *J Clin Oncol* 22: 3408–19.

Berber E, Pelley R, Siperstein A. (2005) Predictors of survival after radiofrequency thermal ablation of colorectal cancer metastases to the liver: a prospective study. *J Clin Oncol* 23: 1358–64.

Bosset J, Calais G, Mineur L *et al.* (2005) Enhanced tumoricidal effect of chemotherapy with preoperative radiotherapy for rectal cancer: preliminary results—EORTC 22921. *J Clin Oncol* 23: 5620.

Buyse M, Zeleniuch-Jacquotte A, Chalmers T. (1988) Adjuvant therapy of colorectal cancer. Why we still don't know. *JAMA* 259: 3571–8.

Camma C, Giunta M, Fiorica F *et al.* (2000) Preoperative radiotherapy for respectable rectal cancer: A meta-analysis. *JAMA* 284: 1008–15.

CCCG. (2001) Adjuvant radiotherapy for rectal cancer: A systematic overview of 8507 patients from 22 randomised trials. Colorectal Cancer Collaborative Group. *Lancet* 358: 1291–1304.

Cunningham D, Humblet Y, Siena S *et al.* (2004) Cetuximab monotherapy and cetuximab plus irinotecan in irinotecan-refractory metastatic colorectal cancer. *N Engl J Med* 351: 337–45.

Decadt B, Siriwardena A. (2004) Radiofrequency ablation of liver tumours: systematic review. *Lancet Oncol* 5: 550–60.

de Gramont A, Figer A, Seymour M *et al.* (2000) Leucovorin and fluorouracil with or without oxaliplatin as first line treatment in advanced colorectal cancer. *J Clin Oncol* 18: 2938–47.

Douillard J, Cunningham D, Roth A *et al.* (2000) Irinotecan combined with fluorouracil alone as first-line treatment for metastatic colorectal cancer: an multicentre randomised trial. *Lancet* 355: 1041–7.

Gerard J, Bonnetain F, Conroy T *et al.* (2005) Preoperative (preop) radiotherapy (RT) + 5FU/folinic acid (FA) in T3–4 rectal cancers: results of the FFCD 9203 randomized trial (abstract). *J Clin Oncol* 23: 247s.

Giacchetti S, Perpoint B, Zidani R *et al.* (2000) Phase III multicenter randomized trial of oxaliplatin added to chronomodulated fluorouracil-leucovorin as first-line treatment of metastatic colorectal cancer. *J Clin Oncol* 18: 136–47.

Goldberg R, Sargent D, Morant R *et al.* (2004) A randomized controlled trial of fluorouracil plus leucovorin, irinotecan and oxaliplatin combinations in patients with previously untreated metastatic colorectal cancer. *J Clin Oncol* 22: 23–30.

Haller D, Catalano P, Macdonald J *et al.* (2005) Phase III study of fluorouracil, leucovorin, and levamisole in high-risk stage II and III colon cancer: final report of Intergroup 0089. *J Clin Oncol* 23: 8671–8.

Hochster H, Hart L, Ramanathan R *et al.* (2006) TREE Study (TREE-2 cohort): TTP and TTF for three bevacizumab and oxaliplatin-fluorpyrimidine regimens. *ASCO Gastrointest Cancer Symp* Abstr 244.

Hohn D, Rayner A, Economou J *et al.* (1986) Toxicities and complications of implanted pump hepatic arterial and intravenous fluxoridine infusion. *Cancer* 57: 465–70.

Hurwitz H, Fehrenbacher L, Novotny W *et al.* (2004) Bevacizumab plus irinotecan, fluorouracil, and leucovorin for metastatic colorectal cancer. *N Engl J Med* 350: 2335–42.

Lembersky B, Wieand H, Petrelli N *et al.* (2006) Oral uracil and tegafur plus leucovorin compared with intravenous fluourouracil and leucovorin in stage II and III carcinoma of the colon: results from National Surgical Adjuvant Breast and Bowel Project Protocol C-06. *J Clin Oncol* 24: 2059–6.

Link K, Sunelaitis E, Kornmann M *et al.* (2001) Regional chemotherapy of nonresectable colorectal liver metastases with mitoxantrone, 5-fluorouracil, folinic acid and mitomycin C may prolong survival. *Cancer* 92: 2746–53.

Meta-analysis Group in Cancer. (1998a) Efficacy of intravenous continuous infusion of fluorouracil compared with bolus administration in advanced colorectal cancer. *J Clin Oncol* 16: 1555–63.

Meta-analysis Group in Cancer. (1998b) Toxicity of fluorouracil in patients with advanced colorectal cancer: effect of administration schedule and prognostic factors. *J Clin Oncol* 16: 3537–41.

Mulier S, Mulier P, Ni Y *et al.* (2002) Complications of radiofrequency coagulation of liver tumors. *Br J Surg* 89: 1206–22.

NIH consensus conference. (1990) Adjuvant therapy for patients with colon and rectal cancer. *JAMA* 264: 1444–50.

Oshowo A, Gillams A, Harrison E *et al.* (2003) Comparison of resection and radiofrequency ablation for treatment of solitary colorectal liver metastases. *Br J Surg* 90: 1240–3.

Registry of Hepatic Metastases. (1988) Resection of the liver for colorectal carcinoma metastases: a multi-institutional study of indications for resection. *Surgery* 103: 278–88.

Saltz L, Cox J, Blanke C *et al.* (2000) Irinotecan plus fluorouracil and leucovorin for metastatic colorectal cancer. Irinotecan Study Group. *N Engl J Med* 343: 905–14.

Sargent D, Niedswiecki D, O'Connell M *et al.* (2001) Recommendations for caution with irinotecan, fluorouracil, and leucovorin for colorectal cancer. *N Engl J Med* 345: 144–5.

Sauer R, Becker H, Hohenberger W *et al.* (2004) Preoperative versus postoperative chemoradiotherapy for rectal cancer. *N Engl J Med* 351: 1731–40.

SRCT. (1997) Improved survival with preoperative radiotherapy in respectable rectal cancer. Swedish Rectal Cancer Trial. *N Engl J Med* 336: 980–7.

Thirion P, Michiels S, Pignon J *et al.* (2004) Modulation of fluorouracil by leucovorin in patients with advanced colorectal cancer: an updated meta-analysis. *J Clin Oncol* 22: 3766–75.

Tournigrand C, Andre T, Achille E. (2004) FOLFIRI followed by FOLFOX6 or the reverse sequence in advanced colorectal cancer: a randomised GERCOR study. *J Clin Oncol* 22: 229–37.

Twelves C, Wong A, Nowacki M *et al.* (2005) Capecitabine as adjuvant treatment for stage III colon cancer. *N Engl J Med* 352: 2696–704.

Van Cutsem E, Hoff P, Harper P *et al.* (2004) Oral capecitabine vs intravenous 5-fluourouracil and leucovorin: integrated efficacy data and novel analyses from two large, randomosed, phase III trials. *Br J Cancer* 90: 1190–7.

Vauthey J, Pawlik T, Ribero D *et al.* (2006) Chemotherapy regimen predicts steatohepatitis and an increase in 90-day mortality after surgery for hepatic colorectal metastastes. *J Clin Oncol* 24: 2065–72.

Wiering B, Krabbe P, Jager G *et al.* (2005) The impact of fluor-18-deoxyglucose-positron emission tomography in the management of colorectal liver metastases. *Cancer* 104: 2658–70.

Wolmark N, Rockette H, Mamounas E *et al.* (1999) Clinical trial to assess the relative efficacy of fluorouracil and leucovorin, fluorouracil and levamisole, and fluorouracil, leucovorin, and levamisole in patients with Duke's B and C carcinoma of the colon: results from the National Surgical Adjuvant Breast and Bowel Project C-04. *J Clin Oncol* 17: 3553–9.

15 Rare Cancers

Edited by Colin McArdle

Gastrointestinal carcinoids

Irvin M. Modlin, Jan Bornschein & Mark Kidd

Introduction

Carcinoids account for 0.5% of all malignancies of the human body. Of these tumors, two-thirds develop within the gastrointestinal (GI) tract and they demonstrate an increasing incidence over the last two decades, probably in some part due to advances in diagnostic procedures (Modlin *et al.* 2006a). Thirty-eight per cent of GI tract carcinoids occur in the small intestine, with the ileum 6.5–8.2 times more frequently affected than the duodenum and the jejunum. Twenty-one per cent of carcinoids occur in the rectum, 18% in the appendix, 12% in the colon and 6% in the stomach. Other GI tract locations exhibit fewer tumors, and the pancreas, esophagus, Meckel's diverticulum, liver, extrahepatic biliary tract system and gallbladder may all develop carcinoid tumors.

Neuroendocrine tumors (NETs = carcinoids) show a significant association with other non-carcinoid tumors, such as GI adenocarcinomas, lymphomas and neoplasms of the breast. This is especially evident for carcinoids located in the ileum (29%) and the rectum (18%) (Modlin *et al.* 2003). Specific GI locations are predisposed to certain types of NETs and associated diseases or tumor entities. Thus, an association with genetic tumor syndromes occurs mainly with gastric and pancreatic lesions (multiple endocrine neoplasia type 1, MEN1) and with duodenal carcinoids (neurofibromatosis type 1 (NF1), MEN1), especially somatostatinomas (ampulla of Vater [NF1]) (Modlin *et al.* 2005). Similarly, type I carcinoids of the stomach (derived from ECL cells) are associated with chronic atrophic gastritis, while type II carcinoids are related to Zollinger-Ellison syndrome and associated with MEN1. As many as one-third of MEN1 patients develop gastric carcinoids (Modlin *et al.* 2005). About 65% of duodenal carcinoids are gastrinomas and 15% somatostatinomas. Non-functioning NETs and poorly differentiated NE carcinomas are rarer and apart from gastrinomas most are located in the periampullary region (Modlin *et al.* 2005).

Gastrointestinal Oncology: A Critical Multidisciplinary Team Approach.
Edited by J. Jankowski, R. Sampliner, D. Kerr, and Y. Fong.

Diagnosis

History

The classical carcinoid syndrome occurs in less than 10% of the patients and is usually associated with an ileal metastatic lesion. The incidence of the syndrome is extremely rare when primaries are located in the colon or rectum (Modlin *et al.* 2005). The carcinoid syndrome is usually apparent if hepatic metastases are present and reflects failure of the liver to adequately degrade bioactive tumor products. Sometimes lesions or metastases draining directly into the systemic circulation (ovary or retroperitoneal deposits) may engender the syndrome. Typical symptoms include cutaneous flushing, gut hypermotility and diarrhea, sweating and bronchospasm, alone or in combination (75%). Flushing occurs mainly in the face, neck and upper chest and may persist for 10–30 minutes before it resolves (in the majority of cases, centrally first) producing gyrate and serpiginous patterns (Modlin *et al.* 2005). The intensity of symptoms is variable and can appear either paroxysmally or be triggered by exercise, serotonin, or tyramine-rich food or drinks, such as alcohol (especially 'young' red wines), cheese and coffee. Frequently, these symptoms, either singly or in combination, are incorrectly diagnosed as an allergy, irritable bowel syndrome, manifestation of a psychological issue, idiosyncratic response to a drug, or menopause-related findings.

Other symptoms related to carcinoids are usually nonspecific and due to local mass effects, tumor invasion or fibrous adhesions. In addition to general symptoms like weight loss and vague or crampy abdominal pain, the tumor can mimic symptoms caused by other malignant entities depending on its localization: altered bowel habits, rectal bleeding and rectal discomfort occurs in cases of a NET located in the colorectal region; dyspeptic symptoms, reflux esophagitis, nausea and vomiting or signs of upper GI bleeding are associated with duodenal or gastric NETs; while jaundice and cholestasis may occur in cases of tumors in the pancreaticobiliary tract or at the ampulla of Vater causing biliary obstruction. Very often however, carcinoids are clinically silent and are only found incidentally during surgical procedures or at autopsies undertaken for other reasons (Berge *et al.* 1977).

Clinical

In the evaluation and the management of NETs, it is important to bear in mind the significant association with synchronous and metachronous non-carcinoid tumors (usually adenocarcinomas of the gut). It is likely that this relationship reflects a common growth factor stimulus and induction of cell proliferation and differentiation of related progenitor cells in different locations by bioactive agents produced and secreted by NETs themselves (Modlin *et al.* 2005).

Apart from coexistent tumor disease, most major clinical symptomatology is due to carcinoid-related fibrosis, either local or distant to the tumor site. Thus, intestinal obstruction with pain and distention is due to adhesive loops, kinking or luminal strictures. Vascular compromise due to peritumoral fibrous tissue may cause mesenteric ischemia and become a major management issue, that can culminate in bowel necrosis (Marshall & Bodnarchuk 1993). The incidence of intestinal obstruction secondary to mesenteric fibrosis associated with midgut carcinoid disease can be as high as 42–66% (Modlin *et al.* 2005).

Two-thirds of the patients with carcinoid syndrome ultimately will demonstrate valvular fibrosis and cardiac disease (Norheim *et al.* 1987). Plaque-like, fibrous endocardial thickening principally involves the right side of the heart and causes retraction and fixation of the leaflets of the tricuspid and pulmonary valves as well as diminished right ventricular function. Heart failure due to right-sided valvular fibrosis now accounts for about 50% of carcinoid-related mortality in some series (Zuetenhorst & Taal 2005). Left-sided carcinoid cardiac disease occurs in less than 10% of patients. Other fibrosis-related events in patients with advanced metastatic disease include pulmonary fibrosis as well as cutaneous manifestations (scleroderma-like lesions), which mostly affect the lower extremities (Modlin *et al.* 2005).

The mechanisms leading to carcinoid-related fibrosis are not completely understood. Associations with cardiac fibrosis include elevated plasma levels of serotonin and its degradatory metabolite 5-HIAA (5-hydroxy-indole-acetic acid) in the urine. The experimental infusion of serotonin results in cardiac and valvular fibrosis (Gustafsson *et al.* 2005). However, treatment with serotonin antagonists or agents that reduce urinary 5-HIAA levels has no effects on amelioration of local and distant fibrosis (Modlin *et al.* 2005). Recent studies support a leading role of TGFβ and related growth factors, e.g. CTGF (connective tissue growth factor) and PDGF (platelet-derived growth factor) secreted by the tumor cells, in the stimulation of fibroblasts as an initial step in the pathogenesis of fibrosis (Waltenberger *et al.* 1993).

Markers for clinical chemistry analysis include urinary 5-HIAA and plasma chromogranin A. Although 5-HIAA can be measured in fasting plasma, it is mostly evaluated in a 24-h collection of urine and has a specificity of 88% (Tormey & FitzGerald 1995). However, this method is cumbersome and has a poor sensitivity (35%) and a large number of drugs and dietary products can interfere with the test result (e.g. ingestion of bananas, tomatoes or eggplant) (Feldman & Lee 1985).

The major screening test is serum CgA, with a sensitivity of 99% (Modlin *et al.* 2006a). CgA levels correlate with the severity of carcinoid disease, i.e. tumor volume and burden (Modlin *et al.* 2006a). Thus, it is a relevant prognostic marker, especially for midgut carcinoids (Modlin *et al.* 2006a). False-positive results can, however, occur with proton pump inhibitor treatment (Modlin *et al.* 2006a). Alternative biochemical markers include other tumor products such as serotonin (predominantly ileal carcinoids), histamine (gastric carcinoids) or substance P, neurotensin, bradykinin, pancreatic polypeptide and human chorionic gonadotropin.

If biochemical results are equivocal for the diagnosis of a GI carcinoid, provocative tests such as pentagastrin injection or alcohol ingestion can be considered (Modlin & Tang 1997). These are potentially dangerous and should be undertaken only under medical surveillance because of the risk of triggering a 'carcinoid crisis'. The latter condition is occasionally engendered by anesthesia, or surgical or radiologic intervention, and manifests in profound flushing, extreme blood pressure fluctuations, bronchoconstriction, tachycardia and arrhythmias culminating in confusion or stupor which may last for hours or days. A high mortality has been reported in the absence of pre-emptive pharmacologic intervention, usually an intravenous bolus of a somatostatin analog (Modlin *et al.* 2005).

Histopathology

Typical carcinoids present with neuroendocrine cells growing in either trabecular, insular or ribbon-like patterns with no or minimal cellular pleomorphism and sparse mitosis (Modlin *et al.* 2005). Atypical carcinoids represent a more aggressive form with poor differentiation, increased mitotic activity and absent or limited necrosis (Modlin *et al.* 2005). A previously much utilized parameter to distinguish different NETs was the reaction to argentaffin or argyrophil staining methods, with gastric and rectal lesions typically being argentaffin negative and small intestinal carcinoids usually argentaffin positive (Modlin *et al.* 2005). Currently, as many as 40 different secretory products are detectable by immunohistochemistry (Delcore & Friesen 1994), of which the most relevant are neuron-specific enolase (NSE), synaptophysin or CgA. Other immunohistochemical markers of interest include carcinoembryonic antigen (CEA) (present in about two-thirds of ileal and jejunal carcinoids) and prostatic acid phosphatase (about 20%), and S-100 protein in 7% (Modlin *et al.* 2005). Several other findings characteristic of GI carcinoid tumors are noted in Table 15.1. Transmural invasion and extensive fibrosis are common features and contribute to the aggressive local behavior of ileal neoplasms. A relatively rare variant of the carcinoid tumor, the so-called adenocarcinoid or goblet cell carcinoma, is found in the appendix and the rectum. It exhibits both neuroendocrine differentiation and mucin production and/or glandular differentiation and tends to behave more aggressively than the pure neuroendocrine tumor (Modlin *et al.* 2005). Immunohistochemical expression of Ki-67 has be used to predict the biologic behavior of GI neuroendocrine tumors and may predict survival (Modlin *et al.* 2005). This is based on the apparently good relationship between Ki-67 staining and mitotic index (Canavese *et al.* 2001). However, other groups have noted that the association between Ki-67 expression and prognosis may be limited (Van Eeden *et al.* 2002).

Imaging and staging

The most useful method for initial imaging of GI NETs is somatostatin receptor scintigraphy (SRS) with ^{111}indium-labeled octreotide ([^{111}In-DTP-d-Phe(10)]-octreotide, 6 mCi administered intravenously). This reflects the fact that octreotide has a particular high affinity for somatostatin receptor (SST_R).subtypes 2 and 5 (Nilsson *et al.* 1998), and more than 70% of gastroenteropancreatic NETs express multiple (SST_R).subtypes with a predominance of 2 and 5 (de Herder & Hofland 2004). Tumors or metastases that fail to express or exhibit low levels of SST_Rs 2 and 5, will not be detected. False positives occur with infection, recent trauma, meningiomas,

Table 15.1 Histopathologic characteristics of GI carcinoids at different localizations. (Data adapted from Modlin *et al.* 2005.)

Localization	Histologic pattern	General markers	Additional markers
Esophagus	Marked cellular atypia; enlarged, pleiomorphic nuclei	NSE, VIP, serotonin Argentaffin +/– Argyrophil +/–	No data
Stomach	Trabecular, gyriform, medullary/solid, glandular/rosette-like ECL-, EC- and X-cells	CgA, synaptophysin, Leu-7, (NSE, serotonin) Argyrophil + Argentaffin +/–	No data
Duodenum	Cribriform, insular, glandular, solid, trabecular	CgA, NSE, Leu-7, (SST, gastrin, serotonin, calcitonin, insulin, PP)	Xenin Psammona bodies (SST-oma)
Ileum	Insular (type I): solid nests/cords Trabecular (type II): narrow cell bands forming ribbons, anastomosing along a vascular network Glandular (III): alveolar, acinar, rosette with cavities/pseudo-cavities undifferentiated and mixed (type IV/V)	CgA, NSE, serotonin, Substance P, Leu-7, (enteroglucagon, PP, peptide YY) Argentaffin + Argyrophil +	Transmural invasion and extended fibrosis common CEA, Prostatic acid phosphatase, S-100
Appendix	Insular EC-cells, L-cells	Serotonin, substance P Argentaffin—(L-cells)	Adenocarcinoids (neuroendocrine and glandular differentiation/ mucin production)
Colon/rectum	Ribbon-like, mixed, acinar Cell clusters, necrosis Colonic carcinoids more undifferentiated	CgA, NSE, (serotonin, SST, glicentin, PP, peptide YY, enkephalin,endorphin) Argentaffin +/– Argyrophil +	Adenocarcinoids (scattered mucus-secreting cells) Prostatic acid phosphatase
Pancreas	Trabecular; granular eosinophilic cytoplasm	CgA, serotonin, synaptophysin, (NSE)	No data
Liver	No data	CgA, NSE, chromostatin, synaptophysin	CEA
Biliary tract	Trabecular/nesting; occasional tubule formation	CgA, (SST, serotonin, synaptophysin, cytokeratin)	No data
Gallbladder	No data	CgA; Argyrophil +	No data

Markers that are rarely expressed are included within ( ).

lymphomas, granulomas or autoimmune disease (Modlin *et al.* 2006a). Sensitivity (80–90%) can be enhanced by simultaneous SPECT (single photon emission computed tomography) and up to 15% more primary lesions can be identified if further imaging methods are applied (e.g. ultrasonography, triple-phase helical CT, MRI, selective mesenteric angiography). However, this protocol is only justified if surgery is considered and a more precise topographic delineation of the lesion is necessary to assure definitive resection or exclude covert metastatic disease (Modlin *et al.* 2005).

γ-detecting handheld probes for intraoperative (abdominal) delineation of small or occult tumors or metastases after injection of ^{111}In-octreotide have to date produced disappointing results due to the relatively low SST_R density compared to the high background uptake in the adjacent kidneys, liver and spleen (Modlin *et al.* 2006a). Scintigraphy with ^{111}In-labeled octreotide or ^{99m}Technetium-MDP can be used for detection of bone metastases, although MRI is probably as effective.

CT and MRI have comparable detection (81%) and sensitivity (80%) rates, although both modalities are inferior to SRS (89%, 84%, respectively) (Modlin & Tang 1997). CT and MRI may therefore be used in precise topographic localization of the tumor and the relation of mass lesions, calcifications and fibrosis to other structures not evident with an isotope scan.

The precise benefit of PET (positron emission tomography) for diagnosis, staging and surveillance of NETs is still under investigation (Table 15.2). FDG-PET (FDG: ^{18}F-2-deoxy-(D)-glucose) is not ideal since most carcinoids are well-differentiated, slow-growing neoplasms with metabolism rates that are too low for FBG to produce adequate imaging. Optimal NET tumor visualization can be obtained using the radioactive labeled serotonin precursor ^{11}C-5HT (5-hydroxytryptamine) and detection rates approaching 100% have been reported (Modlin *et al.* 2005). Other radionuclides that may be considered for NET-imaging include ^{18}F-DOPA, ^{68}Ga- or ^{64}CU-labeled octreotide, ^{123}I-MIBG and additional Tc-labeled isotopes. These have encouraging but not consistent detection rates and sensitivity (Modlin *et al.* 2006a).

Table 15.2 Diagnostic methods. Comparison of the three major methods for NET-imaging evaluating results of 39 studies. SRS (somatostatin receptor scintigraphy using ^{111}In-octreotide): 19 studies; PET (positron emission tomography using the following tracers: FDG, ^{11}C-5HT, F18-DOPA, ^{68}Ga-DOTATOC, ^{64}Cu-TETA-Oct.): 11 studies; CT/MRI (computer tomography and magnetic resonance imaging, including either a single method or combined methods): 9 studies. Values are median (range). (Data adapted from Modlin *et al.* 2006a.)

Modality	Number of patients	Detection (%)	Sensitivity (%)
SRS	17 (5–451)	89 (67–100)	84
PET (FGD)	11 (5–17)	49 (25–73)	29
PET (^{11}C/F18/^{68}Ga/^{64}Cu)	15 (5–18)	100 (100–100)	65
CT	25 (20–80)	81 (76–100)	92
MRI	15 (12–17)	67 (25–81)	72

Angiography is less used currently than in the past and has in most centers been superseded by MRI. It can provide information regarding the degree of tumor vascularity and the sources of its vascular supply as well as delineate the relationship of the tumor (invasion) to adjacent major vascular structures (Modlin *et al.* 2006a). Angiographic changes particularly for small intestinal carcinoids can be distinctive, with narrowing or occlusion of the distal ileal arcade and stenosis of the intramesenteric arteries being a characteristic finding (Modlin *et al.* 2005).

Additional imaging and detection methods can be considered, depending on localization of the lesion. In the stomach, duodenum, colon and rectum, endoscopy with multiple biopsies, as well as endoscopic ultrasound (EUS) is mandatory to determine tumor type and the degree of invasion. EUS is particularly useful in helping determine the extent of hepatic and pancreatic involvement. Enteroscopy is of utility for more distal lesions of the small intestine but is very uncomfortable and time-consuming. More recently, capsule endoscopy (CE) has emerged as having the highest potential for surveillance and detection of small intestinal carcinoids (Gay *et al.* 2004). A meta-analysis comprising 24 studies and including 530 patients compared the diagnostic yield of CE with push enteroscopy, small bowel follow-through (enteroclysis) and colonoscopy with distal ileoscopy (Lewis *et al.* 2005). CE provided a detection rate for small bowel abnormalities of 87%, compared to a mean detection rate of 13% for the other methods. Only 10% of findings were missed (19% were neoplasia) using CE while the other diagnostic modalities failed in 73% (63% were neoplasia) (Lewis *et al.* 2005). CE is the only method that can assess the complete small intestine, while colonoscopy and enteroscopy are primarily limited to either the proximal or the distal part. Double balloon endoscopy is currently under evaluation since it has the potential to overcome this issue (Gay *et al.* 2004). It is likely that enteroclysis (mainly upper GI barium contrast studies) will be abandoned in favor of these techniques, although this modality can yield further information about the location and extension of small intestinal neoplasia, especially if enhanced with CT imaging (Modlin *et al.* 2006a).

ERCP and MRI with dynamic gadolinium enhancement and fat suppression are of use in pancreatic lesions. Individuals with hepatic or pancreatic lesions may benefit from fine needle biopsy of the lesion, especially under US or CT scan control. Portohepatic venous sampling of peptide and amine levels is now only rarely undertaken. For bronchopulmonary or metastatic pulmonary carcinoids bronchoscopy should be considered. Genetic analyses should be undertaken in patients with duodenal location of the NET in Zollinger–Ellison syndrome or von Recklinghausen's disease. It is mandatory that a cardiac echo should be obtained for the assessment of carcinoid-related disease of the heart. Figure 15.1 provides an overview of the currently accepted carcinoid diagnostic algorithm.

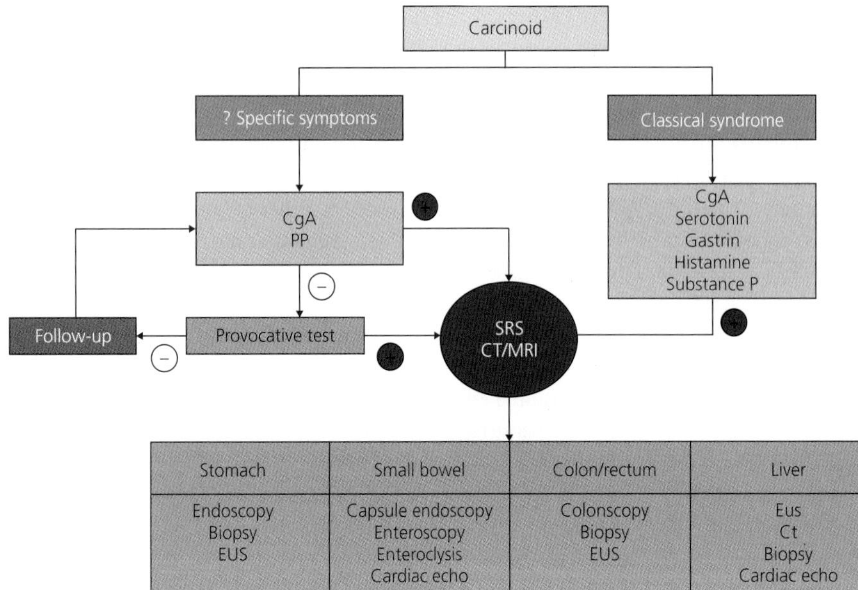

Fig. 15.1 Diagnostic algorithm for gastrointestinal neuroendocrine tumors (carcinoids). SRS, somatostatin receptor scintigraphy; EUS, endoscopic ultrasound. (Adapted from Modlin *et al.* 2006a.)

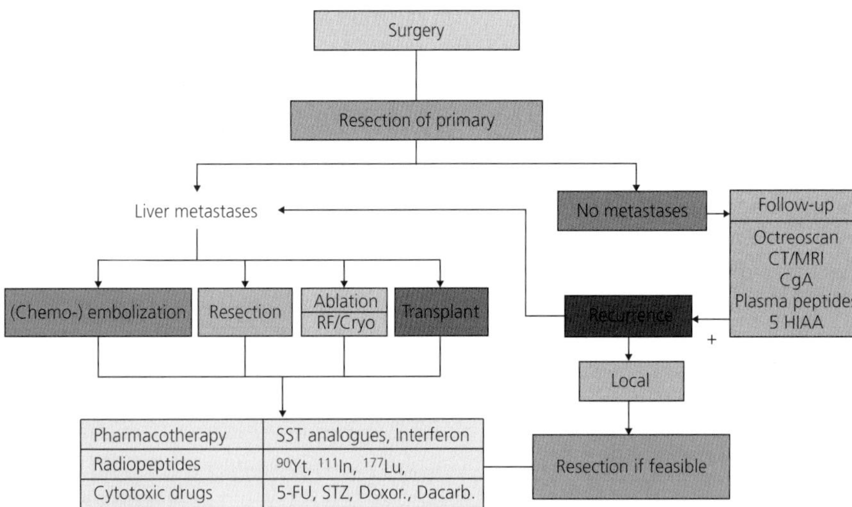

Fig. 15.2 Therapeutic algorithm in the management of gastrointestinal neuroendocrine tumors (carcinoids). RF, radiofrequency ablation; Cryo, cryoablation; 5-FU, 5-fluorouracil; STZ, streptozotocin; Doxor, doxorubicin; Dacarb, dacarbacin. (Adapted from Modlin *et al.* 2006b.)

Treatment

Overview

At this time surgery is the only curative treatment for carcinoid disease (Fig. 15.2). In general there are three main approaches to surgical treatment of carcinoids: (i) adequate (extensive) resection with curative or palliative intent for primary and regional lesions; (ii) surgical resection of regional or distant metastatic disease with cytoreductive intent; and (iii) resection of disease for local symptom palliation without cytoreductive intent.

Chemotherapeutic options (biotherapy) include treatment with somatostatin analogs; depot formulations have proven most effective. Interferons have been used to some advantage but may exhibit substantial adverse effects. A variety of cytotoxic agents have been utilized with inconsistent and mostly disappointing outcomes. A plethora of novel agents targeting angiogenesis, growth stimuli or kinase dependent pathways are under current investigation but to date have exhibited minimal utility (discussed further below).

External radiotherapy is of little use in the management of GI NETs, but internal application of β- or γ-ray emitting radioisotopes linked to SST analogs have produced promising

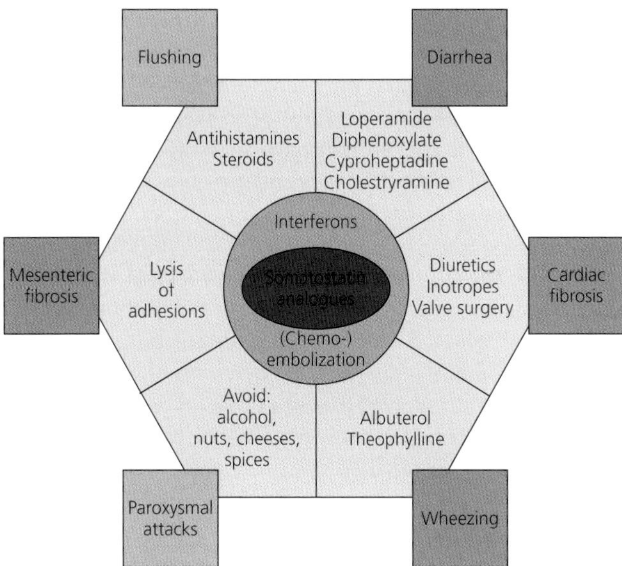

Fig. 15.3 Symptom management for patients with carcinoid disease. (Adapted from Modlin *et al.* 2006b.)

results in terms of disease stability. Tumor regression is however, a far rarer event.

Special techniques including radiofrequency ablation, cryosurgical extirpation, surgical debulking and chemoembolization (bland, cytotoxic impregnated or isotopic spheres) may be considered if hepatic metastatic involvement is evident. Supportive treatment (usually an SST analog) for the major symptoms of carcinoid disease (diarrhea, flushing, cardiac disease) should be included in any treatment algorithm (Fig. 15.3).

Surgery

En bloc resection of the primary tumor and local lymph nodes is the only potentially curative therapy for GI carcinoid tumors. This is usually possible in at most 20% of individuals who present with a small primary tumor and limited local disease (Plockinger *et al.* 2004). Adequate systemic symptomatic palliation can be achieved if more than 90% of the tumor mass is removed, but overt clinical benefit may be evident following tumor debulking, since this may obviate bowel obstruction and ameliorate local mechanical symptoms (Modlin *et al.* 2005).

In general, the surgical approach depends on the localization of the tumor. Gastric carcinoids should be treated according to the type of the lesion. Sporadic aggressive type III NETs of the stomach require gastrectomy, whereas type I and II lesions can often be managed by endoscopic excision, although if widespread and aggressively growing with bleeding, partial gastrectomy may be necessary (Modlin *et al.* 2005). Hypergastrinemia-associated tumors of less than 1 cm in size and less than 3–5 in number (type II carcinoid) should be managed by endoscopic excision of the polypoid lesions, if possible. Local wedge excision should be considered if there is more than one lesion, lesions extend beyon 1 cm or recurrent polypectomy is necessary. In some circumstances, particularly multicentric large tumors in young patients, total gastrectomy might be an option to avoid lifetime endoscopic surveillance (Modlin *et al.* 2005). Antrectomy to remove the gastrin drive was initially proposed but the inability to determine which lesions have attained gastrin autonomy has led to a decline in the use of this procedure. The long-term use of SST analogs to suppress gastrin and ECL cell proliferation has been proposed with some success (D'Adda *et al.* 1996).

Small intestinal carcinoids often present at an advanced stage at diagnosis with multicentric lesions, metastases and associated non-carcinoid malignancies. *En bloc* resection including the mesentery and its lymph nodes is advisable, and should be followed by thorough exploration of the peritoneal cavity and adjacent structures as well as intraoperative ultrasound and biopsy of the liver to identify covert metastases (Modlin *et al.* 2005).

Appendiceal lesions usually have a good prognosis. Right hemicolectomy with mesenteric excision should be undertaken if an appendiceal tumor is greater than 2 cm or multicentric, or other adverse features are present such as cell atypia, presence of mucin (adenocarcinoid) or evidence of invasion, especially in mesoappendiceal vascular or lymphatic structures (Modlin *et al.* 2006b).

Similarly to small intestinal NETs, NETs of the colon have a poor prognosis and patients should undergo a wide resection, including removal of the mesentery and the lymph nodes, followed by peritoneal exploration. For practical purposes, carcinoids of the colon should be managed like adenocarcinomas. Rectal lesions have a better outcome (usually diagnosed earlier by routine colonoscopy or bright red bleeding) and can often be managed by endoscopic or transanal resection since the majority (57–75%) are less than 1 cm in size (Okamoto *et al.* 2004). For rectal tumors 1–2 cm in size without evidence of lymph node metastasis, a wide excision with a meticulous evaluation to exclude muscular invasion is recommended. If the neoplasm is greater than 2 cm or muscular invasion or lymph node metastases are present, radical surgery (low anterior resection with total mesorectal excision or abdominoperineal resection) should be performed. If the lesion is greater than 2 cm, presents with hepatic and lymph node metastases, or exhibits an adenocarcinoid or NE carcinoma phenotype, it should be, like colonic carcinoids, treated as an adenocarcinoma.

Generally, for carcinoids located at rare GI sites, resection is recommended if possible. Hepatic metastases should be resected, when feasible (segment location, number, site, general condition of the patient) since cytoreductive surgery may reduce symptoms, facilitate pharmacologic management and improve survival (Sarmiento *et al.* 2003).

Orthotopic liver transplantation (OLT) for hepatic involvement has a 5-year survival of 36–73% with 24–52% being disease free and 90–100% with symptom relief (Sutcliffe *et al.*

2004). However in a collective review of 103 OLTs undertaken for NETs, 40% exhibited extrahepatic disease at transplantation (Lehnert 1998). High recurrence rates (especially bone and liver metastases) and a procedure-related mortality of 11–28% mandate the use of strict selection criteria (Sutcliffe *et al.* 2004). Currently, the Milan criteria are: (i) confirmed carcinoid histology; (ii) primary tumor drained by the portal system; (iii) <50% of hepatic parenchyma replaced by metastatic/neoplastic tissue; (iv) good response or stable disease during pretransplantation period; and (v) absence of extrahepatic disease (Sutcliffe *et al.* 2004). Cytologic and histologic markers like Ki-67 or MIB-1 are under evaluation to determine their prognostic value in determining the outcome of OLT (Blonski *et al.* 2005).

Abdominal surgery is necessary in case of obstructive bowel symptomatology or gut ischemia due to carcinoid-related fibrosis. These procedures are often technically difficult given the 'cocoon effect' of fibrosis. They have a high morbidity due to both the active fibroblastic process and the 'sclerosis' of the mesenteric vessels with associated poor anastomotic vascularization and consequent high leakage rates (Modlin *et al.* 2004a). Patients with carcinoid cardiac disease should be considered for valvular replacement or at least palliative balloon pulmonary valvuloplasty in conjunction with cardiac catheterization.

Chemotherapy

Somatostatin analogs

The major symptomatic therapy for carcinoid disease is SST analogs (lanreotide, octreotide) with up to 71% experiencing resolution of their main symptoms, i.e. diarrhea or flushing. A further indication, especially for intravenous application of SST analogs, is the management of carcinoid crisis. Although these compounds have demonstrated the ability to inhibit progression of the disease with biochemical or tumor stabilization occurring in 28% and 55% respectively, tumor regression occurs only in isolated patients and is inconsistent and usually absent (Modlin *et al.* 2006b). Patients treated with SST analogs may develop a range of adverse effects. These include nausea, abdominal cramps, loose stools, mild steatorrhea and flatus. Biliary sludge and cholelithiasis can occur in up to 50% (acute symptoms warranting cholecystectomy are rare: 1–5%). Endocrine effects, such as hypothyroidism and hypo- or more commonly hyperglycemia, and cardiac consequences, such as sinus bradycardia, conduction abnormalities and arrhythmias, have also been reported (Schnirer *et al.* 2003; Oberg *et al.* 2004;). Very rarely, gastric atony occurs.

The dosage of octreotide (Sandostatin®) varies from 50 μg to 500 μg subcutaneously three times a day and can be adjusted in accordance with clinical needs. In the event of symptom breakthrough, which may represent tachyphylaxis or increased tumor growth, dosage can be increased (Modlin *et al.* 2005). Repeated subcutaneous injections, however, cause morbidity, are inconvenient and often result in suboptimal symptom control. Compliance and control of carcinoid disease have been facilitated by the introduction of the long-acting SST analog lanreotide (Lanreotide Autogel) and the depot formulation of octreotide (Sandostatin LAR®) with administration every 10–14 days and 4 weeks, respectively. Breakthrough or escape can, however, occur in the last week of the cycle and may require 'rescue' with a short-acting agent (50 or 100 μg octreotide) or by increasing either dose or frequency of the depot injection. Intermediate-acting SST analogs such as Sandostatin® should be used to supplement long-acting agents until a steady state is reached (Oberg *et al.* 2004). An advantageous formulation, Lanreotide Autogel, is administered (120 mg) once a month either subcutaneously or orally. Pooled data of 14 trials of octreotide reflect a median biochemical response rate of 37% (range 0–77%) and a cumulative tumor response rate of 0% (Modlin *et al.* 2006b). Lanreotide (Somatuline®), a long-acting somatostatin analog, has a similar efficacy to octreotide (42% vs. 37%) although the decreased need for injection is advantageous (Modlin *et al.* 2006b). Depot formulations (Lanreotide Autogel®) have similar biochemical responses indicating comparable efficacies for each drug.

Interferons

The second class of therapeutic agents used for the treatment of carcinoid disease is interferons, including IFNα, IFNγ and human leukocyte IFN. The mechanism of action for interferons is not yet completely understood, but appear to be directed at inhibition of cell proliferation, immune cell-mediated cytotoxicity, inhibition of angiogenesis and cell cycle arrest (Modlin *et al.* 2005). Generally, interferons exhibit more favorable tumor responses than SST analogs, but substantial adverse effects are disadvantages. These can vary from fever, fatigue, anorexia and weight loss to alopecia and myelosuppression (Schnirer *et al.* 2003; Oberg *et al.* 2004). The most investigated drug is IFNα, which has a symptom response of ~75% and biochemical and tumor stability of ~40% and ~66%, respectively (Modlin *et al.* 2006b). Results with human leukocyte interferon are comparable, although not as effective as IFNα. Combinations of IFNα with IFNγ (which is not effective as a single agent) or with octreotide have not been demonstrated to produce further benefit.

Cytotoxic agents

'Traditional' (cytotoxic) chemotherapeutic agents such as 5-fluorouracil, doxorubicin, tamoxifen, streptozotocin, dacarbazine or dactinomycin have yielded disappointing clinical results. Responses are inconsistent and unpredictable, with overall rates of only 31% for single-agent administration and up to 39% for combination of drugs (Modlin *et al.* 2006b). Associated adverse events are substantial and significantly diminish quality of life. In general, it is recommended that the use of such agents should be judicious and sparing.

Radiotherapy/radionuclides

The response rate of NETs to external-beam radiation therapy is poor, particularly in the GI tract where usually no 'stationary' target is available (Modlin *et al.* 2006b). In addition, the often indolent proliferative rate of NETs renders them less radiosensitive. Some efficacy of palliative radiotherapy has, however, been reported for the treatment of bone and brain metastases and in the management of spinal cord compression (Modlin *et al.* 2006b).

On the contrary, clinically acceptable responses are associated after intravenous therapy with a variety of different radioisotopes linked to SST analogs—radiopeptide targeted therapy (RPTT). This strategy may produce an acceptable degree of disease stabilization with relatively modest associated adverse events, particularly if the NET has a high expression level of SST_{R}s and exhibits a rapidly growing profile (Table 15.3). Individual isotopes have been considered variously more effective depending on their individual emission spectra of gamma and beta rays or Auger electrons. Nevertheless, substantial renal and bone marrow exposure is a potential safety issue. Kidney irradiation can be significantly decreased by pretherapy amino acid infusion and adequate hydration (Kaltsas *et al.* 2004). Recent data demonstrate that ^{177}Lu bound to [DOTA(0)-Tyr(3)]-octreotate has a three- to fourfold higher uptake in SST_{R}-positive tumors compared to ^{111}In (Breeman *et al.* 2001). Remission rates appear to correlate with high pretherapy uptake of SST analogs and limited hepatic tumor load (Teunissen *et al.* 2004).

Although only limited data are available, the therapeutic effects of ^{90}Y, ^{111}In and ^{131}I-MIBG on tumor stabilization are broadly similar with median tumor response rates ranging from 8 to 15%. Overall, it appears that the benefits of therapeutic protocols using these isotopes may mostly be limited to disease stabilization (Table 15.3). All modalities (indium, yttrium, and iodine) however, appear somewhat effective in achieving biochemical (52–54%) or tumor stability (52–71%). In contrast, the more recent experience with lutetium (^{177}Lu-octreotate) has provided a more promising treatment profile with a tumor response rate of >45% and tumor stabilization in 87% of patients (Kwekkeboom *et al.* 2005).

Table 15.3 Radionuclide therapy. Evaluation of 17 studies investigating the effect of the four radioactive isotopes bound to octreotide that are currently used in the therapy of carcinoids. ^{90}Y: 3 studies; ^{111}In: 6 studies; ^{131}MIBG: 5 studies; ^{177}lutetium: 3 studies. Values are median (range). (Data adapted from de Herder & Hofland 2004.)

Agent	Tumor response (%)	Biochemical stability (%)	Tumor stability (%)
^{90}Yttrium	8 (0–8)	No data	92 (62–100)
^{111}Indium	15 (0–20)	54 (54)	65 (5–89)
^{131}MIBG	11 (0–15)	52 (40–62)	71 (65–74)
^{177}Lutetium	46 (0–48)	No data	82 (79–88)

Ablation

Radiofrequency ablation and cryosurgical debulking have important roles in the downsizing of hepatic carcinoid metastases, but their efficacy requires further rigorous evaluation. Although some palliative symptomatic benefit for the carcinoid syndrome is reported, the effect on outcome is uncertain (Modlin *et al.* 2006b). Both procedures are invasive and serious adverse events (bleeding, bile duct damage) have been reported.

Radiofrequency ablation utilizes a high-frequency alternating current to generate local temperatures of up to 60°C to necrotize metastases. A study using this approach reported 65% decrease in tumor markers, 41% with no further evidence of tumor progression, 13% with local recurrent lesions and 28% with new hepatic foci (Berber *et al.* 2002). Symptom responses were achieved in 95%, with 80% showing significant or complete relief for a mean period of 10 months. Cryoablation involves placing a probe directly into tumor foci and thereafter initiating cycles of freezing and thawing. Symptom relief was attained in 87%, 59% decreased 5-HIAA excretion, but ~90% developed recurrence within 2 years (Chung *et al.* 2001).

Both techniques are of limited use in cases where operative surgical techniques are not applicable, especially if tumors are greater than 35 mm or more than five lesions are present. Median response period for both techniques is 10–11 months (Modlin *et al.* 2006b). *In situ* cryo- or radiofrequency ablations are therefore usually reserved for localized or residual disease, and are often utilized as adjuncts to primary resective surgery.

Chemoembolization

Techniques of hepatic artery occlusion, either by ligation, particle embolization, chemoembolization or isotopic sphere emboli, are utilized in patients with hepatic involvement. The concept is based on the observation that hepatic metastases obtain their major vascular supply from hepatic arteries whereas the portal venous system provides additional blood for normal hepatic parenchyma. The term 'chemoembolization' combines the principle of intra-arterial chemotherapy and hepatic artery embolization, with reduced vascularization and increased anoxia leading to increased local drug concentrations and decreased wash-out times (Ahlman *et al.* 2004). Therapeutic injections should be preceded by superior mesenteric and celiac trunk arteriography to assess normative arterial distribution, portal vein patency and tumor blood flow rates (Modlin *et al.* 2006b). Numerous compounds including gelatin powder, polyvinyl alcohol, gel foam and coils have been used to achieve vascular occlusion. Results are encouraging, with about 75% of patients demonstrating tumor reduction and up to 100%

improvement in symptoms (flushing, diarrhea) (Modlin *et al.* 2006b). However, these effects are relatively short term, and last variably between 14 and 22 months. Substantial adverse events may occur and range from local problems at the site of the arterial puncture (bleeding, pseudoaneurysm) to systemic effects consequent upon tumor necrosis (pain, nausea, fever, fatigue or elevation of liver enzymes—transaminitis or post-embolization syndrome), and massive release of bioactive agents (dramatic fluctuations of blood pressure, circulatory collapse, carcinoid crisis) (Plockinger *et al.* 2004; Modlin *et al.* 2006b). Embolization of branch vessels can lead to ischemia and infection of adjacent organs and structures. Thus, acute ischemic cholycystitis may occur and necessitate cholycystectomy, or liver abscesses may form in necrotic tissue. SST analogs and antibiotics should be given before the procedure to obviate the development of metabolic and infective problems.

Supportive care

Supportive care for patients with carcinoid disease is aimed at improving symptom management by medical and non-medical means (Fig. 15.3).

Diarrhea can be treated with loperamide or diphenoxylate and in individuals who have undergone ileal resection for removal of the primary tumor, further relief from diarrhea may be attained by the use of cholestyramine (bile salt binder). Serotonin antagonists have some utility and may improve anorexia and cachexia ($5HT_2$-antagonist: cyproheptadine) or facilitate gastric emptying and reduce postprandial colonic hypertonic responses ($5HT_3$-antagonist: ondansetron). They have minimal effect on carcinoid-related flushing and exhibit adverse effects, in particular somnolence. Histamine-1 inhibitors, fenoxfenadine or diphenhydramine, can improve skin rashes as may steroids. The latter have substantial adverse effects, particularly in long-term usage. Further treatment targeting the cardiopulmonary system (theophylline or β_2-adrenergens [albuterol]) for bronchospasm or diuretics and inotropes in case of cardiac failure may be of considerable benefit. Generally, patients should be advised to avoid stress and conditions or substances that might precipitate their symptoms (e.g. cheeses, red wine, nuts, certain spices, especially capsaicin-containing foods). There is little evidence to support the use of dietary supplements such as nicotinamide.

Novel agents

Novel agents include newly developed SST analogs like SOM 230. In comparison to octreotide or lanreotide, this derivative has a higher affinity for SST_R 1–3 and 5 and has additional effects on type 4 receptors. A third of patients refractory to lanreotide exhibit symptom response to SOM 230, which also can inhibit the release of growth hormone and IGF1 (Modlin *et al.* 2006b). Results reporting antiproliferative responses to SOM 230 with no side effects, except small changes in plasma glucose levels, are encouraging but remain to be translated into clinical benefit (Bruns *et al.* 2002).

Various drugs, targeting a variety of intracellular pathways, are under investigation (Modlin *et al.* 2006b). Biologic targets include angiogenesis, e.g. bevacizumab a monoclonal antibody against VEGF-A, or proliferation, e.g. inhibition of PDGFR (Imatinib). Other mechanisms are microtubule stabilization (epothilone) and inhibition of topoisomerase I (irinotecan) or of the proteasome complex (bortezomib). Blocking of kinase-dependent pathways by the tyrosine kinase inhibitor gefitinib or the suppression of mTOR (mammalian target of rapamycin) has also been evaluated. In addition, assessment of the pyrimidine antimetabolite gemcitabine and inhibitors of histone deacetylases (e.g. MS-275 and SAHA) and their effect on the cell cycle and the regulation of gene expression are ongoing. Small, highly selected studies suggest initial promising results, with some agents showing induction of disease stability in up to 71% (Modlin *et al.* 2006b). Such agents require rigorous further evaluation before their clinical use can be recommended.

In the treatment of fibrosis, agents that inhibit the CTGF-pathway, including the synthetic prostacyclin analog Iloprost, and human monoclonal antibodies against CTGF (FG-3019) or TGF-β (CAT-192) may have some potential.

Prognosis and follow-up

Well-differentiated carcinoids present with slow proliferation and growth rates and are erroneously considered 'benign' lesions. More aggressive tumors, especially those that require surgical intervention, have a poorer prognosis, albeit usually far better than comparable-stage adenocarcinomas (Table 15.4). Generally, negative prognostic factors for carcinoid disease include multicentricity, evidence of local invasion, a histologically invasive growth pattern, increased cell atypia or high proliferative rates, and demonstrable metastatic spread. Although debulking and resection diminishes or removes symptoms in most patients, symptoms recur in approximately 60% with an overall 5-year survival of 35% (Sarmiento *et al.* 2003). In contrast, resection of the primary tumor may lead to an increase in median survival from 69 to 139 months (Modlin *et al.* 2006b).

In the stomach, hypergastrinemia-associated carcinoids (type I and II) have a good prognosis (~95% 5-year survival) (Modlin *et al.* 2003), since they are generally non-invasive and rarely show metastatic disease, contrary to type III lesions. For the latter, the 5-year survival rate is significantly higher for localized disease (64.3%) than for lesions with regional (29.9%) or distant metastases (10%) (Modlin *et al.* 2004b). After endoscopic or surgical treatment, surveillance endoscopy including biopsy should occur in 6-month intervals (Modlin *et al.* 2005).

Table 15.4 Five-year survival rates and disease extent by site and stage. The data for this figure are derived from the SEER (1973–99) (NCI) registry. Localized: lesion described as *in situ* or confined to organ of origin. Regional: local invasion or lymph node metastasis. Distant: evidence of metastatic invasion of other organs. (Data adapted from Modlin *et al.* 2005.)

Organ site	Localized disease		Regional spread		Distant spread	
	Distribution (%)	5-year SR (%)	Distribution (%)	5-year SR (%)	Distribution (%)	5-year SR (%)
Stomach	61	68	6	35	12	10
Small bowel	30	82	37	60	27	23
Appendix	60	91	27	81	9	28
Colon	26	74	30	51	35	25
Rectum	78	87	4	41	4	25

Small intestinal carcinoids have a particularly poor prognosis compared to other GI carcinoids, especially jejunoileal carcinoids with an overall 5-year survival rate of 60.5%. This outcome is decreased further with hepatic metastases (23%) or in the presence of undifferentiated pattern histology. The latter have a median survival of 6 months, whereas patients with tumors showing an insular or trabecular pattern have a median survival of 2.9 years and 2.5 years, respectively (Modlin *et al.* 2005). The best prognosis is reported for appendiceal carcinoids, especially those <2 cm and with no evidence of invasion. Five-year survival rates for localized lesions, regional spread and distant metastases are 91%, 81% and 28%, respectively (Modlin *et al.* 2005). A similar outcome (87% 5-year survival) occurs with localized rectal carcinoids. In contrast, colonic NETs exhibit amongst the worst prognosis of GI carcinoids with an overall 5-year survival of 33–42% (Modlin *et al.* 2003). At the time of diagnosis, most of these tumors extend beyond 2 cm and have invaded the muscularis propria.

The prognosis in cases of hepatic involvement depends on whether the lesion is of primary or secondary nature. Contrary to the poor prognosis of hepatocellular carcinoma or hepatic carcinoid metastases, primary hepatic lesions appear to exhibit a better prognosis, with survival ranging from several months to 18 years (Modlin *et al.* 2005). Recent reports regarding patients receiving an aggressive regimen with liver resection or orthotopic liver transplants, demonstrate surprisingly positive outcomes with >75% being disease free after 3 years (Fenwick *et al.* 2004). The prognosis of carcinoids at rarer sites (e.g. esophagus, gallbladder) is generally poor, but depends on the predictive factors mentioned above, on tumor extension on presentation and on associated local mass effects.

Although neuroendocrine tumors within the GI tract are overall relatively rare compared to adenocarcinomas, in the small intestine they (carcinoids) are the dominant neoplasm and are being diagnosed in rapidly increasing numbers. These tumors may present with an aggressive biology similar to that of adenocarcinoma and can cause severe and sustained symptoms due to tumor mass effects, fibrosis or the oversecretion of bioactive substances. The delineation of the molecular characteristics of the different NET entities and the identification of robust plasma markers is required to establish an early diagnosis. Elucidation of their fundamental cell biology and the mechanistic basis of neuroendocrine cell proliferation and secretion is necessary to facilitate the development of effective targeted therapeutic modalities.

References

Ahlman H, Nilsson O, Olausson M. (2004) Interventional treatment of the carcinoid syndrome. *Neuroendocrinology* 80 Suppl 1: 67–73.

Berber E, Flesher N, Siperstein AE. (2002) Laparoscopic radiofrequency ablation of neuroendocrine liver metastases. *World J Surg* 26: 985–90.

Berge T, Lundberg S. (1977) Cancer in Malmo 1958–1969. An autopsy study. *Acta Pathol Microbiol Scand Suppl* 1–235.

Blonski WC, Reddy KR, Shaked A, Siegelman E, Metz DC. (2005) Liver transplantation for metastatic neuroendocrine tumor: a case report and review of the literature. *World J Gastroenterol* 11: 7676–83.

Breeman WA, de Jong M, Kwekkeboom DJ *et al.* (2001) Somatostatin receptor-mediated imaging and therapy: basic science, current knowledge, limitations and future perspectives. *Eur J Nucl Med* 28: 1421–9.

Bruns C, Lewis I, Briner U, Meno-Tetang G, Weckbecker G. (2002) SOM230: a novel somatostatin peptidomimetic with broad somatotropin release inhibiting factor (SRIF) receptor binding and a unique antisecretory profile. *Eur J Endocrinol* 146: 707–16.

Canavese G, Azzoni C, Pizzi S *et al.* (2001) p27: a potential main inhibitor of cell proliferation in digestive endocrine tumors but not a marker of benign behavior. *Hum Pathol* 32: 1094–101.

Chung MH, Pisegna J, Spirt M *et al.* (2001) Hepatic cytoreduction followed by a novel long-acting somatostatin analog: a paradigm for intractable neuroendocrine tumors metastatic to the liver. *Surgery* 130: 954–62.

D'Adda T, Annibale B, Delle Fave G, Bordi C. (1996) Oxyntic endocrine cells of hypergastrinaemic patients. Differential response to antrectomy or octreotide. *Gut* 38: 668–74.

de Herder WW, Hofland LJ. (2004) Somatostatin receptors in pheochromocytoma. *Front Horm Res* 31: 145–54.

Delcore R, Friesen SR. (1994) Gastrointestinal neuroendocrine tumors. *J Am Coll Surg* 178: 187–211.

Feldman JM, Lee EM. (1985) Serotonin content of foods: effect on urinary excretion of 5-hydroxyindoleacetic acid. *Am J Clin Nutr* 42: 639–43.

Fenwick SW, Wyatt JI, Toogood GJ, Lodge JP. (2004) Hepatic resection and transplantation for primary carcinoid tumors of the liver. *Ann Surg* 239: 210–19.

Gay G, Delvaux M, Rey JF. (2004) The role of video capsule endoscopy in the diagnosis of digestive diseases: a review of current possibilities. *Endoscopy* 36: 913–20.

Gustafsson BI, Tommeras K, Nordrum I *et al.* (2005) Long-term serotonin administration induces heart valve disease in rats. *Circulation* 111: 1517–22.

Kaltsas GA, Besser GM, Grossman AB. (2004) The diagnosis and medical management of advanced neuroendocrine tumors. *Endocr Rev* 25: 458–511.

Kwekkeboom DJ, Teunissen JJ, Bakker WH *et al.* (2005) Radiolabeled somatostatin analog [177Lu-DOTA0,Tyr3]octreotate in patients with endocrine gastroenteropancreatic tumors. *J Clin Oncol* 23: 2754–62.

Lehnert T. (1998) Liver transplantation for metastatic neuroendocrine carcinoma: an analysis of 103 patients. *Transplantation* 66: 1307–12.

Lewis BS, Eisen GM, Friedman S. (2005) A pooled analysis to evaluate results of capsule endoscopy trials. *Endoscopy* 37: 960–5.

Marshall JB, Bodnarchuk G. (1993) Carcinoid tumors of the gut. Our experience over three decades and review of the literature. *J Clin Gastroenterol* 16: 123–9.

Modlin IM, Tang LH. (1997) Approaches to the diagnosis of gut neuroendocrine tumors: the last word (today). *Gastroenterology* 112: 583–90.

Modlin IM, Lye KD, Kidd M. (2003) A 5-decade analysis of 13,715 carcinoid tumors. *Cancer* 97: 934–59.

Modlin IM, Shapiro MD, Kidd M. (2004a) Carcinoid tumors and fibrosis: an association with no explanation. *Am J Gastroenterol* 99: 2466–78.

Modlin IM, Lye KD, Kidd M. (2004b) A 50-year analysis of 562 gastric carcinoids: small tumor or larger problem? *Am J Gastroenterol* 99: 23–32.

Modlin IM, Kidd M, Latich I, Zikusoka MN, Shapiro MD. (2005) Current status of gastrointestinal carcinoids. *Gastroenterology* 128: 1717–51.

Modlin IM, Latich I, Zikusoka M, Kidd M, Eick G, Chan AK. (2006a) Gastrointestinal carcinoids: the evolution of diagnostic strategies. *J Clin Gastroenterol* 40: 572–82.

Modlin IM, Latich I, Kidd M, Zikusoka M, Eick G. (2006b) Therapeutic options for gastrointestinal carcinoids. *Clin Gastroenterol Hepatol* 4: 526–47.

Nilsson O, Kolby L, Wangberg B *et al.* (1998) Comparative studies on the expression of somatostatin receptor subtypes, outcome of octreotide scintigraphy and response to octreotide treatment in patients with carcinoid tumours. *Br J Cancer* 77: 632–7.

Norheim I, Oberg K, Theodorsson-Norheim E *et al.* (1987) Malignant carcinoid tumors. An analysis of 103 patients with regard to tumor localization, hormone production, and survival. *Ann Surg* 206: 115–25.

Oberg K, Kvols L, Caplin M *et al.* (2004) Consensus report on the use of somatostatin analogs for the management of neuroendocrine tumors of the gastroenteropancreatic system. *Ann Oncol* 15: 966–73.

Okamoto Y, Fujii M, Tateiwa S *et al.* (2004) Treatment of multiple rectal carcinoids by endoscopic mucosal resection using a device for esophageal variceal ligation. *Endoscopy* 36: 469–70.

Plockinger U, Rindi G, Arnold R *et al.* (2004) Guidelines for the diagnosis and treatment of neuroendocrine gastrointestinal tumours. A consensus statement on behalf of the European Neuroendocrine Tumour Society (ENETS). *Neuroendocrinology* 80: 394–424.

Sarmiento JM, Heywood G, Rubin J, Ilstrup DM, Nagorney DM, Que FG.(2003) Surgical treatment of neuroendocrine metastases to the liver: a plea for resection to increase survival. *J Am Coll Surg* 197: 29–37.

Schnirer, II, Yao JC, Ajani JA. (2003) Carcinoid–a comprehensive review. *Acta Oncol* 42: 672–92.

Sutcliffe R, Maguire D, Ramage J, Rela M, Heaton N. (2004) Management of neuroendocrine liver metastases. *Am J Surg* 187: 39–46.

Teunissen JJ, Kwekkeboom DJ, Krenning EP. (2004) Quality of life in patients with gastroenteropancreatic tumors treated with [177Lu-DOTA0,Tyr3]octreotate. *J Clin Oncol* 22: 2724–9.

Tormey WP, FitzGerald RJ. (1995) The clinical and laboratory correlates of an increased urinary 5-hydroxyindoleacetic acid. *Postgrad Med J* 71: 542–5.

Van Eeden S, Quaedvlieg PF, Taal BG, Offerhaus GJ, Lamers CB, Van Velthuysen ML. (2002) Classification of low-grade neuroendocrine tumors of midgut and unknown origin. *Hum Pathol* 33: 1126–32.

Waltenberger J, Lundin L, Oberg K *et al.* (1993) Involvement of transforming growth factor-beta in the formation of fibrotic lesions in carcinoid heart disease. *Am J Pathol* 142: 71–8.

Zuetenhorst JM, Taal BG. (2005) Metastatic carcinoid tumors: a clinical review. *Oncologist* 10: 123–31.

Anorectal melanoma

Gary N. Mann, Shailender Bhatia & John L. Thompson

Introduction

Malignancies of the anal canal are rare, but anorectal melanomas (ARM) are rarer still, making up approximately 4% of all such tumors (Klas *et al.* 1999). While the incidence of cutaneous melanoma is increasing at a greater rate than any other human cancer in the USA, the anorectal site accounts for fewer than 1% of all melanomas. A National Cancer Data Base (NCDB) report on melanoma reported that mucosal melanomas make up 1.3% of all melanomas, with only 24% of these being of the anorectal region (Chang *et al.* 1998). In this NCDB study only 256 cases were reported over a decade.

The majority of tumors are located at or distal to the dentate line, with approximately 24% located more proximally. Presenting symptoms are non-specific: rectal bleeding in 67%, pain in 27%, changes of bowel habits in 22%, a palpable mass in 22%, and 'hemorrhoids' in 13% (Droesch *et al.* 2005). This, together with its rarity, can lead to a delay in the diagnosis, between 4 and 5 months (Cooper *et al.* 1982; Thibault *et al.* 1997), and possibly a more advanced stage of tumor at presentation. This is illustrated by a median tumor size of between 2 and 4 cm, and a median tumor thickness of between 5 and 7 mm (Ballo *et al.* 2002; Droesch *et al.* 2005; Yeh *et al.* 2006).

Once the diagnosis of ARM is made it is important that adequate staging be performed. This would include a full colonoscopy, CT scan of the chest, abdomen and pelvis, and many would feel a bone scan to be appropriate. Imaging of the brain in the absence of symptoms is not likely to be cost-effective. More recently, there has been much interest in the use of PET, and PET-CT fusion imaging. Their role in the staging of ARM is not well established, but it is likely that this modality will play an increasingly important role in the staging of this aggressive malignancy. While used much more extensively in the locoregional staging of anal squamous cell carcinoma and rectal adenocarcinoma, endorectal ultrasound appears to be useful in the T staging (depth) of ARM (Bullard *et al.* 2003). MRI is showing promise in the preoperative staging of anorectal tumors, and there are emerging reports of its use in patients with ARM, demonstrating consistency between the MRI results and pathologic findings (Matsuoka *et al.* 2005). The precise role for these latter two 'local' imaging modalities remains to be established, but they may be used to determine which tumors preclude attempts at local resection (e.g. deeply invasive into sphincters or circumferential).

ARM has a very poor prognosis. In contrast to patients with localized cutaneous melanoma, the majority of patients with apparently localized ARM develop distant metastases, despite initial aggressive surgical measures. The poor outcome in patients with this disease is attributable, in part, to the aforementioned delay in its diagnosis and the unfavorable stage distribution. Consequently, between 26 and 38% of patients have regional nodal or distant metastases at presentation (Wanebo *et al.* 1981; Cooper *et al.* 1982; Goldman *et al.* 1990; Weinstock 1993; Thibault *et al.* 1997). The 5-year overall survival for patients with anorectal melanoma ranges from 4% to 22% (Goldman *et al.* 1990; Slingluff *et al.* 1990; Brady *et al.* 1995; Roumen 1996; Thibault *et al.* 1997). This is in striking contrast to a 5-year overall survival of up to 92% for patients with cutaneous melanoma (Jemal *et al.* 2006). Patients with an advanced stage at diagnosis have a median survival of less than 1 year in most reported series (Goldman *et al.* 1990; Slingluff *et al.* 1990; Weinstock 1993; Roumen 1996; Thibault *et al.* 1997).

Much of the literature on the treatment of ARM has been limited to retrospective single-institution series. While it is clear that the mainstay of therapy is surgical, the poor outcomes of such treatment alone have led to questions regarding the optimal surgical approach, and the desire for improved adjuvant therapies. Unfortunately, no prospective studies of this disease exist. Thus the majority of the data available to guide us are based on these retrospective studies, systematic reviews of such studies, extrapolation from studies of adjuvant therapy for the much more common cutaneous melanoma, and expert opinion. In this chapter we will attempt to interpret the available data objectively, and provide a framework for the treatment of this rare, deadly form of melanoma.

Locoregional therapy for anorectal melanoma

As with most solid tumors, one of the principles governing the surgical therapy of ARM is that a margin-negative resection be obtained. It used to be felt that because of its aggressive nature, ARM required aggressive surgical resection, particularly since the disease is felt to spread proximally via the submucosa, and early via the draining lymphatics. Clearly in the anorectal region an aggressive approach such as this would necessitate an abdominoperineal resection (APR), and a permanent stoma. Several studies have supported this notion, and for many years the gold standard for treatment of ARM was an APR. Despite this, this notion has been challenged by the observation that the majority of patients with ARM ultimately relapsed and died of their disease, despite undergoing a sphincter-sacrificing procedure. Several more contemporary studies have evaluated a less aggressive local resection approach, preserving the anal sphincters, and avoiding the morbidity of a significant procedure such as an APR.

Despite the lack of prospective data, the emerging consensus based on the available data is that, when technically feasible, wide local excision (WLE) of ARM provides equivalent survival to APR. At the Memorial Sloan Kettering Cancer Center (MSKCC) the surgical treatment of ARM has evolved from the radical and morbid APR, to a less aggressive WLE. In their 1995 analysis of the MSKCC experience with 85 ARM patients treated over 64 years, Brady *et al.* (1995) showed that the overall 5-year survival was only 17%, and the median survival was 19 months. Of the 71 patients with resectable disease, those undergoing APR had a superior 5-year disease-free survival of 27%, compared with those undergoing WLE where the corresponding rate was 5%. More recently, Yeh *et al.* (2006) from MSKCC updated these results. They found that there was a dramatic shift in the surgical approach to patients with ARM; prior to 1997 71% of patients underwent APR, whilst after 1997 84% underwent WLE. Despite this there was no increase in local recurrence in their series (21% undergoing APR, 26% undergoing WLE). Indeed, 5-year disease-specific survival was near-identical: 34% following APR, and 35% following WLE. Interestingly, they also performed a multivariate analysis of factors associated with worse outcomes. The only factor associated with poorer survival was the presence of perineural invasion. Factors that one might have expected to predict worse outcome, such as tumor thickness or mural involvement, were not found to be significant.

Numerous, more contemporary, studies have supported the equivalence of these two surgical approaches in terms of patient survival. In contrast to the aforementioned study by Yeh *et al.*, there have been multiple reports of increased local recurrence rates with WLE alone. A combined analysis of multiple studies showed that APR had a local recurrence rate of 35%, half that of the 70% reported after WLE. In spite of this, these same studies failed to demonstrate a survival advantage for APR over

WLE (Ballo *et al.* 2002). This led the MD Anderson Cancer Center to investigate the addition of comprehensive adjuvant radiation therapy to a sphincter-preserving approach in patients with ARM, in an attempt to decrease local recurrence. The dose and fractionation schedule was efficient; 30 Gy in 5 fractions, delivered over 2.5 weeks, delivering a homogenous dose to the primary tumor site and draining lymphatics. Ballo *et al.* reviewed their institution's experience in 23 patients over 12 years, and found that this approach yielded a 5-year overall survival of 31% and a disease-specific survival of 36%, which compares favorably with other centers. Importantly, they found that the local control rate was 74%, and the nodal control rate was 84%, similar to the rates obtained historically with APR.

In order to address the lack of prospective data comparing APR to WLE in treatment of ARM, a recent systematic analysis was performed, in which series were included if they compared these two radically different treatment approaches, and allowed the calculation of median survival (Droesch *et al.* 2005). Although 22 studies over a 40-year period were identified, only 14 were judged suitable for inclusion in the review. A total of 129 patients underwent WLE, and 172 underwent APR. The overall median survival was found to be 21 and 17 months for WLE and APR, respectively, which was not statistically significant (see Table 15.5). Surprisingly, early stage-specific (node-negative) survival was better in those undergoing WLE compared to APR, although the available patient numbers were small. Local recurrence data was available in 100 patients undergoing APR and 96 patients treated by WLE. Respective rates were 23% and 47%, in keeping with the above mentioned doubling of local recurrence with WLE alone.

Other important locoregional issues include the width of surgical margins and management of the regional lymph node basins. There are no definitive data concerning either of these surgical questions. However, based on expert opinion, together with extrapolation from local excision of rectal cancers, as well as the need to avoid functional problems, 1–2-cm radial margins would seem to be adequate in performing a full-thickness WLE. Clearly, WLE would be precluded in tumors that were large and deeply invasive, circumferential, or if salvage therapy for an isolated local recurrence was considered.

Given the changing patterns of surgical treatment, and the rarity of ARM, the precise rate of regional lymph node (perirectal/pelvic and inguinal) metastasis at presentation is unknown, but is likely in the region of 20–30%. Elective lymph node dissection is not recommended in the treatment of ARM, similar to the management of draining nodal basins in cutaneous melanoma (Balch *et al.* 1996). However, we feel that if there is palpable or radiologic evidence of suspicious regional adenopathy, then therapeutic lymph node dissection seems warranted. Certainly, in cutaneous melanoma, there is little doubt as to its efficacy in treatment of documented regional metastasis (Morton *et al.* 2006). Similarly, for regionally metastatic ARM there are several series and reports where therapeutic lymph node dissection has resulted in occasional long-term survivors (Freedman 1984; Thibault *et al.* 1997). The performance of sentinel lymph node biopsy is intriguing, but only isolated case reports are to be found in the literature (Tien *et al.* 2002). Theoretically, it may avoid understaging and afford the patients the opportunity for aggressive treatment such as therapeutic lymph node dissection or systemic chemotherapy or immunotherapy

Table 15.5 Studies comparing wide local excision (WLE) to abdominoperineal resection (APR) and allowing calculation of median survival (months).(From Goldman *et al.* 1990; Mason & Helwig 1966; Abbas *et al.* 1980; Angeras *et al.* 1983; Ward *et al.* 1986; Kantarovsky *et al.* 1988; Ross *et al.* 1990; Antoniuk *et al.* 1993; Konstadoulakis *et al.* 1995; Cooper *et al.* 1982; Slingluff *et al.* 1990; Brady *et al.* 1995; Roumen 1996; Thibault *et al.* 1997.)

Author	Year	Hospital	WLE		APR	
			Number survival	Median	Number survival	Median
Mason *et al.*	1966	Armed Forces Institute	3	18	7	14
Abbas *et al.*	1980	Roswell Park Memorial Institute	7	8	11	20
Cooper *et al.*	1982	University of Virginia	5	17	3	41
Angeras *et al.*	1983	University of Lund	4	14	6	14
Ward *et al.*	1986	Highlands Hospital	3	12	3	8
Kantarovsky *et al.*	1988	Tel Aviv University	5	17	2	16
Goldman *et al.*	1990	University of Uppsala	18	13	15	12
Ross *et al.*	1990	MD Anderson	9	19	13	19
Slingluff *et al.*	1990	Duke University	7	20	13	18
Antoniuk *et al.*	1993	Cleveland Clinic	8	12	4	17
Brady *et al.*	1995	Memorial Sloan-Kettering	28	20	43	22
Konstadoulakis *et al.*	1995	Roswell Park Cancer Institute	5	18	8	14
Roumen	1996	St Joseph Hospital (Netherlands)	16	62	18	16
Thibault *et al.*	1997	Mayo Clinic	11	46	26	26
Total			**129**	**21**	**172**	**17**

(see next section). Its exact role is yet to be determined, but it will likely only have minor impact on this highly aggressive malignancy (Yeh *et al.* 2006), unlike the case for cutaneous melanoma.

Systemic therapy for anorectal melanoma

Given the typical grim outcome of patients with ARM treated with surgical resection alone, there is a rationale for incorporating systemic therapy in their treatment plan. However, no consensus concerning the optimal systemic therapy for ARM exists. As noted, the available literature consists mostly of case series with limited number of patients and retrospective reviews of institutional databases spanning many decades. The details of systemic treatments and clinical responses are often missing, making it impossible to accurately assess the efficacy of various treatments. Due to the paucity of clinic trials for this uncommon malignancy, most systemic therapies tried in patients with ARM have been originally used in patients with cutaneous melanoma. Such extrapolation, however, is fraught with flaws due to likely differences in the biology of these two tumor types. Besides the well-documented differences in clinical course of cutaneous and ARM, there has been some insight into the differences at the molecular level as well. For example, the V600E mutation in *BRAF* gene and mutations in the *NRAS* gene, which are commonly seen in cutaneous melanoma, have been reported to be absent in anorectal or other mucosal melanomas (Edwards *et al.* 2004; Helmke *et al.* 2004; Wong *et al.* 2005). Another report has implicated *KIT* mutations to be oncogenic in some mucosal melanomas and found such mutations to be absent in melanomas on skin without chronic sun damage (Curtin *et al.* 2006).

Various systemic therapies are available for patients with advanced cutaneous melanoma and include cytotoxic chemotherapy, immunotherapy (interferon, interleukin-2), and combination biochemotherapy. Cytotoxic chemotherapy with single-agent dacarbazine (DTIC) or temozolomide has response rates (RR) of approximately 15–20% in patients with metastatic melanoma (Lee *et al.* 2000; Middleton *et al.* 2000). Combination chemotherapy regimens such as CVD (cisplatin, vinblastine, DTIC) or CDBT (cisplatin, DTIC, carmustine, tamoxifen—Dartmouth regimen) have shown higher response rates but increased toxicity and lack of survival benefit, as compared to dacarbazine (Legha *et al.* 1989; Chapman *et al.* 1999). Use of recombinant cytokines such as interferon-α (IFN-α) or interleukin-2 (IL-2) in patients with metastatic cutaneous melanoma has resulted in RR of 15–20%, with complete responses (CR) in 4–6% of patients. Complete responders to therapy with high-dose IL-2 have a median disease-free survival in excess of 10 years and are possibly 'cured' (Atkins *et al.* 1999). However, high-dose IL-2 therapy is toxic and feasible only in patients with good performance status. Attempts to combine cytotoxic chemotherapy with IFN-α or IL-2 or both (biochemotherapy) have resulted in higher RR but have not shown significant survival benefit (Bajetta *et al.* 2006; Rosenberg *et al.* 1999). Many experimental approaches are being investigated in patients with metastatic melanoma including adoptive immunotherapy, cancer vaccines, molecularly targeted therapies, antiangiogenic agents etc. but trials typically exclude patients with ARM.

Many of the treatment approaches described above for cutaneous melanoma have been tried in patients with disseminated ARM. However, it is difficult to assess their efficacy with the limitations of available literature on this rare disease. Immunotherapeutic modalities and chemotherapy alone have been largely ineffective in this disease with an aggressive clinical course. A retrospective report of patients treated with biochemotherapy at MD Anderson Cancer Center showed potential for its use in treatment of unresectable or metastatic ARM (Kim *et al.* 2004). Among 13 patients who received biochemotherapy as first-line systemic therapy, 6 patients (46%) had complete or partial responses, including complete responses in 2 patients (15%). The median time to progression for this group was 6.2 months, and the median overall survival was 12.9 months. On the other hand, there was only 1 partial response observed among 11 patients (9%) treated with systemic therapy other than biochemotherapy as first-line treatment. The limited number of patients and the retrospective nature of this study may make it difficult to generalize these results. However, given the lack of larger prospective studies and any other effective therapy, it is reasonable to consider the use of biochemotherapy in management of patients with advanced ARM. Given the recent detection of *KIT* mutations in some patients with mucosal melanomas, therapy with imatinib is currently being investigated for these patients. Other palliative therapies that have been described in case reports of patients with advanced ARM include chemoembolization or regional chemotherapy for liver metastases or intratumoral IFN injections (Koksal *et al.* 2000; Izawa *et al.* 2002; Ulmer *et al.* 2002). There is an intriguing report of a remarkable response of a patient with metastatic ARM to combination cytotoxic chemotherapy (Yeh *et al.* 2005). After only two cycles of a novel regimen, consisting of cisplatin, temozolomide, and liposomal doxorubicin, the patient had a greater than 50% reduction in tumor size at the primary and metastatic sites, and was even able to have a palliative colostomy reversed. At 12 months there is minimal residual disease in pelvis, liver and lungs. This, and other similar individual responses, has led to the opening of a phase II study of this regimen for advanced mucosal melanomas, the results of which are eagerly awaited.

As mentioned above, the majority of patients with apparently localized ARM eventually succumb to distant metastases, indicating a propensity for early metastasis. ARM may represent a systemic disease at the time of diagnosis in most cases, and use of systemic adjuvant therapy may improve the outcomes for this life-threatening disease. High-dose IFN-α is the only FDA-approved adjuvant therapy, with modest benefit, for patients with stage IIB/III cutaneous melanoma (Kirkwood *et al.* 1996; Kirkwood *et al.* 2000; Kirkwood *et al.* 2001). However, it is fairly toxic, with major side effects including flu-like symptoms, neurocognitive impairment, depression, thyroid dysfunction and hepatotoxicity. Attempts to improve the efficacy of adjuvant therapy include the use of a shorter but more intensive treatment course with biochemotherapy (Kirkwood *et al.* 2006). The ongoing intergroup study S-0008, a phase III trial comparing high dose IFN-α versus biochemotherapy in patients with high-risk cutaneous melanoma in the adjuvant setting, is nearing completion of accrual and the results may influence management of patients with ARM as well. Development of sensitive biomarkers to detect residual disease may also identify the subset of patients most likely to benefit from adjuvant therapies. For example, the use of reverse transcript polymerase chain reaction to detect small numbers of melanoma-associated RNA transcripts in the peripheral blood may have prognostic value in determining early disease recurrence in patients with cutaneous melanoma (Hoon *et al.* 2000).

Conclusions

Anorectal melanoma (ARM) is a rare, highly aggressive malignancy. Diagnosis is often delayed, and patients frequently present with advanced stage of disease. Surgery is the mainstay of therapy and has evolved from the more radical APR, to a less morbid WLE. The rationale is based on the survival equivalence of the two approaches in numerous single-institutional experiences and systematic reviews. The possible increase in local recurrence with the less extensive WLE procedure can potentially be abrogated by an efficient regimen of external-beam radiation therapy.

In those patients with apparently localized ARM survival continues to be poor, since most are likely to harbor occult metastases. The benefit of systemic adjuvant therapy with high-dose IFN-α, a standard therapy in high-risk cutaneous melanoma, is expected to be small. For patients with disseminated disease at presentation, the use of biochemotherapy may cause tumor shrinkage and provide palliative benefit. There is a paramount need to study the biology of this aggressive disease at the molecular level, and to identify prognostic parameters, in order to develop optimal therapeutic approaches and effective targeted therapies. Due to small number of patients, there is also the need for multicenter collaboration and for encouragement of patients to participate in clinical trials. Until then, the systemic management of ARM will continue to be extrapolated from its cutaneous counterpart, and will await the development of novel regimens and/or agents.

References

Abbas JS, Karakousis CP, Holyoke ED. (1980) Anorectal melanoma: clinical features, recurrence and patient survival. *Int Surg* 65: 423–6.

Angeras U, Jonsson N, Jonsson PE. (1983) Primary anorectal malignant melanoma. *J Surg Oncol* 22: 261–4.

Antoniuk PM, Tjandra JJ, Webb BW, Petras RE, Milsom JW, Fazio VW. (1993) Anorectal malignant melanoma has a poor prognosis. *Int J Colorectal Dis* 8: 81–6.

Atkins MB, Lotze MT, Dutcher JP *et al.* (1999) High-dose recombinant interleukin 2 therapy for patients with metastatic melanoma: analysis of 270 patients treated between 1985 and 1993. *J Clin Oncol* 17: 2105–16.

Bajetta E, Del Vecchio M, Nova P *et al.* (2006) Multicenter phase III randomized trial of polychemotherapy (CVD regimen) versus the same chemotherapy (CT) plus subcutaneous interleukin-2 and interferon-alpha2b in metastatic melanoma. *Ann Oncol* 17: 571–7.

Balch CM, Soong SJ, Bartolucci AA *et al.* (1996) Efficacy of an elective regional lymph node dissection of 1 to 4 mm thick melanomas for patients 60 years of age and younger. *Ann Surg* 224: 255–63; discussion 263–6.

Ballo MT, Gershenwald JE, Zagars GK *et al.* (2002) Sphincter-sparing local excision and adjuvant radiation for anal-rectal melanoma. *J Clin Oncol* 20: 4555–8.

Brady MS, Kavolius JP, Quan SH. (1995) Anorectal melanoma. A 64-year experience at Memorial Sloan-Kettering Cancer Center. *Dis Colon Rectum* 38: 146–51.

Bullard KM, Tuttle TM, Rothenberger DA *et al.* (2003) Surgical therapy for anorectal melanoma. *J Am Coll Surg* 196: 206–11.

Chang AE, Karnell LH, Menck HR. (1998) The National Cancer Data Base report on cutaneous and noncutaneous melanoma: a summary of 84,836 cases from the past decade. The American College of Surgeons Commission on Cancer and the American Cancer Society. *Cancer* 83: 1664–78.

Chapman PB, Einhorn LH, Meyers ML *et al.* (1999) Phase III multicenter randomized trial of the Dartmouth regimen versus dacarbazine in patients with metastatic melanoma. *J Clin Oncol* 17: 2745–51.

Cooper PH, Mills SE, Allen MS Jr. (1982) Malignant melanoma of the anus: report of 12 patients and analysis of 255 additional cases. *Dis Colon Rectum* 25: 693–703.

Curtin JA, Busam K, Pinkel D, Bastian BC. (2006) Somatic activation of KIT in distinct subtypes of melanoma. *J Clin Oncol* 24: 4340–6.

Droesch JT, Flum DR, Mann GN. (2005) Wide local excision or abdominoperineal resection as the initial treatment for anorectal melanoma? *Am J Surg* 189: 446–9.

Edwards RH, Ward MR, Wu H *et al.* (2004) Absence of BRAF mutations in UV-protected mucosal melanomas. *J Med Genet* 41: 270–2.

Freedman LS. (1984) Malignant melanoma of the anorectal region: two cases of prolonged survival. *Br J Surg* 71: 164–5.

Goldman S, Glimelius B, Pahlman L. (1990) Anorectal malignant melanoma in Sweden. Report of 49 patients. *Dis Colon Rectum* 33: 874–7.

Helmke BM, Mollenhauer J, Herold-Mende C *et al.* (2004) BRAF mutations distinguish anorectal from cutaneous melanoma at the molecular level. *Gastroenterology* 127: 1815–20.

Hoon DS, Bostick P, Kuo C *et al.* (2000) Molecular markers in blood as surrogate prognostic indicators of melanoma recurrence. *Cancer Res* 60: 2253–7.

Izawa H, Souma I, Fukuchi N *et al.* (2002) [A case of liver metastasis from anorectal malignant melanoma treated by chemoembolization]. *Gan To Kagaku Ryoho* 29: 2350–3.

Jemal A, Siegel R, Ward E *et al.* (2006) Cancer statistics, 2006. *CA Cancer J Clin* 56: 106–30.

Kantarovsky A, Kaufman Z, Zager M, Lew S, Dinbar A. (1988) Anorectal region malignant melanoma. *J Surg Oncol* 38: 77–9.

Kim KB, Sanguino AM, Hodges C *et al.* (2004) Biochemotherapy in patients with metastatic anorectal mucosal melanoma. *Cancer* 100: 1478–83.

Kirkwood JM, Strawderman MH, Ernstoff MS, Smith TJ, Borden EC, Blum RH. (1996) Interferon alfa-2b adjuvant therapy of high-risk resected cutaneous melanoma: the Eastern Cooperative Oncology Group Trial EST 1684. *J Clin Oncol* 14: 7–17.

Kirkwood JM, Ibrahim JG, Sondak VK *et al.* (2000) High- and low-dose interferon alfa-2b in high-risk melanoma: first analysis of intergroup trial E1690/S9111/C9190. *J Clin Oncol* 18: 2444–58.

Kirkwood JM, Ibrahim JG, Sosman JA *et al.* (2001) High-dose interferon alfa-2b significantly prolongs relapse-free and overall survival compared with the GM2-KLH/QS-21 vaccine in patients with resected stage IIB-III melanoma: results of intergroup trial E1694/S9512/C509801. *J Clin Oncol* 19: 2370–80.

Kirkwood JM, Moschos S, Wang W. (2006) Strategies for the development of more effective adjuvant therapy of melanoma: current and future explorations of antibodies, cytokines, vaccines, and combinations. *Clin Cancer Res* 12: 2331s–2336s.

Klas JV, Rothenberger DA, Wong WD, Madoff RD. (1999) Malignant tumors of the anal canal: the spectrum of disease, treatment, and outcomes. *Cancer* 85: 1686–93.

Koksal N, Muftuoglu T, Gunerhan Y, Uskent N. (2000) Complete remission of the liver metastases of anorectal malignant melanoma with regional chemotherapy: a case report. *Hepatogastroenterology* 47: 612–4.

Konstadoulakis MM, Ricaniadis N, Walsh D, Karakousis CP. (1995) Malignant melanoma of the anorectal region. *J Surg Oncol* 58: 118–20.

Lee ML, Tomsu K, Von Eschen KB. (2000) Duration of survival for disseminated malignant melanoma: results of a meta-analysis. *Melanoma Res* 10: 81–92.

Legha SS, Ring S, Papadopoulos N, Plager C, Chawla S, Benjamin R. (1989) A prospective evaluation of a triple-drug regimen containing cisplatin, vinblastine, and dacarbazine (CVD) for metastatic melanoma. *Cancer* 64: 2024–9.

Mason JK, Helwig EB. (1966) Ano-rectal melanoma. *Cancer* 19: 39–50.

Matsuoka H, Nakamura A, Iwamoto K *et al.* (2005) Anorectal malignant melanoma: preoperative usefulness of magnetic resonance imaging. *J Gastroenterol* 40: 836–42.

Middleton MR, Grob JJ, Aaronson N *et al.* (2000) Randomized phase III study of temozolomide versus dacarbazine in the treatment of patients with advanced metastatic malignant melanoma. *J Clin Oncol* 18: 158–66.

Morton DL, Thompson JF, Cochran AJ *et al.* (2006) Sentinel-node biopsy or nodal observation in melanoma. *N Engl J Med* 355: 1307–17.

Rosenberg SA, Yang JC, Schwartzentruber DJ *et al.* (1999) Prospective randomized trial of the treatment of patients with metastatic melanoma using chemotherapy with cisplatin, dacarbazine, and tamoxifen alone or in combination with interleukin-2 and interferon alfa-2b. *J Clin Oncol* 17: 968–75.

Ross M, Pezzi C, Pezzi T, Meurer D, Hickey R, Balch C. (1990) Patterns of failure in anorectal melanoma. A guide to surgical therapy. *Arch Surg* 125: 313–6.

Roumen RM. (1996) Anorectal melanoma in The Netherlands: a report of 63 patients. *Eur J Surg Oncol* 22: 598–601.

Slingluff CL Jr, Vollmer RT, Seigler HF. (1990) Anorectal melanoma: clinical characteristics and results of surgical management in twenty-four patients. *Surgery* 107: 1–9.

Thibault C, Sagar P, Nivatvongs S, Ilstrup DM, Wolff BG. (1997) Anorectal melanoma–an incurable disease? *Dis Colon Rectum* 40: 661–8.

Tien HY, Mcmasters KM, Edwards MJ, Chao C. (2002) Sentinel lymph node metastasis in anal melanoma: a case report. *Int J Gastrointest Cancer* 32: 53–6.

Ulmer A, Metzger S, Fierlbeck G. (2002) Successful palliation of stenosing anorectal melanoma by intratumoral injections with natural interferon-beta. *Melanoma Res* 12: 395–8.

Wanebo HJ, Woodruff JM, Farr GH, Quan SH. (1981) Anorectal melanoma. *Cancer* 47: 1891–900.

Ward MW, Romano G, Nicholls RJ. (1986) The surgical treatment of anorectal malignant melanoma. *Br J Surg* 73: 68–9.

Weinstock MA. (1993) Epidemiology and prognosis of anorectal melanoma. *Gastroenterology* 104: 174–8.

Wong CW, Fan YS, Chan TL *et al.* (2005) BRAF and NRAS mutations are uncommon in melanomas arising in diverse internal organs. *J Clin Pathol* 58: 640–4.

Yeh JJ, Weiser MR, Shia J, Hwu WJ. (2005) Response of stage IV anal mucosal melanoma to chemotherapy. *Lancet Oncol* 6: 438–9.

Yeh JJ, Shia J, Hwu WJ *et al.* (2006) The role of abdominoperineal resection as surgical therapy for anorectal melanoma. *Ann Surg* 244: 1012–7.

Cancer of the anal canal

Matthew Clark & Lincoln Israel

Introduction

Anal cancer is a relatively uncommon tumor of the gastrointestinal tract (Fig. 15.4). Prior to 1995, it was more common in females (Johnson 2004). Since then the incidence in males and females has been similar. There is a strong relationship between anal cancer and incidence of infection with the human papillomaviruses, lifetime number of sexual partners, receptive anal intercourse, and infection with the human immunodeficiency virus (HIV). In the past two decades we have seen an understanding of its etiology paralleled by improvements in treatment (Ryan 2000; Clark 2004). Anal cancer can often be cured by synchronous chemoradiotherapy, which allows preservation of anal continence. Major surgical resection (abdominoperineal resection of the anal canal and rectum with formation of a permanent colostomy) is reserved for recurrent or residual disease after primary chemoradiotherapy. Overall, survival from anal cancer now approaches 80% at 5 years. We may see more of this tumor in the medium-term future due to human papillomavirus and HIV infection, but this may be ultimately balanced by preventative measures, more accurate characterization and treatment of early (*in situ*) disease, and the optimization of chemoradiation regimens.

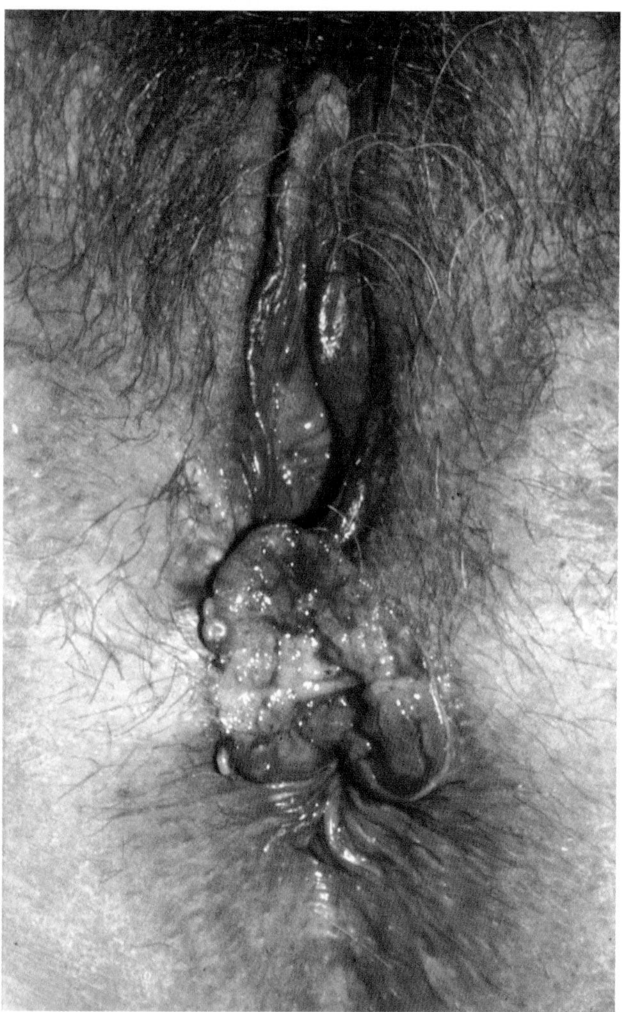

Fig. 15.4 Cancer of the anal canal.

Etiology

A past history of genital warts has been known to predispose to anal cancer, and it is now considered that infection with human papillomavirus (HPV) is the most important etiologic agent (Frisch 1997). HPV can cause anal intraepithelial neoplasia (in the same manner as cervical intraepithelial neoplasia), which may progress to invasive cancer. Current evidence suggests a complex interplay between HPV infection and subsequent DNA integration, and the role of stepwise mutations in tumor suppressor genes in the development of invasive anal cancer (Gervas 2006). Some HPV subtypes are associated with a higher risk of malignant transformation. Immunization against HPV type 16 has been shown to reduce the incidence of cervical neoplasms, and some countries are considering the widespread introduction of such a program. It is possible that this may also protect against the development of anal cancer. Smoking probably increases the risk of anal cancer.

While HPV is the likely causative agent of anal cancer, immune status may determine the time of progression to anal cancer. Therapeutic immunosuppression increases the risk (Patel 2007). The frequency of anal cancer in the presence of HIV infection is increased, but this linkage is confounded by the associated high risk of sexual transmission of HPV in this group of patients.

Incidence

The annual incidence of anal cancer is around 1 per 100,000 in the general population, accounting for around 600 new cases per year in the UK and around 4500 in the USA (American Cancer Society 2007). The peak incidence has been around 60 years, but this has been decreasing since the 1960s due to changes in risk factors. The incidence is up to 35 times higher in men who practice anal-receptive sexual intercourse, and those who are HIV positive have twice the risk of those who are not.

Pathology

The definition and terminology of cancers in the anal region may sometimes be confusing. Squamous tumors of the cutaneous anal margin can be treated like skin lesions with wide excision, resulting in 80% 5-year survival. True anal canal cancer arises from the distal anal canal, which is lined with squamous epithelium, changing to a transitional epithelium near the dentate line and ultimately to non-squamous rectal mucosa. Distal anal tumors tend to have a keratinising squamous morphology, whereas more proximal tumors are less likely to be keratinized (Williams 1994). The latter are sometimes referred to as cloacogenic or basaloid, yet the distinction is of little clinical relevance. Rare anal canal tumors include adenocarcinomas of the anal ducts or glands (which behave almost identically to rectal adenocarcinoma) and anal melanoma, which is very aggressive.

Anal cancer tends to spreads via the lymphatic system initially. Below the dentate line, inguinal and femoral lymph nodes are preferentially involved, whereas the proximal anal canal drains to perirectal nodes. About 10% of patients present with synchronous nodal disease in the groin. Distant metastases (usually to liver and lungs) develop in 10–20% of those who are treated for anal cancer.

Clinical features

Symptoms of anal cancer are not specific. Half of those with anal cancer present with bright red rectal-outlet bleeding, and anal pain occurs in many. Large tumors can interfere with sphincter function and lead to incontinence. A minority of patients have no symptoms. On clinical examination, a mass is usually identified, the median size at diagnosis being in the order of 4 cm. The size and position of the tumor can usually be determined clinically, as can whether the mass is fixed to surrounding structures such as the prostate, vagina, or bony pelvis. Enlarged perirectal lymph nodes are evident on digital examination of the rectum in some patients.

Proctosigmoidoscopy should be performed, as should gynecologic examination in women. Draining nodal basins are checked, and a general examination for distant metastases performed. Some patients may require examination under anesthesia in order to obtain a thorough pelvic examination and facilitate biopsy.

Diagnosis

When a clinically suspicious lesion is found, a diagnosis of anal cancer depends on cytologic or histologic confirmation. Appropriate biopsies with accompanying clinical information should allow the pathologist to confidently diagnose anal cancer.

Staging and other investigations

As the primary treatment for anal cancer is now chemoradiotherapy, the TNM staging system is based upon tumor size and nodal status rather than depth within a surgical specimen (Tables 15.6 & 15.7). Generally, local staging will have little impact on treatment decisions, as most patients will be initially treated with chemoradiotherapy regardless of their stage.

Table 15.6 American Joint Committee on Cancer (AJCC) staging system for anal carcinoma.

Primary tumor (T)	
Tx	Primary tumor cannot be assessed
T0	No evidence of primary tumor
Tis	Carcinoma in situ
T1	Tumor 2 cm or less in greatest dimension
T2	Tumor more than 2 cm but not more than 5 cm in greatest dimension
T3	Tumor more than 5 cm in greatest dimension
T4	Tumor of any size invades adjacent organ(s), e.g., vagina, urethra, bladder (involvement of the sphincter muscle(s) alone is not classified as T4)
Regional lymph nodes (N)	
Nx	Regional lymph nodes cannot be assessed
N0	No regional lymph node metastasis
N1	Metastasis in perirectal lymph node(s)
N2	Metastasis in unilateral internal iliac and/or inguinal lymph nodes
N3	Metastasis in perirectal and inguinal lymph nodes and/or bilateral internal iliac and/or inguinal lymph nodes
Distant metastasis (M)	
Mx	Distant metastasis cannot be assessed
M0	No distant metastasis
M1	Distant metastasis

Table 15.7 Stage grouping.

Stage 0	Tis	N0	M0
Stage I	T1	N0	M0
Stage II	T2	N0	M0
	T3	N0	M0
Stage IIIA	T1	N1	M0
	T2	N1	M0
	T3	N1	M0
	T4	N0	M0
Stage IIIB	T4	N1	M0
	Any T	N2	M0
	Any T	N3	M0
Stage IV	Any T	Any N	M1

Interest has recently focused on nodal staging as questions regarding prophylactic versus targeted inclusion of inguinal nodes in radiation fields are raised.

Locoregional staging relies upon information from both clinical and imaging features. Digital rectal examination will determine tumor size, location and fixity. Clinically involved inguinal nodes should be evaluated with fine needle aspiration, and about 50% of these palpable nodes will contain metastatic deposits. A combination of imaging modalities may then be used, including endoanal ultrasound, CT, MRI, or PET scan.

Staging of the primary tumor

Radiologic techniques most appropriate for staging of the primary tumor include endoanal ultrasound and MRI. Endorectal ultrasound is well proven in the staging of rectal cancer; however, the walls of the anus are not as well defined, and hence for anal cancer ultrasound is primarily confined to detection of T4 cancers invading other structures, and for the detection of perirectal lymph nodes.

An ultrasound-based staging system has been proposed which is defined by depth of invasion into or through the sphincter complex (Taratino 2002). Such staging may influence treatment decisions, especially with local excision possible for early lesions, and may be more discriminatory in trials of different treatment modalities. Studies will be necessary to decide if staging of depth of invasion has any more prognostic significance than that based solely on tumor size.

MRI has been used extensively in the staging of rectal cancer, but few studies have looked at its use in anal cancer. The scan may performed with or without an endorectal coil, with newer units probably not requiring this. In cases where subsequent surgical specimens are available, good correlation with presurgical MRI has been demonstrated (Roach *et al.* 2005). MRI has the advantage of multiplanar visualization. It is less user-dependent than endoanal ultrasound, and many clinicians find the ability to project and compare images (especially follow-up images in questions of recurrence) in a multidisciplinary review extremely useful.

CT of the pelvis is often obtained incidentally during staging for distant disease, but as for rectal cancer it does not reveal the layers of the anorectal region, nor differentiate between tumor and normal pelvic tissues as clearly as MRI.

Staging of lymphatic spread

The presence of nodal disease has important implications for prognosis and may require alterations in treatment. Involvement of perirectal lymph nodes may be more frequent but are clinically less important as such nodes are included in the radiotherapy fields of the primary tumor. In contrast, the diagnosis of involved inguinal or iliac nodes may demand additional radiation to these fields. Any clinically involved groin nodes should be subjected to fine needle aspiration biopsy, and if this is negative an open lymph node biopsy may be considered.

Radiologic nodal assessment usually relies on CT or MRI. CT has a high sensitivity in defining enlarged lymph nodes but these nodes may be enlarged from reactive changes; similarly, normal-sized nodes may be infiltrated by cancer. MRI suffers from the same problems. Functional imaging modalities—specifically 18-fluorodeoxyglucose positron emission tomography (PET) or coregistered CT/PET can identify substantially more abnormal inguinal lymph nodes than CT alone (Cotter 2006). Work in other pelvic malignancies has shown PET to be a highly specific determinant of nodal involvement. However FNA confirmation may still be required to confirm metastatic spread.

Sentinel lymph node biopsy using lymphoscintigraphy and patent blue dye injected around the site of the tumor has been shown to be technically feasible. This sentinel node can then be assessed for microscopic disease. Dissemination to both inguinal lymphatic basins is common in tumors involving the midline of the anal canal. It has been argued that sentinel lymph node biopsy may allow patients with no involvement of inguinal nodes to be spared the morbidity of prophylactic inguinal irradiation. In trials reported to date, around 20% of patients have subclinical lymph node disease at sentinel node biopsy (Damin 2006).

Distant spread

Anal cancer tends to spread hematogenously to the liver and lungs. Contrast-enhanced CT and MRI are the modalities used most often in the detection of metastases to these sites. For cost and efficiency of time we use CT of the chest, abdomen and pelvis primarily for staging of distant disease, and MRI for local staging.

Treatment

The traditional operative treatment for anal cancer, abdominoperineal resection, was a reasonably effective local therapy for early cancer; 5-year survival was in the order of around 70%. However this resulted in a permanent stoma. Such surgery is still required for salvage of residual or recurrent local disease (Nilsson 2002). Radiotherapy alone has also been used in the past in patients for whom surgery was not an option. Combined multimodality treatment has relegated these approaches to historical interest. Of particular note, the success of such treatment, and the implication of appropriate expert multispecialist assessment and treatment, have led to recommendations (such as the NICE guidelines in the UK) that patients should be referred to specialist teams where these exist.

Since Nigro's 1974 publication (Nigro 1974) of pathologic complete responses in two of three patients with anal cancer after low-dose radiotherapy and synchronous mitomycin and fluorouracil (FU) given before abdominoperineal resection, a large number of further studies have determined that primary chemoradiotherapy is appropriate for most patients, with the major benefit of preserved anal sphincter function without an obvious detriment to overall survival. In the 1980s, two studies that compared the results of chemoradiotherapy with historical controls treated by radiotherapy alone suggested improved local control (Cummings *et al.* 1984; Papillon *et al.* 1987).

Two subsequent randomized trials have since confirmed these findings (Table 15.8). In the trial by the European Organisation for Research and Treatment of Cancer (EORTC), 110 patients were randomly assigned radiotherapy alone (45 Gy in 25 fractions, followed 6 weeks later by a boost of 15–20 Gy), or the same radiotherapy schedule with synchronous chemotherapy (mitomycin 15 mg/m^2 on day 1; fluorouracil 750 mg/m^2 on days 1–5 and days 29–33). The combined modality group had better local control (68% vs 55% at 3 years, $p = 0.02$) and colostomy-free interval (72% vs 47% at 3 years, $p = 0.002$) than the radiotherapy group.

In the larger UK Coordinating Committee on Cancer Research (UKCCCR) trial, 585 patients were randomized to radiotherapy (45 Gy in 20 or 25 fractions, followed 6 weeks later by a boost of 15 Gy) or chemoradiotherapy (mitomycin 12 mg/m^2 on day 1; fluorouracil 1 g/m^2 on days 1–4 and days 29–32). Local control at 3 years was better in patients assigned chemoradiotherapy than in those assigned radiotherapy alone (61% vs 39%, $p < 0.0001$). There was no difference in overall survival between chemoradiotherapy and radiotherapy alone in either trial.

Although such trials have established that chemoradiotherapy is more effective than radiotherapy alone in terms of local control, there remains uncertainty as to the most appropriate radiotherapy dosage and fractionation, and the best chemotherapy regimen. Initial studies used doses of 45 Gy in around 20–25 fractions, often with a subsequent 15-Gy boost, and mitomycin and FU. Numerous modifications of both the radiotherapy and chemotherapy arms, including the use of cisplatin and other agents, have also been examined (Eng 2006).

About 5–15% of patients will harbour gross or microscopic residual disease after chemoradiotherapy, and will require abdominoperineal resection. Alternatives include sphincter-sparing resection, second-line chemotherapy, and

Table 15.8 Randomized studies of the treatment of anal cancer.

Studies	No. of patients	Local failure (%)	Colostomy-free survival (%)	Disease-free survival (%)	Overall survival (%)
UKCCR	585				
RT+5-FU		99		61	58
RT+5-FU+mito		36		72	65
		p < 0.0001			NS
EORTC	110				
RT		50	40		52
RT+5-FU+mito		40	73		59
		p = 0.02	p = 0.002		NS
ECOG/RTOG	310				
RT+5-FU			59	51	42
RT+5-FU+mito			71	73	32
			p = 0.014	p = 0.0003	NS

brachytherapy; but these should be considered investigational at this time. Similarly, 10–30% of patients will develop locoregional relapse of disease, and may be treated as above. It is unclear whether residual or recurrent disease carries the worse prognosis, and in both groups the outcome is guarded.

The management of clinically and radiologically negative nodal fields remains uncertain, which is why sentinel node biopsy is conceptually attractive; but generally prophylactic irradiation of the normal groin is not recommended. Involved inguinal nodes at primary diagnosis or as metachronous metastasis after chemoradiotherapy may be treated with therapeutic nodal dissection or radiation (depending on previous dose and fields).

Distant metastatic disease occurs in around 20% of patients, and is treated as appropriate. As the tumor is relatively chemosensitive, chemotherapy is often a treatment component with cisplatin frequently used. Radiotherapy is useful for painful skeletal lesions and brain metastases.

Treatment complications

As with any chemotherapeutic regimen, toxicity may be seen, and death (usually from neutropenic sepsis) may occur in 1–2%. Some severe late side-effects may be seen in those undergoing either radiation treatment or chemoradiotherapy, including bleeding, anal necrosis, skin ulceration, stenosis or fibrosis, and diarrhea; these may be seen in up to 30% of patients. Some patients may elect to undergo colostomy formation with or without anal resection under these circumstances.

Prognosis

Gender, tumor stage, nodal status, and response to chemoradiation are independent prognostic factors for local control and overall survival in anal cancer (Salmon 1986; Johnson 2004). The histologic subtype has little prognostic importance. Patients with well-differentiated tumors have a more favourable outcome than those with poorly differentiated tumors.

References

American Cancer Society. (2007) *Cancer Facts and Figures 2007*. American Cancer Society, Atlanta.

American Joint Committee on Cancer. (1997) *AJCC Cancer Staging Manual*, 5th edn. Lippincott-Raven Publishers, Philadelphia.

Clark MA, Hartley A, Geh JI. (2004) Cancer of the anal canal. *Lancet Oncol* 5: 149–57.

Cotter SE, Perry WG, Siegel BA *et al.* (2006) FDG-PET/CT in the evaluation of anal carcinoma. *Int J Radiat Oncol Biol Phys* 65: 720–25.

Cummings B, Keane T, Thomas G, Harwood A, Rider W. (1984) Results and toxicity of the treatment of anal canal carcinoma by radiation therapy or radiation therapy and chemotherapy. *Cancer* 54: 2062–8.

Damin DC, Rosito MA, Scwartsmann G. (2006) Sentinel lymph node in carcinoma of the anal canal: A review. *Eur J Surg Oncol* 32: 247–52.

Eng C. (2006) Anal cancer: current and future methodology. *Cancer Invest* 24: 535–44.

Frisch M, Glimelius B, Van Den Brule AJC *et al.* (1997) Sexually transmitted infections as a cause of anal cancer. *N Engl J Med* 337: 1350–8.

Gervaz P, Hirschel B, Morel P. (2006) Molecular biology of squamous cell carcinoma of the anus. *Br J Surg* 93: 531–8.

Johnson LG, Madeleine MM, Newcomer LM *et al.* (2004) Anal cancer incidence and survival: the surveillance, epidemiology, and end results experience, 1973–2000. *Cancer* 101(2): 281–8.

Nigro ND, Vaitkevicius VK, Considine B, Jr. (1974) Combined therapy for cancer of the anal canal: a preliminary report. *Dis Colon Rectum* 173: 354–6.

Nilsson PJ, Svensson C, Goldman S, Glimelius B. (2002) Salvage abdominoperineal resection in anal epidermoid cancer. *Br J Surg* 89: 1425–9.

Papillon J, Montbarbon JF. (1987) Epidermoid carcinoma of the anal canal. A series of 276 cases. *Dis Colon Rectum* 30: 324–33.

Patel HS, Silver AR, Northover JM. (2007) Anal cancer in renal transplant patients. *Int J Colorectal Dis* 22: 1–5.

Roach SC, Hulse PA, Moulding FJ, Wilson R, Carrington BM. (2005) Magnetic resonance imaging of anal cancer. *Clin Radiol* 60: 1111–19.

Ryan DP, Compton CC, Mayer RJ. (2000) Carcinoma of the anal canal. *N Engl J Med* 342: 792–800.

Salmon RJ, Zafrani B, Labib A, Asselain B, Girodet J. (1986) Prognosis of cloacogenic and squamous cancers of the anal canal. *Dis Colon Rectum* 29: 336–40.

Tarantino D, Bernsetin MA. (2002) Endoanal ultrasound in the staging and management of squamous-cell carcinoma of the anal canal. Potential implications of a new ultrasound staging system. *Dis Colon Rectum* 45: 16–22.

Williams GR, Talot IC. (1994) Anal carcinoma—a histological review. *Histopathology* 25: 507–16.

Appendiceal epithelial neoplasms

Paul H. Sugarbaker

Diagnosis

History (symptoms)

The preoperative diagnosis in patients with adenocarcinoma of the appendix is usually appendicitis, a right lower quadrant abscess, or tumor mass. Mucinous appendiceal cancer has usually perforated prior to diagnosis (Lyss 1988). This results in tumor spread bilaterally to the ovary, or the tumor may present as peritoneal carcinomatosis within a hernia sac. An aggressive mucinous adenocarcinoma may invade the retroperitoneum and appear as a mucus accumulation in the buttock or thigh. Also, abdominal wall invasion with an enterocutaneous fistula or bladder invasion with an enterovesical fistula may occur. Obstruction of the right ureter by a mucus-containing mass or invasion into the urinary bladder has also occurred.

The symptoms and signs of pseudomyxoma peritonei are quite different from appendiceal adenocarcinoma. The most common symptom in both men and women with pseudomyxoma peritonei syndrome is a gradually increasing abdominal girth (Esquivel & Sugarbaker 2000). In women, the second most common symptom is an ovarian mass, usually on the right side and frequently diagnosed at the time of a routine gynecologic examination. In men, the second most common symptom is a new-onset hernia. The hernia sac is found to be filled by mucin and/or mucinous tumor. In both males and females, the third most common presenting feature is appendicitis. This is the clinical manifestation of rupture of an appendiceal mucocele which contains intestinal bacteria. The patients who present with appendicitis have a higher incidence of more aggressive histology and lymph node involvement.

Clinical signs

Appendiceal epithelial tumors have unique characteristics that result in clinical signs that are in marked contrast to colorectal cancer. Appendiceal neoplasms show varying amounts of invasiveness. About 75% are non-invasive and grow slowly so patients may not appreciate abdominal distention until it is advanced. Patients with minimally aggressive tumors may survive a decade or longer even without specialized treatments. However, some appendiceal tumors (usually signet-ring histologic type) are very invasive, progress rapidly, and can cause death 1–2 years after the initial diagnosis.

A majority of patients with these tumors have peritoneal dissemination at the time of diagnosis. This is a notable contrast with colorectal cancer, in which only about 15% of patients present with carcinomatosis. Progression is usually confined to the peritoneal space, and most patients with minimally invasive tumors die from loss of intestinal function as the mucinous tumors expand within the abdomen and pelvis.

Most patients with appendiceal neoplasms have no lymphatic or hematogenous metastases; 2% of patients have metastases in the lymph nodes and 2% in the liver; thus extensive local–regional treatments can eliminate the disease. Surgical management of the primary tumor is usually appendicectomy or cecectomy, and an appendiceal lymph node dissection is needed to rule out regional lymph-node metastases (Gonzalez-Moreno & Sugarbaker 2004).

Appendiceal mucinous neoplasms spare the small bowel, which qualifies them for aggressive local–regional treatment using peritonectomy. The small bowel and its mesentery are tumor free even though large volumes of mucinous neoplasm are located within the greater and lesser omentum, the space between the liver and the diaphragm, and within the pelvis. Carmignani and colleagues reported that the constant peristaltic activity of the small bowel prevents neoplastic cells from adhering to its surfaces or to the small bowel mesentery, except to the part of the jejunum that is adjacent to the ligament of Treitz and the terminal ileum or ileocecal valve area, which are tethered by a short mesentery to the retroperitoneum (Carmignani *et al.* 2003).

Pseudomyxoma peritonei syndrome

The term pseudomyxoma peritonei is used to describe the less aggressive mucinous appendiceal epithelial neoplasms that show a large volume of mucus and a minimum amount of solid tumor. They have a high propensity for spread to peritoneal surfaces, but almost never metastasize through lymphatic channels into lymph nodes or through venules into the liver. After the tumor ruptures the wall of the appendix (Fig. 15.5), adenomucinosis can progress for months or even years within the abdomen and pelvis without causing other symptoms. As the disease progresses, the peritoneal cavity becomes filled with mucinous neoplasm and mucinous ascites. The greater

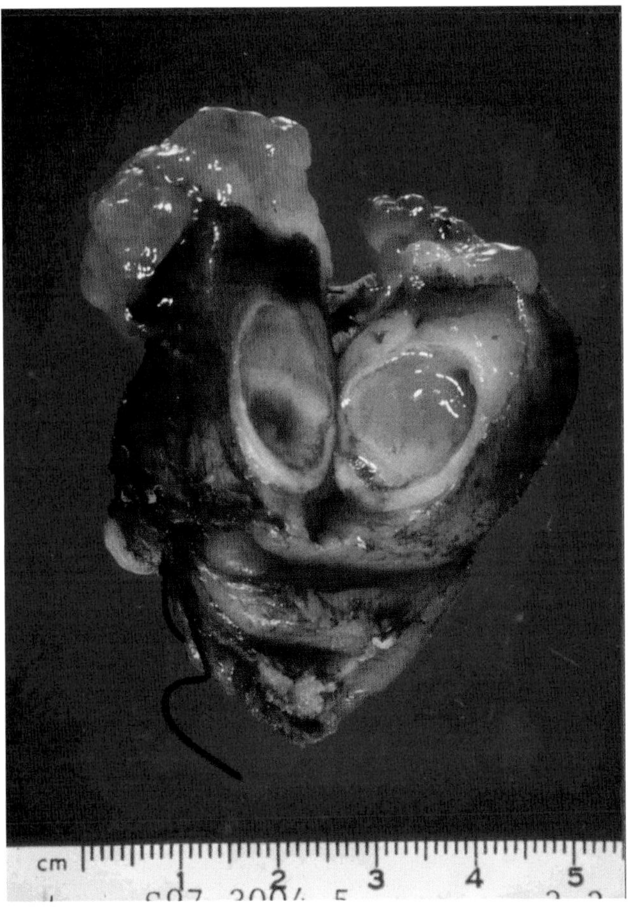

Fig. 15.5 The distal appendix has ruptured from mucin within the mucocele. Adenomatous epithelial cells become widely distributed on peritoneal surfaces. The silk suture is on the base of the appendix.

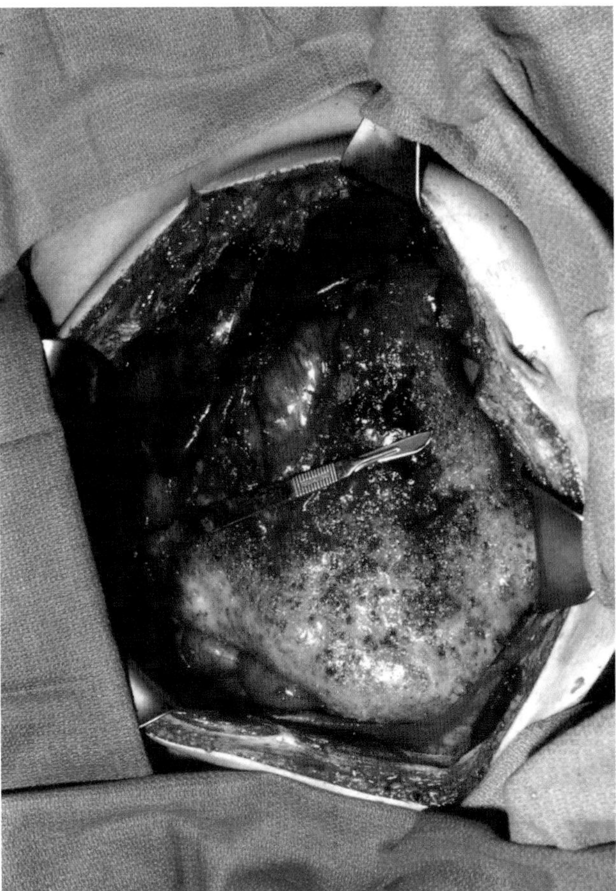

Fig. 15.6 'Omental cake' characteristically present in patients with pseudomyxoma peritonei.

omentum is greatly thickened (omental cake) and extensively infiltrated by tumor (Fig. 15.6). Parts of the abdomen that entrap malignant cells include the undersurface of the right and left hemidiaphragms, the right subhepatic space, the splenic hilus, the right and left abdominal gutters, and the pelvis and cul-de-sac. An important clinical feature of pseudomyxoma peritonei is that tumors spare the mobile portions of the small bowel (Fig. 15.7); consequently, the involved parietal and visceral peritoneal surfaces can thus be resected by visceral resections and by peritonectomy.

Histopathology

Ronnett and colleagues studied the histomorphology of mucinous appendiceal neoplasms and greatly clarified the differences in survival to be expected in this disease process where there is a wide spectrum of aggressive versus non-aggressive neoplasms (Ronnett *et al.* 1997, 2001). In the Ronnett data all patients were treated in a uniform manner with cytoreductive surgery and perioperative intraperitoneal chemotherapy. They separated the mucinous appendiceal neoplasms into three

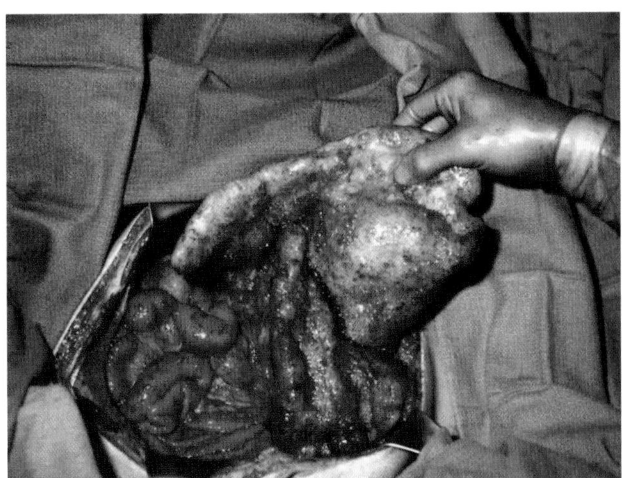

Fig. 15.7 When the omentum is elevated there is a sparing of small bowel by this tumor.

groups: the least aggressive neoplasms were designated disseminated peritoneal adenomucinosis (DPAM), the more aggressive were designated peritoneal mucinous adenocarcinoma (PMCA). Yan and colleagues further classified the PMCA group into well-differentiated, moderately differentiated, and poorly differentiated cancer (Ronnett *et al.* 1995; Yan *et al.* 2001; Sugarbaker 2002; Misdraji *et al.* 2003; Mohamed *et al.* 2004). When survival was assessed using the Ronnett criteria and a uniform treatment plan, these subtypes of mucinous appendiceal neoplasms were associated with statistically different survival.

Imaging and staging

Neoplastic cells existing within copious mucinous fluid which the cancer cells continually produce result in a distinctive pattern of dissemination within the peritoneal cavity that accounts for a unique CT appearance. Physical principles and fluid hydrodynamics predominate in controlling the distribution of the mucinous neoplasms. Tumor accumulation by gravity is into the pelvic and right retrohepatic space. Tumor accumulation within a structure that has the capacity for peritoneal fluid resorption occurs at the greater omentum, lesser omentum, omental appendages, and lymphatic lacunae beneath the right and left hemidiaphragms. Mucinous neoplastic cells recirculating within the peritoneal cavity may become caught within intraperitoneal cul-de-sacs such as the rectovesicle and rectouterine space, omental bursa and subpyloric space, lacunae created by the ligament of Treitz, left paracolic sulcus and inguinal canal.

In contrast to these sites for mucinous neoplasm accumulation some peritoneal surfaces remain clear of tumor accumulation. The movement by peristalsis of the bowel, especially near-continuous peristalsis of the small bowel, spares these structures. Portions of the bowel less mobile because of a lack of mesentery are less spared. The antrum of the stomach and the ileocecal valve region are fixed to the retroperitoneum, and the rectosigmoid colon is fixed within the pelvis causing greater volumes of mucinous neoplasm to accumulate. Tumor that does accumulate on small bowel is often polypoid in nature, reflecting the fact that the adenomatous cells have been frequently moved so that a stalk is created.

These patterns of neoplastic progression that control the gross pathology *in vivo* can be demonstrated by CTs of the abdomen and pelvis. In Fig. 15.8 the greater omentum is infiltrated by a massive tumor accumulation. The small bowel beneath is compartmentalized by the greater omentum plus mucinous ascites and has been spared of large-volume disease.

One additional determinate of *in-vivo* gross pathology needs to be clarified. The surgical management of this disease can have a profound effect upon the distribution of progressive disease within the abdomen and pelvis. These free-floating mucinous tumor cells will become attached to a raw (sticky) tissue surface, implant at that site and progress. This is referred to as tumor cell entrapment. One example is the ruptured Graafian follicle (corpus hemorrhagicum) that causes mucinous neoplastic cells to adhere to the ovary. This accounts for the frequent occurrence of large cystic ovarian masses as a presenting feature of women with this disease. These tumor cells will also attach at sites of a surgical wound such as a laparoscopic trocar site, a right colectomy resection site, or traumatized peritoneal surfaces as a result of handling of a small bowel by the surgeon. Figure 15.9 shows the small bowel and small bowel mesentery in a patient who has had extensive prior debulking procedures. The redistribution of the mucinous tumor away from the small bowel and its mesentery has disappeared. There is now a

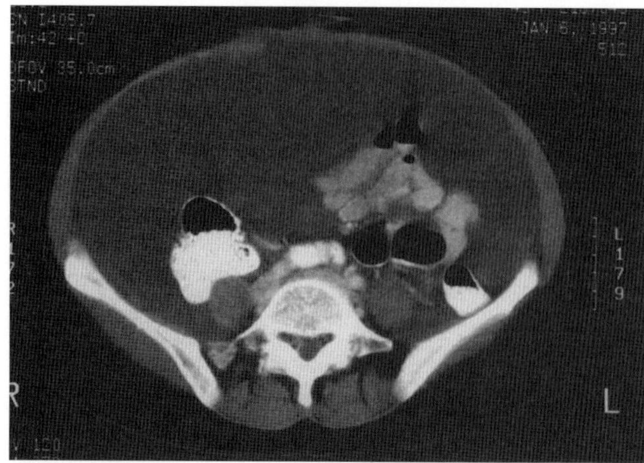

Fig. 15.8 CT through the mid-abdomen shows massive accumulation of tumor within the tissues of the greater omentum. The small bowel along with portions of the ascending and descending colon are compartmentalized by the massive accumulation of mucinous neoplasm and mucinous ascites within the abdomen.

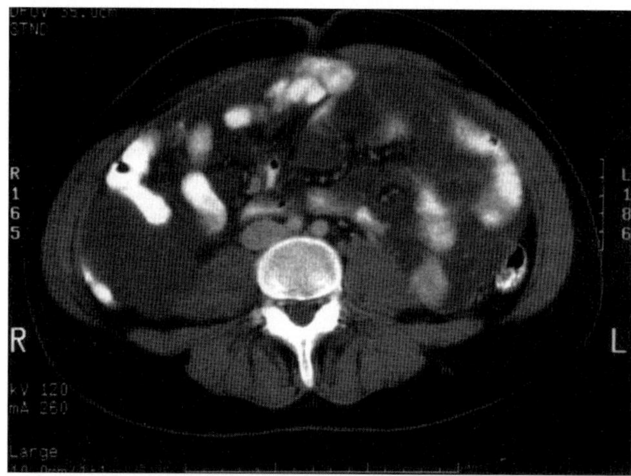

Fig. 15.9 CT through the mid-abdomen showing tumor along with small bowel and small bowel mesentery relatively uniformly distributed throughout the abdomen and pelvis indicating that the bowel is trapped within mucinous tumor masses.

uniform distribution of tumor throughout the mid-abdomen so that the small bowel is no longer compartmentalized but rather entrapped within masses of mucinous tumor.

Treatment

On gross examination at laparoscopy or laparotomy, it may be impossible to distinguish a mucinous tumor of the appendix from a benign mucocele. Both benign and malignant tumors of the appendix are likely to cause appendicitis and there may be mucin collections within the right lower quadrant or throughout the abdominopelvic space in both conditions. Two questions should be answered that will histopathologically separate tumors as inconsequential with complete removal from those capable of causing death from progressive mucinous carcinomatosis (Misdraji *et al.* 2003).

1 Is there invasion through the appendiceal wall by neoplastic glands and perforation?

2 Are atypical epithelial cells found within the extra-appendiceal mucin collection?

If either of these clinical features occur, special follow-up and aggressive treatments may be necessary (Dhage-Ivatury & Sugarbaker 2006).

There is a caveat that should be mentioned regarding the 'benign mucocele' of the appendix. If a mucocele of the appendix is found at the time of a planned laparoscopic appendectomy, then open appendectomy should be performed. Laparoscopic resection of a mucocele is likely to cause rupture of that structure, and pseudomyxoma peritonei syndrome may then result months or even years later. Resection of the appendiceal mass without traumatic rupture and without tumor spillage results in a complete eradication of the disease process (Misdraji *et al.* 2003).

A second caveat regarding the use of laparoscopy in patients with ascites needs to be noted. In all instances, paracentesis or laparoscopy with biopsy should be performed directly within the midline and through the linea alba. These sites can be excised as part of a midline abdominal incision. No lateral puncture sites or port sites should be used, because these will seed the abdominal wall by tumor and greatly interfere with disease eradication. Cytoreductive surgery and intraperitoneal chemotherapy are not effective for tumor within the abdominal wall.

Management of non-mucinous appendiceal adenocarcinoma

In patients with invasive non-mucinous adenocarcinoma of the appendix, although the data are not confirmatory, a right hemicolectomy is suggested to result in nearly twice the survival rate as occurs following routine appendectomy (Hesketh 1963). Therefore, all patients with invasive appendiceal adenocarcinoma, whether or not lymph nodes are involved, should receive a right hemicolectomy either during the same surgical procedure in which the appendectomy is performed or in a subsequent procedure. Certainly, when the surgeon performing an appendectomy finds that the appendix is infiltrated by an aggressive malignant process, emergency cryostat sectioning should be performed. If there is adequate bowel preparation and if a diagnosis of adenocarcinoma can be made definitively, one should proceed without hesitation with a right hemicolectomy procedure. In some patients a cecectomy with preservation of the ileocecal valve has been utilized. This is recommended if the appendiceal lymph nodes are negative by cryostat sectioning.

Management of mucinous tumors with peritoneal dissemination

A majority of patients with mucinous tumors of the appendix show perforation of the appendix at the time of exploration. In most of these patients, peritoneal carcinomatosis or pseudomyxoma peritonei is found at the time of appendectomy. In the past, this was a lethal condition without exception. Recently, peritonectomy procedures combined with intraperitoneal chemotherapy have been employed for the treatment of pseudomyxoma peritonei and peritoneal carcinomatosis (Sugarbaker 1995). The essential features of this approach are diagrammed in Fig. 15.10. The surgeon is responsible for doing as much as possible to remove all tumor on peritoneal surfaces. This is done by a cytoreductive procedure in patients who have gross spread of tumor around the peritoneal cavity. This involves a series of visceral resections including greater and lesser omentectomy, splenectomy and rectosigmoidectomy. This is combined with peritonectomy procedures to strip tumor from the abdominal gutters, pelvis, right subhepatic space, and left subphrenic spaces.

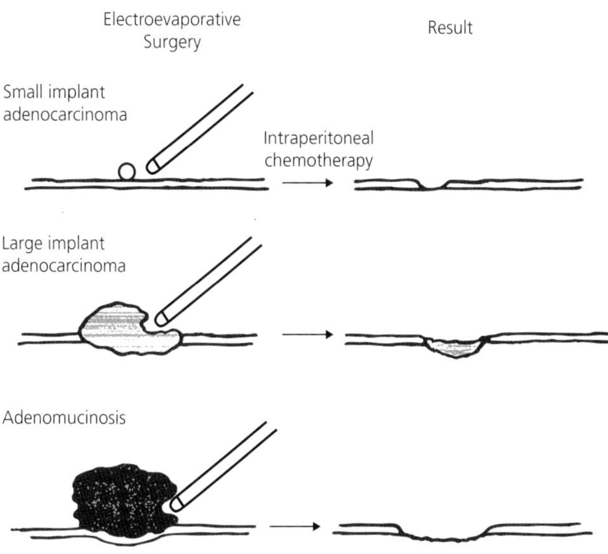

Fig. 15.10 Cytoreductive surgery using the ball tip.

Perioperative intraperitoneal chemotherapy

After the resection, and with the abdomen open, the peritoneal space is extensively washed by a chemotherapy solution and the surgeon's hand using gauze debridement of all surfaces. This is done in the presence of a heated mitomycin C chemotherapy solution (Fig. 15.11). Also, a window of time exists in which all intraperitoneal surfaces are available for intraperitoneal chemotherapy utilizing 5-FU in the early postoperative period. Uniformity of treatment with intraperitoneal chemotherapy to all peritoneal surfaces, including those surfaces dissected by the surgeon, can be achieved if the intraperitoneal chemotherapy is used during the first postoperative week. As the postoperative 5-FU chemotherapy solution is dwelling, distribution is facilitated by turning the patient alternately onto their right and left side as well as into the prone position (Sugarbaker 1999).

This perioperative intraperitoneal chemotherapy (combination of heated intraoperative mitomycin C and early postoperative 5-FU) has been utilized in over 900 patients, and has not been associated with an increased incidence of anastomotic disruptions. In patients who have had extensive prior surgical procedures who require many hours of lysis of adhesions, there is an increased incidence of postoperative bowel perforation. This is presumably a result of the combined effects of damage to small bowel from electrosurgical dissection of adhesions (seromuscular damage) and systemic effects of intraperitoneal chemotherapy on the intestine (mucosa and submucosa damage).

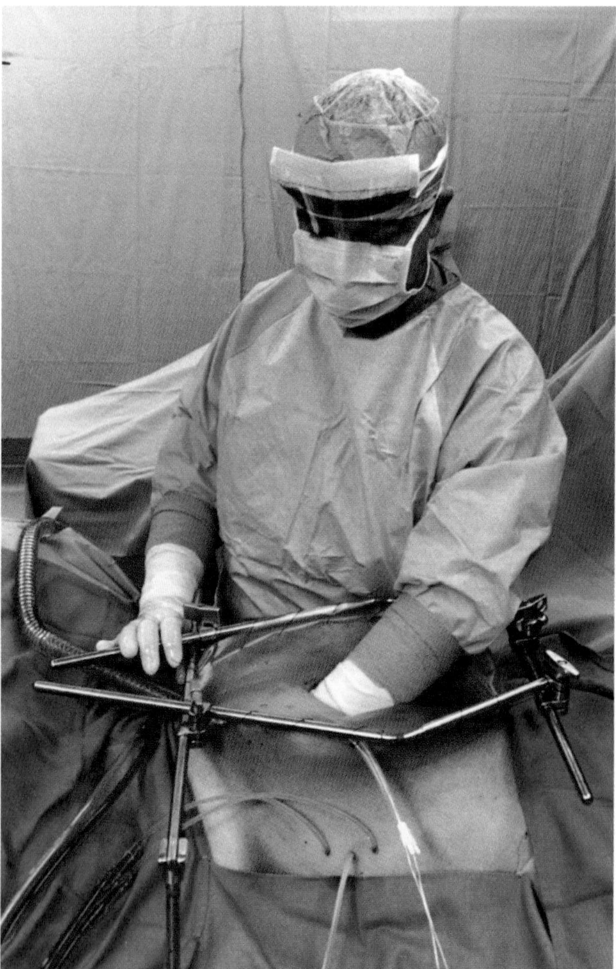

Fig. 15.11 Intraoperative hyperthermic intraperitoneal chemotherapy. The skin edges are suspended on a self-retaining retractor. Warm (41–42°C) chemotherapy solution is perfused while being manually distributed throughout the abdomen and pelvis.

In those patients who have high-grade appendiceal mucinous peritoneal carcinomatosis, intravenous chemotherapy is recommended. Usually, 5-FU, leucovorin and irinotecan for 6 months is appropriate.

In selected patients, usually those who require ostomy closure, at approximately 9 months after the cytoreduction with perioperative chemotherapy a second-look surgery is recommended. If at the staging celiotomy small tumor foci are found in peritoneal fissures in the abdomen or pelvis, the nodules are resected and a final intraperitoneal chemotherapy treatment is performed.

Prior serial debulking jeopardizes definitive cytoreduction

It is important that definitive treatment of peritoneal carcinomatosis or pseudomyxoma peritonei be instituted in a timely fashion. Each non-definitive (debulking) surgical intervention makes potentially curative cytoreductive surgery more difficult. Respect for the peritoneum as the first line of defense of the host against carcinomatosis is a requirement of optimal results using the peritonectomy procedures. Also, the relative sparing of the small bowel seen early in the natural history of peritoneal carcinomatosis and pseudomyxoma peritonei will disappear after several surgical procedures have been performed. The fibrous adhesions that inevitably result will become infiltrated by tumor. This leads to extensive involvement of the small bowel by the malignant process. Eventually it becomes impossible to cytoreduce the tumor safely and the effects of the intraperitoneal chemotherapy by itself are not adequate to keep the patient disease free.

Prognosis and follow-up

The results of these treatments for peritoneal surface dissemination of appendiceal malignancies are unexpectedly good. The results of treatment of 385 patients with prolonged follow-up has been reported (Sugarbaker & Chang 1999).

Survival by completeness of cytoreduction

The mean follow-up of this group of 385 appendix malignancy was 37.6 months; all appendiceal malignancy patients including

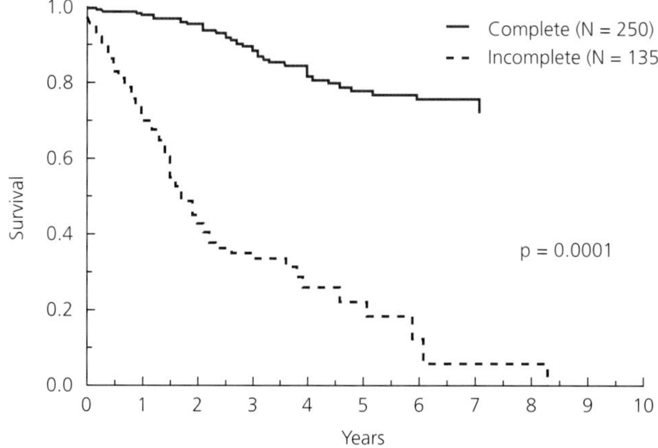

Fig. 15.12 Survival by cytoreduction of appendiceal malignancy with peritoneal dissemination.

adenomucinosis and mucinous adenocarcinoma are included. All patients had documented peritoneal surface disease and a majority had large-volume disease. After the completion of the cytoreductive surgery, all these patients had the abdomen inspected for the presence or absence of residual disease. A completeness of cytoreduction score was obtained for all patients. The completeness of cytoreduction score was based on the size of individual tumor nodules remaining unresected (Jacquet & Sugarbaker 1996). A CC-0 score indicated no visible tumor remaining after surgery. A CC-1 score indicated tumor nodules <2.5 mm. A CC-2 score indicated tumor nodules between 2.5 mm and 2.5 cm. A CC-3 score indicated tumor nodules >2.5 cm or a confluence of implants at any site. In Fig. 15.12, the survival of patients who had a complete cytoreduction (CC-O and CC-1) is compared with those with an incomplete cytoreduction (CC-2 and CC-3). Survival differences were significant with a p value of <0.0001; patients who left the operating room after cytoreductive surgery with tumor nodules <2.5 mm in diameter remaining were much more likely to survive long term than were those with an incomplete cytoreduction. There were no significant differences in survival between patients with CC-2 and CC-3 cytoreductions (data not shown).

Morbidity and mortality

The extensive cytoreductive surgery combined with early postoperative intraperitoneal chemotherapy presents a major physiologic insult. Nevertheless, the mortality rate remains at 2% in this group of patients. Pancreatitis (7.1%) and fistula formation (4.7%) are the major complications. Anastomotic leaks were no more common in this group of patients than in a routine general surgical setting (2.4%). Ten per cent of patients required a return to the operating room. The overall grade III/IV morbidity is 20%. There was no morbidity or mortality directly associated with the intraperitoneal chemotherapy administration. Rather, the incidence of complications depended on the extent of the surgery, number of peritonectomy procedures, and time required to complete the cytoreduction (Stephens *et al.* 1999; Sugarbaker *et al.* 2006).

Follow-up

Follow-up in these patients is important. Approximately 25% of them will require further surgery. Performing surgery in a timely fashion will help minimize the morbidity and mortality of the reoperation.

References

Carmignani CP, Sugarbaker TA, Bromley CM, Sugarbaker PH. (2003) Intraperitoneal cancer dissemination: mechanisms of the patterns of spread. *Cancer Metastasis Rev* 22: 465–72.

Dhage-Ivatury S, Sugarbaker PH. (2006) Update on the surgical approach to mucocele of the appendix. *J Am Coll Surg* 202: 680–4.

Esquivel J, Sugarbaker PH. (2000) Clinical presentation of the Pseudomyxoma peritonei syndrome. *Br J Surg* 87: 1414–18.

Gonzalez-Moreno S, Sugarbaker PH. (2004) Right hemicolectomy does not confer a survival advantage in patients with mucinous carcinoma of the appendix and peritoneal seeding. *Br J Surg* 91: 304–11.

Hesketh KT. (1963) The management of primary adenocarcinoma of the vermiform appendix. *Gut* 4: 158–68.

Jacquet P, Sugarbaker PH. (1996) Current methodologies for clinical assessment of patients with peritoneal carcinomatosis. *J Exp Clin Cancer Res* 15: 49–58.

Lyss AP. (1988) Appendiceal malignancies. *Semin Oncol* 15: 129–37.

Misdraji J, Yantiss RK, Graeme-Cook FM, Balis UJ, Young RH. (2003) Appendiceal mucinous neoplasms: a clinicopathologic analysis of 107 cases. *Am J Surg Pathol* 27: 1089–1103.

Mohamed F, Gething S, Haiba M, Brun EA, Sugarbaker PH. (2004) Clinically aggressive pseudomyxoma peritonei: a variant of a histologically indolent process. *J Surg Oncol* 86: 10–15.

Ronnett BM, Zahn CM, Kurman RJ, Kass ME, Sugarbaker PH, Shmookler BM. (1995) Disseminated peritoneal adenomucinosis and peritoneal mucinous carcinomatosis. A clinicopathologic analysis of 109 cases with emphasis on distinguishing pathologic features, site of origin, prognosis, and relationship to 'pseudomyxoma peritonei'. *Am J Surg Pathol* 19: 1390–1408.

Ronnett BM, Shmookler BM, Sugarbaker PH, Kurman RJ. (1997) Pseudomyxoma peritonei: new concepts in diagnosis, origin, nomenclature, and relationship to mucinous borderline (low malignant potential) tumors of the ovary. *Anat Pathol* 2: 197–226.

Ronnett BM, Yan H, Kurman RJ, Shmookler BM, Wu L, Sugarbaker PH. (2001) Patients with pseudomyxoma peritonei associated with disseminated peritoneal adenomucinosis have a significantly more favorable prognosis than patients with peritoneal mucinous carcinomatosis. *Cancer* 92: 85–91.

Stephens AD, Alderman R, Chang D *et al.* (1999) Morbidity and mortality analysis of 200 treatments with cytoreductive surgery and hyperthermic intraoperative intraperitoneal chemotherapy using the coliseum technique. *Ann Surg Oncol* 6: 790–6.

Sugarbaker PH. (1995) Peritonectomy procedures. *Ann Surg* 221: 29–42.

Sugarbaker PH. (1999) *Intraperitoneal Chemotherapy and Cytoreductive Surgery. A Manual for Physicians and Nurses*, 3rd edn. The Ludan Company, Grand Rapids.

Sugarbaker PH. (2002) The subpyloric space: an important surgical and radiologic feature in pseudomyxoma peritonei. *Eur J Surg Oncol* 28: 443–6.

Sugarbaker PH, Chang D. (1999) Results of treatment of 385 patients with peritoneal surface spread of appendiceal malignancy. *Ann Surg Oncol* 6: 727–31.

Sugarbaker PH, Alderman R, Edwards G *et al.* (2006) Prospective morbidity and mortality assessment of cytoreductive surgery plus perioperative intraperitoneal chemotherapy to treat peritoneal dissemination of appendiceal mucinous malignancy. *Ann Surg Oncol* 13: 635–44.

Yan H, Pestieau SR, Shmookler BM, Sugarbaker PH. (2001) Histopathologic analysis in 46 patients with pseudomyxoma peritonei syndrome: failure versus success with a second-look operation. *Mod Pathol* 14: 164–71.

Diffuse malignant peritoneal mesothelioma

Tristan D. Yan & Paul H. Sugarbaker

Diagnosis

History

Malignant mesothelioma is a highly aggressive primary neoplasm of the serosal lining of the pleura, peritoneum, pericardium, or tunica vaginalis (Battifora & McCaughey 1994). Probably from exposure to asbestos fibers in building materials and in the environment, the incidence of malignant mesothelioma is increasing worldwide. In the United States, there was a steep rise in the mesothelioma incidence through the 1990s, with a recent leveling off of the rate of increase, but no evidence that the peak incidence of mesothelioma has been passed in this country (Spirtas *et al.* 1994; Price & Ware 2003; Weill *et al.* 2004). A similar pattern, with a plateauing of the incidence rate, is present in some European countries that reduced asbestos usage in a similar time frame as the United States (Montanaro *et al.* 2003; Swuste *et al.* 2004; Langard 2005). However, the overall incidence of malignant mesothelioma is increasing worldwide and is not expected to peak for another 5–20 years (Robinson & Lake 2005). The incidence is expected to continue to increase in areas of the world where asbestos use has not been curtailed (Dave & Beckett 2005; Kazan-Allen 2005; Chang *et al.* 2006).

Diffuse malignant peritoneal mesothelioma (DMPM) is the second most common type of malignant mesothelioma (Battifora & McCaughey 1994). A recent analysis of the Surveillance, Epidemiology, and End Results program of the National Cancer Institute estimated approximately 250 new cases of DMPM in the United States each year (Price & Ware 2003). Some studies with an adequate number of cases demonstrated a strong association between occupational exposure to asbestos and the risk of DMPM, especially in males (Antman *et al.* 1983). The overall incidence of this disease is higher in males than females, which may be related to a higher incidence of asbestos-related occupations in men (Welch *et al.* 2005). DMPM has also been reported following radiation therapy, mica exposure, recurrent peritonitis and administration of thorium dioxide (Maurer & Egloff 1975; Riddell *et al.* 1981; Chahinian *et al.* 1982; Peterson 1984; Sugarbaker *et al.* 2003).

Patients who suffer from this disease usually present with abdominal pain or distension. As the disease progresses, they invariably die from intestinal obstruction or terminal starvation within a year. Due to the infrequent occurrence and the lack of understanding of the natural history of DMPM, traditionally there seemed to be a mutual agreement among the medical practitioners that patients with this condition were preterminal. Until recently, few therapeutic advances occurred since the disease was first described by Miller and Wynn in 1908 (Miller & Wynn 1908). Systemic chemotherapy, palliative surgery and/or total abdominal radiation therapy were used selectively, but did not seem to alter the natural history of this disease (Chailleux *et al.* 1988; Antman *et al.* 1988; Sridhar *et al.* 1992; Markman & Kelsen 1992; Yates *et al.* 1997; Neumann *et al.* 1999; Eltabbakh *et al.* 1999).

Clinical presentation

The initial symptoms and signs of DMPM are non-specific, and due to the rarity of the disease, the level of clinical suspicion is relatively low (Acherman *et al.* 2003; Welch *at al.* 2005). Approximately 70% of patients have serous ascites, a product of the tumor nodules. This mixture of fluid and tumor building up under pressure appears to be the major cause of morbidity. Increased abdominal girth (55%), pain (45%), and abdominal or pelvic mass (26%), are the most common predominant initial complaints, which lead the physician to arrange for definitive tests resulting in a diagnosis of DMPM (Table 15.9) (Acherman *et al.* 2003; Chang *et al.* 2006). Unlike pleural mesothelioma, pain has not been found to have a significant negative impact on survival in patients with DMPM. Approximately 13% of patients present with new-onset abdominal wall hernia, which is related to accumulated ascites and increased intraabdominal pressure. Other constitutional symptoms may also be present, such as weight loss (20%) and febrile episodes (10%), which were both associated with a reduced overall survival (Acherman *et al.* 2003). Tejido *et al.* previously reported fever as an initial presentation of DMPM in three patients, and hypothesized that fever constitutes the initial clinical presentation only when the disease remains asymptomatic until it is far advanced (Tejido Garcia *et al.* 1997). In females, approximately 25% seek medical attention, as a result of non-specific gynecologic symptoms, such as pelvic mass or infertility (Welch *et al.*

Table 15.9 Symptoms and signs of diffuse malignant peritoneal mesothelioma.

Symptoms
Abdominal pain (40%)
Abdominal distension (40%)
Constitutional symptoms, such as weight loss and fever (20%)
Incidental finding (10%)
Signs
Ascites (70%)
Abdominal or pelvic mass (30%)
Abdominal wall hernia (10%)
Guarding and rebound tenderness (10%)
Pleural effusion (5%)

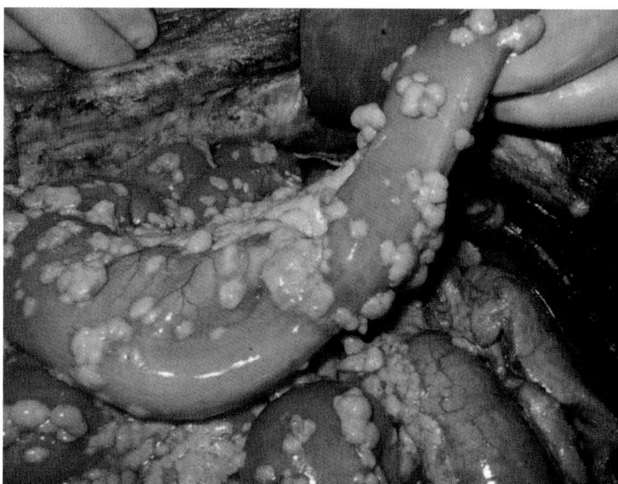

Fig. 15.13 Macroscopically, diffuse malignant peritoneal mesothelioma is characterized by thousands of whitish tumor nodules of variable size and consistency that may coalesce to form plaques or masses or layer out evenly to cover the entire peritoneal surface.

2005). Lymphadenopathy or distant organ metastasis is extremely rare in this disease. Five per cent of patients may present with concomitant pleural effusion.

Diagnosis

Macroscopically, DMPM is characterized by thousands of whitish tumor nodules of variable size and consistency that may coalesce to form plaques or masses or layer out evenly to cover part of or the entire peritoneal surface (Fig. 15.13).

Biopsy

Commonly, a long delay in definitive diagnosis of DMPM is a significant problem for the physician and for the patient. Cytologic examination of ascites fluid removed by paracentesis rarely results in a positive finding (Yu *et al.* 2001). If cells are

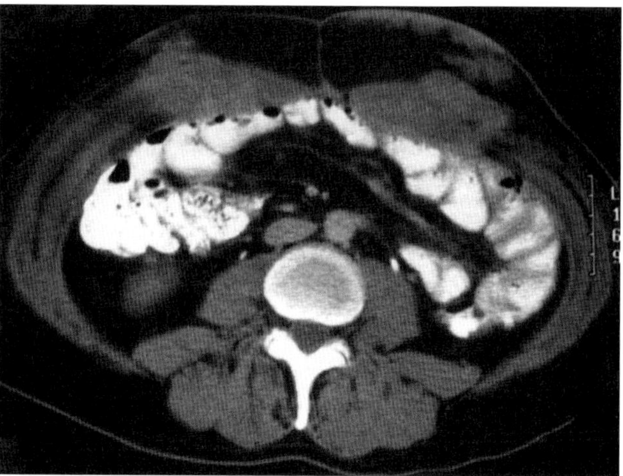

Fig. 15.14 Diffuse malignant peritoneal mesothelioma implantation in the lateral abdominal wall along previous laparoscopic trochar tracts.

recovered in ascites fluid, they frequently resemble hyperplasic mesothelial cells with insufficient atypia present for a confident diagnosis. The state-of-the-art approach to histologic verification of the diagnosis of peritoneal malignancy is a CT-guided biopsy, or a laparoscopy. In a population of 68 consecutive DMPM patients, Sugarbaker *et al.* found very few definitive diagnoses made by paracentesis and cytology (Welch *et al.* 2005). Laparoscopy with biopsy was required in 52%, laparotomy with biopsy in 44%, and a radiologic-guided biopsy in 4% (Welch *et al.* 2005). Eltabbakh and colleagues performed laparotomy or laparoscopy with biopsy as the definitive test for all 15 DMPM patients (Eltabbakh *et al.* 1999). Four of the 15 patients had preoperative paracentesis, but all were reported as adenocarcinoma. The low reliability of cytologic results warrants an invasive procedure to obtain a generous sample of peritoneal tumor in patients with peritoneal surface cancer of uncertain etiology.

However, an important caveat must accompany the recommendation for laparoscopy in the diagnosis of DMPM. In a series of eight patients with DMPM diagnosed by laparoscopy, six patients presented with tumor implantation in the lateral abdominal wall around trochar tracts (Fig. 15.14), resulting in extraperitoneal dissemination, which changed the natural history of the disease (Muensterer *et al.* 1997). Therefore, lateral port sites for laparoscopy must be avoided. Trochars should only be placed within the linea alba, so that port sites can be excised at the time of definitive surgical treatment.

Immunohistochemical stains

A biopsy of the tumor is subjected to a complete histopathologic analysis. However, the distinction of DMPM from adenocarcinoma is subtle both macroscopically and on routine microscopic study. A series of immunohistochemical markers are necessary to differentiate DMPM from adenocarcinoma (Battifora & McCaughey 1994). Calretinin identifies cells as being mesothelial in origin. A positive calretinin, cytokeratins 5/6, WT-1, thrombomodulin, and mesothelin stain, accompanied by a negative B72.3, CEA, CD 15, Leu-M1, and BER-EP4 immunostain is highly suggestive of DMPM.

Histopathology

DMPM has a diversity of cytoarchitectural characteristics that are almost unique among neoplasms originating from a single cell line. The spectrum embraces tumors that are entirely of epithelial or mesenchymal (sarcomatoid) type to a range of biphasic and intermediate forms, as described by Battifora and McCaughey (Battifora & McCaughey 1994).

Seventy-five to 90% of DMPM are of epithelial type, which are characterized by cuboidal or flattened epithelial-like malignant mesothelial cells with ample cytoplasm with distinct cellular membranes, and a relatively uniform, granular to vesicular nuclei (Fig. 15.15a). The subtypes of epithelial DMPM are categorized by the patterns observed for the malignant epithelial component, which are classified as tubulopapillary, solid, deciduoid, storiform-like, fascicular-like, multicystic, papillary, microcystic, and granular.

The sarcomatoid DMPM is composed only of spindle-shaped mesenchymal type cells (Fig. 15.15b). However, the mesenchymal portion can be as diverse as the epithelial component in that the sarcomatous elements may morphologically and immunophenotypically resemble any one of the numerous bone and soft tissue tumors by producing malignant osteoid, cartilage, or other sarcomatous histologies.

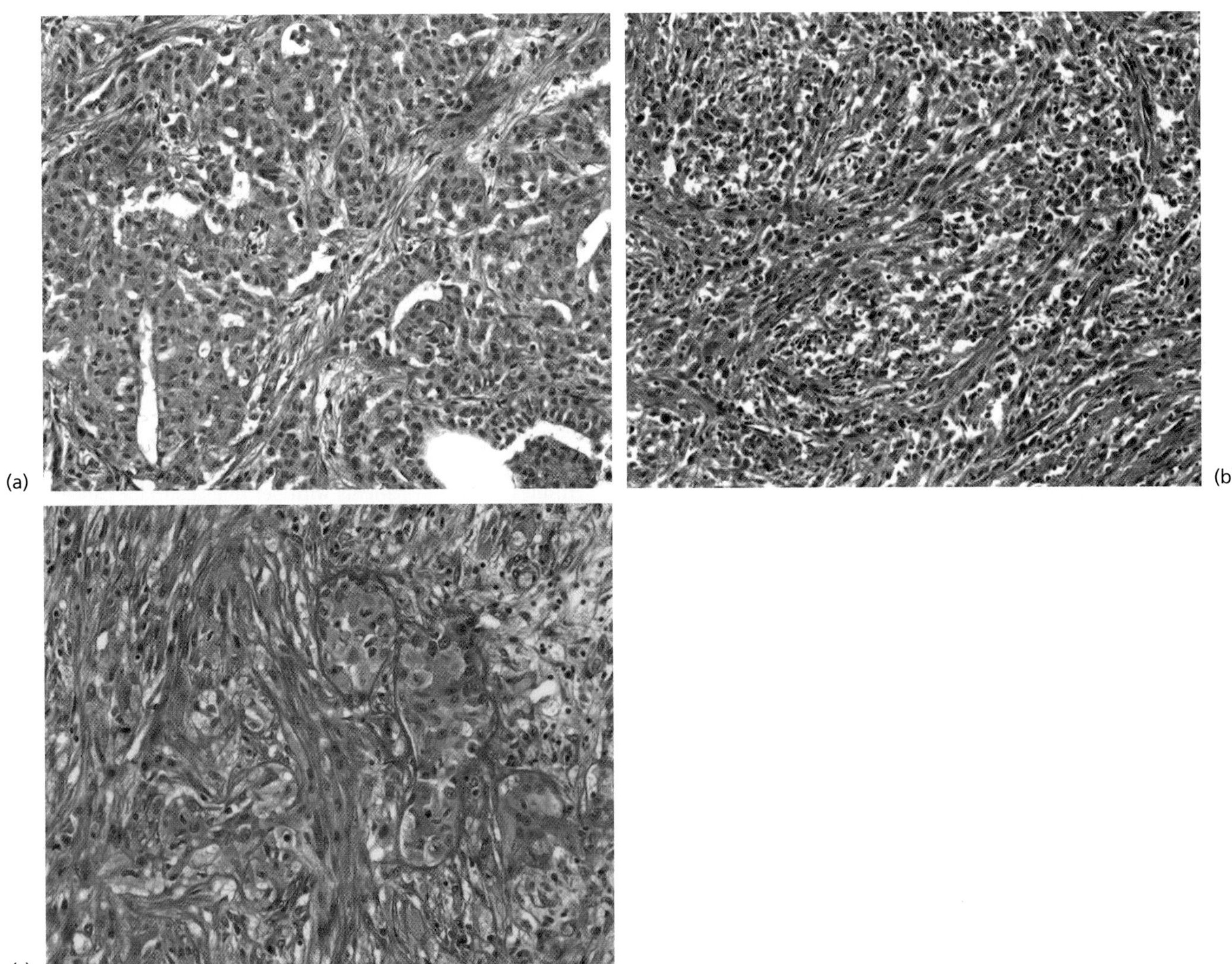

Fig. 15.15 Diffuse malignant peritoneal mesothelioma.(a) Epithelial type, characterized by cuboidal or flattened epithelial-like malignant mesothelial cells (H&E ×20). (b) Sarcomatoid type, characterized by sarcomatous spindle-shaped mesothelial cells (H&E ×20). (c) Biphasic type, characterized by presence of two phenotypes occurring in same tumor, but sometimes they are intimately admixed (H&E ×20).

In biphasic DMPM malignant elements of both epithelial and mesenchymal appearance are present (Fig. 15.15c). Frequently the two phenotypes occur in different parts of the same tumor, but sometimes they are intimately admixed. There is sometimes a high degree of subjectivity involved in the diagnosis of pure sarcomatoid versus biphasic DMPM, which depends on the amount of tissue available and the extent to which it is sampled.

Serum markers

Serum CA-125, a tumor antigen that is present in the majority of patients with ovarian cancer, is also elevated in DMPM. In a study by Kebapci *et al.* CA-125 levels were measured at diagnosis in eight patients with DMPM (Simsek *et al.* 1996; Kebapci *et al.* 2003). Recently, several new tumor markers have been identified for diagnosis of mesothelioma. These studies have mostly involved patients with pleural mesothelioma. However, given the similarity between pleural and peritoneal mesothelioma, it is likely that these tests will also be useful in peritoneal mesothelioma. These new tumor markers include mesothelin, soluble mesothelin-related proteins (SMRP) and osteopontin (Robinson *et al.* 2003; Hassan *et al.* 2004a, 2006; Pass *et al.* 2005).

Radiology

Evolutionary change has occurred in the technology of computed tomography (CT). With administration of adequate intravenous, oral and rectal contrast media multislice CT is the current mainstay imaging tool for patients with DMPM. It allows more precise identification and evaluation of DMPM than sonography. In the past several studies described the radiologic appearances of DMPM in small case series of fewer than 10 patients (Reuter *et al.* 1983; Ros *et al.* 1991; Guest *et al.* 1992).

Yan *et al.* studied preoperative abdominal and pelvic CT scans of 33 DMPM patients in a systematic manner and identified four radiologic characteristics that could be used to distinguish DMPM from other peritoneal carcinomatosis (Yan *et al.* 2005a). First, the authors studied the distribution of DMPM and determined that this disease was diffuse throughout the peritoneal cavity. This lack of a primary site for this disease distinguished it from peritoneal dissemination from gastrointestinal or gynecologic malignancies. Second, the most heavily disease-involved regions were the mid-abdomen and pelvis. In contrast to pseudomyxoma peritonei or other disease causing mucinous carcinomatosis, compartmentalization of the small bowel and a large volume of disease beneath the right hemidiaphragm were absent. Third, the presence of serous ascites rather than mucinous ascites was commonly seen in DMPM. Fourth, none of the patients had extra-abdominal lymph node or distant organ metastasis. One must raise the clinical suspicion of DMPM in patients with serous ascites, no primary tumors and yet a disease process that remains confined to the abdominopelvic cavity.

Prognostic factors and staging

In the past, no uniform treatments were suggested for patients with DMPM and the survival was largely dependent upon the indolent versus aggressive biology of the disease. Several studies reported a reduced survival outcome associated with biphasic or sarcomatoid histologic type, as compared to epithelial type (Sebbag *et al.* 2000; Feldman *et al.* 2003; Welch *et al.* 2005). However, the criterion is not useful as a prognostic indicator, because the majority of DMPM patients show the epithelial type. There was in fact no staging system for DMPM. As more patients are treated with a uniform regimen, a more thorough and precise analysis of clinical, radiologic and histopathologic prognostic parameters are possible (Park *et al.* 1999; Loggie *et al.* 2001; Nonaka *et al.* 2005; Welch *et al.* 2005; Deraco *et al.* 2006; Brigand *et al.* 2006; Yan *et al.* 2006a, 2007).

Gender

Females have been found to show a better prognosis in DMPM, as compared to males (Welch *et al.* 2005). A very real epidemiologic difference between males and females appears to be the likelihood of asbestos exposure. The direct exposure to asbestos was definitely causative in men, but less apparent in women (Antman *et al.* 1983; Spirtas *et al.* 1994). It is possible that this difference in causation is at least in part responsible for the difference in the natural history of DMPM in women. However, other clinical characteristics may contribute to the improved prognosis of females (Yan *et al.* 2006b).

Lymph node metastasis

Lymph node metastasis is uncommon in patients with DMPM, but is associated with a poor prognosis (Yan *et al.* 2006a). In 100 DMPM patients treated at the Washington Cancer Institute, seven patients were found to have positive lymph nodes. The most common sites of a positive lymph node were external, internal, and common iliac lymph nodes and ileocolic lymph nodes. Their median survival was 6 months, with 1- and 2-year survival of 43% and 0%, respectively. Ninety-three patients had absence of lymph node involvement and their median survival was 59 months, with 5- and 7-year survival of 50% and 43%, respectively.

Completeness of cytoreduction

Nearly all treatment centers agree that completeness of cytoreduction is one of the most significant prognostic factors for long-term survival (Park *et al.* 1999; Nonaka *et al.* 2005; Loggie *et al.* 2001; Welch *et al.* 2005; Brigand *et al.* 2006; Deraco *et al.* 2006; Yan *et al.* 2006a, 2007). It is related to the pretreatment tumor load and the surgeon's ability to eradicate gross disease. Unlike pseudomyxoma peritonei or other mucinous adenocarcinoma, DMPM does not spare the peritoneal surfaces of the small intestines. This unfortunately limits the ability to achieve a complete cytoreduction.

Radiologic classifications

There are problems with using completeness of cytoreduction for prognostication, as this clinical information is unavailable preoperatively in the patient selection process. Yan *et al.* described interpretive CT classifications of the small bowel and mesentery, which are useful in determining the operability of a patient with DMPM (Yan *et al.* 2005b). Characteristic interpretative CT appearances of the small bowel and its mesentery are categorized into four classes (class 0–III). In class III disease, configuration of the small bowel and mesentery on CT appears so thickened and grossly distorted that an adequate cytoreduction is almost unable to be achieved.

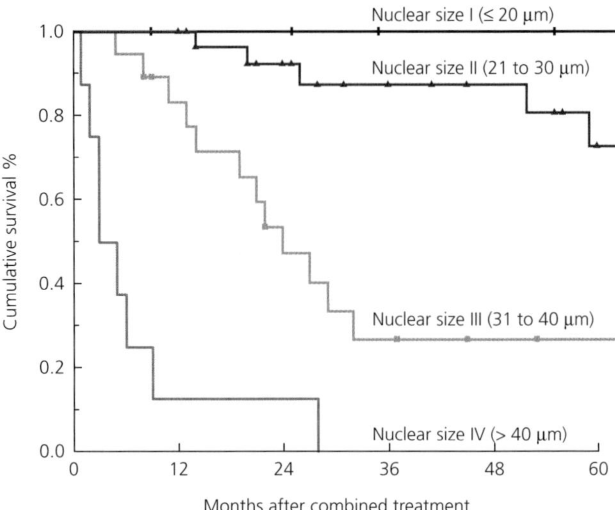

Fig. 15.16 Cumulative survival after cytoreductive surgery and perioperative intraperitoneal chemotherapy for diffuse malignant peritoneal mesothelioma. The prognostic significance of mesothelioma nuclear size was $p < 0.001$.

Histopathologic staging

In 1995, Goldblum and Hart first described a nuclear grading system according to histomorphologic features of DMPM (Goldblum & Hart 1995). In 2001, Kerrigan and colleagues first tested this nuclear grading system in 25 female patients with DMPM who underwent a variety of surgical, chemotherapy, or radiotherapy treatments, and they found that the nuclear grading was not strongly associated with long-term survival (Kerrigan *et al.* 2002). In 2005, Nonaka and coworkers demonstrated that the size of the mesothelioma nucleus was prognostically significant for overall survival in 35 patients who underwent uniform treatment using cytoreductive surgery and perioperative intraperitoneal chemotherapy (Nonaka *et al.* 2005).

In 2006, with a larger sample size, uniform treatment, longer follow-up and more histopathology sections per patients studied, Yan and collaborators found in multivariate analysis that the nuclear size was the only independent prognostic determinant for overall survival in DMPM (Yan *et al.* 2007). The 3-year survival rates with nuclear size of 10–20 μm, 21–30 μm, 31–40 μm and >40 μm were 100%, 87%, 27% and 0%, respectively (Fig. 15.16). The findings may suggest that nuclear size is a surrogate molecular marker of the biologic aggressiveness of DMPM.

Treatment

Overview

Recently, this disease has been re-examined from all aspects of both diagnosis and treatment strategies. This is related to the encouraging reports from numerous centers worldwide on their accumulative experience with a combined local–regional treatment approach using cytoreductive surgery and perioperative intraperitoneal chemotherapy. This new treatment strategy has consistently demonstrated a markedly improved prognosis, achieving a median survival of up to 90 months and a 5-year survival of 60% (Park *et al.* 1999; Loggie *et al.* 2001; Nonaka *et al.* 2005; Welch *et al.* 2005; Yan *et al.* 2007; Brigand *et al.* 2006; Deraco *et al.* 2006; Yan *et al.* 2006a). This significant improvement in treatment means that cure may be an option.

Systemic chemotherapy

Traditionally, there has been an agreement among medical practitioners that DMPM was untreatable and thus a preterminal condition with a rapid progression. The patients were managed with systemic chemotherapy and palliative surgery. However, eventually all patients died from the disease as a result of intestinal obstruction and/or terminal starvation (Chailleux *et al.* 1988; Antman *et al.* 1988; Sridhar *et al.* 1992; Markman & Kelsen 1992; Yates *et al.* 1997; Neumann *et al.* 1999; Eltabbakh *et al.* 1999). The median survival in these patients prior to the year 2000 was less than 1 year. There are now Food and Drug Administration-approved treatment protocols using systemic pemetrexed plus cisplatin (Janne *et al.* 2005).

Intraperitoneal chemotherapy

Several studies have evaluated chemotherapy administered via the intraperitoneal route in an attempt to maximize local–regional cytotoxicity and limit systemic side-effects (Markman

Table 15.10 Recent updates on cytoreductive surgery combined with perioperative intraperitoneal chemotherapy for diffuse malignant peritoneal mesothelioma (NR: median survival was not reached).

Authors	Year	n	Median survival (months)	Survival rates (%)				
				1-year	2-year	3-year	5-year	7-year
Yan *et al.*	2006	100	52	78	64	55	46	39
Feldman *et al.*	2003	49	92	86	77	59	59	–
Deraco *et al.*	2006	49	NR	88	74	65	57	–
Brigand *et al.*	2006	15	36	69	58	43	29	–
Loggie *et al.*	2001	12	34	60	60	50	33	33

1990; Vlasveld *et al.* 1991; Markman & Kelsen 1992). However, intraperitoneal chemotherapy penetrates tumor nodules by passive diffusion; therefore the depth of penetration is limited. In addition, the efficacy of intraperitoneal chemotherapy is reduced due to limited chemotherapy distribution in a grossly diseased abdomen. No studies have demonstrated survival benefit of intraperitoneal chemotherapy alone for DMPM.

Cytoreductive surgery and perioperative intraperitoneal chemotherapy

Recently there has been a reexamination of DMPM treatment, by cytoreductive surgery and perioperative intraperitoneal chemotherapy with intent not to palliate, but to cure (Park *et al.* 1999; Loggie *et al.* 2001; Nonaka *et al.* 2005; Welch *et al.* 2005; Deraco *et al.* 2006; Brigand *et al.* 2006; Yan *et al.* 2006a; Yan *et al.* 2007). There have been already several large studies, including a randomized controlled trial examining the efficacy of this combined procedure for the management of peritoneal carcinomatosis from gastrointestinal and ovarian malignancies (Glehen *et al.* 2003; Verwaal *et al.* 2003; Glehen *et al.* 2004; Verwaal *et al.* 2005; Sugarbaker 2006; Armstrong *et al.* 2006). DMPM remains confined within the peritoneal cavity throughout its clinical course and these patients experience morbidity and mortality almost exclusively as a result of disease progression in the abdominopelvic cavity. The combined locoregional treatment approach has a strong treatment rationale for DMPM patients.

Cytoreductive surgery is an important first step in the combined treatment; it maximally removes peritoneal tumors together with complete lysis of adhesions between the bowel loops (Sugarbaker 1995). This provides an optimal situation for adjuvant intraperitoneal chemotherapy, which is given before the formation of any adhesions, allowing direct chemotherapy and tumor-cell contact, without necessarily increasing systemic toxicity (Sugarbaker *et al.* 1988; Katz & Barone 2003). Hyperthermia has been known to have direct cytotoxic effects in both a temperature and time-dependent manner (Los *et al.* 1992; Armour *et al.* 1993). It also has been shown to allow a greater depth of penetration of the chemotherapy agents into the tumors and synergize the cytotoxic drugs selected for intraperitoneal use at the time of surgery (Los *et al.* 1991; van de Vaart *et al.* 1998; Urano *et al.* 1999; Taub *et al.* 2005).

Prognosis

The most recent phase II study from the National Cancer Institute, Bethesda, USA showed that the median survival of 49 DMPM patients was 92 months, with a 5-year survival rate of 59%, after cytoreductive surgery and intraperitoneal hyperthermic chemotherapy (Feldman *et al.* 2003). The National Cancer Institute of Italy also enrolled 49 patients to undergo the combined treatment and reported that the progression-free survival was 40 months and 5-year survival was 57% (Deraco *et al.* 2006). Washington Cancer Institute, Washington DC, USA recently published an updated series on 100 DMPM patients who underwent the combined treatment, which demonstrated that overall median survival was 52 months, with 5- and 7-year survival of 46% and 39%, respectively (Yan *et al.* 2006a). Table 15.10 demonstrates the most recently published updates from all international treatment centers (Loggie *et al.* 2001; Feldman *et al.* 2003; Brigand *et al.* 2006; Deraco *et al.* 2006; Yan *et al.* 2006a).

Follow-up

Currently, a multi-institutional registry database is required that would collect information on all DMPM patients receiving complete cytoreduction and perioperative intraperitoneal chemotherapy, including chemopathological data, details of the surgical procedure, in-hospital morbidity, and long-term outcome.

References

Acherman YIZ, Welch LS, Bromley CM, Sugarbaker PH. (2003) Clinical presentation of peritoneal mesothelioma. *Tumori* 89: 269–73.

Antman KH, Corson JM, Li FP *et al.* (1983) Malignant mesothelioma following radiation exposure. *J Clin Oncol* 1: 695–700.

Antman K, Shemin R, Ryan L *et al.* (1988) Malignant mesothelioma: prognostic variables in a registry of 180 patients, the Dana-Farber Cancer Institute and Brigham and Women's Hospital experience over two decades, 1965–1985. *J Clin Oncol* 6: 147–53.

Armour EP, McEachern D, Wang Z, Corry PM, Martinez A. (1993) Sensitivity of human cells to mild hyperthermia. *Cancer Res* 53: 2740–4.

Armstrong DK, Bundy B, Wenzel L *et al.* (2006) Intraperitoneal cisplatin and paclitaxel in ovarian cancer. *N Engl J Med* 354: 34–43.

Battifora H, McCaughey W. (1994) *Tumors of the Serosal Membranes*. Armed Forces Institute of Pathology, Washington, DC.

Brigand C, Monneuse O, Mohamed F *et al.* (2006) Malignant peritoneal mesothelioma treated by cytoreductive surgery and intraperitoneal chemohyperthermia: Results of a prospective study. *Ann Surg Oncol* 13: 405–12.

Chahinian AP, Pajak TF, Holland JF, Norton L, Ambinder RM, Mandel EM. (1982) Diffuse malignant mesothelioma–prospective evaluation of 69 patients. *Ann Intern Med* 96: 746–55.

Chailleux E, Dabouis G, Pioche D *et al.* (1988) Prognostic factors in diffuse malignant pleural mesothelioma. A study of 167 patients. *Chest* 93: 159–62.

Chang KC, Leung CC, Tam CM, Yu WC, Hui DS, Lam WK. (2006) Malignant mesothelioma in Hong Kong. *Respir Med* 100: 75–82.

Dave SK, Beckett WS. (2005) Occupational asbestos exposure and predictable asbestos-related diseases in India. *Am J Ind Med* 48: 137–43.

Deraco M, Nonaka D, Baratti D *et al.* (2006) Prognostic analysis of clinicopathologic factors in 49 patients with diffuse malignant peritoneal mesothelioma treated with cytoreductive surgery and intraperitoneal hyperthermic perfusion. *Ann Surg Oncol* 13: 229–37.

Eltabbakh GH, Piver MS, Hempling RE, Recio FO, Intengen ME. (1999) Clinical picture, response to therapy, and survival of women with diffuse malignant peritoneal mesothelioma. *J Surg Oncol* 70: 6–12.

Feldman AL, Libutti SK, Pingpank JF *et al.* (2003) Analysis of factors associated with outcome in patients with malignant peritoneal mesothelioma undergoing surgical debulking and intraperitoneal chemotherapy. *J Clin Oncol* 21: 4560–7.

Freedman RS, Vadhan-Raj S, Butts C *et al.* (2003) Pilot study of Flt3 ligand comparing intraperitoneal with subcutaneous routes on hematologic and immunologic responses in patients with peritoneal carcinomatosis and mesotheliomas. *Clin Cancer Res* 9: 5228–37.

Glehen O, Mithieux F, Osinsky D *et al.* (2003) Surgery combined with peritonectomy procedures and intraperitoneal chemohyperthermia in abdominal cancers with peritoneal carcinomatosis: a phase II study. *J Clin Oncol* 21: 799–806.

Glehen O, Kwiatkowski F, Sugarbaker PH *et al.* (2004) Cytoreductive surgery combined with perioperative intraperitoneal chemotherapy for the management of peritoneal carcinomatosis from colorectal cancer: a multi-institutional study. *J Clin Oncol* 22: 3284–92.

Goldblum J, Hart WR. (1995) Localized and diffuse mesotheliomas of the genital tract and peritoneum in women. A clinicopathologic study of nineteen true mesothelial neoplasms, other than adenomatoid tumors, multicystic mesotheliomas, and localized fibrous tumors. *Am J Surg Pathol* 19: 1124–37.

Guest PJ, Reznek RH, Selleslag D, Geraghty R, Slevin M. (1992) Peritoneal mesothelioma: the role of computed tomography in diagnosis and follow up. *Clin Radiol* 45: 79–84.

Hassan R, Bera T, Pastan I. (2004a) Mesothelin: a new target for immunotherapy.[see comment]. *Clin Cancer Res* 10: 3937–42.

Hassan R, Bullock S, Kindler H, Pastan I. (2004b) Updated results of the phase I study of SS1(dsFv)PE38 for targeted therapy of mesothelin expressing cancers. *Eur J Cancer* 2: 280.

Hassan R, Remaley AT, Sampson ML *et al.* (2006) Detection and quantitation of serum mesothelin, a tumor marker for patients with mesothelioma and ovarian cancer. *Clin Cancer Res* 12: 447–53.

Janne PA, Wozniak AJ, Belani CP *et al.* (2005) Open-label study of pemetrexed alone or in combination with cisplatin for the treatment of patients with peritoneal mesothelioma: outcomes of an expanded access program. *Clin Lung Cancer* 7: 40–6.

Katz MH, Barone RM. (2003) The rationale of perioperative intraperitoneal chemotherapy in the treatment of peritoneal surface malignancies. *Surg Oncol Clin N Am* 12: 673–88.

Kazan-Allen L. (2005) Asbestos and mesothelioma: worldwide trends. *Lung Cancer* 49 Suppl 1:S3–8.

Kebapci M, Vardareli E, Adapinar B, Acikalin M. (2003) CT findings and serum ca 125 levels in malignant peritoneal mesothelioma: report of 11 new cases and review of the literature. *Eur Radiol* 13: 2620–6.

Kerrigan SAJ, Turnnir RT, Clement PB, Young RH, Churg A. (2002) Diffuse malignant epithelial mesotheliomas of the peritoneum in women: a clinicopathologic study of 25 patients. *Cancer* 94: 378–85.

Langard S. (2005) Nordic experience: expected decline in the incidence of mesotheliomas resulting from ceased exposure? *Med Lav* 96: 304–11.

Lenzi R, Rosenblum M, Verschraegen C *et al.* (2002) Phase I study of intraperitoneal recombinant human interleukin 12 in patients with Mullerian carcinoma, gastrointestinal primary malignancies, and mesothelioma. *Clin Cancer Res* 8: 3686–95.

Loggie BW, Fleming RA, McQuellon RP, Russell GB, Geisinger KR, Levine EA. (2001) Prospective trial for the treatment of malignant peritoneal mesothelioma. *Am Surg* 67: 999–1003.

Los G, Sminia P, Wondergem J *et al.* (1991) Optimisation of intraperitoneal cisplatin therapy with regional hyperthermia in rats. *Eur J Cancer* 27: 472–7.

Los G, Smals OA, van Vugt MJ *et al.* (1992) A rationale for carboplatin treatment and abdominal hyperthermia in cancers restricted to the peritoneal cavity. *Cancer Res* 52: 1252–8.

Markman M. (1990) *Intraperitoneal Belly Bath Chemotherapy*, 2nd edn. Percept Press, Chicago.

Markman M, Kelsen D. (1992) Efficacy of cisplatin-based intraperitoneal chemotherapy as treatment of malignant peritoneal mesothelioma. *J Cancer Res Clin Oncol* 118: 547–50.

Maurer R, Egloff B. (1975) Malignant peritoneal mesothelioma after cholangiography with thorotrast. *Cancer* 36: 1381–5.

Miller J, Wynn H. (1908) A malignant tumor arising from the endothelium of the peritoneum and producing a mucoid ascitic fluid. *J Pathol Bacteriol* 12: 267.

Montanaro F, Bray F, Gennaro V *et al.* (2003) Pleural mesothelioma incidence in Europe: evidence of some deceleration in the increasing trends. *Cancer Causes Control* 14: 791–803.

Muensterer OJ, Averbach AM, Jacquet P, Otero SE, Sugarbaker PH. (1997) Malignant peritoneal mesothelioma. Case-report demonstrating pitfalls of diagnostic laparoscopy. *Int Surg* 82: 240–3.

Neumann V, Muller KM, Fischer M. (1999) Peritoneal mesothelioma–incidence and etiology. *Pathologe* 20: 169–76.

Nonaka D, Kusamura S, Baratti D *et al.* (2005) Diffuse malignant mesothelioma of the peritoneum: a clinicopathological study of 35 patients treated locoregionally at a single institution. *Cancer* 104: 2181–8.

Park BJ, Alexander HR, Libutti SK *et al.* (1999) Treatment of primary peritoneal mesothelioma by continuous hyperthermic peritoneal perfusion (CHPP). *Ann Surg Oncol* 6: 582–90.

Pass HI, Lott D, Lonardo F *et al.* (2005) Asbestos exposure, pleural mesothelioma, and serum osteopontin levels. *N Engl J Med* 353: 1564–73.

Peterson JT Jr, Greenberg SD, Buffler PA. (1984) Non-asbestos-related malignant mesothelioma–a review. *Cancer* 54: 951–60.

Price B, Ware A. (2004) Mesothelioma trends in the United States: an update based on Surveillance, Epidemiology, and End Results Program data for 1973 through 2003. *Am J Epidemiol* 159: 107–12.

Reuter K, Raptopoulos V, Reale F *et al.* (1983) Diagnosis of peritoneal mesothelioma: computed tomography, sonography, and fine-needle aspiration biopsy. *AJR* 140: 1189–94.

Riddell RH, Goodman MJ, Moossa AR. (1981) Peritoneal malignant mesothelioma in a patient with recurrent peritonitis. *Cancer* 48: 134–9.

Robinson BWS, Lake RA. 2005) Advances in malignant mesothelioma. *N Engl J Med* 353: 1591–1603.

Robinson BWS, Creaney J, Lake R *et al.* (2003) Mesothelin-family proteins and diagnosis of mesothelioma. *Lancet* 362: 1612–6.

Ros PR, Yuschok TJ, Buck JL, Shekitka KM, Kaude JV. (1991) Peritoneal mesothelioma. Radiologic appearances correlated with histology. *Acta Radiol* 32: 355–8.

Sebbag G, Yan H, Shmookler BM, Chang D, Sugarbaker PH. (2000) Results of treatment of 33 patients with peritoneal mesothelioma. *Br J Surg* 87: 1587–93.

Simsek H, Kadayifci A, Okan E. (1996) Importance of serum CA 125 levels in malignant peritoneal mesothelioma. *Tumour Biol* 17: 1–4.

Spirtas R, Heineman EF, Bernstein L *et al.* (1994) Malignant mesothelioma: attributable risk of asbestos exposure. *Occup Environ Med* 51: 804–11.

Sridhar KS, Doria R, Raub WA Jr, Thurer RJ, Saldana M. (1992) New strategies are needed in diffuse malignant mesothelioma. *Cancer* 70: 2969–79.

Sugarbaker P. (1995) Peritonectomy procedures *Ann Surg* 221: 29–42.

Sugarbaker PH. (2006) New standard of care for appendiceal epithelial neoplasms and pseudomyxoma peritonei syndrome? *Lancet Oncol* 7: 69–76.

Sugarbaker P, Cunliffe W, Belliveau J, Bruin E, Graves T. (1988) Rationale for perioperative intraperitoneal chemotherapy as a surgical adjunct for gastrointestinal malignancy. *Reg Cancer Treat* 66–79.

Sugarbaker PH, Welch LS, Mohamed F, Glehen O. (2003) A review of peritoneal mesothelioma at the Washington Cancer Institute. *Surg Oncol Clin N Am* 12: 605–21.

Swuste P, Burdorf A, Ruers B. (2004) Asbestos, asbestos-related diseases, and compensation claims in The Netherlands. *Int J Occup Environ Health* 10: 159–65.

Taub RN, Hesdorffer ME, Keohan ML. (2005) Combined resection, intraperitoneal chemotherapy, and whole abdominal radiation for malignant peritoneal mesothelioma (MPM). *J Clin Oncol*: 664s.

Tejido Garcia R, Anta Fernandez M, Hernandez Hernandez JL, Bravo Gonzalez J, Gonzalez Macias J. (1997) Fever of unknown origin as the clinical presentation of malignant peritoneal mesothelioma. *An Med Interna* 14: 573–5.

Urano M, Kuroda M, Nishimura Y. (1999) For the clinical application of thermochemotherapy given at mild temperatures. *Int J Hyperthermia* 15: 79–107.

van de Vaart PJ, van der Vange N, Zoetmulder FA *et al.* (1998) Intraperitoneal cisplatin with regional hyperthermia in advanced ovarian cancer: pharmacokinetics and cisplatin-DNA adduct formation in patients and ovarian cancer cell lines. *Eur J Cancer* 34: 148–54.

Verwaal VJ, van Ruth S, de Bree E *et al.* (2003) Randomized trial of cytoreduction and hyperthermic intraperitoneal chemotherapy versus systemic chemotherapy and palliative surgery in patients with peritoneal carcinomatosis of colorectal cancer. *J Clin Oncol* 21: 3737–43.

Verwaal VJ, van Ruth S, Witkamp A, Boot H, van Slooten G, Zoetmulder FAN. (2005) Long-term survival of peritoneal carcinomatosis of colorectal origin. *Ann Surg Oncol* 12: 65–71.

Vlasveld LT, Gallee MP, Rodenhuis S, Taal BG. (1991) Intraperitoneal chemotherapy for malignant peritoneal mesothelioma. *Eur J Cancer* 27: 732–4.

Weill H, Hughes JM, Churg AM. (2004) Changing trends in US mesothelioma incidence. *Occup Environ Med* 61: 438–41.

Welch LS, Acherman YIZ, Haile E, Sokas RK, Sugarbaker PH. (2005) Asbestos and peritoneal mesothelioma among college-educated men. *Int J Occup Environ Health* 11: 254–8.

Yan TD, Haveric N, Carmignani CP, Bromley CM, Sugarbaker PH. (2005a) Computed tomographic characterization of malignant peritoneal mesothelioma. *Tumori* 91: 394–400.

Yan TD, Haveric N, Carmignani CP, Chang D, Sugarbaker PH. (2005b) Abdominal computed tomography scans in the selection of patients with malignant peritoneal mesothelioma for comprehensive treatment with cytoreductive surgery and perioperative intraperitoneal chemotherapy. *Cancer* 103: 839–49.

Yan TD, Yoo D, Sugarbaker P. (2006a) Significance of lymph node metastasis in patients with diffuse malignant peritoneal mesothelioma. *Eur J Surg Oncol* 32: 948–53.

Yan TD, Popa E, Brun EA, Cerruto CA, Sugarbaker PH. (2006b) Sex difference in diffuse malignant peritoneal mesothelioma. *Br J Surg* 93: 1536–42.

Yan TD, Brun EA, Cerruto CA, Haveric N, Chang D, Sugarbaker PH. (2007) Prognostic indicators for patients undergoing cytoreductive surgery and perioperative intraperitoneal chemotherapy for diffuse malignant peritoneal mesothelioma. *Ann Surg Oncol* 14: 41–9.

Yates DH, Corrin B, Stidolph PN, Browne K. (1997) Malignant mesothelioma in south east England: clinicopathological experience of 272 cases. *Thorax* 52: 507–12.

Yu GH, Soma L, Hahn S, Friedberg JS. (2001) Changing clinical course of patients with malignant mesothelioma: implications for FNA cytology and utility of immunocytochemical staining. *Diag Cytopathol* 24: 322–7.

3 Hepatobiliary Cancer

Edited by Yuman Fong

16 Epidemiology of Hepatocellular Carcinoma

Hashem B. El-Serag, Donna L. White & Zhannat Nurgalieva

Global incidence of hepatocellular carcinoma

Overview

Primary liver cancer is the fifth most common cancer worldwide and the third most common cause of cancer mortality (Parkin 2001). Globally, over 560,000 people develop liver cancer each year and an almost equal number, 550,000, die of it. Liver cancer burden, however, is not evenly distributed throughout the world (Fig. 16.1). Most hepatocellular carcinoma (HCC) cases (>80%) occur in either sub-Saharan Africa or in Eastern Asia. China alone accounts for more than 50% of the world's cases (age-standardized incidence rate (ASR) male: 35.2/100,000; female: 13.3/100,000). Other high-rate (>20/100,000) areas include Senegal (male: 28.47/100,000; female: 12.2/100,000), The Gambia (male: 39.67/100,000; female: 14.6/100,000), and South Korea (male: 48.8/100,000; female: 11.6/100,000).

North and South America, Northern Europe and Oceania are low-rate (<5.0/100,000) areas for liver cancer among most populations. Typical incidence rates in these areas are those of the US (male: 4.21/100,000; female: 1.74/100,000), Canada (male: 3.2/100,000; female: 1.1/100,000), Colombia (male: 2.2/100,000; female: 2.0/100,000) UK (male: 2.2/100,000; female: 1.1/100,000), and Australia (male: 3.6/100,000; female: 1.0/100,000). Southern European countries, typified by rates in Spain (male: 7.5/100,000; female: 2.4/100,000), Italy (male: 13.5/100,000; female: 4.6/100,000), and Greece (male: 12.1/100,000; female: 4.6/100,000) are medium rate (5.0–20.0/100,000) (Ferlay 2001).

HCC accounts for between 85% and 90% of primary liver cancer. One noteworthy exception is the Khon Kaen region of Thailand, which has one of the world's highest rates of liver cancer (ASR 1993–1997 male: 88.0/100,000; female: 35.4/100,000) (Parkin 2002). However, due to endemic infestation with liver flukes, the major type of liver cancer in this region is intrahepatic cholangiocarcinoma rather than HCC (Okuda *et al.* 2002).

Encouraging trends in liver cancer incidence have been seen in some of the high-rate areas (McGlynn *et al.* 2001). Between 1978–82 and 1993–97, decreases in incidence were reported among Chinese populations in Hong Kong, Shanghai and Singapore (Parkin 2002). In addition to these areas, Japan also began to experience declines in incidence rates among males for the first time between 1993 and 1997 (Fig. 16.2).

Many high-rate Asian countries now vaccinate all newborns against the hepatitis B virus (HBV) and the effect on HCC rates has already become apparent. In Taiwan, where national newborn vaccination began in 1984, HCC rates among children aged 6–14 years declined significantly from 0.70/100,000 in 1981–1986 to 0.36/100,000 in 1990–1994 (Chang *et al.* 1997). It is too soon yet for HBV vaccination to have had an effect on adult rates, but other public health measures may have contributed to declines in HCC incidence in high-risk areas of China. A Chinese government program started in the late 1980s to shift the staple diet of the Jiangsu Province from corn to rice may have limited exposure to known hepatocarcinogen aflatoxin B_1 (AFB_1) in this area (Yu 1995). Similarly, another Chinese public health campaign initiated in the early 1970s to encourage drinking of well rather than pond or ditch-water, may have decreased consumption of microcystins, cyanobacteria-produced compounds demonstrated to be hepatocarcinogenic in experimental animals.

In contrast, registries in a number of low-rate areas reported increases in HCC incidence between 1978–82 and 1993–97. Included among these registries are those in the US, UK, and Australia. Reasons for both the decreased incidence in high-rate areas and the increased incidence in low-rate areas are not yet clear, suggesting that each area will be an important case study. It has been widely hypothesized, however, that increased incidence in low-rate areas may be related to greater prevalence of hepatitis C virus (HCV) infection in these areas.

Gastrointestinal Oncology: A Critical Multidisciplinary Team Approach.
Edited by J. Jankowski, R. Sampliner, D. Kerr, and Y. Fong.

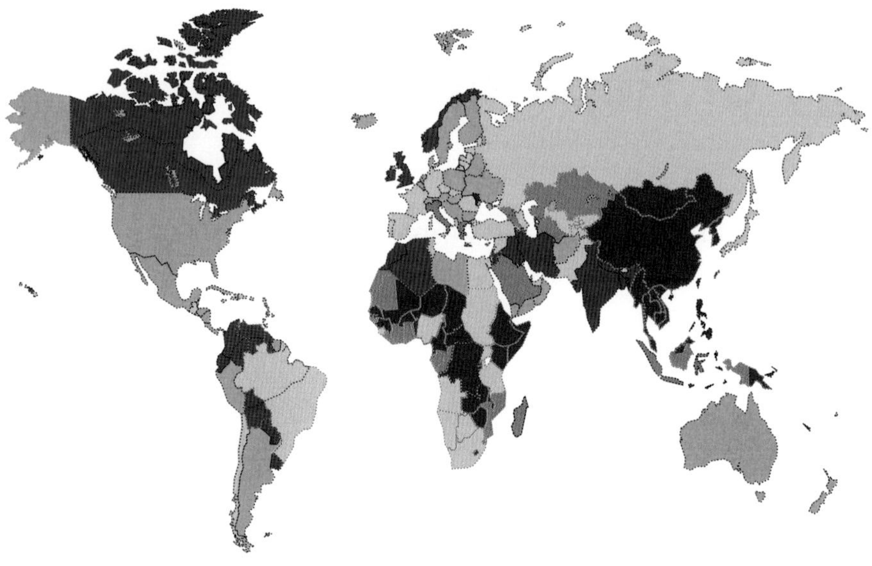

Fig. 16.1 Regional variations in the incidence rates of hepatocellular carcinoma categorized by age-adjusted incidence rates. From Parkin *et al.* (2002).

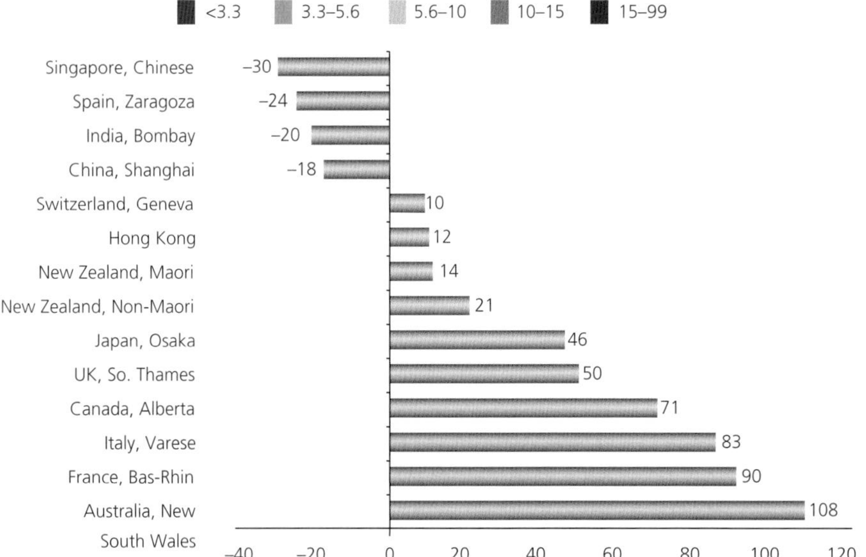

Fig. 16.2 Recent changes in the incidence of HCC. The incidence of HCC has been declining in some 'high-incidence' areas, such as China and Hong Kong. On the other hand, HCC incidence in several 'low- and intermediate-incidence' areas has been increasing. Modified from McGlynn *et al.* (2001).

Race/ethnicity

HCC incidence rates also vary greatly among different populations living in the same region. For example, ethnic Indian, Chinese and Malay populations of Singapore had age-adjusted rates ranging from 21.21/100,000 among Chinese males to 7.86/100,000 among Indian males between 1993 and 1997 (Parkin 2002). The comparable rates for females were 5.13/100,000 among ethnic Chinese and 1.77/100,000 among ethnic Indians. Another example is the US where at all ages and among both genders, HCC rates are two times higher in Asians than in African-Americans, which are themselves two times higher than those in whites. The reason(s) for this interethnic variability likely include differences in prevalence and acquisition time of major risk factors for liver disease and HCC.

Gender

In almost all populations, males have higher liver cancer rates than females, with male : female ratios usually averaging between 2 : 1 and 4 : 1. At present, the largest discrepancies in rates (>4 : 1) are found in medium-risk European populations. Typical among these ratios are those reported from Geneva, Switzerland (4.1 : 1) and Varese, Italy (5.1 : 1). Among 10 French registries listed in Volume VIII of *Cancer in Five Continents* (Parkin *et al.* 2002), nine report male : female ratios > 5 : 1. In contrast, typical ratios currently seen in high-risk populations are those of Qidong, China (3.2 : 1), Osaka, Japan (3.7 : 1), The Gambia (2.8 : 1), and Harare, Zimbabwe (2.4 : 1). Registries in Central and South America report some of the lowest sex ratios for liver cancer. Typical ratios in these regions are reported by Colombia (1.2 : 1) and Costa Rica (1.6 : 1).

The reasons for higher rates of liver cancer in males may relate to gender-specific differences in exposure to risk factors. Men are more likely to be infected with HBV and HCV, consume alcohol, smoke cigarettes, and have increased iron stores. Higher levels of androgenic hormones, body mass index (BMI), and increased genetic susceptibility may also adversely affect male risk.

Age

The global age distribution of HCC varies by region, incidence rate, gender and, possibly, etiology (Parkin 2002). In almost all areas, female rates peak in the age group 5 years older than the peak age group for males. In low-risk populations (e.g. US, Canada, UK), the highest age-specific rates occur among persons aged 75 and older. A similar pattern is seen among most high-risk Asian populations (e.g. Hong Kong, Shanghai). In contrast, male rates in high-risk African populations (e.g. The Gambia, Mali) tend to peak between ages 60 and 65 before declining; while female rates peak between 65 and 70 before declining. These variable age-specific patterns are likely related to differences in the dominant hepatitis virus in the population, the age at viral infection, and the existence of other risk factors. Notably, while most HCV carriers became infected as adults, most HBV carriers became infected at a very young age.

Exceptions to these age patterns occur in Qidong, China, where liver cancer rates are among the world's highest. Age-specific incidence rates among males rise until age 45 and then plateau, while among females, rates rise until age 60 and then plateau. The explanation for these younger peak ages is unclear, but may be due to existence of other hepatocarcinogenic exposures.

Distribution of risk factors

Major risk factors for HCC vary by region. In most high-risk areas, the dominant risk factor is chronic HBV infection. In Asia, HBV infection is largely acquired by maternal–child transmission, while sibling to sibling transmission at young ages is more common in Africa. Consumption of aflatoxin B_1-contaminated foodstuffs is the other major HCC risk factor in most high-rate areas.

Unlike the rest of Asia, the dominant hepatitis virus in Japan is HCV, which began to circulate in Japan shortly after World War II (Yoshizawa 2002). Consequently, HCC rates began to sharply increase in the mid-1970s with an anticipated peak in HCV-related HCC rates projected around 2015, though recent data suggest the peak might have already been reached.

In low-rate HCC areas, increasing numbers of persons living with cirrhosis is the likely explanation for rising HCC incidence. This has resulted from a combination of factors including rising incidence of cirrhosis due to HCV and, to a lesser extent, HBV infection, as well as a general improvement in survival among cirrhosis patients. It has been estimated that HCV began to infect large numbers of young adults in North America and South and Central Europe in the 1960s and 1970s as a result of injection drug use (Armstrong *et al.* 2000). The virus then moved into national blood supplies and circulated until a screening test was developed in 1990, after which time rates of new infection dropped dramatically. Currently, it is estimated that HCV-related HCC in low-rate countries will peak around 2010.

HCC in the United States

Age-adjusted HCC incidence rates increased more than twofold between 1985 and 2002 (El-Serag 2004) (Fig. 16.3). Average annual, age-adjusted rate of HCC verified by histology or cytology increased from 1.3 per 100,000 during 1978–80 to 3.3 per 100,000 during 1999–2001 (El-Serag *et al.* 2003). The increase in HCC started in the mid-1980s with greatest proportional increases occurring during the late 1990s. The largest proportional increases occurred among whites (Hispanics and non-Hispanics), while the lowest proportional increases occurred among Asians. The mean age at diagnosis is approximately 65 years, 74% of cases occur in men, and the racial distribution is 48% white, 15% Hispanic, 13% African-American, and 24% other race/ethnicity (predominantly Asian). During recent years as incidence rates increased, the age-distribution of HCC patients has shifted towards relatively younger ages, with greatest proportional increases between ages 45 and 60.

Four published studies examined secular changes in HCC risk factors in the US (Hassan *et al.* 2002; El Serag & Mason 2000; Davila *et al.* 2004; Kulkarni *et al.* 2004). Two studies were from large, single referral centers where viral risk factor ascertainment was based on serology findings, while the other two were from national databases in which risk factors were ascertained from ICD-9 codes in billing or discharge records. In all four studies, the greatest proportional increases occurred in HCV-related HCC, while HBV-related HCC had the lowest and most stable rates. Overall, between 15 to 50% of HCC patients in the US have no established risk factors.

Risk factors of hepatocellular carcinoma

HCC is unique in that it largely occurs within an established background of chronic liver disease and cirrhosis (~70–90% of all detected HCC cases) (Fig. 16.4). Major causes of cirrhosis in patients with HCC include HBV, HCV, alcoholic liver disease, and possibly, non-alcoholic steatohepatitis.

Hepatitis B virus

Globally, HBV is the most frequent underlying cause of HCC with an estimated 300 million persons with chronic infection worldwide. Case–control studies have demonstrated chronic

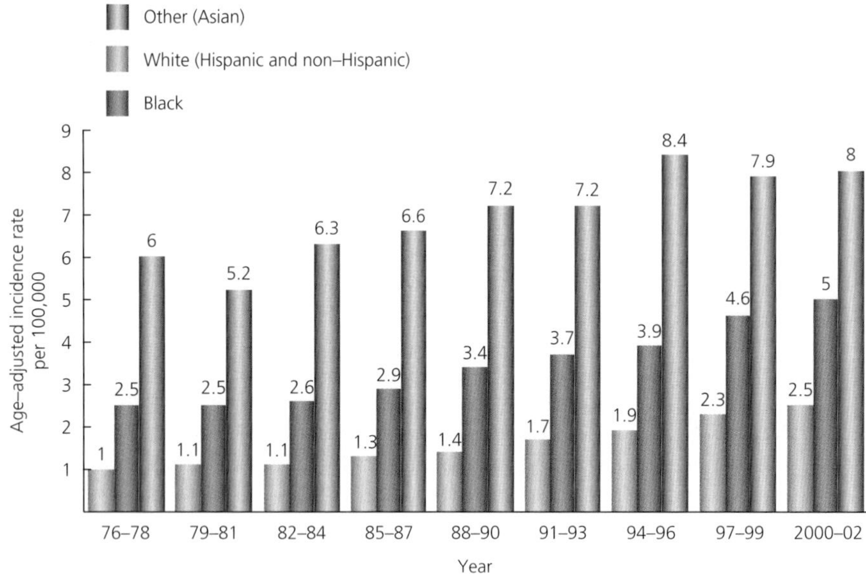

Fig. 16.3 Average yearly, age-adjusted incidence rates for HCC in the United States shown for 3-year intervals between 1975 and 2002. 'White' includes approximately 25% Hispanic while 'Other' is predominantly Asian (88%).

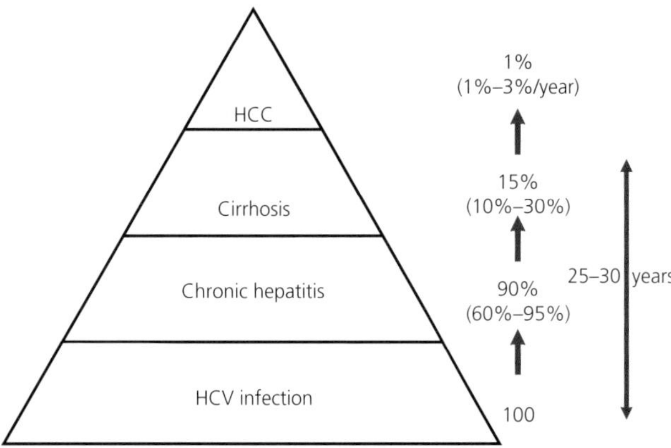

Fig. 16.4 Estimated progression rates to cirrhosis and hepatocellular carcinoma in hepatitis C infection.

HBV carriers have a five- to 15-fold increased risk of HCC compared to the general population.

The great majority, between 70% and 90%, of HBV-related HCC develops in a background of cirrhosis. HBV DNA is found in the host genome of both infected and malignant hepatic cells. HBV may therefore initiate malignant transformation through a direct carcinogenic mechanism by increasing likelihood of viral DNA insertion in or near proto-oncogenes or tumor suppressor genes. However, despite initial excitement accompanying this discovery, subsequent research has failed to show a unifying mechanism by which integration of HBV DNA leads to HCC.

The increased HCC risk associated with HBV infection particularly applies to areas where HBV is endemic. In these areas, it is usually transmitted from mother to newborn (vertical transmission) and up to 90% of infected persons follow a chronic course. This pattern is different in areas with low HCC incidence rates where HBV is acquired in adulthood through sexual and parenteral routes (horizontal transmission) with >90% of acute infections resolving spontaneously. The annual HCC incidence in chronic HBV carriers in Asia ranges between 0.4% and 0.6%. This figure is lower in Alaskan natives (0.26%/year) and lowest in Caucasian HBV carriers (McMahon *et al.* 1990).

Several other factors have been reported to increase HCC risk among HBV carriers including male gender, older age (or longer duration of infection), Asian or African race, cirrhosis, family history of HCC, exposure to aflatoxin, alcohol or tobacco, or coinfection with HCV or HDV. HCC risk is also increased in patients with higher levels of HBV replication, as indicated by presence of HBeAg and high HBV DNA levels. In addition, it has been suggested in Asian studies that genotype C is associated with more severe liver disease than genotype B (Kao *et al.* 2002).

In the natural history of chronic HBV infection, spontaneous or treatment-induced development of antibodies against HBsAg and HBeAg leads to improved clinical outcomes. A meta-analysis of 12 studies with 1187 patients who received interferon and 665 untreated patients followed for 5 years found lower HCC incidence in treated patients (1.9%; 95% confidence interval [CI] 0.8%–3.0%) than untreated patients (3.2%; 95% CI 1.8%–4.5%). However, this difference was not statistically significant (Camma *et al.* 2001).

Using sensitive amplification assays, many studies have demonstrated that HBV DNA persists as 'occult HBV infection' for decades among persons with serological recovery (HBsAg negative) from acute infection. Occult HBV is associated with anti-HBc and/or anti-HBs (Torbenson & Thomas 2002). However, in a significant proportion of individuals, neither anti-HBc nor anti-HBs can be detected. A single multinational investigation found prevalence of occult HBV in liver tissue to be 11% in Italy, 5–9% in Hong Kong, and 0% in the UK. Supporting an association with occult HBV, a high proportion of individuals with HCV infection who develop HCC have demonstrable HBV DNA and proteins in their neoplastic and adjacent non-neoplastic liver tissue. However, although some studies have linked development of HCC in individuals with chronic HCV infection to occult HBV, others have not found an association.

Hepatitis C virus

Chronic HCV infection is a major risk factor for development of HCC. Markers of HCV infection are found in a variable proportion of HCC cases; for example, 44–66% in Italy (Fasani *et al.* 1999; Stroffolini *et al.* 1999), 27–58% in France, 60–75% in Spain, and 80–90% of HCC cases in Japan (Yoshizawa 2002). A higher but undefined proportion of HCC patients might have had HCV detected by PCR testing of liver tissue and/or serum, even if antibody to HCV (anti-HCV) was non-detectable. In a meta-analysis of 21 case–control studies in which second-generation enzyme immunoassay tests for anti-HCV were used, HCC risk was increased 17-fold in HCV-infected patients compared with HCV-negative controls (95% CI 14–22) (Donato *et al.* 2002).

The likelihood of development of HCC among HCV-infected persons is difficult to determine due to the paucity of adequate long-term cohort studies; however, the best estimate is from 1% to 3% after 30 years (Fig. 16.4). HCV increases HCC risk by promoting fibrosis and eventually cirrhosis (Fig. 16.5). Once HCV-related cirrhosis is established, HCC develops at an annual rate of 1–4%; though rates up to 7% have been reported in Japan. Rates of cirrhosis 25–30 years post infection range between 15% and 35% (Freeman *et al.* 2001). The highest incidence rates were observed in HCV-contaminated blood or blood product recipients (14 and 1 per 1000 person-years for cirrhosis and HCC respectively) and in hemophiliacs (5 and 0.7 per 1000 person-years). The lowest rates have been reported in women who received a one-time contaminated anti-D immune globulin treatment (1 and 0 per 1000 person-years respectively).

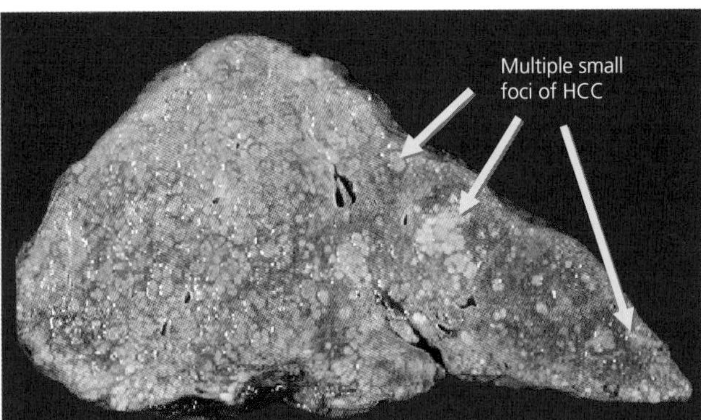

Fig. 16.5 Cirrhosis and hepatocellular carcinoma. Explanted liver showing features of cirrhosis and multiple small foci of HCC throughout the liver in a miliary pattern (arrows).

In HCV-infected patients, factors related to host and environment appear to be more important than viral factors in determining progression to cirrhosis. These factors include older age, older age at the time of acquisition of infection, male gender, heavy alcohol intake (>50 g/day), diabetes, obesity, and coinfection with HIV or HBV (Cramp 1999). There is no strong evidence that HCV viral factors like genotype, load or quasispecies are important in determining the risk of progression to cirrhosis or HCC.

Successful antiviral therapy in patients with HCV-related cirrhosis may reduce future risk of HCC, but the evidence is weak. There is only one prospective, randomized, controlled trial that examined the effects of antiviral therapy on HCC, a Japanese trial in which 100 patients were randomized to receive either 6 million units of interferon alfa three times weekly for 3–6 months or were followed without treatment (Nishiguchi *et al.* 1995). After a 2–7-year follow-up period, HCC was significantly reduced in the treated (4%) compared to the non-treated control group (38%), a 93% reduction in adjusted risk. However, much of this risk reduction was a result of the unusually high HCC rate among these controls. Other studies, mostly retrospective and non-randomized, suggested moderately decreased HCC risk among HCV-infected patients treated with interferon (Imai *et al.* 1998; International Interferon-alpha Hepatocellular Carcinoma Study Group 1998; Niederau *et al.* 1998; Serfaty *et al.* 1998; Ikeda *et al.* 1999; Okanoue *et al.* 1999; Valla *et al.* 1999; Bruno *et al.* 2001).

In general, reported preventive effects of interferon therapy were less marked in European compared to Japanese studies. However, the lack of randomization in most of these studies may exaggerate treatment benefits as it is likely healthier patients tend to get treated more frequently than those with advanced liver disease (who are known to be more likely to develop HCC). In addition to a role in primary prevention of HCC among HCV-infected patients, a few Japanese reports suggest interferon may also be effective for secondary prevention in individuals who have previously undergone resection for HCC.

Alcohol

Heavy alcohol intake, defined as ingestion of >50–70 g/day for prolonged periods, is a well-established HCC risk factor. It is unclear whether risk of HCC is significantly altered in those with low or moderate alcohol intake. Although heavy intake is strongly associated with development of cirrhosis; there is little evidence of a direct carcinogenic effect of alcohol otherwise.

There is also evidence for a synergistic effect of heavy alcohol ingestion with HCV or HBV, with these factors presumably operating together to increase HCC risk by more actively promoting cirrhosis. For example, Donato *et al.* (2002) reported that among alcohol drinkers, HCC risk increased in a linear fashion with daily intake >60 g. However, with concomitant presence of HCV infection, there was an additional twofold increase in HCC risk over that observed with alcohol usage alone (i.e. a positive synergistic effect).

Aflatoxin

Aflatoxin B_1 (AFB_1) is a mycotoxin produced by the *Aspergillus* fungus. This fungus grows readily on foodstuffs like corn and peanuts stored in warm, damp conditions. Animal experiments demonstrated that AFB_1 is a powerful hepatocarcinogen, leading the International Agency for Research on Cancer (IARC) to classify it as carcinogenic (IARC Monographs 1987).

Once ingested, AFB_1 is metabolized to an active intermediate, AFB_1-*exo*-8,9-epoxide, which can bind to DNA and cause damage, including producing a characteristic mutation in the p53 tumor suppressor gene (p53 249^{ser}) (Garner *et al.* 1972). This mutation has been observed in 30–60% of HCC tumors in aflatoxin endemic areas (Bressac *et al.* 1991; Turner *et al.* 2002).

Strong evidence that AFB_1 is a risk factor for HCC has been supplied by person-specific epidemiologic studies performed in the last 15 years. These studies were permitted by development of assays for aflatoxin metabolites in urine, AFB_1-albumin adducts in serum, and detection of a signature aflatoxin DNA mutation in tissues.

Interaction between AFB_1 exposure and chronic HBV infection was revealed in short-term prospective studies in Shanghai, China. Urinary excretion of aflatoxin metabolites increased HCC risk fourfold while HBV infection increased risk sevenfold. However, individuals who both excreted AFB_1 metabolites and were HBV carriers had a dramatic 60-fold increased risk of HCC (Qian *et al.* 1994).

In most areas where AFB_1 exposure is a problem, chronic HBV infection is also highly prevalent. Though HBV vaccination in these areas should be the major preventive tactic, persons already chronically infected will not benefit from vaccination. However, HBV carriers could benefit by eliminating AFB_1 exposure. Efforts to accomplish this goal in China (Yu 1995) and Africa (Turner *et al.* 2002) have been launched.

Non-alcoholic fatty liver disease (NAFLD)

It has been suggested that many cryptogenic cirrhosis and HCC cases represent more severe forms of non-alcoholic fatty liver disease (NAFLD), namely non-alcoholic steatohepatitis (NASH). Studies in the US evaluating risk factors for chronic liver disease or HCC have failed to identify HCV, HBV, or heavy alcohol intake in a large proportion of patients (30–40%). Further, several case–control studies have indicated that HCC patients with cryptogenic cirrhosis tend to have clinical and demographic features suggestive of NASH (predominance of women, diabetes, obesity). However, apart from case reports, there are no prospective studies of HCC in patients with NASH. Moreover, once cirrhosis and HCC are established, it is difficult to identify pathological features of NASH. To date, the most compelling evidence for an association between NASH and HCC comes from studies examining HCC risk with two conditions strongly associated with NASH: obesity and diabetes (described below).

Obesity

In a large prospective cohort study of more than 900,000 individuals in the USA followed for a 16-year period, liver cancer mortality rates were five times greater among persons with the greatest BMI (35–40) (Calle *et al.* 2003) (Fig. 16.6). Several developed countries, most notably the US, are in the midst of a burgeoning obesity epidemic. Although evidence linking obesity to HCC is scant, even small increases in risk related to obesity could translate into a large number of HCC cases.

Diabetes mellitus

Diabetes has been proposed as a risk factor for both chronic liver disease and HCC through development of NAFLD and NASH. In addition, diabetes is associated with increased levels of insulin and insulin-like growth factors, which are potential cancer promoting factors.

Several case–control studies from the USA, Greece, Italy, Taiwan, and Japan examined the association between diabetes, mostly type II, and HCC. At least eight studies found a significant positive association between diabetes and HCC, two found a positive association that did not quite reach significance, and one found a significant negative association. A potential bias in cross-sectional and case–control studies, however, is difficulty in discerning temporal relationships between exposures (diabetes) and outcomes (HCC). This problem is relevant in evaluating HCC risk factors because 10–20% of patients with cirrhosis have overt diabetes and a larger percentage have impaired

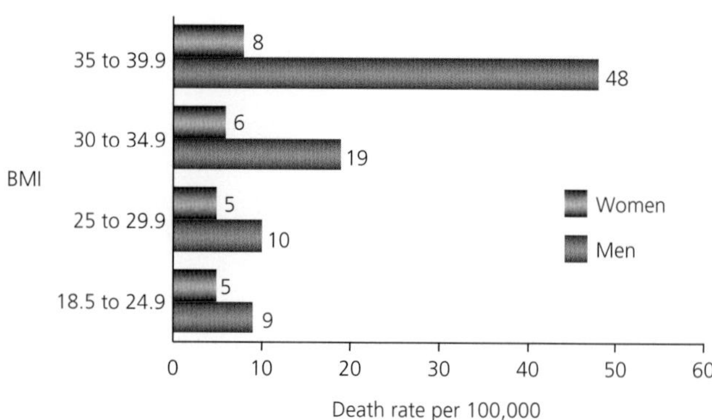

Fig. 16.6 Obesity and liver cancer. In both men and women, a higher body-mass index (BMI) is significantly associated with higher rates of death due to cancer of the liver. Modified from Calle *et al.* (2003).

glucose tolerance. Thus, diabetes may also be the result of cirrhosis.

Cohort studies, which are intrinsically better suited to discern temporal relationships between exposure and disease, have also been conducted. All compared HCC incidence in cohorts of diabetic patients to either the expected incidence given HCC rates in the underlying population or to the observed HCC incidence among a defined cohort without diabetes (El Serag *et al.* 2004). Three studies conducted among younger or smaller cohorts found either no or a low number of HCC cases. At least four other cohort studies examined large numbers of patients for relatively long time periods, with three studies finding significantly increased risk of HCC with diabetes (risk ratios ranging between 2 and 3) (Adami *et al.* 1996; Wideroff *et al.* 1997; El Serag *et al.* 2004). We recently conducted a study of HCC incidence in a large cohort of Department of Veterans Affairs (VA) patients (n = 173,643 with and n = 650,620 without diabetes). The findings of this study indicate HCC incidence doubled among patients with diabetes and was higher among those with longer duration of follow-up (El Serag *et al.* 2004) (Fig. 16.7).

While most studies have been conducted in low-rate areas, diabetes has also been found to be a significant risk factor in areas of high HCC incidence like Japan. Although other underlying risk factors like HCV may confound the association between diabetes and HCC, they do not seem to fully explain observed associations between diabetes and HCC. Taken together, available data suggest diabetes is a moderately strong risk factor for HCC (El-Serag *et al.* 2006). Additional research is required to examine issues related to duration and treatment of diabetes, as well as possible confounding by diet and obesity.

Tobacco

The relationship between cigarette smoking and HCC has been examined in more than 50 studies in both low- and high-rate areas. In almost all countries, both positive association and lack of association findings have been reported. Among studies reporting positive associations, several found effects were limited to population subgroups defined by HBV status, HCV status, a genetic polymorphism or other exposure. Taken together, available evidence suggests that any effect of smoking on HCC is likely to be weak and limited to a subset of the general population. However, because two studies conducted exclusively among women reported positive associations, it has been suggested that attributable risk among women may be higher than that in men (Tanaka *et al.* 1995; Evans *et al.* 2002).

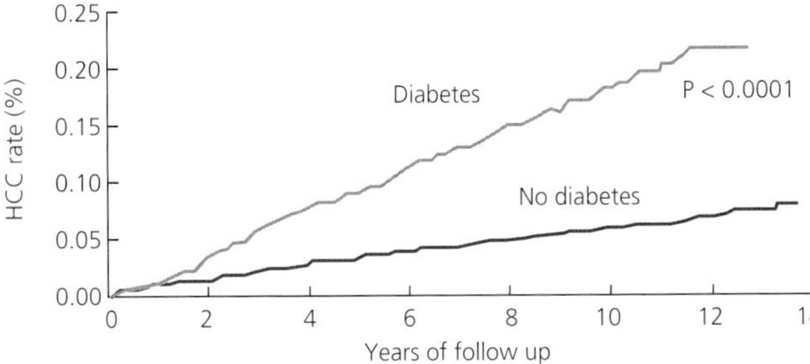

Fig. 16.7 The cumulative incidence of HCC among veteran patients hospitalized between 1985 and 1990. The study examined 173,463 patients with diabetes and 650,620 without diabetes. No patient had acute or chronic liver disease recorded before, during, or within 1 year of their index hospitalization.

Oral contraceptives

The association between oral contraceptive use and HCC risk was examined in at least 12 case–control studies (n = 740 cases and n = 5223 controls) (Maheshwari *et al.* 2007). The pooled estimator was OR = 1.43 (95% CI 0.90–2.26, p = 0.13). Six studies showed a significant two- to 20-fold increase in HCC risk with longer durations (>5 years) of oral contraceptive use. Whether newer, low-dose oral contraceptives convey similar potential risks is currently unknown.

Genetic epidemiology of HCC

Although a very small minority of HCC cases are associated with familial disorders with mendelian inheritance like hereditary hemachromatosis, alpha-1-antitrypsin deficiency or porphyrias, epidemiologic research has convincingly demonstrated that the great majority of adult-onset HCC cases are sporadic (i.e. have no similarly affected first-degree relative) and that many have at least one established non-genetic risk factor like habitual alcohol abuse or chronic infection with hepatitis B or C viruses. However, most people with these known environmental risk factors for HCC never develop cirrhosis or HCC, while a sizable minority of HCC cases develops among individuals without any known risk factors.

Genetic variation has long been suspected to influence the variable risk for HCC observed both within and across populations. It has, however, only recently become possible to perform large-scale epidemiologic studies to evaluate genetic risk factors given rapid advances within the field of genomics, including completion of the Human Genome Project, public accessibility to information on millions of human single nucleotide polymorphisms (SNPs), development of high-throughput DNA microarrays, and a dramatic reduction in the cost of genetic testing. (See the excellent series of review articles in *Lancet* [Burton *et al.* 2005; Cordell & Clayton 2005; Davey *et al.* 2005; Dawn & Barret 2005; Hattersley & McCarthy 2005; Hopper *et al.* 2005] for an overview of the nascent and rapidly evolving field of genetic epidemiology.)

Currently far fewer genetic epidemiologic studies have been reported for HCC than for other more common cancers e.g. lung, prostate or breast cancers, in developed countries. The majority of HCC studies have been case–control studies conducted in populations with high HCC rate (Asian, African) or medium-rate (European). Typically, they have examined only a few polymorphisms in a few genes selected because of: (i) their role in the key liver function of detoxification including phase I and phase II enzymes like cytochrome P450s (CYPs), N-acetyl transferases (NATs), and glutathione S-transferases (GSTs); (ii) their role in biological pathways potentially relevant in chronic liver disease and carcinogenesis including inflammatory response (e.g. interleukins (ILs) 1β, IRN) and DNA repair (e.g. XRCC1); or (iii) their role in mitigating or exacerbating the effects of exposure to specific etiologic risk factors for HCC like alcohol or aflatoxin (e.g. ADH3, ALDH2, EPHX1).

Results from the genetic epidemiology studies evaluating varied polymorphisms as risk factors for HCC, including CYPs (e.g. Yu *et al.* 1995; Yu *et al.* 1999; Wong *et al.* 2000), NATs (e.g. Gelatti *et al.* 2005; Yu *et al.* 2000), GSTs (e.g. Sun *et al.* 2001; Long *et al.* 2006) and ALDH2 (e.g. Kato *et al.* 2003; Sakamoto *et al.* 2006), have largely been equivocal, with findings of a positive association, association only within a limited subset of the population, or no or negative association all reported. The lack of reproducibility is a phenomenon widely reported in the broader field of genetic epidemiology. It has been widely attributed to inadequate sample sizes to reliably detect the likely small effects of individual genes on risk within a background of strong environmental risk factors and polygenic influences on development of disease (Cordell & Clayton 2005; Hattersley & McCarthy 2005). Furthermore, virtually all of these studies have lacked power to detect interactions; it is estimated that several thousand cases and controls are required to adequately assess the effects of gene–gene or gene–environment interactions. Other contributing factors include population stratification or population-based differences in the relative distribution of alleles and among different racial groups risk of disease, use of non-representative control groups, and variable genetic penetrance.

Given genetic epidemiology studies are often highly underpowered, meta-analysis has been recognized as an important tool to more precisely define the effect of individual polymorphisms on relative risk of disease and to identify potentially important sources of between-study heterogeneity (Khoury & Little 2000; Little *et al.* 2003). We recently completed a meta-analysis evaluating the effect of the two most frequently evaluated polymorphisms for HCC risk to date, the dual-deletion GST polymorphisms *GSTM1* (n = 14 studies) and *GSTT1* (n = 13 studies) (White *et al.* 2007). Individual studies for both polymorphisms reported variable findings and therefore the observed heterogeneity necessitated use of a random-effects model. Pooled estimators suggested a possible small excess risk with either *GSTM1* or *GSTT1* null genotypes, though findings approached significance only for *GSTT1* ($OR_{GSTM1} = 1.16$, 95% CI 0.89–1.53; $OR_{GSTT1} = 1.191$, 95% CI 0.99–1.44). Exploratory meta-regressions suggested the source of the controls was a possible source of observed between-study heterogeneity, with greater risk among hospital-based controls for both polymorphisms. Year of publication was an additional source of between-study heterogeneity for *GSTM1* only. Although overall pooled estimators for *GSTM1* and *GSTT1* suggest a possible small excess of HCC with the null genotype, additional studies with larger samples and conducted in other populations are needed to further clarify the role of both polymorphisms in the etiology of HCC and to investigate gene–environment interaction.

A noteworthy recent advance in the field of genetic epidemiology is the development of large-scale cohorts or DNA 'biobank' cohorts that will be prospectively followed for development of disease (e.g. biobanks in the UK (n = 500,000) and Mexico (n = 200,000)) (Davey *et al.* 2005). These large-scale genetic cohort studies offer many important advantages over traditional case–control studies including the ability to validly discern temporal relationships between exposure and disease and the availability of an appropriate control group. However, in spite of their impressive sample size, given the rarity of HCC and the considerable latency until disease onset, they are unlikely to generate enough HCC cases to fully replace genetic case–control and disease-based registry studies.

Overall, as in other areas of genetic epidemiology, results of studies in HCC have fallen short of early expectations that they would rapidly and unequivocally result in identification of genetic variants conveying substantial excess risk of disease and thereby establish the groundwork for effective genetic screening for primary prevention. However, recent identification of genetic risk factors for some chronic diseases such as Alzheimer's disease and breast cancer, as well as multidisciplinary efforts to address the considerable complexity in identifying genetic risk factors, have given rise to 'cautious optimism'(Davey *et al.* 2005) that genetic epidemiology will ultimately provide important information on etiopathogenesis of many chronic diseases, including HCC.

References

Adami HO, Chow WH, Nyren O *et al.* (1996) Excess risk of primary liver cancer in patients with diabetes mellitus. *J Natl Cancer Inst* 88(20): 1472–7.

Armstrong GL, Alter MJ, McQuillan GM, Margolis HS. (2000) The past incidence of hepatitis C virus infection: implications for the future burden of chronic liver disease in the United States. *Hepatology* 31(3): 777–82.

Bressac B, Kew M, Wands J, Ozturk M. (1991) Selective G to T mutations of p53 gene in hepatocellular carcinoma from southern Africa. *Nature* 350(6317): 429–31.

Bruno S, Battezzati PM, Bellati G *et al.* (2001) Long-term beneficial effects in sustained responders to interferon-alfa therapy for chronic hepatitis C. *J Hepatol* 34(5): 748–55.

Burton PR, Tobin MD, Hopper JL. (2005) Key concepts in genetic epidemiology. *Lancet* 366(9489): 941–51.

Calle EE, Rodriguez C, Walker-Thurmond, K *et al.* (2003) Overweight, obesity, and mortality from cancer in a prospectively studied cohort of US adults. *N Engl J Med* 348(17): 1625–38.

Camma C, Giunta M, Andreone P, Craxi A. (2001) Interferon and prevention of hepatocellular carcinoma in viral cirrhosis: an evidence-based approach. *J Hepatol* 34(4): 593–602.

Chang MH, Chen CJ, Lai MS *et al.* (1997) Universal hepatitis B vaccination in Taiwan and the incidence of hepatocellular carcinoma in children. Taiwan Childhood Hepatoma Study Group. *N Engl J Med* 336(26): 1855–9.

Cordell HJ, Clayton DG. (2005) Genetic association studies. *Lancet* 366(9491): 1121–31.

Cramp ME. (1999) HBV + HCV = HCC? *Gut* 45(2): 168–9.

Davey SG, Ebrahim S, Lewis S, Hansell AL, Palmer LJ, Burton PR. (2005) Genetic epidemiology and public health: hope, hype, and future prospects. *Lancet* 366(9495): 1484–98.

Davila JA, Morgan RO, Shaib Y, McGlynn KA, El-Serag HB. (2004) Hepatitis C infection and the increasing incidence of hepatocellular carcinoma: a population-based study. *Gastroenterology* 127(5): 1372–80.

Dawn TM, Barrett JH. (2005) Genetic linkage studies. *Lancet* 366(9490): 1036–44.

Donato F, Tagger A, Gelatti U *et al.* (2002) Alcohol and hepatocellular carcinoma: the effect of lifetime intake and hepatitis virus infections in men and women. *Am J Epidemiol* 155(4): 323–31.

El Serag HB, Mason AC. (2000) Risk factors for the rising rates of primary liver cancer in the United States. *Arch Intern Med* 160(21): 3227–30.

El-Serag HB, Davila JA, Petersen NJ, McGlynn KA. (2003) The continuing increase in the incidence of hepatocellular carcinoma in the United States: an update. *Ann Intern Med* 139(10): 817–23.

El-Serag HB. (2004) Hepatocellular carcinoma: recent trends in the United States. *Gastroenterology* 127(5 Suppl 1): S27–S34.

El Serag HB, Tran T, Everhart JE. (2004) Diabetes increases the risk of chronic liver disease and hepatocellular carcinoma. *Gastroenterology* 126(2): 460–8.

El-Serag HB, Hampel H, Javadi F. (2006) The association between diabetes and hepatocellular carcinoma: a systematic review of epidemiologic evidence. *Clin Gastroenterol Hepatol* 4(3): 369–80.

Evans AA, Chen G, Ross EA, Shen FM, Lin WY, London WT. (2002) Eight-year follow-up of the 90,000-person Haimen City cohort: I. Hepatocellular carcinoma mortality, risk factors, and gender differences. *Cancer Epidemiol Biomarkers Prev* 11(4): 369–76.

Fasani P, Sangiovanni A, De Fazio C *et al.* (1999) High prevalence of multinodular hepatocellular carcinoma in patients with cirrhosis attributable to multiple risk factors. *Hepatology* 29(6): 1704–7.

Ferlay J,Bray F, Pisani P *et al.* (2001) *GLOBOCAN 2000 Cancer Incidence, Mortality and Prevalence Worldwide*, Version 1.0. IARC CancerBase No. 5. IARC Press, Lyon.

Freeman AJ, Dore GJ, Law MG *et al.* (2001) Estimating progression to cirrhosis in chronic hepatitis C virus infection. *Hepatology* 34(4 Pt 1): 809–16.

Garner RC, Miller EC, Miller JA. (1972) Liver microsomal metabolism of aflatoxin B 1 to a reactive derivative toxic to *Salmonella typhimurium* TA 1530. *Cancer Res* 32(10): 2058–66.

Gelatti U, Covolo L, Talamini R *et al.* (2005) N-Acetyltransferase-2, glutathione S-transferase M1 and T1 genetic polymorphisms, cigarette smoking and hepatocellular carcinoma: a case–control study. *Int J Cancer* 115(2): 301–6.

Hassan MM, Frome A, Patt YZ, El Serag HB. (2002) Rising prevalence of hepatitis C virus infection among patients recently diagnosed with hepatocellular carcinoma in the United States. *J Clin Gastroenterol* 35(3): 266–9.

Hattersley AT, McCarthy MI. (2005) What makes a good genetic association study? *Lancet* 366(9493): 1315–23.

Hopper JL, Bishop DT, Easton DF. (2005) Population-based family studies in genetic epidemiology. *Lancet* 366(9494): 1397–1406.

IARC Monographs. (1987) *Overall evaluations of carcinogenicity: An updating of IARC monographs volumes 1–42*, Suppl 7, 83–7. IARC Press, Lyon.

Ikeda K, Saitoh S, Arase Y *et al.* (1999) Effect of interferon therapy on hepatocellular carcinogenesis in patients with chronic hepatitis type C: A long-term observation study of 1,643 patients using statistical bias correction with proportional hazard analysis. *Hepatology* 29(4): 1124–30.

Imai Y, Kawata S, Tamura S *et al.* (1998) Relation of interferon therapy and hepatocellular carcinoma in patients with chronic hepatitis C. Osaka Hepatocellular Carcinoma Prevention Study Group. *Ann Intern Med* 129(2): 94–9.

International Interferon-alpha Hepatocellular Carcinoma Study Group. (1998) Effect of interferon-alpha on progression of cirrhosis to hepatocellular carcinoma: a retrospective cohort study. *Lancet* 351(9115): 1535–9.

Kao JH, Chen PJ, Lai MY, Chen DS. (2002) Genotypes and clinical phenotypes of hepatitis B virus in patients with chronic hepatitis B virus infection. *J Clin Microbiol* 40(4): 1207–9.

Kato S, Tajiri T, Matsukura N *et al.* (2003) Genetic polymorphisms of aldehyde dehydrogenase 2, cytochrome p450 2E1 for liver cancer risk in HCV antibody-positive japanese patients and the variations of CYP2E1 mRNA expression levels in the liver due to its polymorphism. *Scand J Gastroenterol* 38(8): 886–93.

Khoury MJ, Little, J. (2000) Human genome epidemiologic reviews: the beginning of something HuGE. *Am J Epidemiol* 151(1): 2–3.

Kulkarni K, Barcak E, El-Serag H, Goodgame, R. (2004) The impact of immigration on the increasing incidence of hepatocellular carcinoma in the United States. *Aliment Pharmacol Ther* 20(4): 445–50.

Little J, Khoury MJ, Bradley L *et al.* (2003) The human genome project is complete. How do we develop a handle for the pump? *Am J Epidemiol* 157(8): 667–73.

Long XD, Ma Y, Wei YP, Deng ZL. (2006) The polymorphisms of GSTM1, GSTT1, HYL1*2, and XRCC1, and aflatoxin B1-related hepatocellular carcinoma in Guangxi population, China. *Hepatol Res* 36(1): 48–55.

Maheshwari S, Sarraj A, Kramer J, El-Serag HB. (2007) Oral contraception and the risk of hepatocellular carcinoma. *J Hepatol* 47(4): 506–13.

McGlynn KA, Tsao L, Hsing AW, Devesa SS, Fraumeni JF Jr. (2001) International trends and patterns of primary liver cancer. *Int J Cancer* 94(2): 290–6.

McMahon BJ, Alberts SR, Wainwright RB, Bulkow L, Lanier AP. (1990) Hepatitis B-related sequelae. Prospective study in 1400 hepatitis B surface antigen-positive Alaska native carriers. *Arch Intern Med* 150(5): 1051–4.

Niederau C, Lange S, Heintges T *et al.* (1998) Prognosis of chronic hepatitis C: results of a large, prospective cohort study. *Hepatology* 28(6): 1687–95.

Nishiguchi S, Kuroki T, Nakatani S *et al.* (1995) Randomised trial of effects of interferon-alpha on incidence of hepatocellular carcinoma in chronic active hepatitis C with cirrhosis. *Lancet* 346(8982): 1051–5.

Okanoue T, Itoh Y, Minami M *et al.* (1999) Interferon therapy lowers the rate of progression to hepatocellular carcinoma in chronic hepatitis C but not significantly in an advanced stage: a retrospective study in 1148 patients. Viral Hepatitis Therapy Study Group. *J Hepatol* 30(4): 653–9.

Okuda K, Nakanuma Y, Miyazaki M. (2002) Cholangiocarcinoma: recent progress. Part 1: epidemiology and etiology. *J Gastroenterol Hepatol* 17(10): 1049–55.

Parkin DM. (2001) Global cancer statistics in the year 2000. *Lancet Oncol* 2(9): 533–43.

Parkin DM, Whelan SL, Ferlay J, Teppo L, Thomas DB. (2002) *Cancer Incidence in Five Continents*, vol. VIII. IARC Scientific Publications no. 155. IARC Press, Lyon.

Qian GS, Ross RK, Yu MC *et al.* (1994) A follow-up study of urinary markers of aflatoxin exposure and liver cancer risk in Shanghai, People's Republic of China. *Cancer Epidemiol Biomarkers Prev* 3(1): 3–10.

Sakamoto T, Hara M, Higaki Y *et al.* (2006) Influence of alcohol consumption and gene polymorphisms of ADH2 and ALDH2 on hepatocellular carcinoma in a Japanese population. *Int J Cancer* 18(6): 1501–7.

Serfaty L, Aumaitre H, Chazouilleres O *et al.* (1998) Determinants of outcome of compensated hepatitis C virus-related cirrhosis. *Hepatology* 27(5): 1435–40.

Stroffolini T, Andreone P, Andriulli A *et al.* (1999) Gross pathologic types of hepatocellular carcinoma in Italy. *Oncology* 56(3): 189–92.

Sun CA, Wang LY, Chen CJ *et al.* (2001) Genetic polymorphisms of glutathione S-transferases M1 and T1 associated with susceptibility to aflatoxin-related hepatocarcinogenesis among chronic hepatitis B carriers: a nested case–control study in Taiwan. *Carcinogenesis* 22(8): 1289–94.

Tanaka K, Hirohata T, Fukuda K, Shibata A, Tsukuma H, Hiyama T. (1995) Risk factors for hepatocellular carcinoma among Japanese women. *Cancer Causes Control* 6(2): 91–8.

Torbenson M, Thomas DL. (2002) Occult hepatitis B. *Lancet Infect Dis* 2(8): 479–86.

Turner PC, Sylla A, Diallo MS, Castegnaro JJ, Hall AJ, Wild CP. (2002) The role of aflatoxins and hepatitis viruses in the etiopathogenesis of hepatocellular carcinoma: A basis for primary prevention in Guinea-Conakry, West Africa. *J Gastroenterol Hepatol* 17 (Suppl): S441–S448.

Valla DC, Chevallier M, Marcellin P *et al.* (1999) Treatment of hepatitis C virus-related cirrhosis: a randomized, controlled trial of interferon alfa-2b versus no treatment. *Hepatology* 29(6): 1870–5.

White DL, Li D, Nurgelieva Z, El-Serag HB. Genetic variants of glutathione S-transferase as possible rick factors for heptatocellular carcinoma. A HuGE systematic review and meta-analysis. *Am J Epidemiol* in press.

Wideroff L, Gridley G, Mellemkjaer L *et al.* (1997) Cancer incidence in a population-based cohort of patients hospitalized with diabetes mellitus in Denmark. *J Natl Cancer Inst* 89(18): 1360–5.

Wong NA, Rae F, Simpson KJ, Murray GD, Harrison DJ. (2000) Genetic polymorphisms of cytochrome p4502E1 and susceptibility to alcoholic liver disease and hepatocellular carcinoma in a white population: a study and literature review, including meta-analysis. *Mol Pathol* 53(2): 88–93.

Yoshizawa H. (2002) Hepatocellular carcinoma associated with hepatitis C virus infection in Japan: projection to other countries in the foreseeable future. *Oncology* 62 (Suppl 1): 8–17.

Yu MW, Gladek-Yarborough A, Chiamprasert S, Santella RM, Liaw YF, Chen CJ. (1995) Cytochrome P450 2E1 and glutathione S-transferase M1 polymorphisms and susceptibility to hepatocellular carcinoma. *Gastroenterology* 109(4): 1266–73.

Yu MW, Chiu YH, Yang SY *et al.* (1999) Cytochrome P450 1A1 genetic polymorphisms and risk of hepatocellular carcinoma among chronic hepatitis B carriers. *Br J Cancer* 80(3–4): 598–603.

Yu MW, Pai CI, Yang SY, *et al.* (2000) Role of N-acetyltransferase polymorphisms in hepatitis B related hepatocellular carcinoma: impact of smoking on risk. *Gut* 47(5): 703–9.

Yu S. (1995) Primary prevention of hepatocellular carcinoma. *J Gastoenterol Hepatol* 10(6): 674–82.

17 Factors Involved in Carcinogenesis and Prevention in Hepatobiliary Cancer

Paula Ghaneh, William Greenhalf & John P. Neoptolemos

Introduction

The importance of hepatobiliary cancers as a healthcare problem is undeniable. In 2002 there were 626,162 recorded cases of primary liver cancer worldwide and 232,306 pancreatic cancers (http://www-dep.iarc.fr). Estimated incidence figures for the USA for 2007 are: 19,160 for liver and intrahepatic bile duct cancer; 9250 for gallbladder and extrahepatic biliary cancer; and 37,170 for pancreatic cancer (Jemal *et al.* 2007). The etiology and causation vary between each cancer type; in this review we will compare carcinogenesis as it is related to hepatocellular carcinoma, pancreatic ductal adenocarcinoma, cholangiocarcinoma and carcinoma of the gallbladder. Contrasting these different diseases reveals aspects of carcinogenesis that would not be apparent if each form of carcinoma was considered in isolation.

Progression models

In most forms of carcinoma morphologic changes have been identified which are assumed to be intermediate steps in the progression from epithelial cells to invasive carcinoma. The classic example is the polyp, adenoma, carcinoma series in colorectal cancer (Vogelstein *et al.* 1988). These morphologic changes are associated with mutated genes and changes in expression levels. This is clearly a massive oversimplification, but these are working models that function in most forms of carcinoma. In the case of pancreatic ductal adenocarcinoma, pancreatic intraepithelial neoplasia-1 (PanIN) lesions are the most widely accepted precancerous morphologic stages (Maitra *et al.* 2003). PanIN1 are simply elongated mucin-producing cells with little atypia, and these lesions are associated with mutations in the proto-oncogene K-ras (Biankin *et al.* 2003); PanIN-2 exhibit distinct cellular atypia including increased nuclear size and loss of cellular polarity; these are associated with loss of the tumor suppressor p16 (Wilentz *et al.* 1998). PanIN-3 lesions have severe atypia with budding off of cells into the lumen, these are associated with p53 mutations (Biankin *et al.* 2003). In cholangiocarcinomas the equivalent are biliary intraepithelial neoplasias (BilIN1–3) (Zen *et al.* 2005). Again each stage is associated with its own particular profile of mutations. In the gallbladder the morphologic stages are less well established, but a progression from metaplasia to dysplasia and finally carcinoma is assumed with concurrent accumulation of molecular changes (Roa *et al.* 2006). The progression model in hepatocellular carcinoma is the most difficult to establish, but even here it is possible to identify potential premalignant precursor lesions (dysplastic nodules) (Kern *et al.* 2002) and to deduce a progression using comparative genomic hybridization of tumor samples to work backwards through an evolutionary tree to early molecular changes (Poon *et al.* 2006).

Carcinogenesis involves mitogen-independent initiation of cell division, overcoming checkpoint control, suppression of apoptosis and gaining immortality (usually via the expression of telomerase) (Hahn *et al.* 1999, 2002). The order of these changes will determine the morphologic changes seen in precancerous lesions. The simplicity of the morphologic progression models suggests a fixed progression of molecular change; although, as will be discussed, this is a gross oversimplification. Conventionally molecular progression models have been proposed whereby an oncogene is initially mutated allowing cell division, with subsequent loss of tumor suppressors that would control cell growth and loss of chromosomal integrity as the surveillance systems are corrupted, before telomerase is switched on to allow immortality and genes are mutated which allow invasion. Mouse models of hepatobiliary and pancreatic cancers seem to support this as expression of mutant Ras oncogene will result in precancerous lesions in the pancreas (Tuveson *et al.* 2004) and liver (Tuveson *et al.* 2006) and overexpression of the tyrosine kinase receptor ERB-B2 results in cholangiocarcinomas (Kiguchi *et al.* 2001). However, syndromes with inherited predisposition for cancer usually involve germline mutations of tumor suppressor genes or genes involved in maintaining genome stability. It is difficult to prove whether loss of tumor

Gastrointestinal Oncology: A Critical Multidisciplinary Team Approach.
Edited by J. Jankowski, R. Sampliner, D. Kerr, and Y. Fong.

suppressor activity is the first (initiating) event in tumorigenesis, but this does appear likely. Again the example of colorectal cancer is revealing; tumors arising as a result of mutations in mismatch repair genes occur in the absence of multiple polyps (as seen in human non-polyposis colon cancer, HNPCC). The possibility therefore exists that particular progression models are applicable only to tumors that arise after specific classes of initiation event. Surveillance programs for all forms of hepatobiliary and pancreatic cancers are increasingly relying on assumptions based upon progression models, thus, given the previous assumption, are dependent on the nature of the initiating event.

Definitions

In this review the definition of the initiating event will be considered to be separate from the effector of tumorigenesis. The effector of the genetic change that underlies the process of tumorigenesis may be chemical (exposure to mutagens), physical (exposure to radiation), biologic (viral, bacterial or protozoal infection), inherited (a germline mutation passed on from a parent) or indirect (a consequence of another pathology such as inflammation). The initiating event will be a genetic or epigenetic change that defines the cell that will ultimately lead that cell's progeny to become a tumor cell.

The initiating event

The initiating event will vary according to the effector; if a proto-oncogene is mutated the initiating event may be the expression of the mutant protein allowing inappropriate cell division. If a tumor suppressor is mutated then the initiating event may be the loss of a wild-type allele resulting in loss of checkpoint control. Alternatively, even if a mutation in a tumor suppressor is inherited, but the wild-type allele is functional at the time of a mutation of an oncogene, the initiating event is the expression of the mutated oncogene; the germline mutation may well influence tumorigenesis (the cancer would possibly not develop without the subsequent loss of the wild-type allele) but by our definition the germline mutation did not occur at the initiation of tumorigenesis. In Fig. 17.1 three different models are given for development of a carcinoma, differing according to the initiating event. The effectors are given as a thick red arrow; the nature of possible effectors and how they influence the initiating event is discussed below.

Effectors of tumorigenesis

Chemical

Chemical mutagens are the most obvious causes of genetic changes; these may contribute to a progression of mutations and may be the effector of the initiating event. Epidemiologic studies indicate a range of compounds that are associated with hepatobiliary and pancreatic cancers. This implies that these compounds are linked to a limiting step or steps in tumorigenesis; this is likely to include the initiating step. Some chemical entities are directly mitogenic, making an initiating event more likely as a result of mutation during DNA replication; mitogenic compounds are rare, but include anabolic steroids and hormonal components of the contraceptive pill. Oral contraceptives and anabolic steroids are well-established risk factors for hepatocellular carcinoma (Giannitrapani *et al.* 2006); use of anabolic steroids in patients with Fanconi's anemia (discussed later) arguably results in the highest risk of hepatocellular carcinoma (Velazquez & Alter 2004). Sex hormone receptors have been identified in hepatocellular carcinomas, cholangiocarcinomas and pancreatic carcinomas, although epidemiologic evidence for a link between use of hormones and pancreatic cancer has not been convincingly presented. This may reflect a less significant role for sex hormones in the normal physiology of the pancreas; sex hormones may have a significant role in progression, but perhaps not in the initiating event. It is noteworthy that estrogen receptors have been reported in cholangiocytes during biliary cirrhosis and this could provide a sex hormone link between cirrhosis and cholangiocarcinoma (Alvaro *et al.* 2004).

Most chemical effectors of carcinogenesis have clear mechanistic associations with mutation. The question arises as to how particular cells are exposed to these mutagens and what kind of mutations will result. The pattern of tumors caused by different mutagens varies greatly, which may reflect fundamental differences in the process of carcinogenesis in different forms of hepatobiliary cancers. Aflatoxin is produced by species of Aspergillus fungus and is metabolized to toxic compounds which form adducts with DNA. The best-characterized form of aflatoxin is B_1 and the main toxic metabolite is an epoxide derivative produced using cytochrome P450. This forms unstable adducts with guanine residues which breakdown to give apurinic sites in the DNA strand (Smela *et al.* 2001). Aflatoxin is a major risk factor for hepatocellular carcinoma (Jee *et al.* 2004), but although in a model system it has been shown to be toxic to the pancreas, it does not appear to cause pancreatic cancer (Gordis & Gold 1984). The reason for this is likely to be that P450 levels are higher in the liver and so the liver will be more exposed to the carcinogenic aflatoxin metabolites.

Ethanol has been linked to pancreatic cancer (Ekbom & Hunter 2002), cholangiocarcinoma (Shaib *et al.* 2007), and gallbladder cancer (Ji *et al.* 2005). However, the evidence base for the link is open to criticism due to the fact that heavy alcohol users also tend to be heavy smokers and generally to have high-risk lifestyles. The link may also be indirect, for example via inflammatory diseases such as pancreatitis (discussed later). The link between ethanol abuse and hepatocellular carcinoma is much stronger. An annual incidence for hepatocellular carcinoma of over 1% in patients with alcoholic cirrhosis cannot be explained by confounding factors. The mechanism of alcohol-related carcinogenesis is not fully understood, but is

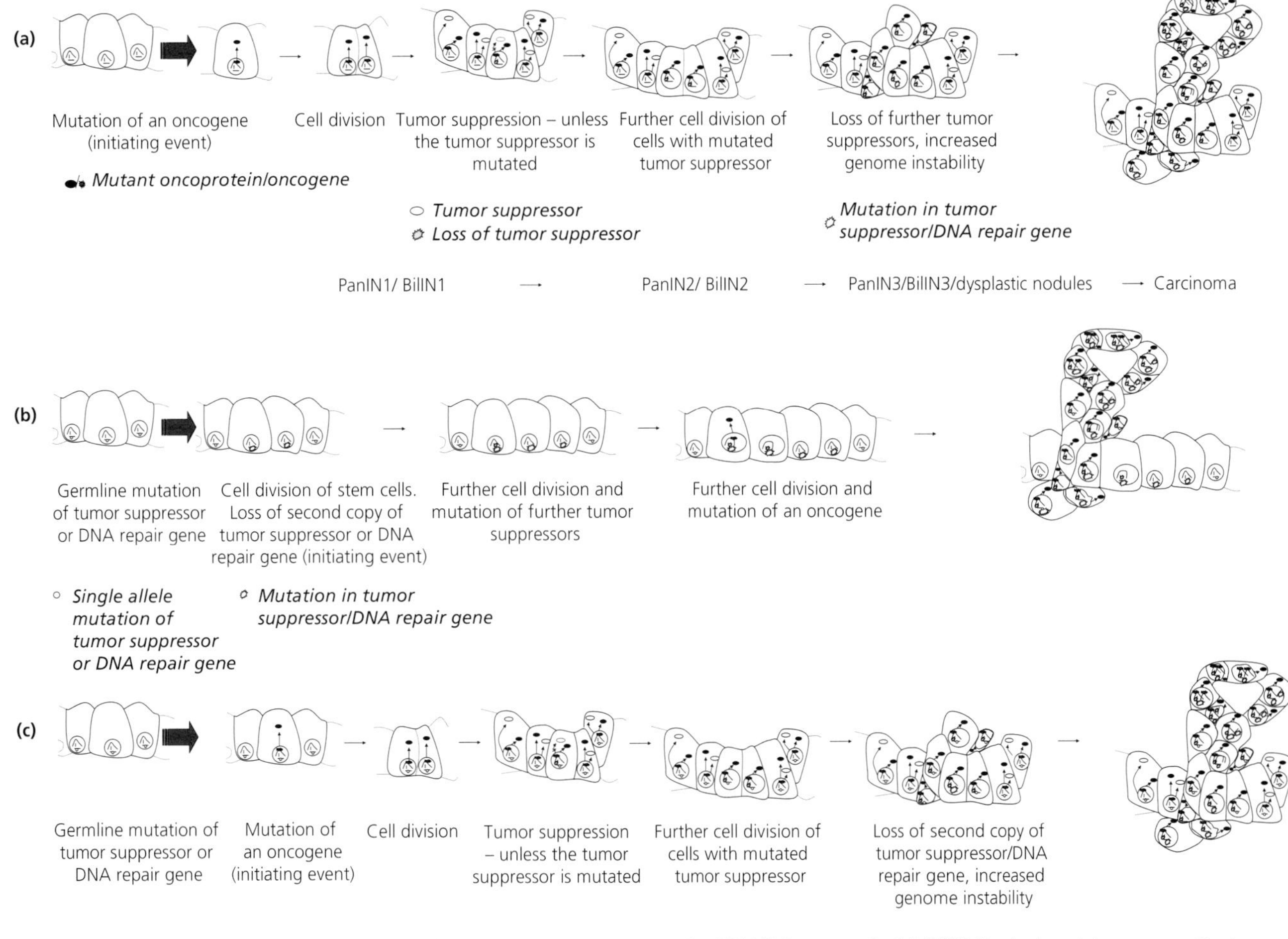

Fig. 17.1 Alternative mechanisms for tumorigenesis. In A the effector of tumorigenesis (large red arrow) causes a mutation in an oncogene and therefore cell division. This causes hyperplasia and lesions that would be consistent with PanIN1 or BilIN1. This would normally lead to senescence or apoptosis, but if a tumor suppressor is subsequently mutated the senescence or apoptotic program is overcome and cell division occurs with further mutation and consequently more advanced lesions (PanIN2/ BilIN2). If the subsequent mutations impair DNA repair the increase in genetic instability will become more rapid; more advanced lesions (PanIN3/BilIN3 or dysplastic nodules) will eventually result in a carcinoma. In B there is a germline mutation in a single allele of a tumor suppressor or DNA repair gene. The effector causes loss of the second allele; this may provoke further mutation or allow the cell to tolerate further genetic instability, giving rise to loss of tumor suppressors and eventually mutation of oncogenes; which will provoke high-grade lesions (PanIN3/ BilIN3/dysplastic nodules) and eventually carcinoma. C is equivalent to A except that it occurs in the background of a germline mutation of a single allele of a tumor suppressor. As a consequence, later loss of this tumor suppressor or DNA repair gene, with consequent progression from precancerous lesions to carcinoma, is more likely.

probably a combination of multiple factors. Alcohol induces hyperplasia and inflammation in the liver which increases the chance of mutation. There is also an increase in oxidative stress due to metabolism of ethanol in the liver combined with impaired antioxidant pathways. Acetaldehyde produced by metabolism of ethanol also directly binds to DNA producing adducts and inhibiting DNA repair systems. Ethanol also affects the expression of numerous genes by diverse mechanisms (directly acting on transcription factors and by interfering with methyl transferases), the consequences of these changes in expression could contribute to carcinogenesis. (Castaneda *et al.* 2006). Finally ethanol effects iron storage (Petersen 2005).

Accumulation of iron in the liver increases oxidative stress; hydroxyl radical formation as a result of iron accumulation causes both DNA base modifications and DNA protein crosslinks. Iron toxicity is normally moderated by binding proteins such as transferrin and the modified bases would normally be repaired by base excision repair, but in conditions which cause an overaccumulation of iron (such as in hereditary hemochromatosis) DNA damage may exceed the body's repair capacity and cell death or cancer may result. As the liver is the main site of iron storage it is not surprising that hepatocellular carcinoma is the main form of cancer associated with this overload. Although iron will also build up in the pancreas, often leading to diabetes mellitus, hemochromatosis is not significantly associated with pancreatic or gallbladder cancer and association with cholangiocarcinoma is at most weak (Kowdley 2004).

Exposure to inorganic arsenic is fortunately rare, but has also been shown to associate with hepatocellular carcinoma, at least in women (Chiu *et al.* 2004). Again the link with cancer is probably via an increase in oxidative stress, and as for iron the specificity for hepatocellular carcinoma probably reflects the pattern of accumulation of the metal.

Tobacco has been linked to all forms of hepatobiliary and pancreatic cancer, but the degree and type of risk varies greatly. The greatest increase in risk is associated with pancreatic cancer, where there is a linear increase in risk of cancer with increased smoking (Lin *et al.* 2002), and some estimates suggest that smoking accounts for nearly one-third of pancreatic cancers (Silverman *et al.* 1994). For gallbladder cancer the increased risk is less certain and probably more marginal (Scott *et al.* 1999). For cholangiocarcinoma and hepatocellular carcinoma the link between smoking and cancer is difficult to establish and even where studies have shown an elevated risk for hepatocellular carcinoma in smokers, the risk is marginal; for example in the large study by Jee *et al.* the relative risk was between 1.3 and 1.6 for men and was not significant for women (Jee *et al.* 2004). What risk there is probably involves increasing the risk of cancer associated with another factor, such as risk of liver cancer-associated hepatitis (Franceschi *et al.* 2006) or cholangiocarcinoma associated with liver fluke infestation (Mitacek *et al.* 1999). This variation in risk suggests either that the different cells have different sensitivities to the carcinogens in tobacco or that exposure is different.

Tobacco smoke contains at least 60 known carcinogens. For simplicity these can be divided into polycyclic aromatic hydrocarbons (PAHs), nitrosamines, aromatic amines and trace metals (Hoffmann & Hoffmann 1997). Naturally most research on the sensitivity of model systems to these agents has focussed on the lung, given that this is the organ most susceptible to tobacco-related cancer; however, it appears that in mouse and other rodent models the liver and biliary tract are exquisitely sensitive to these agents (particularly PAHs) (Von Tungeln *et al.* 1999a,b; Mitacek *et al.* 1999), not surprising considering that PAHs and N-nitrosamines are converted to DNA-damaging agents by components of the P450 system (Guengerich 2000) which is most active in the liver. However, this does not exclude greater resistance to these agents in human liver (compared to human pancreas) as the pattern of expression of DNA repair pathways in humans are significantly different from those in rodents (Hanawalt 2001).

It is also possible that despite processing of PAHs and other tobacco carcinogens in the liver, exposure of the active metabolites is higher in the human pancreas. Exposure is clearly a major factor in explaining why lung cancer is a much greater risk for smokers than liver cancer. Tobacco-related carcinogens do reach the pancreas in humans and do cause damage to DNA (Wang *et al.* 1998; Hecht 1999). However, it is difficult to see why carcinogens taken in through the lungs and processed in the liver should have a greater impact on the pancreas than the liver. In evolutionary terms humans have been smoking for an extremely short time (smoking has only been a significant habit for the last 200 years). However, many of the carcinogens associated with tobacco are also present in cooked foods (albeit at much lower levels) and exposure to these agents through cooked food has a much longer history (greater than 700,000 years: Goren-Inbar *et al.* 2004). It is therefore possible that humans have evolved resistance to these carcinogens, the greatest selective pressure for resistance being in the organs most exposed and thus most likely to suffer carcinogenesis before the reproductive age limit has passed.

Physical

Exposure to ultraviolet light and ionizing radiation are direct causes of mutation and hence carcinogenesis. Due to obvious anatomic reasons hepatobiliary tumors rarely if ever result from exposure to UV; however, the liver is exposed to various ingested radioactive isotopes. The most notorious exposure to such isotopes was the use of Thorotrast as a contrast agent between 1930 and 1960. The radioactive thorium dioxide in Thorotrast concentrates in the liver and emits alpha particles with a half-life of over 20 years. Risk of hepatocellular carcinoma in patients exposed to Thorotrast is 100-fold that in the general population. The risk of other hepatobiliary tumors is significantly lower, consistent with the lower level of exposure (Nyberg *et al.* 2002).

Indirect

Inflammatory diseases

Tumorigenesis can be initiated by mutations occurring during cell division or because of an epigenetic event leading to silencing of a tumor suppressor. Although these are chance events, the likelihood of this occurring may be greatly increased by pathologic conditions, the most obvious being inflammatory diseases (Moss & Blaser 2005). Pancreatitis is associated with pancreatic cancer (Lowenfels *et al.* 1993), particularly the inherited form of pancreatitis (Howes *et al.* 2004); chronic hepatitis is associated with hepatocellular carcinoma (Seitz & Stickel 2006); sclerosing cholangitis is associated with cholangiocarcinoma (Lazaridis & Gores 2006). The links between inflammation and cancer are complex, involving induction of hyperplasia, increased oxidative stress and changes in methyl transferases (Moss & Blaser 2005). Sclerosis or fibrosis resulting from the inflammation is associated with the cancer risk and nearly 90% of hepatocellular carcinomas develop in a background of cirrhosis (Seitz & Stickel 2006).

Diabetes

Diabetes mellitus as a result of hemochromatosis is indirectly linked to hepatocellular carcinoma as discussed above. Pancreatic cancer can cause insulin resistance, as in type 2 diabetes, which is sometimes ameliorated by surgery to remove the tumor (Permert *et al.* 1993; Basso *et al.* 2006). There are also many reports of type 2 diabetes mellitus preceding pancreatic cancer (Silverman *et al.* 1999; Wang *et al.* 2003; Chari *et al.* 2005; Huxley *et al.* 2005). It is unclear in these cases whether diabetes represents an early symptom of pancreatic cancer or whether the onset of diabetes predisposes to tumor development. It is harder to establish a link between type 1 diabetes and pancreatic cancer due to the early onset of diabetes, which meant in the past that few type 1 diabetics reached the age of significant risk of pancreatic cancer. Some reports suggest that type 1 diabetes gives a reduced risk of pancreatic cancer (Zendehdel *et al.* 2003). However, a systematic review of the data does indicate an elevated risk, even in type 1 disease (Stevens *et al.* 2007). Diabetes mellitus is not normally associated with cholangiocarcinomas (Costa *et al.* 2004) but a link with hepatocellular carcinoma is well documented. As for pancreatic cancer it is not clear if this link is direct or is the result of a comorbidity (El-Serag *et al.* 2006).

Biologic

Viral

Over 80% of hepatocellular carcinoma is attributable to infection with hepatitis B (HBV) or hepatitis C (HCV) virus (Bosch *et al.* 1999). The link between hepatitis and hepatocellular carcinoma was discussed previously; however, hepatocellular carcinoma also develops in non-cirrhotic HCV-infected livers (De Mitri *et al.* 1995). HBV-associated hepatocellular carcinomas normally have integrated copies of the virus and this insertion may contribute directly to carcinogenesis by activating oncogenes or inativating tumor suppressors (Paterlini-Brechot *et al.* 2003). In most cases the HBV-X transactivator gene is intact in the integrated virus. HBV-X represses the expression of the p53 tumor suppressor (Lee & Rho 2000) and binds to the DDB1 (XAP-1) protein, significantly reducing the efficiency of nucleotide excision repair (Becker *et al.* 1998). The HCV core protein is a structural homolog of the HBV-X protein (Koike *et al.* 2002); the core protein inhibits DNA repair (van Pelt *et al.* 2004) as well as having a well-characterized role in inhibiting promyelocytic leukemia protein (Herzer *et al.* 2005). The HCV non-structural protein 5A (NS5A) also has multiple oncogenic functions, inhibiting p53-mediated apoptosis and p53 interaction with XPB (ERCC3), a gene essential for nucleotide excision repair (Qadri *et al.* 2002).

Protozoa

Liver flukes, particularly *Opisthorchis viverrini*, seem to specifically sensitize sufferers to cholangiocarcinoma, to such an extent that the normal ratio of hepatocellular carcinoma to cholangiocarcinoma (8:1) is reversed (1:8) (Watanapa & Watanapa 2002). The molecular pathogenesis of cholangiocarcinoma in the presence of the fluke also seems to differ from the normal progression model, in that K-ras mutations are common in the sporadic disease but very rare in the disease associated with flukes. The mechanism of carcinogenesis is not yet known but probably stems from irritation of the biliary tract causing inflammation and hyperplasia. This can lead to increased susceptibility to carcinogenesis as described previously. Inflammatory cells produce nitric oxide which reacts with compounds such as thioproline to produce carcinogens (Watanapa & Watanapa 2002). Flukes also cause activation of P450, either directly or via the inflammatory response, which increases activation of other carcinogens (as described previously) further increasing cancer risk (Watanapa & Watanapa 2002).

DNA repair and carcinogenesis in hepatobiliary cancers

In the absence of mutagens the most common form of potentially cancer-causing mutations is replicative errors; these are normally repaired by replacing the newly synthesized base (mismatch repair). However, in the presence of mutagens the most likely cancer-causing mutations will be by base modification or strand breakage. The carcinogens produced by tobacco cause a range of different DNA damage requiring a range of different repair mechanisms. Direct reversal of the damage is sometimes possible, in particular reversal of alkylation of bases. If this is not possible repair of the lesion can be mediated by base excision or nucleotide excision. Carcinogens may also (directly or indirectly) lead to single or double strand breaks, requiring recombination repair. Differences of the relative sensitivity to tobacco of the liver and pancreas between humans and other animals could reflect different patterns of repair enzymes. Some support for this comes from consideration of the distribution of enzymes used to reverse O6 alkylation of guanine. The enzyme O6-alkylguanine-DNA alkyltransferase (MGMT) repairs this lesion; liver has the highest content of this protein among all tissues in both rats and humans, but human liver has 10-fold more activity than its rodent counterpart (Pegg *et al.* 1982). Furthermore, transgenic mice overexpressing MGMT have a reduced rate of hepatocellular carcinoma (Zhou *et al.* 2001).

If base modification cannot, or is not, reversed then excision repair can still prevent coding changes, although with an increasing level of potential error. In base exision repair (BER) modified bases can be recognized by lesion-specific DNA glycosylases, possibly with the assistance of the XRCC1 protein (Campalans *et al.* 2005). The modified base is then cleaved from the sequence, apurinic or apyrimidinic endonuclease cuts the damaged strand, and then DNA polymerase β removes the deoxyribose phosphate and adds a new base to the free hydroxyl group. The resulting nick is then ligated by a complex of DNA ligase 3 and XRCC1 (Sobol & Wilson 2001). Polymorphisms of XRCC1 which are associated with lower levels of BER are associated with higher incidence of hepatocellular carcinoma, particularly in combination with exposure to aflatoxin (Kirk *et al.* 2005). Although the same polymorphisms do not seem to increase risk of pancreatic cancer in isolation, they do increase risk if associated with particular polymorphisms of MGMT (Jiao *et al.* 2006).

Alternatively, nucleotide excision repair (NER) may be used: Bases with bulky adducts cause distortion of the DNA and this is recognized either by a complex of DDB1, DDB2 and XPC proteins or by RNA polymerase II in combination with the DDB1 protein. In either case TFIIH, XPB (ERCC3) and XPD are then recruited and cause strand separation at the site of the lesion; XPA then recruits replication protein A which stabilizes the single strands. XPG and ERCC1/XPF endonucleases then incise the lesion (de Laat *et al.* 1999; Fousteri *et al.* 2006), and the gap is then repaired by DNA polymerase δ/ε. Mice deficient in XPA have a greater incidence of spontaneous liver cancers and liver cancer induced by aflatoxin (Takahashi *et al.* 2002).

When considering the carcinogenic properties of a compound under given circumstances it is not enough to consider the activity in causing a DNA change. If DNA damage is fatal to the cell it will obviously not result in cancer. Therefore mammalian cells may acquire resistance to killing and to gross chromosomal damage, but not to mutagenesis and propensity to cause cancer. An example of this is methylation tolerance; this results from reduced mismatch repair (Claij & Te Riele 2002). Mismatch repair (MMR) can be induced by base modifications such as alkylation, but as this only repairs the newly synthesized strand the lesion in the original strand is always left behind. Repeated excision of the newly synthesized base will eventually lead to more strand breakage and cellular death. If mismatch repair is compromised, as is seen in families with hereditary non-polyposis colon cancer (HNPCC), the cell will be less likely to die and more likely to undergo tumorigenesis. Germline mutations of mismatch repair genes (such as MLH1 and MSH2) result in greatly elevated risk of pancreatic cancer (Lynch *et al.* 2004) and cholangiocarcinoma (Vernez *et al.* 2006) but do not appear to greatly increase the risk of hepatocellular carcinoma (Chiappini *et al.* 2004). Defects in MMR (HNPCC related or otherwise) will typically give a high level of microsatellite instability (MSI); it is telling that MSI is rare in pancreatic cancer (Yamamoto *et al.* 2001), but where MSI is at high levels K-ras mutations (which are otherwise ubiquitous) are rare, suggesting an alternative pathway of molecular pathogenesis. MSI is also low in hepatocellular and other forms of hepatobilliary carcinoma, but the rare incidences of high MSI in these forms of tumor do not appear to be as distinctive from low-MSI tumors as high-MSI pancreatic cancer is from low-MSI pancreatic cancer (Chiappini *et al.* 2004; Saetta *et al.* 2006; Liengswangwong *et al.* 2006).

Repair of double strand breaks will also impact on survival of the cell as well as carcinogenesis. Failure to repair will cause death, while error-prone repair is more likely to lead to a tumor. There are a number of mechanisms for repairing double strand breaks; these have varying levels of fidelity (Cahill *et al.* 2006). The least error prone is homologous recombination repair (HR); cells deficient in recombination repair will rely more heavily on non-homologous end joining (NHEJ). Therefore, cells deficient in the HR protein BRCA2 are more sensitive to killing by inhibitors of the poly(ADP-ribose)polymerase 1 (PARP1) protein (Bryant *et al.* 2005); which is involved in BER, single strand break repair and a form of NHEJ (Wang *et al.* 2006). A link between somatic mutations and heterozygous germline mutations of genes associated with HR (BRCA1 and Fanconi anemia genes) are well established for pancreatic cancer: Biallelic BRCA2 (FANCD1) mutations are present in approximately 10% of patients with apparently sporadic pancreatic carcinomas (Goggins *et al.* 1996). Germline BRCA2 mutation is found in nearly 20% of familial pancreatic cancer patients (Murphy *et al.* 2002; Hahn *et al.* 2003). There is a nearly fourfold increase in risk of pancreatic cancer in breast and ovarian cancer families with a germline BRCA2 mutation (The Breast Cancer Linkage Consortium 1999) and an approximately twofold increase in breast and ovarian cancers with BRCA1 mutations (Thompson & Easton 2002). Mutations in FANCC and FANCG have been identified in 3/22 (13.6%) patients with early-onset periampullary tumors (two germline and one somatic) (van der Heijden *et al.* 2003). Heterozygous germline mutations of Fanconi anemia genes have also been shown in patients with sporadic pancreatic cancer (van der Heijden *et al.* 2003; van der Heijden *et al.* 2004; Rogers *et al.* 2004): In contrast, heterozygous germline mutation of these genes has not been linked to hepatocellular carcinoma. Homozygous mutations of BRCA2 and other Fanconi anemia genes are associated with the recessive Fanconi anemia syndrome. This is characterized by congenital abnormalities and progressive bone marrow failure (Howlett *et al.* 2002; Tischkowitz & Hodgson 2003); it is also strongly associated with hepatocellular carcinoma but not pancreatic cancer (Alter 2003).

Lessons from comparative studies of hepatobiliary carcinogenesis

From the discussion above it is clear that the liver, biliary system and pancreas have different degrees of susceptibility to different carcinogens. This is only partially explained by different levels of exposure. Basal efficiency of DNA repair pathways are different in the different organs; failure of these repair pathways as a result of germline mutations or viral infection will therefore have different effects on sensitivity to carcinogens and on the molecular progression of the tumors.

Screening

From the discussion above it is clear that some general advice is possible: to avoid these forms of cancer it is wise to not drink or smoke and avoid contact with hepatitis virus or liver flukes (Box 17.1). Any product that will significantly reduce the risk of somatic mutations would also be highly recommended.

Excellent though this advice is, it is unlikely that the majority of the population will be adequately concerned about these forms of cancer to undergo any major lifestyle changes merely on the basis of these suggestions. Advice must therefore be targeted at individuals (Box 17.2) at particularly high risk; Table 17.1 lists the syndromes that would identify such individuals at an increased risk of developing pancreatic cancer. Such individuals would be far more likely to respond to health advice and they might also be suitable for routine screening. It is difficult to know at which point screening will cause more harm than good, but clearly if the consequences of inappropriate treatment are equivalent to the benefits of appropriate treatment then screening requires, at a minimum, that the true-positive to false-positive ratio be >1. In the case of hepatobiliary tumors treatment will inevitably involve surgery; which in all cases will involve a significant risk morbidity and even death, with no guarantee of curing the patient. Balanced against this is the rising risk of death if there is no early treatment; 5-year survival from hepatobiliary tumors if detected late is extremely low. The question is when cost combined with risk of false positives outweigh the benefit derived from screening (Neoptolemos *et al.* 1996) (Box 17.3).

An ideal cancer screening test should be safe, inexpensive and accurate while permitting sufficiently early diagnosis to give an opportunity to cure the disease (Goggins *et al.* 2000). The most common imaging modalities at present are computed tomography (CT) and ultrasound (US) followed by endoluminal ultrasound (EUS) and positron emission tomography (PET) (Kalra *et al.* 2003). Alternatives are magnetic resonance imaging (MRI), endoscopic retrograde cholangiopancreatography (ERCP) and magnetic resonance cholangiopancreatography (MRCP). Little data exist on the sensitivity of these techniques in detecting lesions in asymptomatic individuals. It is likely that no individual imaging technique will offer sufficient accuracy, and combinations of imaging modalities should be employed. To date reliable data on combined efficacy of imaging techniques is limited to a few prospective trials (Soriano *et al.* 2004).

In order to improve specificity for detection of cancers without significantly compromising sensitivity, molecular changes occurring during tumor progression could be exploited. This has been most extensively studied in screening for pancreatic cancer. Yan *et al.* published data on stratification of cancer risk using p53 and K-ras mutation status combined with $p16^{INK4a}$ promoter methylation (Yan *et al.* 2005). They concluded that for individuals in a population with a 1% incidence of cancer, risk could be stratified between negligible and over 50%; exceeding 90% when discriminating patients with malignancy from patients with no pancreatic disease.

Box 17.1 Lifestyle modification.

- Reduce or stop alcohol intake, particularly for risk of hepatocellular carcinoma
- Stop smoking

Box 17.2 Primary screening – identify risk.

Pancreatic cancer
- Family history of pancreatic cancer
- Family history of pancreatitis
- Personal history of pancreatitis
- Late-onset diabetes

Hepatocellular carcinoma
- Personal history of hepatitis
- Cirrhosis
- Exposure to aflatoxin

Cholangiocarcinoma
- Personal history of liver fluke infection

Table 17.1 Hereditary cancer syndromes affecting the pancreas.

Syndrome	Gene mutation	Pancreatic cancer risk—lifetime risk
Familial pancreatic cancer	BRCA2 in up to 20%	Variable dependent on pedigree—up to 50%
Familial atypical multiple mole melanoma (FAMMM)—pancreatic cancer variant	TP16	17%
Familial breast and ovarian cancer syndromes	BRCA1 and BRCA2	Pedigree dependent
Fanconi anemia	FANCA, B, C, D1 (BRCA2), D2, E, F, G	? ~5%
Peutz–Jeghers syndrome	STK11/LKB1	36%
Hereditary pancreatitis	PRSS1 in up to 80%	35%
von Hippel–Lindau disease	VHL	? ~5%
Ataxia telangiectasia	ATM	? ~5%
Li–Fraumeni syndrome	TP53	? ~5%
Cystic fibrosis	CFTR	? ~5%
Familial adenomatous polyposis (FAP)	APC	? ~5%
Hereditary non-polyposis colon cancer (HNPCC)	MLH1, MSH2, MSH6, PMS1, PMS2	? ~5%

Prevention of hepatocellular carcinoma

Infection

Hepatoma is unique among cancers in that the acquired factors are directly responsible for carcinogenesis in the majority of cases. HCV and HBV are the main etiology where infection is prevalent (Omata & Yoshida 2004). This enables efficient screening for HCC development and therefore prevention of HCC by controlling the acquired factor, viral infection. Strategies can be made at two levels: prevention of virus infection and treatment of viral hepatitis (Box 17.4).

Prevention of viral infection

Neonates from HBV-positive mothers can be treated with a combination of hepatitis B vaccination and hepatitis B immune globulin. It effectively prevents infection during delivery. Studies have demonstrated 50% reduction of the incidence of HCC among adolescents as a result of universal immunisation of newborns (Chang *et al.* 1997). There is no current vaccine for the prevention of HCV infection.

Box 17.3 Early symptoms and screening.

Hepatocellular carcinoma
- Vague upper abdominal pain—not fully responding to medication
- Weight loss
- Malaise
- Jaundice
- Fever

Cholangiocarcinoma
- Weight loss
- Jaundice
- Pruritus

Pancreatic cancer
- Vague upper abdominal pain—not fully responding to medication
- Weight loss
- Late-onset diabetes mellitus
- Jaundice (usually at a more advanced stage)

Secondary screening on a research basis via recruitment to the European Registry of Hereditary Pancreatitis and Familial Pancreatic Cancer (EUROPAC), the National Familial Pancreas Tumor Registry at Johns Hopkins or the University of Washington

Box 17.4 Factors important for prevention.

Hepatocellular carcinoma
- Interferon to treat HCV
- Immunization against HBV of neonates from HBV-positive mothers
- Aflatoxin-neutralizing agents

Cholangiocarcinoma
- Praziquantel against liver fluke

Treatment of chronic hepatitis C

The risk of HCC is negligible in asymptomatic healthy carriers and as high as 6% per year in cirrhotic patients. This translates into a 2000 times the incidence of HCC in the population without hepatitis virus infection (Omata & Yoshida 2004). Interferon monotherapy has been shown to be effective against hepatitis C infection. Pretreatment factors predictive for response are serum low virus load and non-1b HCV genotypes. The level of hepatic inflammation and rate of fibrosis varies. The indication of interferon therapy must be considered on the basis of lifetime risk of HCC development and the possibility of achieving sustained virologic response (from viral genotype and load) (Hayashi *et al.* 2002).

Treatment of chronic hepatitis B

The risk ratio can be estimated as one-eighth that of HCV infection. The stage of liver fibrosis and risk of HCC are not as strongly associated in HBV as in HCV. Interferon has been used to treat chronic hepatitis B and does facilitate seroconversion of HBe antigen to HBe antibody, but the efficacy is rather limited. This does not seem to translate into a reduced HCC risk (Yuen *et al.* 2001).

Lamivudine (inhibitor of RNA-dependent DNA polymerase) suppresses the inflammation caused by HBV. HBV-mediated carcinogenesis is associated with the integration of viral DNA into the host genome. Suppression of inflammation and regeneration may diminish the chance of DNA integration but this remains to be confirmed in clinical trials. The use of adefovir dipivoxil also is the focus of further studies (McGlynn & London 2005).

Alcohol

Reduction of alcohol reduces HCC risk in all individuals but is particularly important in HCV-infected individuals.

Aflatoxins

Dietary consumption of aflatoxins is an additional risk factor for HCC in areas with a high prevalence of HBV infection. Synergism between these toxins and HBV has been shown to be instrumental in causing HCC. Chemopreventive agents could neutralize these toxins. Chlorophyllin (binds aflatoxins and impairs their absorption) and oltipraz (induces detoxificant enzymes in the liver) have been tested (Kensler *et al.* 2004). Limiting fungal contamination of crops is another preventative strategy, as is replacing corn (the main source of aflatoxin) with rice as the staple food in high HCC areas.

Chemoprevention

Other strategies for patients with established cirrhosis and premalignant lesions may be the use of herbal medicines and acylic retinoid. There have been some trials to assess these agents (Grau *et al.* 2006).

Prevention of cholangiocarcinoma

Chemoprevention

Excess generation of inducible nitrous oxide (iNOS) has been linked to carcinogenesis, and cyclooxygenase-2 (COX-2) also plays a role in cholangiocarcinogenesis. Selectively targeting iNOS and COX-2, together with altering the composition of the bile acid pool, may provide a strategy for chemoprevention. Ursodeoxycholic acid which is used in the treatment of PSC may reduce colorectal dysplasia but there is no evidence so far that this is also seen in the biliary epithelium. Selective iNOS inhibitors have exhibited chemopreventive effects in rodent models of colorectal cancer but there is no evidence yet for cholangiocarcinoma. Similarly, there are as yet no animal models of chemoprevention of cholangiocarcinoma using COX-2 inhibitors (Sirica 2005). Further *in vivo* studies are warranted.

Primary prevention of cholangiocarcinoma in areas of high liver fluke infestation should involve control of the parasite. Effective treatment is available using drugs such as praziquantel. Unfortunately reinfection occurs rapidly due to persistence of the parasite in the environment. Successful control will require repeated treatment and changes to dietary patterns (Parkin *et al.* 1993).

Prevention of pancreatic cancer

Avoiding alcohol and smoking are obvious preventative measures to reduce the risk of pancreatic cancer (Vimalachandran *et al.* 2004). There are no clinical trials as yet for chemoprevention in pancreatic cancer. The majority of data have been generated in preclinical studies *in vitro* and *in vivo*. Dietary isoprenoids, somatostatin analogs, selective estrogen modulators and antiandrogen agents have shown some effects in preclinical studies. Aspirin, NSAIDs and selective COX-2 inhibitors have also been proposed. The antioxidants associated with green and black tea are also possible agents for chemoprevention. Vitamins C, E and selenium are also potential chemopreventative agents (Doucas *et al.* 2006). The majority of the evidence for these compounds is based on *in vitro* studies and therefore much work is still needed (Lowenfels & Maisonneuve 2006).

Conclusion

Hepatobiliary cancers are not a single entity and should not be considered as such. Identifying high-risk groups for each form of cancer will allow targeted application of screening and chemoprevention in multiple parallel research programs; this will allow best practice to be adopted for each set of high-risk individuals and offer insight for the prevention and treatment of the more common sporadic diseases. The conclusions of each of these parallel research programs and the lessons learnt along the way should be placed in the context of the molecular pathology of the individual cancer type.

References

Alter BP. (2003) Cancer in Fanconi anemia, 1927–2001. *Cancer* 97: 425–40.

Alvaro D, Invernizzi P, Onori P *et al.* (2004) Estrogen receptors in cholangiocytes and the progression of primary biliary cirrhosis. *J Hepatol* 41: 905–12.

Basso D, Greco E, Fogar P *et al.* (2006) Pancreatic cancer-derived S-100A8 N-terminal peptide: A diabetes cause? *Clin Chim Acta* 373: 120–8.

Becker SA, Lee TH, Butel JS, Slagle BL. (1998) Hepatitis B virus X protein interferes with cellular DNA repair. *J Virol* 72: 266–72.

Biankin AV, Kench JG, Dijkman FP, Biankin SA, Henshall SM. (2003) Molecular pathogenesis of precursor lesions of pancreatic ductal adenocarcinoma. *Pathology* 35: 14–24.

Bosch FX, Ribes J, Borras J. (1999) Epidemiology of primary liver cancer. *Semin Liver Dis* 19: 271–85.

Bryant HE, Schultz N, Thomas HD *et al.* (2005) Specific killing of BRCA2-deficient tumours with inhibitors of poly(ADP-ribose) polymerase. *Nature* 434: 913–7.

Cahill D, Connor B, Carney JP. (2006) Mechanisms of eukaryotic DNA double strand break repair. *Front Biosci* 11: 1958–76.

Campalans A, Marsin S, Nakabeppu Y, O'Connor TR, Boiteux S, Radicella JP. (2005) XRCC1 interactions with multiple DNA glycosylases: a model for its recruitment to base excision repair. *DNA Repair (Amst)* 4: 826–35.

Castaneda F, Rosin-Steiner S, Jung K. (2006) Functional genomics analysis of low concentration of ethanol in human hepatocellular carcinoma (HepG2) cells. Role of genes involved in transcriptional and translational processes. *Int J Med Sci* 4: 28–35.

Chang MH, Chen CJ, Lai MS *et al.* (1997) Universal hepatitis B vaccination in Taiwan and the incidence of hepatocellular carcinoma in children. Taiwan Childhood Hepatoma Study Group. *N Engl J Med* 336: 1855–9.

Chari ST, Leibson CL, Rabe KG, Ransom J, De Andrade M, Petersen GM. (2005) Probability of pancreatic cancer following diabetes: a population-based study. *Gastroenterology* 129: 504–11.

Chiappini F, Gross-Goupil M, Saffroy R *et al.* (2004) Microsatellite instability mutator phenotype in hepatocellular carcinoma in non-alcoholic and non-virally infected normal livers. *Carcinogenesis* 25: 541–7.

Chiu HF, Ho SC, Wang LY, Wu TN, Yang CY. (2004) Does arsenic exposure increase the risk for liver cancer? *J Toxicol Environ Health A* 67: 1491–500.

Claij N, Te Riele H. (2002) Methylation tolerance in mismatch repair proficient cells with low MSH2 protein level. *Oncogene* 21: 2873–9.

Costa DB, Chen AA, Marginean EC, Inzucchi SE. (2004) Diabetes mellitus as the presenting feature of extrahepatic cholangiocarcinoma in situ: case report and review of literature. *Endocr Pract* 10: 417–23.

De Laat WL, Jaspers NG, Hoeijmakers JH. (1999) Molecular mechanism of nucleotide excision repair. *Genes Dev* 13: 768–85.

De Mitri MS, Poussin K, Baccarini P *et al.* (1995) HCV-associated liver cancer without cirrhosis. *Lancet* 345: 413–5.

Doucas H, Garcea G, Neal CP, Manson MM, Berry DP. (2006) Chemoprevention of pancreatic cancer: a review of the molecular pathways involved, and evidence for the potential for chemoprevention. *Pancreatology* 6: 429–39.

Ekbom A, Hunter D. (2002) Pancreatic cancer. In: Adami H, Hunter D, Trichopoulos D, eds. *Textbook of Cancer Epidemiology*, pp. 233–47. Oxford University Press, New York.

El-Serag HB, Hampel H, Javadi F. (2006) The association between diabetes and hepatocellular carcinoma: a systematic review of epidemiologic evidence. *Clin Gastroenterol Hepatol* 4: 369–80.

Fousteri M, Vermeulen W, Van Zeeland AA, Mullenders LH. (2006) Cockayne syndrome A and B proteins differentially regulate recruitment of chromatin remodeling and repair factors to stalled RNA polymerase II in vivo. *Mol Cell* 23: 471–82.

Franceschi S, Montella M, Polesel J *et al.* (2006) Hepatitis viruses, alcohol, and tobacco in the etiology of hepatocellular carcinoma in Italy. *Cancer Epidemiol Biomarkers Prev* 15: 683–9.

Giannitrapani L, Soresi M, La Spada E, Cervello M, D'Alessandro N, Montalto G. (2006) Sex hormones and risk of liver tumor. *Ann N Y Acad Sci* 1089: 228–36.

Goggins M, Canto M, Hruban R. (2000) Can we screen high-risk individuals to detect early pancreatic carcinoma? *J Surg Oncol* 74: 243–48.

Goggins M, Schutte M, Lu J *et al.* (1996) Germline BRCA2 gene mutations in patients with apparently sporadic pancreatic carcinomas. *Cancer Res* 56: 5360–4.

Gordis L, Gold EB. (1984) Epidemiology of pancreatic cancer. *World J Surg* 8: 808–21.

Goren-Inbar N, Alperson N, Kislev ME *et al.* (2004) Evidence of hominin control of fire at Gesher Benot Ya'aqov, Israel. *Science* 304: 725–7.

Grau MV, Rees JR, Baron JA. (2006) Chemoprevention in gastrointestinal cancers: current status. *Basic Clin Pharmacol Toxicol* 98: 281–7.

Guengerich FP. (2000) Metabolism of chemical carcinogens. *Carcinogenesis* 21: 345–51.

Hahn SA, Greenhalf B, Ellis I *et al.* (2003) BRCA2 germline mutations in familial pancreatic carcinoma. *J Natl Cancer Inst* 95: 214–21.

Hahn WC, Counter CM, Lundberg AS, Beijersbergen RL, Brooks MW, Weinberg RA. (1999) Creation of human tumour cells with defined genetic elements. *Nature* 400: 464–8.

Hahn WC, Dessain SK, Brooks MW *et al.* (2002) Enumeration of the simian virus 40 early region elements necessary for human cell transformation. *Mol Cell Biol* 22: 2111–23.

Hanawalt PC. (2001) Revisiting the rodent repairadox. *Environ Mol Mutagen* 38: 89–96.

Hayashi K, Kumada T, Nakano S *et al.* (2002) Incidence of hepatocellular carcinoma in chronic hepatitis C after interferon therapy. *Hepatogastroenterology* 49: 508–12.

Hecht SS. (1999) DNA adduct formation from tobacco-specific N-nitrosamines. *Mutat Res* 424: 127–42.

Herzer K, Weyer S, Krammer PH, Galle PR, Hofmann TG. (2005) Hepatitis C virus core protein inhibits tumor suppressor protein promyelocytic leukemia function in human hepatoma cells. *Cancer Res* 65: 10830–7.

Hoffmann D, Hoffmann I. (1997) The changing cigarette, 1950–1995. *J Toxicol Environ Health* 50: 307–64.

Howes N, Lerch MM, Greenhalf W *et al.* (2004) Clinical and genetic characteristics of hereditary pancreatitis in Europe. *Clin Gastroenterol Hepatol* 2: 252–61.

Howlett NG, Taniguchi T, Olson S *et al.* (2002) Biallelic inactivation of BRCA2 in Fanconi anemia. *Science* 297: 606–9.

Huxley R, Ansary-Moghaddam A, Berrington De Gonzalez A, Barzi F, Woodward M. (2005) Type-II diabetes and pancreatic cancer: a meta-analysis of 36 studies. *Br J Cancer* 92: 2076–83.

Jee SH, Ohrr H, Sull JW, Samet JM. (2004) Cigarette smoking, alcohol drinking, hepatitis B, and risk for hepatocellular carcinoma in Korea. *J Natl Cancer Inst* 96: 1851–6.

Jemal A, Siegel R, Ward E, Murray T, Xu J, Thun MJ. (2007) Cancer statistics, 2007. *CA Cancer J Clin* 57: 43–66.

Ji J, Couto E, Hemminki K. (2005) Incidence differences for gallbladder cancer between occupational groups suggest an etiological role for alcohol. *Int J Cancer* 116: 492–3.

Jiao L, Bondy ML, Hassan MM *et al.* (2006) Selected polymorphisms of DNA repair genes and risk of pancreatic cancer. *Cancer Detect Prev* 30: 284–91.

Kalra MK, Maher MM, Mueller PR, Saini S. (2003) State-of-the-art imaging of pancreatic neoplasms. *Br J Radiol* 76: 857–65.

Kensler TW, Egner PA, Wang JB *et al.* (2004) Chemoprevention of hepatocellular carcinoma in aflatoxin endemic areas. *Gastroenterology* 127: S310–8.

Kern MA, Breuhahn K, Schirmacher P. (2002) Molecular pathogenesis of human hepatocellular carcinoma. *Adv Cancer Res* 86: 67–112.

Kiguchi K, Carbajal S, Chan K *et al.* (2001) Constitutive expression of ErbB-2 in gallbladder epithelium results in development of adenocarcinoma. *Cancer Res* 61: 6971–6.

Kirk GD, Turner PC, Gong Y *et al.* (2005) Hepatocellular carcinoma and polymorphisms in carcinogen-metabolizing and DNA repair enzymes in a population with aflatoxin exposure and hepatitis B virus endemicity. *Cancer Epidemiol Biomarkers Prev* 14: 373–9.

Koike K, Tsutsumi T, Fujie H, Shintani Y, Kyoji M. (2002) Molecular mechanism of viral hepatocarcinogenesis. *Oncology* 62 Suppl 1: 29–37.

Kowdley KV. (2004) Iron, hemochromatosis, and hepatocellular carcinoma. *Gastroenterology* 127: S79–86.

Lazaridis KN, Gores GJ. (2006) Primary sclerosing cholangitis and cholangiocarcinoma. *Semin Liver Dis* 26: 42–51.

Lee SG, Rho HM. (2000) Transcriptional repression of the human p53 gene by hepatitis B viral X protein. *Oncogene* 19: 468–71.

Liengswangwong U, Karalak A, Morishita Y *et al.* (2006) Immunohistochemical expression of mismatch repair genes: a screening tool for predicting mutator phenotype in liver fluke infection-associated intrahepatic cholangiocarcinoma. *World J Gastroenterol* 12: 3740–5.

Lin Y, Tamakoshi A, Kawamura T *et al.* (2002) A prospective cohort study of cigarette smoking and pancreatic cancer in Japan. *Cancer Causes Control* 13: 249–54.

Lowenfels AB, Maisonneuve P. (2006) Epidemiology and risk factors for pancreatic cancer. *Best Pract Res Clin Gastroenterol* 20: 197–209.

Lowenfels AB, Maisonneuve P, Cavallini G *et al.* (1993) Pancreatitis and the risk of pancreatic cancer. International Pancreatitis Study Group. *N Engl J Med* 328: 1433–7.

Lynch HT, Deters CA, Lynch JF, Brand RE. (2004) Familial pancreatic carcinoma in Jews. *Fam Cancer* 3: 233–40.

Maitra A, Adsay NV, Argani P *et al.* (2003) Multicomponent analysis of the pancreatic adenocarcinoma progression model using a pancreatic intraepithelial neoplasia tissue microarray. *Mod Pathol* 16: 902–12.

Mcglynn KA, London WT. (2005) Epidemiology and natural history of hepatocellular carcinoma. *Best Pract Res Clin Gastroenterol* 19: 3–23.

Mitacek EJ, Brunnemann KD, Hoffmann D *et al.* (1999) Volatile nitrosamines and tobacco-specific nitrosamines in the smoke of Thai cigarettes: a risk factor for lung cancer and a suspected risk factor for liver cancer in Thailand. *Carcinogenesis* 20: 133–7.

Moss SF, Blaser MJ. (2005) Mechanisms of disease: inflammation and the origins of cancer. *Nat Clin Pract Oncol* 2: 90–7.

Murphy KM, Brune KA, Griffin C *et al.* (2002) Evaluation of candidate genes MAP2K4, MADH4, ACVR1B, and BRCA2 in familial pancreatic cancer: deleterious BRCA2 mutations in 17%. *Cancer Res* 62: 3789–93.

Neoptolemos JP, Lemoine NR, Ching CH, Rhodes JM. (1996) Cancer of the pancreas and ampulla of Vater. In: Fielding JWL, Allum WH, eds. *Premalignancy And Early Cancer In General Surgery,* pp. 66–100. Oxford University Press, Oxford.

Nyberg U, Nilsson B, Travis LB, Holm LE, Hall P. (2002) Cancer incidence among Swedish patients exposed to radioactive thorotrast: a forty-year follow-up survey. *Radiat Res* 157: 419–25.

Omata M, Yoshida H. (2004) Prevention and treatment of hepatocellular carcinoma. *Liver Transpl* 10: S111–4.

Parkin DM, Ohshima H, Srivatanakul P, Vatanasapt V. (1993) Cholangiocarcinoma: epidemiology, mechanisms of carcinogenesis and prevention. *Cancer Epidemiol Biomarkers Prev* 2: 537–44.

Paterlini-Brechot P, Saigo K, Murakami Y *et al.* (2003) Hepatitis B virus-related insertional mutagenesis occurs frequently in human liver cancers and recurrently targets human telomerase gene. *Oncogene* 22: 3911–6.

Pegg AE, Roberfroid M, Von Bahr C *et al.* (1982) Removal of O6-methylguanine from DNA by human liver fractions. *Proc Natl Acad Sci U S A* 79: 5162–5.

Permert J, Adrian TE, Jacobsson P, Jorfelt L, Fruin AB, Larsson J. (1993) Is profound peripheral insulin resistance in patients with pancreatic cancer caused by a tumor-associated factor? *Am J Surg* 165: 61–6; discussion 66–7.

Petersen DR. (2005) Alcohol, iron-associated oxidative stress, and cancer. *Alcohol* 35: 243–9.

Poon TC, Wong N, Lai PB, Rattray M, Johnson PJ, Sung JJ. (2006) A tumor progression model for hepatocellular carcinoma: bioinformatic analysis of genomic data. *Gastroenterology* 131: 1262–70.

Qadri I, Iwahashi M, Simon F. (2002) Hepatitis C virus NS5A protein binds TBP and p53, inhibiting their DNA binding and p53 interactions with TBP and ERCC3. *Biochim Biophys Acta* 1592: 193–204.

Roa I, De Aretxabala X, Araya JC, Roa J. (2006) Preneoplastic lesions in gallbladder cancer. *J Surg Oncol* 93: 615–23.

Rogers CD, Van Der Heijden MS, Brune K *et al.* (2004) The genetics of FANCC and FANCG in familial pancreatic cancer. *Cancer Biol Ther* 3: 167–9.

Saetta AA, Gigelou F, Papanastasiou PI *et al.* (2006) High-level microsatellite instability is not involved in gallbladder carcinogenesis. *Exp Mol Pathol* 80: 67–71.

Scott TE, Carroll M, Cogliano FD, Smith BF, Lamorte WW. (1999) A case-control assessment of risk factors for gallbladder carcinoma. *Dig Dis Sci* 44: 1619–25.

Seitz HK, Stickel F. (2006) Risk factors and mechanisms of hepatocarcinogenesis with special emphasis on alcohol and oxidative stress. *Biol Chem* 387: 349–60.

Shaib YH, El-Serag HB, Nooka AK *et al.* (2007) Risk factors for intrahepatic and extrahepatic cholangiocarcinoma: a hospital-based case-control study. *Am J Gastroenterol* 102: 1016–21.

Silverman DT, Dunn JA, Hoover RN *et al.* (1994) Cigarette smoking and pancreas cancer: a case-control study based on direct interviews. *J Natl Cancer Inst* 86: 1510–6.

Silverman DT, Schiffman M, Everhart J *et al.* (1999) Diabetes mellitus, other medical conditions and familial history of cancer as risk factors for pancreatic cancer. *Br J Cancer* 80: 1830–7.

Sirica AE. (2005) Cholangiocarcinoma: molecular targeting strategies for chemoprevention and therapy. *Hepatology* 41: 5–15.

Smela ME, Currier SS, Bailey EA, Essigmann JM. (2001) The chemistry and biology of aflatoxin B(1): from mutational spectrometry to carcinogenesis. *Carcinogenesis* 22: 535–45.

Sobol RW, Wilson SH. (2001) Mammalian DNA beta-polymerase in base excision repair of alkylation damage. *Prog Nucleic Acid Res Mol Biol* 68: 57–74.

Soriano A, Castells A, Ayuso C *et al.* (2004) Preoperative staging and tumor resectability assessment of pancreatic cancer: prospective study comparing endoscopic ultrasonography, helical computed tomography, magnetic resonance imaging, and angiography. *Am J Gastroenterol* 99: 492–501.

Stevens RJ, Roddam AW, Beral V. (2007) Pancreatic cancer in type 1 and young-onset diabetes: systematic review and meta-analysis. *Br J Cancer* 96: 507–9.

Takahashi Y, Nakatsuru Y, Zhang S *et al.* (2002) Enhanced spontaneous and aflatoxin-induced liver tumorigenesis in xeroderma pigmentosum group A gene-deficient mice. *Carcinogenesis* 23: 627–33.

The Breast Cancer Linkage Consortium. (1999) Cancer risks in BRCA2 mutation carriers. *J Natl Cancer Inst* 91: 1310–1316.

Thompson D, Easton DF. (2002) Cancer Incidence in BRCA1 mutation carriers. *J Natl Cancer Inst* 94: 1358–65.

Tischkowitz MD, Hodgson SV. (2003) Fanconi anaemia. *J Med Genet* 40: 1–10.

Tuveson DA, Shaw AT, Willis NA *et al.* (2004) Endogenous oncogenic K-ras(G12D) stimulates proliferation and widespread neoplastic and developmental defects. *Cancer Cell* 5: 375–87.

Tuveson DA, Zhu L, Gopinathan A *et al.* (2006) Mist1-KrasG12D knock-in mice develop mixed differentiation metastatic exocrine pancreatic carcinoma and hepatocellular carcinoma. *Cancer Res* 66: 242–7.

Van Der Heijden MS, Brody JR, Gallmeier E *et al.* (2004) Functional defects in the Fanconi anemia pathway in pancreatic cancer cells. *Am J Pathol* 165: 651–7.

Van Der Heijden MS, Yeo CJ, Hruban RH, Kern SE. (2003) Fanconi anemia gene mutations in young-onset pancreatic cancer. *Cancer Res* 63: 2585–8.

Van Pelt JF, Severi T, Crabbe T *et al.* (2004) Expression of hepatitis C virus core protein impairs DNA repair in human hepatoma cells. *Cancer Lett* 209: 197–205.

Velazquez I, Alter BP. (2004) Androgens and liver tumors: Fanconi's anemia and non-Fanconi's conditions. *Am J Hematol* 77: 257–67.

Vernez M, Hutter P, Monnerat C, Halkic N, Gugerli O, Bouzourene H. (2006) A case of Muir-Torre syndrome associated with mucinous hepatic cholangiocarcinoma and a novel germline mutation of the MSH2 gene. *Fam Cancer.*

Vimalachandran D, Ghaneh P, Costello E, Neoptolemos JP. (2004) Genetics and prevention of pancreatic cancer. *Cancer Control* 11: 6–14.

Vogelstein B, Fearon ER, Hamilton SR *et al.* (1988) Genetic alterations during colorectal-tumor development. *N Engl J Med* 319: 525–32.

Von Tungeln LS, Xia Q, Bucci T, Heflich RH, Fu PP. (1999a) Tumorigenicity and liver tumor ras-protooncogene mutations in CD-1 mice treated neonatally with 1- and 3-nitrobenzo[a]pyrene and their trans-7,8-dihydrodiol and aminobenzo[a]pyrene metabolites. *Cancer Lett* 137: 137–43.

Von Tungeln LS, Xia Q, Herreno-Saenz D, Bucci TJ, Heflich RH, Fu PP. (1999b) Tumorigenicity of nitropolycyclic aromatic hydrocarbons in the neonatal B6C3F1 mouse bioassay and characterization of ras mutations in liver tumors from treated mice. *Cancer Lett* 146: 1–7.

Wang F, Herrington M, Larsson J, Permert J. (2003) The relationship between diabetes and pancreatic cancer. *Mol Cancer* 2: 4.

Wang M, Abbruzzese JL, Friess H *et al.* (1998) DNA adducts in human pancreatic tissues and their potential role in carcinogenesis. *Cancer Res* 58: 38–41.

Wang M, Wu W, Wu W *et al.* (2006) PARP-1 and Ku compete for repair of DNA double strand breaks by distinct NHEJ pathways. *Nucleic Acids Res* 34: 6170–82.

Watanapa P, Watanapa WB. (2002) Liver fluke-associated cholangiocarcinoma. *Br J Surg* 89: 962–70.

Wilentz RE, Geradts J, Maynard R *et al.* (1998) Inactivation of the p16 (INK4A) tumor-suppressor gene in pancreatic duct lesions: loss of intranuclear expression. *Cancer Res* 58: 4740–4.

Yamamoto H, Itoh F, Nakamura H *et al.* (2001) Genetic and clinical features of human pancreatic ductal adenocarcinomas with widespread microsatellite instability. *Cancer Res* 61: 3139–44.

Yan L, Mcfaul C, Howes N *et al.* (2005) Molecular analysis to detect pancreatic ductal adenocarcinoma in high-risk groups. *Gastroenterology* 128: 2124–30.

Yuen MF, Hui CK, Cheng CC, Wu CH, Lai YP, Lai CL. (2001) Long-term follow-up of interferon alfa treatment in Chinese patients with chronic hepatitis B infection: The effect on hepatitis B e antigen seroconversion and the development of cirrhosis-related complications. *Hepatology* 34: 139–45.

Zen Y, Aishima S, Ajioka Y *et al.* (2005) Proposal of histological criteria for intraepithelial atypical/proliferative biliary epithelial lesions of the bile duct in hepatolithiasis with respect to cholangiocarcinoma: preliminary report based on interobserver agreement. *Pathol Int* 55: 180–8.

Zendehdel K, Nyren O, Ostenson CG, Adami HO, Ekbom A, Ye W. (2003) Cancer incidence in patients with type 1 diabetes mellitus: a population-based cohort study in Sweden. *J Natl Cancer Inst* 95: 1797–800.

Zhou ZQ, Manguino D, Kewitt K *et al.* (2001) Spontaneous hepatocellular carcinoma is reduced in transgenic mice overexpressing human O6- methylguanine-DNA methyltransferase. *Proc Natl Acad Sci U S A* 98: 12566–71.

18 Molecular Biology of Hepatobiliary Cancer

Knut Ketterer & Helmut Friess

Introduction

Over the past two decades, research into the molecular mechanisms of carcinogenesis of malignant diseases has met with great success. An understanding of the genetic code, the principle of transcription to RNA and translation to protein has formed the basis for modern molecular research. Techniques for detection and quantification of DNA, RNA and proteins were established and introduced in oncology research in the 1980s. Later, techniques were developed for *in vitro* studies and for genetic manipulation in cell culture experiments and in animal models. As a result of those developments, scientific knowledge about molecular alterations in cancer has increased exponentially. It has become difficult to present an overview of the at times very distinct findings and to put them into context. At the latest, from the beginning of the microarray era, an overview of all acquired expression data seems to be possible only with computer-based programs.

On the other hand, some mechanisms of molecular carcinogenesis are remarkably well characterized and understood. These are either common mechanisms exhibited by different types of cancers or specific changes observed in distinct tumor entities. Malignant cells are characterized by their capacity for uncontrolled proliferation, their resistance to apoptosis, their ability to invade local tissues and vessels, and their capacity to separate from their organized assembly of cells and grow after settling in an alien site. The development of a fast-growing and metastasizing carcinoma cell is a multistep process with many—perhaps 10 or more—consecutive genetic mutations and a much larger number of epigenetic changes in the cell's expression profile. New molecular therapies have evolved from this knowledge, and are proving encouraging.

Gastrointestinal Oncology: A Critical Multidisciplinary Team Approach.
Edited by J. Jankowski, R. Sampliner, D. Kerr, and Y. Fong.

Pancreatic cancer

Pancreatic cancer is a devastating disease with an overall mortality close to 100%. It ranks as the fourth most common cause of cancer mortality. Authors who describe pancreatic cancer are usually referring to pancreatic ductal adenocarcinoma (PDAC), which comprises 90% of all pancreatic malignancies. We will also focus on PDAC here.

Smoking is a commonly accepted risk factor for pancreatic cancer, whereas the influence of dietary factors is not conclusive. It seems that both type II diabetes and chronic pancreatitis are associated with an increased risk of pancreatic cancer.

Not long ago, histopathologic precursor lesions that lead to the development of malignant epithelial neoplasms were identified (Hruban *et al.* 2001). These were named *pancreatic intraepithelial neoplasia* (PanIN 1–3). In brief, PanIN-1A consists of a flat mucosa of tall columnar mucinous cells, and PanIN-1B includes a papillary structure with a mucinous epithelium. PanIN-2 lesions are flat or mostly papillary, and the cells show some nuclear abnormalities but no atypical mitoses. The papillary or micropapillary architecture in PanIN-3 is more complex, with severe cellular atypia but without invasion through the basement membrane. Therefore an adenoma–carcinoma sequence seems to exist in pancreatic cancer as well as in colon cancer, for example.

Accompanying genetic alterations have been identified, so that the basic structure of a tumor progression model has been established. However, there are still no exact data on the time frame over which PDAC develops from early lesions to invasive carcinoma. It is currently believed that PDAC develops in a multistep process, with at least three mutations necessary to develop an invasive carcinoma. Furthermore, other than the very few genetic alterations with high incidence in pancreatic cancer, the genetic background is not uniform. In addition to oncogenic activation and inactivated tumor suppressor genes, a huge variety of epigenetic changes, including overexpression of growth factors, chemokines and cytokines, is considered to play a crucial role in the fast growth and metastasis of this cancer. Indeed, although most common ductal adenocarcino-

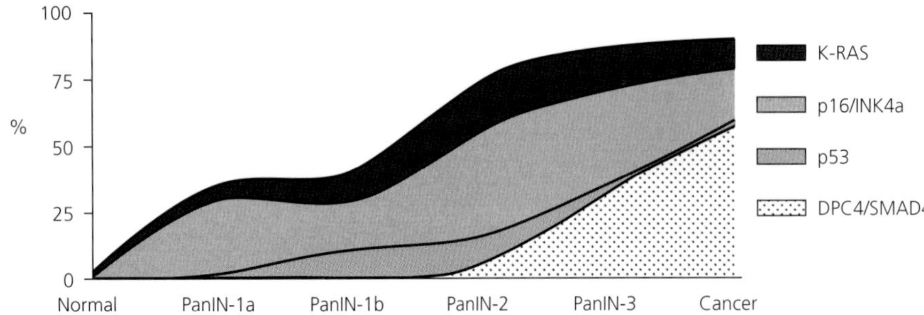

Fig. 18.1 Frequency of major genetic alterations in pancreatic ductal adenocarcinoma and pancreatic intraepithelial neoplasias (PanIN). PanINs are premalignant lesions evolving in a progression model to invasive carcinoma. The graph shows activating K-RAS point mutations, inactivation of the p16/INK4 locus, mutation of p53, and deletion of DPC4/SMAD4.

mas are relatively uniform clinically and pathologically, there are distinct genetic differences, and tumors exhibit variable gene expression profiles on the molecular level. There is hope that these genetic subtypes could be applied in the clinical management of the disease in terms of adjusted chemotherapy protocols.

The earliest presently known event in the carcinogenesis of ductal adenocarcinoma is the mutation of the proto-oncogene K-RAS in codon 12. It is mutated in more than 90% of all ductal adenocarcinomas, with mutation rates of 30–44% in PanIN-1 lesions and about 70% in PanIN-2 lesions, and is the most frequent genetic alteration in these precursor lesions. This mutation results in a constitutively active RAS protein. *RAS* genes in general mediate the signals arising from binding of growth factors and major mitogen-activated protein kinase pathways. However, in epithelial cells, mutated *RAS* genes alone are not sufficient for oncogenic transformation and are also found in benign diseases of the pancreas—such as chronic pancreatitis (Fig. 18.1).

In the pancreatic cancer progression model, presumably the next genetic alterations are the homozygous deletion of the $p16^{INK4A}/p14^{ARF}$ locus and p53 mutations. Both are also found in PanIN-2 and PanIN-3 lesions. Around 95% of the cancers harbor p16/p14 deletions, and 50–75% have p53 mutations (Fig. 18.1). $p16^{A}$ and p14 are two related tumor suppressor genes. Whereas p16 is an inhibitor of the cyclin-dependent kinase complex in the G1 phase, p14 facilitates MDM2/HDM2 degradation, leading to p53 accumulation. p53 regulates an essential growth check point that protects against genomic rearrangements or DNA mutations. DNA damage or other genomic aberrations lead to p53 activation and consecutive p53 accumulation. p53 can induce cell cycle arrest and DNA repair, or can induce apoptosis of the damaged cell. Loss of p53 function through inactivated mutations is associated with aneuploidy and genomic instability (Schneider & Schmid 2003).

SMAD4/DPC4 is deleted or mutated in over 50% of pancreatic carcinomas, an event occurring late in the tumor progression model. Approximately 30% of PanIN-3 lesions exhibit its inactivation (Fig. 18.1). SMAD4 is a signaling molecule downstream from TGF-β which is a potent inhibitor of cell growth, mediated by a cell cycle G1 arrest. Restoration of SMAD4 in human pancreatic cancer cells was found to suppress tumor formation *in vivo* in animal models.

The BRCA2 protein is involved in the repair of DNA strand breaks and is found as germline mutations in patients with breast and pancreatic cancer. Nonetheless, BRCA2 mutations do not convey a high penetrance for malignant disease, and often families carrying the BRCA2 mutation do not stand out with accumulated cancers. Indeed, only 5–7% of patients presenting clinically with sporadic pancreatic cancers exhibit BRCA2 germline mutations.

Other genetic alterations with lower incidence in ductal adenocarcinoma of the pancreas are LKB1/STK11 (homozygously deleted in 4%), AKT2 (amplified in 10–20%), MYB (amplified in 10%), MKK4 (homozygously deleted in 4%), and TGFBR1 and TGFBR2 (Maitra *et al.* 2006).

Here it should be noted that for hereditary chronic pancreatitis in which the *PRSS1* gene (cationic trypsinogen) is mutated, the penetrance of pancreatic ductal adenocarcinoma is greater than 50% among gene carriers. Since *PRSS1* is neither an oncogene nor a tumor suppressor gene, it has been suggested that the tremendously increased cell division cycle in combination with the chronic inflammation and continued reparative process increases the incidence of mutations, and consequently cancer development.

The tumor biology of an aggressively infiltrating and fast metastasizing tumor cannot be explained only by genetic changes; there must also be numerous epigenetic changes. It is a generally accepted theory that cancer cells develop a gene expression profile as a result of clonal selection in order to maintain growth advantages. In the following sections, major aspects and established theories will be demonstrated.

Growth factors are expressed in many different cell types, and exert their effects via autocrine and paracrine mechanisms. Their biological effects are varied. They can stimulate or inhibit cell division, differentiation and resistance against apoptosis, but also regulate cell migration, infiltration, angiogenesis, extracellular matrix synthesis, and local immune system functions.

Several studies have established that pancreatic cancers overexpress multiple tyrosine kinase growth factor receptors and their ligands. This enhances mitogenesis and loss of responsiveness to the growth-inhibitory signals of members of the transforming growth factor beta (TGFβ) family, and therefore contributes to the biological aggressiveness of pancreatic ductal adenocarcinoma.

One of the best characterized epigenetic phenomena is human pancreatic cancer's overexpression of the epidermal growth factor receptor family (EGFR, c-erb-B2, c-erb-B3 and c-erb-B4) and of six ligands that bind directly to EGFR (EGF, TGF-α, HB-EGF, betacellulin, epiregulin and amphiregulin). These cancers also overexpress several members of the fibroblast growth factor family (FGF), keratinocyte growth factor (KGF), platelet-derived growth factor B (PDGF B), insulin-like growth factor-I (IGF-I), the EGF-like growth factor cripto, hepatocyte growth factor (HGF), vascular endothelial growth factor (VEGF), all transforming growth factor beta (TGFβ) isoforms, bone morphogenetic protein-2 (BMP-2) and activin βA. Many but not all of the corresponding receptors are concomitantly overexpressed. For example, there is overexpression of PDGF receptor α and β, the IGF-1 receptor, MET (the receptor that binds HGF), the FGF receptor 1 (FGFR-1), and the type 2 TGFβ receptor (TGFBR2), whereas the type 1 TGFβ receptor (TGFBR1) is underexpressed. Thus, there is selective overexpression of specific receptors and their ligands, and this concomitant overexpression leads to the creation of aberrant paracrine and autocrine signaling pathways, conferring a distinct growth advantage on pancreatic cancer cells.

These findings also have clinical implications, since the concomitant presence in the cancer cells of EGFR and either EGF or TGF-α is associated with disease progression and decreased survival, and the overexpression of c-erbB3, FGF-2 or TGFβ is associated with diminished patient survival. Inhibition of either EGFR or FGFR-1 attenuates pancreatic cancer cell growth *in vitro* (Friess *et al.* 1999).

Among other things, the downstream intracellular signaling pathway of the above-mentioned growth factor receptors consists of non-receptor intracellular SRC tyrosine kinases and mitogen-activated protein kinases (MAPKs), PI3K with activation of the PKB/AKT pathway, c-JUN N-terminal protein kinase, and p38 MAPK, all of which can also be targeted in new molecular therapy approaches (Fig. 18.2). Several cell culture studies and animal models have attempted the selective inhibition of these kinases, and have resulted in impressive tumor growth reduction. The advantage of these target molecules is that a common trunk of a variety of growth factor-mediated signaling in the end of the signaling cascade is blocked. On the other hand, this mechanism is not specific for tumor cells, and the clinical use of these substances needs to be tested, especially with regard to side-effects.

Secretion of growth factors not only leads to autocrine stimulation of cell growth and division of the tumor cells themselves, but also has effects on neighboring cells and tissues, such as stromal cells, nerves and blood vessels. Growth-promoting effects on cancer cells by neurotrophic growth factors transmitted from nerves are one example of the complex mechanisms involved in the network of different cell types interacting with each other (Ketterer *et al.* 2003).

Several angiogenic growth factors have been found to play a role in pancreatic cancer (e.g. VEGF and the proangiogenic chemokines). In general, vascular endothelial growth factor A (VEGF A) is considered to be the most potent factor in angiogenesis. Pancreatic cancer cells produce different isoforms of VEGF, which stimulate endothelial cell proliferation through binding to the VEGF receptors 1 and 2 on the surface of endothelial cells. Several studies have reported a positive correlation between blood vessel density, tumor VEGF-A levels, and disease progression in pancreatic ductal adenocarcinoma. Specific drugs blocking the VEGF receptor or experimental studies blocking VEGF signaling through modern molecular technologies have come up. For example, adenoviral infection of cell lines with vectors carrying sequences for soluble VEGF receptors that bind and neutralize VEGF ligands without initializing signaling, inhibit the growth and metastasis of pancreatic cancers in mouse models.

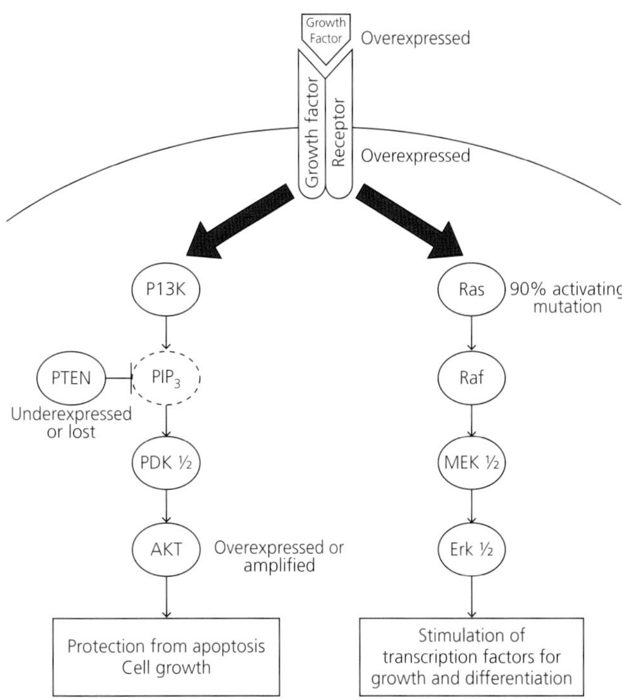

Fig. 18.2 Typical downstream signaling of growth factor receptors. Pancreatic and other cancers use this pathway for uncontrolled proliferation by overexpression of growth factors and their receptors, activating mutations of RAS, inactivation of the inhibitor PTEN, and overexpression of AKT.

Neuropilin-1 and neuropilin-2, originally identified as neuronal guidance molecules, act as coreceptors for VEGF and are overexpressed in pancreatic cancers as well as in other gastrointestinal cancers. Neuropilins bind to VEGF receptors and strengthen VEGF signaling (Korc 2003).

Tumor invasion and metastasis is a complex process. Cancer cells or cell islands must invade the surrounding stroma and vessels and disrupt their adhesive connections by disrupting their junctional contacts. Circulating cancer cells then need to adhere to different organs and to survive in the foreign tissue environments.

One widely observed alteration in cell-to-environment interaction in pancreatic cancer involves E-cadherin, which couples adjacent cells by E-cadherin bridges. The cytoplasmic domain of E-cadherin is associated with catenins, which link the cadherins with the actin-based cytoskeleton. In a majority of pancreatic tumors, E-cadherin function is lost and β-catenin-mediated signal transduction mechanisms that regulate cell growth and differentiation are activated. Several mechanisms for activating this pathway have been reported which result in accumulation and translocation of β-catenin to the nucleus and subsequent activation of proliferate gene transcription (e.g. cyclin D1 and C-MYC).

Interestingly, many genetic alterations seen frequently in other cancers, such as inactivated mutations of the glycogen synthase kinase-3β or genetic inactivation of the *APC* or *axin* genes, are rare in pancreatic cancer. Instead, β-catenin activation seems to be an epigenetic effect resulting from activation of the WNT pathway and growth factor signaling (Al Aynati *et al.* 2004).

The expression level and the pattern of cell adhesion molecules and integrins is changed in malignant pancreatic cancer. Neural cell adhesion molecule (N-CAM) undergoes a switch to poorly adhesive isoforms, and is expressed at lower levels. Other cell adhesion molecules, such as intercellular adhesion molecule-1 (ICAM-1) and vascular cell adhesion molecule-1 (VCAM-1), have been found to be overexpressed in human pancreatic cancer tissues.

Malignant tumors have a capacity to degrade the extracellular matrix (ECM) by controlled proteolysis. Degradation of connective tissue is associated with high expression of different types of matrix metalloproteases (especially MMP-2, -7, -9) of the cancer cells. Hypoxia—often found in a tumor environment—induces the expression of MMPs, as well as other proteases and C-MET (the receptor of HGF that enhances invasiveness), via HIF-α (hypoxia-inducible factor-α), promoting several invasive and angiogenic mechanisms. TIMP (tissue inhibitor of metalloproteinase) antagonizes matrix metalloproteinase activity and can suppress tumor growth, angiogenesis, invasion, and metastasis. TIMP-3 was found to be methylated and therefore underexpressed in several pancreatic adenocarcinomas.

In addition to the MMP family, the plasminogen activator system has been implicated in tumor invasion and metastasis through activation of plasmin, which is able to degrade fibrin and numerous other components of the extracellular matrix. uPA (urokinase plasminogen activator) and tPA (tissue plasminogen activator) are both overexpressed and active in pancreatic cancer. PAI (plasminogen activator inhibitor), a protease inhibitor which is correlated with metastasis and poor prognosis, is also highly expressed. Direct mechanisms leading to cell detachment and inhibition of cell adhesion seem to be responsible for this. In animal models, targeting the uPA/uPAR system with inhibitory antibodies was able to decrease pancreatic tumor growth and hepatic metastasis, and completely inhibited retroperitoneal invasion (Keleg *et al.* 2003).

Recent studies point to the importance of cyclooxygenase and 5-lipoxygenase (5-LOX) in cancer development. Both enzymes are highly expressed in ductal adenocarcinomas of the pancreas, and this overexpression is also present in PanINs (Fig. 18.3). Especially 5-LOX is absent from all normal ductal epithelial cells of the pancreas but is already expressed in all PanIN-1 lesions. *In vitro*, the 5-LOX metabolites 5(S)-HETE and LTB_4 stimulate pancreatic cancer cell proliferation, whereas 5-LOX inhibitors inhibit cell proliferation and can induce apoptosis. 5-LOX inhibitors have been introduced into the clinic for treatment of chronic inflammatory diseases. Whether these substances could be helpful in the therapy or prevention of pancreatic cancer has not yet been answered (Hennig *et al.* 2005).

Apoptosis is the programmed cell death necessary to maintain balanced tissue homeostasis. Because chemotherapy and radiotherapy act primarily by inducing apoptosis, defects in the apoptotic pathway can cause cancer cell resistance. Resistance to apoptosis upon detachment from the extracellular matrix—so-called anoikis—is a fundamental characteristic of malignant epithelial cancer cells.

Except genetic alterations like p53 or SMAD4, which influence apoptosis in the endpoint, no mutations in the apoptosis-related genes are known, and in general the system is functional. Nevertheless, deregulation of apoptotic proteins and pathways leads to resistance to apoptosis and consequently to reduced apoptosis rates in pancreatic cancer.

Pancreatic cancer cells can evade apoptosis by downregulation of the FAS receptor and upregulation of FAP-1 (FAS-associated phosphatase), which blocks the function of FAS. Moreover, pancreatic cancer cells overexpress SODD (silencer of death domains), which suppresses TNFα-induced cell death.

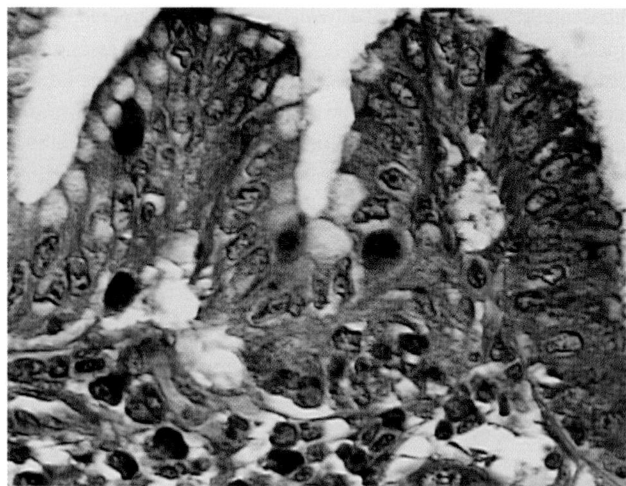

Fig. 18.3 Immunohistochemical analysis of 5-LOX in a human PanIN-3 lesion. Strong staining in ductal cells is a sign of early overexpression of this gene in the carcinogenesis of pancreatic ductal adenocarcinoma. Ducts in normal tissue do not stain for 5-LOX. (Image kindly provided by R. Hennig.)

Pancreatic cancer cells highly express TRAIL (tumor necrosis factor-related apoptosis-inducing ligand) receptors, but TRAIL-mediated apoptosis is blocked downstream in the apoptotic pathway. Antiapoptotic factors, such as BCL-2, BCL-XL and cIAP2 (cellular inhibitor of apoptosis protein 2), are overexpressed in pancreatic cancer, and expression of the pro-apoptotic BAX in pancreatic cancers has been associated with longer survival (Westphal & Kalthoff 2003).

Neuroendocrine tumors of the pancreas

Endocrine tumors of the pancreas are rare, accounting for about 1–2% of all pancreatic masses. Earlier they were also named neuroendocrine tumors of the pancreas, indicating the intimate relationship to neural elements and the frequent immunoreactivity for general neuroendocrine markers. Since histologic diagnosis can be difficult, the immunohistochemical detection of the expression of general neuroendocrine markers, such as the cytosolic markers NSE (neuron-specific enolase) and PGP 9.5 (protein gene product 9.5), small vesicle-associated markers (e.g. synaptophysin, synapsin, and synaptotagmin) or secretory granule-associated markers, such as chromogranin A and HISL-19, is routinely used to differentiate adenocarcinomas of the pancreas. Increased circulating levels of the α-subunits of hCG (human chorionic gonadotropin) have been implicated as a sign of malignancy of endocrine pancreatic tumors. It should be mentioned that there are also mixed ductal-endocrine tumors, but these are not the subject of this chapter (Oberg & Eriksson 2005).

The origin of these endocrine tumors is still under discussion. Either they evolve from the islets of Langerhans or they arise from pluripotent stem cells in the ductal epithelium (Vortmeyer *et al.* 2004). Many tumors retain the capability to produce a particular hormone, and the overproduction of insulin, glucagons, somatostatin, gastrin, or VIP (vasoactive polypeptide) is often adequate to cause clinical manifestations. The tumors might also express pancreatic polypeptide, neurotensin, cytokeratin 8, 18 and 19, and vesicle monoamine transporter proteins 1 and 2 (VMAT-1 and VMAT-2).

A number of studies have revealed that the common tumor suppressor genes (p53, retinoblastoma susceptibility gene) and oncogenes like RAS, SRC, MYC, FOS and JUN do not play dominant roles in the molecular genetics of neuroendocrine tumors. On the other hand, mutations of SMAD4/DPC4, p16/p14, and the MEN1 genes have been reported in spontaneous endocrine tumors.

As for ductal adenocarcinomas, growth factors and their receptors seem to be crucial in the biology of these tumors as well. Overexpression of the insulin-like growth factor, vascular endothelial growth factor, platelet-derived growth factor, fibroblast growth factor and transforming growth factors α and β, as well as several growth factor receptors, which leads to autocrine or paracrine growth stimulation, has been reported. Many endocrine tumors express different isoforms of the somatostatin receptors, with the somatostatin receptor 2 being predominant. Somatostatin inhibits production of multiple hormones, blocks autocrine and paracrine growth-promoting factors, and even induces apoptosis. These physiologic effects are the basis for the therapeutic use of stable analogs in these tumors. While the hormone-related symptoms can be controlled in a high percentage of patients, the clinical inhibitory effect on tumor growth has not been very satisfactory, with only 5–10% of the patients showing a measurable response.

Some of the endocrine pancreatic tumors are part of the multiple endocrine neoplasia 1 syndrome (MEN1). This syndrome exhibits an autosomal dominant pattern of inheritance. MEN1 syndrome is associated with mutations in the *menin* gene on chromosome 11q13. Menin is a tumor suppressor gene interacting as a nuclear protein with JUN D and API transcription factor. About 20% of the spontaneous endocrine neoplasms exhibit MEN1 mutations, and up to 68% show loss of heterozygosity.

A second syndrome involving hereditary endocrine tumors of the pancreas is von Hippel–Lindau disease (VHL). Five to 10 per cent of VHL patients develop pancreatic tumors, most commonly non-secretory islet cell tumors. The *VHL* gene has been localized on chromosome 3 p 25-26, and more than 250 germline mutations have been described. The VHL protein interacts with the regulatory alpha subunit of HIF and targets it for oxygen-dependent polyubiquitylation. Mutations in the VHL tumor suppressor gene lead to stabilization and inappropriate expression of HIF-1 and HIF-2 and activation of hypoxic gene response pathways.

Liver cancer

Hepatocellular carcinoma

Hepatocellular carcinoma is a malignancy affecting approximately one million people around the world every year. The incidence is low in North America and western Europe, and high in locations such as Southeast Asia and parts of Africa. Hepatocellular carcinoma (HCC) primarily affects old people, reaching its highest prevalence among those aged 65–69 years. The major etiology is chronic infection by the hepatitis B and hepatitis C viruses. Other risk factors are cirrhosis, alcohol abuse, obesity, hemochromatosis, α_1-antitripsin deficiency, and toxins similar to aflatoxin and vinyl chloride.

As for most types of cancer, hepatocarcinogenesis is a multi-step process involving multiple genetic alterations which finally ends in a malignant transformation of hepatocytes. But in contrast to some other cancers, the carcinogenesis of HCC is still poorly understood, and the morphologic and also the molecular structure of HCC is rather heterogeneous. The spectrum of etiological factors results in chronic liver injury, leading to enhanced regeneration, with liver cell turnover and development of cirrhosis. Chronic liver injury and chronic inflammation lead to oxidative stress and DNA damage. Mutations take place, activating oncogenes and deactivating tumor suppressor genes. In addition, genomic instability, DNA mismatch repair defects, and impaired chromosomal segregation promote malignant transformation. Furthermore, growth factors and proangiogenic factors are overexpressed in livers with chronic injury and regeneration, which is considered at least as a cofactor in carcinogenesis (Moradpour & Blum 2005).

The strong correlation of HCC with chronic hepatitis B infection (40% of all HCCs worldwide occur in patients infected with hepatitis B virus, HBV) suggests that the HBV directly influences DNA and carcinogenesis. Viral hepatitis induces liver injury and hepatocyte death, and promotes hepatocarcinogenesis. It is still not clear whether it is the virus infection causing the tumor initiation or whether it is the subsequent inflammation leading to liver regeneration and cirrhosis, which acts as a tumor promotor in hepatocarcinogenesis.

The genome of the HBV consists of a double-strand DNA (Fig. 18.4). For replication the virus is able to reverse transcribe an RNA intermediate. Integration of HBV DNA is not part of the virus life cycle, but rather occurs as an epiphenomenon of HBV replication. Integrated HBV DNA sequences have been found in chronic hepatitis as well as in most HBV-related HCCs.

HBV integration sites are often mutated, and chromosomal rearrangements such as translocations, deletions, and inverted duplications are frequent. Many different HBV integration sites have been documented, and these seem to be randomly distributed in the genome. Only a few integration sequences that seem to have direct oncogenic potential have been found. One example is the insertion of a hepatitis B DNA sequence in the retinoic acid receptor β (RAR-β) locus. These tumors overexpress a truncated RAR-β with altered functions. Another interesting integration site is within the cyclin A gene, resulting in a pre-S2/S–cyclin A fusion protein with increased stability. Accumulation of the cyclin A gene causes increased proliferation. However, these cases are notable exceptions and there is no specific and common integration site for hepatitis DNA in HCC. Moreover, HBV seems to be a non-selective insertional mutagen agent, and secondary chromosomal rearrangements associated with HBV DNA integration have been reported. Enhanced frequency of translocations or deletions has also been reported, suggesting that increased chromosomal instability is associated with HBV infection (Cougot *et al.* 2005).

The HBV contains a transcriptional transactivator gene called *X* gene; its gene product is referred to as X protein or HBx. This gene generally supports viral replication, and *X* gene mutations lead to substantial block in viral DNA synthesis. Although the precise role played by *X* gene remains unclear, in several models it could be shown that the X protein has oncogenic potential. HBx is a multifunctional viral regulator that modulates transcription, protein degradation, and signaling pathways. These modulations affect viral replication and viral proliferation. HBx also affects cell cycle checkpoints, cell death, and carcinogenesis.

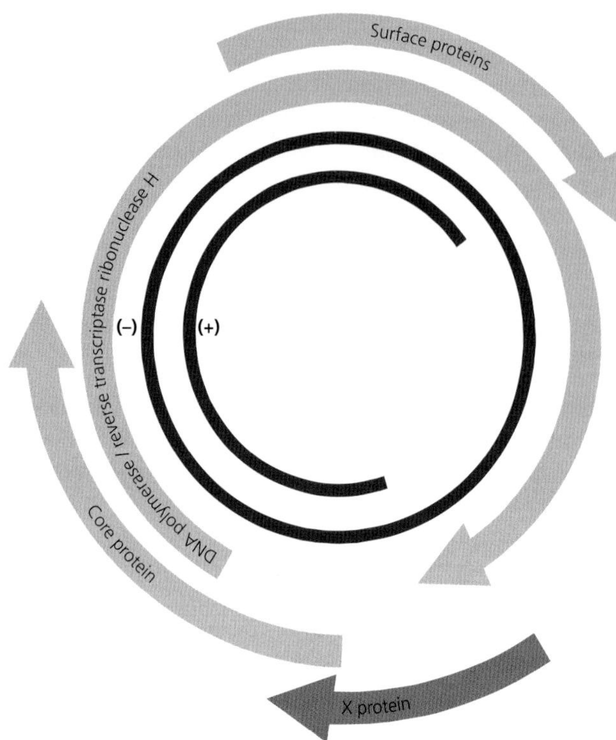

Fig. 18.4 The ~3 kbp HBV DNA in its partially double-stranded form contains at least four partially overlapping open reading strands. The viral envelope is composed of three isoforms of the surface protein, and the core protein builds the nucleocapsid. The viral polymerase can act through its different domains either as a DNA polymerase, as a reverse transcriptase, or as ribonuclease H. The X protein is a generally transcriptional transactivator and is thought to be involved in HCC carcinogenesis.

HBx activates reporter genes driven by a variety of promoters. Most HBx-responsive promoters harbor binding sites for particular transcription factors, such as AP-1, AP-2, CREB, NF-κB, c/EBP or NFAT. Besides having these direct transcriptional functions, HBx also seems to influence different signaling pathways in the cytosol of the cells, somehow activating the RAS/RAF pathway or the kinase PYK2. The detailed mechanism is not clear so far. Ca^{2+} influx is one possibility which has been considered. In addition, HBx binds to p53 and inactivates p53-dependent activities, such as p53-dependent transcriptional activity, and blocks p53-mediated apoptosis (Wang *et al.* 2002).

Like hepatitis B, hepatitis C is also a leading cause of chronic hepatitis and of the development of cirrhosis. Chronic liver injury, regeneration, and fibrosis, as mentioned above, are conditions promoting liver cell carcinogenesis. Direct mechanisms by the hepatitis C virus (HCV) leading to malignant transformation are postulated, but the evidence is not as clearly documented as for hepatitis B. Various viral proteins (e.g. 'Core' and NS5A) have been implicated in carcinogenesis of hepatocytes, but further investigations are needed to confirm this role of HCV.

Chronic hepatitis and chronic inflammatory and oxyradical disorders, including Wilson disease and hemochromatosis, generate reactive oxygen/nitrogen species that can activate signal transduction pathways, resulting in the transcriptional induction of growth-competence-related oncogenes (e.g. C-FOS, C-JUN and C-MYC). In addition, reactive oxygen species can damage DNA, resulting in mutations. A variety of genetic alterations have been found in hepatocellular carcinoma. Mutations of hepatocyte nuclear factor 1α (HNF1α), β-catenin, axin, APC, K-RAS and p53, as well as inactivation of p16 by promoter hypermethylation (75% of the HCCs) and inactivation of RB1, are common mechanisms (Laurent-Puig & Zucman-Rossi 2006).

The tumor suppressor gene *p53* plays a major role in the carcinogenesis of HCC as well as many other tumors. p53 is found mutated in more than 30% of HCCs. Interestingly, there is a large spectrum of different p53 mutations, and the specific hot spots in different tumor types make it possible to draw conclusions about environmental carcinogens. In HCC there is a point mutation at the third position of codon 249 that is atypical in other types of human cancers. It has been shown that aflatoxin B_1 (AFB_1) exposure and codon 249^{ser} mutations in HCC are correlated. Aflatoxin B_1 is a potent mutagen that is enzymatically activated by human hepatocytes, and *in vitro* binding of the AFB_1 oxide to codon 249 has been demonstrated. *HBx* gene expression increases the frequency of 249^{ser} mutations in cells exposed to AFB_1 *in vitro*. 249^{ser} mutations are also found in non-malignant hepatocytes, and the frequency is associated with dietary intake of aflatoxin B_1. Especially in areas with high AFB_1 intake, p53 mutation is an early event in carcinogenesis. On the other hand, in areas with minimal AFB_1 intake, p53 mutations may occur as a later event in tumor progression. Several studies have shown clear growth advantages and increased cell survival for p53 249^{ser} mutants. In addition to AFB1 exposure, oxidative stress in chronic inflammations, such as in patients with hemochromatosis and Wilson disease, is also associated with p53 mutations (Staib *et al.* 2003).

Cholangiocellular carcinoma

Cholangiocarcinoma is the collective term used to describe cancers arising within the intrahepatic and extrahepatic biliary tract. More than 90% of these cancers are histologically adenocarcinomas; one-third are intrahepatic, two-thirds are ductal cholangiocarcinomas. The histologic carcinogenesis ranges from hyperplastic biliary epithelium to carcinoma *in situ* and invasive cholangiocarcinoma. For most patients no conclusive risk factors can be established. Only a few patients exhibit primary sclerosing cholangitis, Caroli's disease, congenital choledochal cyst, chronic intrahepatic lithiasis, or intraductal parasitic infestation (*Clonorchis sinensis*, *Opisthorchis viverrini*), all of which are clearly associated with increased incidence of cholangiocellular carcinoma. Specific mechanisms of cancer development in association with *Opisthorchis* infection, as seen frequently in Asian countries, are rare. One study showed frequent *hMLH1* gene inactivation in liver fluke-related cholangiocarcinoma (Berthiaume & Wands 2004).

The above-mentioned chronic bile duct diseases serve as the basis for a model of cholangiocellular cancer development, with all of them leading to chronic inflammation associated with the generation of cytokines, increased reactive oxygen species, and enhanced proliferation of cholangiocytes. Eventually under these conditions accumulation of unrepaired genomic damage leads to malignant transformation of the biliary epithelial cells.

Under these conditions, interleukin (IL)-6 and hepatocyte growth factor (HGF) are upregulated, resulting in an activated MAPK-pathway via the IL-6 receptor (gp80/gp130) and the concomitantly overexpressed C-MET receptor for HGF. It has been shown that the proliferatory effect of IL-6 on biliary epithelial cells can be attenuated by phospholipase A2 and cyclooxygenase-2 (COX-2) inhibitors, suggesting that the downstream arachidonic acid/eicosanoid pathways may be important in this signaling cascade. COX-2 is overexpressed in cholangiocellular carcinomas, and expression is also seen in inflamed and dysplastic areas, as well as in neoplastic cells. *In vitro* exposure of a cholangiocarcinoma cell line to bile acids induces COX-2 expression (Wu, 2005).

The expression of other growth factor receptors, such as EGFR and c-erb-B2, plays a prominent role in the multistep process of cholangiogenesis as well. Normal and reactive biliary epithelial cells, as well as cholangiocellular cancer cells, express the EGF receptor, while normal bile ducts are usually negative for c-erb-B2, and its expression is associated with advanced tumor grades. Gene amplifications for c-erb-B2 have also been reported.

Mutations of the signaling molecule K-RAS, described above for pancreatic cancers, occur frequently in cholangiocellular carcinoma as well. The incidence is reported to be up to 100%, while the rate in countries with a large proportion of cholangiocellular cancers related to *Opisthorchis* infections seems to be much lower. Vascular endothelial growth factor (VEGF), which is thought to be the main player in paracrine stimulation of neoangiogenesis, is strongly expressed in the generally highly vascularized cholangiocarcinomas.

Mutations and inactivation of p53, as observed in many other cancers, are also common in cholangiocellular cancers. Mutation rates for p53 in cholangiocellular cancers are reported with a frequency of 20–80%. Furthermore, other alterations of the p53 pathway, such as inactivation of p21/WAF, p16 or elevated MDM2 protein levels, occur frequently in this tumor type (Berthiaume & Wands 2004).

The β-catenin pathway is activated, as shown by reduced membranous and enhanced cytoplasmic and nuclear location, in about half of the cancers. One study found axin 1 mutations in 40%, while mutations in the β-catenin and adenomatous polyposis coli genes are seldom in this type of cancer. Furthermore, cyclin D1, C-MYC and urinary-type plasminogen activator receptor, which are downstream target genes in the WNT signaling pathway, were overexpressed.

Cholangiocarcinoma cells are more resistant to apoptosis than non-transformed bile duct epithelial cells. While the FAS receptor remains expressed on these cells, the signaling molecule FLIP is upregulated. FLIP is thought to inhibit the activation of procaspase 8, which forwards the downstream signaling from the death receptor. As a second mechanism, nitric oxide is proposed to directly inhibit apoptosis. In some studies the antiapoptotic proteins BCL-2, BCL-XL and MCL-1 have been shown to be overexpressed and were presumed responsible for inhibition of apoptosis. However, there was some controversy between different studies. As mentioned before, COX-2 is overexpressed in cholangiocellular carcinomas, and in several *in vitro* studies COX-2 serves as an inhibitor of apoptosis. Finally, growth factor receptors such as EGFR and c-erb-B2, which signal with the RAS/RAF as well as the PI3K pathway, are antiapoptotic in general. This is a significant aspect of cancer biology not only in cholangiocellular cancers but also in many other systems (Celli & Que 1998).

References

Al Aynati MM, Radulovich N, Riddell RH, Tsao MS. (2004) Epithelial-cadherin and beta-catenin expression changes in pancreatic intraepithelial neoplasia. *Clin Cancer Res* 10(4): 1235–40.

Berthiaume EP, Wands J. (2004) The molecular pathogenesis of cholangiocarcinoma. *Semin Liver Dis* 24(2): 127–37.

Celli A, Que FG. (1998) Dysregulation of apoptosis in the cholangiopathies and cholangiocarcinoma. *Semin Liver Dis* 18(2): 177–85.

Cougot D, Neuveut C, Buendia MA. (2005) HBV-induced carcinogenesis. *J Clin Virol* 34(Suppl 1): S75–S78.

Friess H, Guo XZ, Nan BC, Kleeff O, Buchler MW. (1999) Growth factors and cytokines in pancreatic carcinogenesis. *Ann NY Acad Sci* 880: 110–21.

Hennig R, Grippo P, Ding XZ *et al.* (2005) 5-Lipoxygenase, a marker for early pancreatic intraepithelial neoplastic lesions. *Cancer Res* 65(14): 6011–16.

Hruban RH, Adsay NV, Albores-Saavedra J *et al.* (2001) Pancreatic intraepithelial neoplasia: a new nomenclature and classification system for pancreatic duct lesions. *Am J Surg Pathol* 25(5): 579–86.

Keleg S, Buchler P, Ludwig R, Buchler MW, Friess H. I(2003) nvasion and metastasis in pancreatic cancer. *Mol Cancer* 2: 14.

Ketterer K, Rao S, Friess H, Weiss J, Buchler MW, Korc M. (2003) Reverse transcription-PCR analysis of laser-captured cells points to potential paracrine and autocrine actions of neurotrophins in pancreatic cancer. *Clin Cancer Res* 9(14): 5127–36.

Korc M. (2003) Pathways for aberrant angiogenesis in pancreatic cancer. *Mol Cancer* 2: 8.

Laurent-Puig P, Zucman-Rossi J. (2006) Genetics of hepatocellular tumors. *Oncogene* 25(27): 3778–86.

Maitra A, Kern SE, Hruban RH. (2006) Molecular pathogenesis of pancreatic cancer. *Best Pract Res Clin Gastroenterol* 20(2): 211–26.

Moradpour D, Blum HE. (2005) Pathogenesis of hepatocellular carcinoma. *Eur J Gastroenterol Hepatol* 17(5): 477–83.

Oberg K, Eriksson B. (2005) Endocrine tumours of the pancreas. *Best Pract Res Clin Gastroenterol* 19(5): 753–81.

Schneider G, Schmid RM. (2003) Genetic alterations in pancreatic carcinoma. *Mol Cancer* 2: 15.

Staib F, Hussain SP, Hofseth LJ, Wang XW, Harris CC. (2003) TP53 and liver carcinogenesis. *Hum Mutat* 21(3): 201–16.

Vortmeyer AO, Huang S, Lubensky I, Zhuang Z. (2004) Non-islet origin of pancreatic islet cell tumors. *J Clin Endocrinol Metab* 89(4): 1934–8.

Wang XW, Hussain SP, Huo TI *et al.* (2002) Molecular pathogenesis of human hepatocellular carcinoma. *Toxicology* Dec 27:181–182: 43–47.

Westphal S, Kalthoff H. (2003) Apoptosis: targets in pancreatic cancer. *Mol Cancer* 2: 6.

Wu T. (2005) Cyclooxygenase-2 and prostaglandin signaling in cholangiocarcinoma. *Biochim Biophys Acta* 1755(2): 135–50.

19 Primary Liver Cancer

Edited by Charlie Pan & Theodore Lawrence

Diagnosis

History and clinical

Jorge A. Marrero & Charlie Pan

Hepatic tumors may originate from the liver (hepatocytes, bile duct epithelium or mesenchymal tissue), or spread to the liver from primary lesions in other organs. This section will concentrate on the clinical aspects of a diagnosis of hepatocellular carcinoma (HCC), the most common primary hepatic neoplasm.

Hepatocellular carcinoma is the fifth most common solid tumor worldwide (Parkin *et al.* 2001), and the incidence in the United States is increasing (El Serag & Mason 1999). In the United States, it is currently the tumor with the second highest increase in incidence and the one with the highest increase in death rates over the last 10 years in the United States (www.seer.gov). It has been estimated that the number of cases of HCC will continue to increase by 81%, from a baseline of about 18,000 in 2005 based on the Surveillance Epidemiology and End Result Program, by the year 2020. Despite advances in medical technology, the 5-year survival between 1981 and 1998 improved only 3%, likely due to the fact that the majority of patients with HCC are diagnosed at advanced stages leading to an overall 1-year survival of 25% in the United States (El Serag & Mason 2001). To understand the clinical aspects in the diagnosis of HCC, it is important to understand the patients at risk for developing this tumor.

Population at risk

One of the issues that separates HCC from other solid organ tumors is that the majority of patients have underlying liver disease. Table 19.1 shows the risk factors for the development of HCC. The largest concentration of cases of liver cancer in the world is in Asia, followed by Africa, Europe, North and South America (Fattovich *et al.* 2004). In Japan, Europe and America about 60% of cases of HCC are attributed to chronic hepatitis C (HCV) infection, while 20% are attributed to chronic hepatitis B (HBV) infection, and about 20% to cryptogenic and alcoholic liver disease (Fattovich *et al.* 2004). In high HBV prevalence areas such as Eastern Asia, China and Africa, about 8% of the population is chronically infected, due to vertical (mother-to-child) or horizontal (child-to-child) transmission, resulting in about 80% of patients with HCC having underlying chronic HBV infection. The broad traits of the epidemiology of HCC can be traced to the prevalence of hepatotropic viral infections.

More than 80% of the cases of HCC occur in the setting of cirrhosis (Kao *et al.* 2000). The risk of HCC in persons with HBV increases from asymptomatic carriers, inactive carriers and chronic hepatitis without cirrhosis (all with an incidence <1 per 100 person-years), to 2.2–4.3 per 100 person-years in compensated cirrhotics (Kao *et al.* 2000). One important feature of HCC in patients with chronic HBV infection is that about 20% of patients present without evidence of cirrhosis. Risk for development of HCC is also related to a high degree of viral replication, viral genotype, and concomitant use of alcohol and tobacco (Donato *et al.* 1998; Donato *et al.* 2002; Chen *et al.* 2003; Franceschi *et al.* 2006).

The risk of HCC among patients with chronic HCV infection occurs mainly in the setting of patients with cirrhosis. In the United States and Europe, the summary incidence rate in cirrhotic patients with HCV infection has been shown to be 3.7 per 100 person-years, whereas it was zero for patients with chronic hepatitis without cirrhosis (Kao *et al.* 2000). The 5-year cumulative incidence rate for HCC in patients with cirrhosis was 17% in Europe and the United States, while it was 30% in Japan. The incidence of HCC among those patients with the other causes of cirrhosis listed in Table 19.1 is slightly lower than those with chronic HCV infection. Among patients with cirrhosis, alcohol use, tobacco use, obesity, diabetes, older age

Gastrointestinal Oncology: A Critical Multidisciplinary Team Approach. Edited by J. Jankowski, R. Sampliner, D. Kerr, and Y. Fong.

Table 19.1 Risk factors for developing hepatocellular carcinoma.

Host related factors
Older age
Male gender
Severity of liver disease
Obesity
Diabetes
Chronic liver disease
Hepatitis B
Hepatitis C
Alcoholic liver disease
Hereditary hemochromatosis
Non-alcoholic fatty liver disease
Primary biliary cirrhosis
Autoimmune hepatitis
External factors
Alcohol
Tobacco
Aflatoxin
Thorotrast
Androgenic steroids

and male gender increase the risk for the development of HCC (Kao *et al.* 2000; Calle *et al.* 2003; El-Serag *et al.* 2004; Lazaridis & Gores 2005; Marrero *et al.* 2005).

Screening

Criteria have been developed, first promoted by the World Health Organization, to assure the benefits of screening for a specific disease (Sarasin *et al.* 1996). HCC meets these criteria for performing screening. Several decision analysis models have shown that the surveillance of HCC is a cost-effective strategy, and these studies also showed that an incidence rate of HCC of at least 1.5% per year should trigger surveillance (Trevisani *et al.* 2001). Patients with cirrhosis have an incidence rate >1.5% per year, and therefore they are the target population for performing surveillance for HCC.

Since the goal of screening is to reduce mortality by detecting patients with occult disease, patients with cirrhosis (regardless of the cause) present a unique opportunity for screening for HCC. The most commonly used screening test for HCC is the alpha-fetoprotein (AFP). It has been shown that the optimal balance of sensitivity and specificity is achieved by a cut-off level of 20 ng/mL (Bruix & Sherman 2005). However, this cut-off leads to sensitivities between 41% and 60% and specificities between 80% and 94% (Zhang *et al.* 2004). The other surveillance test that is commonly used is ultrasound (US) of the liver. The sensitivity and specificity of US has been shown to be between 58% and 78% and 93% and 98%, respectively (Zhang *et al.* 2004). A recent randomized controlled study of screening for HCC has been performed in China (Llovet *et al.* 1999). This study compared US and AFP versus no screening in 18,818 HBV carriers and it achieved a compliance rate of 60%. It showed that screening led to a reduction of 37% in mortality compared to no screening. This is the first evidence that the strategy of surveillance for HCC with AFP and US improves mortality. The recent guidelines by the American Association for the Study of Liver Disease recommended the surveillance to involve US and AFP at a frequency of 6–12 months (Zhang *et al.* 2004).

History and clinical symptoms

When evaluating a patient, one must determine any predisposing factors for HCC, such as history of hepatitis or jaundice, blood transfusion, or use of intravenous drugs. A detailed review of any family history, specifically of HCC or hepatitis, and a detailed social history should be performed.

Because screening for HCC in patients with cirrhosis has been shown to reduce overall mortality, many patients are now diagnosed with asymptomatic, occult disease (small tumors). It has been shown that about 23% of patients with HCC are diagnosed at the asymptomatic stage while 32% have abdominal pain, 8% have jaundice, 10% have anorexia and weight loss, and 6% general malaise (Koprowski *et al.* 1979). Other symptoms include abdominal swelling or vomiting. It is important to point out that these symptoms are not specific of HCC and mainly indicate the presence of significant tumor burden. Because the majority of patients with HCC have underlying liver disease, a significant proportion of patients do present with hepatic decompensation at the time of diagnosis. These include variceal hemorrhage, development of ascites and hepatic encephalopathy, and jaundice.

Common physical signs include hepatomegaly, hepatic bruit, ascites, splenomegaly, jaundice, wasting, and fever. Hepatomegaly is the most frequent physical sign, occurring in 50–90% of patients. Especially in endemic areas, livers may be massive. Abdominal bruits arising from the HCC, presumably from the associated vascularity, occur in 5–25%. Ascites occur in 30–60% of patients, and this is usually due to underlying liver disease. Occasionally, this may be caused by hemoperitoneum.

Serologic assays

AFP level is elevated in approximately 70% of individuals in Asian countries with HCC, while it is only increased in approximately 50% of patients in the United States and Europe (Piper 1992). In a patient who presents with a new hepatic mass, AFP should be drawn. Additionally, carcinoembryonic antigen (CEA), prothrombin time, partial thromboplastin time, albumin level, transaminases, lactate dehydrogenase, and alkaline phosphatases should be measured. Platelet count and white blood cell count decreases may reflect portal hypertension and associated hypersplenism. Serologic testing for hepatitis A, B, C, and D viruses should be performed.

References

Bruix J, Sherman M. (2005) Management of hepatocellular carcinoma. *Hepatology* 42: 1208–36.

Calle EE, Rodriguez C, Walker-Thurmond K, Thun MJ. (2003) Overweight, obesity, and mortality from cancer in a prospectively studied cohort of U.S. adults. *N Engl J Med* 348: 1625–38.

Chen Z, Liu B, Boreham J, Wu Y, Chen J, Peto R. (2003) Smoking and liver cancer in China: case-control comparison of 36,000 liver cancer deaths vs. 17,000 cirrhosis deaths. *Int J Cancer* 107: 106–12.

Donato F, Boffetta P, Puoti M. (1998) A metaanalysis of epidemiological studies on the combined effects of hepatitis B and C virus in causing hepatocellular carcinoma. *Int J Cancer* 75: 347–54.

Donato F, Tagger A, Gelatti U, Parrinello G, Bofetta P, Albertini A. (2002) Alcohol and hepatocellular carcinoma: the effect of lifetime intake and viral hepatitis infection in men and women. *Am J Epidemiol* 155: 323–31.

El Serag H, Mason A. (1999) Rising incidence of hepatocellular carcinoma in the United States. *N Engl J Med* 340: 745–50.

El Serag H, Mason A. (2001) Trends in survival of patients with hepatocellular carcinoma between 1977 and 1996 in the United States. *Hepatology* 33: 62–5.

El-Serag HB, Tran T, Everhart JE. (2004) Diabetes increases the risk of chronic liver disease and hepatocellular carcinoma. *Gastroenterology* 126: 460–8.

Fattovich G, Stroffolini T, Zagni I, Donato F. (2004) *Gastroenterology* 127: S35–S50.

Franceschi S, Montella M, Polese LJ *et al.* (2006) Hepatitis viruses, alcohol, and tobacco in the etiology of hepatocellular carcinoma in Italy. *Cancer Epidemiol Biomarkers Prev* 15: 683–9.

Kao J, Chen P, Lai M, Chen D. (2000) Hepatitis B genotypes correlate with clinical outcomes in patients with chronic hepatitis B. *Gastroenterology* 118: 554–9.

Koprowski H, Steplewski Z, Mitchell K, Herlyn M, Herlyn D, Fuhrer P. (1979) Colorectal carcinoma antigens detected by hybridoma antibodies. *Somatic Cell Genet* 5: 957–71.

Lazaridis KN, Gores GJ. (2005) Cholangiocarcinoma. *Gastroenterology* 128: 1655–67.

Llovet JM, Bru C, Bruix J. (1999) Prognosis of hepatocellular carcinoma: the BCLC staging classification. *Semin Liver Dis* 19: 329–38.

Marrero JA, Fontana RJ, Fu S, Conjeevaram HS, Su GL, Lok AS. (2005) Alcohol, tobacco and obesity are synergistic risk factors for hepatocellular carcinoma. *J Hepatol* 42: 218–24.

Parkin D, Bray F, Ferlay J, Pisani P. (2001) Estimating the world cancer burden: Globocan 2000. *Int J Cancer* 94: 153–6.

Piper M. (1992) Alpha-fetoprotein (AFP) and des-gamma-carboxyprothombin (DCP) in hepatocellular carcinoma (HCC) and chronic liver diseases. *Hepatology* 16: 538.

Sarasin FP, Giostra E, Hadengue A. (1996) Cost-effectiveness of screening for detection of small hepatocellular carcinoma in western patients with Child-Pugh class A cirrhosis. *Am J Med* 101: 422–34.

Trevisani F, D'intino PE, Morselli-Labate AM *et al.* (2001) Serum alpha-fetoprotein for diagnosis of hepatocellular carcinoma in patients with chronic liver disease: influence of HBsAg and anti-HCV status. *J Hepatol* 34: 570–5.

Zhang BH, Yang BH, Tang ZY. (2004) Randomized controlled trial of screening for hepatocellular carcinoma. *J Cancer Res Clin Oncol* 130: 417–22.

Histopathology

Rebecca F. Harrison & Angus H. McGregor

Histopathology of hepatocellular carcinoma

This section deals with the most common of hepatic primary malignancies, hepatocellular carcinoma (HCC). HCC is one of the three most common cancers worldwide. The most important etiologic factors are hepatitis B virus (HBV) and hepatitis C virus (HCV) infection, with up to 80% of HCC worldwide being related to one or another of these viruses. Accordingly, the distribution of these infections reflects the incidence of HCC, being commonest in East Asia, South Africa and sub-Saharan Africa, with lower rates in northern Europe and Australia (Hirohashi *et al.* 2000). HBV exerts its effects by integration into the host genome; HCV, of which there are at least six major subtypes, does not integrate into the host genome but exerts its effects via chronic inflammation and proinflammatory cytokines resulting in fibrosis and cirrhosis. However, evidence is accumulating that HCV may also contribute directly to HCC by influencing oncogenic pathways such as Wnt signalling/beta-catenin pathway (Levrero 2006). In Western countries the presence of cirrhosis due to whatever cause is a risk factor for HCC, with 80% of HCCs developing on a background of cirrhosis, but alcohol-induced liver injury is the commonest cause of HCC. Other diseases with a strong association with development of HCC are hemochromatosis, secondary hemosiderosis and tyrosinemia. Other well-documented risk factors for HCC include ingestion of aflatoxin B_1 produced by the mould *Aspergillus* on grain and peanuts.

Pathologic features

HCC is most commonly seen arising in the cirrhotic liver, but in the West, the background liver is frequently non-cirrhotic. Macroscopically, and most commonly, HCC may be solitary (Fig. 19.1), often possessing a fibrous capsule, or may present as nodules of varying sizes; typically there are intrahepatic satellite nodules. Grossly the tumors are soft and bulge from the fresh cut surface; they may appear yellowish-green due to bile production within the tumor, but if there is little or no bile production they appear greyish-pink.

The macroscopic assessment of a hepatectomy specimen containing HCC should include the size, color and consistency of the tumor and its relationship to portal structures, gallbladder bed, resection margins and liver capsule. Blocks of each tumor and the interface between tumor and uninvolved liver should be sampled for histologic examination. Background liver should also be sampled, as this is important for assessment of the pre-existing liver disease and any portal vein invasion, which is characteristic of HCC. Biopsy specimens are of the

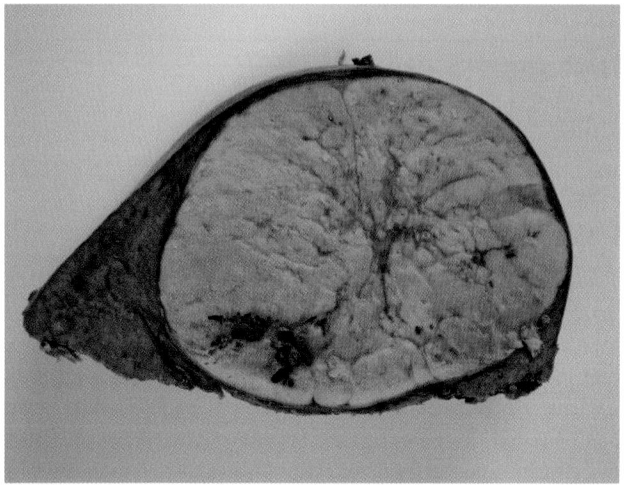

Fig. 19.1 Hepatocellular carcinoma in a cirrhotic liver.

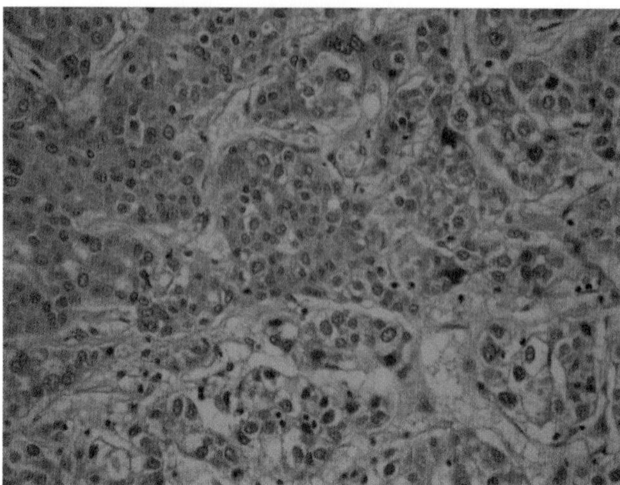

Fig. 19.2 Hepatocellular carcinoma composed of trabeculae and groups of eosinophilic cells resembling hepatocytes.

transcutaneous needle type or transjugular, the latter generally being smaller specimens and more difficult to interpret.

There have been several attempts at gross classification of HCC. Of these, Eggel's classification (Eggel) is still probably the most utilitarian; it describes tumors as being 'massive' (single large mass), with or without satellite nodules; nodular (multiple nodules), and diffuse, when there are many, often ill-defined nodules throughout the liver. However, despite other terms such as infiltrating, pushing and expansive, none of these classifications has been of any proven prognostic significance. Several other macroscopic patterns, however, do appear to have some relationship to prognosis, including the encapsulated and pedunculated varieties; it is thought that this morphology is a result of somewhat slower growth and therefore a better prognosis is associated with them. With the advent of transplantation, so-called 'small HCC' (Leoni *et al.* 2006) has been recognised. Such tumors are 2 cm or less in size and are often multifocal in a background cirrhotic liver, but they do not appear to differ significantly from other types of HCC.

Microscopically, most commonly the tumor cells of HCC mimic normal hepatocytes and may form trabecula or pseudoacini (Fig. 19.2). Tumor cells can also contain many of the features seen in non-neoplastic hepatocytes such as fat, Mallory's hyalin, fibrinogen, and alpha-1 antitrypsin globules. Other recognised growth patterns include a scirrhous type characterised by extensive fibrosis, pleomorphic cell variant with bizarre giant cells, a clear cell variant where tumor cells have abundant clear cytoplasm containing glycogen, and a sarcomatoid change where the cells become more spindled (Ishak *et al.* 2001). Bile production seen as canalicular plugs or intracytoplasmic granules in tumor cells, is pathognomonic of HCC, but is not often seen.

A particularly important subcategory of HCC is the fibrolamellar variant which occurs mainly in young people in the West. Microscopically and macroscopically, fibrolamellar hepatoma has a distinctive appearance: tumor cells are large, polygonal with abundant pink cytoplasm, and grow in short trabecula or sheets separated by septa of fibrous tissue. There are often pale-pink globular intracytoplasmic inclusions which stain positively on immunohistochemistry for fibrinogen. The cytoplasmic granularity seen is due to an abundance of mitochondria which can be demonstrated on electron microscopy. Macroscopically, there is characteristically a central stellate fibrous scar, which because of its morphologic similarity to that found in focal nodular hyperplasia was at one time thought to possibly relate to these two entities. Fibrolamellar HCC is also distinguished by its more favorable prognosis and slower growth when compared to other subtypes of HCC.

Edmondson and Steiner first proposed a grading system for HCC in which well-differentiated tumors indistinguishable from hepatic adenomas were classified as grade 1, and anaplastic, pleomorphic tumors were classified as grade 4 (Edmondson & Steiner 1954). This system has formed the basis for many studies up to the present day, ranging from survival studies to correlation with molecular biomarkers. However, there are a number of problems with grading HCCs, not the least being that a range of differentiations can occur within a single tumor. Other systems, including detailed nuclear assessments and modifications of the original grading system, have been performed but there are opposing views as to the prognostic utility of grading at all.

Combined tumors

In 1–2% cases an HCC may exhibit the features of both hepatocellular and cholangiocellular differentiation, so-called combined hepatocellular cholangiocarcinoma. The latter component can be distinguished by its biliary epithelial-type appearance and/or production of luminal/intracytoplasmic mucin seen on PAS–D/Alcian blue staining. The acinar differentiation seen in HCC should not be confused with this and is surrounded by neighbouring hepatocytes and lacks surrounding stroma. Such tumors may be genuine single tumors, though occasionally they can result from the 'collision' of separate HCC and cholangiocarcinoma (Ishak *et al.* 2001).Very rarely HCC has a sarcomatous element which may show differentiation to recognisable elements such as bone or cartilage. Undifferentiated sarcomatous areas are vimentin positive and occasionally cytokeratin positive on immunohistochemistry.

Hepatocellular dysplasia

HCC is believed to evolve from hepatocellular dysplasia which causes a number of problems in terms of diagnostic accuracy and nomenclature. Small foci of dysplasia can be seen on biopsy but are usually invisible on imaging. Large cell dysplasia was always considered to be the most likely precursor lesion for hepatocellular carcinoma, but there is now controversy over this. Some evidence has suggested a four- to fivefold increased risk for HCC, but it may represent a reactive process to cholestasis or a change in normal liver cell polyploidy. Small cell liver cell dysplasia, or small cell change, refers to hepatocytes that have an increased nuclear: cytoplasmic ratio, contrasting with large cell dysplasia, in which this ratio is normal. In fact the nuclei are larger than those of normal hepatocytes. Morphologic studies (Edmondson & Steiner 1954) suggest that this type of dysplasia may be the real precursor lesion to liver cancer.

With regard to discrete dysplastic lesions, the preferred terminology is of dysplastic nodules; synonyms include the older terms macroregenerative nodule, adenomatous hyperplasia and atypical adenomatous hyperplasia. Dysplastic nodules can show low- or high-grade dysplasia. It can be difficult to distinguish high-grade dysplastic nodules from early HCC, the latter being often indistinct and well differentiated in chronic liver disease. However, such nodules larger than 1.5 cm in diameter are generally regarded as small hepatocellular carcinomas. In hemachromatosis, foci of hepatocytes containing much less iron than the cells in the surrounding liver, and having an expanding nature as seen on reticulin staining, are thought to be preneoplastic.

Differential diagnosis

One of the major problematic areas in differential diagnosis is distinguishing well-differentiated HCC from hepatocellular adenoma. It should be emphasized that such a distinction cannot be accomplished by frozen section, as it is problematical even on paraffin sections. Indeed, the role of frozen section in the intraoperative identification of hepatocellular nodules is limited; distinguishing focal nodular hyperplasia, hepatic adenoma, HCC, dysplastic nodules and macroregenerative nodules is not in the scope of the frozen section investigation. In distinguishing hepatic adenoma from HCC, absence of pericellular reticulin staining in HCC is often helpful (Scheuer & Lefkowitch 2000). In focal nodular hyperplasia, there are 'pseudoportal tracts' with transformed ductular structures which are absent in HCC. Hepatoid adenocarcinoma arising from a gastrointestinal or Mullerian origin can be a convincing mimic of primary HCC and may even produce bile and express AFP.

Table 19.2 Immunohistochemical markers useful in the differential diagnosis of the three commonest hepatic malignancies.

Antibody	HCC	Cholangiocarcinoma	Metastatic adenocarcinoma
CK7	–	+++	–
CK20	–	+	+++
CD10	++	–	+/–
CEA-polyclonal	+++	–	–
EMA	–	+++	+++
HepPAR1	+++	–	–
CA19-9	–	+++	+++
CK19	–	+++	+++
AFP	+	–	–
AE1	+	+++	+

Immunohistochemistry in differential diagnosis

Table 19.2 illustrates antibodies which may be useful in assessment of HCC. CD10 and polyclonal carcinoembryonic antigen (CEA) stain the brush border of neocanaliculae. This contrasts with diffuse cytoplasmic staining as in other epithelial tumor types; this pattern of staining is specific and can aid greatly in differential diagnosis between metastatic adenocarcinoma, cholangiocarcinoma and HCC. HepPar1 is highly specific for hepatocellular differentiation but is only expressed in around 75% of HCC and also stains non-neoplastic hepatocytes. In routine use, it is much less helpful in poorly differentiated tumors, which is precisely when additional diagnostic modalities are needed. Alpha-fetoprotein (AFP) is detectable by immunohistochemistry in less than 40% of tumors and its routine use has been abandoned by some pathologists. Differential cytokeratin stains are frequently used in diagnostic pathology. They are especially useful when dealing with a metastasis from an unknown primary. Cytokeratins 7 and 20 (CK7 and CK20) are most commonly used in the field of gastrointestinal pathology. CK20 is a good marker for adenocarcinomas arising in the colon, and CK7 is similarly useful to suggest a pancreaticobiliary or lung origin. By way of contrast, HCC is negative for CK7 and CK20. CD34 is a marker of capillarized endothelium that is expressed in the vasculature of HCC but not in normal liver sinusoidal endothelium; however it cannot help distinguish HCC from hepatic adenoma or focal nodular hyperplasia.

Patterns of metastasis

HCC metastasizes chiefly via the hematogenous route. Portal vein invasion with thrombosis is seen in 65–75% and hepatic vein thrombosis in 20–25% of cases. Extension into the vena cava and right heart is described. Around 5% of cases have bile duct invasion. Sixty per cent of tumors show intrahepatic metastases, but if the tumor is greater than 5 cm in diameter, this increases to 95%. Local invasion in advanced disease may involve the diaphragm, gallbladder and peritoneum.

Molecular pathology

A wide range of molecular markers have been assessed in HCC with the intention of relating their expression to differentiation and prognosis, including p53, CD81, heat shock proteins (HSP) and p21. It is becoming recognised that HCC may have several different biologic phenotypes. Evidence for this comes from several papers. In one, which subtypes hepatocellular carcinoma according to patterns of CK7 and CK19 expression, it has been shown that cytokeratin 7/19 positivity was associated with poorer prognosis, elevated serum AFP, less parenchymal fibrosis and higher recurrence rate. This type of tumor is potentially derived from hepatic progenitor cells, as they express both CK7 and CK19 (Durnez *et al.* 2006). In another, tumors which shared their gene expression pattern with fetal hepatoblasts had a poorer prognosis; the same markers were identified in hepatic oval cells, also suggesting an origin from hepatic progenitor cells (Lee *et al.* 2006). The oncogene *met* signaling pathway is often associated with tumor progression, and in hepatocellular carcinoma, expression of this pathway is significantly associated with increased microvascular density, increased vascular invasion and reduced mean survival (Kaposi-Novak *et al.* 2006). Increased VEGF expression and microvascular density correlate with invasiveness and likelihood of extrahepatic metastasis and recurrence (Yao *et al.* 2005). HSP expression (implicated in the regulation of apoptosis) is frequently upregulated in HCC (Edmondson & Steiner 1954). In HBV-associated HCC, HSP expression increased from dysplastic nodules to overt malignancy.

References

Durnez A, Verslype C, Nevens F. (2006) The clinicopathological and prognostic relevance of cytokeratin 7 and 19 expression in hepatocellular carcinoma. A possible progenitor cell origin. *Histopathology* 49: 138–51.

Edmondson HA, Steiner P. (1954) Primary carcinoma of the liver: a study of 100 cases among 48,900 necropsies. *Cancer* 7: 462–503.

Eggel H. (1910) Uber das primare Carcinom der Leber. *Beitr z path Anat z allg Path*: 506–604.

Hirohashi S, Ishal KG, Kojiro M. (2000) Hepatocellular carcinoma. In: Hamilton SR, Aaltonen LA, eds. *WHO Classification of Tumours: Tumours of the Digestive System*, pp. 158–81. IARC Press, Lyon.

Ishak KA, Goodman ZD, Stocker J. (2001) Hepatocellular carcinoma. In: *Tumours of the liver and bile ducts*, pp. 199–230. Armed Forces Institute Publishing, Washington.

Kaposi-Novak P, Lee J, Gomez-Quiroz L, Coulouarn C, Factor V, Thorgeirsson S. (2006) Met-regulated expression signature defines a subset of human hepatocellular carcinomas with poor prognosis and aggressive phenotype. *J Clin Invest* 116: 1582–95.

Lee J, Heo J, Libbrecht L. (2006) A novel prognostic subtype of human hepatocellular carcinoma derived form hepatic progenitor cells. *Nature Medicine*: 410–6.

Leoni S, Piscaglia F, Righini R, Bolondi L. (2006) management of small hepatocellular carcinoma. *Acta Gastroenterol Belg* 69: 230–55.

Levrero M. (2006) Viral hepatitis and liver cancer: the case of hepatitis C. *Oncogene* 25: 3834–47.

Scheuer P, Lefkowitch JH. (2000) *Neoplasms and Nodules in Liver Biopsy Interpretation*, 6th edn. WB Saunders, Philadelphia.

Yao D, Wu X, Zhu Y. (2005) Quantitative analysis of vascular endothelial growth factor, microvascular density and their clinicopathologic features in human hepatocellular carcinoma. Hepatobiliary pancreatic. *Disease International* 4: 220–6.

Imaging and staging

Jonathon Willatt & Hero K. Hussain

Introduction

The imaging of hepatocellular carcinoma (HCC) can be divided into three steps: diagnosis, staging, and surveillance following locoregional treatment. This review of imaging will discuss the roles of ultrasound, CT and MRI in the context of these three stages.

For many years the diagnosis of HCC was dependent on percutaneous biopsy. Tumor staging required invasive procedures such as angiography and lipiodol CT. Although non-invasive imaging techniques are now generally used for both the detection and the staging of HCC, imaging in cirrhosis remains challenging.

The development of HCC in the cirrhotic liver is described either as de novo hepatocarcinogenesis or as a multistep progression from regenerative nodule (RN) to low-grade dysplastic nodule (DN) to high-grade dysplastic nodule, dysplastic nodule with microscopic foci of HCC, small HCC, and finally to overt carcinoma. Patients with high-grade dysplastic nodules are at the greatest risk for HCC. It is because of the multistep process that the imaging features of these nodules overlap, particularly with regard to differentiation of dysplastic nodules and small HCC. The imaging features during the progression to cancer can be largely explained by the changes in the nature of the blood supply to the nodule. Studies based on findings at CT during arterial portography (CTAP) and CT during hepatic arteriography (CTHA) with pathologic correlation have shown that as the grade of malignancy within the nodules evolves, there is gradual reduction of the normal hepatic arterial and portal venous supply to the nodule followed by an increase in the abnormal arterial supply via newly formed abnormal arteries (neoangiogenesis). Histopathologically, this corresponds to a diminution in the portal tracts (portal vein and hepatic artery) which are virtually absent in HCC.

An RN is defined as a hepatocellular nodule containing more than one portal tract located in a liver that is otherwise abnormal due to either cirrhosis or other severe disease. These nodules are present in all cirrhotic livers and are surrounded by fibrous septa (Baron & Peterson 2001). The blood supply of an RN continues to be largely from the portal vein, with minimal contribution from the hepatic artery. This vascular supply dynamic explains why there is no enhancement during the hepatic arterial phase. Regenerative nodules can become large and mimic a mass.

A DN is defined as a nodule of hepatocytes of at least 1 mm in diameter with dysplasia of low or high grade but no histologic criteria for malignancy, usually found in a cirrhotic liver. Low-grade DN (LG-DN) are composed of liver cells with minimally increased nuclear : cytoplasmic ratio, nuclear atypia, and absent mitosis (Ishak *et al.* 2001b). These nodules are not premalignant. High-grade DN (HG-DN) display moderate atypia and occasional mitosis. They may even express AFP but are not frankly malignant. They are considered premalignant, and development of HCC within a DN has been documented within as little as 4 months (Sakamoto *et al.* 1991). Occasionally, DN can be larger than 2 cm in size.

HCC is defined as a malignant neoplasm composed of cells that differentiate in some way in the manner of hepatocytes (Ishak *et al.* 2001a). Macroscopically HCC is classified as 'massive' when there is a single large mass with or without small satellite nodules; as 'nodular' when there are multiple, fairly discrete nodules throughout the liver; or as 'diffuse' when there are multiple, minute indistinct nodules throughout the liver (Ishak *et al.* 2001a).

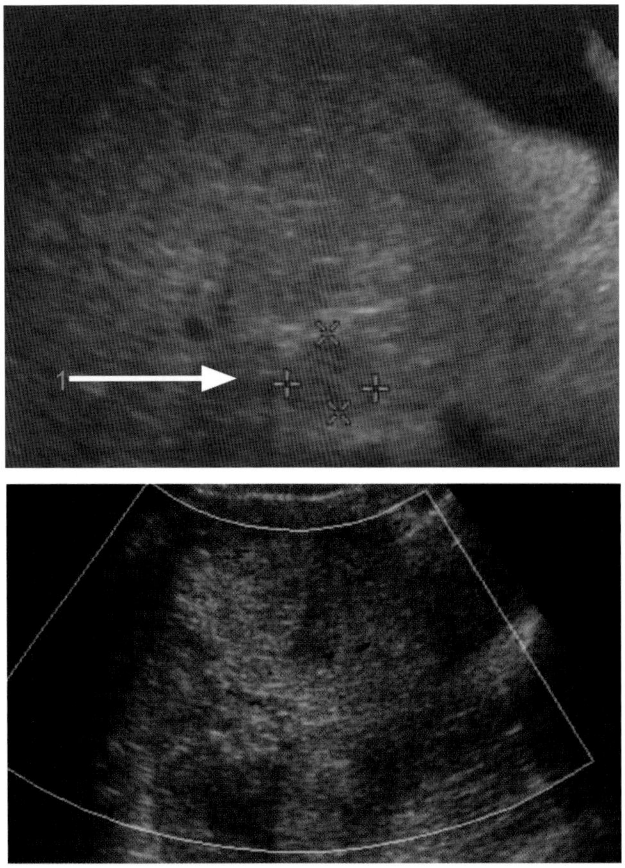

(a)

(b)

Fig. 19.3 (a) Greyscale ultrasound shows a 2-cm hypoechoic HCC in the right hepatic lobe. (b) In a different patient there is a diffusely heterogenous appearance consistent with a large HCC. Arterial flow is shown on color Doppler.

Ultrasound

The advantages of ultrasound include its cost, availability, and ability to guide biopsy. Owing to its global availability, ultrasound has received considerable attention as a tumor-screening technique and is still often quoted as the main imaging screening modality (Bruix *et al.* 2001). Ultrasound is able to characterize common benign lesions (cysts, hemangiomas). It is also non-invasive unless ultrasound contrast agents are used. Its weaknesses include its inability to image the entire liver in some patients and its operator dependence. Larger patient body habitus can also be a limiting factor.

The gray-scale appearance of HCC is variable. Smaller lesions can appear hyperechoic, isoechoic, or hypoechoic (Dodd *et al.* 1992) (Fig. 19.3). In a patient with multinodular HCC the liver appears nodular and the tumor has irregular or blurred margins. Necrotic areas will appear hypoechoic and hemorrhagic areas will vary in their complexity depending on the chronicity. It is difficult to differentiate tumors from metastases or benign lesions on gray-scale imaging. With the help of color Doppler equipment, blood flow within liver tumors can be identified and the pattern of flow on spectral analysis can be used to characterize lesions.

Sonography is not a reliable screening technique for HCC. Prospective studies with explant correlation have shown a sensitivity for detection of malignancy of around 50% and a sensitivity for individual lesion detection of only 45% (Dodd *et al.* 1992). Retrospective studies have shown lesion detection sensitivities of 20–67% (Liu *et al.* 2003). In all of these studies detectability was significantly affected by tumor size, the sensitivity being the least with the smaller lesions.

The introduction of contrast agents will open new opportunities for ultrasound specialists (Fracanzani *et al.* 2001). HCC shows strong intratumoral enhancement in the arterial phase followed by rapid washout with an isoechoic or hypoechoic appearance in the portal and delayed phases. Regenerative and dysplastic nodules do not show early contrast uptake. Contrast agents are limited, however, in assessing the whole of the liver as the dynamic nature of the agent inhibits full review of all segments of the liver following a single injection.

CT and MRI

The advent of spiral and multidetector CT and of rapid MR imaging sequences has enabled radiologists to scan the whole of the liver in a single breath-hold. Multiplanar imaging capability is no longer an issue following the advent of multidetector CT. The liver can be scanned in the different phases of contrast enhancement to facilitate characterization of hepatic lesions. Images can be reviewed in axial, sagittal and coronal planes. Both dynamic contrast-enhanced helical CT and MRI using a bolus injection of contrast material play an important role in the detection and staging of HCC. The timing of the arterial phase is crucial as HCC classically enhances in the arterial phase and demonstrates hypointensity or hypoattenuation in the delayed phase. Although variability in the arrival of the arterial phase of contrast is well recognized, imaging at around 10–15 seconds following the trigger from bolus tracking creates the optimal tumor to liver attenuation difference. However, given the variability in cardiovascular dynamics, there is concern that tumors can be missed and up to six arterial phases have been proposed to minimize this (Ito 2006). Optimal venous imaging is at 45 seconds. Delayed phase imaging can be performed at 180–210 seconds from the start of the injection.

The process of neoangiogenesis or arterial recruitment dictates the main imaging feature of HCC, which is arterial enhancement (Marrero *et al.* 2005). Arterial enhancement is considered an essential characteristic of HCC and is used as the only radiologic feature for the non-invasive diagnosis of HCC by the United Network for Organ Sharing (UNOS) (Sharing 2005). Arterial enhancement is heterogeneous in large lesions and homogeneous in small lesions (Yamashita *et al.* 1996).

HCC becomes isodense or hypodense to the liver on the venous phase of CT as the remainder of the liver enhances most avidly and homogeneously during this phase. However, the delayed phase is also useful as tumors will have lost most of their contrast by this stage whilst the liver parenchyma will still retain contrast during this interstitial equilibrium phase. HCC will therefore characteristically appear as hypodense during the delayed phase (Yamashita *et al.* 1996) (Fig. 19.4). A small proportion of dysplastic nodules receive their supply from the hepatic artery and the delayed phase can therefore play a role in distinguishing these precancerous nodules from HCC.

Large tumors present a mosaic appearance on contrast-enhanced CT, which reflects tumor composed of multiple internal regions of hemorrhage, necrosis, fatty metamorphosis, and fibrosis. Calcifications are seen in up to 28% of large tumors. A thin surrounding capsule is often seen which is of low attenuation on unenhanced imaging, of low or intermediate attenuation on arterial phase imaging, and of high attenuation on the delayed phases (Peterson & Baron 2001). Satellite lesions are often seen.

Apart from the main distinguishing features of arterial enhancement and delayed hypoattenuation, and a hypoattenuating rim on the arterial phase which becomes hyperattenuating

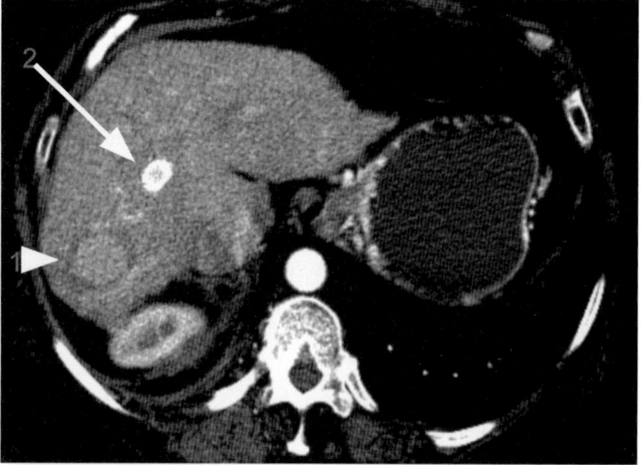

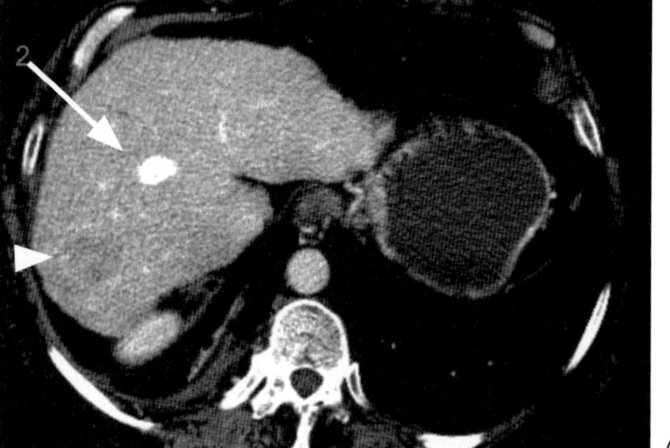

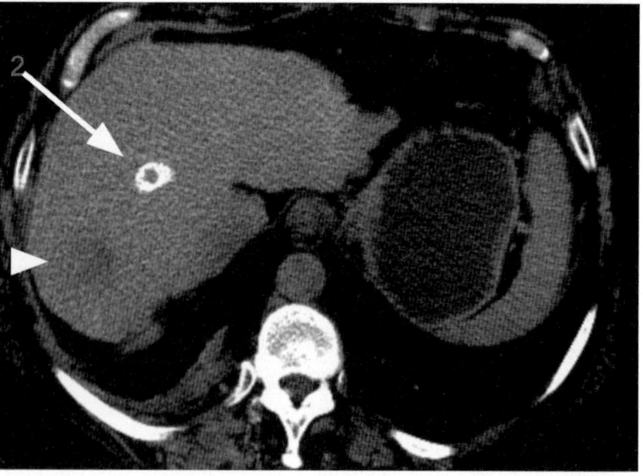

Fig. 19.4 A 3.5-cm HCC (arrow 1) in the right hepatic lobe which shows arterial enhancement (a) and hypoattenuation on the venous and delayed phases (b and c). There is a TIPS shunt (arrow 2).

on the delayed phase, invasion of portal vein branches is also helpful when identified.

The reported sensitivity of CT, however, remains poor. Lencioni (Lencioni *et al.* 2005) summarizes six series of lesion-by-lesion imaging pathologic correlations in explanted livers. The sensitivity of spiral CT in the detection of HCC ranges from

52% to 79%. Only 10–43% of lesions smaller than 1 cm and 44–65% of lesions measuring 1–2 cm were identified. The specificity of CT is also limited, as benign lesions such as adenoma, hemangioma, focal nodular hyperplasia, as well as regenerative and dysplastic nodules can demonstrate arterial enhancement (Freeny *et al.* 2003).

Although the most common appearance of HCC on MRI is hypointensity on T1-weighted imaging, hyperintensity on T2-weighted imaging, and diffuse heterogeneous arterial enhancement with venous washout, small HCCs measuring equal or less than 1.5 cm are frequently isointense on T1-weighted and T2-weighted imaging and are only detected in the arterial phase (Kelekis *et al.* 1998). Occasional high signal intensity on T1-weighted imaging is attributed to intratumoral fat, copper or glycogen in the surrounding parenchyma. Fat content leads to signal loss on opposed phase imaging (Mitchell *et al.* 1991).

Enhancement in the arterial phase is the main distinguishing feature. Tumors usually become hypointense in the portal venous and delayed phases (Fig. 19.5) and often have a delayed enhancing capsule. Occasionally, however, early-stage HCC, especially tumors smaller than 2 cm, can be isointense or hypointense in the arterial phase. This probably reflects the stage of carcinogenesis within the nodule where there has been partial or complete loss of the normal portal tract with no associated increased arterialization to cause hyperintensity in the arterial phase (Ito 2006).

Histologically and radiologically it can be difficult to differentiate some dysplastic nodules and small HCC. Radiologic criteria favoring malignancy are larger than 3 cm in size, hyperintensity on T2-weighted imaging, delayed hypointensity 'washout', delayed enhancing tumor capsule, and rapid interval growth (Krinsky & Lee 2000).

Large HCC is characterized by a more variable pattern. The mosaic pattern of confluent nodules separated by fibrous septa and areas of necrosis is usually of high signal on T2-weighted imaging and enhances heterogeneously. Large HCCs (>2 cm) do not pose a diagnostic problem. Diffuse-type HCC constitutes up to 13% of cases of HCC and appears as an extensive, heterogeneous permeative hepatic tumor with portal venous tumor thrombosis, often associated with elevated serum AFP. These tumors have a patchy or nodular early enhancement pattern and can be difficult to detect on T1-weighted or T2-weighted imaging. They become hypointense in the late phases of enhancement.

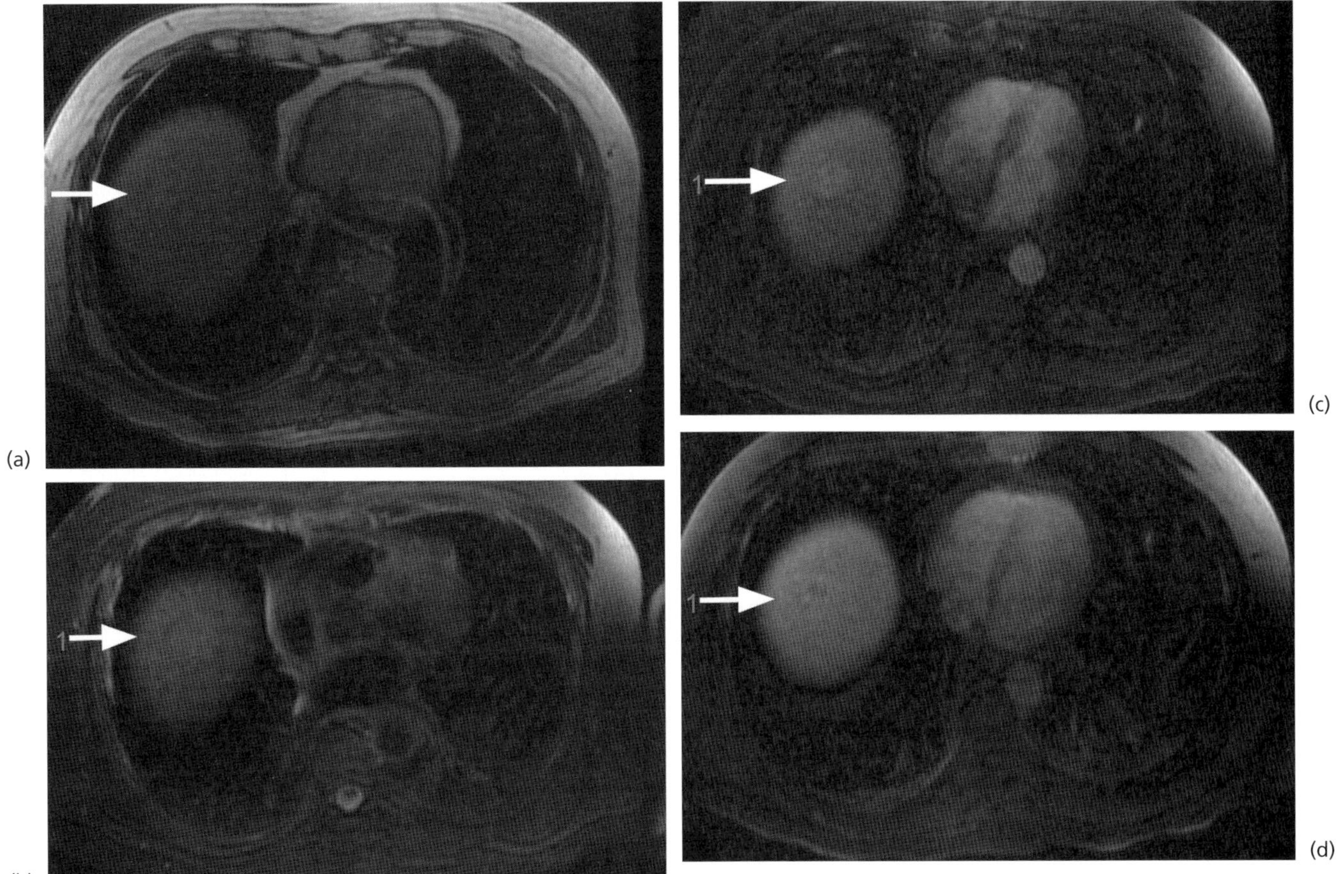

Fig. 19.5 A 3-cm HCC in the right hepatic lobe shows mild hyperintensity on T1-weighted (T1-w) imaging (a), hyperintensity on T2-w imaging (b), arterial enhancement (c), and hypointensity on the delayed phase (d).

The main difficulty in imaging the cirrhotic liver is determining the etiology of small (<2 cm) arterially enhancing lesions. The advantage of MRI over CT is excellent tissue contrast. With the use of fat suppression techniques, the conspicuity of small enhancing lesions in the liver parenchyma is increased. By using a combination of unenhanced T1-weighted imaging, T2-weighted imaging, in- and out-of-phase chemical shift imaging, and dynamic gadolinium enhancement, characterization of a large proportion of hepatic nodules in the context of cirrhosis is possible. The advantage of CT is mainly temporal. With imaging acquisition possible within 5 seconds using 16- and 64-slice CT scanners, it is now possible to acquire both early arterial phase imaging, which can be used for mapping the hepatic arteries for surgical planning, and late arterial phase imaging which is optimal for the detection of HCC. The other advantage of dual arterial phase imaging is that the optimal time for catching the enhancement of small HCC is rarely missed.

Accuracies of ultrasound, CT, and MRI

Two studies, both published since 2001, have compared the sensitivities of ultrasound, CT and MRI and show that contrast-enhanced MRI is the most sensitive technique for detecting liver nodules (Table 19.3)(Rode *et al.* 2001; Libbrecht *et al.* 2002). Their conclusions were that currently used imaging techniques cannot correctly determine the exact tumor burden in some cirrhotic patients, that lesions smaller than 1 cm are never seen on ultrasound, and that lesions smaller than 5 mm are never shown on CT or MRI. Because of these shortcomings patients undergo transplantation even though they exceed the tumor number limit and patients are explanted despite having no malignant lesion.

Colli *et al.*(Colli *et al.* 2006) performed a systematic review of 30 studies comparing ultrasound, spiral CT and MRI, as well as alpha-fetoprotein (AFP), and found that although ultrasound is highly specific, it is insufficiently sensitive to support an effective surveillance program. MRI was found to be the most sensitive of the three tests.

The role of imaging in HCC

Imaging plays an increasingly important role in the detection and staging of HCC, as well as in the assessment of response to treatment. Although ultrasound has been the mainstay of screening in the past, it has been shown that this technique is too insensitive. Therefore, depending on availability, either spiral CT or MRI should be used as the imaging techniques for screening of HCC in the cirrhotic patient. If HCC is suspected on CT, MRI should be used to stage the patient. Following locoregional treatment or transplant, MRI should then remain the primary imaging technique given its greater sensitivity. CT should be limited to those patients who are unable to undergo MRI for technical reasons.

Staging of HCC

Several staging systems have been proposed for HCC. The United Network for Organ Sharing (UNOS) uses the modified tumor/node/metastasis (TNM) staging system for HCC to determine eligibility for liver transplantation. Patients with TNM stage II HCC (a single tumor 2–5 cm or up to three tumors, all ≤3.0 cm) with no extrahepatic spread and/or macrovascular involvement (i.e. porta or hepatic veins) are eligible for liver transplantation. The modified TNM classification is based on the Milan criteria for HCC, which has been widely used as the guideline for selection of patients for transplantation. The Milan criteria were embraced after a study by Mazzaferro et al. (Mazzaferro *et al.* 1996) showed excellent overall and recurrence-free survival rates of 85% and 92%, respectively, at 4 years after orthotopic liver transplantation in patients with solitary HCC not exceeding 5 cm in maximal diameter, and no more than three tumors with none greater than 3 cm.

However, unlike most cancers, staging of HCC is not simply a process of measuring tumor extent, nodal involvement and metastasis, or of assessing the aggressiveness of the tumor by its histologic characteristics. The staging of HCC, particularly in the context of assessment for resection or for transplantation, is complicated by the fact that it is almost always found on the background of cirrhosis and therefore liver function has to be taken into account. For this reason the staging process is complicated and several different systems have been proposed.

The best staging system for HCC has been shown to include tumor burden, hepatic function, and overall patient health and has a link to treatment. The only staging system that includes these criteria is the Barcelona Clinic Liver Cancer (BCLC)

Table 19.3 Sensitivity and specificity of imaging modalities.

Study	Ultrasound		CT		MRI	
	Sensitivity (%)	Specificity (%)	Sensitivity (%)	Specificity (%)	Sensitivity (%)	Specificity (%)
Rode *et al.* (69 nodules)	46	95	54	93	77	57
Libbrecht *et al.* (49 patients)	40	100	50	79	70	82

system, which was recently endorsed by the 2005 European Association for the Study of the Liver (EASL) and the American Association for the study of Liver Disease (AASLD).

The BCLC staging system is linked to an evidence-based treatment strategy: radical approaches including resection and transplantation are offered to patients at stage 0 (HCC <2 cm without vascular invasion or spread) and stage A (solitary tumor of up to 5 cm or up to three nodules ≤3 cm). If radical therapies are not feasible, patients are evaluated for percutaneous ablative treatments. With this strategy the expected 5-year survival is between 50% and 75%. Chemoembolization is offered to stage B patients (large or multinodular HCC without vascular invasion, extrahepatic spread, or cancer-related symptoms), particularly those with compensated cirrhosis. The expected 3-year survival in these patients may exceed 50%. Patients with stage C disease (advanced tumor with vascular involvement, extrahepatic spread, or physical impairment) are entered into research trials to assess new antitumoral agents. Their survival is less than 10% at 3 years. Finally, patients at stage D (with impaired physical status or excessive tumor burden and severe liver impairment) receive symptomatic treatment to minimize suffering. Their survival at 1 year is also usually less than 10%.

References

Baron RL, Peterson MS. (2001) From the RSNA refresher courses: screening the cirrhotic liver for hepatocellular carcinoma with CT and MR imaging: opportunities and pitfalls. *Radiographics* 21 Spec No: S117–32.

Bruix J, Sherman M, Llovet JM *et al.* (2001) Clinical management of hepatocellular carcinoma. Conclusions of the Barcelona-2000 EASL conference. European Association for the Study of the Liver. *J Hepatol* 35: 421–30.

Colli A, Fraquelli M, Casazza G *et al.* (2006) Accuracy of ultrasonography, spiral CT, magnetic resonance, and alpha-fetoprotein in diagnosing hepatocellular carcinoma: a systematic review. *Am J Gastroenterol* 101: 513–23.

Dodd GD 3rd, Miller WJ, Baron RL, Skolnick ML, Campbell WL. (1992) Detection of malignant tumors in end-stage cirrhotic livers: efficacy of sonography as a screening technique. *AJR Am J Roentgenol* 159: 727–33.

Fracanzani AL, Burdick L, Borzio M *et al.* (2001) Contrast-enhanced Doppler ultrasonography in the diagnosis of hepatocellular carcinoma and premalignant lesions in patients with cirrhosis. *Hepatology* 34: 1109–12.

Freeny PC, Grossholz M, Kaakaji K, Schmiedl UP. (2003) Significance of hyperattenuating and contrast-enhancing hepatic nodules detected in the cirrhotic liver during arterial phase helical CT in pre-liver transplant patients: radiologic-histopathologic correlation of explanted livers. *Abdom Imaging* 28: 333–46.

Ishak K, Goodman Z, Stocker J. (2001a) Hepatocellular carcinoma. In: Rosai J, ed. *Atlas of Tumor Pathology. Tumors of the Liver and Intrahepatic Bile Ducts*, Third series Washington DC, Armed Forces Institute of Pathology, 199–230.

Ishak K, Goodman Z, Stocker J. (2001b) Putative precancerous lesions. In: Rosai J, ed. *Atlas of Tumor Pathology. Tumors of the Liver and Intrahepatic Bile Ducts*, Third series Washington DC, Armed Forces Institute of Pathology, 185–198.

Ito K. (2006) Hepatocellular carcinoma: conventional MRI findings including gadolinium-enhanced dynamic imaging. *Eur J Radiol* 58: 186–99.

Kelekis NL, Semelka RC, Worawattanakul S *et al.* (1998) Hepatocellular carcinoma in North America: a multiinstitutional study of appearance on T1-weighted, T2-weighted, and serial gadolinium-enhanced gradient-echo images. *AJR Am J Roentgenol* 170: 1005–13.

Krinsky GA, Lee VS. (2000) MR imaging of cirrhotic nodules. *Abdom Imaging* 25: 471–82.

Lencioni R, Cioni D, Della Pina C, Crocetti L, Bartolozzi C. (2005) Imaging diagnosis. *Semin Liver Dis* 25: 162–70.

Libbrecht L, Bielen D, Verslype C *et al.* (2002) Focal lesions in cirrhotic explant livers: pathological evaluation and accuracy of pretransplantation imaging examinations. *Liver Transpl* 8: 749–61.

Liu WC, Lim JH, Park CK *et al.* (2003) Poor sensitivity of sonography in detection of hepatocellular carcinoma in advanced liver cirrhosis: accuracy of pretransplantation sonography in 118 patients. *Eur Radiol* 13: 1693–8.

Marrero JA, Hussain HK, Nghiem HV, Umar R, Fontana RJ, Lok AS. (2005) Improving the prediction of hepatocellular carcinoma in cirrhotic patients with an arterially-enhancing liver mass. *Liver Transpl* 11: 281–9.

Mazzaferro V, Regalia E, Doci R *et al.* (1996) Liver transplantation for the treatment of small hepatocellular carcinomas in patients with cirrhosis. *N Engl J Med* 334: 693–9.

Mitchell DG, Palazzo J, Hann HW, Rifkin MD, Burk DL Jr, Rubin R. (1991) Hepatocellular tumors with high signal on T1-weighted MR images: chemical shift MR imaging and histologic correlation. *J Comput Assist Tomogr* 15: 762–9.

Peterson MS, Baron RL. (2001) Radiologic diagnosis of hepatocellular carcinoma. *Clin Liver Dis* 5: 123–44.

Rode A, Bancel B, Douek P *et al.* (2001) Small nodule detection in cirrhotic livers: evaluation with US, spiral CT, and MRI and correlation with pathologic examination of explanted liver. *J Comput Assist Tomogr* 25: 327–36.

Sakamoto M, Hirohashi S, Shimosato Y. (1991) Early stages of multistep hepatocarcinogenesis: adenomatous hyperplasia and early hepatocellular carcinoma. *Hum Pathol* 22: 172–8.

United Network for Organ Sharing. http://www.unos.org/policiesandbylaws/policies.asp?resources-true. Accessesed December 11, 2007.

Yamashita Y, Mitsuzaki K, Yi T, Ogata I, Nishiharu T, Urata J, Takahashi M. (1996) Small hepatocellular carcinoma in patients with chronic liver damage: prospective comparison of detection with dynamic MR imaging and helical CT of the whole liver. *Radiology* 200: 79–84.

Treatment

Overview

Charlie Pan

Treatment of hepatocellular carcinoma (HCC) is complex, because of both the number of treatment options and the underlying liver disease that affects the majority of HCC patients. Because the natural history of HCC is variable, from approximately 5 months median survival for advanced tumors (vascular invasions, symptoms, extrahepatic spread) to a more prolonged survival even without treatment (Llovet *et al.* 1999), treatment results in the literature can be difficult to interpret. This is in part due to the profound effect on overall survival of the underlying liver disease, which therefore must be taken into account when making clinical management choices. A multidisciplinary team, including a hepatologist, surgical oncologist, transplant surgeon, interventional radiologist, radiation oncologist, and medical oncologist, is important for the comprehensive management of HCC patients.

For early-stage tumors, treatment options include surgical resection, local ablation (radiofrequency ablation), local injection therapies (ethanol injection), and radiation therapy. Additionally, as many patients have underlying liver disease and may not tolerate a significant loss of normal hepatic parenchyma due to treatment, these patients may also be eligible for liver transplantation. One principle to follow in the treatment of early-stage HCC is maximal sparing of normal hepatic parenchyma.

For intermediate-stage tumors, surgical or local therapy options are usually unavailable. In patients without cirrhosis, a major hepatectomy is feasible and provides the best chance of long-term survival, although prognosis is poor. Preoperative portal vein occlusion to induce compensatory hypertrophy may improve the tolerability of a major hepatectomy in these patients. Although this approach is unproven, neoadjuvant treatment approaches such as chemoembolization may decrease the size of the primary tumor to allow for less surgery. Successful regional therapies may also make patients eligible for transplantation.

Advanced-stage and metastatic patients have limited options. Prognosis is especially poor for these patients, and no surgical treatment is recommended. These patients should be enrolled onto clinical trials testing novel agents or managed symptomatically.

A guideline from the American Association for the Study of Liver Disease (AASLD) (Bruix & Sherman 2005) provides a reasonable algorithm for therapy (Fig. 19.6). In this algorithm, patients who have a single lesion can be offered surgical resection if they are non-cirrhotic or have cirrhosis but still have well preserved liver function, normal bilirubin and hepatic vein pressure gradient < 10 mmHg. Liver transplantation is an effective option for patients with HCC corresponding to the Milan criteria: solitary tumor < 5 cm or up to three nodules < 3 cm. Living donor transplantation should be considered for HCC if the waiting time for a cadaveric transplantation is long enough to result in tumor progression leading to exclusion from the waiting list. Preoperative therapy can be considered if the waiting list exceeds 6 months. Local ablation is safe and effective therapy for patients who cannot undergo resection, or as a bridge to transplantation. Alcohol injection and radiofrequency are equally effective for tumors < 2 cm. However, the necrotic effect of radiofrequency is more predictable in all tumor sizes and, in addition its efficacy is clearly superior to that of alcohol injection in larger tumors.

For patients without curative options, transarterial chemoembolization (TACE) is recommended as first line non-curative therapy for non-surgical patients with large/multifocal HCC who do not have vascular invasion or extrahepatic spread. Tamoxifen, antiandrogens, octreotide or hepatic artery ligation/embolization are not recommended. Other options such as radiolabeled yttrium-90 glass beads, radiolabeled lipiodol, or immunotherapy cannot currently be recommended as standard therapy for advanced HCC outside of clinical trials. Systemic chemotherapy is also not recommended outside of clinical trials.

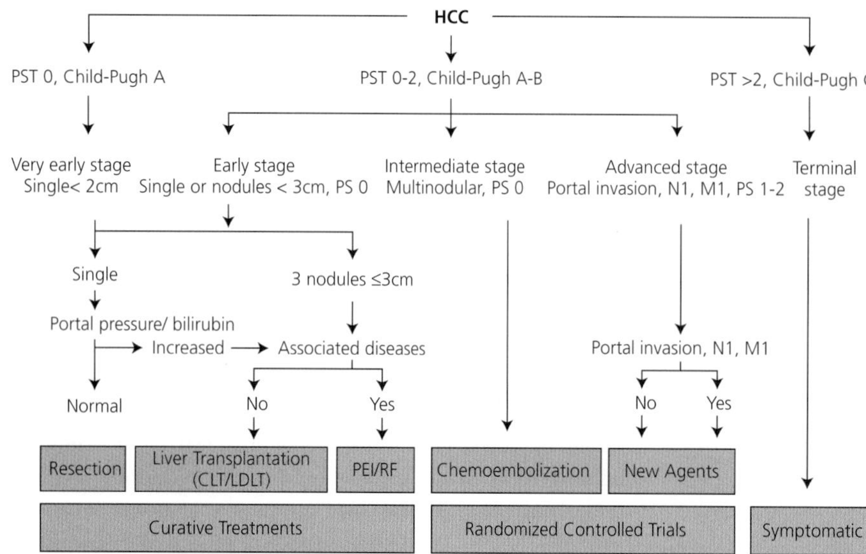

Fig. 19.6 Strategy for staging and treatment assignment in patients diagnosed with HCC according to the BCLC proposal.

References

Bruix J, Sherman M. (2005) Management of hepatocellular carcinoma. *Hepatology* 42: 1208–36.

Llovet JM, Bustamante J, Castells A *et al.* (1999) Natural history of untreated nonsurgical hepatocellular carcinoma: rationale for the design and evaluation of therapeutic trials. *Hepatology* 29: 62–7.

Surgery

Shawn J. Pelletier & James A. Knol

Introduction

Historically, patients with primary liver tumors generally would present with advanced disease and were not candidates for surgical resection. With advancements in imaging and screening, an increasing proportion of primary liver cancers are now being identified at an earlier stage. This may increase the number of patients eligible for therapies offering a high rate of potential cure using surgical resection or liver transplantation (Llovet *et al.* 2003). At present, the data used to develop treatment strategies for patients with primary liver cancers are limited to cohort investigations with few randomized controlled trials. In this section, discussion for surgical treatment will be limited to HCC.

Most patients with HCC represent a challenging population for surgical resection, largely related to underlying liver disease, usually cirrhosis. Although not true for the fibrolamellar variant, most patients with HCC have cirrhosis associated with hepatitis B infection worldwide, or, increasingly in the United States, hepatitis C virus infection, with a smaller proportion due only to alcohol. Because of decreased hepatic reserve and risk of bleeding from portal hypertension, surgical resection in patients with cirrhosis can be more difficult and is associated with an increased morbidity and mortality. In general, the first line of therapy for HCC remains surgical resection. However, in patients with cirrhosis there is a high rate of recurrent cancer, and resection can only be performed safely in selected patients because many present with decompensated cirrhosis, with multifocal HCC, or with tumors requiring an extensive resection in the setting of limited hepatic reserve. For patients with decompensated cirrhosis and with a solitary cancer not invading major hepatic vasculature or with early multifocal disease (up to three lesions, none larger than 3 cm) (Mazzaferro *et al.* 1996), the best option may be liver transplantation (Llovet *et al.* 2003). For patients with solitary tumors and well-compensated cirrhosis not requiring a major hepatic resection (four or more segments), the optimal treatment strategy is likely to be resection, but the best treatment is still under debate (Llovet *et al.* 2000).

Surgical resection for HCC

Surgical resection is clearly the treatment of choice for HCC in non-cirrhotic patients. One of the major limitations on resection of HCC is imposed by the presence of cirrhosis, and absence of cirrhosis allows much larger liver resections to achieve cure. The operative mortality and morbidity are also much lower than in those patients with cirrhosis. In the West, about 60% of patients with HCC do not have cirrhosis, whereas in Asia and among emigrant Asians, only about 25% of patients with HCC do not have underlying cirrhosis (Vauthey *et al.* 1995). Five-year survival after resection of HCC in patients without cirrhosis is about 40%, which is similar to the 5-year survival in patients with cirrhosis; however, the average size of resected tumors in patients without cirrhosis tends to be larger than in resected patients with cirrhosis (Vauthey *et al.* 1995). Patient selection influences the survival rate, illustrated by series that report that in selected patients with cirrhosis, 5-year survival after resection can exceed 50–70% (Takayama *et al.* 1998; Fong *et al.* 1999; Arii *et al.* 2000; Grazi *et al.* 2001). Therefore, preoperative evaluation is needed to determine the extent of fibrosis and hepatic reserve, to determine if compensated cirrhosis is present, and to determine the extent of portal hypertension.

Preoperative evaluation

For cirrhotic patients undergoing any major surgical procedure, the risk of liver decompensation leading to death is a major concern. Multiple preoperative criteria have been developed to predict which cirrhotic patients are likely to tolerate liver resection (Table 19.4). Preoperative evaluation of cirrhotics has, classically, included determination of Child–Pugh classification (Pugh *et al.* 1973). However, patients with Child–Pugh Class A cirrhosis may have portal hypertension, mild elevations in bilirubin, or fluid retention, all of which can be features of advanced disease (D'Amico *et al.* 1986; Gines *et al.* 1987). Child–Pugh classification alone does not accurately predict which patients will tolerate surgical resection, nor the extent of

Table 19.4 Guidelines to predict which cirrhotic patients with resectable HCC will tolerate surgical resection.

No evidence of portal hypertension

1 Platelet count >100,000/mm^3
2 No evidence of ascites
3 No evidence of esophageal varices
4 Hepatic venous pressure gradient ≤10 mmHg

Adequate liver functional reserve

1 Normal bilirubin
2 Normal coagulation studies
3 Indocyanine green retention rate ≤20% after 15 minutes
4 Tumor not requiring extensive resection such as right hepatic lobectomy or trisegmentectomy

such resection. In Japan, indocyanine green retention has been used to determine the extent of resection expected to be tolerated (Torzilli *et al.* 1999). In the United States and Europe, the extent of portal hypertension has been used as a guide to help predict the ability to tolerate resection. Portal hypertension can be suspected if esophageal varices or ascites are present. Also, clinically significant portal hypertension can be suspected if platelet counts $< 100{,}000/\mu L$ are associated with splenomegaly (Bruix & Sherman 2005). In indeterminate cases, the difference in pressure between the right atrium and the wedged hepatic vein, termed the corrected sinusoidal pressure, can be measured using hepatic vein catheterization, with portal hypertension defined as corrected sinusoidal pressure > 10 mmHg. In patients with a normal total bilirubin and no portal hypertension, the risk for decompensation is low and a 5-year survival >70% can be achieved in patients resected for HCC (Bruix *et al.* 1996; Llovet *et al.* 1999). In the short term, despite an initially increased operative risk, patients with cirrhosis who have adequate hepatic reserve may fare as well as patients who do not have cirrhosis (Vauthey *et al.* 1995).

Liver resection and surgical margin

For compensated cirrhotic patients eligible for resection, the least amount of liver possible should be resected. In most cases, this will involve a wedge or a segmental anatomic resection according to Couinaud criteria. With current techniques, in selected patients with cirrhosis, segmental resections can be performed safely and the need for blood transfusion occurs only in about 10% and mortality related to surgery may be as low as 1–3% (Rees *et al.* 1996; Llovet *et al.* 1999; Torzilli *et al.* 1999). Neoadjuvant therapies including transarterial chemoembolization (TACE) prior to resection do not appear beneficial in decreasing tumor size such that the needed size of resection is decreased (Yamasaki *et al.* 1996). Whereas a left hepatic lobectomy may be possible in selected patients with cirrhosis, a right hepatic lobectomy is more likely to result in postoperative liver failure. Volumetric analysis of the proposed liver resection is useful for more extensive resections (Torzilli *et al.* 1999). However, there are minimal data regarding safe resection with respect to ratio of remnant liver volume to functional liver volume in patients with cirrhosis. When an extensive resection is necessary and adequate hepatic reserve is questionable, portal vein embolization (PVE) of the involved hepatic lobe (future surgical specimen) can be performed several weeks preoperatively to induce compensatory hypertrophy in the unaffected lobe (surgical remnant) (Tanaka *et al.* 2000; Farges *et al.* 2003). However, no randomized studies have been performed to confirm that PVE is beneficial, particularly in patients with cirrhosis. Concerns include the delay that PVE requires from patient presentation until resection, that PVE may induce hepatic decompensation, and the theoretical possibility that malignant hepatocytes may respond to the stimulus for proliferation.

The importance of ensuring a wide surgical margin in resections of HCC is controversial. One of the characteristics of larger HCC tumors is the frequent presence of satellite tumors scattered about the neighborhood of the large tumor. Some reports have shown that a clearance of less than 1 cm is associated with higher rates of intrahepatic recurrence, but other reports have not confirmed that contention (Belghiti *et al.* 1991; Arii *et al.* 1992; Chen *et al.* 1994). Moreover, the usefulness of the 1-cm margin has been challenged. The frequent detection of synchronous tumors in the residual liver suggests recurrence near the surgical site may be due to an undetected synchronous tumor as much as from an incomplete resection or failure to encompass satellite lesions. In general, our practice is to attempt to obtain a 1-cm margin around all detectable tumor, but a negative pathologic margin is considered acceptable.

Treatment of recurrence

The rate of relapse after surgical resection for hepatocellular carcinoma may be as high as 70% at 5 years (Shirabe *et al.* 1991; Okada *et al.* 1994; Adachi *et al.* 1995; Llovet *et al.* 1999; Poon *et al.* 1999; Minagawa *et al.* 2003) and is most likely to be detected within the first 3 years (Imamura *et al.* 2003). The strongest predictors of recurrence following resection are vascular invasion and multifocal disease (Shirabe *et al.* 1991; Nagasue *et al.* 1993; Okada *et al.* 1994; Adachi *et al.* 1995; Llovet *et al.* 1999; Poon *et al.* 1999; Minagawa *et al.* 2003). For surgical resection, tumor size alone is not a limiting factor. Although risk of vascular invasion or dissemination increases with tumor size (Nakashima *et al.* 2003) some tumors may grow to be relatively large without vascular invasion and have the same prognosis after resection as smaller tumors (Okada *et al.* 1994; Llovet *et al.* 1999). Although several strategies have been explored, adjuvant therapy has not been demonstrated to reduce the rate of recurrence (Schwartz *et al.* 2002).

Although recurrent solitary tumors may benefit from re-resection, most patients with recurrence of HCC after resection will present with multifocal disease (Takayasu *et al.* 1989; Poon *et al.* 2002; Minagawa *et al.* 2003). Approximately 60% of those with recurrence may be candidates for salvage liver transplantation (Majno *et al.* 2000; Tanaka *et al.* 2005). Some have proposed that those with a high likelihood for recurrence, as determined by post-resection pathology, should be listed for liver transplantation immediately after resection (Sala *et al.* 2004). The life expectancy for patients undergoing primary resection followed by salvage transplantation has been calculated to be 7.8 years (Majno *et al.* 2000).

Liver transplantation for HCC

Because of poor recipient selection, liver transplantation for HCC in the 1980s resulted in a high recurrence rate and poor survival. Since 1996 and the publication of the Milan criteria by Mazzaferro *et al.* (Mazzaferro *et al.* 1996) HCCs meeting those criteria have become a standard indication for liver transplantation. The post-transplant patient survival rates in those selected patients are now similar to those in liver recipients without cancer. Compared to liver resection, liver transplantation has the advantage of not only widely resecting the primary tumor or tumors, but also removing the remaining cirrhotic liver that has a propensity for recurrent HCC. It restores normal liver function, and can resolve portal hypertension. However, these advantages are offset by the need for lifelong immunosuppression and a relative shortage of deceased organ donors.

The Milan criteria are based on tumor morphology and require either a solitary tumor <5 cm in diameter, or multifocal HCC with three or fewer tumors each measuring <3 cm in diameter. Recipients with preoperative HCC meeting Milan criteria were found to have a 4-year actuarial and disease-free survival of 75% and 83%, respectively (Mazzaferro *et al.* 1996). While studies have tried to identify other patient populations that may have satisfactory outcomes after transplantation using more liberal criteria for tumors than in the Milan criteria (Yao 2006), no such criteria modifications have yet reached general acceptance.

Since February 2002, the deceased-donor liver allocation system in the United States has used severity of illness as determined by the model for end-stage liver disease (MELD) score rather than waiting time. Candidates with HCC within Milan criteria are given an increased-exception MELD score (currently 22 points), so that more than half of liver candidates with HCC meeting Milan criteria are transplanted within 90 days of listing. However, suspicious tumors <2 cm diameter have been found to have a relatively high false positive rate for HCC and also have generally shown a slow progression of tumor growth. Because of those findings, candidates with a single suspicious nodule or even biopsy-proven HCC <2 cm are no longer given an exception MELD score. Most candidates with HCC have relatively low MELD scores when compared to other liver transplant candidates, who usually have hepatic decompensation associated with their being listed. These patients with HCC without the added exception score, because of tumors beyond Milan criteria or with a solitary nodule <2 cm in diameter, are effectively excluded from having a liver allocated from the deceased-donor waiting list. Despite being counter to general principles of treating cancer, candidates with small tumors essentially need to wait for transplant until the tumor size has increased to 2 cm or greater in diameter. Tumors <2 cm in diameter can be treated with other therapeutic options including radiofrequency ablation, TACE, or, if a living liver donor was available, living donor liver transplantation.

When considering all candidates listed for liver transplant, approximately 20% will die or otherwise be removed from the waiting list because of becoming too sick or from tumor progression (Llovet *et al.* 1999). Because of this, strategies have been developed as a 'bridge' to transplantation; these are principally RFA and TACE. However, for those who undergo transplant within 6 months of listing, pretransplant therapies, including TACE and RFA, have not been shown to have a significant effect (Shiffman *et al.* 2002; Porrett *et al.* 2006). Availability of a living donor essentially eliminates the risk of dying while on the waiting list, and living-donor transplant is a reasonable option for those with a solitary tumor <2 cm in diameter.

Conclusion

With improved methods of imaging and screening for HCC in patients with cirrhosis or with a history of hepatitis B or C, an increasing proportion of patients are expected to be identified with early-stage tumors that will be amenable to surgical resection or liver transplantation. For patients with no cirrhosis, surgical resection is the established best treatment, when possible. For patients with well-compensated cirrhosis, adequate hepatic reserve, and no clinical evidence of portal hypertension, partial hepatectomy may also be the best option for therapy. For patients with tumors within Milan criteria and with evidence of decompensated cirrhosis, multifocal disease, or requiring too extensive a resection, liver transplantation is the treatment of choice.

References

Adachi E, Maeda T, Matsumata T *et al.* (1995) Risk factors for intrahepatic recurrence in human small hepatocellular carcinoma. *Gastroenterology* 108: 768–75.

Arii S, Tanaka J, Yamazoe Y *et al.* (1992) Predictive factors for intrahepatic recurrence of hepatocellular carcinoma after partial hepatectomy. *Cancer* 69: 913–9.

Arii S, Yamaoka Y, Futagawa S *et al.* (2000) Results of surgical and nonsurgical treatment for small-sized hepatocellular carcinomas: a retrospective and nationwide survey in Japan. The Liver Cancer Study Group of Japan. *Hepatology* 32: 1224–9.

Belghiti J, Panis Y, Farges O, Benhamou JP, Fekete F. (1991) Intrahepatic recurrence after resection of hepatocellular carcinoma complicating cirrhosis. *Ann Surg* 214: 114–7.

Bruix J, Sherman M. (2005) Management of hepatocellular carcinoma. *Hepatology* 42: 1208–36.

Bruix J, Castells A, Bosch J *et al.* (1996) Surgical resection of hepatocellular carcinoma in cirrhotic patients: prognostic value of preoperative portal pressure. *Gastroenterology* 111: 1018–22.

Chen MF, Hwang TL, Jeng LB, Wang CS, Jan YY, Chen SC. (1994) Postoperative recurrence of hepatocellular carcinoma. Two hundred five consecutive patients who underwent hepatic resection in 15 years. *Arch Surg* 129: 738–42.

D'Amico G, Morabito A, Pagliaro L, Marubini E. (1986) Survival and prognostic indicators in compensated and decompensated cirrhosis. *Dig Dis Sci* 31: 468–75.

Farges O, Belghiti J, Kianmanesh R *et al.* (2003) Portal vein embolization before right hepatectomy: prospective clinical trial. *Ann Surg* 237: 208–17.

Fong Y, Sun RL, Jarnagin W, Blumgart LH. (1999) An analysis of 412 cases of hepatocellular carcinoma at a Western center. *Ann Surg* 229: 790–9; discussion 799–800.

Gines P, Quintero E, Arroyo V *et al.* (1987) Compensated cirrhosis: natural history and prognostic factors. *Hepatology* 7: 122–8.

Grazi GL, Ercolani G, Pierangeli F *et al.* (2001) Improved results of liver resection for hepatocellular carcinoma on cirrhosis give the procedure added value. *Ann Surg* 234: 71–8.

Imamura H, Matsuyama Y, Tanaka E *et al.* (2003) Risk factors contributing to early and late phase intrahepatic recurrence of hepatocellular carcinoma after hepatectomy. *J Hepatol* 38: 200–7.

Llovet JM, Fuster J, Bruix J. (1999) Intention-to-treat analysis of surgical treatment for early hepatocellular carcinoma: resection versus transplantation. *Hepatology* 30: 1434–40.

Llovet JM, Bruix J, Gores GJ. (2000) Surgical resection versus transplantation for early hepatocellular carcinoma: clues for the best strategy. *Hepatology* 31: 1019–21.

Llovet JM, Burroughs A, Bruix J. (2003) Hepatocellular carcinoma. *Lancet* 362: 1907–17.

Majno PE, Sarasin FP, Mentha G, Hadengue A. (2000) Primary liver resection and salvage transplantation or primary liver transplantation in patients with single, small hepatocellular carcinoma and preserved liver function: an outcome-oriented decision analysis. *Hepatology* 31: 899–906.

Mazzaferro V, Regalia E, Doci R *et al.* (1996) Liver transplantation for the treatment of small hepatocellular carcinomas in patients with cirrhosis. *N Engl J Med* 334: 693–9.

Minagawa M, Makuuchi M, Takayama T, Kokudo N. (2003) Selection criteria for repeat hepatectomy in patients with recurrent hepatocellular carcinoma. *Ann Surg* 238: 703–10.

Nagasue N, Uchida M, Makino Y *et al.* (1993) Incidence and factors associated with intrahepatic recurrence following resection of hepatocellular carcinoma. *Gastroenterology* 105: 488–94.

Nakashima Y, Nakashima O, Tanaka M, Okuda K, Nakashima M, Kojiro M. (2003) Portal vein invasion and intrahepatic micrometastasis in small hepatocellular carcinoma by gross type. *Hepatol Res* 26: 142–7.

Okada S, Shimada K, Yamamoto J *et al.* (1994) Predictive factors for postoperative recurrence of hepatocellular carcinoma. *Gastroenterology* 106: 1618–24.

Poon RT, Fan ST, Lo CM, Liu CL, Wong J. (1999) Intrahepatic recurrence after curative resection of hepatocellular carcinoma: long-term results of treatment and prognostic factors. *Ann Surg* 229: 216–22.

Poon RT, Fan ST, Lo CM, Liu CL, Wong J. (2002) Long-term survival and pattern of recurrence after resection of small hepatocellular carcinoma in patients with preserved liver function: implications for a strategy of salvage transplantation. *Ann Surg* 235: 373–82.

Porrett PM, Peterman H, Rosen M *et al.* (2006) Lack of benefit of pre-transplant locoregional hepatic therapy for hepatocellular cancer in the current MELD era. *Liver Transpl* 12: 665–73.

Pugh RN, Murray-Lyon IM, Dawson JL, Pietroni MC, Williams R. (1973) Transection of the oesophagus for bleeding oesophageal varices. *Br J Surg* 60: 646–9.

Rees M, Plant G, Wells J, Bygrave S. (1996) One hundred and fifty hepatic resections: evolution of technique towards bloodless surgery. *Br J Surg* 83: 1526–9.

Sala M, Fuster J, Llovet JM *et al.* (2004) High pathological risk of recurrence after surgical resection for hepatocellular carcinoma: an indication for salvage liver transplantation. *Liver Transpl* 10: 1294–300.

Schwartz JD, Schwartz M, Mandeli J, Sung M. (2002) Neoadjuvant and adjuvant therapy for resectable hepatocellular carcinoma: review of the randomised clinical trials. *Lancet Oncol* 3: 593–603.

Shiffman ML, Brown RS Jr, Olthoff KM *et al.* (2002) Living donor liver transplantation: summary of a conference at The National Institutes of Health. *Liver Transpl* 8: 174–88.

Shirabe K, Kanematsu T, Matsumata T, Adachi E, Akazawa K, Sugimachi K. (1991) Factors linked to early recurrence of small hepatocellular carcinoma after hepatectomy: univariate and multivariate analyses. *Hepatology* 14: 802–5.

Takayama T, Makuuchi M, Hirohashi S *et al.* (1998) Early hepatocellular carcinoma as an entity with a high rate of surgical cure. *Hepatology* 28: 1241–6.

Takayasu K, Muramatsu Y, Moriyama N *et al.* (1989) Clinical and radiologic assessments of the results of hepatectomy for small hepatocellular carcinoma and therapeutic arterial embolization for postoperative recurrence. *Cancer* 64: 1848–52.

Tanaka H, Hirohashi K, Kubo S, Shuto T, Higaki I, Kinoshita H. (2000) Preoperative portal vein embolization improves prognosis after right hepatectomy for hepatocellular carcinoma in patients with impaired hepatic function. *Br J Surg* 87: 879–82.

Tanaka H, Kubo S, Tsukamoto T *et al.* (2005) Recurrence rate and transplantability after liver resection in patients with hepatocellular carcinoma who initially met transplantation criteria. *Transplant Proc* 37: 1254–6.

Torzilli G, Makuuchi M, Inoue K *et al.* (1999) No-mortality liver resection for hepatocellular carcinoma in cirrhotic and noncirrhotic patients: is there a way? A prospective analysis of our approach. *Arch Surg* 134: 984–92.

Vauthey JN, Klimstra D, Franceschi D *et al.* (1995) Factors affecting long-term outcome after hepatic resection for hepatocellular carcinoma. *Am J Surg* 169: 28–34; discussion 34–5.

Yamasaki S, Hasegawa H, Kinoshita H *et al.* (1996) A prospective randomized trial of the preventive effect of pre-operative transcatheter arterial embolization against recurrence of hepatocellular carcinoma. *Jpn J Cancer Res* 87: 206–11.

Yao FY. (2006) Expanded criteria for hepatocellular carcinoma: downstaging with a view to liver transplantation—yes. *Semin Liver Dis* 26: 239–47.

Ablation

James A. Knol

Ablation methods have achieved importance in the management of patients with hepatocellular cancer (HCC), for several reasons. The first is that although cure of HCC can be achieved only by resection, less than 20% of patients with HCC are candidates for resection. Cirrhosis is present in the majority of patients with HCC and limits the extent of liver resection because of the risk of liver failure. Multicentricity of HCC is also frequent in patients with cirrhosis, also limiting resection options. A second reason for importance of ablation methods is that other treatments for unresectable disease have been limited to transcatheter arterial chemoembolization (TACE). There has been almost no role played by systemic chemotherapy, radiotherapy, or immunotherapy. A third factor increasing the importance of tumor ablation more recently is that, in circumstances where there is the option of liver transplantation for HCC (see Surgery section), use of ablation to control/destroy even resectable tumors to maintain the patient's disease within the Milan criteria as a bridge to transplant has become necessary and widely practiced.

Tumor ablation methods use a variety of methods to directly destroy individual tumors, as much as possible, in order to achieve cure or to prolong survival. Ablative approaches to the liver are divided into percutaneous and operative approaches; operative approaches are subdivided into open and laparoscopic approaches. The currently available ablative methods are based upon injection of an agent directly into and around the tumor or upon application of thermal energy directly to the tumor (Lau *et al.* 2003). Injection methods include the injection of the chemicals ethanol or acetic acid; the injection of radioactive isotopes, such as yttrium-90 microspheres; injection of hyperthermic saline or hyperthermic distilled water at up to 60°C; or direct injection of chemotherapeutic agents within a gel that inhibits rapid dispersion of the agent. The ablative methods which use thermal energy include methods which supply heat through a probe or a needle inserted into the tumor and include radiofrequency ablation (RFA), microwave coagulation, and interstitial laser photocoagulation. Thermal coagulation of tumor can also be performed without device insertion using high-intensity focused ultrasound ablation (Wu *et al.* 2005). Cryoablation uses probes to rapidly freeze the tumor and adjacent margin of liver causing intracellular ice crystals, destroying the cells by dehydration and disruption of cellular structures.

There are some conditions which are required for all the ablative therapies for HCC. These include the presence of unresectable lesions or refusal of surgery, or, in the case of conditions appropriate for liver transplantation, a desire to avoid resection of individual lesions. It is desirable to treat all of the lesions present by some modality, either concurrently or sequentially. Ablative therapies also require the ability to adequately image the lesions in real time (most often requiring ultrasonographic imaging).

Contraindications to the use of ablative therapies include uncorrectable coagulopathy or thrombocytopenia; the presence of extrahepatic metastases; large infiltrative tumors; tumor thrombosis of the main portal vein or one of the main hepatic veins; and obstructive jaundice with the risk of bile leak and bile peritonitis. For the percutaneous approaches, contraindications also include significant ascites at the time of the procedure, and tumors adjacent to the surface of the liver (increased risk of seeding of the peritoneal cavity and of bleeding). For the thermal methods, tumor adjacent to other organs (esophagus, colon, stomach, duodenum, gallbladder) contraindicates the percutaneous approach, whereas these organs can often be treated without injury by a laparoscopic or open operative approach. Thermal ablation, including cryoablation, of tumor adjacent to central bile ducts is also contraindicated because of the likelihood of bile duct stricture at the site of thermal injury.

Imaging plays an essential role in the utilization of ablative techniques. Because each of the techniques requires interpretation and action based upon real-time events, the imaging must be real time, and therefore ultrasonography is the principal imaging modality. Using the percutaneous approach, probes or needles have been positioned using CT, but monitoring the ongoing progress of a percutaneous treatment is less than optimal with CT; using an imaging modality other than ultrasound within an operative approach is nearly impossible. Therefore, in general, lesions which are not able to be imaged by ultrasound are not candidates for ablative therapy. Moreover, the surgeon who intends to utilize ablative techniques must be facile in the use of ultrasound in imaging and in positioning the ablative instruments with reference to the tumor.

Imaging also plays an essential role in the follow-up monitoring of treated lesions. CT or MRI using IV contrast is generally performed at about 1 month following completion of treatment, with successful ablation indicated by replacement of the tumor by a uniform low-density region. The treated lesion, on follow-up scans, is typically somewhat larger than the initial tumor diameter, without any regions of contrast enhancement. Any area of contrast enhancement indicates a likely area of residual viable tumor.

Ethanol injection therapy

Ethanol injection therapy has been utilized for the longest time of any of the ablation methods, and has continued to be the most frequently and widely utilized worldwide. Use of ethanol as the injection agent far exceeds the use of other agents such as acetic acid or hyperthermic saline. The effect of the alcohol on the tumor is through cellular dehydration and protein denaturation and by small vessel thrombosis. Cirrhosis, when present, tends to confine the infiltration of the ethanol to the area of the relatively softer tumor, aiding effectiveness of the treatment. The injection is usually administered percutaneously, usually in the outpatient setting, using local anesthesia. The method uses a fine needle directed into the tumor under ultrasound guidance. Absolute ethanol is injected slowly into the tumor under ultrasound monitoring until the entire area of the tumor appears hyperechoic. The volume of the tumor and the volume of ethanol injected have a correspondence, but more ethanol may be required in some cases because of leakage into vasculature or bile ducts associated with the tumor. Ethanol injection is usually repeated twice per week for up to six to eight sessions, based upon tumor size. At 1 month following the course of treatment, the effect of treatment is assessed with contrast CT or MRI.

The best candidates for ethanol injection are patients with tumors 3 cm or smaller in diameter, and three or fewer tumors (Poon *et al.* 2002). Tumor necrosis has been shown to be complete in almost 100% of tumors smaller than 2 cm, and up to

70% of tumors smaller than 3 cm, but becomes less effective as the tumor size increases. Local recurrence rates range from 14% (Ikeda *et al.* 2001) to 20% at 1 year (Lin *et al.* 2004).

Ethanol injection is safe when limited to small tumors, with a treatment-related mortality rate of about 0.1%, and a severe complication rate of 1.7–3.2% (Poon *et al.* 2002). Severe complications include liver abscess, liver failure, intraperitoneal hemorrhage, hemobilia, and cholangitis. There is also a 1% incidence of tumor seeding along the needle track (Poon *et al.* 2002). In contrast to the limitations with treatment around the central bile ducts associated with the thermal ablation methods, no similar injury seems to occur to the bile ducts by ethanol injection into tumors adjacent to bile ducts. Mild complications include pain, fever, and rise in liver function tests.

Thermal ablation methods

Thermal ablation methods utilize a heat source or cold source to cause cell death by denaturation of proteins and coagulative necrosis in the treated tissue and tumor. Currently, radiofrequency ablation is the most utilized of these methods. The other heat-producing methods include microwave, laser, and high-frequency focused ultrasound (Wu *et al.* 2005). Except for the last method, each method requires insertion of a probe into the tumor. Geometry of the tumor and of the lesion produced by the individual application of the heat or cold source are important considerations in the effectiveness of tumor ablation with these methods, increasingly critical as the size of the tumor approaches or exceeds the dimensions of the individual treatment-induced lesion. The goal of the ablation is to exceed the outside margin of the tumor by a minimum of 5 mm in all directions. For small tumors 2 cm or smaller, each of the probe methods can usually reliably ablate the lesion with a single accurate probe placement. Less effective ablation will occur with lesions adjacent to a large vessel (more than 5 mm diameter), which will act as a heat or cold sink (Lu *et al.* 2005)

For tumors greater than 2 cm with laser and microwave, and greater than 3 cm with RFA and cryoablation, multiple probe placements are likely to be required. Intraoperative monitoring of treatment margin versus tumor margin then becomes critical. Each of the methods has problems in this regard. Although the edge of the iceball with cryoablation is easily discerned, the iceball blocks ultrasound, so that the relationship of the iceball to the tumor margin requires ultrasound placement from a number of different directions, not always possible with a laparoscopic, or the infrequent percutaneous, approach. Moreover, with multiple sequential probe placement, the margins of the receding iceball and the edge of tumor become indistinguishable. For the heating methods, the hyperechoic margin of treated tumor and liver may become indistinguishable from the margin of a hyperechoic tumor. In addition, microbubbles that often form during the course of the RFA treatment obscure ultrasound visualization of the tumor margins, and the hyperechoic margin of treatment which appears during the heating may disappear or become much less distinct once heating ceases. Mathematical models for multiple probe placements have been advanced as a means to completely ablate large lesions, but even expert application of that system in patients with tumors ranging from 3.6 to 7.0 cm resulted in 12% failure of complete ablation (Chen *et al.* 2004). Follow-up at 1 month with contrast CT or MRI is performed for assessment of completeness of ablation.

The best candidates for thermal ablation are patients with tumors 3 cm or smaller in diameter, but larger tumors can be effectively ablated in many cases (Poon *et al.* 2004). Most centers limit treatment to patients with four or fewer tumors and tumors less than 8 cm in diameter, and exclude patients with Child–Pugh C cirrhosis (Poon *et al.* 2004), although other centers will treat patients with Child–Pugh C cirrhosis percutaneously (Curley *et al.* 2000). Tumors cannot be located close to the central bile ducts. Tumors located close to intra-abdominal organs preclude a percutaneous approach. Complete ablation of tumors smaller than 3–5 cm after a single treatment with RFA is 80–90% (Poon *et al.* 2002). Similar rates of ablation have been reported in HCC of up to 8 cm, in experienced hands (Poon *et al.* 2004).

RFA is a safe procedure, with a mortality rate of less than 0.3–0.9% for percutaneous treatment and up to 2.4% for intraoperative treatment (de Baère *et al.* 2003; Livraghi *et al.* 2003), and a major complication rate of 2.2–12.7% (Curley *et al.* 2000; de Baère *et al.* 2003; Livraghi *et al.* 2003). Major complications include liver abscess, highly related to the presence of biliary–enteric anastomoses (de Baère *et al.* 2003); intra-abdominal bleeding; intestinal perforation; acute renal failure (myoglobinuria is common after large ablations); and needle tract seeding (Livraghi *et al.* 2003). After larger ablations (greater than 4.5 cm diameter), postablation syndrome consisting of fever, malaise, chills, delayed pain, and nausea, may occur in about a third of patients (Dodd *et al.* 2005).

Comparison of ablation techniques

There are two goals with ablative therapy for HCC: effectiveness of ablation with the aim of elimination of all hepatic tumor; and applicability to a maximum number of patients who cannot undergo resection. For ethanol ablation of small tumors, the reported effectiveness is similar to that achieved by RFA. The mortality and morbidity for ethanol ablation in retrospective studies appear to be better than those for RFA. An advantage of ethanol injection is that it does not require costly equipment, and its applicability for tumors less than 3 cm in diameter is similar or more comprehensive than for thermal ablative methods.

With respect to thermal methods for ablation for HCC, RFA is currently the preferred technology, overall. Compared with RFA, microwave coagulation therapy and laser coagulation therapy are more limited in the volume of ablation resulting from an individual treatment, and equipment is much more expensive. Although ultrasonographic monitoring of the progress of treatment volume and tumor margins may be more clear with microwave or laser ablation, the limitations and major complications associated with these treatments are similar to those of RFA. In a prospective but non-randomized comparison of cryoablation with RFA for treatment of hepatic malignancies, cryoablation had a much higher complication and local recurrence rate (Pearson *et al.* 1999).

There are three randomized studies comparing percutaneous ethanol ablation with RFA (Lin *et al.* 2004, 2005; Shiina *et al.* 2005). Each of these studies found a significantly smaller local recurrence rate for RFA as compared to ethanol injection. Although survival and tumor-free survival are also recorded as endpoints in these studies, propensity toward multicentricity, number of lesions treated per individual patient, and presence and stage of cirrhosis are confounding variables. None of the studies were large enough to stratify the patients such that the effect of the ablation technique can be tested as a fully independent variable for survival or tumor-free survival. Nevertheless, in each of the studies, tumor-free survival and overall survival are also significantly better for patients treated with RFA as compared to percutaneous ethanol injection.

References

Chen M-H, Yang W, Yan K *et al.* (2004) Large liver tumors: protocol for radiofrequency ablation and its clinical application in 110 patients—mathematic model, overlapping mode, and electrode placement process. *Radiology* 232: 260–71.

Curley S, Izzo F, Ellis L, Vauthey J, Vallone P. (2000) Radiofrequency ablation of hepatocellular cancer in 110 patients with cirrhosis. *Ann Surg* 232: 381–91.

De Baère T, Risse O, Kuoch V *et al.* (2003) Adverse events during radiofrequency treatment of 582 hepatic tumors. *AJR* 181: 695–700.

Dodd GI, Napier D, Schoolfield J, Hubbard L. (2005) Percutaneous radiofrequency ablation of hepatic tumors: postablation syndrome. *AJR* 185: 41–57.

Ikeda M, Okada S, Ueno H, Okusaka T, Kuriyama H. (2001) Radiofrequency ablation and percutaneous ethanol injection in patients with small hepatocellular carcinoma: a comparative study. *Jpn J Clin Oncol* 31: 322–6.

Lau W, Leung T, Yu S, Ho S. (2003) Percutaneous local ablative therapy for hepatocellular carcinoma: a review and look into the future. *Ann Surg* 237: 171–9.

Lin S-M, Lin C-J, Lin C-C, Hsu C-W, Chen Y-C. (2004) Radiofrequency ablation improves prognosis compared with ethanol injection for hepatocellular carcinoma ≤4 cm. *Gastroenterology* 127: 1714–23.

Lin S-M, Lin C-J, Lin C-C, Hsu C-W, Chen Y-C. (2005) Randomised controlled trial comparing percutaneous radiofrequency thermal ablation, percutaneous ethanol injection, and percutaneous acetic acid injection to treat hepatocellular carcinoma of 3 cm or less. *Gut* 54: 1151–6.

Livraghi T, Solbiati L, Meloni M, Gazelle G, Halpern E, Goldberg S. (2003) Treatment of focal liver tumors with percutaneous radio-frequency ablation: complications encountered in a multicenter study. *Radiology*: 441–51.

Lu D, Yu N, Raman S *et al.* (2005) Radiofrequency ablation of hepatocellular carcinoma: treatment success as defined by histologic examination of the explanted liver. *Radiology*: 954–60.

Pearson A, Izzo F, Fleming R *et al.* (1999) Intraoperative radiofrequency ablation or cryoablation for hepatic malignancies. *Am J Surg* 178: 592–9.

Poon R-P, Fan S-T, Tsang F-F, Wong J. (2002) Locoregional therapies for hepatocellular carcinoma: a critical review from the surgeon's perspective. *Ann Surg* 235: 466–86.

Poon R, Ng K, Lam C-M, Ai V, Yuen J, Fan S-T. (2004) Effectiveness of radiofrequency ablation for hepatocellular carcinomas larger than 3 cm in diameter. *Arch Surg* 139: 281–7.

Shiina S, Teratiani T, Obi S *et al.* (2005) A randomized controlled trial of radiofrequency ablation with ethanol injection for small hepatocellular carcinoma. *Gastroenterology* 129: 122–30.

Wu F, Wang Z-B, Chen W-Z *et al.* (2005) Advanced hepatocellular carcinoma: treatment with high-intensity focused ultrasound ablation combined with transcatheter arterial embolization. *Radiology* 235: 659–67.

Radiotherapy

Charlie Pan & Theodore Lawrence

The whole-liver tolerance to radiation, estimated to be approximately 30 Gy (Emami *et al.* 1991), historically limited the use of radiation as an effective treatment modality for tumors within the liver, as tumorcidal doses for solid tumors typically require a minimum of 50 Gy. Techniques that selectively irradiate an intrahepatic tumor while sparing adequate normal liver tissue have recently been developed and have shown some success.

External-beam radiotherapy

The development of three-dimensional radiation therapy treatment planning (3D-CRT) has allowed for increased use of external-beam radiotherapy for patients with intrahepatic malignancies. A series of prospective controlled studies at the University of Michigan have demonstrated the safety of delivering doses well above the whole-liver tolerance dose to focal lesions (Robertson *et al.* 1997; McGinn *et al.* 1998; Dawson *et al.* 2000; Ben-Josef *et al.* 2005). To deliver these high doses, a normal-tissue complication probability (NTCP) model that quantitatively described the relationship between dose and volumes irradiated and the probability of developing radiation-induced liver disease (RILD) was developed. A phase I/II trial was conducted to test the safety of the model parameters and to begin to develop efficacy data at the maximum tolerated dose (Dawson *et al.* 2000). Individual radiation dose was determined based upon the volume of normal liver that could be spared. Each individual received the maximal possible dose associated with an estimated NTCP not exceeding 15%. Prescribed doses ranged from 40 Gy to 90 Gy (median 60.75 Gy). Floxuridine (0.2 mg/kg/day) was also delivered concurrently via a hepatic arterial catheter. A phase II trial followed, involving a total of 81 patients with HCC or cholangiocarcinoma, and with a median follow-up of 16 months (26 months in living patients). The median overall survival of HCC patients was 15 months ($p < 0.0001$, compared to 8 months for historical controls). Total radiation dose was the most important predictor of survival in a multivariate analysis. The pattern of failure analysis revealed a tendency of HCC tumors to progress locally, with 64% occurring within the liver. Together, these findings emphasize the need to develop more intensive liver-directed therapies.

Radiation dose-limiting organs

The major dose-limiting organ for irradiation to the hepatobiliary system is the liver. Radiation-induced liver disease (RILD) typically occurs 4–8 weeks after the completion of radiation therapy (Lawrence *et al.* 1995). Patients complain of fatigue and may have vague right upper quadrant discomfort. They may have signs and symptoms of anicteric ascites, with rapid weight gain and increased abdominal girth. Laboratory studies show a large increase in alkaline phosphatase to 3–10 times normal, moderate elevations of the transaminases, but little to no increase in bilirubin or lactic dehydrogenase (LDH) at first presentation. Evaluation includes an abdominal CT scan and paracentesis of the ascetic fluid to rule out recurrent disease, though differentiation on CT scan of recurrent disease versus radiation change within the liver is often difficult. The pathological finding in RILD is that of veno-occlusive disease, with thrombosis occurring in the central veins of the liver. This is consistent with the clinical syndrome of posthepatic occlusion. RILD is treated conservatively using diuretics and steroids, as with benign liver dysfunction, although some have suggested anticoagulation as well. It is possible that defibrotide, which has been shown to have effectiveness in the treatment of veno-occlusive disease secondary to bone marrow transplantation, may also have some effectiveness in the treatment of RILD.

The risk for RILD is highly dependent on the volume of the liver irradiated. Irradiation of the whole liver in a normal patient to a total dose of 30 Gy in 2 Gy fractions or less has minimal risk of a complication. Risk for RILD rises steeply above a dose of 33 Gy, and it has been estimated that at 42 Gy, there is an approximately 50% risk of symptoms. However, partial liver volumes can be safely irradiated to very high doses without clinically relevant toxicity. Trials at the University of Michigan using 3D-CRT have shown that approximately one-third of the normal liver can tolerate over 70 Gy (Jackson *et al.* 1995; Dawson *et al.* 2002). Accumulated data in these trials now allow for an estimation of an individual's risk for complication based on the distribution of the radiation dose within the liver. While the use of concurrent hepatic arterial fluorodeoxyuridine was not found to increase the risk of RILD, case reports suggest that previous alkylator therapy increases the chances of RILD (Lawrence *et al.* 1995). Finally, for patients with pre-existing liver disease, Xu *et al.* recently reported on a series of patients with Child–Pugh grade A and B cirrhosis and found that radiation tolerance was significantly less in these patients (Xu *et al.* 2006).

Other dose-limiting organs within the upper abdomen include the kidneys, stomach, and small bowel. A major portion of the right kidney is often exposed, and special care needs to be taken to spare the left kidney. Dosimetric criteria used at the University of Michigan include that when more than half of one kidney needs to receive 20 Gy or more, then no more than 10% of the other kidney can receive greater than 18 Gy. The stomach and duodenum are also of concern, especially when the tumors involve the left lobe of the liver or the extrahepatic biliary tract. The maximum doses to the stomach and duodenum currently allowed are 60 Gy and 68 Gy, respectively. Improvements in technology, specifically with intensity-modulated radiation therapy (IMRT), allow for both dose escalation of tumors as well as improved sparing of these critical organs.

External-beam radiotherapy technique

Palliative liver irradiation may be indicated for both locally advanced hepatic tumors and metastatic disease. While irradiation of locally unresectable hepatocellular cancers to doses above the whole-liver tolerance requires 3D treatment planning, palliative liver radiation can be accomplished with simple opposed anteroposterior fields or tangential approaches, as doses do not exceed whole-liver tolerance. Appropriate dose and schedule for palliation was examined in a prospective, non-randomized trial of over 100 patients with symptomatic liver metastases (Borgelt *et al.* 1981). Six different dose and fractionation options, ranging from 21 Gy in 7 fractions to 25.6 Gy in 16 fractions were tested. Palliation of pain was achieved in 55% of patients, with no difference among the treatment regimens. Although radiation-induced liver disease was not reported with any of the dose fractionation options, the short median survival of this patient group and the problem distinguishing this complication from progressive disease make interpretation of this finding difficult.

If doses above the whole-liver tolerance are to be used for irradiation of locally unresectable hepatic tumors, three-dimensional treatment planning is required. The gross tumor volume is typically defined as the radiographically abnormal area seen on the CT scan. Additional information from MRI can also be used. The clinical target volume that receives the highest dose is defined as the gross tumor volume. A second CTV that receives a dose adequate to control microscopic disease can also be delineated, which represents the GTV plus 1 cm based on surgical reports that at least a 1-cm resection margin is necessary for a successful partial hepatectomy (Ozawa *et al.* 1991). The planning target volume includes the clinical target volume plus 0.5 cm for daily patient set-up variation and between 0.5 and 2.5cm (determined under fluoroscopy) in the cranial–

caudal dimension to account for liver motion resulting from breathing. This additional breathing motion can be excluded if the liver is localized using active breathing control (ABC) (Dawson *et al.* 2001). The normal liver is defined as the gross tumor volume subtracted from the total liver volume. With this technique, patients' tumors have been safely treated with up to 90 Gy in 1.5 Gy fractions (Ben-Josef *et al.* 2005).

While 3D-CRT entails sophisticated shaping of the dose distribution by collimation design (or shaping of the fields) and the selection of beam directions and beam weights based on 3D images of the patient, IMRT improves on the dose conformality by enabling variations of the radiation intensity within each beam and beamlet. An example case is seen in Fig. 19.7. IMRT plans give the physician improved ability to shape the dose, allowing for avoidance of excessive dose to organs at risk as well as dose escalation to the tumors. In cases in which the tumor is adjacent to the stomach or duodenum, IMRT permits an increase in the dose to the tumor by 11 Gy while maintaining the same dose to the critical structure (Thomas *et al.* 2005).

External-beam radiotherapy with transcatheter arterial chemoembolization

Another strategy involves using lower doses of radiation with transcatheter arterial chemoembolization (TACE) in unresectable HCC, as reported by many Asian investigators (Guo *et al.* 2000; Li *et al.* 2003; Seong *et al.* 2003; Zeng *et al.* 2004). The stated rationale for combining 3D-CRT and TACE included the multifocal nature of HCC and the ability of iodized oil injection by TACE to improve tumor delineation by sharpening the GTV margin and highlighting previously unidentified lesions on post-TACE CT scan. However, as TACE may also decrease perfusion to the tumor and hence result in areas of radioresistance due to hypoxia, the optimal sequence of TACE and 3D-CRT remains to be determined.

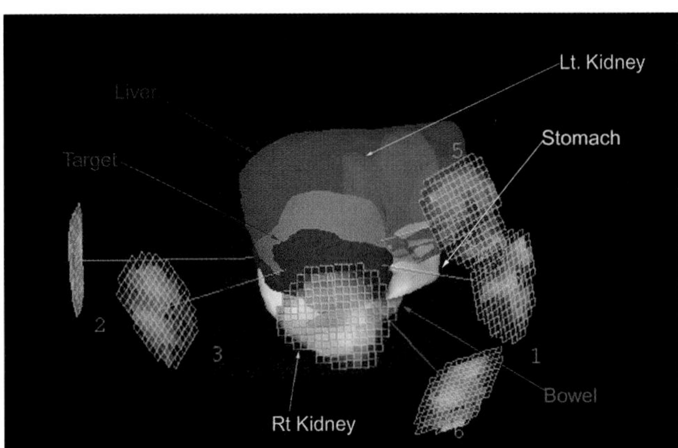

Fig. 19.7 IMRT treatment for a patient with unresectable hepatocellular carcinoma. The solid-surface reconstruction of the target volume (red), liver (purple), right and left kidneys (yellow), stomach (white), and bowel (blue) are shown, along with the projections of six IMRT fields, with the dose intensity in each beamlet represented by gray-scale.

Zeng *et al.* reported on retrospective series of 203 patients treated with TACE, with 54 patients also receiving 3D-CRT. These patients were free of tumor thrombus, lymph node involvement, severe cirrhosis, and extrahepatic metastasis. Selection for radiotherapy was primarily driven by unsatisfactory lipiodol uptake or worsening of liver function after TACE. In comparison with patients who were treated with TACE alone, patients who were treated with TACE and 3D-CRT had superior response rates (76% vs 31%, $p < 0.001$) and 3-year survival (24% vs 11.1%).

Other reports are summarized in Table 19.5. In general, response rates are between 50% and 90% with median survival between 10 and 23 months. These retrospective studies vary in patient selection and treatment details, making interpretation of these results difficult. However, similar to the University of Michigan experience, a common finding was that radiotherapy dose significantly affected survival.

Stereotactic body radiation therapy

Stereotactic body radiation therapy (SBRT) is a technique (sometimes called stereotactic radiosurgery) where a single or limited number of high-dose radiation fractions are delivered to a small, precisely defined target by using multiple radiation beams. The beams converge precisely on the target lesion, minimizing radiation exposure to adjacent normal tissue. This targeting has been used in the treatment of tumors less than about 5 cm in diameter in extracranial sites. Stereotactic approaches to RT are increasingly being used for treatment of metastatic liver tumors.

Experience with stereotactic body radiotherapy for primary liver tumors is limited but increasing (Schefter *et al.* 2005; Wulf *et al.* 2006; Dawson *et al.* 2006; Mendez Romero *et al.* 2006; Lin *et al.* 2006). In one series, 20 patients with primary hepatocel-

Table 19.5 Results of low- to intermediate-dose radiotherapy with transcatheter arterial chemoembolization in unresectable hepatocellular carcinoma.

Study	Mean tumor size (range)	No. of patients	Treatment	Median survival (months)
Zeng *et al.* (2004)		54	TACE + 36–60 Gy	20
Seong *et al.* (2003)	9.0 cm (6–12)	158	TACE + 40–56 Gy	10
Li *et al.* (2003)	8.5 cm (4–13)	45	TACE + 50.4 Gy	23.5
Guo & Yu (2000)	10.2 cm (5–18)	107	TACE + 25–55 Gy	18

lular carcinoma (average tumor size 3.8 cm, range 2–6.5cm) underwent fractionated SBRT (50 Gy in 5 or 10 fractions) (Choi *et al.* 2006). After a median follow-up of 23 months, four patients (20%) had a complete response, 12 (60%) a partial response, and 4 (20%) had stable disease. The 2-year survival and disease-free survival rates were 43% and 33%, respectively. There were no instances of grade 3 or 4 toxicity.

This approach seems most applicable to patients with relatively small hepatocellular carcinomas who are either inoperable or who refuse operation. Whether SBRT is a more effective or less toxic approach than radiofrequency ablation or other local therapies in these patients remains to be determined. The RTOG is planning a multi-institutional clinical trial to determine the efficacy of SBRT for hepatocellular carcinomas.

Selective internal radiation with radioactive isotopes

An alternative means of delivering focal radiation involves radioactive isotopes, either glass microspheres incorporating yttrium-90 (^{90}Y) or iodine-131 (^{131}I)-labeled lipiodol, delivered selectively to the tumor via the hepatic artery. Early reports suggest that radioembolization using intrahepatic artery administration of ^{90}Y microspheres is safe and induces objective responses in patients with unresectable hepatocellular carcinomas (Kennedy *et al.* 2004; Sarfaraz *et al.* 2004; Salem *et al.* 2005). In a series of 43 patients with hepatocellular carcinoma treated with ^{90}Y microspheres, 20 patients (47%) had an objective response, and median survival was 21 and 14 months for Child class A and B/C, respectively. No life-threatening adverse events related to treatment were reported in this series (Salem *et al.* 2005). The lack of prospective trials using this technique makes it difficult to judge the efficacy of treatment. Additional experience and longer follow-up is needed for this technique.

Future directions

A number of avenues for improvement with the application of radiation to patients with hepatocellular carcinomas are currently being pursued. Better physical dose delivery with heavy ions such as protons may help to improve the therapeutic index by decreasing the dose to normal liver. Experience from Japan with 162 patients treated to 72 Gy in 16 fractions resulted in a 5-year overall survival rate of 24% (Chiba *et al.* 2005). It is not clear at this time whether these results, which are typically obtained in patients with tumors of <5 cm, are superior to stereotactic body radiation using photons. While the cost of protons may restrict this modality to select patients, this experience demonstrates the importance of dose conformality when treating tumors to high radiation doses.

Improved imaging techniques may also be helpful in both tumor definition as well as predicting radiation-induced liver toxicity. Additionally, a better understanding of radiation-induced liver disease may ultimately permit the toxicity of treatment to be decreased. While advances in this area have been hampered by the lack of an animal model, data suggest that cytokines such as transforming growth factor may at least participate in the process leading to veno-occlusive disease (Anscher *et al.* 1993).

Another method of improving the therapeutic ratio could include the more standard use of radiation sensitizers or radioprotectors. Agents could be administered either systemically or via the hepatic artery, which is particularly attractive given that the dual blood supply of the liver permits selective perfusion of tumors by this route. Along this concept, radioprotectors such as amifostine, while primarily administered systemically, could be given through the portal vein and produce selective protection of the normal liver and also improve the therapeutic index. Preclinical studies have shown that amifostine protects the normal liver, but not tumor, from radiation (Symon *et al.* 2001).

In addition to these methods of increasing effective tumor dose without producing hepatic toxicity, future investigations need to address non-hepatic toxicities, which can sometimes limit radiation doses that can be delivered to patients with intrahepatic cancers.

References

Anscher MS, Peters WP, Reisenbichler H, Petros WP, Jirtle RL. (1993) Transforming growth factor beta as a predictor of liver and lung fibrosis after autologous bone marrow transplantation for advanced breast cancer. *N Engl J Med* 328(22): 1592–8.

Ben-Josef E, Normolle D, Ensminger WD *et al.* (2005) Phase II trial of high-dose conformal radiation therapy with concurrent hepatic artery floxuridine for unresectable intrahepatic malignancies. *J Clin Oncol* 23(34): 8739–47.

Borgelt BB, Gelber R, Brady LW, Griffin T, Hendrickson FR. (1981) The palliation of hepatic metastases: results of the Radiation Therapy Oncology Group pilot study. *Int J Radiat Oncol Biol Phys* 7(5): 587–91.

Chiba T, Tokuuye K, Matsuzaki Y *et al.* (2005) Proton beam therapy for hepatocellular carcinoma: a retrospective review of 162 patients. *Clin Cancer Res* 11(10): 3799–805.

Choi BO, Jang HS, Kang KM *et al.* (2006) Fractionated stereotactic radiotherapy in patients with primary hepatocellular carcinoma. *Jpn J Clin Oncol* 36(3): 154–8.

Dawson LA, McGinn CJ, Normolle D *et al.* (2000) Escalated focal liver radiation and concurrent hepatic artery fluorodeoxyuridine for unresectable intrahepatic malignancies. *J Clin Oncol* 18(11): 2210–8.

Dawson LA, Brock KK, Kazanjian S *et al.* (2001) The reproducibility of organ position using active breathing control (ABC) during liver radiotherapy. *Int J Radiat Oncol Biol Phys* 51(5): 1410–21.

Dawson LA, Normolle D, Balter JM, McGinn CJ, Lawrence TS, Ten Haken RK. (2002) Analysis of radiation-induced liver disease using the Lyman NTCP model. *Int J Radiat Oncol Biol Phys* 53(4): 810–21.

Dawson LA, Eccles C, Craig T. (2006) Individualized image guided iso-NTCP based liver cancer SBRT. *Acta Oncol* 45(7): 856–64.

Emami B, Lyman J, Brown A *et al.* (1991) Tolerance of normal tissue to therapeutic irradiation. *Int J Radiat Oncol Biol Phys* 21(1): 109–22.

Guo WJ, Yu EX. (2000) Evaluation of combined therapy with chemoembolization and irradiation for large hepatocellular carcinoma. *Br J Radiol* 73(874): 1091–7.

Jackson A, Ten Haken RK, Robertson JM, Kessler ML, Kutcher GJ, Lawrence TS. (1995) Analysis of clinical complication data for radiation hepatitis using a parallel architecture model. *Int J Radiat Oncol Biol Phys* 31(4): 883–91.

Kennedy AS, Nutting C, Coldwell D, Gaiser J, Drachenberg C. (2004) Pathologic response and microdosimetry of (90)Y microspheres in man: review of four explanted whole livers. *Int J Radiat Oncol Biol Phys* 60(5): 1552–63.

Lawrence TS, Robertson JM, Anscher MS, Jirtle RL, Ensminger WD, Fajardo LF. (1995) Hepatic toxicity resulting from cancer treatment. *Int J Radiat Oncol Biol Phys* 31(5): 1237–48.

Li B, Yu J, Wang L *et al.* (2003) Study of local three-dimensional conformal radiotherapy combined with transcatheter arterial chemoembolization for patients with stage III hepatocellular carcinoma. *Am J Clin Oncol* 26(4):e92–9.

Lin CS, Jen YM, Chiu SY *et al.* (2006) Treatment of portal vein tumor thrombosis of hepatoma patients with either stereotactic radiotherapy or three-dimensional conformal radiotherapy. *Jpn J Clin Oncol* 36(4): 212–7.

McGinn CJ, Ten Haken RK, Ensminger WD, Walker S, Wang S, Lawrence TS. (1998) Treatment of intrahepatic cancers with radiation doses based on a normal tissue complication probability model. *J Clin Oncol* 16(6): 2246–52.

Mendez Romero A, Wunderink W, Hussain SM *et al.* (2006) Stereotactic body radiation therapy for primary and metastatic liver tumors: A single institution phase i-ii study. *Acta Oncol* 45(7): 831–7.

Ozawa K, Takayasu T, Kumada K *et al.* (1991) Experience with 225 hepatic resections for hepatocellular carcinoma over a 4-year period. *Am J Surg* 161(6): 677–82.

Robertson JM, McGinn CJ, Walker S *et al.* (1997) A phase I trial of hepatic arterial bromodeoxyuridine and conformal radiation therapy for patients with primary hepatobiliary cancers or colorectal liver metastases. *Int J Radiat Oncol Biol Phys* 39(5): 1087–92.

Salem R, Lewandowski RJ, Atassi B *et al.* (2005) Treatment of unresectable hepatocellular carcinoma with use of 90Y microspheres (TheraSphere): safety, tumor response, and survival. *J Vasc Interv Radiol* 16(12): 1627–39.

Sarfaraz M, Kennedy AS, Lodge MA, Li XA, Wu X, Yu CX. (2004) Radiation absorbed dose distribution in a patient treated with yttrium-90 microspheres for hepatocellular carcinoma. *Med Phys* 31(9): 2449–53.

Schefter TE, Kavanagh BD, Timmerman RD, Cardenes HR, Baron A, Gaspar LE. (2005) A phase I trial of stereotactic body radiation therapy (SBRT) for liver metastases. *Int J Radiat Oncol Biol Phys* 62(5): 1371–8.

Seong J, Park HC, Han KH, Chon CY. (2003) Clinical results and prognostic factors in radiotherapy for unresectable hepatocellular carcinoma: a retrospective study of 158 patients. *Int J Radiat Oncol Biol Phys* 55(2): 329–36.

Symon Z, Levi M, Ensminger WD, Smith DE, Lawrence TS. (2001) Selective radioprotection of hepatocytes by systemic and portal vein infusions of amifostine in a rat liver tumor model. *Int J Radiat Oncol Biol Phys* 50(2): 473–8.

Thomas E, Chapet O, Kessler ML, Lawrence TS, Ten Haken RK. (2005) Benefit of using biologic parameters (EUD and NTCP) in IMRT optimization for treatment of intrahepatic tumors. *Int J Radiat Oncol Biol Phys* 62(2): 571–8.

Wulf J, Guckenberger M, Haedinger U *et al.* (2006) Stereotactic radiotherapy of primary liver cancer and hepatic metastases. *Acta Oncol* 45(7): 838–47.

Xu ZY, Liang SX, Zhu J *et al.* (2006) Prediction of radiation-induced liver disease by Lyman normal-tissue complication probability model in three-dimensional conformal radiation therapy for primary liver carcinoma. *Int J Radiat Oncol Biol Phys* 65(1): 189–95.

Zeng ZC, Tang ZY, Fan J *et al.* (2004) A comparison of chemoembolization combination with and without radiotherapy for unresectable hepatocellular carcinoma. *Cancer J* 10(5): 307–16.

Chemotherapy

Charlie Pan & William D. Ensminger

Systemic chemotherapy

Unresectable or metastatic hepatocellular carcinoma (HCC) carries a poor prognosis, and systemic therapy with cytotoxic agents has not been very successful. Many clinical studies, both controlled and uncontrolled, have been completed for most of the major classes of chemotherapy, given as a single agent or in combination. Unfortunately, no single agent or combination of agents given systemically has been found to reproducibly result in greater than a 25% response rate or have a significant effect on survival.

Hepatocellular cancer has therefore been considered to be a relatively chemotherapy-refractory tumor. This may be due in part to the high rate of expression of multidrug resistance genes, including p-glycoprotein, glutathione-S-transferase, heat shock proteins, and mutations in p53 (Huang *et al.* 1992; Kuo *et al.* 1992; Soini *et al.* 1996; Caruso *et al.* 1999; Kato *et al.* 2001). Additionally, benefit from chemotherapy is difficult to assess in patients with advanced HCC, as survival is often influenced more by the degree of hepatic dysfunction and not by tumor aggressiveness or the impact of a systemic treatment. Systemic chemotherapy is usually not well tolerated by patients with significant underlying hepatic dysfunction. Due to these limitations, clinical investigations of chemotherapy in advanced HCC have involved diverse patient populations. By comparison, Asian patients tend to be significantly younger, with well-compensated cirrhosis due to chronic hepatitis B or C, while patients from North America or Europe are typically over 60, with alcoholic cirrhosis and comorbid illnesses. The difference in pre-existing hepatic dysfunction not only interferes with chemotherapy tolerance, dose, and the reported side-effect profile, but in studies applying strict entry criteria, those results may be applicable only to the small minority of Western patients who have well-preserved hepatic function. Finally, chemotherapy may also have less efficacy in patients with significant cirrhosis. For instance, in this one study of 147 patients, there were no objective responders among patients with either a poor performance status, ascites, portal vein tumor thrombus, or serum bilirubin >2.0 mg/dL (Nagahama *et al.* 1997).

Given these limitations, several single agents and combinations have been studied. These agents include doxorubicin, 5-fluorouracil, mitoxantrone, VP-16, cisplatin, epirubicin, gemcitabine, and paclitaxel. Table 19.6 summarizes the results with single agents. Table 19.7 summarizes the results with combination regimens. As no single agent or combination of these drugs has been associated with significant survival advantage over untreated controls, treatments with single or combination agents should be done preferably within the setting of a cancer clinical trial.

Table 19.6 Single agent systemic chemotherapy for hepatocellular carcinoma.

Study	Drug	Response rate (%)
Johnson *et al.* (1978)	Doxorubicin	32
Sciarrino *et al.* (1985)	Doxorubicin	0
Ravry *et al.* (1986)	Cisplatin	0
Falkson *et al.* (1987)	Cisplatin	17
Falkson *et al.* (1987)	Mitoxantrone	8
Lai *et al.* (1989)	Mitoxantrone	0
Melia *et al.* (1983)	VP-16	18
Chao *et al.* (1998)	Paclitaxel	0
Patt *et al.* (2004)	Capecitabine	11
Yang *et al.* (2000)	Gemcitabine	18
Fuchs *et al.* (2002)	Gemcitabine	0
O'Reilly *et al.* (2001)	Irinotecan	7
Halm *et al.* (2000)	Pegylated liposomal doxorubicin	0
Stuart *et al.* (1999)	Nolatrexed	8

Table 19.7 Combination regimens of systemic chemotherapy for hepatocellular carcinoma.

Study	Drug	Response rate (%)
Ravry *et al.* (1984)	Doxorubicin + bleomycin	16
Al-Idrissi *et al.* (1985)	Doxorubicin + 5-FU + mitomycin C	13
Patt *et al.* (2003)	5-FU + IFN	14
Ji *et al.* (1996)	Cisplatin + IFN	13
Ikeda *et al.* (2005)	Cisplatin + Mitoxantrone + 5-FU	27
Leung *et al.* (1999)	Cisplatin + IFN + doxorubicin + 5-FU (PIAF)	26
Lee *et al.* (2004)	Cisplatin + doxorubicin	19
Taieb *et al.* (2003)	Gemcitabine + oxaliplatin	19
Bobbio-Pallavicini *et al.* (1997)	Epirubicin + etoposide	39

Regional chemotherapy

The results of regional chemotherapy, as delivered by hepatic arterial infusions, are much more encouraging than systemic agents. The blood supply of HCC allows for the regional chemotherapy to be successful. At very early stages, HCC is not highly vascularized and its blood supply comes from the portal vein. As an HCC tumor grows, the blood supply becomes progressively arterialized, so that even well-differentiated HCC is mostly dependent on the hepatic artery for blood. This provides the rationale to support arterial obstruction as an effective therapeutic option. The procedure requires the advancement of the catheter into the hepatic artery and then to lobar and segmental branches aiming to be as selective as possible so as to induce only minimal injury to the surrounding non-tumorous liver.

Drugs such as cisplatin, doxorubicin, mitomycin C, and possibly neocarzinostatin have been found to produce substantial objective responses when administered regionally. These regional chemotherapies are often used with an embolizing agent such as lipiodol, gelatin, starch, microspheres, or polyvinyl alcohol, which in combination with chemotherapy (TACE), results in higher objective response rates than any form of systemic chemotherapy.

Initial trials previously did not demonstrate any survival benefit with TACE (Groupe d'Etude et de Traitement du Carcinome Hepatocellulaire 1995; Pelletier *et al.* 1998, 1990; Bruix *et al.* 1998). However, two recent randomized trials have demonstrated a survival benefit in a group of selected patients with unresectable HCC treated with TACE (Lo *et al.* 2002; Llovet *et al.* 2002). In a trial from Asia, 80 patients were randomized between TACE and symptomatic treatment, with a variable dose of an emulsion of cisplatin in lipiodol and gelatin-sponge particles injected through the hepatic artery. Chemoembolization was repeated every 2–3 months unless there was evidence of contraindications or progressive disease. Chemoembolization resulted in a marked tumor response, and the 2-year actuarial survival was significantly better in the chemoembolization group (31%) than in the control group (11%), $p = 0.002$ (Lo *et al.* 2002). In a trial from Europe, 112 patients of Child–Pugh class A or B and Okuda stage I or II were randomized between regularly repeated TACE (gelatin sponge plus doxorubicin), arterial embolization only (gelatin sponge), or conservative treatment. TACE in this population induced a 35% objective response rate. Two-year survival was 63% for TACE, 50% for embolization, and 27% for conservative treatment (Llovet *et al.* 2002). The data from these two trials, and results of a recent meta-analysis (Llovet & Bruix 2003) support the use of TACE as an treatment option for patients with unresectable disease and good performance status who do not have portal vein thrombosis, vascular invasion or extrahepatic spread.

Hormonal therapy

Hormone receptors are present in HCC, and this has led many investigators to examine the role of hormonal manipulation.

Some evidence suggests a possible association between estrogen and HCC. Estrogen receptors are known to be expressed in normal human liver, chronic hepatitis, benign hepatic tumor tissues, and HCC (Eagon *et al.* 1991; Claviere *et al.* 1998). Additionally, in animal models, estrogens have been shown to stimulate hepatocyte proliferation *in vitro* and may promote liver tumor growth *in vivo*, and tamoxifen appeared to inhibit the estrogen effect (Francavilla *et al.* 1989). Tamoxifen also may inhibit hepatoma cells through an estrogen receptor-independent mechanism (Jiang *et al.* 1995), as it may function as a potential inhibitor of p-glycoprotein.

Numerous studies involving tamoxifen have been performed. Three small, earlier studies demonstrated a significantly longer survival time in patients treated with tamoxifen (Farinati *et al.* 1990; Martinez Cerezo *et al.* 1994; Elba *et al.* 1994). However, five large, randomized studies (four of which were double-blinded) with a total of 1144 patients failed to demonstrate longer survival with tamoxifen (Castells *et al.* 1995; Manesis *et al.* 1995; CLIP Group 1998; Riestra *et al.* 1998; Liu *et al.* 2000). Results of a European Organization for Research and Treatment of Cancer trial of the antiandrogen nilutamide (Anandron) and the luteinizing hormone-releasing hormone agonist goesrelin (Zoladex) were disappointing (Grimaldi *et al.* 1998). Reponses with octreotide, megestrol, and lanreotide have also been disappointing. While there exist some preliminary data suggesting benefit, larger trials are necessary to determine if there is truly any benefit with these agents.

References

Al-Idrissi HY, Ibrahim EM, Abdel Satir A, Satti MB, Al-Kasem S, Al-Qurain A. (1985) Primary hepatocellular carcinoma in the eastern province of Saudi Arabia: treatment with combination chemotherapy using 5-fluorouracil, Adriamycin and mitomycin-C. *Hepatogastroenterology* 32(1): 8–10.

Bobbio-Pallavicini E, Porta C, Moroni M *et al.* (1997) Epirubicin and etoposide combination chemotherapy to treat hepatocellular carcinoma patients: a phase II study. *Eur J Cancer* 33(11): 1784–8.

Bruix J, Llovet JM, Castells A *et al.* (1998) Transarterial embolization versus symptomatic treatment in patients with advanced hepatocellular carcinoma: results of a randomized, controlled trial in a single institution. *Hepatology* 27(6): 1578–83.

Caruso ML, Valentini AM. (1999) Overexpression of p53 in a large series of patients with hepatocellular carcinoma: a clinicopathological correlation. Anticancer Res 19(5B): 3853–6.

Castells A, Bruix J, Bru C *et al.* (1995) Treatment of hepatocellular carcinoma with tamoxifen: a double-blind placebo-controlled trial in 120 patients. *Gastroenterology* 109(3): 917–22.

Chao Y, Chan WK, Birkhofer MJ *et al.* (1998) Phase II and pharmacokinetic study of paclitaxel therapy for unresectable hepatocellular carcinoma patients. *Br J Cancer* 78(1): 34–9.

Claviere C, Bronowicki JP, Hudziak H, Bigard MA, Gaucher P. (1998) [Role of sex steroids and their receptors in the pathophysiology of hepatocellular carcinoma]. *Gastroenterol Clin Biol* 22(1): 73–86.

CLIP Group (Cancer of the Liver Italian Programme). (1998) Tamoxifen in treatment of hepatocellular carcinoma: a randomised controlled trial. *Lancet* 352(9121): 17–20.

Eagon PK, Francavilla A, DiLeo A *et al.* (1991) Quantitation of estrogen and androgen receptors in hepatocellular carcinoma and adjacent normal human liver. *Dig Dis Sci* 36(9): 1303–8.

Elba S, Giannuzzi V, Misciagna G, Manghisi OG. (1994) Randomized controlled trial of tamoxifen versus placebo in inoperable hepatocellular carcinoma. *Ital J Gastroenterol* 26(2): 66–8.

Falkson G, Ryan LM, Johnson LA *et al.* (1987) A random phase II study of mitoxantrone and cisplatin in patients with hepatocellular carcinoma. An ECOG study. *Cancer* 60(9): 2141–5.

Farinati F, Salvagnini M, de Maria N *et al.* (1990) Unresectable hepatocellular carcinoma: a prospective controlled trial with tamoxifen. *J Hepatol* 11(3): 297–301.

Francavilla A, Polimeno L, DiLeo A *et al.* (1989) The effect of estrogen and tamoxifen on hepatocyte proliferation in vivo and in vitro. *Hepatology* 9(4): 614–20.

Fuchs CS, Clark JW, Ryan DP *et al.* (2002) A phase II trial of gemcitabine in patients with advanced hepatocellular carcinoma. Cancer 94(12): 3186–91.

Grimaldi C, Bleiberg H, Gay F *et al.* (1998) Evaluation of antiandrogen therapy in unresectable hepatocellular carcinoma: results of a European Organization for Research and Treatment of Cancer multicentric double-blind trial. *J Clin Oncol* 16(2): 411–7.

Groupe d'Etude et de Traitement du Carcinome Hepatocellulaire. (1995) A comparison of lipiodol chemoembolization and conservative treatment for unresectable hepatocellular carcinoma. *N Engl J Med* 332(19): 1256–61.

Halm U, Etzrodt G, Schiefke I *et al.* (2000) A phase II study of pegylated liposomal doxorubicin for treatment of advanced hepatocellular carcinoma. *Ann Oncol* 11(1): 113–4.

Huang CC, Wu MC, Xu GW *et al.* (1992) Overexpression of the MDR1 gene and P-glycoprotein in human hepatocellular carcinoma. *J Natl Cancer Inst* 84(4): 262–4.

Ikeda M, Okusaka T, Ueno H, Takezako Y, Morizane C. (2005) A phase II trial of continuous infusion of 5-fluorouracil, mitoxantrone, and cisplatin for metastatic hepatocellular carcinoma. *Cancer* 103(4): 756–62.

Ji SK, Park NH, Choi HM *et al.* (1996) Combined cis-platinum and alpha interferon therapy of advanced hepatocellular carcinoma. *Korean J Intern Med* 11(1): 58–68.

Jiang SY, Shyu RY, Yeh MY, Jordan VC. (1995) Tamoxifen inhibits hepatoma cell growth through an estrogen receptor independent mechanism. *J Hepatol* 23(6): 712–9.

Johnson PJ, Williams R, Thomas H, Sherlock S, Murray-Lyon IM. (1978) Induction of remission in hepatocellular carcinoma with doxorubicin. *Lancet* 1(8072): 1006–9.

Kato A, Miyazaki M, Ambiru S *et al.* (2001) Multidrug resistance gene (MDR-1) expression as a useful prognostic factor in patients with human hepatocellular carcinoma after surgical resection. *J Surg Oncol* 78(2): 110–5.

Kuo MT, Zhao JY, Teeter LD, Ikeguchi M, Chisari FV. (1992) Activation of multidrug resistance (P-glycoprotein) mdr3/mdr1a gene during the development of hepatocellular carcinoma in hepatitis B virus transgenic mice. Cell Growth Differ 3(8): 531–40.

Lai KH, Tsai YT, Lee SD *et al.* (1989) Phase II study of mitoxantrone in unresectable primary hepatocellular carcinoma following hepatitis B infection. *Cancer Chemother Pharmacol* 23(1): 54–6.

Lee J, Park JO, Kim WS *et al.* (2004) Phase II study of doxorubicin and cisplatin in patients with metastatic hepatocellular carcinoma. *Cancer Chemother Pharmacol* 54(5): 385–90.

Leung TW, Patt YZ, Lau WY *et al.* (1999) Complete pathological remission is possible with systemic combination chemotherapy for inoperable hepatocellular carcinoma. *Clin Cancer Res* 5(7): 1676–81.

Liu CL, Fan ST, Ng IO, Lo CM, Poon RT, Wong J. (2000) Treatment of advanced hepatocellular carcinoma with tamoxifen and the correlation with expression of hormone receptors: a prospective randomized study. *Am J Gastroenterol* 95(1): 218–22.

Llovet JM, Real MI, Montana X *et al.* (2002) Arterial embolisation or chemoembolisation versus symptomatic treatment in patients with unresectable hepatocellular carcinoma: a randomised controlled trial. *Lancet* 359(9319): 1734–9.

Llovet JM, Bruix J. (2003) Systematic review of randomized trials for unresectable hepatocellular carcinoma: Chemoembolization improves survival. *Hepatology* 37(2): 429–42.

Lo CM, Ngan H, Tso WK *et al.* (2002) Randomized controlled trial of transarterial lipiodol chemoembolization for unresectable hepatocellular carcinoma. *Hepatology* 35(5): 1164–71.

Manesis EK, Giannoulis G, Zoumboulis P, Vafiadou I, Hadziyannis SJ. (1995) Treatment of hepatocellular carcinoma with combined suppression and inhibition of sex hormones: a randomized, controlled trial. *Hepatology* 21(6): 1535–42.

Martinez Cerezo FJ, Tomas A, Donoso L *et al.* (1994) Controlled trial of tamoxifen in patients with advanced hepatocellular carcinoma. *J Hepatol* 20(6): 702–6.

Melia WM, Johnson PJ, Williams R. (1983) Induction of remission in hepatocellular carcinoma. A comparison of VP 16 with adriamycin. *Cancer* 51(2): 206–10.

Nagahama H, Okada S, Okusaka T *et al.* (1997) Predictive factors for tumor response to systemic chemotherapy in patients with hepatocellular carcinoma. *Jpn J Clin Oncol* 27(5): 321–4.

O'Reilly EM, Stuart KE, Sanz-Altamira PM *et al.* (2001) A phase II study of irinotecan in patients with advanced hepatocellular carcinoma. *Cancer* 91(1): 101–5.

Patt YZ, Hassan MM, Lozano RD *et al.* (2003) Phase II trial of systemic continuous fluorouracil and subcutaneous recombinant interferon Alfa-2b for treatment of hepatocellular carcinoma. *J Clin Oncol* 21(3): 421–7.

Patt YZ, Hassan MM, Aguayo A *et al.* (2004) Oral capecitabine for the treatment of hepatocellular carcinoma, cholangiocarcinoma, and gallbladder carcinoma. *Cancer* 101(3): 578–86.

Pelletier G, Roche A, Ink O *et al.* (1990) A randomized trial of hepatic arterial chemoembolization in patients with unresectable hepatocellular carcinoma. *J Hepatol* 11(2): 181–4.

Pelletier G, Ducreux M, Gay F *et al.* (1998) Treatment of unresectable hepatocellular carcinoma with lipiodol chemoembolization: a multicenter randomized trial. Groupe CHC. *J Hepatol* 29(1): 129–34.

Ravry MJ, Omura GA, Bartolucci AA. (1984) Phase II evaluation of doxorubicin plus bleomycin in hepatocellular carcinoma: a Southeastern Cancer Study Group trial. Cancer Treat Rep 68(12): 1517–8.

Ravry MJ, Omura GA, Bartolucci AA, Einhorn L, Kramer B, Davila E. (1986) Phase II evaluation of cisplatin in advanced hepatocellular carcinoma and cholangiocarcinoma: a Southeastern Cancer Study Group Trial. *Cancer Treat Rep* 70(2): 311–2.

Riestra S, Rodriguez M, Delgado M *et al.* (1998) Tamoxifen does not improve survival of patients with advanced hepatocellular carcinoma. *J Clin Gastroenterol* 26(3): 200–3.

Sciarrino E, Simonetti RG, Le Moli S, Pagliaro L. (1985) Adriamycin treatment for hepatocellular carcinoma. Experience with 109 patients. *Cancer* 56(12): 2751–5.

Soini Y, Virkajarvi N, Raunio H, Paakko P. (1996) Expression of P-glycoprotein in hepatocellular carcinoma: a potential marker of prognosis. *J Clin Pathol* 49(6): 470–3.

Stuart K, Tessitore J, Rudy J, Clendennin N, Johnston A. (1999) A Phase II trial of nolatrexed dihydrochloride in patients with advanced hepatocellular carcinoma. *Cancer* 86(3): 410–4.

Taieb J, Bonyhay L, Golli L *et al.* (2003) Gemcitabine plus oxaliplatin for patients with advanced hepatocellular carcinoma using two different schedules. *Cancer* 98(12): 2664–70.

Yang TS, Lin YC, Chen JS, Wang HM, Wang CH. (2000) Phase II study of gemcitabine in patients with advanced hepatocellular carcinoma. *Cancer* 89(4): 750–6.

Novel agents

Charlie Pan & William D. Ensminger

Hepatocellular carcinoma is very complex, and nearly every carcinogenic mechanism is altered to some degree in this malignancy. Hepatocarcinogenesis is a multifactorial, multistep process in which numerous factors induce genetic changes in mature hepatocytes leading to cellular proliferation, cell death, and the production of monoclonal populations (Table 19.8). There is no consistent pattern of genetic damage that has been characterized for HCC, as the molecular pathways leading to each individual HCC likely differ according to etiology. Several reviews summarize the most common and important molecular aberrations in HCC (Sheu 1997; Nagai *et al.* 1997; Thorgeirsson & Grisham 2002; Lee *et al.* 2005).

These molecular changes are often found within both the cells of underlying cirrhosis and inflammatory activity as well as in dysplastic nodules and the HCC tumors. Changes in

Table 19.8 Carcinogenic mechanisms in HCC and potential targeted therapies.

Mechanism	Target	Potential therapy
Growth factor dysregulation	EGFR	Gefitinib
	Overexpression of EGFR ligands (EGF, HGF, TGFβ, IGF) mitogenic for hepatocytes and implicated in hepatocarcinogenesis; upregulated in HCC cell lines, dysplastic nodules, and HCC tumors	Erlotinib
	Her2/neu expression low in HCC	Cetuximab
Intracellular signaling pathways	MAPK/ERK pathway activated in HCC	Sorafenib
Angiogenesis	VEGF	Bevacizumab

growth factor expression, protease and matrix metalloproteinase (MMP) expression, increased expression of cyclooxygenase enzymes, reduced apoptosis, somatic mutations, and oncogene expression are often seen in early chronic hepatitis. These alterations generally become more prominent and involved as liver injury progresses through fibrosis, cirrhosis, dysplastic foci, nodules, and finally into HCC.

HCC cells have many genetic defects, which occur at varying frequencies. These genetic alterations accumulate during the progression to HCC by repeated damage and regeneration of hepatocytes. Aneuoploidy is seen, as is considerable loss of heterozygosity involving numerous chromosomes, including 1p, 4q, 6q, 8p, 8q, 9p, 13q, 16p, 16q, and 17p. Key genes with mutations include *p53, p73, Rb, APC, DLC-1, p16, PTEN, IGF-2, BRCA2, SOCS-1, Smad2, Smad4, β-catenin, c-myc*, and *cyclin D1*. Considering all these involved genes, there appear to be multiple pathways for HCC formation. While knowledge of these possible targets can help to guide future therapies, the diversity of targets will most likely require multiple agents.

Growth factors, growth factor receptors, and angiogenesis

Agents that inhibit EGFR or VEGFR function include antibodies to the extracellular receptor domain and small molecules that bind to and inhibit the intracellular receptor tyrosine kinase domain. The EGFR-inhibiting agents gefitinib and erlotinib have been approved for the treatment of lung cancer, and cetuximab is approved for metastatic colorectal cancer. These agents have some *in vitro* activity on HCC (Hopfner *et al.* 2004; Huether *et al.* 2005a,b) and may have a role in treatment of HCC. A recent phase II study suggests some clinical benefit with erlotinib in patients with advanced HCC, with 32% progression-free survival at 6 months and acceptable toxicity (Philip *et al.* 2005). Further studies are needed to determine the true benefit of these agents for HCC.

Sorafenib is an oral multikinase inhibitor that targets two classes of kinases known to be involved in cell proliferation (tumor cell growth) and angiogenesis (tumor vasculature), including RAF kinase, VEGFR-1, VEGFR-2, VEGFR-3, PDGFR-B, KIT, FLT-3, and RET. A phase II study involving 137 patients demonstrated a partial or minor response and stable disease for at least 16 weeks in 8% and 34% of the patients (Abou-Alfa *et al.* 2006). Median time to progression was 4.2 months, and median overall survival was 9.2 months. A recent phase III trial using sorafenib vs. placebo in patients with advanced hepatocellular carcinoma demonstrated improved survival (Sorafenib 2007). Grade 3/4 adverse events were 38% for sorafenib versus 28% for placebo. Sorafenib should play a role in multimodality therapy for HCC in the future.

Bevacizumab is a monoclonal antibody that interferes with VEGFR signaling and the angiogenesis pathway. A phase II study of gemcitabine and oxaliplatin with bevacizumab was carried out on 30 patients with advanced HCC (Zhu *et al.* 2006). The objective response rate was 20%, and 27% of patients had stable disease. Median progression-free survival and overall survival were 5.3 months and 9.6 months, respectively.

Identification of appropriate targets and effective targeted therapies in HCC patients is a significant challenge, given the heterogeneity of HCC tumors. These early studies of targeted therapies for HCC, while promising, are faced with the limitation of focusing on one potential therapeutic target at a time. Future strategies of identifying each tumor's appropriate target and choosing the appropriate combination of targeted therapies need to be developed.

References

Abou-Alfa GK, Schwartz L, Ricci S *et al.* (2006) Phase II study of sorafenib in patients with advanced hepatocellular carcinoma. *J Clin Oncol* 24(26): 4293–300.

Hopfner M, Sutter AP, Huether A, Schuppan D, Zeitz M, Scherubl H. (2004) Targeting the epidermal growth factor receptor by gefitinib for treatment of hepatocellular carcinoma. *J Hepatol* 41(6): 1008–16.

Huether A, Hopfner M, Baradari V, Schuppan D, Scherubl H. (2005a) EGFR blockade by cetuximab alone or as combination therapy for growth control of hepatocellular cancer. *Biochem Pharmacol* 70(11): 1568–78.

Huether A, Hopfner M, Sutter AP, Schuppan D, Scherubl H. (2005b) Erlotinib induces cell cycle arrest and apoptosis in hepatocellular cancer cells and enhances chemosensitivity towards cytostatics. *J Hepatol* 43(4): 661–9.

Lee JS, Grisham JW, Thorgeirsson SS. (2005) Comparative functional genomics for identifying models of human cancer. *Carcinogenesis* 26(6): 1013–20.

Nagai H, Pineau P, Tiollais P, Buendia MA, Dejean A. (1997) Comprehensive allelotyping of human hepatocellular carcinoma. *Oncogene* 14(24): 2927–33.

Philip PA, Mahoney MR, Allmer C *et al.* (2005) Phase II study of erlotinib (OSI-774) in patients with advanced hepatocellular cancer. *J Clin Oncol* 23(27): 6657–63.

Sheu JC. (1997) Molecular mechanism of hepatocarcinogenesis. *J Gastroenterol Hepatol* 12(9–10): S309–13.

Sorafenib HCC. (2007) Assessment randomized protocol (SHARP) trial. *J Clin Oncol* 25: 518.

Thorgeirsson SS, Grisham JW. (2002) Molecular pathogenesis of human hepatocellular carcinoma. *Nat Genet* 31(4): 339–46.

Zhu AX, Blaszkowsky LS, Ryan DP *et al.* (2006) Phase II study of gemcitabine and oxaliplatin in combination with bevacizumab in patients with advanced hepatocellular carcinoma. *J Clin Oncol* 24(12): 1898–903.

Prognosis and follow-up

Charlie Pan

Prognosis

The prognosis of patients with hepatocellular carcinoma is

Table 19.9 Summary of treatment options and outcomes for HCC.

Treatment option	Survival	Comments
Liver transplantation	5-year—57–75% (Llovet *et al.* 2005; Hemming *et al.* 2001)	Improved survival over historically low survival rates (20–36%) likely related to adoption of Milan criteria at transplantation centers
Surgical resection	5-year—30–50% (Llovet *et al.* 2005)	Majority of patients develop recurrences or second primary tumors Resection in cirrhotic patients carries higher morbidity and mortality
TACE	1-year—57–82% (Camma *et al.* 2002; Llovet & Bruix 2003)	Objective tumor responses and slowed tumor progression seen, but questionable survival benefit Greatest benefit in patients with preserved liver function, absence of vascular invasion, and smallest tumors
Radiation therapy	5-year—9–19% Median survival—10–25 months (Ben-Josef *et al.* 2005; Hawkins & Dawson 2006)	Local control range from 40 to 90% Potential survival benefit of RT remains to be tested in randomized controlled trials
Percutaneous ablation (ethanol injections, RFA)	Ethanol injection (Lin *et al.*2004) 3-year—36–70% RFA 3-year—62–78%	PEI and RFA well tolerated Recurrence rates similar to those for postresection
Chemotherapy and hormonal therapy		Little evidence for survival benefit over supportive care Targeted therapies may hold some promise
Best supportive care	5-year—0–9% Median survival—5–8 months (Llovet *et al.* 1999)	

dependent on the tumor, underlying liver dysfunction, and treatment. Table 19.9 is a summary of treatment options for HCC and their outcomes. Overall, patients with early-stage tumors that can be treated with surgical therapy have the best survival. Those with intermediate- to advanced-stage tumors who receive non-surgical therapy have comparatively worse survival. Development of strategies combining neoadjuvant or adjuvant therapies (TACE, RFA, radiation therapy, chemotherapy, and/or targeted agents) with surgical resection or transplantation may help to improve the outcomes of patients with HCC.

Follow-up

Follow-up schedule should be based upon the clinical situation. Generally, patients should be evaluated at a minimum of every 3–6 months for the first 2 years, then annually, in the outpatient clinic with clinical examination and blood tests, including AFP if initially elevated. Radiographic imaging with either dynamic CT or MRI should be performed with similar frequency (Benson *et al.* 2006). Patients presenting with liver decompensation during follow-up should receive the same treatment as patients with non-neoplastic liver disease. Pain should be treated, but non-steroidal anti-inflammatory agents should be avoided.

References

Ben-Josef E, Normolle D, Ensminger WD *et al.* (2005) Phase II trial of high-dose conformal radiation therapy with concurrent hepatic artery floxuridine for unresectable intrahepatic malignancies. *J Clin Oncol* 23: 8739–47.

Benson AB 3rd, Bekaii-Saab T, Ben-Josef E *et al.* (2006) Hepatobiliary cancers. Clinical practice guidelines in oncology. *J Natl Compr Canc Netw* 4: 728–50.

Camma C, Schepis F, Orlando A *et al.* (2002) Transarterial chemoembolization for unresectable hepatocellular carcinoma: meta-analysis of randomized controlled trials. *Radiology* 224: 47–54.

Hawkins MA, Dawson LA. (2006) Radiation therapy for hepatocellular carcinoma: from palliation to cure. *Cancer* 106: 1653–63.

Hemming AW, Cattral MS, Reed AI, Van Der Werf WJ, Greig PD, Howard RJ. (2001) Liver transplantation for hepatocellular carcinoma. *Ann Surg* 233: 652–9.

Lin SM, Lin CJ, Lin CC, Hsu CW, Chen YC. (2004) Radiofrequency ablation improves prognosis compared with ethanol injection for hepatocellular carcinoma < or =4 cm. *Gastroenterology* 127: 1714–23.

Llovet JM, Bruix J. (2003) Systematic review of randomized trials for unresectable hepatocellular carcinoma: chemoembolization improves survival. *Hepatology* 37: 429–42.

Llovet JM, Bustamante J, Castells A *et al.* (1999) Natural history of untreated nonsurgical hepatocellular carcinoma: rationale for the design and evaluation of therapeutic trials. *Hepatology* 29: 62–7.

Llovet JM, Schwartz M, Mazzaferro V. (2005) Resection and liver transplantation for hepatocellular carcinoma. *Semin Liver Dis* 25: 181–200.

20 Metastatic Liver Cancer

Edited by Yuman Fong

Treatment

Overview

Yuman Fong

The liver is the most common site for blood-borne metastasis from colorectal cancers. Until the early 1980s, it was generally accepted that hepatic metastases from colorectal cancer represented just one site in a wide systemic dissemination of tumor, and hepatectomy was rarely used as treatment. Since then, numerous studies have shown that resection can prolong survival and potentially provide cure. Surgical excision for hepatic metastases from colorectal cancer is now considered standard therapy for patients with metastases isolated to the liver. In the next section, we will summarize the data supporting such therapies, as well as clinical parameters that influence outcome.

Since acceptance of surgery as a local therapy for this disease, a number of other local therapies have emerged as effective treatment options for hepatic metastases. The data supporting use of radiotherapy will be presented, as well as recent data documenting outcome of treatment with ablative therapies such as radiofrequency ablation and cryoablation. These tissue-sparing local treatments for hepatic colorectal metastases have further extended treatment possibilities.

Recent advancements in chemotherapies and biologic therapies have also contributed to effective treatment for hepatic colorectal metastases and extended the possibility for cure. As many as 5% of patients previously beyond curative therapies are being converted by systemic therapies to resectable. Those not resectable for cure are effectively treated by systemic and regional therapies to achieve extension of life. In the following sections we will present the current approach of palliative and adjuvant chemotherapy. The use of systemic and regional chemotherapy as neoadjuvant therapy prior to hepatectomy will also be discussed.

The combined advances in surgery, systemic therapies, and regional ablative therapies have transformed this disease from uniformly and immediately fatal to increasingly curable.

Gastrointestinal Oncology: A Critical Multidisciplinary Team Approach.
Edited by J. Jankowski, R. Sampliner, D. Kerr, and Y. Fong.

Surgical therapy for hepatic colorectal metastases

Darren Carpizo & Yuman Fong

Introduction

The liver is a common site for metastasis from colorectal cancers. One-quarter of patients will be found to have hepatic metastases synchronous with their colorectal primary, and nearly half of patients will develop metachronous liver metastasis after colorectal resection (Ekberg *et al.* 1987). Untreated colorectal metastasis to the liver uniformly results in death within months (Oxley & Ellis 1969). Even with the best current systemic chemo- and biologic therapies, median survival of unresected disease is less than 2 years (Saltz *et al.* 2000; Hurwitz *et al.* 2004; Cunningham *et al.* 2004).

Abundant data accumulated over the last decades have definitively demonstrated that hepatectomy is a potentially curative treatment of colorectal metastases (Wilson & Adson 1976; Wagner *et al.* 1984). We will review these data in this chapter. The patient selection criteria, preoperative work-up, and clinical determinants of outcome will be presented in the context of current multimodality treatment. While the bulk of discussion on chemotherapy will be presented in the chapter on systemic and regional therapy for this cancer, we will summarize the issues related to perioperative use of chemotherapy as it relates to surgical outcome and conduct.

Table 20.1 Natural history of liver metastasis from colorectal cancer.

Study	Number of patients	Median (months)	1 yr %	3 yr %	5 yr %
Bengmark 1968 (Bengmark & Hafstrom 1969)	173	–	5.7	0	0
Oxley 1969 (Oxley & Ellis 1969)	640	–	27	4	1
Wood 1976 (Wood *et al.* 1976)	113	6.6	15	3	1
Wagner 1984 (Wagner *et al.* 1984)	252	–	49	7	2
Scheele 1990 (Scheele *et al.* 1990)	921	–	–	–	0

– Data not specified.

Natural history of hepatic colorectal metastases

Many studies in the 20th century had examined the outcome of untreated hepatic colorectal metastases. Median survival is 5–10 months. Outcome is clearly related to tumor burden (Bengmark & Hafstrom 1969; Wood *et al.* 1976; Bengtsson *et al.* 1981) (Table 20.1). While the 1-year survival was only 5.7% for patients with widespread liver disease, 60% of patients with solitary metastasis were alive at 1 year and these patients with solitary metastases had a mean survival of 25 months (Wood *et al.* 1976). Wood *et al.* compared the survival of 13 unresected patients with technically resectable disease with 100 patients with unresectable disease. For these 13, the 1-, 3-, and 5-year survival was 77%, 23%, and 8%, compared with 15%, 0, and 0 for the unresectable group (Wood *et al.* 1976). Wagner *et al.* reported the 3- and 5-year survival for untreated resectable disease to be 14% and 2%, compared with 4% and 0 for unresectable disease (Wagner *et al.* 1984). Regardless of tumor burden, 5-year survival for untreated disease is extremely rare.

Similar conclusions were found in case–control studies. Wilson and Adson (Wilson & Adson 1976) compared 60 patients with resection to 60 patients with a comparable number of lesions and extent of disease not subjected to resection. The 5- and 10-year survivals of resected patients were 25% and 19%, while no unresected patient survived 5 years. Two other case–control studies had almost identical results (Wagner *et al.* 1984; Scheele *et al.* 1991). These data, combined with extensive data documenting long-term survival after hepatectomy, have led to general acceptance of hepatectomy as an effective treatment for liver colorectal metastases, even though no randomized trial had ever been performed.

Results of resection for colorectal liver metastases

Many studies have been published over the last three decades demonstrating resection of liver metastases from colorectal primaries to be safe and effective (Simmonds *et al.* 2006). Initially, the reports were retrospective in nature. More recently, results are from prospectively gathered data (Nordlinger *et al.* 1996; Fong *et al.* 1999; Wei *et al.* 2006) (Table 20.2). Even without randomized controlled trial data, it is well accepted that hepatectomy is superior to medical management. The reason is that virtually no-one under medical management lives more than 5 years. Since all major series have demonstrated that hepatectomy results in long-term survival in approximately one-third of patients, these data are so compelling that randomized trials are both unethical and unnecessary.

Of note, the mortality in most series is 3–5% and the 5-year survival is approximately 35%. These numbers have changed little over the last two decades. This does not mean that we have not made progress. As safety of hepatectomy has improved, clinicians have been increasingly willing to perform ever more extensive resections to eradicate tumor. In addition, as long-term outcomes improve due to improving adjuvant therapies, clinicians have been extending the indications for resection. Whereas trisectorectomies and resections of more than four tumors were unusual a decade ago, these are now routine. This explains the fact that operative mortality and long-term survival has plateaued. Most clinicians are willing to perform an operation with a 5% mortality if one-third of these patients can be cured from an otherwise fatal condition.

Following is a review of the peri-operative and long-term outcomes over the last three decades.

Perioperative mortality and morbidity

Recent advances in understanding of liver anatomy, in resectional techniques and in anesthetic care have translated into favorable survival rates for even the most extensive resections. The mortality associated with an elective liver resection for colorectal metastases is less than 5% in most recent series (Busuttil 1974; Foster 1978; Hughes *et al.* 1986; Schlag *et al.* 1990; Doci *et al.* 1991; Younes *et al.* 1991; Rosen *et al.* 1992; Scheele *et al.* 1995; Nordlinger *et al.* 1996; Jamison *et al.* 1997; Fong *et al.* 1999; Minagawa *et al.* 2000; Choti *et al.* 2002; Belli *et al.* 2002; Kato *et al.* 2003; Mutsaerts *et al.* 2005; Wei *et al.* 2006) (Table 20.2). The majority of the deaths occur from peri-operative hemorrhage, liver failure, or sepsis.

Table 20.2 Results of hepatic resection for metastatic colorectal cancer.

Study	Number of patients	Operative mortality %	1 year survival %	3 year survival %	5 year survival %	10 year survival %	Median months
Foster 1978 (Foster, 1978)	78	5	–	–	22	–	–
Adson 1984 (Adson *et al.* 1984)	141	3	80	42	25	–	–
Fortner 1984 (Busuttil, 1974)	75	7	89	57	35	–	–
Hughes 1986 (Hughes *et al.* 1986)	607	–	–	–	33	–	–
Schlag 1990 (Schlag *et al.* 1990)	122	4	85	40	30	–	32
Doci 1991 (Doci *et al.* 1991)	100	5	–	28	–	28	–
Younes 1991 (Younes *et al.* 1991)	133	–	91	–	–	–	–
Rosen 1992 (Rosen *et al.* 1992)	280	4	84	47	25	–	–
Scheele 1995 (Scheele *et al.* 1995)	434	4	85	45	33	20	40
Jamison 1997 (Jamison *et al.* 1997)	280	4	84	–	27	20	33
Nordlinger 1995 (Nordlinger *et al.* 1996)	1568	2	–	–	28	–	–
Fong 1999 (Fong *et al.* 1999)	1001	2.8	89	57	36	22	42
Minagawa 2000 (Minagawa *et al.* 2000)	235	0.85	–	51	38	26	
Choti 2002 (Choti *et al.* 2002)	226	1	93	57	40	26	46
Belli 2002 (Belli *et al.* 2002)	181	–	91.2	55.3	39.8	–	–
Kato 2003 (Kato *et al.* 2003)	585	0*	–	–	33	–	–
Mutsaerts 2005 (Mutsaerts *et al.* 2005)	102	3	–	–	29	–	–
Wei 2006 (Wei *et al.* 2006)	423	2	93	–	47	28	53

* Patients who died perioperatively were excluded from study.
– Not specified.

Complication rates remain high because of the physiologic stress of removing a significant portion of such a metabolically and immunologically important organ as the liver. The reported complication rates vary between 20 and 50% (Table 20.3). Pulmonary complications are frequent and reflect the pulmonary compromise produced by a combination of a large upper abdominal incision and the significant sympathetic pleural effusion that occurs postoperatively. In fact, 5–10% of pleural effusions may be sufficiently symptomatic to require tube thoracostomy (Coppa *et al.* 1985). Pneumonia occurs in 5–22% (Schlag *et al.* 1990). Pulmonary embolism (Scheele *et al.* 1991; Cunningham *et al.* 1994) or myocardial infarction each occur only in approximately 1% of patients but may result in mortality (Scheele *et al.* 1991).

Among the liver-specific complications, liver failure is the most dreaded and occurs in 3–8% of all major resections (Schlag *et al.* 1990; Scheele *et al.* 1991). Bilary leak and fistula occur in approximately 4% (Schlag *et al.* 1990; Scheele *et al.* 1991). Perihepatic abscess occurs in 2–10% (Schlag *et al.* 1990; Scheele *et al.* 1991). Significant hemorrhage is rare (1–3%) but is a major cause of perioperative mortality.

Of note, complications do not always translate to prolonged hospital stays or mortality. If rapidly and appropriately treated, most complications do not result in poor outcome. The usual hospital stay in major centers after a major liver resection is generally less than 2 weeks (Fong *et al.* 2005).

Long-term results

Five-year survival after hepatectomy for colorectal metastases is 25–40% and a 33–46 month median survival can be expected (Fong *et al.* 1999; Younes *et al.* 1991; Choti *et al.* 2002). (Table 20.2) A number of series now have sufficiently long follow-up for us to be confident that 10-year survival after hepatectomy can be expected in 20–30% of patients (Fong *et al.* 1999; Minagawa *et al.* 2000; Wei *et al.* 2006). Not only is there no doubt that resection prolongs survival, resection can produce cure from this stage IV cancer. Surgical resection has therefore become standard therapy and treatment of choice for metastatic colorectal cancer isolated to the liver.

Sites of recurrence

The patterns of recurrence in patients who are not cured by hepatectomy have also been well documented (Table 20.4). The liver is the most common site of recurrence. It is the first site of recurrence in 50% of cases. The lung is the first site of recurrence in 25%. Recurrence in the colon or rectum occurs in 10–20% of cases. This is the reason that follow-up consists of abdominal CT, chest X-ray, and colonoscopy.

Re-resection for recurrence after resection

Since the liver is the most common site for recurrence after hepatectomy, treatment of such recurrences constitutes an

Table 20.3 Complications of liver resection.

	Scheele (Scheele *et al.* 1991)	Schlag (Schlag *et al.* 1990)	Doci (Doci *et al.* 1991)	Mala (Mala *et al.* 2002)	Jarnagin (Jarnagin *et al.* 2002)	Cady (Cady *et al.* 1998) (%)
Total resections	219	122	100	146	1803	244
Liver-related complications						
Hemorrhage	7 (3)		3	4* (3)	18 (1)	1
Bile fistula	8 (4)	5 (4)	4	2 (1)		2
Perihepatic abscess	4 (2)	11 (9)	5		110 (6)	1
Liver failure	17 (8)		3		99 (5)	1
Renal failure	3 (1)		1			
Portal vein thrombosis				1 (<1)	9 (.5)	
Infections						
Wound		7 (6)			94 (5)	2
Sepsis		3 (2)	2	3 (2)	39 (2)	2
General complications						
GI bleed					21 (1)	0
DVT	2 (1)				24 (1)	<1
Pulmonary embolism	4 (2)					<1
Cardiac/MI	2 (1)	6 (5)	1	1 (<1)	21 (1)	3
Pneumonia		10 (8)	22	13 (9)	54 (2)	1
Pleural effusion					154 (9)	2

* One patient reoperated twice for hemorrhage.
n (%)

Table 20.4 Sites of initial recurrence after liver resection for colorectal metastasis.

Study	n	Recurrences	Liver	Liver and other	Lung	Lung and other	Colon/rectum
Hughes (Maeda *et al.* 1992)	607	424	149 (35)	42 (10)	73 (17)	–	33 (8)
Schlag (Hohenberger *et al.* 1990)	122	80	17 (14)	55 (45)	–	–	–
Butler (Butler *et al.* 1986)	62	30	10 (33)	10 (33)	–	–	–
Ekberg (Ekberg *et al.* 1987)	68	53	19 (28)	25 (47)	3 (6)	12 (23)	8 (15)
Bozetti (Bozzetti *et al.* 1987)	45	28	11 (39)	5 (18)	5 (17)	–	–
Nordlinger (Nordlinger *et al.* 1987)	80	51	21 (42)	13 (26)	11 (22)	–	11 (22)
Fortner (Fortner, 1988)	69	45	8 (12)	–	16 (23)	–	–
Suzuki (Suzuki *et al.* 1997)	64	45	31 (48)	–	16 (25)	–	–

n = number of patients (%).

important part of the overall treatment plan for patients. Approximately one-third of patients with hepatic recurrence will be candidates for further resection (Fortner 1988). As liver surgeons have become increasingly comfortable with liver resections, an increasing number of repeat hepatectomies are being performed as treatment for recurrent disease. Table 20.5 summarizes the data for such repeat hepatectomies (Stone *et al.* 1990; Bozzetti *et al.* 1992; Vaillant *et al.* 1993; Elias *et al.* 1993; Que & Nagorney 1994; Fong *et al.* 1994; Yamamoto *et al.* 1999; Muratore *et al.* 2001; Suzuki *et al.* 2001; Petrowsky *et al.* 2002; Shaw *et al.* 2006).

These repeat hepatectomies are quite safe, with operative mortalities much lower than series for first-time hepatectomies. In the 432 patients summarized in Table 20.5 there were only 8 reported operative deaths, an operative mortality of less than 2%. Complication rates are comparable to first-time resections and have been reported to be 15–50% (Lange *et al.* 1989). In the most recent series, 5-year survival after second resection is reported to be over 40% (Petrowsky *et al.* 2002; Shaw *et al.* 2006). In a report examining 10-year survivors after liver resection, nearly half of these patients required a second liver resection to achieve long-term survival (D'Angelica *et al.* 1997). Thus, patients with resectable recurrences in the liver should be considered for repeat hepatectomy, and patients with limited but unresectable disease isolated to the liver should be considered for thermoablation (see section on ablative therapy).

Table 20.5 Results of repeat hepatic resections.

Author	Year	Resected	Mortality	2-year survival	5-year survival
Stone (Stone *et al.* 1990)	1990	10	0/10	25	–
Bozzetti (Bozzetti *et al.* 1992)	1992	10	1/11	23	–
Vaillant (Vaillant *et al.* 1993)	1993	16	1/16	33	–
Elias (Elias *et al.* 1993)	1993	28	1/28	30	–
Que (Que & Nagorney, 1994)	1994	21	1/21	41	–
Fong (Fong *et al.* 1994)	1994	25	0/25	30	–
Yamamoto (Yamamoto *et al.* 1999)	1999	75	0/75	–	23
Muratore (Muratore *et al.* 2001)	2001	29	1/29	–	–
Suzuki (Suzuki *et al.* 2001)	2001	26	0/26	–	31
Petrowsky (Petrowsky *et al.* 2002)	2002	126	2/126	–	43
Shaw (Shaw *et al.* 2006)	2006	66	1/66	–	44

– Data not specified.

Table 20.6. Predictors of recurrence after hepatic resection for metastatic colorectal cancer.

Study	Patient age	Primary stage	Metastases					Chemo	Surgical margin	CEA
			Synchronous	Size	Number	Bilobar	Satellite			
Foster 1978 (Foster 1978)	–	N	N	Y	Y	–	–	–	–	–
Fortner 1984 (Fortner *et al.* 1984b)	N	Y	–	N	N	–	–	N	–	N
Iwatsuki 1986 (Pagana 1986)	N	Y	N	Y	Y	–	–	Y	–	–
Hughes 1988 (Hughes *et al.* 1988b)	–	Y	Y	Y	Y	Y	–	Y	Y	Y
Schlag 1990 (Schlag *et al.* 1990)	–	–	Y	–	–	–	–	–	–	–
Doci 1991 (Doci *et al.* 1991)	N	Y	N	N	N	N	–	–	–	N
Scheele 1991 (Scheele *et al.* 1991)	N	Y	Y	N	N	N	Y	–	Y	–
Younes 1991 (Younes *et al.* 1991)	–	N	N	Y	Y	–	–	–	–	Y
Cady 1992 (Cady *et al.* 1992a)	N	N	N	N	Y	–	–	–	Y	Y
Rosen 1992 (Rosen *et al.* 1992)	–	N	N	N	N	–	Y	–	N	–
Nordlinger 1995 (Nordlinger *et al.* 1996)	Y	Y	Y	Y	Y	N	–	–	Y	Y
Scheele 1995 (Scheele *et al.* 1995)	N	Y	Y	Y	N	N	Y	–	Y	Y
Fong 1999 (Fong *et al.* 1999)	N	Y	Y	Y	Y	Y	–	–	Y	Y

Prognostic variables

Over the years, investigators have also attempted to determine the clinical prognostic factors that govern long-term outcome. Identifying parameters that predict poor cancer outcome allows for selection of patients for adjuvant or neoadjuvant therapy. In addition, such parameters allow for patient stratification in clinical trials.

Investigators have also attempted to synthesize the resilient prognostic factors into staging systems for classifying patients with metastatic colorectal cancer. This is necessary because the traditional TNM staging systems classify all patients with hepatic colorectal metastases in the same category: stage IV. Clearly, the patient with a solitary metastasis found 4 years after resection of a node-negative primary is very different from a patient found with bilobar multiple metastases synchronous to discovery of a node-positive primary.

In the following paragraphs, we will summarize the factors that do and do not influence outcome (Table 20.6). These parameters are further divided into (i) variables associated with the primary cancer; (ii) variables associated with the presentation of the liver metastases; and (iii) pathologic characteristics of the liver metastases.

Factors influencing outcome

Characteristics of the primary tumor

The stage of the primary is a major determinant of outcome (Hughes *et al.* 1986; Doci *et al.* 1991). In particular, regional nodal positivity is a powerful predictor of recurrence (Hughes *et al.* 1989; Scheele *et al.* 1995; Nordlinger *et al.* 1996; Fong *et al.* 1999). Synchronous presentation of liver metastases also predicts poor outcome (Ballantyne & Quin 1993). Patients with symptoms related to metastatic disease also do not fare as well as asymptomatic patients (Hughes *et al.* 1986, 1988b).

Clinical characteristics of the liver metastases

Short disease-free interval between primary cancer and hepatic metastases is associated with poor outcome (Hughes *et al.* 1986; Rosen *et al.* 1992). Other parameters associated with poor outcome include large size of tumor (Hughes *et al.* 1986; Stephenson *et al.* 1988), multiple tumors (Hughes *et al.* 1986; Rosen *et al.* 1992), bilateral tumors (Ekberg *et al.* 1987), and high carcinoembryonic antigen (CEA) levels (Hughes *et al.* 1986; Nordlinger *et al.* 1996).

Operative and pathologic characteristics of the liver metastases

An overwhelming predictor of recurrence is involvement of the resection margin by tumor (Cady & McDermott 1985; Hughes *et al.* 1986). Anatomic resections are associated with better outcome than wedge resections, probably due to a significantly lower rate of positive margins (DeMatteo *et al.* 2000). The operative finding most influential on long-term survival however, is extrahepatic disease (Fortner *et al.* 1984b; Adson *et al.* 1984; Cady & McDermott 1985; Hughes *et al.* 1986; Ekberg *et al.* 1987; Rosen *et al.* 1992). Although selected patients with limited numbers of lung nodules (Miller *et al.* 2007), adrenal metastases, or patients with great response of extrahepatic disease to systemic chemotherapy may have favorable outcome after hepatectomy, most patients with extrahepatic disease do poorly. The existence of extrahepatic disease should be considered a relative contraindication to liver resection. Satellite lesions are also a poor prognostic factor (Gayowski *et al.* 1994; Scheele *et al.* 1995).

Factors not influencing outcome

In most series, age has not been found to have prognostic significance (Hughes *et al.* 1988a; Cady *et al.* 1992b; Ballantyne & Quin 1993). This likely reflects the successful medical selection criteria for hepatectomy, and the superior perioperative care delivered by anesthesiologists and surgeons at major centers. Gender has not been found to be a consistent predictor of outcome (Adson 1987; Holm *et al.* 1989). The location of primary cancer also does not seem to influence outcome, there being no significant differences between rectal and colon cancers (Adson 1987; Doci *et al.* 1991). Whether the primary tumor is poorly differentiated also has not been shown to influence outcome (Doci *et al.* 1991).

Clinical risk score

It is clear that numerous factors have been found to be important in categorizing this disease. Most of the factors identified, however, cannot by themselves be considered a complete contraindication to resection. For example, even when the number of tumors is above four, complete removal of all tumors has been shown to be better than medical management (Fortner *et al.* 1984a,b; Hughes *et al.* 1986; Cady *et al.* 1992b). Thus, investigators have attempted to combine the various prognostic variables into a scoring or staging system for use. Until recently, most reports attempting to identify clinical prognostic factors were of insufficient size to allow for definitive recommendations for a multivariable staging system.

Recently, two very large patient series have allowed for robust multivariate analysis of prognostic variables. Results from both series were very similar. Nordlinger *et al.* reported a multicenter collected series of over 1500 patients subjected to hepatectomy for colorectal metastases (Nordlinger *et al.* 1996). Memorial Sloan-Kettering Cancer Center (MSKCC) reported a single institutional series of 1001 patients that allowed analysis for independent predictors of poor outcome (Fong *et al.* 1999). Seven parameters were found to be independent predictors of prognosis. These were (i) positive resection margin, (ii) extrahepatic disease, (iii) nodal metastases from primary cancer, (iv) short disease-free interval, (v) largest tumor greater than 5 cm, (vi) more than one liver metastasis, and (vii) CEA over 200 ng/mL. Data for the first two of these are not available preoperatively. Furthermore, no surgeon would go to the operating room expecting a positive margin, and extrahepatic disease is considered a relative contraindication to resection. Thus, using the last five criteria, a clinical risk score (CRS) system was created (Table 20.7) counting each criterion as one point. This CRS is a simple, easily remembered staging system for classifying patients with liver-exclusive stage IV colorectal cancer. This CRS has proven useful for comparing results from diverse centers, for selection of patients for neoadjuvant and adjuvant therapy, for surgical and ablative therapies, and as stratification of patients for trials.

Current use of clinical risk score

The clinical risk score has proven to be a useful guide in the delivery of multimodality therapy for hepatic colorectal metastases. A score of 2 or less places a patient in a good prognostic group, for whom resection or other local therapies is ideal. For scores of 3 or higher, outcome is less favorable and patients should be considered for aggressive trials of adjuvant therapy.

The clinical risk score has been verified by independent investigators from Norway (Mala *et al.* 2002). Thus, it is not just pertinent to a large tertiary American center. Recent data from Asia also indicate that the CRS is useful for predicting outcome after ablative therapy of liver metastases.

Table 20.7 Prognostic scoring system for hepatic colorectal metastases. Sum of points with one point assigned for each positive criteria. Score ≤ 2 represents a good prognosis.

Node-positive primary tumor
Disease-free interval less than 12 months between colon resection and appearance of metastases
Size of largest lesion >5 cm
More than one tumor
Carcinoembryonic antigen >200 ng/mL

This clinical risk score has also proven useful in helping select the extent of preoperative assessment. A high clinical risk score justifies both FDG-PET scanning and laparoscopy as preoperative tests (Jarnagin *et al.* 2001; Schussler-Fiorenza *et al.* 2004). Given the high cost of these tests, having a way of choosing patients who would benefit provides a data-driven approach that would optimize patient outcome while minimizing cost.

Perioperative use of chemotherapy

Potential role of adjuvant therapy

Most patients surviving after liver resection die of recurrent disease resulting from microscopic residual cancer not detected at the time of hepatectomy (Ekberg *et al.* 1987; Bozzetti *et al.* 1987; Maeda *et al.* 1992). A full chapter in this book addresses the theory and practice of chemotherapy for hepatic colorectal metastases. For details of the various agents and use, the reader is referred to that chapter. In the following section, we will summarize data regarding use of adjuvant systemic and regional chemotherapy in attempts to prevent recurrence, and preoperative use of chemotherapy to convert patients with unresectable disease to resectable. This section is meant to put into focus the current use of perioperative chemotherapy.

Adjuvant systemic chemotherapy

Until recently, little prospective data examined the utility of adjuvant systemic chemotherapy after complete resection of liver tumors. Data from early retrospective studies were equivocal, due likely to the patient selection process for chemotherapy. There were suggestions that chemotherapy may improve outcome. Iwatsuki *et al.* (Pagana 1986) and Hughes *et al.* (Hughes *et al.* 1988b) found that patients who received chemotherapy had a significantly better survival than patients who did not. The differences found in these studies were small, and insufficient details were given to allow determination of whether comparable groups were studied.

Recently, two studies were almost simultaneously published that clearly indicated adjuvant chemotherapy to improve survival. The first, a two-center retrospective study, examined the utility of adjuvant 5-fluorouracil (5-FU) and leucovorin after hepatectomy (Park *et al.* 2007). In this study, investigators examined outcomes of patients from Memorial Sloan-Kettering Cancer Center, where adjuvant chemotherapy is often administered, and patients from the Edinburgh Royal Infirmary, where adjuvant chemotherapy was not often given. 518 patients treated with no chemotherapy were compared with 274 patients treated with 5-FU-based adjuvant chemotherapy. Patient survival analysis was performed with stratification by the clinical risk score. Patients subjected to adjuvant chemotherapy had improved survival ($p=0.007$, log-rank test). In every clinical risk score category, patients subjected to adjuvant chemotherapy had a higher chance of survival.

Meanwhile, Portier *et al.* 2006 reported a multicenter trial that randomized 173 patients after hepatectomy for colorectal cancer to surgery alone or to surgery followed by 6 months of systemic adjuvant chemotherapy with fluorouracil and folinic acid. The 5-year disease-free survival rate was 34% for patients subjected to chemotherapy compared to 27% for patients in the control group ($p=0.03$). Adjuvant intravenous systemic chemotherapy provided a significant disease-free survival benefit for patients with resected liver metastases from colorectal cancer and was an independent predictor of outcomes.

At present there are clearly many more choices for systemic therapy than 5-FU and leucovorin. However, more sophisticated regimens do not always translate to better outcome in the adjuvant setting since patients are also in the process of recovering from a major operation. In the situation of adjuvant chemotherapy after resection of colorectal primaries, for example, a large randomized trial demonstrated that patients subjected to irinotecan, 5-FU, and leucovorin has significantly higher toxicity without any benefit in survival when compared to patients treated with 5-FU and leucovorin (Saltz *et al.* 2004).

At present, data would support use of 5-FU and leucovorin as adjuvant therapy after liver resection if patients have not previously failed this regimen. Thus, for patients with synchronous disease or who did not receive adjuvant therapy after a prior resection for colorectal cancer, this would be the regimen of choice. For those who have previously failed this regimen, an oxaliplatin- or irinotecan-containing regimen should be considered but this approach has not been substantiated by data.

Adjuvant intra-arterial chemotherapy (hepatic arterial infusion, HAI)

Since the liver is the most common site for tumor recurrence after hepatectomy, there have been numerous studies examining the use of chemotherapy directed regionally at the liver. The theory underlying this type of chemotherapy as well as in depth details of various clinical trials will be discussed extensively in the subsequent chapter on chemotherapy.

Studies reported in the 1990s were prospective single-arm trials demonstrating safety and feasibility of adjuvant regional hepatic chemotherapy (Marcove *et al.* 1977; Moriya *et al.* 1991; Goodie *et al.* 1992; Curley *et al.* 1993). Recently, two positive adjuvant regional chemotherapy trials were completed (Nagino *et al.* 1995; Kemeny *et al.* 1999), clearly demonstrating that administration of floxuridine administered directly to the liver was highly effective at controlling liver disease.

With availability of irinotecan, oxaliplatin, and bevacizumab, there is now opportunity to combine use of these systemic therapies with regional FUDR. Such a strategy combines use of the most effective systemic therapy with the most effective regional therapy. Clinical data suggest this will not only optimize treatment by targeting all sites, there also seems to be synergy of action at the liver site. Response rate of non-resectable hepatic colorectal metastases to CPT-11/HAI FUDR is 75% (Kemeny *et al.* 2001), even if the patients had previously failed systemic

CPT-11. Results from studies examining combined systemic oxaliplatin and HAI FUDR are similar (Kemeny *et al.* 2005). Strong consideration should be given to using such combined regimens in patients who had previously failed systemic chemotherapy, since the likelihood of responding to other systemic regimens is only of the order of 15–20%.

Chemotherapy to downstage patients who present with non-resectable disease

The clinical approval of CPT-11 and oxaliplatin ushered in a new era in the treatment of patients with metastatic colorectal cancer and has resulted in improved palliative treatment of patients with this disease. Since early use of oxaliplatin, there were reports that such chemotherapy may convert non-resectable cases to resectable. Henri Bismuth and his colleagues published this observation in 2000, reporting on 330 consecutive patients presenting to their institution with non-resectable disease. They found that oxaliplatin-based chemotherapy converted 53 of these patients to resectable disease. Adam *et al.* recently updated this series, reporting on 701 patients with non-resectable disease treated with oxaliplatin/5-FU/LV. Ninety-three of these patients (13.6%) had a significant response and proceeded to liver resection. The 5-year survival following liver resection was 34% (Adam *et al.* 2001). This indicates that even patients with incurable disease can be converted by response to chemotherapy to a favorable outcome.

There is also recent data that suggest that HAI chemotherapy may also convert unresectable liver metastases to resectable. Clavien *et al.* reported that of a series of 23 patients treated with regional FUDR chemotherapy, 6 patients were converted to resectable (Clavien *et al.* 2002). With improving systemic and regional chemotherapy, it is likely that an increasing number of patients with unresectable disease will become surgical candidates.

Neoadjuvant use of chemotherapy

Some clinicians have argued that since the current generation of chemotherapy is so good at killing cancer, neoadjuvant use of chemotherapy should be considered. This is the use of chemotherapy in the preoperative setting for a patient with clearly resectable disease, and must be distinguished from the use of chemotherapy to downstage an otherwise unresectable patient. The theoretical benefits of neoadjuvant therapy are many. Preoperative treatment may allow potential eradication of microscopic disease even prior to resection. Treatment while the liver tumors are in place allows *in vivo* determination of effectiveness of the chosen regimen. A delay to surgery allows declaration of occult disease. Finally, reducing the tumor size may allow easier resection or ablation. These theoretical benefits are largely unproven. Furthermore, there are certainly detrimental effects to preoperative use of chemotherapy. First and foremost is clear documentation that chemotherapies may produce liver damage and detrimentally affect recovery after hepatectomy. Costs can also be considerable. A 6-month neoadjuvant course of chemotherapy can cost as much as $180,000.

The approach we recommend is a selective use of neoadjuvant chemotherapy. For patients presenting shortly after resection of the colorectal primary who have not sufficiently recovered from the first operation to tolerate a liver resection, neoadjuvant therapy should be considered. For patients with a high risk of recurrence, such as those with a high clinical risk score, particularly patients with synchronous disease discovered during resection of a lymph-node positive primary, neoadjuvant therapy can be justified.

Chemotherapy-associated steatohepatitis (CASH)

There has been a long history of reports supporting the notion that most chemotherapeutic agents, even 5-FU, can cause hepatic damage (Peppercorn *et al.* 1998). While the most recently approved chemotherapies such as irinotecan, oxaliplatin, and bevacizumab (Avastin) have produced great impact upon the survival of patients (Leonard *et al.* 2005), these agents clearly have a higher propensity for liver damage (Karoui *et al.* 2006). It is now common that patients are subjected to a number of chemotherapies prior to hepatectomy. The hepatic surgeon is therefore increasingly challenged by postoperative management of the patient with hepatic damage from use of these agents.

Another factor contributing to these difficulties is the number of different chemotherapies that are available. Many patients subjected to second- and third-line therapies remain candidates for liver resection, whereas in years past, most patients failing first-line therapy were unlikely to be offered surgery. Thus, chemotherapy-associated steatohepatitis (CASH) has become commonplace.

It is important for the clinician to recognize CASH. The clinical triad is hepatic fatty infiltration, splenomegaly from portal hypertension, and refractory thrombocytopenia (Fig. 20.1). The damage can progress to fibrosis and cirrhosis of the liver. The thrombocytopenia is consumptive and not related to bone marrow suppression. Therefore, it is not corrected even when chemotherapy is stopped.

Preoperative portal vein embolization to improve perioperative outcome

Detection of CASH is not purely academic. Recognition of CASH may lead to active interventions to improve outcome. One such potential intervention is use of preoperative portal vein embolization (PVE) to grow the remnant liver before resection. This technique involves a percutaneous, interventional radiologic approach for depriving portal blood flow to the liver tissues in the planned resection. Over a period of 3–4 weeks, atrophy of the embolized liver occurs with contralateral

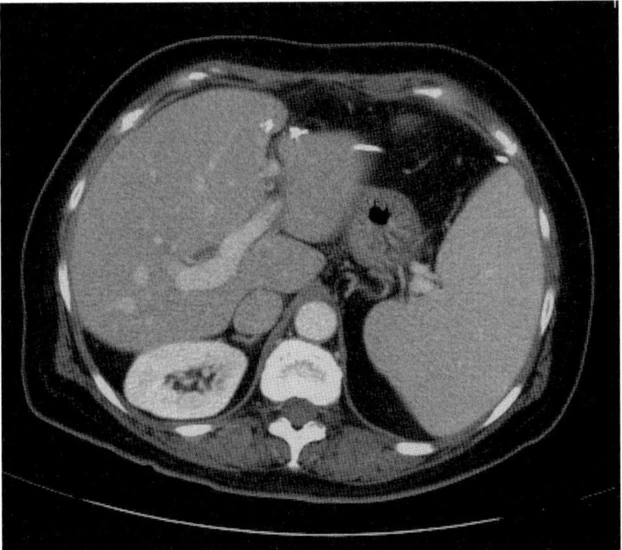

Fig. 20.1 Typical radiologic findings for chemotherapy-associated steatohepatitis (CASH). CT of the abdomen demonstrates steatosis of the liver as indicated by the liver being darker than the spleen. Splenomegaly is also seen. The third part of the triad that characterizes this syndrome is a thrombocytopenia due to increased clearance of platelets by the spleen.

remnant liver hypertrophy. Makuuchi first proposed using PVE to produce atrophy on the side of liver to be resected and hypertrophy of the contralateral remnant liver (Makuuchi *et al.* 1990). Originally, clinicians suggested using this technique when the planned remnant liver after resection is less than 25% of total functional liver (Hemming *et al.* 2003). The presence of CASH would encourage consideration of such portal vein embolizations even when the remnant is more than 25% (Beal *et al.* 2006). The PVE can act as a 'stress test' for the liver, allowing preoperative determination of capacity for regeneration. PVE also seems to enhance recovery. Use of PVE will likely expand as increasing numbers of patients present with damaged parenchyma.

Preparation of the patient for surgery

Preparation of the patient for hepatectomy can be divided into medical preparation and tumor staging/technical surgical planning.

Preoperative medical preparation

In general, preoperative preparation involves the correction of anemia and of coagulopathy and appropriate single-dose antibiotic prophylaxis. All patients with a history of cardiorespiratory disease and all patients over the age of 65 are submitted to full cardiorespiratory investigation.

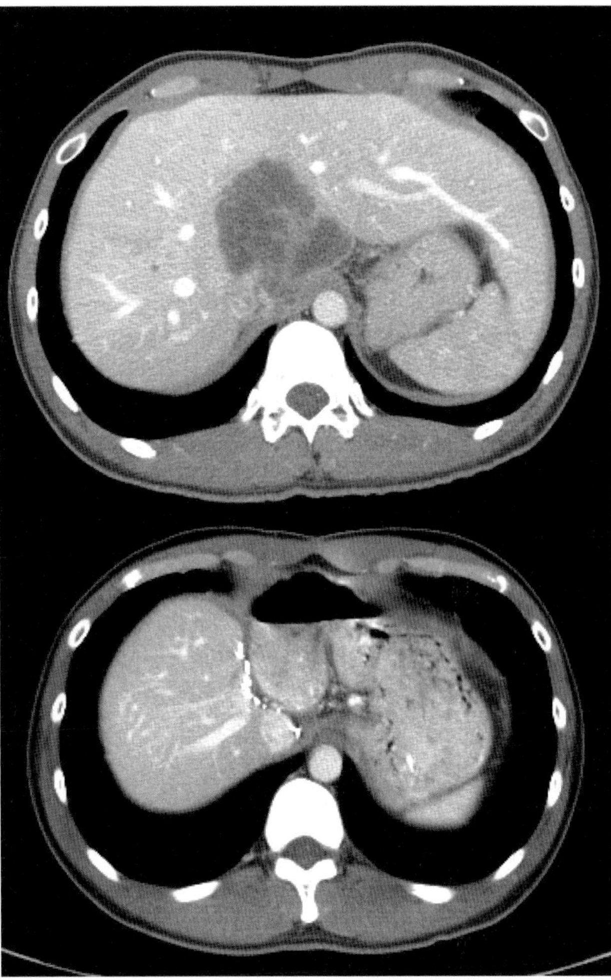

Fig. 20.2 Large tumor in immediate adjacency of the vena cava. This poorly placed metastatic lesion located in the back of segment IV and extending onto the caudate lobe was pressing against the vena cava for a long length but not invaded. Below is the scan performed over 2 years after resection showing a disease-free patient.

Preoperative imaging for staging and surgical planning

Many sophisticated imaging techniques are now available to define number and location of liver lesions, and determine the presence or absence of extrahepatic disease.

A computed tomographic (CT) scan is the standard scan for evaluating extent of liver disease. Current generation helical CT with contrast enhancement of vasculature is invaluable in determining number of lesions, relationship to lesions of vascular structures, and potential involvement of neighboring organs. Metastatic colorectal cancer in the liver tends to respect intersegmental planes and the liver capsule, and push structures away rather than directly invade them (Baer *et al.* 1989). Thus, even very large lesions that are in close proximity to the inferior vena cava most often do not invade the adjacent vessels and usually can be resected (Fig. 20.2).

Magnetic resonance imaging (MRI) can also give the same information as a CT scan but is much more expensive. Routine use of MRI is unnecessary. We recommend its use in patients with hepatic steatosis. In fatty livers, small lesions may not be apparent on CT. MRI is far superior for imaging of lesions in a fatty liver.

Hepatic angiography and inferior vena cavography are rarely needed given the quality of vascular imaging possible in current generation CT or MRI.

^{18}F-fluorodeoxyglucose positron emission tomography (FDG-PET) is the most important recent innovation influencing surgical treatment of patients with metastatic colorectal cancer. This scan uses the glucose analog ^{18}F-FDG, and exploits the glucose-avid nature of colorectal cancers to image tumor. Using this to stage patients increases yield of staging, and improves patient selection, resulting in improved survival of patients (Strasberg *et al.* 2001). Patients with hepatic colorectal metastases who were assessed by FDG-PET prior to liver resection had higher resectability, lower recurrence, and improved long-term survival (Strasberg *et al.* 2001). The PET scan is particularly good at detection of extrahepatic disease, such as nodal, peritoneal, lung, or bone metastases (Fig. 20.3). It is inferior to CT or MRI for detection of liver lesions because the normal liver is also a glucose-avid tissue and therefore the background is too high (Akhurst *et al.* 2005). Fewer than 20% of subcentimeter metastases in the liver are visible by PET. In fact, since chemotherapy also reduces tumor glucose uptake, fewer than 5% of subcentimeter tumors are visible by PET when the patient is on chemotherapy.

Recommendation for scanning: For patients being considered for liver resection, CT of the abdomen and pelvis, and FDG-PET scanning should be performed. During every whole-body PET-CT, a non-contrast CT of the chest is performed and therefore a separate scan is not necessary. If patient has a very fatty liver, MRI should be considered. With current use of PET, bone scans are rarely necessary.

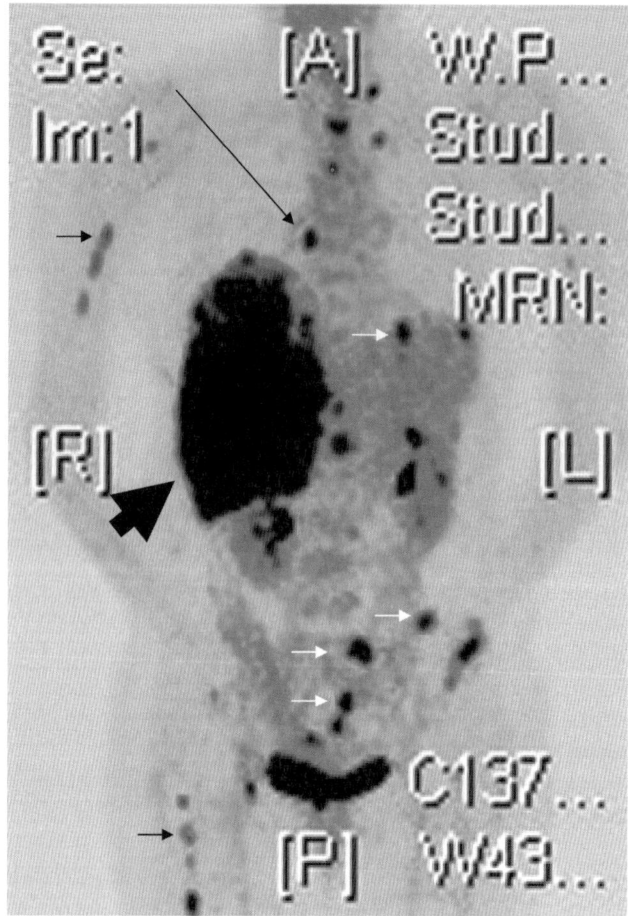

Fig. 20.3 FDG-PET scan demonstrating widespread disease in this patient with a very large hepatic metastasis (large arrow). Peritoneal metastases (white arrows), bone metastases (small black arrows), and mediastinal nodal metastases (long black arrows) are demonstrated.

Summary

Data gathered over the last decades have proven liver resection to be the treatment of choice for patients with resectable metastatic colorectal cancer to the liver. Resections are now routinely performed and may produce cure in this otherwise fatal disease that is still classified as stage IV. The clinical parameters that govern long-term survival are now well known, and have been combined into a clinical risk score that can be used to stratify patients according to risk. Although a number of clinical or pathologic factors clearly predict worse outcome, the only absolute contraindications to liver resection are prohibitively poor general health, or clear evidence of wide dissemination of disease. Major advances have also been made recently concerning chemotherapeutic treatments for this disease. There is no doubt that systemic therapies are effective adjuvants to surgery, and may also be used as upfront therapy to convert some patients from being unresectable to resectable. There is also no doubt that regional chemotherapy can provide successful and durable treatment of liver disease. The important areas for future study include the combined use of systemic and regional therapies as adjuvant therapy.

References

Adam R, Avisar E, Ariche A *et al.* (2001) Five-year survival following hepatic resection after neoadjuvant therapy for nonresectable colorectal [liver] metastases. *Ann Surg Oncol* 8: 347–53.

Adson MA. (1987) Resection of liver metastases. When is it worthwhile? *World J Surg* 11: 511–20.

Adson MA, Van Heerden JA, Adson MH. (1984) Resection of hepatic metastases from colorectal cancer. *Arch Surg* 119: 647–51.

Akhurst T, Kates TJ, Mazumdar M *et al.* (2005) Recent chemotherapy reduces the sensitivity of [18F]fluorodeoxyglucose positron emission tomography in the detection of colorectal metastases. *J Clin Oncol* 23: 8713–16.

Baer HU, Gertsch P, Matthews JB *et al.* (1989) Resectability of large focal liver lesions. *Br J Surg* 76: 1042–4.

Ballantyne GH, Quin J. (1993) Surgical treatment of liver metastases in patients with colorectal cancer. *Cancer* 71: 4252–66.

Beal IK, Anthony S, Papadopoulou A *et al.* (2006) Portal vein embolisation prior to hepatic resection for colorectal liver metastases and the effects of periprocedure chemotherapy. *Br J Radiol* 79: 473–8.

Belli G, D'Agostino A, Ciciliano F, Fantini C, Russolillo N, Belli A. (2002) Liver resection for hepatic metastases: 15 years of experience. *J Hepatobiliary Pancreat Surg* 9: 607–13.

Bengmark S, Hafstrom L. (1969) The natural history of primary and secondary malignant tumors of the liver. *Cancer* 23: 198–202.

Bengtsson G, Carlsson G, Hafström L, Jonsson PE. (1981) Natural history of patients with untreated liver metastases from colorectal cancer. *Am J Surg* 141: 586–9.

Bozzetti F, Bignami P, Morabito A, Doci R, Gennari L. (1987) Patterns of failure following surgical resection of colorectal cancer liver metastases. *Ann Surg* 205: 264–70.

Bozzetti F, Bignami P, Montalto R *et al.* (1992) Repeated hepatic resection for recurrent metastases from colorectal cancer. *Br J Surg* 79: 146–8.

Busuttil A. (1974) Ectopic adrenal within the gall-bladder wall. *J Pathol* 113: 231–3.

Butler J, Attiyeh FF, Daly JM. (1986) Hepatic resection for metastases of the colon and rectum. *Surg Gynecol Obstet* 162: 109–13.

Cady B, McDermott WV. (1985) Major hepatic resection for metachronous metastases from colon cancer. *Ann Surg* 201: 204–9.

Cady B, Jenkins RL, Steele GD Jr *et al.* (1998) Surgical margin in hepatic resection for colorectal metastasis: a critical and improvable determinant of outcome. *Ann Surg* 227: 566–71.

Cady B, Stone MD, McDermott WV *et al.* (1992a) Technical and biological factors in disease-free survival after hepatic resection for colorectal cancer metastases. *Arch Surg* 127: 561–9.

Cady B, Stone MD, McDermott WV *et al.* (1992b) Technical and biological factors in disease-free survival after hepatic resection for colorectal cancer metastases. *Arch Surg* 127: 561–9.

Choti MA, Sitzmann JV, Tiburi MF *et al.* (2002) Trends in long-term survival following liver resection for hepatic colorectal metastases. *Ann Surg* 235: 759–66.

Clavien PA, Selzner N, Morse M, Selzner M, Paulson E. (2002) Downstaging of hepatocellular carcinoma and liver metastases from colorectal cancer by selective intra-arterial chemotherapy. *Surgery* 131: 433–42.

Coppa GF, Eng K, Ranson JH, Gouge TH, Localio SA. (1985) Hepatic resection for metastatic colon and rectal cancer. An evaluation of preoperative and postoperative factors. *Ann Surg* 202: 203–8.

Cunningham JD, Fong Y, Shriver C, Melendez J, Marx WL, Blumgart LH. (1994) One hundred consecutive hepatic resections: blood loss, transfusion and operative technique. *Arch Surg* 129: 1050–6.

Cunningham D, Humblet Y, Siena S *et al.* (2004) Cetuximab monotherapy and cetuximab plus irinotecan in irinotecan-refractory metastatic colorectal cancer. *N Engl J Med* 351: 337–45.

Curley SA, Roh MS, Chase JL, Hohn DC. (1993) Adjuvant hepatic artery infusion chemotherapy after curative resection of colorectal liver metastases. *Am J Surg* 166: 743–8.

D'Angelica M, Brennan MF, Fortner JG, Cohen AM, Blumgart LH, Fong Y. (1997) Ninety-six five-year survivors after liver resection for metastatic colorectal cancer. *J Am Coll Surg* 185: 554–9.

DeMatteo RP, Palese C, Jarnagin WR, Sun RL, Blumgart LH, Fong Y. (2000) Anatomic segmental hepatic resection is superior to wedge resection as an oncologic operation for colorectal liver metastases. *J Gastrointest Surg* 4: 178–84.

Doci R, Gennari L, Bignami P, Montalto F, Morabita A, Bozzetti F. (1991) One hundred patients with hepatic metastases from colorectal cancer treated by resection: Analysis of prognostic determinants. *Br J Surg* 78: 797–801.

Ekberg H, Tranberg KG, Andersson R *et al.* (1987) Pattern of recurrence in liver resection for colorectal secondaries. *World J Surg* 11: 541–7.

Elias D, Lasser P, Hoang JM *et al.* (1993) Repeat hepatectomy for cancer. *Br J Surg* 80: 1557–62.

Fong Y, Blumgart LH, Cohen A, Fortner J, Brennan MF. (1994) Repeat hepatic resections for metastatic colorectal cancer. *Ann Surg* 220: 657–62.

Fong Y, Fortner J, Sun RL, Brennan MF, Blumgart LH. (1999) Clinical score for predicting recurrence after hepatic resection for metastatic colorectal cancer: analysis of 1001 consecutive cases. *Ann Surg* 230: 309–18.

Fong Y, Gonen M, Rubin D, Radzyner D, Brennan MF. (2005) Long-term survival is superior after resection for cancer in high volume centers. *Ann Surg* 242: 540–7.

Fortner JG. (1988) Recurrence of colorectal cancer after hepatic resection. *Am J Surg* 155: 378–82.

Fortner JG, Silva JS, Cox EB, Golbey RB, Gallowitz H, Maclean BJ. (1984a) Multivariate-analysis of a personal series of 247 patients with liver metastases from colorectal-cancer .2. Treatment by intrahepatic chemotherapy. *Ann Surg* 199: 317–24.

Fortner JG, Silva JS, Maj MC, Golbey RB, Cox EB, Maclean BA. (1984b) Multivariate analysis of a personal series of 247 consecutive patients with liver metastases from colorectal cancer. *Ann Surg* 199: 306–16.

Foster JH. (1978) Survival after liver resection for secondary tumors. *Am J Surg* 135: 389–94.

Gayowski TJ, Iwatsuki S, Madariaga JR *et al.* (1994) Experience in hepatic resection for metastatic colorectal cancer: analysis of clinical and pathological risk factors. *Surgery* 116: 703–11.

Goodie DB, Horton MD, Morris RW, Nagy LS, Morris DL. (1992) Anaesthetic experience with cryotherapy for treatment of hepatic malignancy. *Anaesth Intensive Care* 20: 491–6.

Hemming AW, Reed AI, Howard RJ *et al.* (2003) Preoperative portal vein embolization for extended hepatectomy. *Ann Surg* 237: 686–91.

Hohenberger P, Schlag P, Schwarz V, Herfarth C. (1990) Tumor recurrence and options for further treatment after resection of liver metastases in patients with colorectal cancer. *J Surg Oncol* 44: 245–51.

Holm A, Bradley E, Aldrete JS. (1989) Hepatic resection of metastasis from colorectal-carcinoma - morbidity, mortality, and pattern of recurrence. *Ann Surg* 209: 428–34.

Hughes KS, Simon R, Songhorabodi S *et al.* (1986) Resection of the liver for colorectal carcinoma metastases: a multi-institutional study of patterns of recurrence. *Surgery* 100: 278–84.

Hughes KS, Rosenstein RB, Songhorabodi S *et al.* (1988a) Resection of the liver for colorectal carcinoma metastases. A multi-institutional study of long-term survivors. *Dis Colon Rectum* 31: 1–4.

Hughes KS, Simons R, Songhorabodi S, Adson MA *et al.* (1988b) Resection of the liver for colorectal carcinoma metastases: a multi-institutional study of indications for resection. *Surgery* 103: 278–88.

Hughes K, Scheele J, Sugarbaker PH. (1989) Surgery for colorectal cancer metastatic to the liver. *Surg Clin N Am* 69: 339–59.

Hurwitz H, Fehrenbacher L, Novotny W *et al.* (2004) Bevacizumab plus irinotecan, fluorouracil, and leucovorin for metastatic colorectal cancer. *N Engl J Med* 350: 2335–42.

Jamison RL, Donohue JH, Nagorney DM, Rosen CB, Harmsen WS, Ilstrup DM. (1997) Hepatic resection for metastatic colorectal cancer results in cure for some patients. *Arch Surg* 132: 505–11.

Jarnagin WR, Conlon K, Bodniewicz J *et al.* (2001) A clinical scoring system predicts the yield of diagnostic laparoscopy in patients with potentially resectable hepatic colorectal metastases. *Cancer* 91: 1121–8.

Jarnagin WR, Gonen M, Fong Y *et al.* (2002) Improvement in perioperative outcome after hepatic resection: analysis of 1,803 consecutive cases over the past decade. *Ann Surg* 236: 397–406.

Karoui M, Penna C, Amin-Hashem M *et al.* (2006) Influence of preoperative chemotherapy on the risk of major hepatectomy for colorectal liver metastases. *Ann Surg* 243: 1–7.

Kato T, Yasui K, Hirai T *et al.* (2003) Therapeutic results for hepatic metastasis of colorectal cancer with special reference to effectiveness of hepatectomy: analysis of prognostic factors for 763 cases recorded at 18 institutions. *Dis Colon Rectum* 46: S22–S31.

Kemeny N, Huang Y, Cohen AM *et al.* (1999) Hepatic arterial infusion of chemotherapy after resection of hepatic metastases from colorectal cancer. *N Engl J Med* 341: 2039–48.

Kemeny N, Gonen M, Sullivan D *et al.* (2001) Phase I study of hepatic arterial infusion of floxuridine and dexamethasone with systemic irinotecan for unresectable hepatic metastases from colorectal cancer. *J Clin Oncol* 19: 2687–95.

Kemeny N, Jarnagin WR, Paty P *et al.* (2005) Phase I trial of systemic oxaliplatin combination chemotherapy with hepatic arterial infusion in patients with unresectable liver metastases from colorectal cancer. *J Clin Oncol* 23: 4888–96.

Lange JF, Leese T, Castaing D, Bismuth H. (1989) Repeat hepatectomy for recurrent malignant tumors of the liver. *Surg Gynecol Obstet* 169: 119–26.

Leonard GD, Brenner B, Kemeny NE. (2005) Neoadjuvant chemotherapy before liver resection for patients with unresectable liver metastases from colorectal carcinoma. *J Clin Oncol* 23: 2038–48.

Maeda T, Hasebe Y, Hanawa S *et al.* (1992) Trial of percutaneous hepatic cryotherapy: preliminary report. *Nippon Geka Gakkai Zasshi – J Japan Surg Soc* 93: 666.

Makuuchi M, Thai BL, Takayasu K *et al.* (1990) Preoperative portal embolization to increase safety of major hepatectomy for hilar bile duct carcinoma: A preliminary report. *Surgery*, 107: 521–7.

Mala T, Bohler G, Mathisen O, Bergan A, Soreide O. (2002) Hepatic resection for colorectal metastases: can preoperative scoring predict patient outcome? *World J Surg* 26: 1348–53.

Marcove RC, Searfoss RC, Whitmore WF, Grabstald H. (1977) Cryosurgery in the treatment of bone metastases from renal cell carcinoma. *Clin Orthop* 127: 220–7.

Miller G, Biernacki P, Kemeny NE *et al.* (2007) Outcomes after resection of synchronous or metachronous hepatic and pulmonary colorectal metastases. *J Am Coll Surg* 205: 231–8.

Minagawa M, Makuuchi M, Torzilli G *et al.* (2000) Extension of the frontiers of surgical indications in the treatment of liver metastases from colorectal cancer: long-term results. *Ann Surg* 231: 487–99.

Moriya Y, Sugihara K, Hojo K, Makuuchi M. (1991) Adjuvant hepatic intra-arterial chemotherapy after potentially curative hepatectomy for liver metastases from colorectal cancer: a pilot study. *Eur J Surg Oncol* 17: 519–25.

Muratore A, Polastri R, Bouzari H, Vergara V, Ferrero A, Capussotti L. (2001) Repeat hepatectomy for colorectal liver metastases: A worthwhile operation? *J Surg Oncol* 76: 127–32.

Mutsaerts EL, van RS, Zoetmulder FA, Rutgers EJ, Hart AA, van CF. (2005) Prognostic factors and evaluation of surgical management of hepatic metastases from colorectal origin: a 10-year single-institute experience. *J Gastrointest Surg* 9: 178–86.

Nagino M, Nimura Y, Kamiya J *et al.* (1995) Changes in hepatic lobe volume in biliary tract cancer patients after right portal vein embolization. *Hepatology* 21: 434–9.

Nordlinger B, Parc R, Delva E, Quilichini M, Hannoun L, Huguet C. (1987) Hepatic resection for colorectal liver metastases. *Ann Surg* 205: 256–63.

Nordlinger B, Guiguet M, Vaillant JC *et al.* (1996) Surgical resection of colorectal carcinoma metastases to the liver. A prognostic scoring system to improve case selection, based on 1568 patients. Association Francaise de Chirurgie. *Cancer* 77: 1254–62.

Oxley EM, Ellis H. (1969) Prognosis of carcinoma of the large bowel in the presence of liver metastases. *Br J Surg* 56: 149–52.

Pagana TJ. (1986) A new technique for hepatic infusional chemotherapy. *Semin Surg Oncol* 2: 99–102.

Park R, Gonen M, Kemeny N *et al.* (2007) Adjuvant chemotherapy improves survival after resection of hepatic colorectal metastases: analysis of data from two continents. *J Am Coll Surg* 204: 753–61.

Peppercorn PD, Reznek RH, Wilson P, Slevin ML, Gupta RK. (1998) Demonstration of hepatic steatosis by computerized tomography in patients receiving 5-fluorouracil-based therapy for advanced colorectal cancer. *Br J Cancer* 77: 2008–11.

Petrowsky H, Gonen M, Jarnagin W *et al.* (2002) Second liver resections are safe and effective treatment for recurrent hepatic metastases from colorectal cancer: a bi-institutional analysis. *Ann Surg* 235: 863–71.

Portier G, Elias D, Bouche, O *et al.* (2006) Multicenter randomized trial of adjuvant fluorouracil and folinic acid compared with surgery alone after resection of colorectal liver metastases. *J Clin Oncol* 24: 4976–82.

Que FG, Nagorney DM. (1994) Resection of 'recurrent' colorectal metastases to the liver. *Br J Surg* 81: 255–8.

Rosen CB, Nagorney DM, Taswell HF *et al.* (1992) Perioperative blood transfusion and determinants of survival after liver resection for metastatic colorectal carcinoma. *Ann Surg* 216: 492–505.

Saltz LB, Cox JV, Blanke C *et al.* (2000) Irinotecan plus fluorouracil and leucovorin for metastatic colorectal cancer. Irinotecan Study Group. *N Engl J Med* 343: 905–14.

Saltz LB, Niedzwiecki D, Hollis D *et al.* (2004) Irinotecan plus fluorouracil/leucovorin (IFL) versus fluorouracil/leucovorin alone (FL) in stage III colon cancer (intergroup trial CALGB C89803). (Abstract). *J Clin Oncol* 22: 246.

Scheele J, Strangl R, Altendor-Hofman A. (1990) Hepatic metastases from colorectal carcinoma: impact of surgical resection on natural history. *Br J Surg* 77: 1241–6.

Scheele J, Stangl R, Altendorf-Hofmann A, Gall FP. (1991) Indicators of prognosis after hepatic resection for colorectal secondaries. *Surgery* 110: 13–29.

Scheele J, Stang R, Altendorf-Hofmann A, Paul M. (1995) Resection of colorectal liver metastases. *World J Surg* 19: 59–71.

Schlag P, Hohenberger P, Herfarth CH. (1990) Resection of liver metastases in colorectal cancer-competitive analysis of treatment results in synchronous versus metachronous metastases. *Eur J Surg Oncol* 16: 360–5.

Schussler-Fiorenza CM, Mahvi DM, Niederhuber J, Rikkers LF, Weber SM. (2004) Clinical risk score correlates with yield of PET scan in patients with colorectal hepatic metastases. *J Gastrointest Surg* 8: 150–7.

Shaw IM, Rees M, Welsh FK, Bygrave S, John TG. (2006) Repeat hepatic resection for recurrent colorectal liver metastases is associated with favourable long-term survival. *Br J Surg* 93: 457–64.

Simmonds PC, Primrose JN, Colquitt JL, Garden OJ, Poston GJ, Rees M. (2006) Surgical resection of hepatic metastases from colorectal cancer: a systematic review of published studies. *Br J Cancer* 94: 982–99.

Stephenson KR, Steinberg SM, Hughes KS, Vetto JT, Sugarbaker PH, Chang AE. (1988) Perioperative blood transfusions are associated with decreased time to recurrence and decreased survival after resection of colorectal liver metastases. *Ann Surg* 208: 679–87.

Stone MD, Cady B, Jenkins RL, McDermott WV, Steele GD Jr. (1990) Surgical therapy for recurrent liver metastases from colorectal cancer. *Arch Surg* 125: 718–21; discussion.

Strasberg SM, Dehdashti F, Siegel BA, Drebin JA, Linehan D. (2001) Survival of patients evaluated by FDG-PET before hepatic resection for metastatic colorectal carcinoma: a prospective database study. *Ann Surg* 233: 293–9.

Suzuki S, Nakamura S, Ochiai H *et al.* (1997) Surgical management of recurrence after resection of colorectal liver metastases. *J Hepatobiliary Pancreat Surg* 4: 103–12.

Suzuki S, Sakaguchi T, Yokoi Y *et al.* (2001) Impact of repeat hepatectomy on recurrent colorectal liver metastases. *Surgery* 129: 421–8.

Vaillant JC, Balladur P, Nordlinger B *et al.* (1993) Repeat liver resection for recurrent colorectal metastases. *Br J Surg* 80: 340–4.

Wagner JS, Adson MA, Van Heerden JA, Adson MH, Ilstrup DM. (1984) The natural history of hepatic metastases from colorectal cancer. a comparison with resective treatment. *Ann Surg* 199: 502–8.

Wei AC, Greig PD, Grant D, Taylor B, Langer B, Gallinger S. (2006) Survival after hepatic resection for colorectal metastases: a 10-year experience. *Ann Surg Oncol* 13: 668–76.

Wilson SM, Adson MA. (1976) Surgical treatment of hepatic metastases from colorectal cancers. *Arch Surg* 111: 330–4.

Wood CB, Gillis CR, Blumgart LH. (1976) A retrospective study of the natural history of patients with liver metastases from colorectal cancer. *Clin Oncol* 2: 285–8.

Yamamoto J, Kosuge T, Shimada K, Yamasaki S, Moriya Y, Sugihara K. (1999) Repeat liver resection for recurrent colorectal liver metastases. *Am J Surg* 178: 275–81.

Younes RN, Rogatko A, Brennan MF. (1991) The influence of intraoperative hypotension and perioperative blood transfusion on disease-free survival in patients with complete resection of colorectal liver metastases. *Ann Surg* 214: 107–13.

Systemic chemotherapy

Nancy Kemeny

For nearly four decades the treatment of choice for colorectal cancer was 5-FU and leucovorin (LV). The average response rate was 20% and the average median survival was 12 months (Saltz *et al.* 2000). In the 1980s, a topoisomerase inhibitor, irinotecan (CPT-11), demonstrated tumor responses in pretreated patients with colorectal cancer. Then two studies comparing 5-FU with or without CPT-11 in chemotherapy-naïve patients reported higher response rates and a significant survival advantage for the CPT-11-containing regimens (Rougier *et al.* 1998; Douillard *et al.* 2000). The first study used bolus 5-FU with LV and CPT-11 and obtained a median survival of 14.8 months with the three drugs versus 12.6 months with the two drugs (Rougier *et al.* 1998). The second study, using a continuous infusion 5-FU with LV and CPT-11, reported a median survival of 17 months with the three drugs (Douillard *et al.* 2000).

The next new drug to show activity in treating colorectal cancer was oxaliplatin. Infusion of 5-FU and LV combined with oxaliplatin (FOLFOX) as first-line therapy produced response rates of approximately 50% (de Gramont *et al.* 2000; Giacchetti *et al.* 2000). In an intergroup phase III trial (Goldberg *et al.* 2004), metastatic colorectal cancer patients were randomized to FOLFOX versus CPT-11/bolus 5-FU/LV (IFL). The study demonstrated a significant increase in response rate, time to progression and median survival for FOLFOX versus IFL with 45% responding to FOLFOX with a 19.5 months median survival (Goldberg *et al.* 2004).

It is still under consideration in what order these new drugs should be administered. In the Tournigand study, FOLFOX followed by FOLFIRI (infusional of 5-FU/LV/CPT-11) compared to FOLFIRI followed by FOLFOX produced similar median survivals of 21.5 and 20.6 months, respectively (Tournigand *et al.* 2004) (Table 20.8). Another trial exploring the order of drugs was the Focus trial. Patients were randomized to three treatment arms: (i) 5-FU/LV followed by CPT-11, (ii) 5-FU/LV followed by CPT-11/5-FU/LV or FOLFOX, or (iii) initial

Table 20.8 Systemic chemotherapy in previously untreated patients.

Regimen	Response	1-year survival	2-year survival
5-FU + LV (Kemeny *et al.* 2004)	20%	56	27
CPT-11 + 5-FU + LV (Saltz *et al.* 2000)	39%	54	25
FOLFIRI (Douillard *et al.* 2000)	41%	72	32
FOLFOX (Goldberg *et al.* 2004)	45%	72	35
IFL + Bev (Hurwitz *et al.* 2004)	45%	72	39

LV, leucovorin; 5-FU, 5-fluorouracil; IFL, irinotecan/bolus 5-FU/leucovorin; Bev, bevacizumab; FOLFOX, 5-FU/leucovorin/oxaliplatin; FOLFIRI, infusional 5-FU/leucovorin/irinotecan.

FOLFOX or CPT-11/5-FU/LV. There was no significant difference in survival within the three arms and 2-year survival was around 28–30% (Seymour *et al.* 2005).

A number of growth factors are increased in colorectal cancer tumor specimens. Recent development of targeted agents against epidermal growth factor (EGFR) and vascular endothelial growth factor (VEGF) have produced new agents that can be used to treat metastases from colorectal cancer. Antibodies to EGFR, such as cetuximab in combination with CPT-11, produced a 23% response rate in patients whose tumor had progressed on CPT-11 (Cunningham *et al.* 2004). Bevacizumab (Bev), a monoclonal antibody that inhibits VEGF, has activity when combined with chemotherapy. In a randomized study of IFL with or without Bev as first-line therapy, response was 45% versus 35%, and median survival 20.3 versus 15.6 months, for IFL+Bev versus IFL, respectively (Hurwitz *et al.* 2004).

The advances with systemic chemotherapy have improved overall survival, but 2-year survival is still only 30–39%, even with the new agents in combination with 5-FU (Table 20.8).

Second-line therapy—systemic

In the second-line setting, irinotecan (CPT-11) has a response rate of 14% and a median survival of 9.9 months (Rothenberg *et al.* 1999). Second-line CPT-11 in FOLFOX-4 refractory patients has demonstrated a 5% response rate. FOLFOX administered in CPT-11-refractory patients produces a 9.9% response rate with a median survival of 9.8 months (Table 20.9) (Rothenberg *et al.* 2003). Cetuximab (C225) can produce a 10% response rate as second-line therapy, increasing to 23% when combined with CPT-11 (Cunningham *et al.* 2004).

In the chemotherapy-naïve patient, a number of regimens can now be used exploring the new drugs and new inhibitors of VEGF. For patients who have progressed on systemic chemotherapy, another systemic therapy has only a small benefit (Table 20.10).

Table 20.9 Systemic therapy in previously treated patients.

Regimen	Number of patients	1-Year Survival	% Response
CPT-11 (Rothenberg *et al.* 1999)	205	46%	11%
CPT-11 + Erbitux (Cunningham *et al.* 2004)	218	–	23%
FOLFOX (Rothenberg *et al.* 1999)	289	40%	20%
FOLFOX + Bev (Hurwitz *et al.* 2004)	290	55%	–
CPT-11 + Erbitux + Bev (Saltz *et al.* 2005)	45	35%	35%

FOLFOX, 5-FU leucovorin oxaliplatin; Bev, bevacizumab.

Hepatic arterial infusion

The rationale for hepatic arterial chemotherapy is based on the following factors. Liver metastases are perfused almost exclusively by the hepatic artery, while the normal liver hepatocytes derive their blood supply mostly from the portal vein (Breedis & Young 1954). Additionally, certain drugs are largely extracted by the liver during the first pass through the arterial circulation, which results in high local concentrations of the drug with minimal systemic toxicity. In 1978, Ensminger and colleagues demonstrated that 94–99% of floxuridine (FUDR) is extracted by the liver during the first pass, compared to 19–55% of 5-FU. Drugs with a high total body clearance and short plasma half-life are more useful for hepatic infusion (Ensminger *et al.* 1978).

The liver is often the first and only site of metastatic disease and it is possible that hematogenous spread occurs via the portal vein to the liver, and then from the liver to other organs. Therefore, aggressive treatment of metastases confined to the liver may prolong survival.

Regional hepatic arterial therapy can be delivered using either an intra-arterial catheter connected to an external pump or a totally implantable pump. Early studies with percutaneously placed hepatic artery catheters produced high response rates, but clotting of the catheters or the hepatic artery, duodenal ulcers, and bleeding from around the catheters (Tandon *et al.* 1973) led physicians to abandon this method. The development of a totally implantable pump allowed long-term hepatic artery infusion (HAI) with a lower incidence of complications (Ensminger *et al.* 1981) (Table 20.11). One study comparing:

Table 20.10 Rationale for hepatic arterial infusion (HAI).

1 Liver metastases perfused by hepatic artery; normal liver by portal vein.
2 Some drugs extracted by liver during first pass; less systemic toxicity.
3 Liver may be only site of metastatic disease; stepwise pattern of metastatic progression.

Table 20.11 Drugs for hepatic arterial infusion (HAI).

Drug	Half-life (min)	Estimated increased exposure via HAI
Fluorouracil (5-FU)	10	5–10-fold
5-fluoro-2-deoxyuridine (FUDR)	<10	100–400-fold
Bischlorethylnitrosourea (BCNU)	<5	6–7-fold
Mitomycin C	<10	6–8-fold
Cisplatin	20–30	4–7-fold
Adriamycin (doxorubicin hydrochloride)	60	2-fold

(i) surgical placement of a hepatic artery port catheter, (ii) percutaneous placement of the port catheter, and (iii) surgical placement of a pump, reported the ability to administer chemotherapy in days as 31, 25, and 115 days, respectively (Yasuda *et al.* 1990).

The first seven trials comparing HAI to systemic therapy all showed an increase in response rate and a number showed an increase in time to progression for the HAI study arms (Table 20.12). Most of the trials contain relatively few patients, so the power to observe differences in survival was low. Because of the early successes with HAI, some of these studies allowed patients in the systemic arm to cross over to HAI therapy after tumor progression on systemic therapy. This crossover may have negated any difference in survival between the two groups. The studies do demonstrate a survival advantage for the groups who received subsequent hepatic arterial treatment, with a mean 1-year survival of 69% for the patients who had crossed over from systemic therapy to HAI versus 35% for the group who did not cross over. In a meta-analysis combining the results of the seven earlier trials, the use of HAI FUDR produced a significantly better response rate of 41% with HAI, a 14% response rate with systemic 5-FU, and median survival time of 16 versus 13 months, respectively (Meta-analysis Group in Cancer 1996). The data of some of these trials have been subjected to two different meta-analyses (Meta-analysis Group in Cancer 1996; Harmantas *et al.* 1996). Each meta-analysis confirmed the trends that were apparent in the individual studies; namely, that response rates were greater with HAI therapy.

Recently there have been three new large trials. In an English trial, patients were randomized to HAI 5-FU/LV or systemic 5-FU/LV (Kerr *et al.* 2003). Of patients randomized to the HAI therapy, 37% did not receive HAI therapy and all these patients are included in the survival analysis. No analysis was done on patients who actually received treatment which may be necessary in a trial where 37% of the patients were not treated with the assigned treatment. Amongst the patients who did receive HAI therapy, 29% of patients received fewer than six cycles due to catheter failure (Kerr *et al.* 2003). A port rather than a pump was used, which may account for the failure to be able to continue treatment.

Table 20.12 Randomized trials of HAI chemotherapy for unresectable liver metastases.

Study	Arms	n	% in HAI arm receiving Tx	Crossover to HAI	OR (CR+PR)	Median OS(mo)
MSKCC (Kemeny *et al.* 1987)	HAI	48	94%	Yes	50%*	17
	IV	51			20%	12
NCI (Chang *et al.* 1987)	HAI	32	66%	No	62%*	17†
	IV	32			17%	12†
NCOG (Hohn *et al.* 1989)	HAI	67	75%	Yes	42%*	16.5
	IV	76			10%	15.8
City of Hope (Wagman *et al.* 1990)	HAI	31	100%	Yes	55%*	13.8
	IV	10			20%	11.6
NCCTG (Martin *et al.* 1990)	HAI	39	85%	No	48%	12.6
	IV	35			12%	10.5
French (Rougier *et al.* 1992)	HAI	81	87%	No	44%*	15*
	IV	82			9%	11
English (Allen-Mersh *et al.* 1994)	HAI	51	96%	No	NR	13.5*
	IV	49			NR	7.5
MRC/EORTC (Kerr *et al.* 2003)	HAI[a]	145	63%	No	22%‡	14.7
	IV	145			19%	14.8
German (Lorenz and Muller, 2000)	HAI[b]	54	69%	No	43%*	12.7
	IV	57			20%	17.6
CALGB (Kemeny *et al.* 2006)	HAI	68	87%	No	48%*	24*
	IV	67			25%	20

* $p<0.05$
† Based on published Kaplan–Meier curves.
‡ Responses were calculated at a single time point (12 weeks).
n = number of patients (%)
a All trials used HAI FUDR except this study, which used HAI 5-FU.
b This study had two groups of HAI therapy. The group using HAI 5-FU is not listed in this table.
HAI, hepatic arterial infusion; IV, intravenous; Tx, treatment; CR, complete response: PR, partial response; OS, overall survival; 5-FU, 5-fluorouracil; FUDR, floxuridine; MSKCC, Memorial Sloan-Kettering Cancer Center; NCI, National Cancer Institute; NCOG, Northern California Oncology Group; NCCTG, North Central Cancer Treatment Group; MRC/EORTC, UK Medical Research Council/European Organization for Research and Treatment of Cancer; CALGB, Cancer and Leukemia Group B.

A German Cooperative Group randomized colorectal cancer patients to three arms: (i) HAI 5-FU/LV, (ii) HAI FUDR and (iii) intravenous 5-FU/LV (Lorenz & Muller 2000). Despite the statistically significant doubling of the response rates of the HAI chemotherapy arms compared to the intravenous 5-FU/LV arm, this did not translate into a statistically significant survival advantage. Again, a number of patients assigned to HAI FUDR were not treated (31%) (Lorenz & Muller 2000).

In the American trial conducted by the Cancer and Leukemia Group B (CALGB), metastatic colorectal cancer patients were randomized to either HAI FUDR, LV, and dexamethasone, or to intravenous 5-FU plus LV (Kemeny *et al.* 2006). The primary endpoint of the CALGB trial was survival. Other endpoints concerned correlation of survival with tumor biology, assessment of clinical response and toxicity, and economic analysis (Kemeny *et al.* 2003). Quality of life using the Rand 36-Item Health Status Profile, Memorial Symptom Assessment Scale, and other instruments demonstrated an improvement in physical functioning in the HAI group. A statistically significant survival advantage was seen with HAI relative to systemic 5-FU/LV (24 vs. 20 months, p=0.0034). The response rate was also higher in the HAI arm at 48% versus 25% (p=0.001), as was the hepatic disease-free survival (9.8 vs. 7.3 months, p=0.034) (Kemeny *et al.* 2006).

Table 20.13 Hepatic arterial infusion in previously treated patients.

Regimen	No. of patients	Partial response	Alive at 1 year
HAI alone			
FUDR alone (Kemeny *et al.* 1993)	49	33%	67%
FUDR+Mit+BCNU (Kemeny *et al.* 1993)	45	47%	70%
FUDR+LV+Dex (Kemeny etal. 1994)	29	52%	66%
Mit+FUDR+Dex (Kemeny *et al.* 2005a)	37	65%	77%
HAI + SYS			
FUDR+Dex & SYS CPT (Kemeny *et al.* 2001)	56	84%	74%
FUDR+Dex & SYS Oxal (Kemeny *et al.* 2005c)	36	86%	80%

HAI, hepatic arterial infusion; FUDR, floxuridine; MIT, mitomycin C; BCNU, carmustine (Bischlorethylnitrosourea); LV, leucovorin; Dex, dexamethasone; SYS, systemic; Oxal, oxaliplatin.

Second-line therapy—HAI + systemic

HAI-based therapy in previously treated patients refractory to first-line systemic therapy with 5-FU has produced much higher response rates (Table 20.12). Trials using HAI-FUDR, LV and dexamethasone (Kemeny *et al.* 1994), or HAI-FUDR and dexamethasone and mitomycin C through the pump side port (Kemeny *et al.* 1995), have shown response rates of 52% and 70%, respectively, with median survivals of 13.5 and 19 months from the start of HAI therapy after progression on systemic therapy. A phase I study of HAI FUDR combined with systemic single agent CPT-11 in previously treated patients (16/38 patients had received prior CPT-11) reported a response rate of 74%, time to progression of 8.1 months, and a median survival of 20 months (Kemeny *et al.* 2001). Thirteen of the 16 patients with prior CPT-11 exposure responded to this regimen (Kemeny *et al.* 2001). Oxaliplatin combinations and concurrent HAI in 36 previously treated patients (74% had received prior irinotecan) produced response rates of 86% and 1-year survival of 80% with a median survival of 36 months (Table 20.13) (Kemeny *et al.* 2005b).

Toxicity of hepatic arterial FUDR infusion

The most common problems with HAI are hepatic toxicity and gastric ulcerations. Myelosuppression, nausea, vomiting, and diarrhea do not occur with HAI therapy using FUDR. If diarrhea does occur, shunting to the bowel should be suspected (Gluck *et al.* 1985). Clinically, biliary toxicity is manifested as elevations of aspartate transaminase (AST), alkaline phosphatase, and bilirubin. In the early stages, hepatic enzyme elevations will return to normal when the drug is withdrawn and the patient is given a rest period, while in more advanced cases, it does not resolve. Therefore careful monitoring of liver function tests is necessary to avoid this toxicity. The bile ducts derive their blood supply almost exclusively from the hepatic artery (Northover & Terblanche 1979), and thus are also perfused with high doses of chemotherapy by using HAI therapy.

In patients who develop jaundice, an endoscopic retrograde cholangiopancreatogram (ERCP) may demonstrate lesions resembling idiopathic sclerosing cholangitis in 5–29% of patients treated by experienced clinicians. The strictures may be focal and present at the hepatic duct bifurcation, and therefore drainage procedures either by ERCP or by transhepatic cholangiogram may be helpful. Duct obstruction from metastases or bile duct strictures from surgery can also be causes of elevated bilirubin.

Rationale for HAI in the adjuvant setting

Once metastases grow beyond 3 mm, they obtain their blood supply from arterial circulation, while the normal hepatocytes continue to receive blood flow from the portal vein. With hepatic resection of liver metastases, residual disease, if present, may be 2–3 mm in diameter, and therefore derive its blood supply from the hepatic artery.

Randomized trials of adjuvant therapy after liver resection

There are four large randomized trials addressing the question of whether adjuvant therapy with HAI is useful after liver resection. At Memorial Sloan-Kettering Cancer Center (MSKCC) (Kemeny *et al.* 1999), patients were randomized after liver resection to HAI FUDR plus dexamethasone and systemic 5-FU+/–LV, or systemic chemotherapy alone. The endpoint was 2-year survival. Patients were stratified according to the number of liver metastases (1, 2–4, >4) and type of chemotherapy (none, 5-FU+/–levamisole, or 5-FU+LV) (Kemeny *et al.* 1999). Numerous other parameters, including molecular markers, were comparable in both treatment groups.

Survival at 2 years was significantly increased with HAI plus systemic (86% vs. 72%, p=0.03). An update with a median follow-up time of 10 years revealed a 10-year survival of 40% for the HAI + systemic group and 27% for the systemic-alone group. The 2-year time to hepatic recurrence was also increased in patients treated with HAI plus systemic therapy and was 90% and 60%, respectively (Kemeny & Gonen 2005). Median time to hepatic recurrence had not been reached in the HAI + systemic therapy arm, but was 32.5 months in patients treated with systemic therapy (p=0.01). The overall progression-free survival was 31.3 months versus 17.2 months (p=0.02) (Kemeny & Gonen 2005).

The Eastern Cooperative Oncology Group (ECOG) and Southwest Oncology Group (SWOG) conducted a prospective trial of hepatic resection alone versus resection followed by HAI (FUDR) and systemic infusional 5-FU (Kemeny *et al.* 2002). Only patients with three or less hepatic metastases were enrolled and 109 patients were randomized prior to resection. Because of the timing of the randomization, 29 patients were found not to be eligible at the time of liver resection. For the 75 patients who actually entered the study, 4-year disease-free survival was significantly longer with HAI plus systemic therapy versus resection alone, 58% and 34%, respectively (p=0.039). The primary endpoint of the study was disease-free survival and the study was not powered for overall survival. The 5-year survival was 58% for the HAI and systemic group and 40% for the resection-only group (Table 20.14) (Kemeny *et al.* 2002).

In a German, multicenter randomized trial of hepatic resection versus hepatic resection plus adjuvant HAI 5-FU/LV, patients were stratified according to number of liver metastases (1–2, 3–6) and the site of the primary tumor (colon or upper rectum, mid- or lower rectum) (Lorenz *et al.* 1998). 113 patients were assigned to each group. Despite initial randomization, only 87 (77%) were actually treated in the HAI+SYS group, for various reasons including extrahepatic disease and technical complications. Of the 113 patients randomized, 73 (64.6%) had chemotherapy data available, and only 34 patients (30%) completed the assigned protocol, possibly due to the use of ports and 5-FU therapy. No survival advantage was seen. In the secondary analysis comparing the actual 'treated patients' (n=87) to those receiving no therapy (n=114), median survival was 44.8 versus 39.7 months, respectively. Median time to liver progression doubled in the group receiving HAI 5-FU/LV: 44.8 versus 23.3 months, and median time to progression was 20 versus 12.6 months, respectively (Lorenz *et al.* 1998).

A prospective randomized study from Greece used interoperative randomization to regional liver therapy plus systemic versus systemic alone (Lygidakis *et al.* 2001). The regional group received mitomycin-C, 5-FU, and LV with IL-2 via a hepatic arterial catheter and also received IV injections of the same drugs. In the systemic group, this therapy was given by IV only. 143 patients were randomized, 5 died during the post-operative period, and 16 were lost to follow-up, leaving 122 in the follow-up groups. The 2-year survivals were 80% and 71% respectively, and 5-year survival was 73% and 60% respectively, in the regional plus systemic versus systemic alone groups (p=0.004). Five-year hepatic-free recurrence was also significantly increased in the HAI group at 82%, versus 49% in the systemic-alone group (p<0.001).

Table 20.14 Randomized trials of HAI versus systemic therapy (SYS) or control: survival.

	No. of patients	3-year survival		5-year survival	
		HAI	SYS or control	HAI	SYS or control
Kusonoki *et al.* 2000	58	78%	30%	60%	30%
Tono *et al.* 2000	19	78%	50%	78%	50%
Kemeny *et al.* 1999	156	70%	60%	59%	46%
Lorenz *et al.* 1998	201*	50%	50%	50%	30%
Kemeny *et al.* 2002	75†	70%	70%	60%	35%‡
Lygidakis *et al.* 2001	122	80%	71%	73%	60%
Asahara *et al.* 1998	38	100%	60%	100%	47%§

* Treated patients, not everyone randomized.
† Patients entered in study, not everyone randomized.
‡ Updated figures.
§ 4-year survival.
HAI, hepatic arterial infusion; SYS, systemic.

In 2003, Tono *et al.* randomized 19 patients to continuous infusion of 5-FU, 500 mg/day for 4 days via HAI for 6 weeks. Though this is an extremely small study, there was an increase in survival with 5-year survival of 77.8% for the regional group versus 50% for the control group. This was not significant, but significance would almost be impossible with 19 patients. Three-year disease-free survival was 66.7% for the regional group and 20% for the control group ($p=0.045$) (Tono *et al.* 2003).

In a non-randomized study from Japan, 58 patients who had radical resection of metastatic colorectal carcinoma could select whether they wanted HAI after surgery (Kusunoki *et al.* 2000). The HAI therapy was 5-FU, 600 mg/m^2/day for 2 days with oral UFT (tegafur and uracil) for 5 days, 200 mg twice daily. The systemic group received oral UFT. The 5-year survival was significantly increased for the hepatic arterial group with 5-year survival of 59% for the HAI group versus 27% for the systemic group ($p<0.001$) (Kusunoki *et al.* 2000). There was also significant reduction in hepatic recurrence. The difference was 7% recurrence for the HAI group and 57% recurrence for the systemic group ($p<0.001$) (Kusunoki *et al.* 2000). Another small Japanese study of 38 patients had two groups, one receiving 5-FU infusion for 3 weeks and the other no further treatment after hepatic resection. Four-year survival was 100% versus 47% for the HAI and control groups ($p=0.05$) (Asahara *et al.* 1998). A meta-analysis by Clancy suggests no increase in survival when 1- and 2-year survivals were reported (Clancy *et al.* 2005). However, looking at these same studies and reporting 3- and 5-year survivals show different results (Table 20.14).

Neoadjuvant chemotherapy

Neoadjuvant chemotherapy has been evaluated as a way to decrease hepatic tumor burden in order to proceed with hepatic resection. In 1999, Giacchetti and colleagues conducted a retrospective review of 151 patients with unresectable liver-only metastases from colorectal cancer who were treated with 5-FU/LV and oxaliplatin followed by attempted liver resection. The criteria used to define unresectability were: (i) > 4 liver metastases, (ii) single tumor > 5 cm, (iii) tumor in both hepatic lobes, (iv) invasion of the intrahepatic vascular structures, and (v) high percentage of liver involvement (> 25% liver involvement). The 5-year survival rate for the 77 patients who underwent hepatic resection was 50%. Of the completely resected patients, median overall survival was not reached, but 72% had relapsed within a median of 12 months.

A prospective trial is under way at the Mayo clinic (Alberts *et al.* 2005) enrolling patients considered unresectable due to: (i) involvement of all three major hepatic veins, the portal vein bifurcation, or the retrohepatic vena cava; (ii) involvement of the main right or main left portal vein and the main hepatic vein of the opposite lobe; (iii) disease requiring more than a right or left trisegmentectomy; or (iv) six or more metastatic lesions distributed diffusely in both lobes of the liver. In the presence of any of the above, patients were treated with 5-FU, LV, and oxaliplatin (FOLFOX). Seventeen out of 44 patients with the above criteria were able to undergo a resection, but 73% recurred in the liver. Median survival was 26 months (Alberts *et al.* 2005).

References

Alberts SR, Horvath WL, Sternfeld WC *et al.* (2005) Oxaliplatin, fluorouracil, and leucovorin for patients with unresectable liver-only metastases from colorectal cancer: A North Central Cancer Treatment Group Phase II Study. *J Clin Oncol* 23(36): 9243–9.

Allen-Mersh TG, Earlam S, Fordy C, Abrams K, Houghton J. (1994) Quality of life and survival with continuous hepatic-artery floxuridine infusion for colorectal liver metastases. *Lancet* 344(8932): 1255–60.

Asahara T, Kikkawa M, Okajima M *et al.* (1998) Studies of postoperative transarterial infusion chemotherapy for liver metastasis of colorectal carcinoma after hepatectomy. *Hepatogastroenterology* 45(21): 805–11.

Breedis C, Young G. (1954) The blood supply of neoplasms in the liver. *Am J Pathol* 30(5): 969–77.

Chang AE, Schneider PD, Sugarbaker PH, Simpson C, Culnane M, Steinberg SM. (1987) A prospective randomized trial of regional versus systemic continuous 5-fluorodeoxyuridine chemotherapy in the treatment of colorectal liver metastases. *Ann Surg* 206(6): 685–93.

Clancy TE, Dixon E, Perlis R, Sutherland FR, Zinner MJ. (2005) Hepatic arterial infusion after curative resection of colorectal metastases: a meta-analysis of prospective clinical trials. *J Gastrointest Surg* 9(2): 198–206.

Cunningham D, Humblet Y, Siena S *et al.* (2004) Cetuximab montherapy and cetuximab plus irinotecan-refractory metastatic colorectal cancer. *N Engl J Med* 351(4): 337–45.

Douillard JY, Cunningham D, Roth AD *et al.* (2000) Irinotecan combined with fluorouracil compared with fluorouracil alone as first-line treatment for metastatic colorectal cancer: a multicentre randomised trial. *Lancet* 355(9209): 1041–7.

de Gramont A, Figer A, Seymour M *et al.* (2000) Leucovorin and fluorouracil with or without oxaliplatin as first-line treatment in advanced colorectal cancer. *J Clin Oncol* 18(16): 2938–47.

Ensminger WD, Rosowsky A, Raso V *et al.* (1978) A clinical-pharmacological evaluation of hepatic arterial infusions of 5-fluoro-2′-deoxyuridine and 5-fluorouracil. *Cancer Res* 38(11 Pt 1): 3784–92.

Ensminger W, Niederhuber J, Dakhil S, Thrall J, Wheeler R. (1981) Totally implanted drug delivery system for hepatic arterial chemotherapy. *Cancer Treat Rep* 65(5–6): 393–400.

Giacchetti S, Itzhaki M, Gruia G *et al.* (1999) Long-term survival of patients with unresectable colorectal cancer liver metastases following infusional chemotherapy with 5-fluorouracil, leucovorin, oxaliplatin and surgery. *Ann Oncol* 10(6): 663–9.

Giacchetti S, Perpoint B, Zidani R *et al.* (2000) Phase III multicenter randomized trial of oxaliplatin added to chronomodulated fluorouracil-leucovorin as first-line treatment of metastatic colorectal cancer. *J Clin Oncol* 18(1): 136–47.

Gluck WL, Akwari OE, Kelvin FM, Goodwin BJ. (1985) A reversible enteropathy complicating continuous hepatic artery infusion chemotherapy with 5-fluoro-2-deoxyuridine. *Cancer* 56(10): 2424–7.

Goldberg RM, Sargent DJ, Morton RF *et al.* (2004) A randomized controlled trial of fluorouracil plus leucovorin, irinotecan, and oxaliplatin combinations in patients with previously untreated metastatic colorectal cancer. *J Clin Oncol* 22(1): 23–30.

Harmantas A, Rotstein LE, Langer B. (1996) Regional versus systemic chemotherapy in the treatment of colorectal carcinoma metastatic to the liver. Is there a survival difference? Meta-analysis of the published literature. *Cancer* 78(8): 1639–45.

Hohn DC, Stagg RJ, Friedman MA *et al.* (1989) A randomized trial of continuous intravenous versus hepatic intraarterial floxuridine in patients with colorectal cancer metastatic to the liver: the Northern California Oncology Group trial. *J Clin Oncol* 7(11): 1646–54.

Hurwitz H, Fehrenbacher L, Novotny W *et al.* (2004) Bevacizumab plus irinotecan, fluorouracil, and leucovorin for metastatic colorectal cancer. *N Engl J Med* 350(23): 2335–42.

Lorenz M, Muller HH. (2000) Randomized, multicenter trial of fluorouracil plus leucovorin administered either via hepatic arterial or intravenous infusion versus fluorodeoxyuridine administered via hepatic arterial infusion in patients with nonresectable liver metastases from colorectal carcinoma. *J Clin Oncol* 18(2): 243–54.

Lorenz M, Muller HH, Schramm H *et al.* (1998) Randomized trial of surgery versus surgery followed by adjuvant hepatic arterial infusion with 5-fluorouracil and folinic acid for liver metastases of colorectal cancer. German Cooperative on Liver Metastases (Arbeitsgruppe Lebermetastasen). *Ann Surg* 228(6): 756–62.

Kemeny NE, Gonen M. (2005) Hepatic arterial infusion after liver resection. *N Engl J Med* 352(7): 734–5.

Kemeny N, Daly J, Reichman B, Geller N, Botet J, Oderman P. (1987) Intrahepatic or systemic infusion of fluorodeoxyuridine in patients with liver metastases from colorectal carcinoma. A randomized trial. *Ann Intern Med* 107(4): 459–65.

Kemeny N, Cohen A, Seiter K *et al.* (1993) Randomized trial of hepatic arterial floxuridine, mitomycin, and carmustine versus floxuridine alone in previously treated patients with liver metastases from colorectal cancer. *J Clin Oncol* 11(2): 330–5.

Kemeny N, Conti JA, Cohen A *et al.* (1994) Phase II study of hepatic arterial floxuridine, leucovorin, and dexamethasone for unresectable liver metastases from colorectal carcinoma. *J Clin Oncol* 12(11): 2288–95.

Kemeny NE, Conti JA, Blumgart L *et al.* (1995) Hepatic arterial infusion of floxuridine (FUDR), dexamethasone (Dex) and high dose mitomycin C (Mit C): comparable response to FUDR/leucovorin/Dex but with greater toxicity. Abstract #480 In: 1995 ASCO Annual Meeting, Los Angeles, CA, USA. *Am Soc Clin Oncol.*

Kemeny N, Huang Y, Cohen AM *et al.* (1999) Hepatic arterial infusion of chemotherapy after resection of hepatic metastases from colorectal cancer. *N Engl J Med* 341(27): 2039–48.

Kemeny N, Gonen M, Sullivan D *et al.* (2001) Phase I study of hepatic arterial infusion of floxuridine and dexamethasone with systemic irinotecan for unresectable hepatic metastases from colorectal cancer. *J Clin Oncol* 19(10): 2687–95.

Kemeny MM, Adak S, Gray B *et al.* (2002) Combined-modality treatment for resectable metastatic colorectal carcinoma to the liver: surgical resection of hepatic metastases in combination with continuous infusion of chemotherapy—an intergroup study. *J Clin Oncol* 20(6): 1499–505.

Kemeny NE, Niedzwiecki D, Hollis DR *et al.* (2003) Hepatic arterial infusion (HAI) versus systemic therapy for hepatic metastases from colorectal cancer; a CALGB randomized trial of efficacy, quality of life (QOL), cost effectiveness, and molecular markers. *Proc Am Soc Clin Oncol* 22: 252a, #1010.

Kemeny N, Kemeny MM, Lawrence TS. (2004) Liver metastases. In: Abeloff MD, Armitage JO, Niederhuber JE, Kastan MB, McKenna WG, eds. *Clinical Oncology*, 3rd edn, pp. 1141–78. Elsevier, Philadelphia.

Kemeny N, Eid A, Stockman J *et al.* (2005a) Hepatic arterial infusion of floxuridine and dexamethasone plus high-dose mitomycin C for patients with unresectable hepatic metastases from colorectal carcinoma. *J Surg Oncol* 91(2): 97–101.

Kemeny N, Jarnagin W, Paty P *et al.* (2005b) Phase I trial of systemic oxaliplatin combination chemotherapy with hepatic arterial infusion in patients with unresectable liver metastases from colorectal cancer. *J Clin Oncol* 23(22): 4888–96.

Kemeny NE, Niedzwiecki D, Hollis DR *et al.* (2006) Hepatic arterial infusion versus systemic therapy for hepatic metastases from colorectal cancer: a randomized trial of efficacy, quality of life, and molecular markers (CALGB 9481). *J Clin Oncol* 24(9): 1395–403.

Kerr DJ, McArdle CS, Ledermann J *et al.* (2003) MRC/EORTC Colorectal Cancer Study Group. Intrahepatic arterial versus intravenous fluorouracil and folinic acid for colorectal cancer liver metastases: a multicentre randomised trial. *Lancet* 361(9355): 368–73.

Kusunoki M, Yanagi H, Noda M, Yoshikawa R, Yamamura T. (2000) Results of pharmacokinetic modulating chemotherapy in combination with hepatic arterial 5-fluorouracil infusion and oral UFT after resection of hepatic colorectal metastases. *Cancer* 89(6): 1228–35.

Lorenz M, Muller HH, Schramm H *et al.* (1998) Randomized trial of surgery versus surgery followed by adjuvant hepatic arterial infusion with 5-fluorouracil and folinic acid for liver metastases of colorectal cancer. German Cooperative on Liver Metastases (Arbeitsgruppe Lebermetastasen). *Ann Surg* 228(6): 756–62.

Lygidakis NJ, Sgourakis G, Vlachos L *et al.* (2001) Metastatic liver disease of colorectal origin: the value of locoregional immunochemotherapy combined with systemic chemotherapy following liver resection. Results of a prospective randomized study. *Hepatogastroenterology* 48(42): 1685–91.

Martin JK Jr, O'Connell MJ, Wieand HS *et al.* (1990) Intra-arterial floxuridine vs systemic fluorouracil for hepatic metastases from colorectal cancer. A randomized trial. *Arch Surg* 125(8): 1022–7.

Meta-Analysis Group in Cancer. (1996) Reappraisal of hepatic arterial infusion in the treatment of nonresectable liver metastases from colorectal cancer. *J Natl Cancer Inst* 88(5): 252–8.

Northover JM, Terblanche J. (1979) A new look at the arterial supply of the bile duct in man and its surgical implications. *Br J Surg* 66(6): 379–84.

Rothenberg ML, Cox JV, DeVore RF *et al.* (1999) A multicenter, phase II trial of weekly irinotecan (CPT-11) in patients with previously treated colorectal carcinoma. *Cancer* 85(4): 786–95.

Rothenberg ML, Oza AM, Bigelow RH, *et al.* (2003) Superiority of oxaliplatin and fluoroacil-leucovorin compared with either therapy alone in patients with progressive colorectal cancer after irinotecan and fluorouracil-leucovorin: interim results of a phase II trial. *J Clin Oncol* 21(11): 2059–69.

Rougier P, Laplanche A, Huguier M *et al.* (1992) Hepatic arterial infusion of floxuridine in patients with liver metastases from colorectal carcinoma: long-term results of a prospective randomized trial. *J Clin Oncol* 10(7): 1112–8.

Rougier P, Van Cutsem E, Bajetta E *et al.* (1999) Randomised trial of irinotecan versus fluorouracil by continuos infusion after fluorouracil failure in patients with metastatic colorectal cancer. *Lancet* 352(9138): 1407–12.

Saltz LB, Cox JV, Blanke C *et al.* (2000) Irinotecan plus fluorouracil and leucovorin for metastatic colorectal cancer. Irinotecan Study Group. *N Engl J Med* 343(13): 905–14.

Saltz LB, Lenz HJ, Hochster H *et al.* (2005) Randomized phase II trial of cetuximab/bevacizumab/irinotecan (CBI) versus cetuximab/bevacizumab (CB) in irinotecan-refractory colorectal cancer. *Proc Am Soc Clin Oncol* 23(16S): 248s.

Seymour MT, Group UNCCS. (2005) Fluorouracil, oxaliplatin and CPT-11 (irinotecan), use and sequencing (MRC FOCUS): A 2135-patient randomized trial in advanced colorectal cancer (ACRC). *J Clin Oncol* (Abstracts) 23(16 Suppl): 3518.

Tandon RN, Bunnell IL, Cooper RG. (1973) The treatment of metastatic carcinoma of the liver by the percutaneous selective hepatic artery infusion of 5-fluorouracil. *Surgery* 73(1): 118–21.

Tono T, Hasuike Y, Ohzato H, Takatsuka Y, Kikkawa N. (2000) Limited but definite efficacy of prophylactic hepatic arterial infusion chemotherapy after curative resection of colorectal liver metastases: A randomized study. *Cancer* 88(7): 1549–56.

Tournigand C, Andre T, Achille E *et al.* (2004) FOLFIRI followed by FOLFOX6 or the reverse sequence in advanced colorectal cancer: a randomized GERCOR study. *J Clin Oncol* 22(2): 229–37.

Wagman LD, Kemeny MM, Leong L *et al.* (1990) A prospective, randomized evaluation of the treatment of colorectal cancer metastatic to the liver. *J Clin Oncol* 8(11): 1885–93.

Yasuda S, Noto T, Ikeda M *et al.* (1990) [Hepatic arterial infusion chemotherapy using implantable reservoir in colorectal liver metastasis]. *Gan To Kagaku Ryoho* 17(8 Pt 2): 1815–9.

Ablative therapy

Anne M. Covey

Introduction

The American Cancer Society estimates that 145,290 new cases of colorectal cancer will be diagnosed in 2005, accounting for more cancer deaths than any other tumor except lung cancer (American Cancer Society 2005). The liver is the most common site of distant metastases from colorectal cancer, occurring in up to 50% of patients. In most cases, liver failure secondary to tumor involvement is the direct cause of death (Wagner *et al.* 1984). Unlike other histologies, in 20–30% of patients with metastatic colorectal cancer, metastases are commonly limited to the liver. Between 20 and 30% of patients have disease amenable to curative resection, and in the remaining 70–80% regional therapy has been shown to prolong overall survival (Kemeny *et al.* 2006).

A 1988 Registry of Hepatic Metastases evaluated 859 patients from 24 institutions who underwent hepatic metastectomy for colorectal cancer between 1948 and 1985. The analysis showed a 5-year actuarial survival of 33% and 5-year actuarial disease-free survival of 21%. Poor prognostic indicators included the presence of known extrahepatic disease, margin of < 1 cm and resection of more than three tumors. In 1996, Nordlinger *et al.* reported their results on 1568 patients who underwent hepatic metastectomy for colorectal carcinoma. Following complete resection, they demonstrated 3- and 5-year survivals of 40% and 28%, respectively (Nordlinger *et al.* 1996). Together, these studies validate an aggressive approach to the treatment of isolated liver metastases from colorectal cancer. Over two-thirds of patients are not candidates for resection and even the minority that do undergo 'curative' resection have a 50% recurrence rate, most within 2 years (Nordlinger *et al.* 1996). Therefore, the need for parenchyma-sparing treatments is enormous.

Today, there are several options in addition to surgical resection to effect local control of liver metastases including hepatic artery chemoinfusion, chemoembolization, bland embolization, and ablation. In this section, we will focus on ablation of liver metastases from colorectal cancer.

Ablation refers to the application of extreme temperature or direct injection of chemical agents to effect tumor cell death. The concept of thermal ablation is by no means new. There are descriptions in papyri from Ancient Egypt of heat being used over 3500 years ago to minimize operative bleeding and to cauterize superficial tumors. Modern ablation methods include the application of heat using radiofrequency ablation (RFA), laser interstitial thermotherapy (LITT), and microwave ablation (MWA). At the opposite end of the spectrum, cryotherapy causes tumor necrosis by alternating cycles of freezing and thawing. High-intensity focused ultrasound (HIFU) is the only extracorporeal method; it uses mechanical agitation delivered transcutaneously to cause heat and cavitation leading to cell death. Chemical ablation with absolute ethanol or acetic acid is commonly used to treat hepatocellular carcinoma (HCC). Although chemical ablation has been attempted in colorectal metastases (Salim 1993), it has shown little promise in practice. Unlike HCC, which is a relatively soft tumor occurring most often in the setting of a cirrhotic (hard) liver, colorectal metastases are firm lesions in the setting of a soft liver, making direct injection difficult and adequate dispersion of the agent within the tumor poor.

Modalities

The choice of modality depends on several factors, including tumor histology, the location, number and geometry of lesion(s) and perhaps most importantly, institutional preference. Whereas RFA is the most widespread modality in use in the US, LITT is common in Europe, MWA in Japan and HIFU in China; each uses varying frequencies along the electromagnetic spectrum to effect tumor kill.

Radiofrequency ablation

In 1891 d'Arsonval noted that radiofrequency waves passed through tissue caused an elevation in temperature. Ultimately this led to the development of an alternating electric current generator in the range of radiofrequency (200–1200 MHz): the

Bovie electrocautery device. In RFA, a high-energy alternating current is applied via an exposed electrode placed directly into a target lesion. Alternating current causes agitation of intracellular ions constantly trying to align with the direction of current. This in turn causes frictional heat resulting in desiccation of cells, protein denaturation, microvascular thrombosis, and ultimately coagulative necrosis.

Malignant cells are more resistant to freezing than normal cells, but are more sensitive to hyperthermic damage. Thermal injury occurs at 42°C; as the temperature is increased the time needed to cause cell death decreases. At lethal temperatures of 60°C and over, protein denaturation, tissue coagulation, and vascular thrombosis result in a zone of complete ablation. On the periphery of the ablation, a rim of partial tissue destruction up to 8 mm in diameter can be seen surrounding the zone of coagulation (Curley *et al.* 2002).

In clinical practice, the RITA device (RITA Medical Systems, Inc, Freemont, CA) is the only generator that uses temperature (target 100°C as measured at the tines) as a surrogate marker for cell death. If exceedingly high temperatures are reached (>110°C) in the tissue surrounding the electrode, tissue charring results. Charring increases the local impedence and therefore decreases energy transfer to surrounding tissues, ultimately resulting in a smaller zone of ablation.

The LeVeen RF ablation system (RadioTheraputics, Mountain View, CA) uses impedence-based feedback in the tissue near the tip of the electrode to adjust the delivered power (Fig. 20.4a,b). When the tissue is completely coagulated, the impedence rises exponentially and the current stops, a phenomenon known as 'roll-off,' the endpoint of ablation with this device.

The third device in use in the United States is the Cool-tip electrode (Valleylab, Boulder, CO), an insulated hollow needle or cluster of three needles for larger needles (Fig. 20.4c) with two channels to allow for internal circulation of cool water to minimize charring. Similar to the RadioTheraputics device, there is a feedback loop to adjust power when impedence at the tip rises. With this device, energy is delivered for a set time of 12 minutes.

The first liver RFA was performed in the early 1990s in the treatment of small hepatocellular cancer (Rossi *et al.* 1995). In 2001, Ikeda *et al.* (Ikeda *et al.* 2001) demonstrated that RFA provided similar survival to percutaneous ethanol injection for solitary HCC but in fewer treatment sessions, popularizing this modality. It should be noted that most of the early studies using RFA were in the treatment of HCC, not metastases. The ability to extrapolate the experience in treating HCC to liver metastases is limited because the cirrhotic liver acts like an insulator, potentiating the heat deposited within the tumor, known as the 'oven effect.' In addition, metastases are more likely to have microscopic tumor surrounding the imaged tumor, increasing the risk of treatment failure and recurrence at the periphery of a lesion.

In vitro, the size of the ablation zone is dependent on both radiant and conductive properties, and is proportional to the

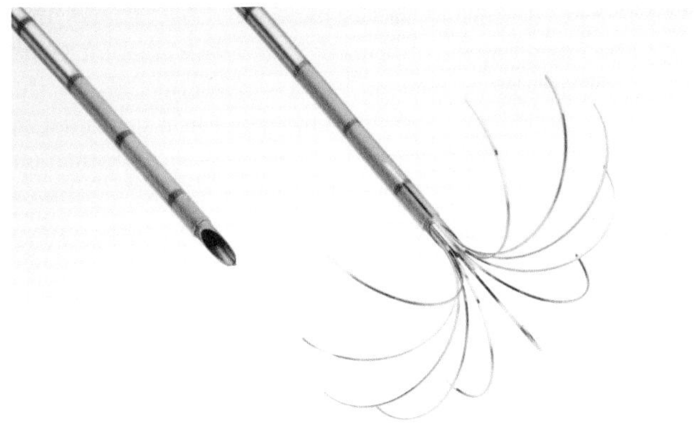

(a)

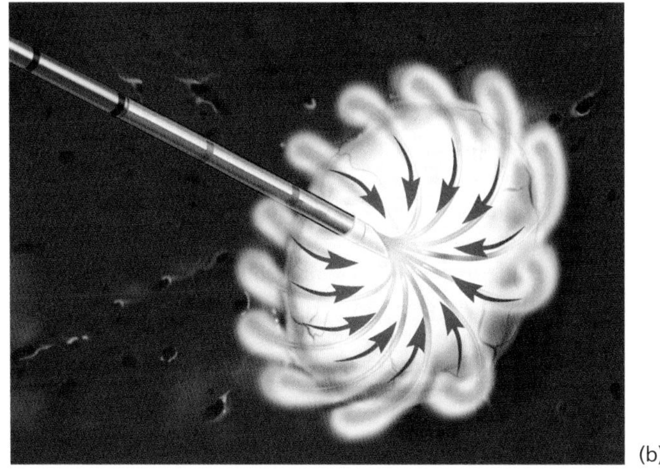

(b)

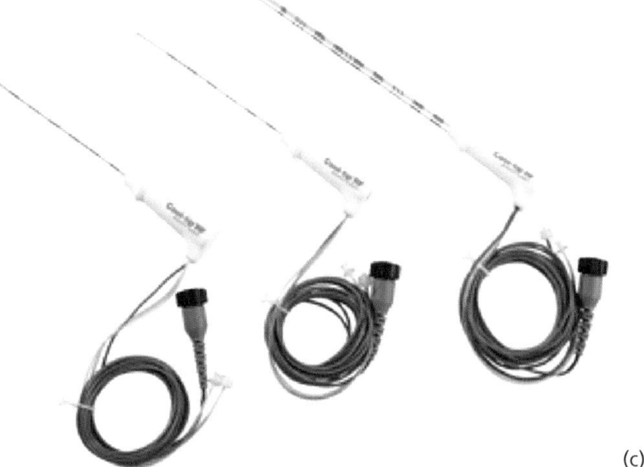

(c)

Fig. 20.4 Multitined ablation needles include the RITA (not shown) and LeVeen electrodes (a). Each uses feedback from near the tip of the electrodes (b) to adjust delivered power based on temperature (RITA) or impedance (LeVeen). The Cool-Tip electrode (c) is a hollow needle or cluster of three needles with internal channels for circulation of cool water to minimize charring around the electrode.

square of the RF current. *In vivo*, however, other factors come in to play, including the presence of large vessels adjacent to the target ablation zone. Flowing blood, while protective of the vascular endothelium, limits the amount of heat deposited in portions of tumor abutting large vessels—a phenomenon known as 'heat sink.' It has been suggested that RF combined with temporary hepatic inflow occlusion—in surgery with a Pringle maneuver (Denys *et al.* 2001) or by percutaneous balloon occlusion (Yamasaki *et al.* 2002)—can enlarge the ablation zone and increase the likelihood of ablating tumor on the vascular margin.

Large bile ducts do not have the same protection from thermal injury that blood vessels have, because the flow of bile does not remove the applied heat in the same way that flowing blood does. Therefore, lesions at the hilar plate (where the common bile duct enters the liver) and adjacent to the falciform ligament (where the left hepatic duct lies) should be treated with caution, as ablation of these ducts can lead to biliary fistula or stricture. It has been suggested that placement of biliary catheters for cool saline infusion during RFA may decrease the incidence of biliary complications (Stippel *et al.* 2005) but this has been attempted in few patients and further studies are needed. For lesions adjacent to the gallbladder or bowel, carbon dioxide, sterile water or a balloon catheter can be injected or inserted to provide a safe window. Saline as an injectate should be avoided because it is an ionic fluid and can counterproductively conduct RF energy to the structure intended to be protected.

There are few prospective studies and several retrospective reports on disease-free survival and survival following RFA of colorectal metastases. In 2001, Solbiati *et al.* (Solbiati 2001a) reported median disease-free and overall survival was 12 months and 36 months respectively, with 1-, 2-, and 3-year actuarial survival of 93%, 69% and 46% respectively after treating 179 tumors in 117 patients. Seventy (39%) patients developed local recurrence during follow-up, almost all within 1 year. Local recurrence was less common (22%) in lesions <2.5 cm, and survival was not dependent on the number of lesions treated (Solbiati *et al.* 2001a). Similar survival was reported by Gilliams and Lees (2005). They treated 73 patients with lesions <5 in number and <5 cm with a median survival of 38 months and 5-year survival of 25% after treatment.

In 2004, Abdalla *et al.* reported on 358 patients treated with either surgery alone, RFA alone or a combination of the two. Overall and disease-free survival was significantly better following resection versus RFA, but survival after RFA in non-operative candidates was found to be superior to chemotherapy alone.

In 2005, Berber *et al.* prospectively studied 135 patients after laparoscopic RFA. Median survival was 28.9 months following treatment, an improvement over their historical controls receiving chemotherapy alone in which survival was 11–14 months. Improved survival was with lesions <3 cm. Neither the presence of extrahepatic disease (present in 30% of their cohort), nor number of lesions treated was a predictor of poor survival (Berber *et al.* 2005).

Laser interstitial thermotherapy

Also known as photodynamic laser therapy, laser thermal ablation and laser photocoagulation, LITT causes thermal destruction of tumor by the conversion of laser (light) energy to heat. The most common laser used in the treatment of liver tumors is neodymium:yttrium-aluminum-garnet (Nd:YAG), with a wavelength of 1064 nm. This is a bare quartz or sapphire-tipped laser fiber, the latter allowing for less carbonization or charring around the applicator. Individual 0.5–2.5-mm diameter laser fibers can produce ablation zones of 10–36 mm depending on shape of crystal, and modifications such as scattering and cool-tip applicators. Unlike most RF devices (the exception being the switching controller of the Valleylab generator that allows up to three simultaneous electrodes to be used), multiple fiber systems (beam splitters) may be used simultaneously, allowing for a synergistic effect in treating larger tumors. Nd:YAG lasers have tissue penetration of 10–12 mm, somewhat larger than diode lasers with wavelengths of 800–980 nm, as optical penetration increases with increasing wavelength (similar to AM vs. FM radio signal).

Prolonged heating at low power (3–20 W) in continuous mode for 2–20 minutes (slow, low power to avoid char near fiber) produces an enlarging zone of conductive tissue heating as photons from low-intensity laser energy interact with molecular chromophores (hemoglobin, myoglobin, bilirubin and cytochrome pigments). In the future, it is conceivable that the efficacy of LITT may be enhanced by the concomitant use of photosensitizers as in other medicinal applications of laser therapy.

In the largest published series using LITT for treatment of non-operative colorectal liver metastases, 603 non-operative candidates with 1801 colorectal metastases <5 cm in size, Vogl *et al.* (2004) reported a mean survival of 3.8 years and local tumor control of 95.6–98.8 (depending on the size of the lesion) at 6-month follow-up.

Microwave ablation/microwave coagulation therapy

Microwave radiation is between infrared and radiowaves on the electromagnetic spectrum, with frequencies of 900–2450 MHz. In MWA, a 14.5-gauge microwave antenna is placed directly into the tumor and a generator emits electromagnetic waves through the non-insulated portion of the antenna. A microwave at 920 MHz changes charge nearly 2 billion times per second, causing rapid vibration of nearby dipoles (water) in tissue, resulting in dielectric heat and thermal coagulation (Simon *et al.* 2005).

Currently, the only clinically available system in the United States is made by Vivant Medical (Mountain View, CA); it delivers 60 W to each generator at 915 MHz. Potential advantages of MWA include large and rapid ablation with concomitant use of multiple transmitters and no need for grounding pads. Perhaps most significant in clinical practice, MWA has a larger zone of active heating—up to 2 cm—compared to millimeters with RF and LITT, the latter two relying more on thermal conduction within tissue for effect. The reliance on more active heating results in a consistently high intratumoral temperature and less heat sink effect (Simon *et al.* 2005), and charring is less likely.

Clinical experience with MWA is limited, but promising. In 2000, Shibata *et al.* randomized 30 patients to MWA versus surgical resection. Mean survival was 27 and 25 months respectively; 3-year survival following MWA was 14% versus 23% in the resection group (Shibata *et al.* 2000). A randomized controlled trial comparing RFA to MWA in the treatment of HCC demonstrated treatment success in 96% of patients treated with RF and 89% with MWA, but no similar data is available for metastases (Shibata *et al.* 2002).

High-intensity focused ultrasound (HIFU)

Ultrasound refers to mechanical vibrations, or sound waves, that are above the threshold of human hearing (16kHz). Most diagnostic ultrasound equipment is in the range of 1–10 MHz. In HIFU a high-amplitude, low-frequency ultrasound beam emitted from a specialized concave ultrasound transducer is focused onto a target lesion. The energy delivered is converted to heat in the target zone leading to coagulative necrosis as in RFA. A second mechanism causing cell injury and death involves cavitation. The high-amplitude sound wave of HIFU causes tissues to vibrate, resulting in alternating compression and rarefaction. A phase change from water to gas results and microbubbles are released from intracellular water. When these bubbles collapse, mechanical stress results in cavitation.

The Model JC HIFU system (HAIFU Technology Company, Chongqing, People's Republic of China) has a 12-cm diameter single element piezoceramic transducer operating at 0.8–1.6 MHz with variable focal lengths of 9–15 cm. A diagnostic transducer is mounted coaxially for real-time imaging during ablation. Ablations of up to 3.3 cm in the path of the beam and 1 cm perpendicular to the beam can be achieved.

Although the non-invasive nature of HIFU minimizes risks of bleeding and tract seeding, the need for a path clear of any structures between the skin and target that absorb or reflect the ultrasound beam limit the ability to treat lesions in the dome of the liver. With current technology, the ability to treat lesions > 10 cm deep to skin are limited. Finally, treatment times are a major limitation—treatment of a superficial 2–3 cm lesion takes approximately 2 hours.

HIFU is currently performed almost exclusively in China, and clinical experience with this technique is limited, but promising. Wu *et al.* (2001) reported on 30 patients with solid carcinomas metastatic to liver. Lesions 2–10 cm in diameter were treated with HIFU and underwent definitive resection within 2 weeks. In all lesions they achieved complete necrosis with no pathologic evidence of residual tumor at the ablation site.

Cryoablation

The mechanism of action of cryoablation, which uses alternating cycles of freezing and thawing, is markedly different from the other thermal ablation methods. A cryoprobe cooled with liquid nitrogen or argon is placed into a tumor. Whereas heat causes coagulative necrosis, freezing causes phase changes from liquid (water) to solid (ice) that destroy cell membranes and organelles. Both non-neoplastic and neoplastic cells are sensitive to cold temperatures; hepatocytes die at –15–20°C, and tumor cells at –30–40°C. Maximum cell death occurs with slow (<2°C/min) or rapid (>50°C/min) cooling. With slow cooling, the relatively solute-poor extracellular fluid freezes before the intracellular fluid, creating an osmotic gradient across the cell membrane. Intracellular fluid flows out of the cell across the gradient, resulting in cellular dehydration, protein denaturation and loss of the integrity of the cell membrane. Because the cell membrane is disrupted, surviving but injured cells are killed during thaw, when the osmotic gradient is returned to normal as the extracellular ice melts. In rapid cooling intracellular fluid freezes before cells become dehydrated. Ice crystals coalesce, causing direct injury to cell organelles and membranes, resulting in cell death. The cycle is usually repeated two or more times, each subsequent cycle producing a larger ice ball due to increased conductivity from the prior freeze (Polk *et al.* 1995).

Similar to LITT, multiple cryoprobes may be placed simultaneously to enlarge the iceball to treat larger lesions. Percutaneous probes are 1.7 or 2.4 mm in diameter and a single probe can create an iceball of up to 3 × 5 cm.

The data on cryotherapy in the treatment of unresectable colorectal metastases are more mature than for other methods because it has been in clinical practice longer. Reports of 1-year survival ranges from 77% to 95% and 2-year survival from 52% to 78% has been reported. A study of 58 patients with 209 lesions comparing percutaneous RFA to cryotherapy demonstrated 1- and 2-year survival of 93% and 75% for RFA, and 76% and 61% for cryotherapy, respectively (not significantly). For lesions <4 cm, RFA and cryotherapy both had local recurrence of 6%, but cryotherapy was associated with a higher complication rate (30% vs. 11%) (Joosten *et al.* 2005).

Indications

Percutaneous ablation is a relatively new technology and the indications are in evolution and differ from country to country, institution to institution and practitioner to practitioner. Although local ablation is considered a palliative procedure, the goal of treatment is to effect a cure. Today, patients with isolated liver metastases from colorectal cancer who can be resected, should be. While short-term data are promising, all ablative techniques lack the long-term follow-up from prospective studies to establish comparable long-term disease-free and survival rates.

Generally accepted inclusion criteria for ablation are patients who are not surgical candidates based on either lesion location (adjacent vital structures, precluding margin negative resection, bilobar disease), hepatic reserve or comorbid disease. Intraoperative ablation may also be performed in concert with hepatic resection, broadening the criteria for resectability to include more patients with bilobar disease. Patients should have liver-only or liver-dominant metastases amenable to ablation based on location, number (<4) and size (<5 cm). Although acceptable size criteria vary greatly, it is known that local recurrence and treatment failure are higher with larger lesions due to incomplete ablation at the periphery. Solbiati *et al.* (2001b) treated 172 lesions in 109 patients and achieved local control in 70% of lesions. Local recurrence was seen in only 16.5% of patients with lesions <3 cm and 56% in patients with lesions ≥3 cm.

The largest device currently available is the StarBurst XL from RITA, which creates a 7-cm ablation using saline dripped through each of nine electrodes. If perfectly centered, the largest tumor that the StarBurst XL can treat with a single ablation is 5 cm, allowing for a 1-cm margin of normal liver. Based on computer modeling, with a 5-cm ablation six optimally positioned overlapping ablations are required to adequately treat a 4.25-cm tumor. In light of this, reported local recurrence of percutaneous ablated lesion up to 40% in lesions larger than 4 cm is not surprising.

There are some instances in which ablation may be considered in patients who are candidates for resection, including patients who refuse surgery or warrant a 'test of time' (Livraghi *et al.* 2003a). In the 'test of time' approach, patients with resectable disease undergo ablation and short-interval follow-up. If no disease progression (i.e. new lesions) is detected within 3–6 months, resection is performed (Livraghi *et al.* 2003a). If new lesions are detected, the patient is spared a surgery that would not have been curative due to the presence of micrometastatic disease. In this way, the 'test of time' or 'wait and see' approach is a selection criterion to determine which patients are most likely to benefit from resection. Solbiati *et al.* (2003a) treated 119 lesions in 88 patients with resectable disease (<3 lesions and <4 cm). Over 18–75 months follow-up, 70% developed new lesions and in 29 patients, new metastases precluded resection. Absolute contraindications to ablation are few, and include uncorrectable coagulopathy and life expectancy <6 months.

Imaging during ablation

Percutaneous ablation may be performed using ultrasound, CT or MR guidance. In most centers, ultrasound is the modality of choice because it is relatively inexpensive, readily available, does not use ionizing radiation and allows for real-time visualization of probe placement and ablation. CT is useful in targeting lesions difficult to see with ultrasound. Most commonly it is used for lesions in the dome, because air in the base of the lung reflects the ultrasound beam, limiting the utility of ultrasound to see this area. CT also offers superior visualization of the ablation zone during and immediately following ablation. Ultrasound during ablation shows an hyperechoic ball that makes assessment of the ablation zone and the need to reposition the probe to treat large lesions difficult because of shadowing.

Our protocol is to evaluate patients after ablation with CT (or MR) at 1 month for evidence of complete ablation. The normal appearance at this time is an ablation zone larger than the treated lesion (Fig. 20.5), often with a smooth enhancing hypervascular rim of inflammatory tissue. Any nodularity or asymmetry of the hyperemia should raise the suspicion of tumor. Successful retreatment of incompletely ablated or recurrent lesions has been shown to provide similar survival benefit than if the lesion is completely treated in one session. The hyperemic rim usually resolves by the next imaging study at 3 months. Imaging is obtained every 3 months for 1 year, every 6 months for the next 2 years, and yearly thereafter. Other modalities, including dynamic MR, microbubble ultrasound and PET, have also been used to evaluate for recurrence and progression. Finally, MR thermometry has been used during RFA, LITT and MWA to monitor the ablation, but MR availability limits the clinical utility.

Complications

Complications common to RFA, LITT and MWA include bleeding, tract seeding, sepsis, and intestinal perforation. Tract seeding is an important consideration when evaluating patients with hepatocellular carcinoma for percutaneous intervention in the era of liver transplantation. Llovet *et al.* (2001) reported an incidence of 12.5% of tract seeding following RFA for HCC, all in patients who had previously undergone percutaneous biopsy. Livraghi *et al.* (2005) had 12 cases of tract seeding in 1314 patients who underwent RFA. Although the risk of tract seeding from treatment of colorectal metastases is less well known, at least one case has been reported (Bonatti *et al.* 2003).

In an multicenter study, Livraghi *et al.* (2003b) reported complications following RFA in 3554 lesions. Six deaths (0.3%) were reported; one case each of sepsis, massive hemorrhage, and liver failure; two caused by multiorgan failure following intestinal perforation; and one case of sudden death of uncertain cause 3 days after the procedure. Major complications were reported in 50 patients (2.2%) including intraabdominal hemorrhage requiring treatment (12, 24%), tract seeding (12, 24%), liver abscess (6,12%), intestinal perforation, cardiac arrest, pulmonary embolism, pneumothorax, biloma, and cholecystitis. Increased RF sessions were related to higher rates of major complications ($p<0.01$) (Livraghi *et al.* 2003b), whereas when electrode type or tumor size was compared, the number of complications was not significantly different (Livraghi *et al.* 2003b). In less than 5% of patients minor complications were

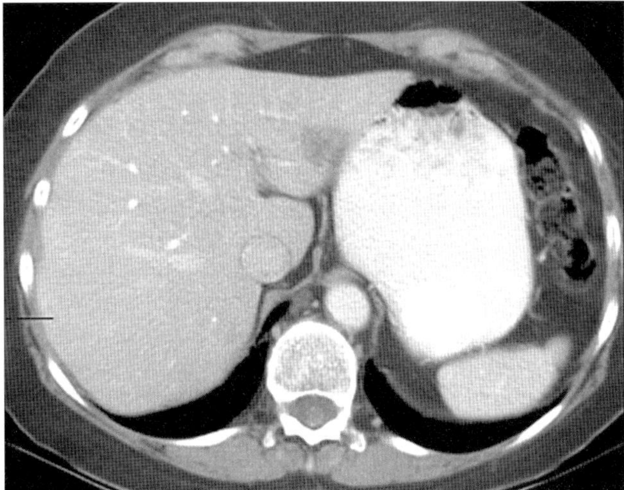
(a)

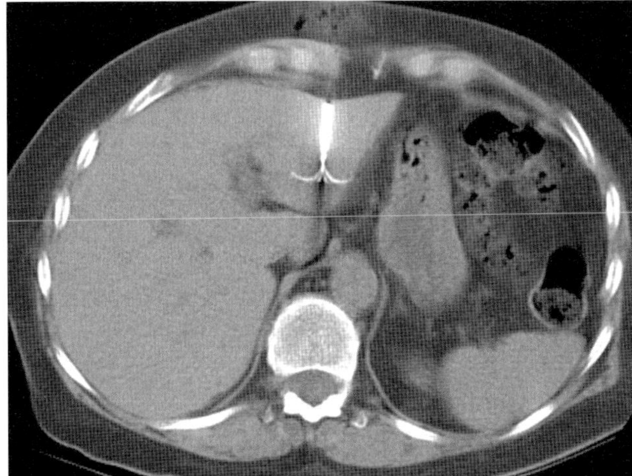
(b)

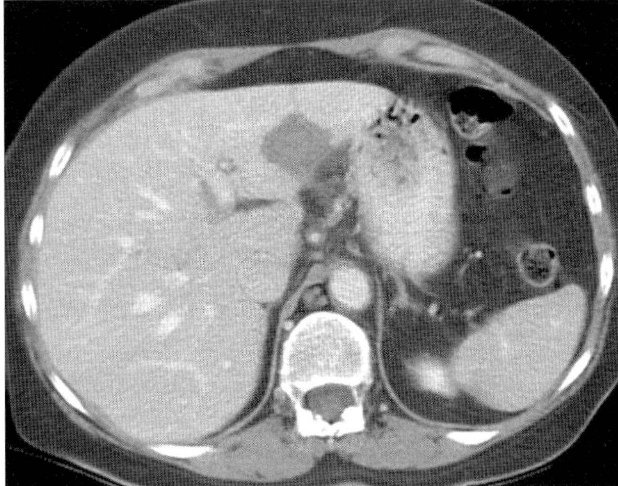
(c)

Fig. 20.5 A solitary lesion in the left lateral segment (a) in a patient with a short disease-free interval was treated with RFA (b) using a multitined electrode. Contrast enhanced CT 4 weeks later demonstrates a hypovascular ablation zone larger than the treated tumor with no residual hypervascularity.

observed including skin burn, self-limited bleeding, arterioportal and bilioportal fistula, biloma, pain, and biliary stricture.

Complications unique to cryoablation include 'cryoshock,' hypothermia and organ fracture. Cryoshock is a systemic reaction that occurs in 1% of patients following cryoablation (Weber & Lee 2005) and consists of intravascular hemolysis, disseminated intravascular coagulation, and multisystem organ failure. It has been hypothesized that liberation of interleukin-6 and tumor necrosis factor into the systemic circulation from cells with disrupted membranes cause the systemic response (Seifert *et al.* 1999). The incidence of cryoshock is higher in patients who undergo large-volume ablations. Like cryoshock, the incidence of hypothermia is higher in patients who undergo large ablations. Hypothermia can lead to cardiac depression and arrhythmia. For cases in which a large volume is to be ablated, application of Bair Huggers or other warming devices may be used. Organ fracture due to freezing has been reported in the surgical literature. It is conceivable that the risk of fracture is less with percutaneous cryoablation because the chest wall limits the motion of the probe and there is normal liver surrounding the tract of the probe that can serve to tamponade the probe. In addition, the air–iceball interface is absent (Weber & Lee 2005).

Conclusion

The search for a reliable, minimally invasive way to treat isolated liver metastases in patients who are unable to undergo surgical resection is ongoing. Multiple thermal ablation techniques have been developed and introduced into modern medical practice in the past two decades. To date, prospective studies with long-term follow-up to evaluate recurrence, disease-free and overall survival rates are limited, accounting for the fact that no single modality has become the standard of care.

References

Abdalla EK, Vauthey JN, Ellis LM *et al.* (2004) Recurrence and outcomes following hepatic resection, radiofrequency ablation, and combined resection/ablation for colorectal liver metastases. *Ann Surg* 239(6): 818–25.

American Cancer Society. (2005) *Colorectal Cancer Facts and Figures.* American Cancer Society, Atlanta, GA.

Berber E, Pelley R, Siperstein AE. (2005) Predictors of survival after radiofrequency thermal ablation of colorectal cancer metastases to the liver: a prospective study. *J Clin Oncol* 23(7): 1358–64.

Bonatti H, Bodner G, Obrist P, Bechter O, Wetscher G, Oefner D. (2003) Skin implant metastasis after percutaneous radio-frequency ablation therapy of liver metastasis of a colorectal carcinoma. *Am Surg* 69(9): 763–5.

Curley SA, Cusack JC Jr., Tanabe KK, Stoelzing O, Ellis LM. (2002) Advances in the treatment of treatment of liver tumors. *Curr Probl Surg* 39(5): 449–571.

D'Arsonval MA. (1891) Action physiologique des courants alternatifs. *CR Soc Biol* 43: 283–6.

Denys AL, De Baere T, Mahe C *et al.* (2001) Radio-frequency tissue ablation of the liver: effects of vascular occlusion on lesion diameter and biliary and portal damages in a pig model. *Eur Radiol* 11(10): 2102–8.

Dodd GD, III, Frank MS, Aribandi M, Chopra S, Chintapalli KN. (2001) Radiofrequency thermal ablation: computer analysis of the size of the thermal injury created by overlapping ablations. *AJR Am J Roentgenol* 177(4): 777–82.

Gillams AR, Lees WR. (2005) Radiofrequency ablation of colorectal liver metastases. *Abdom Imaging* 30(4): 419–26.

Ikeda M, Okada S, Ueno H, Okusaka T, Kuriyama H. (2001) Radiofrequency ablation and percutaneous ethanol injection in patients with small hepatocellular carcinoma: a comparative study. *Jpn J Clin Oncol* 2001: 31(7): 322–6.

Joosten J, Jager G, Oyen W, Woobes T, Ruers T. (2005) Cryosurgery and radiofrequency ablation for unresectable colorectal liver metastases. *Eur J Surg Oncol* 31(10): 1152–9.

Kemeny NE, Niedzwiecki D, Hollis DR *et al.* (2006) Hepatic arterial infusion versus systemic therapy for hepatic metastases from colorectal cancer: a randomized trial of efficacy, quality of life, and molecular markers (CALGB 9481). *J Clin Oncol* 24(9): 1395–403.

Livraghi T, Solbiati L, Meloni F, Ierace T, Goldberg SN, Gazelle GS. (2003a) Percutaneous radiofrequency ablation of liver metastases in potential candidates for resection: the 'test-of-time approach'. *Cancer* 97(12): 3207–35.

Livraghi T, Solbiati L, Meloni MF, Gazelle GS, Halpern EF, Goldberg SN. (2003b) Treatment of focal liver tumors with percutaneous radio-frequency ablation: complications encountered in a multicenter study. *Radiology* 226(2): 441–51.

Livraghi T, Lazzaroni S, Meloni F, Solbiati L. (2005) Risk of tumor seeding after percutaneous radiofrequency ablation for hepatocellular carcinoma. *Br J Surg* 92(7): 856–8.

Llovet JM, Vilana R, Bru C *et al.* (2001) Barcelona Clinic Liver Cancer (BCLC) Group. Increased risk of tumor seeding after percutaneous radiofrequency ablation for a single hepatocellular carcinoma. *Hepatology* 33(5): 1124–9.

Nordlinger B, Guiguet M, Vaillant JC *et al.* (1996) Surgical resection of colorectal carcinoma metastases to the liver. A prognostic scoring system to improve case selection, based on 1568 patients. Association Francaise de Chirurgie. *Cancer* 77(7): 1254–62.

Polk W, Fong Y, Karpeh M, Blumgart LH. (1995) A technique for the use of cryosurgery to assist hepatic resection. *J Am Coll Surg* 180(2): 171–6.

Registry of Hepatic Metastases. (1988) Resection of the liver for colorectal carcinoma metastases: A multi-institutional study of indications for resection. *Surgery* 103(3): 278–88.

Rossi S, Di SM, Buscarini E *et al.* (1995) Percutaneous radiofrequency interstitial thermal ablation in the treatment of small hepatocellular carcinoma. *Cancer J Sci Am* 1(1): 73.

Salim AS. (1993) Pilot study on alcohol-induced chemonecrosis of hepatic metastases from colonic cancer. A new approach for percutaneous localized dynamic destruction of the hepatic spread. *HPB Surgery* 7(1): 33–9.

Seifert JK, Stewart GJ, Hewitt PM, Bolton EJ, Juninger T, Morris DL. (1999) Interleukin-6 and tumor necrosis factor-alpha levels following hepatic cryotherapy: association with volume and duration of freezing. *World J Surg* 23(10): 1019–26.

Shibata T, Niinobu T, Ogata N, Takami M. (2000) Microwave coagulation therapy for multiple hepatic metastases from colorectal carcinoma. *Cancer* 89(2): 276–84.

Shibata T, Iimuro Y, Yamamoto Y *et al.* (2002) Small hepatocellular carcinoma: comparison of radio-frequency ablation and percutaneous microwave coagulation therapy. *Radiology* 223(2): 331–7.

Simon CJ, Dupuy DE, Mayo-Smith WW. (2005) Microwave ablation: principles and applications. *Radiographics* 25 Suppl 1: S69–S83.

Stippel DL, Banguard C, Kasper HU, Fischer JH, Holscher AH, Grossman A. (2005) Experimental bile duct protection by intraductal cooling during radiofrequency ablation. *Br J Surg* 92(7): 849–55.

Solbiati L, Livraghi T, Goldberg SN *et al.* (2001a) Percutaneous radio-frequency ablation of hepatic metastases from colorectal cancer: Long-term results in 117 patients. *Radiology* 221(1): 159–66.

Solbiati I, Ierace T, Tonolini M, Osti V, Cova L. (2001b) Radiofrequency thermal ablation of hepatic metastases. *Eur J Ultrasound* 13(2): 149–58.

Vogl TJ, Straub R, Eichler K, Sollner O, Mack MG. (2004) Colorectal carcinoma metastases in liver: laser-induced interstitial thermotherapy—local tumor control rate and survival data. *Radiology* 230(2): 450–8.

Wagner JS, Adson MS, Van Heeden JA, Adson MH, Illstrup DM. (1984) The natural history of hepatic metastases from colorectal cancer. A comparison with resective treatment. *Ann Surg* 199(5): 502–8.

Weber SM, Lee FT Jr. (2005) Expanded treatment of hepatic tumors with radiofrequency ablation and cryoablation. *Oncology (Williston Park)* 19(11 Suppl 4): 27–32.

Wu F, Chen WZ, Bai J *et al.* (2001) Pathological changes in human malignant carcinoma treated with high-intensity focused ultrasound. *Ultrasound Med Biol* 27(8): 1099–106.

Yamasaki T, Kurokawa F, Shirahashi H, Kusano N, Hironaka K, Okita K. (2002) Percutaneous radiofrequency ablation therapy for patients with hepatocellular carcinoma during occlusion of hepatic blood flow. Comparison with standard percutaneous radiofrequency ablation therapy. *Cancer* 95(11): 2353–60.

Radiation therapy

Christopher Willett & Brian G. Czito

Introduction

Over the past 10 years, innovative approaches employing radiation therapy have been developed in the treatment of patients with hepatic metastases from colorectal cancer. These treatment strategies have included conformal radiation therapy, stereotactic body radiation therapy, and hepatic artery infusion (HAI) of radioactive spheres. Given the limited tolerance of the liver to radiation therapy, the common goal of these therapeutic approaches has been to deliver tumoricidal doses of radiation therapy to the hepatic lesion(s) while minimizing irradiation of surrounding uninvolved liver. Phase I and II studies utilizing these treatment approaches are under way, exploring the feasibility, indications, results, and potential efficacy of these strategies. This section will review these therapeutic methods and results.

Conformal radiation therapy

In the past, radiation therapy has been used infrequently in the treatment of liver malignancies secondary to the limited tolerance of the whole liver to radiation (Ben-Josef *et al.* 2005a). Radiation-induced liver disease, a syndrome characterized by anicteric hepatomegaly, ascites, and impaired liver tests, develops in 5% of patients receiving 30–35 Gy to the whole liver. Three-dimensional (3D) conformal treatment planning permits treatment of the tumor while minimizing dose to the uninvolved liver, and allows a quantitative understanding of the relationships of dose, volume, and probability of complication (Ben-Josef *et al.* 2005a).

Employing this technology, investigators from the University of Michigan demonstrated that higher radiation doses than the traditional 30–35 Gy could control some tumors and that these doses could be safely administered contingent upon the dose and volume of normal liver irradiated. In their initial phase I study, these investigators reported the preliminary results of 43 patients with unresectable intrahepatic tumors (primary hepatobiliary cancer, 27 patients and colorectal metastases, 16 patients) treated to a median dose of 58.5 Gy (range, 28.5–90 Gy) with 1.5-Gy fractions administered twice daily with concurrent continuous infusion hepatic arterial fluorodeoxyuridine (Dawson *et al.* 2000). The response rate in 25 assessable patients was 68%. With a median potential follow-up period of 26.5 months, the median times to progression for all tumors, liver metastases and hepatobiliary cancer were 6, 8, and 3 months, respectively. The median survival times of all patients, patients with liver metastases, and patients with hepatobiliary cancer were 16, 18, and 11 months, respectively. On multivariate analyses, escalated RT dose was independently associated with improved progression-free and overall survival. The median survival of patients treated with 70 Gy or more had not been reached (16.4 months+) compared with 11.6 months in patients treated with lower RT doses.

Following completion of the phase I study, these investigators continued to explore these techniques in the phase II setting. The combined results of these studies have been recently published (Ben-Josef *et al.* 2005b). Of the 128 patients with unresectable intrahepatic tumors enrolled in both studies, a large number of patients (47) were treated for metastases arising from colorectal cancer. With a median follow-up time of 16 months (26 months in patients who were alive), the median survival time of all 128 patients was 15.8 months, significantly longer than in the historical controls. The 3-year actuarial survival was 17%. The total dose of radiation therapy was the only significant predictor of survival. Local failure (as measured by first site of disease progression) was seen in 24/42 (57%) of patients with colorectal cancer. Primary hepatobiliary tumors had a significantly greater tendency to remain confined to the liver than did colorectal cancer metastases. Overall toxicity was acceptable, with 27 patients (21%) and 11 patients (9%) developing grade 3 and 4 toxicity, respectively (Ben-Josef *et al.* 2005b). Given the high rates of extrahepatic progression in patients treated for colorectal cancer metastases, these investigators recommend integration of this approach with newer systemic therapy for these patients.

Stereotactic body radiation therapy

Recent technological advances have made it possible to deliver high tumoricidal doses of radiation therapy to small tumors in one or a small number of fractions (Kavanagh *et al.* 2006). This treatment paradigm has been studied extensively in patients with intracranial metastases. Intracranial stereotactic radiosurgery (SRS) has become a routine treatment option for patients with metastases to the brain. This work has evolved from single-institution experiences to multicenter and cooperative group trials. In the past 5 years, prospective randomized trials have helped to define the proper role of SRS in patients with intracranial metastases.

Along the similar theme of SRS, stereotactic body radiation therapy (SBRT) is a treatment method to deliver a high dose of radiation to the target, utilizing either a single dose or a small number of fractions with a high degree of precision within the body. In contrast to the University of Michigan protocols using twice-daily radiation treatments administered over many weeks, SBRT employs high-dose radiation usually delivered over one to three treatments. With this technique, control rates in excess of 80% have been achieved in selected patients with metastases from lung, breast, renal and other cancers (Kavanagh *et al.* 2006). Similar control rates may be feasible using SBRT for defined patients with inoperable hepatic metastases. In contrast to intracranial radiosurgery, the application of SBRT has been handicapped by two problems (Kavanagh *et al.* 2006). First, tumors in the liver are subject to motion related to respiration. Second, because the treatments are highly focused, it is required that the target extent be confidentially and reproducibly defined by diagnostics and treatment planning imaging. As such, image guidance during therapy is required to ensure that selected patients are properly treated with limited fields and that the target extent can be determined accurately. Over the past 10 years, significant technological advances in defining tumor motion through image guidance have overcome these challenges and have permitted the concepts of SRS to be extrapolated to extracranial sites, including the liver (Figs 20.6 and 20.7).

The few reported studies of SBRT for liver tumors have included both single-fraction and multiple-fraction regimens. Herfarth and colleagues at Heidelberg University applied single-fraction SBRT to primary and metastatic liver lesions and safely escalated the dose from 14 to 26 Gy (Herfath *et al.* 2004). Thirty-seven patients were enrolled with a median tumor volume of 10 mL (range, 1–132 mL). A total of 60 lesions were treated, 4 primary liver tumors, and 56 metastases. No patients experi-

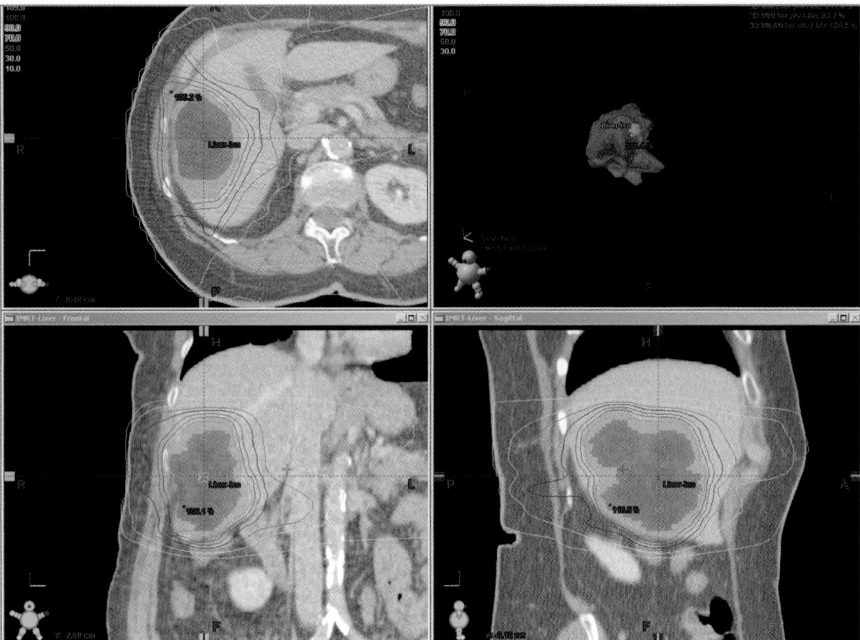

Fig. 20.6 Axial, sagittal, coronal radiation isodose distribution of stereotactic treatment of hepatic metastasis (courtesy of Dr Fang Fang Yin and Dr Lawrence Marks, Duke University Medical Center).

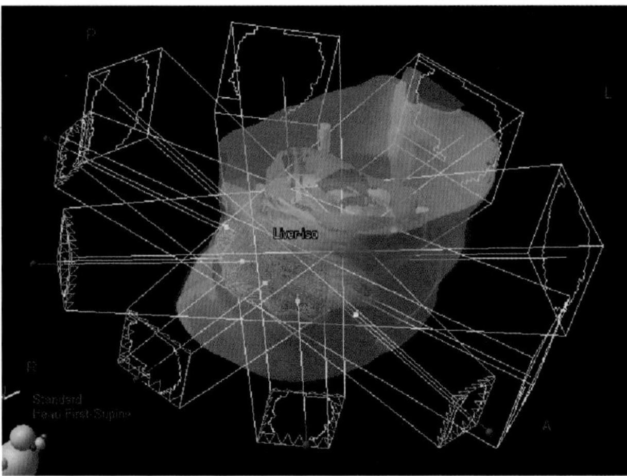

Fig. 20.7 Field arrangements of stereotactic body radiation therapy for hepatic metastasis (courtesy of Dr Fang Fang Yin and Dr Lawrence Marks, Duke University Medical Center).

enced radiation-induced liver disease. The actuarial freedom from local failure at 18 months for the entire group was 67%; failures occurred mainly in the patients with the lower doses. These same investigators have also characterized the transient radiographic changes typically observed after liver SBRT. A sharp demarcated hypodense area surrounds the treated tumor in non-enhanced CT scans, potentially obscuring evaluation of response within the first few months after treatment before resolving (Herfath *et al.* 2004). Based on these results, a multicenter trial comparing single-dose to hypofractionated (three fraction) SBRT in patients with prospective nonoperable liver metastases has been undertaken.

Blomgren and colleagues at the Karolinska Institute administered 20–45 Gy in two to four fractions to a group of 17 patients with 21 hepatic metastases (Blomgren *et al.* 1998). Only one patient developed a serious toxicity (hemorrhagic gastritis in a patient with a previous history of gastritis) possibly attributable to SBRT. Of the 21 lesions treated, only one instance of local tumor progression was observed after a mean follow-up interval of 9.6 months (Blomgren *et al.* 1998).

Wulf and colleagues at the University of Wurzburg used fractionated SBRT, typically 30 Gy in three fractions, in 23 patients with solitary liver lesions and observed no grade 3 or higher acute or late toxicity from treatment (Wulf *et al.* 2001). After treatment, the actuarial rates of local control at 1 and 2 years were 76% and 61%, respectively.

A multicenter study from the University of Colorado, University of Texas-Southwestern, and University of Indiana recently reported the results of a phase I trial of SBRT for liver metastases (Schefter *et al.* 2005). Eligible patients had one to three liver metastases, tumor diameter <6 cm, and adequate liver function. The first patient cohort received 36 Gy delivered over three fractions to the target volume. Subsequent cohorts received progressively higher doses up to a maximum of 60 Gy in three fractions. Eighteen patients were enrolled and the most common primary site was colorectal cancer. No patients experienced dose-limiting toxicity and dose was escalated to 60 Gy in three fractions without reaching maximum tolerated dose. The authors concluded that biologically potent doses of SBRT are well tolerated in patients with liver metastases. These investigators are pursuing a phase II study of 60 Gy over three fractions for liver metastases.

Resin yttrium microspheres

Resin microspheres containing yttrium, a high energy beta-emitting isotope, have also been used in the treatment of patients with hepatic metastases from colorectal cancer (Lim *et al.* 2005; Kennedy *et al.* 2006). The yttrium resin microspheres are embolized into the hepatic artery where they become lodged within the tumor microvasculature. The treatment is relatively selective as hepatic tumors derive their blood supply almost exclusively from the hepatic artery whereas normal liver parenchyma is supplied by the portal circulation. Animal studies suggest that the yttrium microspheres allow on average 200–300 Gy to be delivered to liver tumors.

A retrospective multicenter analysis of 208 patients with unresectable colorectal liver metastases that were refractory to chemotherapy treated with yttrium microspheres was recently reported (Kennedy *et al.* 2006). Patients were selected from seven institutions for treatment after screening defined vascular access to all the tumors and imaging confirmed microspheres would be implanted only in the liver tumors. Median follow-up was 13 months (range, 1–42 months). Computed tomography partial response rate was 35%; positron emission tomography (PET) response rate was 91%, and reduction in CEA of 70% of patients was achieved. Median survival was 10.5 months for responding patients but only 4.5 months in non-responding patients. No treatment-related procedure deaths or radiation-related venoocclusive liver failures were found.

A prospective study from three Australian centers evaluated the efficacy and safety of yttrium microspheres in 30 patients with inoperable liver metastases who had failed 5-FU-based chemotherapy (Lim *et al.* 2005). There were 10 partial responses with the median duration of response of 8.3 months (range 2–18 months) and median time to progression of 5.3 months. Response rates were lower (21%) and progression-free survival shorter (3.9 months) in patients who had received all standard chemotherapy options. No responses were seen in patients with a poor performance status (n=3) or extrahepatic disease (n=6). Overall treatment-related toxicity was acceptable; however, significant late toxicity included four cases of gastric ulceration. These investigators recommend further studies to better define the subsets of patients most likely to respond.

Conclusion

Recent technological advances in radiation therapy have provided the means to deliver tumoricidal doses of radiation therapy to patients with inoperable colorectal cancer metastases to the liver. These techniques include fractionated conformal chemoradiation, stereotactic body radiation therapy, and hepatic artery infusion of radioactive spheres. Studies employing these approaches are in their infancy, limited to single- or multi-institution retrospective or phase I and II trials. The ultimate efficacy of these approaches has yet to be defined and will be based on results of future studies and the appropriate integration with new effective systemic therapies.

References

Ben-Josef E, Lawrence TS. (2005a) Radiotherapy for unresectable hepatic malignancies. *Semin Radiat Oncol* 15(4): 273–8.

Ben-Josef E, Normolle D, Ensminger WD *et al.* (2005b) Phase II trial of high-dose conformal radiation therapy with concurrent hepatic artery floxuridine for unresectable intrahepatic malignancies. *J Clin Oncol* 23(34): 8739–47.

Blomgren J, Lax, I Göranson H *et al.* (1998) Radiosurgery for tumors in the body: Clinical experience using a new method. *J Radiosurg* 1: 63–74.

Dawson LA, McGinn CJ, Normolle D *et al.* (2000) Escalated focal liver radiation and concurrent hepatic artery fluorodeoxyuridine for unresectable intrahepatic malignancies. *J Clin Oncol* 18(11): 2210–8.

Herfarth KK, Debus J, Wannenmacher M. (2004) Stereotactic radiation therapy of liver metastases: update of the initial phase-I/II trial. *Front Radiat Ther Oncol* 38: 100–5.

Kavanagh BD, McGarry RC, Timmerman RD. (2006) Extracranial radiosurgery (stereotactic body radiation therapy) for oligometastases. *Semin Radiat Oncol* 16(2): 77–84.

Kennedy AS, Coldwell D, Nutting C *et al.* (2006) Resin (90)Y-microsphere brachytherapy for unresectable colorectal liver metastases: Modern USA experience. *Int J Radiat Oncol Biol Phys* 65(2): 412–25.

Lim L, Gibbs P, Yip D *et al.* (2005) A prospective evaluation of treatment with selective internal radiation therapy (SIR-spheres) in patients with unresectable liver metastases from colorectal cancer previously treated with 5-FU based chemotherapy. *BMC Cancer* 5: 132.

Schefter TE, Kavanagh BD, Timmerman RD, Cardenes HR, Baron A, Gaspar LE. (2005) A phase I trial of stereotactic body radiation therapy (SBRT) for liver metastases. *Int J Radiat Oncol Biol Phys* 62(5): 1371–8.

Wulf J, Hadinger U, Oppitz U, Thiele W, Ness-Dourdoumas R, Flentje M. (2001) Stereotactic radiotherapy of targets in the lung and liver. *Strahlenther Onkol* 177(12): 645–55.

21 Primary Pancreatic Adenocarcinoma

Edited by Christopher L. Wolfgang

Diagnosis

Epidemiology, history and clinical findings

Timothy M. Pawlik

Epidemiology and history

Pancreatic adenocarcinoma is the fourth leading cause of cancer mortality in the United States and the sixth leading cause in Europe (Greenlee *et al.* 2000; Michaud 2004) with 1- and 5-year survival rates of 25% and 5%, respectively (Ries *et al.* 2003). In most developed countries the rate of mortality from pancreatic cancer has remained the same in women and has decreased slightly in men over the past two decades (Sahmoun *et al.* 2003). In 2005, the estimated number of pancreatic cancer cases in the United States was 32,180 and the number of estimated deaths was 31,180 (American Cancer Society 2005). As such, pancreatic adenocarcinoma is considered to be one of the deadliest malignancies with a death to incidence ratio of approximately 0.99 (Devesa *et al.* 1995). Although there has been only modest improvement in the overall survival of patients with pancreatic adenocarcinoma, the morbidity and mortality associated with surgical treatment of this disease has improved dramatically. This section focuses on the epidemiology, predisposing factors, as well as history and clinical characteristics of patients with pancreatic adenocarcinoma. Accurate identification of high-risk cohorts, as well as early detection of patients with signs and symptoms of pancreatic carcinoma, may lead to better diagnosis and treatment of this disease.

Age, gender and race

Pancreatic adenocarcinoma is primarily a disease of patients older than 60 years of age. In fact, approximately half of patients diagnosed with pancreatic cancer in the United States are older than 75 years of age and only 13% of patients are diagnosed before the age of 60 (Ries *et al.* 2003). Pancreatic cancer also occurs more frequently in males than females (Lin *et al.* 2001; Michaud 2004). In developed countries men have a higher incidence and mortality than women (incidence of 8.5 per 100,000 in men versus 5 per 100,000 in women; mortality of 2.4 per 100,000 in men versus 1.6 per 100,000 in women) (Parkin *et al.* 1999).

In the United States incidence rates and mortality from pancreatic cancer are higher among blacks than whites for both men and women (Gold & Goldin 1998; Chang *et al.* 2005). Chang *et al.* (2005) attributed this higher incidence to two known risk factors for pancreatic cancer: a history of diabetes and smoking. In the same study blacks were also found to be less likely to undergo surgery for a mass in the pancreas (Chang *et al.* 2005). There is much speculation about the reason for the increased incidence and mortality of pancreatic cancer among blacks in the United States (Chang *et al.* 2005; Hayanga 2005). Some studies have called into question the reported higher mortality rate among black Americans (Bach *et al.* 2002; Saif *et al.* 2005). Eloubeidi *et al.* (Eloubeidi *et al.* 2006) found that in Alabama's Statewide Cancer Registry race had no effect on overall survival when one adjusted for stage at presentation, type of therapy received, age at diagnosis, and site of primary tumor. The investigators did note that black patients were less likely to receive therapy, but also were more likely to refuse the indicated therapy (Eloubeidi *et al.* 2006).

On a molecular level black Americans have more frequent K-ras mutations than American whites (Pernick *et al.* 2003). Similarly, Chinese patients appear to have different expressions of K-ras and p53 than Western or Japanese patients (Dong *et al.* 2000; Song *et al.* 2000). Longernecker *et al.* (Longnecker *et al.* 2000) used population-based data collected in Hawaii,

Gastrointestinal Oncology: A Critical Multidisciplinary Team Approach.
Edited by J. Jankowski, R. Sampliner, D. Kerr, and Y. Fong.
© 2008 Blackwell Publishing, ISBN: 978-1-4501-2783-7

San Francisco, and Seattle and found that Asians diagnosed with pancreatic cancer had longer survival than did whites. Of note, Asian patients as a group, and Japanese patients in particular, were more likely to have tumors diagnosed as intraductal papillary mucinous neoplasms (IPMNs) or mucinous cystic carcinomas compared with white patients. Since patients with IPMNs and mucinous cystic carcinomas have an improved survival compared with patients diagnosed with ductal adenocarcinoma, this may explain the apparent race-based differences in survival. In support of this theory was the finding that the survival advantage of Japanese patients over white patients diminished significantly after adjusting for grade, stage, and tumor histologic subtype. This suggests that the pathologic characteristics of the pancreatic tumor—rather than race *per se*—are the most important prognostic factors with regard to long-term survival (Longnecker *et al.* 2000).

Genetic factors

Less than 10% of pancreatic adenocarcinoma cases can be accounted for by hereditary genetic factors. Germline mutations in PRSS1, STK11, CDKN2a, BRCA2, or mismatch repair genes may account for up to 20% of inherited pancreatic adenocarcinomas (Rieder & Bartsch 2004). Several genetic syndromes have been associated with an increased risk of pancreatic cancer including hereditary pancreatitis, hereditary non-polyposis colorectal cancer, ataxia telangiectasia, Peutz–Jeghers syndrome, familial breast cancer, and familial atypical multiple-mole melanoma (Table 21.1) (Hruban *et al.* 1998; Klein *et al.* 2001). Hereditary pancreatitis also has been found to increase the risk of pancreatic adenocarcinoma. Specifically, the estimated relative risk of pancreatic cancer for patients with hereditary pancreatitis is 100 compared with the general population, with a lifetime risk of about 40%.

Familial pancreatic cancer is a separate, albeit very heterogeneous clinical entity, with the majority of underlying genetic defects still unknown. Familial pancreatic cancer syndrome is generally defined as a patient who has at least two first-degree relatives with pancreatic adenocarcinoma and who does not meet the criteria of other hereditary cancer syndromes. Recent data have suggested that the risk of developing pancreatic cancer among first-degree relatives of familial pancreatic cancer patients is increased about 19-fold, and may be even higher in patients with a history of more than one affected family member (Tersmette *et al.* 2001). Patients suspected of being part of a familial pancreatic carcinoma kindred should undergo genetic counseling and a detailed analysis of their family tree. Such individuals should also be enrolled in annual screening, which should begin at least 10 years below the youngest age of onset of pancreatic cancer in the family. Screening options include endoscopic ultrasound, helical computed tomography, or magnetic resonance imaging.

Table 21.1 Risk factors associated with pancreatic adenocarcinoma.

Hereditary factors	Environmental/ other factors
Hereditary pancreatitis	Smoking
Hereditary non-polyposis colorectal cancer	Chronic pancreatitis
Ataxia telangiectasia	Obesity
Peutz–Jeghers syndrome	Diabetes
Familial breast cancer	
Atypical multiple-mole melanoma	

Pre-existing disease

Pre-existing chronic pancreatitis has been associated with a 10–20-fold increased risk of pancreatic cancer (Lowenfels *et al.* 1993, 1994). Specifically, a multicenter cohort study of 2000 patients with chronic pancreatitis recently reported a 16-fold increased risk of pancreatic adenocarcinoma (Lowenfels *et al.* 1993). In a separate study, patients with chronic pancreatitis had a sevenfold increase in the risk of developing adenocarcinoma, but this risk declined to a twofold risk after a decade of follow-up (Karlson *et al.* 1997). In general, the cumulative 25-year risk for patients with chronic pancreatitis is about 4% (Lillemoe *et al.* 2000). The increased risk of pancreatic adenocarcinoma in patients with chronic pancreatitis suggests that a common risk factor for both diseases may exist; however, some forms of chronic pancreatitis may actually be an indolent form of pancreatic cancer that was initially misdiagnosed (Lillemoe *et al.* 2000).

Other studies have linked the development of diabetes to pancreatic cancer. These data, however, are inconsistent. A study from California reported that patients with diabetes who had been treated with oral diabetes medication or insulin for 5 or more years were not at higher risk for pancreatic cancer; in contrast, those patients with newly diagnosed diabetes who had been treated with insulin for fewer than 5 years had a 6.8-fold increased risk for pancreatic cancer (Everhart & Wright 1995). The authors concluded that diabetes, although not causally related to pancreatic cancer, may be a complication or an early marker of pancreatic cancer (Everhart & Wright, 1995). La Vecchia *et al.* (1990) similarly demonstrated that the risk of pancreatic cancer decreased with time following the initial diagnosis of diabetes. The relative risk declined from 3.2 in the first 5 years after diagnosis of diabetes to 1.3 after 10 or more years from diagnosis (La Vecchia *et al.* 1990).

Behavior and environmental factors

Smoking has been consistently and convincingly linked to a marked increased risk of pancreatic cancer (Li *et al.* 2004). In fact, studies have shown a specific dose–response effect with an incremental increase in the risk of pancreatic cancer as the number of cigarettes smoked increases (Gold & Goldin 1998). In general, cigarette smoking has been estimated to account for roughly 25–29% of the overall incidence of pancreatic cancer in the United States (Rulyak *et al.* 2003; Lowenfels & Maisonneuve 2005; Maisonneuve *et al.* 2005).

The association of other lifestyle and dietary factors with the risk of pancreatic cancer has been examined; however, the data are much less compelling compared with the data linking smoking to pancreatic cancer. Two prospective cohort studies suggested that obesity significantly increased the risk of pancreatic cancer, while physical activity appeared to be associated with a protective effect (Michaud *et al.* 2001). The association between pancreatic cancer, coffee, and alcohol consumption has also been studied. Data from a large cohort studies revealed no overall association between coffee or alcohol intake and pancreatic cancer (Lin *et al.* 2002).

Occupational risk factors may also increase one's risk of pancreatic adenocarcinoma. Some studies have shown an association between pancreatic cancer and certain occupations (e.g. chemical workers, coal gas workers, aluminum metal workers, textile workers, and workers in the tanning industries) (Pietri *et al.* 1990Mikoczy *et al.* 1996; Iaia *et al.* 2006; ; Veyalkin & Gerein 2006). An Italian study (Ronneberg *et al.* 1999; Carta *et al.* 2004) of aluminum smelter workers revealed that after controlling for cigarette smoking, occupational exposure in an anodes factory was associated with a significant increased risk of pancreatic cancer. Although occupational exposure needs to be considered, the impact of occupational exposure on the incidence of pancreatic cancer is likely no more than 5% (Lowenfels & Maisonneuve 2004).

Table 21.2 Presenting symptoms associated with adenocarcinoma (DiMagno 1992).

Symptom	Percentage (%)	
	Head of pancreas	Tail of pancreas
Weight loss	92	100
Jaundice	82	87
Abdominal pain	72	43
Anorexia	64	33
Nausea, vomiting	42	41
Light stool/dark urine	62	n/a
Overall weakness/fatigue	35	42
Pruritus	20	n/a

Adapted in part from DiMagno EP. (1992) Cancer of the pancreas and biliary tract. In: Winawer SJ, ed. *Management of Gastrointestinal Diseases*. Gower Medical Publishing, New York.

Clinical findings

With the aforementioned risk factors in mind, a full detailed history should be obtained from each patient. In addition, the physician also needs to assess and catalog presenting signs and symptoms that may suggest an underlying pancreatic neoplasm.

The presenting clinical features of pancreatic adenocarcinoma depend on the size and location of the tumor. Most patients initially present with non-specific symptoms (Table 21.2) and therefore most pancreatic cancers—especially those in the tail—are either diagnosed incidentally or late in their clinical course. Tumors in the head of the pancreas often present with symptoms caused by compression of associated structures, such as the common bile duct. Biliary duct obstruction frequently causes jaundice with marked elevation in conjugated bilirubin levels. As such, patients may present with dark urine as a result of the high level of conjugated bilirubin and the absence of urobilinogen in the urine. For similar reasons, patients may also have pale-appearing stool due to the lack of stercobilinogen in the bowel. Severely elevated bilirubin levels may also cause pruritus, which can be quite significant and clinically symptomatic.

If jaundice is not present, symptoms are usually non-specific. Many patients may experience abdominal or back pain either before or concurrently with the development of jaundice. Patients with tumors in the body and tail of the pancreas are more likely to present with non-specific pain and weight loss without jaundice, as body and tail tumors are much less likely to cause obstructive signs and symptoms. Regardless of location of the pancreatic mass, the pain is typically described as dull and constant. The pain is usually 'nagging' in nature, with less than one-third of patients presenting with pain that they would characterize as severe (Lillemoe *et al.* 2000). The pain is usually localized to the epigastric area or the mid- to upper back area and may be worse in the supine position but improved by leaning forward (Lillemoe *et al.* 2000). In addition to pain, patients may also describe anorexia, fatigue, and weight loss. Other symptoms can include new-onset diabetes (endocrine insufficiency) or malabsorption (exocrine insufficiency) (Li *et al.* 2004). Malabsorption usually is manifested by foul-smelling, steatotic stools that may float in the toilet. Frank diarrhea is much less common. In rare cases, patients may present with pancreatitis (Lin & Feller 1990).

On physical exam, weight loss and jaundice are the most common findings. Subtle jaundice can be detected by examining the sclera. An examination of the relevant lymph node basins should be performed, as patients with advanced disease may be found to have left supraclavicular lymphadenopathy (Virchow's node). In most cases, examination of the abdomen is unremarkable. However, some jaundiced patients (about one-third) may present with a distended, palpable but non-tender gallbladder (Courvoisier's sign). Courvoisier's sign has been reported to be 80–90% specific, but only 25–50% sensitive for malignant obstruction of the bile duct (McGee 1995). As such, although an interesting physical finding, its absence does not rule out malignant obstruction of the bile duct. In patients with advanced metastatic disease, and who are unlikely candidates for surgical resection, the abdominal exam may reveal hepatomegaly, ascites, and spider angiomas.

Following the history and physical examination, laboratory tests should be obtained. Perturbations in laboratory values will depend on the location of the mass within the pancreatic parenchyma. Tumors in the head of the pancreas usually results in an elevated total bilirubin, alkaline phosphatase, ψ-glutamyl transpeptidase and, possibly, mild elevations in the hepatic aminotransferases. In contrast, patients with lesions in the tail of the pancreas frequently will have a normal biochemical profile.

The serum tumor marker cancer antigen (CA) 19-9 may help confirm the diagnosis in patients suspected of harboring a pancreatic malignancy (Malesci *et al.* 1992; McGee 1995). In addition, some investigators have suggested that preoperative CA19-9 levels may be a useful marker for determining preoperatively which patients have unresectable disease despite the demonstration on computed tomography of resectable disease (Kilic *et al.* 2006). As such, patients who are otherwise candidates for surgical resection, but who have markedly elevated CA19-9 levels, may be best served with an initial diagnostic laparoscopy at the time of surgery to rule out occult intraperitoneal metastases. CA19-9 levels have also been linked to prognosis following pancreatectomy. Specifically, both a postoperative decrease in CA19-9 and a postoperative CA19-9 value of less than 200 U/mL have been reported to be strong independent predictors of survival, even after adjusting for stage (McGee 1995; Ferrone *et al.* 2006). Despite its clinical and prognostic applications, CA19-9 lacks sufficient sensitivity (50–75%) and specificity (83%) to warrant its use as a general screening tool for pancreatic adenocarcinoma.

References

American Cancer Society. (2005) *Cancer Facts and Figures 2005*. American Cancer Society, Atlanta.

Bach PB, Schrag D, Brawley OW, Galaznik A, Yakren S, Begg CB. (2002) Survival of blacks and whites after a cancer diagnosis. *JAMA* 287: 2106–13.

Carta P, Aru G, Cadeddu C *et al.* (2004) Mortality for pancreatic cancer among aluminium smelter workers in Sardinia, Italy. *G Ital Med Lav Ergon* 26: 83–9.

Chang KJ, Parasher G, Christie C, Largent J, Anton-Culver H. (2005) Risk of pancreatic adenocarcinoma: disparity between African Americans and other race/ethnic groups. *Cancer* 103: 349–57.

Devesa SS, Blot WJ, Stone BJ, Miller BA, Tarone RE, Fraumeni JF Jr. (1995) Recent cancer trends in the United States. *J Natl Cancer Inst* 87: 175–82.

DiMagno EP. (1992) Cancer of the pancreas and biliary tract. In: Winawer SJ, ed. *Management of Gastrointestinal Disease*. Gower Medical Publishing, New York.

Dong M, Nio Y, Tamura K *et al.* (2000) Ki-ras point mutation and p53 expression in human pancreatic cancer: a comparative study among Chinese, Japanese, and Western patients. *Cancer Epidemiol Biomarkers Prev* 9: 279–84.

Eloubeidi MA, Desmond RA, Wilcox CM *et al.* (2006) Prognostic factors for survival in pancreatic cancer: a population-based study. *Am J Surg* 192: 322–9.

Everhart J, Wright D. (1995) Diabetes mellitus as a risk factor for pancreatic cancer. A meta-analysis. *JAMA* 273: 1605–9.

Ferrone CR, Finkelstein DM, Thayer SP, Muzikansky A, Fernandez-Delcastillo C, Warshaw AL. (2006) Perioperative CA19-9 levels can predict stage and survival in patients with resectable pancreatic adenocarcinoma. *J Clin Oncol* 24: 2897–902.

Gold EB, Goldin SB. (1998) Epidemiology of and risk factors for pancreatic cancer. *Surg Oncol Clin N Am* 7: 67–91.

Greenlee RT, Murray T, Bolden S, Wingo PA. (2000) Cancer statistics, 2000. *CA Cancer J Clin* 50: 7–33.

Hayanga AJ. (2005) Risk of pancreatic adenocarcinoma: disparity between African Americans and other race/ethnic groups. *Cancer* 104: 2530–1; author reply 2531.

Hruban RH, Petersen GM, Ha PK, Kern SE. (1998) Genetics of pancreatic cancer. From genes to families. *Surg Oncol Clin N Am* 7: 1–23.

Iaia TE, Bartoli D, Calzoni P *et al.* (2006) A cohort mortality study of leather tanners in Tuscany, Italy. *Am J Ind Med* 49: 452–9.

Karlson BM, Ekbom A, Josefsson S, Mclaughlin JK, Fraumeni JF Jr, Nyren O. (1997) The risk of pancreatic cancer following pancreatitis: an association due to confounding? *Gastroenterology* 113: 587–92.

Kilic M, Gocmen E, Tez M, Ertan T, Keskek M, Koc M. (2006) Value of preoperative serum CA 19-9 levels in predicting resectability for pancreatic cancer. *Can J Surg* 49: 241–4.

Klein AP, Hruban RH, Brune KA, Petersen GM, Goggins M. (2001) Familial pancreatic cancer. *Cancer J* 7: 266–73.

La Vecchia C, Negri E, D'avanzo B *et al.* (1990) Medical history, diet and pancreatic cancer. *Oncology* 47: 463–6.

Li D, Xie K, Wolff R, Abbruzzese JL. (2004) Pancreatic cancer. *Lancet* 363: 1049–57.

Lillemoe KD, Yeo CJ, Cameron JL. (2000) Pancreatic cancer: state-of-the-art care. *CA Cancer J Clin* 50: 241–68.

Lin A, Feller ER. (1990) Pancreatic carcinoma as a cause of unexplained pancreatitis: report of ten cases. *Ann Intern Med* 113: 166–7.

Lin Y, Tamakoshi A, Kawamura T *et al.* (2001) An epidemiological overview of environmental and genetic risk factors of pancreatic cancer. *Asian Pac J Cancer Prev* 2: 271–80.

Lin Y, Tamakoshi A, Kawamura T *et al.* (2002) Risk of pancreatic cancer in relation to alcohol drinking, coffee consumption and medical history: findings from the Japan collaborative cohort study for evaluation of cancer risk. *Int J Cancer* 99: 742–6.

Longnecker DS, Karagas MR, Tosteson TD, Mott LA. (2000) Racial differences in pancreatic cancer: comparison of survival and histologic types of pancreatic carcinoma in Asians, blacks, and whites in the United States. *Pancreas* 21: 338–43.

Lowenfels AB, Maisonneuve P. (2004) Epidemiology and prevention of pancreatic cancer. *Jpn J Clin Oncol* 34: 238–44.

Lowenfels AB, Maisonneuve P. (2005) Risk factors for pancreatic cancer. *J Cell Biochem* 95: 649–56.

Lowenfels AB, Maisonneuve P, Cavallini G *et al.* (1993) Pancreatitis and the risk of pancreatic cancer. International Pancreatitis Study Group. *N Engl J Med* 328: 1433–7.

Lowenfels AB, Maisonneuve P, Cavallini G *et al.* (1994) Prognosis of chronic pancreatitis: an international multicenter study. International Pancreatitis Study Group. *Am J Gastroenterol* 89: 1467–71.

Maisonneuve P, Lowenfels AB, Mullhaupt B *et al.* (2005) Cigarette smoking accelerates progression of alcoholic chronic pancreatitis. *Gut* 54: 510–14.

Malesci A, Montorsi M, Mariani A *et al.* (1992) Clinical utility of the serum CA 19-9 test for diagnosing pancreatic carcinoma in symptomatic patients: a prospective study. *Pancreas* 7: 497–502.

McGee S. (1995) Percussion and physical diagnosis: separating myth from science. *Dis Mon*: 641–92.

Michaud DS. (2004) Epidemiology of pancreatic cancer. *Minerva Chir* 59: 99–111.

Michaud DS, Giovannucci E, Willett WC, Colditz GA, Stampfer MJ, Fuchs CS. (2001) Physical activity, obesity, height, and the risk of pancreatic cancer. *JAMA* 286: 921–9.

Mikoczy Z, Schutz A, Stromberg U, Hagmar L. (1996) Cancer incidence and specific occupational exposures in the Swedish leather tanning industry: a cohort based case-control study. *Occup Environ Med* 53: 463–7.

Parkin DM, Pisani P, Ferlay J. (1999) Estimates of the worldwide incidence of 25 major cancers in 1990. *Int J Cancer* 80: 827–41.

Pernick NL, Sarkar FH, Philip PA, Arlauskas P, Shields AF, Vaitkevicius VK, Dugan MC, Adsay NV. (2003) Clinicopathologic analysis of pancreatic adenocarcinoma in African Americans and Caucasians. *Pancreas* 26: 28–32.

Pietri F, Clavel F, Auquier A, Flamant R. (1990) Occupational risk factors for cancer of the pancreas: a case-control study. *Br J Ind Med* 47: 425–8.

Rieder H, Bartsch DK. (2004) Familial pancreatic cancer. *Fam Cancer* 3: 69–74.

Ries LAG, Eisner MP, Kosary CL *et al.*, eds. (2003) *SEER Cancer Statistics Review, 1975–2000*. National Cancer Institute. Bethesda MD. http://seer.cancer.gov/csr/1975_2000

Ronneberg A, Haldorsen T, Romundstad P, Andersen A. (1999) Occupational exposure and cancer incidence among workers from an aluminum smelter in western Norway. *Scand J Work Environ Health* 25: 207–14.

Rulyak SJ, Lowenfels AB, Maisonneuve P, Brentnall TA. (2003) Risk factors for the development of pancreatic cancer in familial pancreatic cancer kindreds. *Gastroenterology* 124: 1292–9.

Sahmoun AE, D'Agostino RA Jr, Bell RA, Schwenke DC. (2003) International variation in pancreatic cancer mortality for the period 1955–1998. *Eur J Epidemiol* 18: 801–16.

Saif MW, Sviglin H, Carpenter M. (2005) Impact of ethnicity on outcome in pancreatic carcinoma. *JOP—Journal of the Pancreas* 6: 246–54.

Song MM, Nio Y, Dong M *et al.* (2000) Comparison of K-ras point mutations at codon 12 and p21 expression in pancreatic cancer between Japanese and Chinese patients. *J Surg Oncol* 75: 176–85.

Tersmette AC, Petersen GM, Offerhaus GJ *et al.* (2001) Increased risk of incident pancreatic cancer among first-degree relatives of patients with familial pancreatic cancer. *Clin Cancer Res* 7: 738–44.

Veyalkin I, Gerein V. (2006) Retrospective cohort study of cancer mortality at the Minsk Leather Tannery. *Ind Health* 44: 69–74.

Histopathology

Ralph H. Hruban

Introduction

While a broad spectrum of neoplasms has long been recognized in the pancreas, recent evidence-based medicine has helped define precursor lesions to infiltrating adenocarcinoma, as well as distinct clinicopathologic entities in which characteristic tumor morphologies are associated with distinct prognostic outcomes. This section will provide an overview of the histopathology of the common malignancies of the pancreas and their precursor lesions.

Infiltrating ductal adenocarcinoma

The most common malignancy of the pancreas is the infiltrating ductal adenocarcinoma. Infiltrating ductal adenocarcinoma, commonly known as 'pancreatic cancer,' is defined as an invasive malignant epithelial neoplasm with glandular (ductal) differentiation (Hruban *et al.* 2006). The majority (60–70%) of pancreatic cancers arise in the head of the gland, most are solitary, and most are firm, poorly defined, white-yellow, and they obscure the normal lobular architecture of the pancreas (Hruban *et al.* 2006). Infiltrating ductal adenocarcinomas have two remarkable features at the microscopic level. First, they elicit an intense desmoplastic reaction (Fig. 21.1). As a result, most of the cells that comprise the mass produced by a pancreatic cancer are non-neoplastic fibroblasts, lymphocytes and macrophages. Second, despite the highly lethal nature of pancreatic cancer, most of these neoplasms are remarkably well-differentiated. Indeed, some pancreatic cancers are so well differentiated that they cannot be distinguished from benign reactive glands in

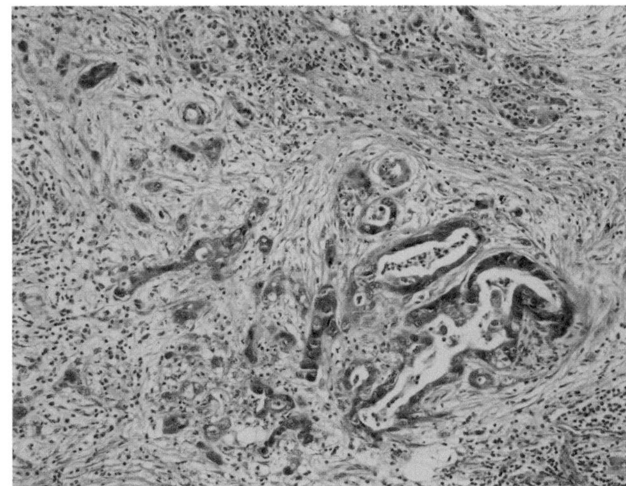

Fig. 21.1 Infiltrating ductal adenocarcinoma with desmoplastic stroma.

small biopsies. Well-defined criteria therefore need to be rigorously employed in the interpretation of biopsies of the pancreas. Features supportive of a diagnosis of pancreatic cancer include perineural invasion, vascular invasion, a haphazard arrangement of the glands, nuclear pleomorphism, the presence of a gland immediately adjacent to a muscular artery, and luminal necroses. Immunohistochemical labeling can be used to characterize the direction of differentiation of the neoplastic cells. Most pancreatic cancers express cytokeratin (CK7, 8, 13, 18 and 19), carcinoembryonic antigen (CEA), carcinoma antigen 19-9 (CA19-9), B72.3, CA125, and DUPAN 2 (Hruban *et al.* 2006). Adenocarcinomas of the pancreas express several high molecular weight glycoproteins (mucins) including MUC1 (a pan-epithelial mucin), MUC3, MUC4, and MUC5AC (a gastric foveolar mucin) (Hruban *et al.* 2006). The *DPC4/MADH4* gene is deleted in 55% of pancreatic cancers and these cancers show loss of immunolabeling for the Dpc4 protein (Wilentz *et al.* 2000b). It is anticipated that new markers of pancreatic cancer will be developed through global analyses of gene expression, and that these new markers will enhance our screening, diagnostic and prognostic capabilities (Iacobuzio-Donahue *et al.* 2003).

Common variants of infiltrating ductal adenocarcinoma

A number of phenotypically distinct variants of pancreatic cancer have been identified and several have distinct clinical features.

Adenosquamous carcinoma

Adenosquamous carcinoma is a malignant epithelial neoplasm with significant squamous and glandular differentiation (Hruban *et al.* 2006). Adenosquamous carcinomas need to be distinguished clinically from squamous cell carcinoma metastatic to the pancreas, and they appear to have a very poor prognosis with few patients surviving beyond 1 year (Hruban *et al.* 2006).

Colloid carcinoma

Colloid carcinomas are malignant gland-forming epithelial neoplasms characterized by copious mucin production and the formation of large extracellular pools of mucin (Fig. 21.2) (Hruban *et al.* 2006). Typically the neoplastic cells can be seen 'floating' within the mucin pools. Almost all colloid carcinomas arise in association with an intraductal papillary mucinous neoplasm (IPMN) and patients with colloid carcinomas appear to have a better prognosis than do patients with a standard infiltrating ductal adenocarcinoma of the pancreas (Seidel *et al.* 2002).

Hepatoid carcinoma

Hepatoid carcinomas of the pancreas are extremely rare neoplasms that have liver differentiation as evidenced by a morphologic resemblance to the normal liver and the production

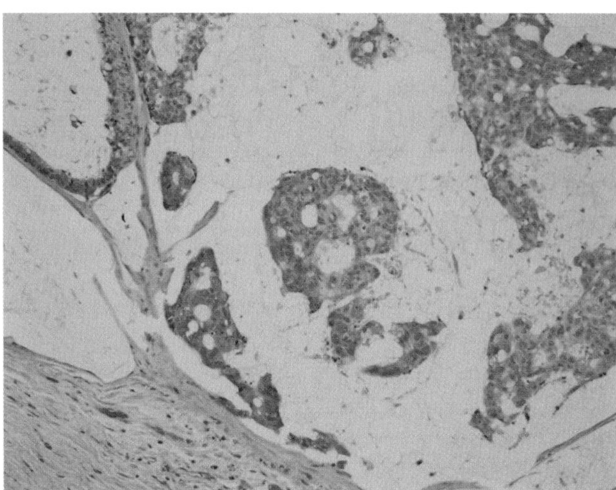

Fig. 21.2 Colloid carcinoma with abundant extracellular mucin production.

of markers of liver differentiation (Hruban *et al.* 2006). For example, these neoplasms label with the hepatocyte paraffin-1 (Hep Par-1) antibody (Hruban *et al.* 2006). Imaging can be used to distinguish hepatoid carcinomas of the pancreas from primary hepatocellular carcinoma of the liver metastatic to the pancreas.

Medullary carcinoma

Medullary carcinoma of the pancreas is a malignant epithelial neoplasm characterized by poor differentiation, pushing borders, a syncytial growth pattern and necrosis (Wilentz *et al.* 2000a; Hruban *et al.* 2006). Medullary carcinomas are important to recognize because they often have microsatellite instability and may be associated with the hereditary non-polyposis coli (HNPCC) syndrome (Wilentz *et al.* 2000a). Patients with medullary carcinomas of the pancreas also appear to have a better prognosis than do patients with a standard infiltrating ductal adenocarcinoma of the pancreas (Wilentz *et al.* 2000a; Hruban *et al.* 2006).

Signet-ring cell carcinoma

Signet-ring cell carcinoma is a malignant epithelial neoplasm of the pancreas composed of infiltrating round non-cohesive (isolated) cells containing intracytoplasmic mucin (Hruban *et al.* 2006). Some signet-ring cell carcinomas show loss of E-cadherin expression. Endoscopy can be used to distinguish signet-ring cell carcinomas of the pancreas from the more common primary gastric signet-ring cell carcinomas. Patients with signet-ring cell carcinomas of the pancreas have a poor prognosis, with many patients surviving only a few months (Hruban *et al.* 2006).

Undifferentiated carcinoma

This malignant epithelial neoplasm lacks glandular structures or other features to indicate a definite direction of differentiation (Fig. 21.3) (Hruban *et al.* 2006). Instead, these high-grade carcinomas show a spectrum of morphologies ranging from pleomorphic epithelioid mononuclear cells containing abundant eosinophilic cytoplasm admixed with bizarre frequently multinucleated giant cells, to relatively monomorphic spindle cells (Hruban *et al.* 2006). Needless to say, patients with these carcinomas have an extremely poor prognosis with a mean survival of only 5 months (Hruban *et al.* 2006).

Undifferentiated carcinoma with osteoclast-like giant cells

These are distinctive malignant epithelial neoplasms composed of benign-appearing multinucleated giant cells admixed with atypical neoplastic mononuclear cells (Fig. 21.4) (Westra *et al.* 1998; Hruban *et al.* 2006). The multinucleated giant cells are believed to be non-neoplastic reactive cells. Patients with undifferentiated carcinomas with osteoclast-like giant cells were once felt to have a better prognosis, but a growing body of evidence suggests that the average patient survives only 12 months (Hruban *et al.* 2006).

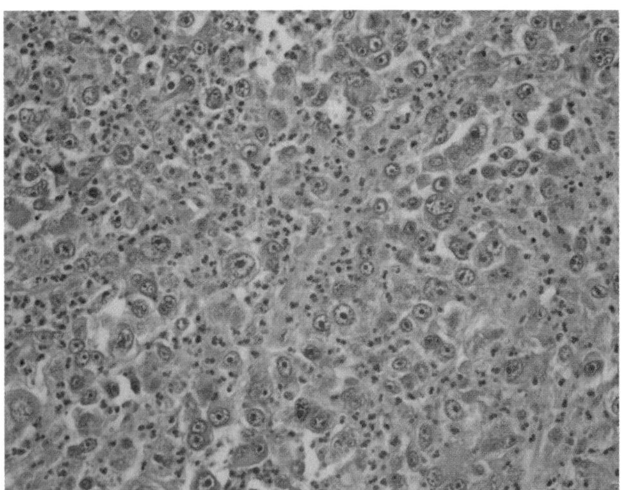

Fig. 21.3 Undifferentiated carcinoma lacking a definitive direction of differentiation.

Precursors to infiltrating ductal adenocarcinoma

A number of distinct histologic precursors to infiltrating adenocarcinoma of the pancreas have recently been characterized. These include *pancreatic intraepithelial neoplasia* (PanIN), *intraductal papillary mucinous neoplasms (IPMNs)*, and *mucinous cystic neoplasms (MCNs)*.

Evidence linking these precursor lesions to invasive pancreatic cancer includes the morphologic association of these precursor lesions with infiltrating adenocarcinomas, anecdotal case reports in which patients with one of these precursor lesions later develop an infiltrating adenocarcinoma of the pancreas, and molecular analyses of these precursor lesions which demonstrate that they harbor many of the same genetic alterations as are found in infiltrating adenocarcinoma (Hruban *et al.* 2006). PanINs are microscopic non-invasive epithelial proliferations within the smaller pancreatic ducts (Fig. 21.5), IPMNs are macroscopic non-invasive epithelial proliferations within the larger pancreatic ducts (Fig. 21.6), and MCNs have a distinctive ovarian type of stroma (Fig. 21.7).

Less common neoplasms

Several of the less common neoplasms of the pancreas deserve note.

Acinar cell carcinoma

Acinar cell carcinoma is a malignant epithelial neoplasm with an acinar growth pattern that demonstrates evidence of exo-

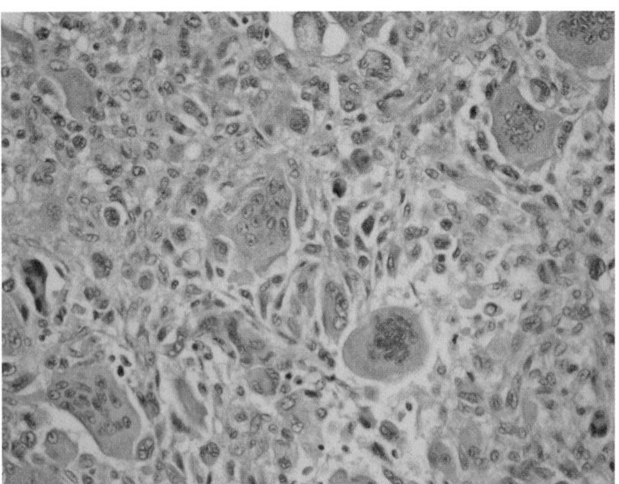

Fig. 21.4 Undifferentiated carcinoma with osteoclast-like giant cells.

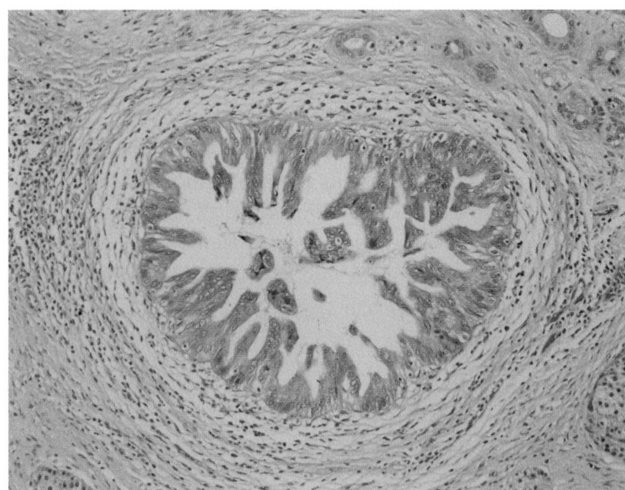

Fig. 21.5 Pancreatic intraepithelial neoplasia (PanIN-3).

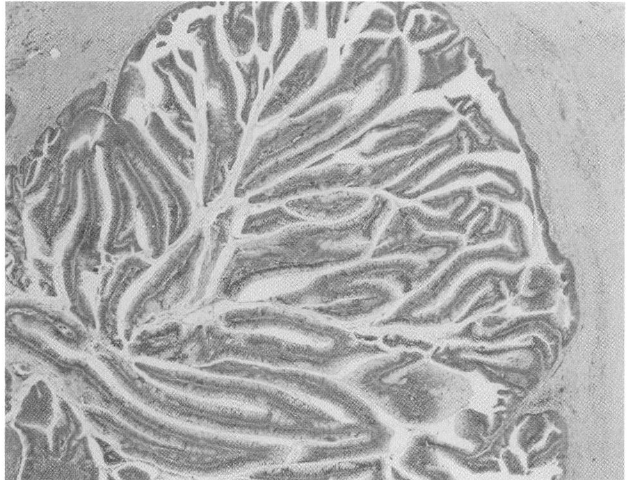

Fig. 21.6 Intraductal papillary mucinous neoplasm.

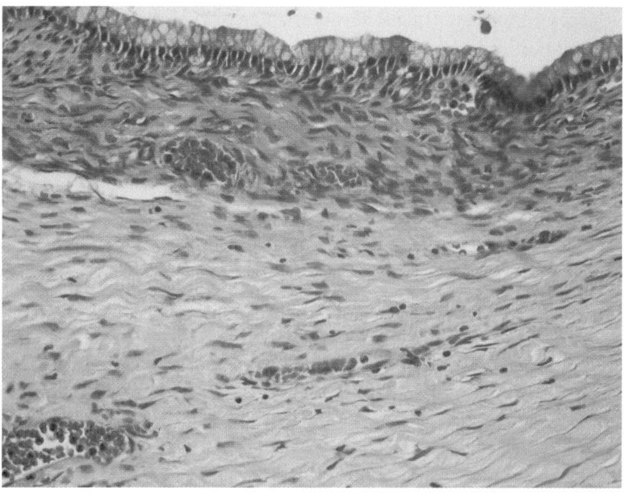

Fig. 21.7 Mucinous cystic neoplasm. Note the 'ovarian-type' stroma.

crine enzyme production by the neoplastic cells (Fig. 21.8) (Hruban *et al.* 2006). The exocrine enzymes produced by these neoplasms can be released into the blood producing a distinctive syndrome characterized by foci of subcutaneous fat necrosis, polyarthralgia, and peripheral blood eosinophilia (Hruban *et al.* 2006).

Pancreatoblastoma

These distinctive neoplasms occur primarily in children and histologically show cells with acinar differentiation and squamoid nests (Fig. 21.9).

Serous cystic neoplasms

These benign epithelial neoplasms are composed of uniform cuboidal glycogen-rich cells that form numerous small cysts containing serous fluid (Fig. 21.10) (Hruban *et al.* 2006).

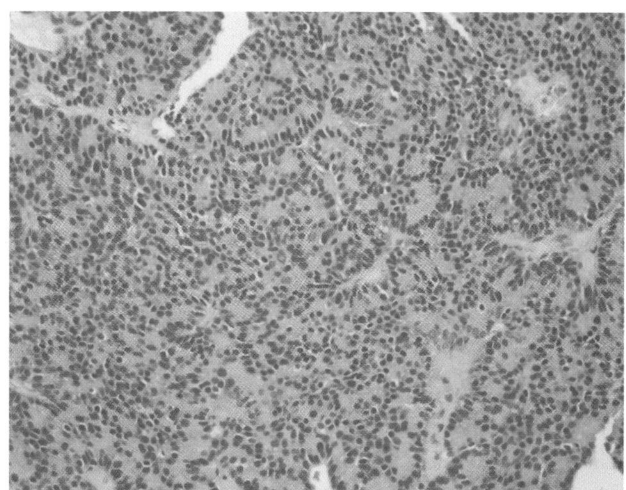

Fig. 21.8 Acinar cell carcinoma.

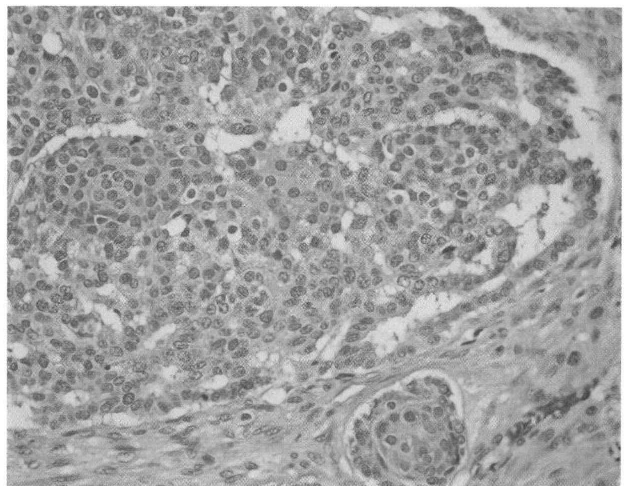

Fig. 21.9 Pancreatoblastoma with squamoid nests.

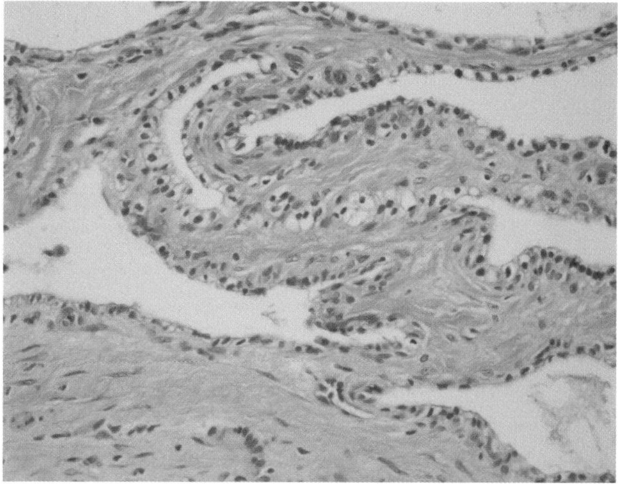

Fig. 21.10 Serous cystadenoma.

Extremely rare examples with extrapancreatic metastases have been reported.

Solid pseudopapillary neoplasms

These distinctive neoplasms occur predominantly in women in their twenties (Hruban *et al.* 2006). They are composed of discohesive polygonal cells that surround delicate blood vessels and form solid masses and degenerative cysts (Hruban *et al.* 2006). The neoplastic cells harbor mutations in the β-*catenin* gene and, as a result, most show an abnormal nuclear pattern of labeling with antibodies to the β-catenin protein (Fig. 21.11).

Well-differentiated pancreatic endocrine neoplasms

These neoplasms, also known as *islet cell tumors*, are histologically characterized by organoid growth of cells cytologically resembling normal islet cells (Fig. 21.12) (Hruban *et al.* 2006).

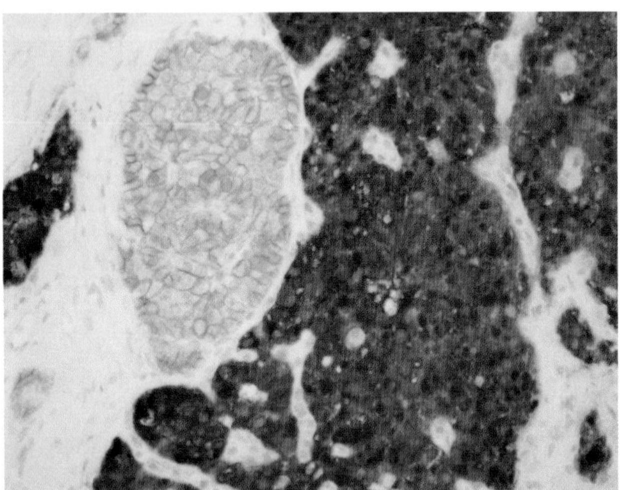

Fig. 21.11 Solid pseudopapillary neoplasm immunolabeled for beta-catenin. Note the nuclear labeling of the neoplastic cells (right) and the membranous pattern of labeling of the normal cells (upper left).

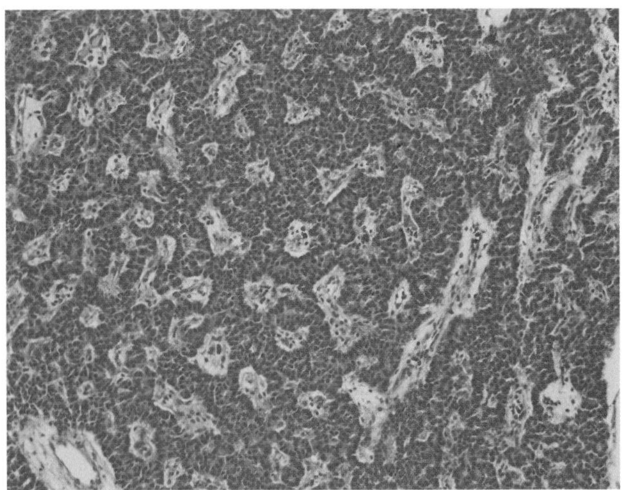

Fig. 21.12 Well-differentiated pancreatic endocrine neoplasm.

The cells have a relatively low mitotic rate (up to 10 mitoses per 10 high-power microscopic fields). Pancreatic endocrine neoplasms (PENs) can release their hormones into the blood producing distinctive clinical syndromes (i.e. insulinomas) (Hruban *et al.* 2006). The prognosis for patients with a PEN is significantly better than the prognosis for patients with an infiltrating ductal adenocarcinoma.

Poorly differentiated endocrine neoplasms

Although extremely rare, poorly differentiated small cell carcinomas and poorly differentiated large cell endocrine carcinomas of the pancreas have been reported. These are associated with an extremely poor prognosis.

References

Hruban RH, Klimstra DS, Pitman MB. (2006) *Atlas of Tumor Pathology. Tumors of the Pancreas*, 4th Series edn. Armed Forces Institute of Pathology, Washington, DC.

Iacobuzio-Donahue CA, Ashfaq R, Maitra A *et al.* (2003) Highly expressed genes in pancreatic ductal adenocarcinomas: a comprehensive characterization and comparison of the transcription profiles obtained from three major technologies. *Cancer Research* 63(24): 8614–22.

Seidel G, Zahurak M, Iacobuzio-Donahue CA *et al.* (2002) Almost all infiltrating colloid carcinomas of the pancreas and periampullary region arise from in situ papillary neoplasms: a study of 39 cases. *Am J Surg Pathol* 26(1): 56–63.

Westra WH, Sturm PJ, Drillenburg P *et al.* (1998) K-ras oncogene mutations in osteoclast-like giant cell tumors of the pancreas and liver: genetic evidence to support origin from the duct epithelium. *Am J Surg Pathol* 22(10): 1247–54.

Wilentz RE, Goggins M, Redston M *et al.* (2000a) Genetic, immunohistochemical, and clinical features of medullary carcinoma of the pancreas: a newly described and characterized entity. *Am J Pathol* 156(5): 1641–51.

Wilentz RE, Su GH, Dai JL *et al.* (2000b) Immunohistochemical labeling for Dpc4 mirrors genetic status in pancreatic adenocarcinomas: a new marker of DPC4 inactivation. *Am J Pathol* 156: 37–43.

CT imaging in pancreatic cancer

Karen M. Horton & Elliot K. Fishman

Introduction

Spiral CT has been shown to be an excellent imaging modality for the diagnosis and staging of pancreatic adenocarcinoma. Recent advancements in CT technology including the development of multidetector CT scanners (MDCT) have allowed unprecedented imaging capability (Horton *et al.* 2002). New scanners allow thin collimation and rapid scanning. When this is coupled with newly developed real-time 3D imaging software, the ability of CT to detect and accurately stage pancreatic adenocarcinoma has continued to improve. CT is an essential tool to detect suspected pancreatic lesions and is routinely performed once the diagnosis is made to accurately stage the patient in an attempt to identify patients who would benefit from attempted curative resection.

High-quality CT imaging of the pancreas is greatly dependent on the type of scanner utilized, the use of appropriate CT protocols, and the availability of experienced radiologists and 3D imaging software. This chapter will discuss the role of state of the art MDCT in the detection of pancreatic cancer, staging pancreatic cancer, and follow-up after surgery.

Technique

Accurate pancreatic cancer detection, staging and follow-up require careful attention to CT technique, including CT scanner parameters, oral contrast selection, intravenous (IV) contrast administration and 3D imaging.

CT scanner parameters

CT scanners have undergone significant advancements in the last decade. This represents a progression from old dynamic scanners to high-powered spiral CT scanners. Early single-slice spiral CT scanners demonstrated significant potential to improve pancreatic cancer diagnosis and staging by allowing faster scanning and thinner collimation. Early single-slice spiral CT scanners typically allowed slices in the 2–3 mm range.

However, the introduction of MDCT in the late 1990s truly revolutionized CT imaging of the abdomen and pelvis (Horton *et al.* 2002). Current MDCT scanners allow submillimeter slices and extremely rapid scanning. For example, the state of the art scanner today is 64-slice MDCT. Our 64-slice MDCT (Siemens Sensation 64) allows 0.6 mm collimation with a rotation speed of 0.33 s. Therefore, the abdomen can be scanned with unprecedented resolution, in under 10 seconds. Faster scanning speeds coupled with faster IV injection rates have significantly improved our ability to visualize the peripancreatic vasculature by specifically timing the scan to maximize enhancement of these vessels.

Intravenous contrast

Using today's scanners, our typical protocol would include injection of 120 cc of non-ionic iodinated contrast injected at rate of 3–5 cc per second. For comprehensive imaging of the pancreas the patient is usually scanned in the arterial and venous phases. Over the years, multiple multiphase CT protocols have been described in the literature but most were based on single detector CT scanners. Most centers utilize a fixed injection rate of between 3 and 6 cc per second (Hollett *et al.* 1995; Bonaldi *et al.* 1996; Graf *et al.* 1997). However, other authorities advocate a fixed duration of injections since the injection duration is usually the most important factor affecting the time to peak contract enhancement (Bae 2003; Goshima *et al.* 2006). At our institution, we typically scan the patient at 30–35 s after the start of the injection (Horton & Fishman 2002b). This corresponds to the arterial phase of enhancement and results in excellent opacification of the celiac access, superior mesenteric artery, and peripancreatic arteries. This is crucial when staging pancreatic cancer. The second phase obtained is at 50 s after the start of injection, which corresponds to a portal venous phase of injection (Horton & Fishman 2002a). During this phase, the superior mesenteric vein, splenic vein and portal vein are well opacified and the pancreas itself is better enhanced to allow identification pancreatic adenocarcinoma, which will typically appear hypodense on this phase.

Oral contrast

When performing CT of the pancreas it is important to choose a low-density or neutral oral contrast agent. Traditional CT oral contrast agents consist of either dilute barium solutions or dilute iodinated solutions which opacify the stomach and GI tract and appear white on a CT scan. However, when imaging the pancreas and performing 3D analysis, it is important that a low-density contrast agent be administered, as a high-density agent will interfere with 3D visualization of the vessels and will require extensive post-process editing (Horton & Fishman 2002a,b). However, the use of water or other commercially available low-density agent will result in good distention of the GI tract and will not interfere with the visualization of the enhanced vessels (Megibow *et al.* 2006; Mitka 2007). At our institution, we currently use water as oral contrast and administer approximately 500 cc 20 minutes prior to the study and another 250 cc immediately prior to the study. This extra cup of water just before the scan starts is important to make sure the stomach and duodenum is well distended.

Three-dimensional imaging

Once the data is obtained, MDCT scanners allow reconstruction of the data at various slice thicknesses. For example, for our 3D imaging portion of the exam, the data is reconstructed at 0.75 mm every 0.5 mm. This is a large dataset consisting of approximately of 600–700 images per acquisition. This is transferred to a dedicated 3D imaging computer for analysis. The data are also reconstructed at 3–5 mm slices for review of the extrapancreatic structures.

3D imaging is essential when diagnosing and staging pancreatic adenocarcinoma. Even with single-detector CT, investigators found that 3D imaging of the peripancreatic vasculature was more accurate than axial images alone in revealing resectable disease (Raptopoulos *et al.* 1997). In a study by Raptopoulus, published in 1997 and using single-detector CT scanners, the investigators found that by adding 3D imaging of the vessels, the negative predictive value of a resectable tumor was 96% compared for 76% for axial images alone (Raptopoulos *et al.* 1997). A more recent study in 2004 by House *et al.* using 16-slice MDCT again demonstrated that 3D imaging resulted in high accuracy in determining cancer invasion of the superior mesenteric vessels (House *et al.* 2004). Therefore, today's standard of care requires visualization of the dataset using 3D imaging software.

A comprehensive CT examination in patients with suspected or known pancreatic cancer requires review of both the vasculature and the pancreas. Initial evaluation of the CT dataset usually begins with scrolling through the thin axial imaging to evaluate the pancreas and adjacent vessels. However, the axial plane is not optimal to evaluate all the peripancreatic vessels, or even the entire pancreas given its anatomy. Therefore, the ability to view the data in multiple planes is essential. The thin collimation obtainable with MDCT allows multiplanar reconstructions to be created while maintaining the same high resolution as the original axial images. When visualizing the celiac access and superior mesenteric artery, the ability to view the data in the sagittal and coronal planes is essential (Horton & Fishman 2002b). Current 3D imaging software varies by vendor, but all systems usually include a combination of multiplanar reconstruction, volume rendering and maximum intensity projection (MIP) (Fishman *et al.* 2006). Mutliplanar reconstructions are the simplest to use and allow visualization of the dataset in any plane. However, for full analysis of the pancreas and the peripancreatic vessels, volume rendering is the most widely used tool. Volume rendering allows the brightness, opacity, window width and window level to be adjusted in real time in order to accentuate the peripancreatic vessels and to optimize visualization of the pancreatic tumor (Fishman *et al.* 2006). Manipulating trapezoidal transfer functions interactively modifies the image contrast and the related pixel attenuations in the final image. This function allows color and opacity assignments to each voxel and can be adjusted to alter the display instantaneously (Johnson *et al.* 1998). With volume rendering, all the voxels are incorporated into the display. Although initial volume rendering software was somewhat labor intensive, today's software packages are simple to use and can be adjusted in real time. Also, the process can be simplified by creating presets, which can be applied quickly and then only minor adjustments are needed. MIP is a projection technique in which the brightest voxel is displayed along a ray (Fishman *et al.* 2006). This can be valuable using thin slabs of data to accentuate small vessels.

Currently, review of our 3D datasets when either diagnosing or staging pancreatic cancer can be completed in approximately 5 minutes. At our institution, the radiologists perform the post processing.

CT imaging

Tumor detection

Despite the development of other imaging modalities such as magnetic resonance imaging and endoscopic ultrasound, CT is still considered the imaging modality of choice to detect suspected pancreatic neoplasms. With improvements in CT resolution and improvement in contrast administration, it is now possible to detect even smaller tumors using current technology. Studies using MDCT have demonstrated an accuracy of detecting pancreatic cancer using CT in the 95% range (McNulty *et al.* 2001; House *et al.* 2004).

In order to detect small tumors, maximum enhancement of the pancreatic parenchyma is essential in order to increase tumor conspicuity (Graf *et al.* 1997). Since the normal pancreas enhances greater than pancreatic adenocarcinoma, tumors will appears lower in density compared to the adjacent normal pancreas (Fig. 21.13). In addition to identifying the pancreatic

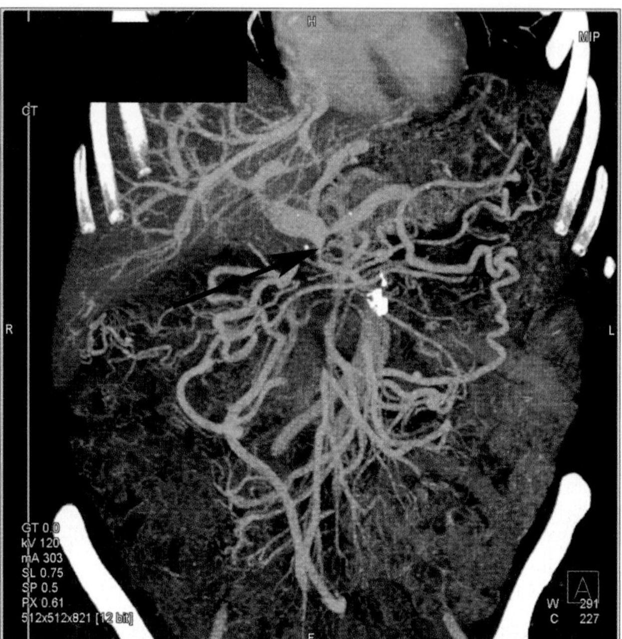

(a)

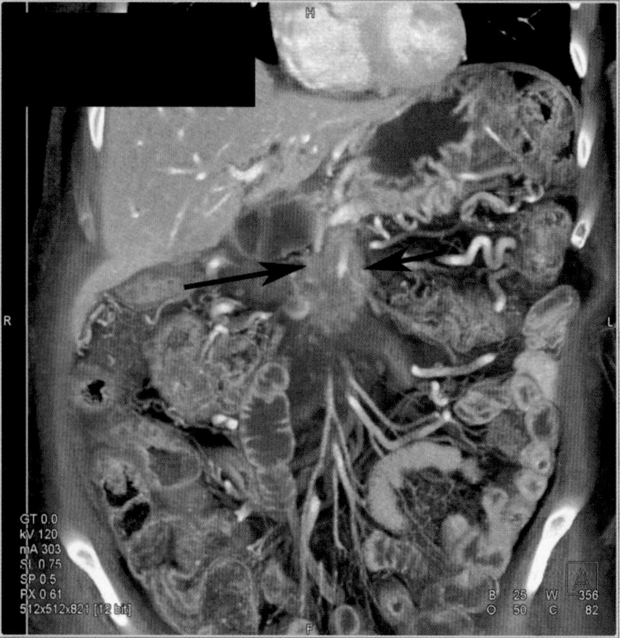

(b)

Fig. 21.13 A 68-year-old female presenting with pain and weight loss. (a) Axial contrast-enhanced MDCT demonstrates a 2.5-cm mass (arrow) in the body of the pancreas with distal pancreatic ductal dilatation and atrophy of the distal pancreas. (b) Coronal multiplanar reconstruction also demonstrates the mass (arrow).

mass, secondary signs can be useful. For example, most pancreatic cancers will result obstruction of the pancreatic duct distal to the tumor. The pancreas, distal to the tumor, also usually appears atrophic. Lesions located in the pancreatic head will result in the obstruction of the common duct as well as the pancreatic duct (Figs 21.14 & 21.15).

Smaller tumors may be confined to the gland and when less than 2 cm, may be difficult to detect. In a study by Bronstein *et al.*, the sensitivity of triple-phase helical CT for the detection of pancreatic masses less than 2 cm was 77% with a specificity of 100%. As the tumor grows, it typically infiltrates the peripancreatic structures and results in encasement of adjacent vasculature and in some cases, adjacent organs. Pancreatic cancers can occasionally appear cystic or necrotic and in rare cases, can contain calcium. Based on its enhancement pattern, when a tumor is identified in the pancreas it is often possible to distinguish pancreatic adenocarcinoma from other primary pancreatic lesions. For example, pancreatic neuroendocrine tumors typically demonstrate increased enhancement and are best seen on the arterial phase (Horton *et al.* 2006). Unlike pancreatic adenocarcinoma, neuroendocrine tumors typically do not result in ductal obstruction. Therefore, based on the CT

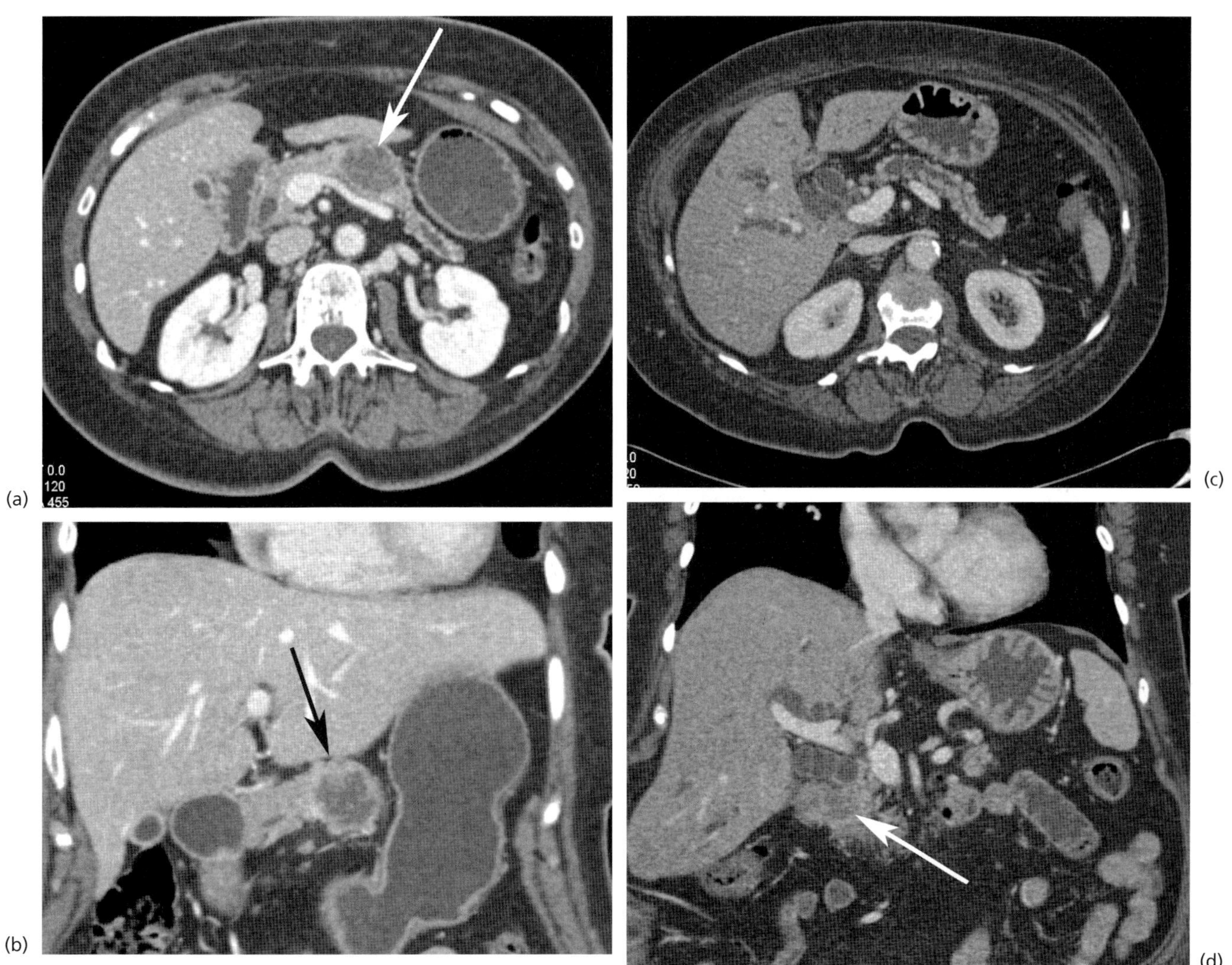

Fig. 21.14 A 71-year-old female with jaundice. (a) Axial contrast-enhanced CT demonstrates atrophy of the body and tail of the pancreas as well as biliary ductal dilation and pancreatic ductal dilatation. (b) Coronal multiplanar reconstruction demonstrates the low-density mass in the head of the pancreas (arrow). This is resulting in dilatation of the common bile duct. (c) Sagittal volume rendered CT angiogram demonstrates a normal-caliber celiac access and SMA. (d) Coronal volume rendered image demonstrates normal appearance of the superior mesenteric vein, splenic vein, and portal vein as well as the celiac access and SMA branches. The patient underwent a successful Whipple surgery, which demonstrated a 1.4-cm infiltrating moderate to poorly differentiated adenocarcinoma in the head of the pancreas. Surgical margins were negative and 19/19 nodes were negative.

(a)

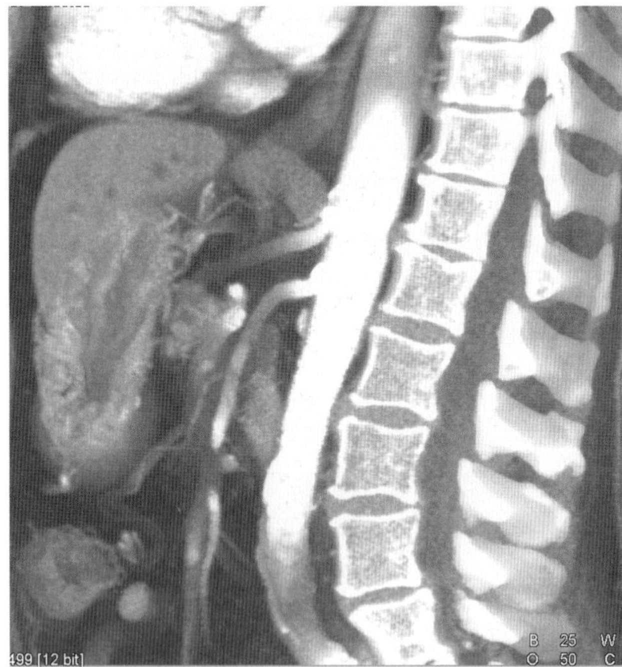

(b)

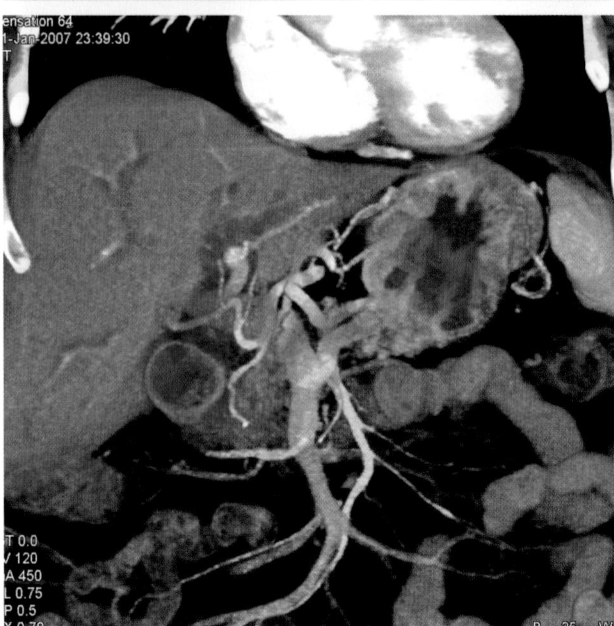

Fig. 21.15 A 74-year-old female presenting with abdominal pain. (a) Coronal volume rendered CT image demonstrates a low-density mass in the neck of the pancreas (arrow). This is resulting in obstruction of the distal pancreatic duct. (b) Coronal multiplanar reconstruction demonstrates focal invasion of the portal vein (arrowhead). Additional low-density tumor is seen surrounding the common hepatic artery (arrow) Biopsy demonstrated adenocarcinoma. Patient was deemed unresectable and therefore, received chemotherapy and radiation therapy.

enhancement characteristics of the lesion and the presence or absence of other secondary findings, the CT is often able to distinguish the various histologies based on the CT appearance.

Tumor staging

Once a pancreatic cancer has been diagnosed, CT is the modality of choice for preoperative staging and to identify patients for a possible curative resection. The role of CT is to attempt to detect any contraindications to surgical resection. For example, it is the role of CT to detect any distant metastasis, usually to the liver or peritoneal structures, to detect any distant lymph node metastasis and to identify vascular encasement. CT has been shown to have a high predictive value of unresectiblity (90–100%) with a slightly lower predictive value of resectability (76–90%) (Lu *et al.* 1997; Raptopoulos *et al.* 1997; Arslan *et al.* 2001; Nakayama *et al.* 2001; House *et al.* 2004). This is usually due to CT's inability to detect tiny liver metastasis or minimal peritoneal spread (Valls *et al.* 2002). These numbers are a marked improvement from conventional CT, which was only in the accuracy range of 44–73% (Rosch *et al.* 1992; Vellet *et al.* 1992; Megibow *et al.* 1995). The value of MDCT and 3D imaging is improved staging of peripancreatic involvement and vascular involvement but its ability to detect the tiny peritoneal and liver metastasis is probably not much improved over earlier scanners.

Due to the lack of distinct pancreatic capsule, adenocarcinoma of the pancreas easily infiltrates the adjacent tissues including the peripancreatic fat and vessels. Involvement of important arterial structures will make surgical resection impossible (Figs 21.15 & 21.16). Therefore, it is the goal of CT to identify any possible vascular involvement. Typically, involvement of the celiac artery, hepatic artery or SMA will indicate unresectable disease. Involvement of venous structures is somewhat more controversial. Usually, significant involvement of the portal vein (PV) or superior mesenteric vein (SMV) will make surgical resection impossible. However, at some centers, focal involvement of the portal vein near the confluence or minimal involvement of the SMV near the confluence is not considered unresectable as skilled surgeons can perform vascular reconstruction (Alexakis *et al.* 2004).

In 1997, an article by Lu, *et al.* described a CT grading system to identify vascular involvement in patients with pancreatic cancer (Lu *et al.* 1997). Those authors suggested that when more than 50% of a vessel's circumference (arteries or veins) is in contact with the tumor it would be unresectable (Lu *et al.* 1997). Using this criterion, the sensitivity for resectability was 84% with 98% specificity (Lu *et al.* 1997). This was even with early single-detector CT scanners. In 2001, Nakayama applied the same criteria as Lu, but felt that although this criterion worked well for the veins, it did not work as well for the arteries, as sometimes arteries are surrounded by fibrous tissue or

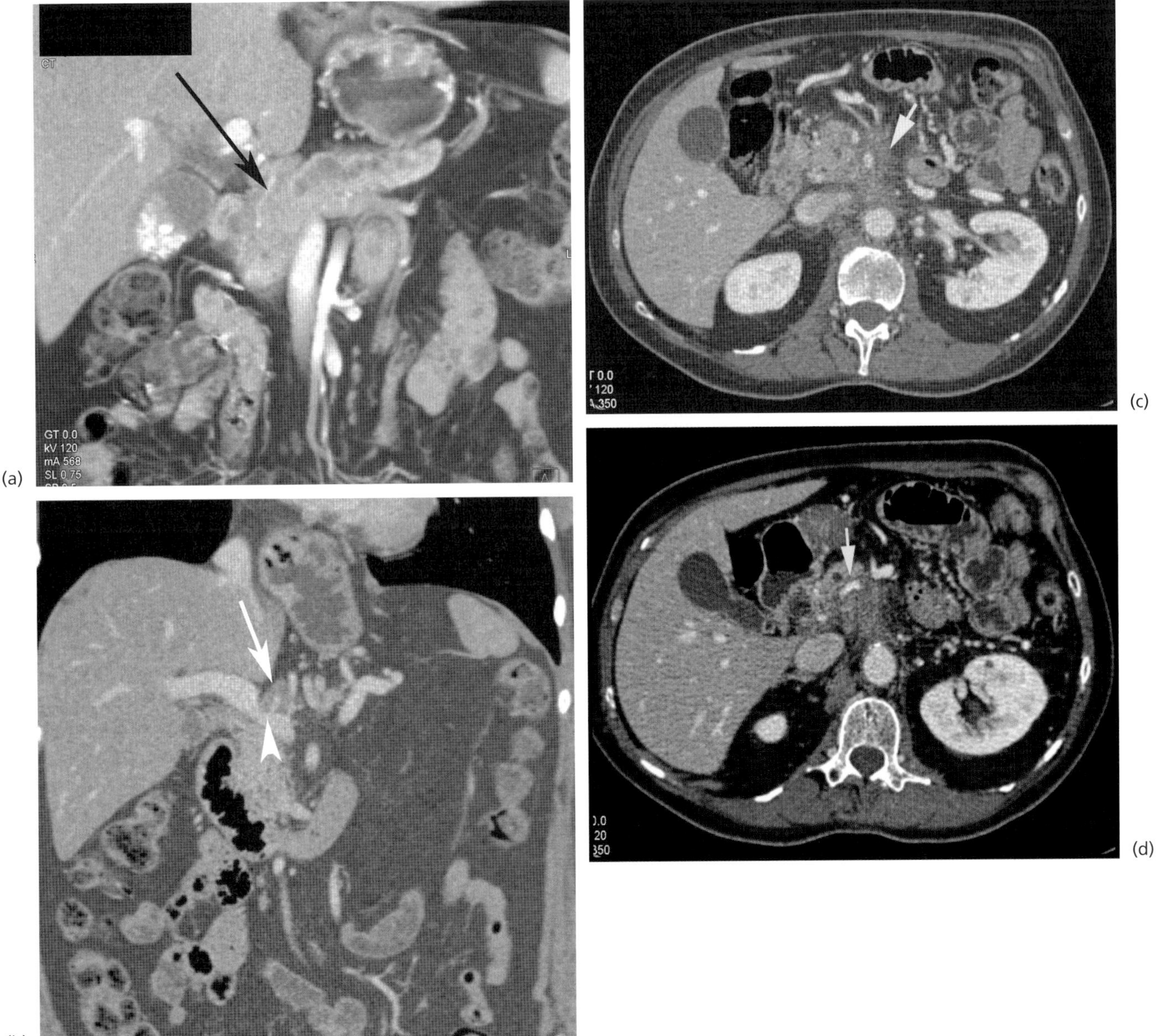

Fig. 21.16 A 63-year-old female presenting with back pain. (a) Axial contrast-enhanced image demonstrates tumor infiltration (arrow) around the SMA and SMV. (b) Axial contrast-enhanced image demonstrates compression of the superior mesenteric vein (arrow). (c) Sagittal volume rendered CT angiogram demonstrates narrowing of the proximal SMA (arrow), compatible with tumor encasement. (d) Coronal maximum intensity projection image demonstrates marked narrowing at the portal confluence (arrow) compatible with tumor encasement. Extensive venous collaterals are also noted. Based on the CT scan, the patient was deemed unresectable. A biopsy confirmed pancreatic adenocarcinoma and the patient went on to receive chemotherapy.

inflammatory stranding that can be mistaken for tumor involvement (Nakayama *et al.* 2001).

More recently, investigators have looked beyond a circumferential grading system to determine whether or not there is a vascular involvement. For example, investigators use 3D imaging of the vessel itself to determine whether there is any compression or direct invasion of the vessel or change in vessel caliber, which would confirm vascular involvement (Horton & Fishman 2002b). Also, the presence of collaterals is a good indication that a venous structure is truly encased. Investigators typically get an accuracy rate of greater than 90% for determining vascular invasion (Arslan *et al.* 2001). In a study from 2004, using MDCT and 3D imaging, 3D CT was shown to be 95% accurate in determining cancer invasion of the superior mesenteric vessels (House *et al.* 2004). Identifying vascular involvement is crucial in the staging of pancreatic cancer, as it will triage patients to either surgical resection versus chemotherapy and radiation or other experimental therapies.

In addition to determining vascular encasement in patients with pancreatic cancer, CT will also attempt nodal staging (Fig. 21.17). The criteria used by radiologists to determine possible nodal involvement by cancer relies on an arbitrary size criterion. However, this is not always accurate, as even tiny nodes can harbor malignancy and large nodes can simply be reactive. In a study by Roche, 62 patients with pancreatic cancer were analyzed (Roche *et al.* 2003). Twenty-eight of these patients underwent surgery and 9 patients had detailed nodal classification, including radiologic, surgical, and pathologic correlation. In total 40 nodes were prospectively identified (Roche *et al.* 2003). After analysis, 2 of 23 nodes which measured less than 5 mm were malignant, whereas 1/6 nodes greater than 10 mm was malignant (Roche *et al.* 2003). Four of eleven nodes in the 5–10 mm range were malignant (Roche *et al.* 2003). Therefore, this study confirms that that using a specific size criterion is not always adequate. When applying a greater than 10 mm size to detected nodes, that study showed a sensitivity of only 14% to identify malignant nodes with a specificity of 85%. This resulted in a positive predictor value of 17% and a negative predictor value of 82% (Roche *et al.* 2003). In addition to size, sometimes the morphology of a node may help to suggest if there is tumor involvement. An ovoid shape, clustering of nodes or the absence of a fatty hilum can be a helpful indication of a malignant node but is usually not that evident. Therefore, when determining resectability of ductal adenocarcinoma, CT is not accurate overall for the prediction of nodal involvement. In a patient deemed resectable by other standards, the presence of peripancreatic lymph nodes should not prevent attempted curative resection.

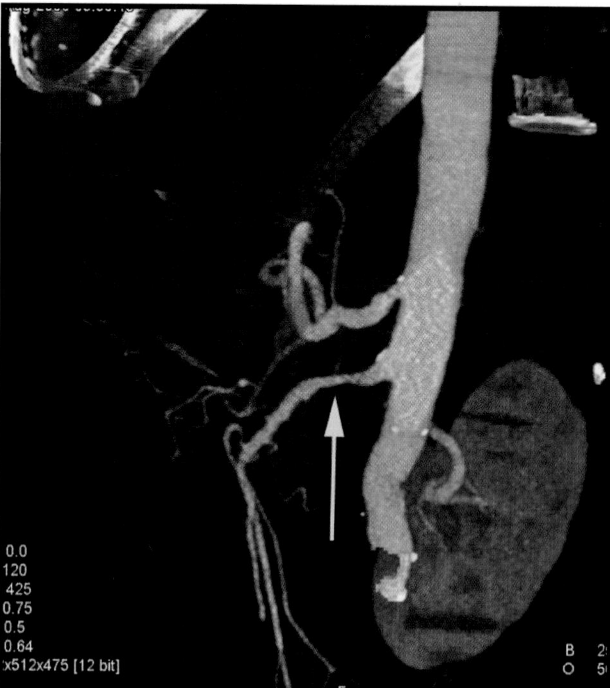

Fig. 21.17 A 75-year-old male with known pancreatic cancer. Axial contrast-enhanced image demonstrates a mass in the body of the pancreas (arrow). Low-density adenopathy is present in the porta (arrowheads). Liver metastases are also seen.

In addition to local staging of adjacent vessels as well as detecting possible nodal involvement, CT is the modality of choice to detect distant metastasis. In patients with pancreatic cancer, the liver is the most common organ involved with metastases. CT is excellent at detecting liver metastasis. These typically appear low density on the portal venous phase of the study. There is a size limitation for CT detection of metastasis in the liver. Even normal patients commonly have a few small-density lesions in the liver thought to represent tiny cysts, hemangiomas or bile duct hamartomas. Therefore, the presence of a few tiny lesions in the liver would not necessarily indicate metastases. Larger lesions in the liver can be confidently diagnosed as metastasis. However, there is still the limitation of CT and some patients determined to be resectable by other criteria are sometimes found to be unresectable at surgery and small liver and peritoneal implants are seen which are below the resolution of CT (Valls *et al.* 2002).

In summary, once CT detects the pancreatic tumor, accurate staging is performed. This involves a careful 3D analysis of the pancreatic vasculature to determine possible arterial or venous encasement. CT is also used to identify obvious distant nodal metastasis or distant metastasis to other organs, such as the liver or the adrenal gland.

Recurrent disease

CT is also the imaging modality of choice for following patients after surgery for pancreatic cancer (Johnson *et al.* 2002). The postoperative appearance after a Whipple procedure in particular can be complex, especially in the early postoperative period. The diagnosis of recurrent disease can be further complicated by normal changes as a result of postoperative radiation and chemotherapy. Therefore, accurate interpretation of these postoperative examinations and follow-up is important to detect recurrent disease. For example, after Whipple surgery, the pancreatic jejunostomy can be difficult to identify particularly when the remnant pancreatic gland becomes atrophic (Johnson *et al.* 2002). Often oral contrast will not opacify this bowel loop and therefore this loop of bowel can be mistaken for recurrent tumor. Small lymph nodes are common in the postoperative period and over time usually regress. Soft tissue stranding in the mesenteric fat in the immediate postoperative period is common and is related to postsurgical changes. This should be followed over time. If this progresses, then tumor recurrence is likely (Fig. 21.18). Radiation changes after Whipple surgery include thickening of the gastric antrum, gastrojejunostomy and fatty infiltration of the left lobe of the liver as well as the stranding

(a)

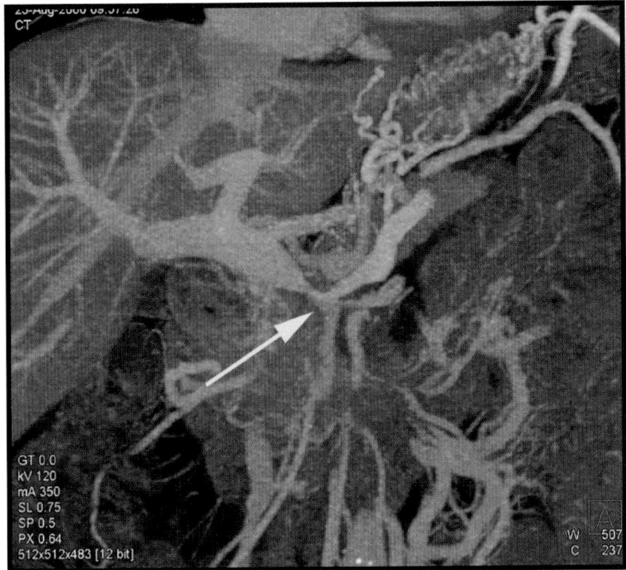

(b)

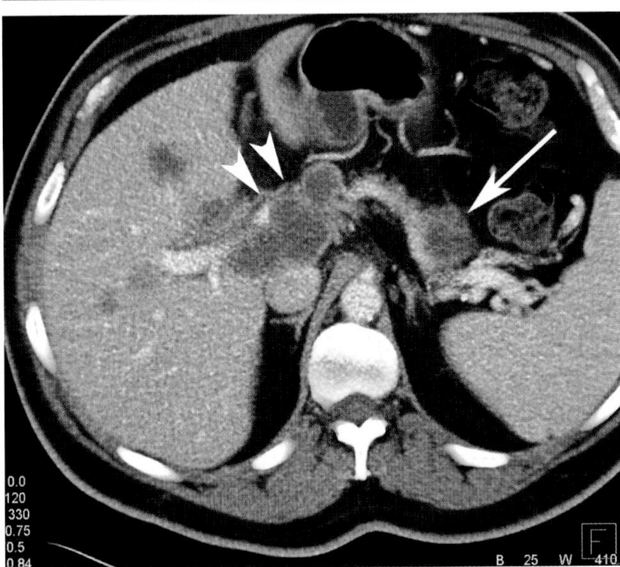

Fig. 21.18 A 67-year-old female 2 years after surgical resection of a 2.2-cm adenocarcinoma in the pancreatic head. The surgical margins were negative at surgery, although 2/7 nodes were positive. (a) Coronal volume rendered images shows tumor recurrence in the surgical bed encasing the SMA and occluding the SMV. (b) Coronal MIP image shows occlusion of the SMV (arrow) and extensive collaterals.

of the mesenteric fat (Johnson *et al.* 2002). This should not be mistaken for tumor recurrence.

Postpancreatic surgery patients will be followed over time. CT can detect the appearance of distant metastasis to the liver or other organs. In addition, CT is also useful to detect recurrence in the surgical bed, which often appears as soft tissue density in the region of the SMA or the celiac axis. For accurate detection of recurrent disease, we utilize a CT protocol similar to our staging protocol. That is, dual phase imaging is performed to the pancreas using IV contrast and water as oral contrast, as well as thin collimation and 3D imaging.

Conclusions

CT is considered to be the imaging modality of choice for detection and staging of patients with pancreatic adenocarcinoma. Recent advancements in CT technology, as well as development of real-time volume rendering software, have significantly improved our ability to both detect and accurately stage pancreatic cancers. CT is also essential in the postoperative period for those patients who undergo attempted curative resection. After pancreatic surgery, patients will be followed routinely with CT in order to detect the development of metastasis or recurrence within the surgical bed.

References

Alexakis N, Halloran C, Raraty M, Ghaneh P, Sutton R, Neoptolemos JP. (2004) Current standards of surgery for pancreatic cancer. *Br J Surg* 91: 1410–27.

Arslan A, Buanes T, Geitung JT. (2001) Pancreatic carcinoma: MR, MR angiography and dynamic helical CT in the evaluation of vascular invasion. *Eur J Radiol* 38: 151–9.

Bae KT. (2003) Peak contrast enhancement in CT and MR angiography: when does it occur and why? Pharmacokinetic study in a porcine model. *Radiology* 227: 809–16.

Bonaldi VM, Bret PM, Atri M, Garcia P, Reinhold C. (1996) A comparison of two injection protocols using helical and dynamic acquisitions in CT examinations of the pancreas. *AJR Am J Roentgenol* 167: 49–55.

Fishman EK, Ney DR, Heath DG, Corl FM, Horton KM, Johnson PT. (2006) Volume rendering versus maximum intensity projection in CT angiography: what works best, when, and why. *Radiographics* 26: 905–22.

Goshima S, Kanematsu M, Kondo H *et al.* (2006) Pancreas: optimal scan delay for contrast-enhanced multi-detector row CT. *Radiology* 241: 167–74.

Graf O, Boland GW, Warshaw AL, Fernandez-Del-Castillo C, Hahn PF, Mueller PR. (1997) Arterial versus portal venous helical CT for revealing pancreatic adenocarcinoma: conspicuity of tumor and critical vascular anatomy. *AJR Am J Roentgenol* 169: 119–23.

Hollett MD, Jorgensen MJ, Jeffrey RB Jr. (1995) Quantitative evaluation of pancreatic enhancement during dual-phase helical CT. *Radiology* 195: 359–61.

Horton KM, Fishman EK. (2002a) Adenocarcinoma of the pancreas: CT imaging. *Radiol Clin North Am* 40: 1263–72.

Horton KM, Fishman EK. (2002b) Multidetector CT angiography of pancreatic carcinoma: part 2, evaluation of venous involvement. *AJR Am J Roentgenol* 178: 833–6.

Horton KM, Sheth S, Corl F, Fishman EK. (2002) Multidetector row CT: principles and clinical applications. *Crit Rev Comput Tomogr* 43: 143–81.

Horton KM, Hruban RH, Yeo C, Fishman EK. (2006) Multidetector row CT of pancreatic islet cell tumors. *Radiographics* 26: 453–64.

House MG, Yeo CJ, Cameron JL *et al.* (2004) Predicting resectability of periampullary cancer with three-dimensional computed tomography. *J Gastrointest Surg* 8: 280–8.

Johnson PT, Curry CA, Urban BA, Fishman EK. (2002) Spiral CT following the Whipple procedure: distinguishing normal postoperative findings from complications. *J Comput Assist Tomogr* 26: 956–61.

Johnson PT, Fishman EK, Duckwall JR, Calhoun PS, Heath DG. (1998) Interactive three-dimensional volume rendering of spiral CT data: current applications in the thorax. *Radiographics* 18: 165–87.

Lu DS, Reber HA, Krasny RM, Kadell BM, Sayre J. (1997) Local staging of pancreatic cancer: criteria for unresectability of major vessels as revealed by pancreatic-phase, thin-section helical CT. *AJR Am J Roentgenol* 168: 1439–43.

McNulty NJ, Francis IR, Platt JF, Cohan RH, Korobkin M, Gebremariam A. (2001) Multi-detector row helical CT of the pancreas: effect of contrast-enhanced multiphasic imaging on enhancement of the pancreas, peripancreatic vasculature, and pancreatic adenocarcinoma. *Radiology* 220: 97–102.

Megibow AJ, Zhou XH, Rotterdam H *et al.* (1995) Pancreatic adenocarcinoma: CT versus MR imaging in the evaluation of resectability—report of the Radiology Diagnostic Oncology Group. *Radiology* 195: 327–32.

Megibow AJ, Babb JS, Hecht EM *et al.* (2006) Evaluation of bowel distention and bowel wall appearance by using neutral oral contrast agent for multi-detector row CT. *Radiology* 238: 87–95.

Mitka M. (2007) Milk shows potential as CT contrast agent. *JAMA* 297: 353.

Nakayama Y, Yamashita Y, Kadota M *et al.* (2001) Vascular encasement by pancreatic cancer: correlation of CT findings with surgical and pathologic results. *J Comput Assist Tomogr* 25: 337–42.

Raptopoulos V, Steer ML, Sheiman RG, Vrachliotis TG, Gougoutas CA, Movson JS. (1997) The use of helical CT and CT angiography to predict vascular involvement from pancreatic cancer: correlation with findings at surgery. *AJR Am J Roentgenol* 168: 971–7.

Roche CJ, Hughes ML, Garvey CJ *et al.* (2003) CT and pathologic assessment of prospective nodal staging in patients with ductal adenocarcinoma of the head of the pancreas. *AJR Am J Roentgenol* 180: 475–80.

Rosch T, Braig C, Gain T *et al.* (1992) Staging of pancreatic and ampullary carcinoma by endoscopic ultrasonography. Comparison with conventional sonography, computed tomography, and angiography. *Gastroenterology* 102: 188–99.

Valls C, Andia E, Sanchez A *et al.* (2002) Dual-phase helical CT of pancreatic adenocarcinoma: assessment of resectability before surgery. *AJR Am J Roentgenol* 178: 821–6.

Vellet AD, Romano W, Bach DB, Passi RB, Taves DH, Munk PL. (1992) Adenocarcinoma of the pancreatic ducts: comparative evaluation with CT and MR imaging at 1.5 T. *Radiology* 183: 87–95.

Treatment

Overview

Christopher L. Wolfgang

The outlook of individuals with pancreatic adenocarcinoma (pancreatic cancer) is dismal as described by the following statistics. The overall survival for patients diagnosed with pancreatic cancer is only 4%. It is the 10th most common cancer but the fourth most fatal (Jemal *et al.* 2006). Over 80% of patients with pancreatic adenocarcinoma have advanced disease at the time of diagnosis and are not candidates for a potentially curative resection. In this group of patients, approximately 20% will have locally advanced disease with a median survival of 8–12 months and 50% will have metastatic disease with median survival of 3–6 months (Brennan 1993). Of the remaining patients who undergo a resection, the chance of long-term survival is low; 80–90% will go on to have recurrence. One-half of patients undergoing a potentially curative resection will be dead of disease in 18 months and less than 20% will be alive at 5 years (Winter *et al.* 2006). Certain pathologic features such as a tumor size less than 2 cm, absence of spread to regional lymph nodes, and a surgical margin free of carcinoma are good prognostic indicators (Brennan 1993; Wenger *et al.* 2000). Under ideal circumstances, in which all of these factors are favorable, 5-year survival is achieved in only 43% (Winter *et al.* 2006). The major factors contributing to the lethality of this disease are the inability to detect early cancers and ineffective systemic therapy.

The only chance for long-term survival in patients with pancreatic cancer is with surgical resection. However, since the majority of patients have occult systemic disease at the time of resection, cure relies on systemic therapy. Currently no systemic therapy has been identified that has potent biologic activity against pancreatic cancer. Three major prospective randomized clinical trials (phase III) have been conducted regarding the efficacy of adjuvant therapy: Gastrointestinal Tumor Study Group (GITSG), European Organization for Research and Treatment of Cancer (EORTC), and European Study Group for Pancreatic Cancer (ESPAC). These are described in detail in the sections on chemotherapy and radiotherapy in this chapter. Each one of these trials has significant limitations that have resulted in unclear interpretation of the data. As a result no unified treatment regimen exists for pancreatic cancer. The overall consensus of the current literature points toward a small but significant benefit to adjuvant therapy of some sort. Definitive advances in the treatment of pancreatic cancer will likely develop only with more efficacious chemotherapeutics. The section on novel agents in this chapter reviews several new compounds that have made it to clinical trials.

In no other type of cancer is management by a multidisciplinary team more important. This statement is supported by the fact that our most effective therapy for what is essentially a systemic disease is surgery. Numerous factors such as accurate preoperative staging, surgical margins and minimizing morbidity for the timely institution of adjuvant therapy have a major impact on outcome. The fact remains, however, that resection is not definitive for the vast majority of individuals with pancreatic cancer, since most will go on to die from their disease. The progression to this ultimate fate by those who have undergone a potentially curative resection, and those who will only undergo palliative therapy, requires the ongoing attention of clinicians experienced in the management of this disease. This is best accomplished by a coordinated effort of a multidisciplinary team. Perhaps the one of the most significant contributions of this team is the improved efficiency of patient accrual to clinical trials, accelerating the pace to early diagnosis and improved therapy.

References

Brennan MF. (1993) Cancer of the pancreas. In: DeVita V, ed. *Principles and Practice of Oncology*, 5th edn, pp. 849–882. J.B. Lippencott, Philadelphia.

Jemal A, Siegel R, Ward E *et al.* (2006) Cancer statistics, 2006. *CA Cancer J Clin.* 56(2): 106–30.

Wenger FA, Peter F, Zieren J, Steiert A, Jacobi CA, Muller JM. (2000) Prognosis factors in carcinoma of the head of the pancreas. *Dig Surg* 17(1): 29–35.

Winter JM, Cameron JL, Campbell KA *et al.* (2006) 1423 pancreaticoduodenectomies for pancreatic cancer: A single-institution experience. *J Gastrointest Surg* 10(9): 1199–1210.

Surgery

Robert A. Meguid & Christopher L. Wolfgang

Introduction

The long-term survival of patients with pancreatic adenocarcinoma (pancreatic cancer) is only possible through complete resection of the primary lesion. Unfortunately, since most patients have occult metastatic disease at the time of surgery, long-term survival following a potentially curative operation is uncommon. Furthermore, most patients (80%) with pancreatic cancer are diagnosed at an advanced stage and thus are not candidates for a potentially curative operation (Brennan 1993). These facts emphasize the importance of the multidisciplinary care of patients with this disease. Within this team, the primary responsibility of the surgeon is determining which patients are candidates for a potentially curative resection and performing this operation in a manner that renders the patient free of disease and in a condition suitable to undergo adjuvant therapy. The literature suggests that outcomes for pancreatic surgery are superior at high-volume centers (Birkmeyer *et al.* 1999).

The purpose of this section is to provide a surgical perspective on the management of pancreatic cancer to non-surgical members of the multidisciplinary team. In particular, this section will focus on three general areas:

1 preoperative management
2 operative management
3 outcomes and common postoperative complications.

Preoperative management

Staging

The clinically relevant staging of pancreatic cancer is aimed at determining resectability. Further classification along the lines of the American Joint Commission on Cancer (2002) is important for uniform communication and comparison of therapies, but has little bearing on directing treatment. Accurately determining resectability is critical, since this will stratify patients into those who will undergo potentially curative therapy versus those who will receive palliative treatment. Thus, inadequate assessment of the extent of disease may result in inappropriate denial of potentially curative therapies, or in an unnecessarily high rate of non-therapeutic laparotomies.

Resectability is based on both systemic and local factors. The presence of clinically apparent metastasis (M1 disease) is a contraindication to an attempt at a curative resection. In the absence of disseminated disease, the relationship of the tumor to the superior mesenteric artery (SMA) and celiac axis, and the extent of involvement of the superior mesenteric vein (SMV) and portal vein (PV) defines resectability. The determination of resectability has evolved from principally an intraoperative assessment to one based on preoperative studies. The finding of unexpected abdominal metastasis or locally advanced disease at the time of laparotomy has become an uncommon occurrence at most high-volume centers. The main advance that has made more accurate staging possible is improved imaging, in particular the advancement of MDCT technology (House *et al.* 2004; O'Malley *et al.* 1999). In addition, the selective use of laparoscopic exploration (Conlon & Brennan 2000), endoscopic retrograde cholangiopancreatography (ERCP), endoscopic ultrasound (Gress *et al.* 1999), ^{18}fluorodeoxyglucose positron emission tomography (PET) (Rose *et al.* 1999), and magnetic resonance imaging (MRI) (Sheridan *et al.* 1999) contribute additional useful information in a subset of patients.

Assessment of systemic disease

Clinically apparent metastatic disease is present in over 50% of patients at the time of diagnosis (Brennan 1993). Unlike colon cancer, in which recent advances in systemic therapy have resulted in a dramatic improvement in control of metastatic disease, no such therapy exists for pancreatic cancer. As a result, the presence of metastatic disease is a contraindication to an attempt at a curative resection.

The determination of metastasis relies heavily on imaging studies and the selective use of staging laparoscopy. The finding of palpable supraclavicular, periumbilical or pelvic nodes is uncommon. Other frequent sites of metastasis such as liver, peritoneum and lung are not accurately assessed by physical exam. A contrast-enhanced CT scan of the abdomen and pelvis is the primary modality for the initial assessment of metastatic disease. In some institutions a chest CT is added for the evaluation of the thorax. The presumed advantage of a chest CT over a plain film is an improved ability to identify pulmonary lesions and enlarged thoracic and cervical lymph nodes. The cost effectiveness of this approach and translation into improved patient selection has not been reported in the literature.

Liver metastases appear as hypodense lesions with peripheral enhancement on contrast-enhanced CT. The ability to identify metastatic disease to the liver by CT is related to size and diminishes significantly for lesions less than 2 cm (Megibow *et al.* 1995). As a result, it is not uncommon to be faced with an indeterminate lesion within the liver based on CT findings. In small lesions of uncertain diagnosis it is unlikely that percutaneous biopsy will be successful in obtaining tissue for diagnosis. As with CT, the ability of PET to distinguish metastatic disease from benign lesions is limited by small size (Rose *et al.* 1999; Diederichs *et al.* 2000). Consequently, further characterization in this subset of patients requires surgical exploration preferably in the form of laparoscopy.

The majority of patients with pancreatic cancer are found to have metastasis to regional lymph nodes following resection (N1) (Winter *et al.* 2006). Regional lymph node involvement is associated with a significant reduction in long-term survival in comparison to node-negative patients, but is not a contraindication to an attempt at a curative resection (Wenger *et al.* 2000; Richter *et al.* 2003; Winter *et al.* 2006). Therefore the preoperative assessment of these nodes is inconsequential in the determination of resectability. Spread of cancer to more distant nodes is considered M1 disease and is not amenable to surgery. The ability of CT scan to accurately detect nodal disease is relatively poor (Roche *et al.* 2003). The sensitivity for CT scan in determining nodal metastasis ranges from only 14 to 37%. Moreover, the finding of enlarged nodes does not strictly correlate with cancer involvement. Normal-sized nodes are often found to contain cancer, while some enlarged nodes may be reactive. The enlarged lymph nodes found on CT scan should be assessed for cancer using additional methods only if it will influence the management of the patient. In the absence of definitive proof of distant nodal spread, patients should be offered a potentially curative resection.

A major limitation of MDCT in the staging of pancreatic cancer is the ability to detect peritoneal dissemination (M1 disease). As a result, several studies have evaluated the effectiveness of laparoscopic exploration for assessment of peritoneal spread (Conlon *et al.* 1996; Conlon & Brennan 2000; Jimenez *et al.* 2000; Pisters *et al.* 2001b). This technique has the potential advantage of allowing direct inspection of peritoneal surfaces while avoiding the morbidity associated with a laparotomy. Laparoscopic staging is performed prior to conversion to laparotomy or as a separate procedure. The yield of laparoscopic staging in identifying CT-occult peritoneal disease is related to the quality of the preoperative imaging. Early studies, in which laparoscopy was added to evaluation with single-detector CT, demonstrated upstaging due to peritoneal M1 disease in as many as one-third of patients (Conlon *et al.*1996; Jimenez *et al.* 2000). With the improvement of imaging technology the utility of laparoscopy has declined (Pisters *et al.* 2001b). For example, using MDCT (Pisters *et al.* 2001b; House *et al.* 2004) it was found that less than 10% of patients with presumed resectable tumors by MDCT scan were found to have M1 disease at surgery. This finding is consistent with other published reports that used similar technology in staging of pancreatic cancer. Therefore, using state-of-the-art CT imaging one could expect upstaging by laparoscopy in, at best, approximately 10% of patients initially thought to have M0 disease. This view is supported by recent studies which estimate no more than 13% of patients will be spared laparotomy following high-quality CT imaging (Friess *et al.* 1998; Steinberg *et al.* 1998). As a result most surgeons have adopted a selective approach to the use of laparoscopic exploration. In this paradigm patients at highest risk for occult M1 disease undergo laparoscopy prior to formal laparotomy and resection. Patients at increased risk for peritoneal dissemination include those with locally advanced primary tumors (Jimenez *et al.* 2000; Pisters *et al.* 2001b), body and tail lesions (Jimenez *et al.* 2000; Pisters *et al.* 2001b), or a profoundly elevated CA19-9 (>100 units/mL)(Karachristos *et al.* 2005). Additionally, laparoscopy should also be applied when CT findings are suggestive, but not conclusive, of peritoneal spread.

The role of PET in the preoperative staging of pancreatic cancer is evolving. The ability of PET to identify malignancy relies on the glucose-avid nature of transformed cells in relation to that of normal cells. The theoretical advantage is the ability to differentiate between benign and malignant lesions. Based on this premise, there are reports of PET scans identifying CT-occult *primary* pancreatic cancers in patients with unclear etiology of painless jaundice (Rose *et al.* 1999; Diederichs *et al.* 2000). Its application for this use however is limited, since most of these patients will be offered resection based on clinical suspicion for malignancy regardless of PET results. The main application of PET in the evaluation of patients with pancreatic cancer has been for the clarification of M status. PET has the ability to evaluate the entire body, making it a potentially useful survey for M1 disease. Several studies have reported PET to be more sensitive than CT alone in identifying metastatic disease (Rose *et al.* 1999; Diederichs *et al.* 2000). In a study aimed at assessing the role of PET in the management of patients with pancreatic adenocarcinoma, Rose *et al.* (1999) reported identification of CT-occult metastatic disease in 5 of 65 patients. A separate group reported the sensitivity of PET in detecting liver metastasis from pancreatic cancer was 68%. In this study the ability to detect liver metastasis was dependent on size. For lesions larger than 1 cm PET had a detection rate of 97%, while the detection rate for less than 1 cm was only 43%. As a result, PET scanning does not offer an advantage over MDCT for lesions < 1 cm. Although PET is able to identify M1 disease in sites other than liver, its efficacy in relation to other modalities has not been established in this regard. In our practice PET is infrequently employed in the preoperative setting. It is used to *clarify* the status of indeterminate pulmonary nodules or enlarged lymph nodes outside of the peripancreatic region not amenable to biopsy. In addition, it is used to evaluate suspect pulmonary and hepatic lesions.

Assessment of local disease

In the absence of identifiable M1 disease the resectability of a pancreatic cancer is determined by the extent of local invasion. Local criteria for resectability include the absence of celiac axis or SMA involvement and a patent PV–SMV confluence. A curative resection should only be considered when a high probability of achieving a resection with a margin free of cancer (R0 resection) exists. In practice this determination is relatively imprecise. Even in high-volume centers with experience in preoperative assessment of resectability, 20–40% of patients are left with microscopically identifiable cancer at the margin (Tseng *et al.* 2004; Winter *et al.* 2006). The most effective method of evaluating the relationship of tumor with vessels is by using contrast-enhanced 3D CT. Using this technology, the ability to predict a margin-negative resection (R0) is of the order of 73% (House *et al.* 2004). The determination of resectablity at laparotomy should be avoided since it subjects the patient to a non-therapeutic operation associated with significant morbidity. In addition, adequate intraoperative assessment of the tumor's relationship with the SMA is difficult prior to the division of the pancreatic neck and mobilization of the PV–SMVconfluence. At this point in the operation one is essentially committed to proceeding with a pancreaticoduodenectomy. It should be noted that patients that undergo a pancreaticoduodenectomy leaving gross tumor at the uncinate margin (R2) have a median survival of less than 6 months (Willett *et al.* 1993; Sohn *et al.* 2000a).

In order to consistently evaluate tumor resectability based on the relationship of the tumor to the vessels, standardized nomenclatures have been proposed for the interpretation of CT scan images (Loyer *et al.* 1996; Lu *et al.* 1997; Sohn *et al.* 2000a). Separation of the vessel from the tumor by a well-defined fat plane indicates no involvement by the tumor and a high likelihood of achieving a margin-negative resection. Borderline resectable patients have tumor that extend to either the SMA or celiac axis but have less than 180° circumferential involvement. Patients with borderline resectable disease may potentially undergo a margin-negative resection and should be offered a potentially curative surgery. Patients with cancer that involves greater than 180° of arterial circumference are said to have encasement and have essentially no chance at an R0 resection. This is considered a T4 lesion and designates the patient as unresectable (stage III, locally advanced).

Invasion of the PV–SMV does not preclude a pancreaticoduodenectomy as long as the vessel is patent and venous resection and reconstruction is possible based on anatomic constraints (Tseng *et al.* 2004). Complete occlusion of the PV–SMV is a contraindication for an attempt at a curative resection since it is often associated with encasement of the SMA (Tseng *et al.* 2004). The largest published experience on venous resection comes from the M.D. Anderson Cancer Center (Tseng *et al.* 2004). In their series, 141 patients underwent pancreaticoduodenectomy with *en bloc* venous resection (PV, SMV or PV–SMV confluence). Venous reconstruction was accomplished by primary anastomosis, vein patch or internal jugular interposition graft. The retroperitoneal margin-positivity rate in patients undergoing venous resection was 20%. The median survival for patients requiring venous resection was comparable to that for historical controls undergoing standard pancreaticoduodenectomies (23 months vs. 26 months). These results demonstrate that patients requiring PV–SMV resection to undergo a potentially curable resection do as well as similar patients not requiring venous resection.

Preoperative tissue biopsy

A tissue diagnosis of adenocarcinoma is not required prior to an attempt at a curative resection in all cases. The presentation of jaundice and weight loss along with a pancreatic mass or stricture of the distal bile duct should be considered carcinoma until proven otherwise in a patient with appropriate risk factors. In addition to periampullary cancers, the differential diagnosis in these patients includes benign conditions such as choledocholithiasis, benign biliary strictures and chronic pancreatitis. No single test will definitively rule out carcinoma in such patients. This includes a 'negative' or indeterminate biopsy of the mass which can a carry a false negative rate of 15% (Varadarajulu & Wallace 2004). Therefore in a patient with the appropriate history, the decision to offer a curative resection is not altered by the biopsy result.

Several exceptions to this paradigm exist. Patients undergoing neoadjuvant therapy require a tissue diagnosis prior to the institution of therapy. In addition, the diagnosis of adenocarcinoma may be uncertain in the work-up of a pancreatic mass. Neuroendocrine cancers, lymphomas, cystic lesions and even non-neoplastic conditions may not appear distinct on MDCT imaging. In these cases endoscopic ultrasound guided fine-needle aspiration may yield a tissue diagnosis and alter the therapeutic management.

Tissue diagnosis is also important in the conformation of M1 disease suggested on other studies such as MDCT. A patient with a pancreatic mass consistent with adenocarcinoma and a worrying lesion in the liver should undergo a percutaneous biopsy of the *liver* lesion. A biopsy positive for adenocarcinoma confirms the presence of stage IV disease and eliminates consideration for curative resection. In the event that a biopsy of a potential M1 lesion is negative for carcinoma or indeterminate, a healthy patient should be given the benefit of the doubt and proceed to an attempt at curative resection.

Preoperative biliary decompression

Obstructive jaundice is a predominant feature in many patients with adenocarcinoma involving the head of the pancreas. It was previously felt that the rate of operative complications was increased in jaundiced patients. Indeed, the original description of the Whipple operation was that of a two-stage procedure with the first stage aimed at relieving the obstructive jaundice prior to pancreatic resection (Whipple 1963). This has been supplanted by using either endoscopically or percutaneously placed biliary stents.

The practice of preoperative biliary decompression has recently come into question based on the results of several studies. Povoski *et al.* (1999) reported preoperative stenting is associated with an increase in perioperative mortality and morbidity. Other retrospective studies have demonstrated that only wound infections are increased in patients undergoing preoperative biliary decompression (Sohn *et al.* 2000b; Pisters *et al.* 2001a). The largest series on this topic comes from the Johns Hopkins Hospital (Sohn *et al.* 2000b). In their analysis of 567 patients, only the risk of wound infection was increased in patients undergoing preoperative biliary decompression. Mortality was equivalent in both the stented and unstented groups. Similar results were found in another large series of 300 patients from M.D. Anderson (Pisters *et al.* 2001a).

Biliary decompression is not a requisite prior to performing a pancreaticoduodenectomy in jaundice patients. However, many factors make the use of preoperative biliary decompression necessary. This includes treatment of patients with neoadjuvant therapy, organization of referral to specialist and limited operating room availability at high-volume centers. In light of the need for preoperative biliary decompression under these circumstances, it is generally considered that the utility of this practice is not outweighed by the manageable associated risks.

Operative management

The operation necessary to resect pancreatic cancer depends on the location of the tumor. Adenocarcinomas arising in the uncinate or head of the pancreas require a pancreaticoduodenectomy, while those in the tail require a distal pancreatectomy with an *en bloc* splenectomy. Lesions located in the neck and body may require a pancreaticoduodenectomy, distal pancreatectomy or even a total pancreatectomy for complete extirpation. This decision is often made intraoperatively. A central pancreatectomy is not performed for pancreatic adenocarcinoma since it is an inadequate operation with respect to oncologic principles. The contention that a total pancreatectomy is a more appropriate oncologic operation than a pancreaticoduodenectomy has been studied. Several independent studies have demonstrated no survival benefit for patients undergoing total pancreatectomy in comparison to those undergoing pancreaticoduodenectomy (Sarr *et al.*1993; Karpoff *et al.* 2001). Patients who have had their pancreas completely resected are committed to a life of brittle diabetes and a risk of fatal hypoglycemia. In light of these results total pancreatectomy is reserved for patients with lesions in the body of the pancreas that cannot be adequately removed by either a pancreaticoduodenectomy or a distal pancreatectomy.

With the emergence of non-operative biliary decompression and endoscopically directed therapies such as duodenal wall-stents, the need for surgical palliation has decreased. However, in certain instances surgery plays an important role in palliation of patients with terminal disease.

The following is a description of a pancreaticoduodenectomy and a distal pancreatectomy performed for curative intent. In addition, the role of surgical palliation will be discussed.

Pancreaticoduodenectomy (Whipple operation)

The abdomen is entered through either a large midline or chevron incision and a self-retaining retractor is placed. The operation begins with a careful exploration of the peritoneal surface for implants. The liver is inspected both visually for surface lesions and by palpation for deeper lesions. Alternatively, intraoperative ultrasonography may be used to assess the liver parenchyma. As outlined above, patients at high risk for peritoneal dissemination should undergo these initial steps laparoscopically.

Exposure of the pancreatic head is initiated by first mobilizing the right colon. A complete Cattell–Braasch maneuver may be performed, but is not necessary in all cases. The transverse mesocolon is dissected free from the head of the pancreas by dividing the loose areolar attachment with electrocautery. At this point the middle colic vein is identified and can be dissected down to the anterior surface of the SMV. The gastroepoploic vein is usually identified at this point as either a second tributary of the SMV or arising as a common tributary with the middle colic vein called the gastrocolic trunk. The middle colic, gastroepoploic vein or common gastrocolic trunk are divided to avoid a traction injury to the SMV. The lesser sac is entered by continued medial dissection and division of the gastrocolic ligament between the antrum and proximal transverse colon. A Kocher maneuver is performed by dividing the retroperitoneal attachments of the duodenum laterally. The fibroadipose tissue of the retroperitoneum is kept in continuity with the specimen thus cleanly exposing the inferior vena cava, both renal veins, gonadal veins, the right ureter and the medial edge of the left kidney. At this point the anterior exposure of the SMV can be completed by excising the remaining peritoneal covering laterally. The first jejunal venous tributary of the SMV is also exposed at its posterolateral insertion on the SMV.

With the duodenum fully Kocherized the surgeon carefully assesses for anomalous arterial vasculature. The most common anomaly is a replaced right hepatic artery arising as the first branch off the SMA. A replaced right hepatic artery courses laterally and inferiorly in the porta hepatis. Other common anomalies include an accessory right hepatic and replaced common hepatic arteries. The identification of anomalous arterial anatomy is important, since ligation of a major hepatic artery can result in fatal hepatic necrosis.

The lymph node bundle lateral to the portal vein and common bile duct is divided near the level of the cystic duct and swept inferiorly to be removed with the specimen. This maneuver often exposes the right lateral edges of the common bile duct and PV. The peritoneal attachments of the hepatoduodenal ligament are divided and tied. The peritoneal covering of the common bile duct are divided anteriorly and the cystic duct is identified, cleared and encircled with a tie. The cystic artery is divided and the gallbladder is excised from the gall bladder fossa using electrocautery. The cystic duct is then ligated and divided and the gall bladder is handed from the field.

The common bile duct is next encircled with a vesseloop. Separation of the posterior wall of the common bile duct from the anterior wall of the PV can be difficult in patients with a history of cholangitis. The bile duct is divided near its junction with the cystic duct stump. The gastroduodenal artery (GDA) is identified close to the superior edge of the first portion of the duodenum. Complete mobilization of the neck of the pancreas requires division of the GDA. Prior to dividing the GDA it is clamped and flow through the proper hepatic artery is confirmed. In patients with celiac stenosis hepatic circulation is fed from the SMA through retrograde flow from the GDA.

If a pylorus-preserving pancreaticoduodenectomy will be performed the first portion of the duodenum is transected using a linear GIA stapler at least 1.5 cm distal to the pylorus. If a standard pancreaticoduodenectomy is to be performed the stomach is divided proximal to the antrum with several firings of a linear GIA stapler. In general, small adenocarcinomas of the pancreatic head and unciate process, ampullary cancinomas and distal cholangocarinomas can be adequately removed while preserving the pylorus. On the other hand, larger lesions of the head uncinate and neck often require *en bloc* distal gastrectomy (standard pancreaticoduodenectomy).

The jejunum is divided approximately 20–30 cm distal to the ligament of Treitz with a linear stapler. The intervening mesentery is divided between ties until the jejunum and third and fourth portions of the duodenum can be passed beneath the superior mesenteric vessels to the right upper quadrant. At this point, the tunnel is developed posterior to the neck of the pancreas. Figure-of-eight stitches are placed superiorly and inferiorly on both sides of the intented area of pancreatic transection to control bleeding from the superior and inferior pancreaticoduodenal arteries. Identification of a small pancreatic duct is facilitated by dividing the pancreas with a knife as opposed to electrocautery. At this point the pancreatic neck and common bile duct margins should be sent for intraoperative frozen section evaluation.

Once the neck is transected the pancreatic head and duodenum are retracted to the right and the PV and SMV can be easily mobilized to the patient's left. Retraction of the PV and SMV to the left is necessary for adequate exposure of the uncinate process and SMA. The division of the uncinate process from the SMA in order to achieve a clear margin is often the most difficult step in the operation. This is best achieved by dividing the uncinate process, starting proximally on the SMA and working distally. Dominant arterial branches are individually ligated and divided. The plane of dissection should result in a completely skeletonized right lateral border of the SMA. Failure to transect the uncinate tissue in this manner may result in an unnecessary positive margin. The uncinate should be appropriately marked with a suture or ink in order for proper analysis by pathology. Histologically it will be difficult for the pathologist to determine a microscopically positive margin (R1) versus a grossly positive margin (R2). This determination is best made by operative assessment and should be documented in the operative notes. The significance of the margin status is discussed in more detail elsewhere. Extent of lymph node dissection has been studied in a prospective randomized trial. It has been shown that an extended lymphadenectomy adds no survival benefit to a standard pancreaticoduodenectomy (Sarr *et al.* 1993; Yeo *et al.* 2002). Moreover, extended lymphadenectomy was associated with increased morbidity.

The re-establishment of enteric, biliary and pancreatic continuity requires the construction of three anastomoses; pancreaticojejunostomy, hepaticojejunostomy and gastrojejunostomy for a standard pancreaticoduodenectomy, or duodenojejunostomy for the pylorus-preserving version. These anastomoses are created in a limb of jejunum passed retrocolic and to the right of the middle colic vessels. Diverse variations of the pancreaticojejunostomy exist but generally fall into two categories: invagination or duct to mucosa. The pancreaticojejunostomy is the most prone of the three anastomoses to leak. At our institution a duct to mucosa is most commonly used. This consists of an inner layer of interrupted absorbable suture that approximates the pancreatic duct to the jejunal mucosa. The outer layer imbricates the jejunal serosa onto the surface of the pancreas. The hepaticojejunostomy is fashioned as a single layered anastomosis using interrupted absorbable suture downstream from the pancreaticojejunostomy. The duodenojejunostomy or gastrojejunostomy consists of an inner layer of running absorbable suture and an outer layer of silk Lembert inverting sutures.

Drains are placed in the vicinity of the pancreaticojejunostomy to identify and control leakage from this anastamosis. An additional drain is typically placed in the area of the hepaticojejunostomy.

Distal pancreatectomy

The abdomen is entered though a midline incision and a self-retaining retractor is placed. The abdomen is explored as described for the pancreaticoduodenectomy. Patients with body and tail lesions are more commonly found to have peritoneal spread (M1) disease at the time of surgery. Therefore consideration should be given to performing a laparoscopic exploration prior to laparotomy.

Following exploration the lesser sac is entered by removing the gastrocolic ligament from the transverse colon through the avascular plane using electrocautery. This line of dissection is carried to the descending colon, and the proximal white line of Toldt is lysed. The stomach is further mobilized by dividing the short gastric vessels (vasa brevia). This dissection is carried to the superior pole of the spleen. Once the stomach is fully mobilized it is retracted superiorly along with the omentum to provide wide exposure of the anterior surface of the pancreas. The general location of the tumor should be noted at this point. The peritoneum is divided along the inferior edge of the pancreas using electrocautery. Care is taken to identify and avoid injury of the inferior mesenteric vein (IMV) which joins the splenic vein posterior to the body of the pancreas or less commonly directly joining the SMV.

The splenic artery which sends multiple branches to the superior edge of the pancreas prior to terminating in the spleen is identified and encircled near its origin at the celiac. Once a test clamp is performed and preservation of flow to the hepatic artery is confirmed the splenic artery is divided. The splenic artery stump should be further secured with a non-absorbable suture ligature. After medially retracting the spleen toward the spine electrocautery is used to incise the peritoneal reflection starting at the previously made incision at the inferior edge of the pancreas and extending this incision laterally and superiorly to finally meet up with the site of transection of the splenic artery. The spleen and tail of the pancreas are mobilized out of the retroperitoneum using electrocautery or sharp dissection. Care must be taken to remain anterior to the left adrenal gland and Gerota's fascia of the left kidney. The splenic vein is intimately involved with the pancreas laterally. Once the junction of the IMV is reached, the splenic vein can usually be separated from the pancreatic parenchyma and divided lateral to this junction. If the lesion is in the body of the pancreas, it may necessary to divide the splenic vein near its junction with the SMV–PV confluence. Transection of the pancreas can be accomplished with a knife, electocautery, linear stapler or harmonic scalpel. The development of a postoperative pancreatic fistula may occur in up to 25% of patients. Only direct ligation of the pancreatic duct and the perioperative use of octreotide have been shown to reduce the rate of postoperative pancreatic fistulas. If a stapler is not used to transect the pancreas the remnant is oversewn in two layers with absorbable suture. A surgical drain is placed before closure in order to identify and control a pancreatic fistula.

Cancer of the body of the pancreas can be the most difficult lesion to manage surgically. By virtue of this location extension superiorly beyond the pancreas often results in involvement of the celiac trunk, common hepatic artery and base of the splenic artery at its take-off from the celiac trunk. Growth slightly to the right and posterior will involve the medial wall of the PV or SMV and may also infiltrate the junction of the splenic vein with the PV–SMV confluence. In these patients, considerable complexity is added to a distal pancreatectomy. The determination of resectability in these patients is based on the extent of involvement of the celiac axis. Therefore dissection should begin at the common hepatic artery and be carried toward the celiac axis. If a clear margin is achievable then the tumor is resectable. Involvement of the PV–SMV may require *en bloc* resection and portal vein reconstruction to achieve a negative margin.

Surgical palliation

The majority of patients diagnosed with pancreatic cancer will not be candidates for a curative resection; 50% will have metastatic disease and 20% will have locally advanced cancers. In these patients the goal of all interventions is the improvement of quality of life. The symptoms amenable to surgical interventions include (i) obstructive jaundice, (ii) duodenal obstruction, and (iii) intractable cancer-associated pain. The importance of surgery for the management of these symptoms has diminished with the emergence of effective non-operative alternatives. In certain subsets of patients operative intervention continues to provide the most effective means of palliation. For a comprehensive review of palliation for patients with periampullary cancers see Lillemoe (1998), Yeo *et al.* (2002), House & Choti (2004), and Koninger *et al.* (2007).

Prolonged obstructive jaundice is associated with significant sequelae that interfere with quality of life and may actually shorten an already reduced life-span. Severe pruritus, malabsorption diarrhea and malnutrition may result from distal biliary tract obstruction. Prolonged biliary stasis can also lead to bouts of cholangitis and hepatic failure. The appropriate treatment of obstructive jaundice depends on the clinical circumstances. In patients that are clearly not candidates for curative resection non-operative measures should be considered as the primary mode of therapy. This can be accomplished by the placement of endoprosthetic or percutaneous biliary stents. An endoscopic stent should be attempted as the first-line therapy since it carries a high chance of successful placement and is effective in biliary decompression without the need for an external catheter (Lichtenstein & Carr-Locke 1995; Arguedas *et al.* 2002). There are two general types of stents: silastic endoprosthetic stents and permanent metallic wallstents. Endoprosthetic stents are often placed at the time of initial management of jaundice prior to the determination of resectability. In patients that are subsequently found to be unresectable these stents tend to malfunction over time as a result of occlusion. Therefore in patients undergoing endoscopic biliary decompression in the setting of known unresectable disease a wallstent may provide a longer period of patency. It should be noted that the placement of a wallstent does not preclude an attempt at a curative resection (Mullen *et al.* 2005). This situation is often seen at major referral centers in which a patient was thought to be unresectable by inadequate staging at the primary institution.

In 10% of jaundiced patients endoscopic biliary decompression is unsuccessful. This is often the case with large bulky primary tumors that invade the duodenum (House & Choti 2004). In these patients percutaneous transhepatic cholangiography and external biliary drainage is an alternative. In many cases the interventional radiologist is able to cross the obstruction into the duodenum with the stent thus allowing internal drainage of biliary secretions. If this is not possible bile is drained externally. Although this will result in resolution of jaundice it does not correct the problem of malabsorption and malnutrition. As with endoscopic biliary decompression, the percutaneous approach can be used to place a biliary wallstent.

The main indication for surgical biliary decompression is in patients found to have unresectable disease at laparotomy. Patients found to have unresectable disease at laparotomy that are felt to have at least a 6-month life expectancy as a result of minimal or no metastatic disease should be considered for biliary bypass (House & Choti 2004). The benefit of surgical bypass is less certain in patients that are felt to have less than 6 months' survival based on the extent of disease. Many of these patients are likely to already have stents in place which will provide adequate palliation for the remainder of their life. Biliary bypass in this setting is surgeon dependent and may depend on the anticipated difficulty of dissection of the porta hepatis. Surgical biliary decompression is accomplished by either a roux-en-Y or loop gastrojejenostomy.

Approximately 20% of patients may have impingement of the duodenum by pancreatic cancer that results in significant duodenal obstruction at the time of diagnosis (Lillemoe 1998). The effectiveness of endoscopic therapy in these patients is not well established. Patients with significant comorbidities making surgery prohibitive or those with a life expectancy of 3–6 months may be considered for placement of duodenal wallstent. However, very little data exist on the long-term effectiveness of this intervention. In our practice patients found to be unresectable at laparotomy undergo an isoperistalitic loop gastrojejenostomy 30–40 cm distal to the ligament of Treitz. This adds no additional morbidity or mortality over that of a laparotomy (Lillemoe *et al.* 1999). Patients with known unresectable disease with symptomatic duodenal obstruction corroborated by contrast fluoroscopy should undergo a surgical gastrojejunostomy if they are expected to have significant life expectancy and are able to tolerate anesthesia.

Despite the notion that pancreatic cancer most often presents as painless jaundice, at least 80% of patients will have significant cancer-associated pain throughout the course of their disease. This is often manageable through aggressive use of medical management. In addition, patients with pain refractory to this type of management are well served by percutaneous celiac plexus block. In patients found unresectable at laparotomy celiac plexus block (chemical splenectomy) has been shown to significantly reduce cancer-associated pain in a prospective randomized trial (Lillemoe *et al.* 1993). This effect appears to last the life of the patient. Interestingly, this same trial demonstrated that patients with significant preoperative pain were actually found to have a significant increase in survival.

Complications

Through the 1970s, the mortality rate associated with pancreaticoduodenectomies was as high as 30%. This has been reduced to less than 2% over the subsequent three decades (Winter *et al.* 2006). However, the morbidity rate associated with pancreaticoduodenectomy has remained between 30% and 45%, even at institutions where the procedure is performed regularly. As reported in a recent analysis of 1423 patients undergoing pancreaticoduodenectomy for pancreatic cancer at the Johns Hopkins Hospital, the most common postoperative morbid complication is delayed gastric emptying (DGE), occurring in 15% of patients, followed by wound infection (8%), pancreatic fistula (5%), cardiac morbidity (4%), abdominal abscess (4%), cholangitis (2%), sepsis (2%), bile leak (2%) and several other complications occurring in less than 2% of patients.

Outcomes

While mortality rates associated with pancreatic cancer resection have improved dramatically over the past three decades, improvements in long-term outcomes have been less clear. Surgical resection with the intent to cure is currently the only long-term survival option for patients with pancreatic adenocarcinoma. Pancreatic resection and pancreaticoduodenectomy are highly effective modes of treatment for the various non-adenocarcinoma tumors of the pancreas and distal biliary tree; however, several considerations must be taken with pancreatic adenocarcinoma.

A margin-negative resection is achieved in 60–80% of operations (Neoptolemos *et al.* 2001; Richter *et al.* 2003; Wagner *et al.* 2004; Winter *et al.* 2006). However, while these patients are considered cleared of all known disease, their long-term survival remains poor. Even in the setting of margin-negative resections (R0 resections), the 5-year survival rate is 25%, and the 10-year survival rate is less than 10% (Richter *et al.* 2003). Studies correlating lymph node status with survival reveal that survival is improved for lymph node-negative patients. Wagner *et al.* report a median survival time of 26 months in lymph node-negative patients as compared to 16 months in lymph node-positive patients (Wagner *et al.* 2004). However, it should be noted that there is a wide range in survival times in both patient populations.

The subset of patients with the most favorable outcome are those with tumors less than 2–3 cm in diameter and with lymph nodes negative for disease (Wagner *et al.* 2004). While this constitutes approximately one-third of all patients undergoing surgery for pancreatic adenocarcinoma, this proportion is increasing over time, suggesting that more patients are being detected at an earlier stage (Winter *et al.* 2006). Other factors associated with improved prognosis include R0 resection and moderately to well-differentiated tumor grades.

Selective studies do report an improvement in overall survival of patients receiving treatment for pancreatic cancer over recent decades. In the largest single-institution series to date, that of the Johns Hopkins Hospital constituting 1423 patients undergoing pancreaticoduodenectomies for pancreatic cancer, the 2-year survival rate for the 2000s is 42%, as compared to 35% during the 1990s. However, since the 1990s, the 5-year survival for patients who underwent surgery for pancreatic cancer, with and without perioperative chemotherapy, has remained at 20% (Winter *et al.* 2006).

References

American Joint Committee on Cancer (2002) Exocrine pancreas. In: *AJCC Staging Manual*, 6th edn. Springer, New York.

Arguedas MR, Heudebert GH, Stinnett AA, Wilcox CM. (2002) Biliary stents in malignant obstructive jaundice due to pancreatic carcinoma: a cost-effectiveness analysis. *Am J Gastroenterol* 97(4): 898–904.

Birkmeyer JD, Finlayson SR, Tosteson AN, Sharp SM, Warshaw AL, Fisher ES. (1999) Effect of hospital volume on in-hospital mortality with pancreaticoduodenectomy. *Surgery* 125(3): 250–6.

Brennan MF. (1993) Cancer of the pancreas. In: DeVita V, ed. *Principles and Practice of Oncology*, 5th edn, pp. 849–82. J.B. Lippencott, Philadelphia.

Conlon KC, Brennan MF. (2000) Laparoscopy for staging abdominal malignancies. *Adv Surg* 34: 331–50.

Conlon KC, Dougherty E, Klimstra DS, Coit DG, Turnbull AD, Brennan MF. (1996) The value of minimal access surgery in the staging of patients with potentially resectable peripancreatic malignancy. *Ann Surg* 223(2): 134–40.

Diederichs CG, Staib L, Vogel J *et al.* (2000) Values and limitations of 18F-fluorodeoxyglucose-positron-emission tomography with pre-operative evaluation of patients with pancreatic masses. *Pancreas* 20(2): 109–16.

Friess H, Kleeff J, Silva JC, Sadowski C, Baer HU, Buchler MW. (1998) The role of diagnostic laparoscopy in pancreatic and periampullary malignancies. *J Am Coll Surg* 186(6): 675–82.

Gress FG, Hawes RH, Savides TJ *et al.* (1999) Role of EUS in the preoperative staging of pancreatic cancer: a large single-center experience. *Gastrointest Endosc* 50(6): 786–91.

House MG, Choti MA. (2004) Palliative therapy for pancreatic/biliary cancer. *Surg Oncol Clin N Am* 13(3): 491–503.

House MG, Yeo CJ, Cameron JL *et al.* (2004) Predicting resectability of periampullary cancer with three-dimensional computed tomography. *J Gastrointest Surg* 8(3): 280–8.

Jimenez RE, Warshaw AL, Rattner DW, Willett CG, McGrath D, Fernandez-del CC. (2000) Impact of laparoscopic staging in the treatment of pancreatic cancer. *Arch Surg* 135(4): 409–14.

Karachristos A, Scarmeas N, Hoffman JP. (2005) CA 19–9 levels predict results of staging laparoscopy in pancreatic cancer. *J Gastrointest Surg* 9(9): 1286–92.

Karpoff HM, Klimstra DS, Brennan MF, Conlon KC. (2001) Results of total pancreatectomy for adenocarcinoma of the pancreas. *Arch Surg* 136(1): 44–7.

Koninger J, Wente MN, Muller MW, Gutt CN, Friess H, Buchler MW. (2007) Surgical palliation in patients with pancreatic cancer. Langenbecks *Arch Surg* 392(1): 13–21.

Lichtenstein DR, Carr-Locke DL. (1995) Endoscopic palliation for unresectable pancreatic carcinoma. *Surg Clin North Am* 75(5): 969–88.

Lillemoe KD. (1998) Palliative therapy for pancreatic cancer. *Surg Oncol Clin N Am* 7(1): 199–216.

Lillemoe KD, Cameron JL, Kaufman HS, Yeo CJ, Pitt HA, Sauter PK. (1993) Chemical splanchnicectomy in patients with unresectable pancreatic cancer. A prospective randomized trial. *Ann Surg* 217(5): 447–55.

Lillemoe KD, Cameron JL, Hardacre JM *et al.* (1999) Is prophylactic gastrojejunostomy indicated for unresectable periampullary cancer? A prospective randomized trial. *Ann Surg* 230(3): 322–8.

Loyer EM, David CL, Dubrow RA, Evans DB, Charnsangavej C. (1996) Vascular involvement in pancreatic adenocarcinoma: reassessment by thin-section CT. *Abdom Imaging* 21(3): 202–6.

Lu DS, Reber HA, Krasny RM, Kadell BM, Sayre J. (1997) Local staging of pancreatic cancer: criteria for unresectability of major vessels as revealed by pancreatic-phase, thin-section helical CT. *AJR Am J Roentgenol* 168(6): 1439–43.

Megibow AJ, Zhou XH, Rotterdam H *et al.* (1995) Pancreatic adenocarcinoma: CT versus MR imaging in the evaluation of resectability—report of the Radiology Diagnostic Oncology Group. *Radiology* 195(2): 327–32.

Mullen JT, Lee JH, Gomez HF *et al.* (2005) Pancreaticoduodenectomy after placement of endobiliary metal stents. *J Gastrointest Surg* 9(8): 1094–1104.

Neoptolemos JP, Stocken DD, Dunn JA *et al.* (2001) Influence of resection margins on survival for patients with pancreatic cancer treated by adjuvant chemoradiation and/or chemotherapy in the ESPAC-1 randomized controlled trial. *Ann Surg* 234(6): 758–68.

O'Malley ME, Boland GW, Wood BJ, Fernandez-del CC, Warshaw AL, Mueller PR. (1999) Adenocarcinoma of the head of the pancreas: determination of surgical unresectability with thin-section pancreatic-phase helical CT. *AJR Am J Roentgenol* 173(6): 1513–18.

Pisters PW, Hudec WA, Hess KR *et al.* (2001a) Effect of preoperative biliary decompression on pancreaticoduodenectomy-associated morbidity in 300 consecutive patients. *Ann Surg* 234(1): 47–55.

Pisters PW, Lee JE, Vauthey JN, Charnsangavej C, Evans DB. (2001b) Laparoscopy in the staging of pancreatic cancer. *Br J Surg* 88(3): 325–37.

Povoski SP, Karpeh MS Jr, Conlon KC, Blumgart LH, Brennan MF. (1999) Association of preoperative biliary drainage with postoperative outcome following pancreaticoduodenectomy. *Ann Surg* 230(2): 131–42.

Richter A, Niedergethmann M, Sturm JW, Lorenz D, Post S, Trede M. (2003) Long-term results of partial pancreaticoduodenectomy for ductal adenocarcinoma of the pancreatic head: 25-year experience. *World J Surg* 27(3): 324–9.

Roche CJ, Hughes ML, Garvey CJ *et al.* (2003) CT and pathologic assessment of prospective nodal staging in patients with ductal adenocarcinoma of the head of the pancreas. *AJR Am J Roentgenol* 180(2): 475–80.

Rose DM, Delbeke D, Beauchamp RD *et al.* (1999) 18-Fluorodeoxyglucose-positron emission tomography in the management of patients with suspected pancreatic cancer. *Ann Surg* 229(5): 729–37.

Sarr MG, Behrns KE, van Heerden JA. (1993) Total pancreatectomy. An objective analysis of its use in pancreatic cancer. *Hepatogastroenterology* 40(5): 418–21.

Sheridan MB, Ward J, Guthrie JA *et al.* (1999) Dynamic contrast-enhanced MR imaging and dual-phase helical CT in the preoperative assessment of suspected pancreatic cancer: a comparative study with receiver operating characteristic analysis. *AJR Am J Roentgenol* 173(3): 583–90.

Sohn TA, Yeo CJ, Cameron JL *et al.* (2000a) Resected adenocarcinoma of the pancreas-616 patients: results, outcomes, and prognostic indicators. *J Gastrointest Surg* 4(6): 567–79.

Sohn TA, Yeo CJ, Cameron JL, Pitt HA, Lillemoe KD. (2000b) Do preoperative biliary stents increase postpancreaticoduodenectomy complications? *J Gastrointest Surg* 4(3): 258–67.

Steinberg WM, Barkin J, Bradley EL, III, Dimagno E, Layer P. (1998) Workup of a patient with a mass in the head of the pancreas. *Pancreas* 17(1): 24–30.

Tseng JF, Raut CP, Lee JE *et al.* (2004) Pancreaticoduodenectomy with vascular resection: margin status and survival duration. *J Gastrointest Surg* 8(8): 935–49.

Varadarajulu S, Wallace MB. (2004) Applications of endoscopic ultrasonography in pancreatic cancer. *Cancer Control* 11(1): 15–22.

Wagner M, Redaelli C, Lietz M, Seiler CA, Friess H, Buchler MW. (2004) Curative resection is the single most important factor determining outcome in patients with pancreatic adenocarcinoma. *Br J Surg* 91(5): 586–94.

Wenger FA, Peter F, Zieren J, Steiert A, Jacobi CA, Muller JM. (2000) Prognosis factors in carcinoma of the head of the pancreas. *Dig Surg* 17(1): 29–35.

Whipple AO. (1963) A reminiscence: pancreaticduodenectomy. *Rev Surg* 20: 221–5.

Willett CG, Lewandrowski K, Warshaw AL, Efird J, Compton CC. (1993) Resection margins in carcinoma of the head of the pancreas. Implications for radiation therapy. *Ann Surg* 217(2): 144–8.

Winter JM, Cameron JL, Campbell KA *et al.* (2006) 1423 pancreaticoduodenectomies for pancreatic cancer: A single-institution experience. *J Gastrointest Surg* 10(9): 1199–1210.

Yeo CJ, Cameron JL, Lillemoe KD *et al.* (2002) Pancreaticoduodenectomy with or without distal gastrectomy and extended retroperitoneal lymphadenectomy for periampullary adenocarcinoma, part 2: randomized controlled trial evaluating survival, morbidity, and mortality. *Ann Surg* 236(3): 355–66.

Chemotherapy

Daniel Laheru

Introduction

There is unfortunately no universally accepted standard treatment for resected or advanced pancreatic cancer. This section will describe the current treatment recommendations as well as highlight the most recent treatment advances for resected and advanced disease.

Therapy for adjuvant disease

The current standard of 5-fluorouracil (5-FU)-based combined modality chemoradiotherapy is originally based on data from the Gastrointestinal Tumor Study Group (GITSG). This study was the first to document that adjuvant therapy following surgical resection for pancreatic surgery prolonged survival (Kalser & Ellenberg 1985).

A number of groups have further developed this approach and have generally utilized 5-FU-based chemotherapy (Kalser & Ellenberg 1985; Klinkenbijl *et al.* 1999; Neoptolemos *et al.* 2001; Picozzi *et al.* 2003; Regine *et al.* 2006) (Table 21.3).

Recently the Virginia Mason Medical Center published their experience of 53 patients with resected pancreatic adenocarcinoma who received combined radiotherapy (external beam at

Table 21.3 Selected adjuvant studies in pancreatic cancer.

Adjuvant study	Number of patients	EBRT dose (Gy)	Chemotherapy	Median survival (mo)	1-year survival	2-year survival	5-year survival
GITSG (1985)	22 pts surgery alone	None	None	11	49%	15%	NR
(Kalser & Ellenberg, 1985)	21 pts to chemorad	40 split course	5-FU bolus	20 p = 0.01	63%	42%	NR
RTOG 9704 (2006)	270 pts 5-FU based chemo	54	5-FU	16.9	NR	NR	N/A
(Regine *et al.* 2006)	288 pts gemzar based chemo	54	Gem	20.3 p = 0.03	NR	NR	N/A
Picozzi (2003)	53	45–50	5-FU CI with cisplatin and IFN-alpha	46	88%	53%	49%
EORTC (1999)	54 pts surgery alone	None	None	12.6	40% (est)	23%	10%
(Klinkenbijl *et al.* 1999)	60 pts chemorad	40	5-FU bolus	17.1 p = 0.099	65% (est)	37%	20%
ESPAC1 (2001)	200 pts surgery alone	None	None	16.1	N/A	N/A	NR
(Neoptolemos *et al.* 2001)	103 pts chemorad	40 split course	None	15.5	N/A	N/A	NR
	166 pts chemo alone	none	5-FU bolus	19.7	60% (est)	39% (est)	16% (est)
	72 pts chemorad with additional chemo	40 split course	5-FU bolus	N/A	N/A	N/A	NR

a dose of 45–54 Gy in standard fractions d1–35) and chemotherapy (5-FU 200 mg/m^2/day as continuous infusion, weekly cisplatin 30 mg/m^2 intravenous bolus, interferon-alpha 3 million units SQ every other day) during radiation or GITSG-type chemotherapy with radiation therapy. Following combined-modality chemoradiotherapy, chemotherapy alone was administered (5-FU 200 mg/m^2/day as continuous infusion) in two 6-week courses during weeks 9–14 and 17–22. There were significant grade III/IV gastrointestinal toxicities including vomiting, mucositis, diarrhea and gastrointestinal bleeding in the interferon-based chemotherapy requiring hospitalization in 43% of patients. However, the majority of patients were still able to receive > 80% of planned therapy. The median survival and 2-year survival were 46 months and 53% respectively for the interferon-based chemoradiotherapy (Picozzi *et al.* 2003). The American College of Surgery Oncology Group (ACOSOG) has recently completed a multi-institutional phase II study to test this regimen in patients with pancreatic adenocarcinoma who are candidates for resection. We are awaiting the final results.

The Radiation Therapy Oncology Group (RTOG) recently reported on a phase III study of 518 resected pancreatic cancer patients randomized to either 5-FU continuous infusion (250 mg/m^2/day for 3 weeks), followed by 5-FU continuous infusion (250 mg/m^2/day) during radiation therapy (50.4 Gy in 1.8-Gy fractions), followed by two cycles of 5-FU continuous infusion, versus gemcitabine 1000 mg/m^2 weekly × 3, followed by 5-FU continuous infusion during radiation therapy, followed by three cycles gemcitabine alone (Regine *et al.* 2006). While there was a higher incidence of grade III or IV neutropenia for patients in the gemcitabine arm, the median survival was 20.3 months for gemcitabine-treated patients versus 16.3 months for 5-FU-treated patients ($p = 0.03$) (Regine *et al.* 2006).

However, adjuvant chemoradiation has not been universally accepted as standard of care. One of the criticisms has been that none of these studies included an observation-only arm. There have been two major studies that have demonstrated contrasting conclusions.

A European Organization for Research and Treatment of Cancer (EORTC) trial randomized 218 patients with pancreatic and non-pancreatic periampullary adenocarcinoma 2–8 weeks following potentially curative resection to either observation or to combined radiotherapy (40 Gy using a 3- or 4-field technique in 2-Gy fractions with a 2-week break at mid-treatment) and chemotherapy (5-FU administered as a continuous infusion 25 mg/kg/day during first week of each 2-week radiation therapy module only) (Klinkenbijl *et al.* 1999). No postradiation chemotherapy was administered. Median progression-free survival was 16 months in the observation arm versus 17.4 months in the treatment arm ($p = 0.643$). Median survival was 19 months in the observation group versus 24.5 months in the treatment group, but was not statistically significant ($p = 0.737$). For the subgroup of patients with pancreatic adenocarcinoma ($n = 114$), the median survival was 12.6 months in the observation group versus 17.1 months in the treatment arm but was not statistically significant ($p = 0.099$). Therefore, this study could be better described as an underpowered positive study (Klinkenbijl *et al.*1999) .

Recently, the European Study Group for Pancreatic Cancer (ESPAC) randomized 541 patients with pancreatic adenocarcinoma in a four-arm design based on a two-by-two factorial design:

(a) observation

(b) concomitant chemoradiotherapy alone: 20 Gy in 10 fractions over 2 weeks with 500 mg/m^2 5-FU intravenous bolus during the first 3 days of radiation therapy (Neoptolemos *et al.* 2001); the module is repeated after a planned 2-week break followed by no additional chemotherapy

(c) chemotherapy alone (leucovorin 20 mg/m^2 bolus followed by 5-FU 425 mg/m^2 administered for 5 consecutive days repeated every 28 days for 6 cycles)

(d) chemoradiotherapy followed by chemotherapy (Neoptolemos *et al.* 2001).

There was no significant difference in survival between patients assigned to chemoradiotherapy (median survival 15.5 months) versus observation (median survival 16.1 months, $p = 0.24$). The survival data were similar in the subset ($n = 285$ patients) randomized through the two-by-two design. In contrast, there was a survival advantage for those patients treated with chemotherapy alone (median survival 19.7 months) versus the observation arm (median survival 14 months, $p = 0.0005$). For the same subset randomized through the original two-by-two design, survival demonstrated a trend towards survival for chemotherapy alone (median survival 17.4 months) versus observation alone (15.9 months) but was not statistically significant ($p = 0.19$). Multivariate analysis for known prognostic factors including margin status, lymph node involvement, tumor grade and size did not alter the effect for chemoradiotherapy treatment. The study authors concluded that there was no survival benefit for adjuvant chemoradiotherapy. In addition, the authors concluded that a potential benefit existed for adjuvant chemotherapy alone following surgical resection (Neoptolemos *et al.* 2001).

While this was a randomized study consisting of over 500 patients, the conclusions of the study should be carefully measured. In order to encourage maximal patient recruitment, the study was modified in that 68 patients were assigned separately and randomized to either chemoradiotherapy or observation. In addition, 188 patients were subsequently assigned separately and randomized to either chemotherapy alone or observation. In a sense, three randomizations were possible for inclusion into the same study. Also, patients in the additional two randomizations could have potentially received 'background chemotherapy or chemotherapy' which was not specifically defined. The background treatment was not known in 82 eligible patients. Of note, these patients were still assigned into an arm of the study despite lack of definitive knowledge of prior therapy.

Finally, 25 of the eligible 541 patients refused to accept their randomization and an additional 25 patients withdrew secondary to treatment toxicities.

As the debate continues, there are several studies that have recently opened or have been proposed by either the cooperative groups or through single institutions. These future studies will be characterized by the addition of multiagent chemotherapy to irradiation at the co-operative group level, by the addition of gemcitabine to the period of chemoradiation, and by the use of conformal, 3D-planned irradiation planned to patient-specific anatomic and surgical pathologic data.

Role of neoadjuvant therapy

Neoadjuvant therapy is a potentially attractive alternative to current standard adjuvant chemoradiation for several reasons: (i) radiation is more effective on well-oxygenated cells that have not been devascularized by surgery; (ii) contamination and subsequent seeding of the peritoneum with tumor cells secondary to surgery could theoretically be reduced; (iii) patients with metastatic disease on restaging following adjuvant therapy would not need to undergo definitive resection and might benefit from palliative intervention; (iv) the risk of delaying adjuvant therapy would be eliminated since it would be delivered in the neoadjuvant setting.

There are significant published data primarily from M.D. Anderson Cancer Center and Fox Chase Cancer Center using chemoradiotherapy in a neoadjuvant approach for resectable pancreas cancer. To date, the current data demonstrate that while neoadjuvant chemoradiotherapy can be administered safely, there is no clear advantage to this strategy compared to postoperative therapy. In patients with marginally resectable disease, it remains to be seen whether there is a meaningful cohort of patients for whom this approach may represent an important therapeutic advantage based on 'downstaging' and improved surgical outcomes.

Treatment of advanced disease

In patients with metastatic disease, the current standard of care is single-agent gemcitabine. Burris and colleagues randomized 126 patients with unresectable pancreatic cancer to either gemcitabine (1000 mg/m^2 weekly over a 30-min infusion ×7 followed by 1 week rest then weekly ×3 every 4 weeks) or 5-FU (600 mg/m^2 weekly). Although the primary endpoints were issues related to quality of life (performance status, weight gain, analgesic consumption and pain), median survival was 5.7 months in the gemcitabine arm compared to 4.4 months in the 5-FU arm (Burris *et al.* 1997). In addition, 1-year survival was 18% in the gemcitabine arm compared to 2% in the 5-FU arm ($p = 0.0025$) with median time to progression also favoring gemcitabine (9 weeks compared to 4 weeks in the 5-FU arm, $p = 0.0002$). Gemcitabine was well tolerated, with the majority of side-effects related to grade III or IV neutropenia (26%) without associated infections, low-grade fevers (30%), and nausea and vomiting (9.5% and 3.2%) (Burris *et al.* 1997). Based on this study, gemcitabine was approved for the treatment of patients with advanced pancreatic cancer in the USA and many other countries and is currently considered the standard agent for the treatment of this disease as well as the accepted control with which to compare new drugs and interventions.

Recent efforts have focused on developing strategies that would enhance the efficacy of gemcitabine and ultimately improve on median survival. These strategies include identifying alternative dosing schedules of gemcitabine that might both enhance drug delivery to tumor cells as well as identifying synergistic combinations with other chemotherapeutic agents. Tempero and colleagues randomized 92 patients to either gemcitabine (2200 mg/m^2) over the standard 30-min infusion or gemcitabine (1500 mg/m^2) at a rate of 10 mg/m^2/min. Patients on the fixed-dose rate had a higher response rate (11.6 vs. 4.1%), median survival (8 months vs. 5 months, $p = 0.013$) and 1-year survival (23.8% vs. 7.3%) than patients treated on the

Table 21.4 Selected studies in advanced pancreatic cancer.

Study	Patient no.	Chemotherapy	PR/CR rate	Median survival (mo)		1-year survival
Burris (1997)	63	5-FU bolus	0 (0%)	4.4		2%
	63	Gemcitabine	3 (5.4%)	5.7	p = 0.0025	18%
Tempero (2003)	49	Gem standard infusion	2 of 22 (9.1%)	5		9%
	43	Gem fixed infusion	1 of 17 (5.9%)	8	p = 0.013	28.8%
Moore (2005)	260	Gem	8.7	5.9		20%
	261	Gem+erlotinib	7.9	6.4	p = 0.025	26%
Cunningham (2005)	266	Gem	7%	6		19%
	267	Gem+capecitabine	14%	7.4	p = 0.025	26%
ECOG 6201 (2006)	279	Gem	5%	4.9		17%
	277	Gem FDR	10%	6		21%
	276	Gem + oxaliplatin	9%	5.9		21%

conventional schedule (Tempero *et al.* 2003). This strategy was recently tested in a phase III study of 832 patients with advanced disease randomized to gemcitabine alone at standard dose and infusion, gemcitabine at fixed-dose infusion and gemcitabine at fixed-dose infusion and oxaliplatin. Unfortunately, the overall survival was similar for all three arms (Poplin *et al.* 2006).

Other potentially synergistic agents that have been used with gemcitabine include small molecule targets such as the oral tyrosine kinase inhibitor erlotinib. A recent phase III study of 569 patients treated with gemcitabine alone or with gemcitabine and erlotinib (100 mg/day) demonstrated a survival benefit (6.4 months vs. 5.9 months, $p = 0.025$) with improvement in 1-year survival (26% vs. 20%) in favor of gemcitabine + erlotinib although the clinical significance has been questioned (Moore *et al.* 2005). While erlotinib was approved in the USA in November 2005, it is not approved in Europe. Also, a phase III study of 569 patients randomized to gemcitabine plus capecitabine versus gemcitabine alone demonstrated a survival advantage for the combination over gemcitabine as a single agent (7.4 months vs. 6 months, $p = 0.05$) (Cunningham *et al.* 2005).

New drugs in pancreatic cancer

During the last few years, an increasing number of new drugs, many of them targeted to specific alterations in malignant cells, have been tested in pancreatic cancer. The rationale to develop these drugs in pancreatic cancer comes from the better understanding of the biologic basis of the disease that have made possible the identification and validation of some of these targets in pancreatic cancer. To date, targeted drugs such as the matrix metalloproteinase inhibitors (marimastat and Bay12-9566), inhibitors of angiogenesis (bevacizumab), agents targeted to the Ras oncogene (R115777 and lonafarnib), and inhibitors of the EGFR family of membrane receptors (trastuzumab [Herceptin], cetuximab), immunotherapy and gene therapy have been evaluated in this patient population with mixed results.

In summary, gemcitabine is currently the only internationally approved chemotherapeutic agent that has demonstrated significant antitumor effects in advanced pancreatic cancer. Although the efficacy of gemcitabine may be augmented by innovative dosing schedules or by the use of synergistic drug combinations such as erlotinib, the standard regimen to date remains single-agent gemcitabine. Combinations of gemcitabine with other agents including cisplatin, irinotecan, oxaliplatin, bevacizumab, and fluoropyrimidines have not consistently resulted in significant improvement in survival or quality of life in studies available thus far and should not be considered standard of care at the present time though this could change as the result of randomized studies are available. Given the data with conventional treatments, enrolment in a clinical trial should still be the preferred approach for these patients.

References

Burris HA, Moore MJ, Anderson J *et al.* (1997) Improvements in survival and clinical benefit with gemcitabine as first-line therapy for patients with advanced pancreas cancer: a randomized trial. *J Clin Oncol* 15(6): 2403–13.

Cunningham D, Chau I, Stockten D *et al.* (2005) Phase III randomized comparison of gemcitabine versus gemcitabine plus capecitabine in patients with advanced pancreatic cancer. *Eur J Cancer* 34: 4.

Kalser MH, Ellenberg SS. (1985) Pancreatic cancer: adjuvant combined radiation and chemotherapy following curative resection. *Arch Surg* 120: 899–903.

Klinkenbijl JH, Jeekel J, Sahmoud T *et al.* (1999) Adjuvant radiotherapy and 5-Fluorouracil after curative resection of cancer of the pancreas and periampullary region. *Ann Surg* 230(6): 776–84.

Moore MJ, Goldstein D, Hamm J *et al.* (2005) Erlotinib plus gemcitabine compared to gemcitabine alone in patients with advanced pancreatic cancer. A phase III trial of the National Cancer Institute of Canada Clinical Trials Group (NCIC-CTG). *Proc ASCO* 23: 1s: abstract 1.

Neoptolemos JP, Dunn JA, Stocken DD *et al.* (2001) Adjuvant chemoradiotherapy and chemotherapy in resectable pancreatic cancer: a randomized controlled trial. *Lancet* 358: 1576–85.

Picozzi VJ, Kozarek RE, Traverso LW. (2003) Interferon-based adjuvant chemoradiation therapy after pancreaticoduodenectomy for pancreatic adenocarcinoma. *Am J Surg* 185: 476–80.

Poplin, E, Levy D, Berlin J *et al.* (2006) Phase III trial of gemcitabine (30 minute infusion) versus gemcitabine (fixed dose rate) versus gemcitabine + oxaliplatin in patients with advanced pancreatic cancer. *Proc ASCO* 24: 180S: late breaking abstract 4.

Regine WF, Winter KW, Abrams R *et al.* (2006) RTOG 9704 a phase III study of adjuvant pre-and post chemoradiation 5FU versus gemcitabine for resected pancreatic adenocarcinoma. *Proc ASCO* 24: 180s: abstract 4007.

Tempero M, Plunkett W, van Haperan VR *et al.* (2003) Randomized phase II comparison of dose-intense Gemcitabine: thirty-minute infusion and fixed dose rate infusion in patients with pancreatic adenocarcinoma. *J Clin Oncol* 21(18): 1–7.

Radiotherapy

Joseph Herman

Background

Radiation treatment recommendations differ for resectable, borderline resectable, unresectable, and metastatic pancreatic cancer (www.nccn.org). The standard of care and only potentially curative treatment for resectable pancreatic cancer is surgery (Cameron *et al.* 2006). Since both local and systemic recurrences are common after resection of pancreatic cancer, adjuvant treatment is indicated for these patients (Foo *et al.* 1993). Whether patients should receive adjuvant chemoradiation (CRT) or chemotherapy alone is currently controversial (Garofalo *et al.* 2006). Several US trials have demonstrated a survival advantage with the use of adjuvant CRT after definitive surgery (Gastrointestinal Tumor Study Group 1987; Kalser *et al.* 1985). Trials in Europe have not confirmed a survival benefit favoring CRT, and some European studies suggest a detriment in survival with CRT compared with chemotherapy alone (Neoptolemos *et al.* 2004). Ongoing and future clinical trials should serve to optimize adjuvant therapy after curative resection for pancreatic cancer.

Recent studies suggest neoadjuvant CRT in resectable patients increases the proportion of patients receiving CRT and undergoing R0 resections when compared to adjuvant CRT (Crane *et al.* 2006b). Patients with borderline resectable or unresectable pancreatic cancer are often treated with chemoradiation or more recently, chemotherapy alone. Advances in the delivery of radiation therapy allow for dose escalation and sparing of normal tissues which may lead to improved outcomes (Ben-Josef *et al.* 2004). Although little progress has been made in the past 30 years for this commonly fatal disease, immunotherapy, novel chemotherapeutic agents, and targeted therapies offer new promise (Picozzi *et al.* 2003; Laheru *et al.* 2005a; Crane *et al.* 2006a).

Radiation therapy methods

The majority of trials discussed in this section utilize standard fractionated (1.8–2.0-Gy) external-beam radiation therapy (EBRT) delivered either continuously (daily over 5–6 weeks) or in a split course (2-week break during radiation). The advent of 3D conformal radiation (3DRT) and intensity-modulated radiation therapy (IMRT) allows for more specific irradiation to the tumor/tumor bed and lymph nodes while limiting the dose to normal structures including the kidneys, liver, and bowel (Ben-Josef *et al.* 2004). Treatment with IMRT appears to result in decreased toxicity and improved quality of life compared with conventional treatment methods (Milano *et al.* 2004). Because of these advances, split-course radiation has been abandoned and efforts have been made to shorten the course of radiation by hypofractionation (increasing the daily dose of radiation). M.D. Anderson has reported that 30 Gy delivered over 10 treatments has equivalent efficacy to conventional radiation delivered over 5–6 weeks (50.4 Gy) for palliation of locally advanced disease (Wong *et al.* 2005).

Stereotactic body radiation therapy (SBRT) delivers high single-dose fractions (15–25 Gy) of radiation to the pancreatic tumor. Used alone or as a boost to conventional chemoradiation, SBRT appears to be safe; however long-term toxicity is unknown (Koong *et al.* 2004, 2005). Intraoperative radiation therapy (IORT) is radiation delivered at the time of surgery. Intraoperative electron beam radiation therapy (IOERT) has been more widely used and results in improved local control with some studies suggesting a survival benefit (Gunderson *et al.* 1987; Sindelar *et al.*1999; Crane *et al.* 2003). High dose rate (HDR) and low dose rate (LDR) intraoperative radiation therapy utilize catheters which are placed in the tumor bed during surgery. LDR sources are administered after surgery is completed and are placed by the radiation oncologist. HDR-IORT uses a flexible applicator (Freiburg flap) which is placed in the tumor bed. I^{192} wires pass through the catheters imbedded in the flap. The dose and dose rate can be altered based on the number of catheters and catheter dwell times and positions. While earlier trials used only high doses of IORT, more recent studies add IORT (10–20 Gy) as a boost to neoadjuvant or adjuvant CRT (Willett *et al.* 2005). Combinations of these delivery methods can be used to escalate the dose of radiation to the tumor or tumor bed. Additional studies are necessary to determine optimal combinations of EBRT, IORT/IOERT, and SBRT with systemic therapies.

Adjuvant therapy

US trials: GITSG, RTOG, Johns Hopkins, and others

The *Gastrointestinal Tumor Study Group* (GITSG) conducted a prospective phase III trial in which patients were randomized after curative resection to observation or radiation plus 5-FU (40 Gy in a 6-week split course technique with 5-FU 500 mg/m^2 days 1–3 of each sequence followed by weekly 5-FU for 2 years) (Kalser *et al.* 1985). Radiation fields included the tumor bed and major nodal areas at risk. Compared to surgery alone, patients who received adjuvant 5-FU and radiation demonstrated significant improvements in median survival (20 months versus 11 months), 2-year survival (42% versus 15%), and 5-year survival (19% versus 5%, $p = 0.05$). Subsequently, the GITSG registered an additional 30 patients to receive adjuvant 5-FU and radiation as delivered in the experimental arm of the study and confirmed the improved survival seen in the randomized comparison to surgery alone (Gastrointestinal Tumor Study Group 1987).

The GITSG study was criticized for its 8-year time to accrual, small power, and delay to initiation of adjuvant therapy (25% >10 weeks). In spite of these limitations, the GITSG study established adjuvant CRT as the standard of care for resectable pancreatic cancer.

Between 1991 and 1995, the Johns Hopkins Medical Institute reported a prospective single-institution series of 174 patients who were offered three options after surgical resection: observation ($n = 53$), and standard EBRT plus concurrent and maintenance bolus 5-FU either with ($n = 99$), or without ($n = 21$) prophylactic liver irradiation (Yeo *et al.* 1997). Patients receiving postoperative CRT had an improvement in median survival (20 vs.14 months) and 2-year survival (40 vs. 31%) when compared to observation ($p = 0.003$). Liver irradiation resulted in more toxicity and no improvement in median survival when compared to standard 5-FU and radiation (17.5 vs. 21 months). Swartz *et al.* presented an update to the Johns Hopkins University experience at ASTRO (American Society for Therapeutic Radiology and Oncology) in 2006. Between August 8 1993 and

February 28 2005, 902 patients underwent pancreaticoduodenectomy for pancreatic ductal adenocarcinoma at Johns Hopkins Hospital. Of the 409 patients who received adjuvant therapy, 190 patients were treated elsewhere and 219 patients were treated at Johns Hopkins Hospital. Since 63 patients received an experimental vaccine, they were excluded from the analysis. At a median follow-up of 5.8 years, the median, 2-year, and 5-year overall survival were significantly improved in those patients who received adjuvant 5-FU-based CRT (50.4 Gy) compared with observation (21 vs. 16 months, 45% vs. 36%, and 25% vs. 16%). This relationship persisted after controlling for age, margin status, tumor size, and postoperative complications.

The RTOG 97–04 trial was designed to evaluate whether gemcitabine before and after adjuvant 5-FU-based CRT was superior to a 5-FU-based adjuvant regimen. This intergroup trial included patients with pancreatic adenocarcinoma who underwent a gross total resection (pathologic stage T1–4, N0–1, M0). Patients were initially stratified by nodal status (uninvolved vs. involved), primary tumor diameter (<3 cm vs. ≥3 cm) and surgical margins (negative vs. positive vs. unknown). Continuous-infusion (CI) 5-FU was delivered at 250 mg/m^2/day. Gemcitabine was given 1000 mg/m^2 IV weekly. Both were given over 3 weeks pre- and 12 weeks post CRT. Patients received a total of 50.4 Gy (1.8-Gy fractions) to the tumor bed and adjacent lymph nodes with CI 5-FU (250 mg/m^2/day). The results were presented in abstract form at ASCO (American Society of Clinical Oncology) 2006 (Regine *et al.* 2006). Of 538 patients enrolled, 442 were eligible and analysable. In a preplanned analysis of patients with pancreatic head tumors (n = 380), the median and 3-year survival were 18.8 months and 31% for the gemcitabine arm. This was significantly superior to the median and 3-year survival seen in the 5-FU arm: 16.7 months and 21% (p = 0.047; HR 0.79, CI 0.63–0.99). There was no significant difference in non-hematologic grade ≥3 toxicity. The ability to complete chemotherapy and radiation were similar in both groups. This trial supports the use of maintenance gemcitabine with 5-FU-based CRT in patients with resected pancreatic cancer.

Blackstock *et al.* evaluated the efficacy of twice-weekly gemcitabine (40 mg m^2) for 5 weeks concurrent with radiation (50.4 Gy) in patients with resected pancreatic cancer (Blackstock *et al.* 2006). Weekly gemcitabine (1000 mg/m^2) was given for two cycles following chemoradiation. Of 46 evaluable patients 73% had stage T3 or T4 disease, and 70% were node positive. Grade III/IV gastrointestinal or hematologic toxicities were infrequent. The median survival was 18.3 months. Twenty-four per cent of patients were alive at 3 years. Only six of 34 patients with progression experienced local regional relapse as a component of the first site of failure. These results confirm the feasibility of twice-weekly gemcitabine-based CRT in the adjuvant setting.

Picozzi *et al.* published a single-institution experience using radiation, 5-FU, and alpha-interferon following surgery (Picozzi *et al.* 2003). At a mean follow-up of 31.9 months, 67% of the patients were alive. Actuarial overall survival for the 1-, 2-, and 5-year periods was 95%, 64%, and 55%. Although promising, 42% of patients required hospitalization because of gastrointestinal toxicity. This regimen was tested in a phase III trial through ACOSOG (American College of Surgeons Oncology Group) and has completed accrual. The results are pending.

In an attempt to improve survival rates and reduce toxicity, Laheru *et al.* developed a novel pancreatic granulocyte/macrophage colony-stimulating factor (GM-CSF)-secreting tumor vaccine (Laheru *et al.* 2005b). It incorporates two irradiated pancreatic cell lines that elicit immune responses against pancreatic tumors (Disis & Cheever 1988; Greten & Jaffee 1999; Wang & Rosenberg 1999). In phase I/II trials involving patients with resected pancreatic cancer, a combination of the GM-CSF vaccine with CRT resulted in a 2-year survival of 76% with less toxicity than traditional therapies (Laheru *et al.* 2005a).

European trials: EORTC, ESPAC-1

The *EORTC trial* was a randomized phase III trial comparing observation with postoperative CRT (EBRT as per GITSG, plus CI 5-FU during weeks 1 and 3 of radiation) (Klinkenbijl *et al.* 1999).Compared with observation (n = 54), patients receiving adjuvant CRT (60) had a borderline significant improvement in survival (median overall survival 17.1 vs. 12.6 months, 2-year overall survival (37 vs 23%), 3-year overall survival (20 vs. 10%). Patients in the adjuvant CRT arm did not receive maintenance chemotherapy, a major change from the GITSG trial.

The *ESPAC-1 trial* consisted of three separate phase III trials run concurrently to test the value of both adjuvant chemotherapy and CRT in 541 patients with grossly resected pancreas cancer (positive resection margins 18%) (Neoptolemos *et al.* 2001). EBRT plus 5-FU were given as per the GITSG trial. In the adjuvant chemotherapy arm, 5-FU/leucovorin was given for 6 cycles (425 mg/m^2 for 5 days each month). The trial with a 2 × 2 factorial design randomized 285 patients from multiple centers into four arms (surgery alone, adjuvant EBRT+5-FU, adjuvant 5-FU/leucovorin, adjuvant EBRT/5-FU plus maintenance 5-FU/leucovorin). Clinicians could also randomize patients into one of the main treatment comparisons: chemotherapy versus no chemotherapy (n = 188), or CRT versus no CRT (n = 68). Background therapy was allowed before patients entered the trial and radiation was given according to the standard of the individual institutions. In the initial analysis, an advantage for adjuvant chemotherapy could be obtained only by merging data from the three separate randomized trials in a pooled analysis (median SR 19.7 months in 238 patients randomized to adjuvant chemotherapy vs. 14.0 months in 235 patients randomized to no adjuvant chemotherapy; p = 0.005).

The latest report of the ESPAC-1 trial describes an analysis of 289 patients randomized into a 2 × 2 factorial design: observation (n = 69), EBRT plus 5-FU (n = 73), 5-FU/leucovorin (n = 75), or EBRT/5-FU plus maintenance 5-FU/lecucovorin (n = 72) (Neoptolemos *et al.* 2004). Patients randomized to receive 6 months of adjuvant 5-FU/leucovorin had a survival advantage over those who did not receive prolonged adjuvant chemotherapy (Table 21.5). Local recurrence was a component of relapse in 99 patients (34% of 289 patients at risk, 63% of 158 patients with relapse). The authors concluded that adjuvant CRT was inferior to chemotherapy because it delayed the administration of chemotherapy. The results of this study have been criticized because of the lack of centralized quality assurance, standardization of radiation fields, allowance for physician selection bias, and allowance for background therapy (Garofalo *et al.* 2006). For these reasons, the standard of care in the United States is still adjuvant chemoradiation using 5-FU or gemcitabine followed by maintenance gemcitabine. In Europe, EORTC 40013 randomizes patients with resected pancreatic cancer to gemcitabine followed by gemcitabine with radiation (50.4 Gy) versus gemcitabine alone. Based on the ESPAC-1 results, the ESPAC-3 (v2) trial has abandoned radiation therapy and randomizes patients with resected pancreatic cancer to 5-FU plus folinic acid or gemcitabine. Recently, Oettle *et al.* reported preliminary results from a phase III randomized trial (n = 368) of adjuvant gemcitabine versus observation (CONKO-001). The results show improved disease-free survival with adjuvant gemcitabine compared to observation (www.egms.de/en/meetings/dkk2006/06dkk230.shtml.

Table 21.5 Phase III results of adjuvant therapy in pancreatic cancer series of patients.

	No. of patients	Marg/node positive (%)	Post-CRT chemotherapy	Local recurrence (%)	Median survival (months)	2-yr survival (%)	p-value
GTSG (phase III)			Yes				
Surgery alone	22	0/29		86*	11	15	
Postop EBRT + 5-FU	21	0/30		71	20	43	<0.05
Postop EBRT/5FU (registered)	30				18	46	
EORTC (phase III)			No				
Surgery alone	54	24/54 (panc)		22.1 (all)	12.6 (panc)	23 (panc)	
Postop EBRT + 5-FU	60	19/47 (panc)		22.3 (all)	17.1 (panc)	37 (panc)	0.099
ESPAC-1 (phase III 2 × 2 design)†		16–19/73–82	Yes/No	35‡			
Surgery alone no adjuv CT	69				16.9	30	
Postop EBRT + 5-FU	73				13.9		
Postop EBRT/5-FU; 5-FU/leucovorin	72				19.9	40 adjuv CT	0.009, adjuv
CT vs no adjuv CT							
Postop 5-FU/ leucovorin (6 mo)	75				21.6		
RTOG 97-04 (phase III)§	380	N/A¶	Yes	N/A			
5-FU→5-FU/RT→5-FU					16.7	21 (3 yr)	
Gem→5-FU/RT→Gem					18.8	31 (3 yr)	0.047

* Represents total recurrence; 50% of patients with recurrence had liver metastases. Eight patients (4 each group) had recurrence found at the time of autopsy.

† The ESPAC-1 trial was three separate phase III trials, only 2 × 2 data are shown; background therapy was allowed before randomization, thus resulting in the equivalent of a non-randomized trial with regard to selection of patients and treatment options. Margin and node-positive numbers reflect a range between the groups of patients receiving chemoradiotherapy and/or chemotherapy.

‡Of 158 patients who had recurrence in all arms, 35% of patients had local recurrence only. Local recurrence alone was not reported for each treatment group.

§ Data represent patients with pancreatic head tumors. When analysis included patients with body/tail tumors there was no significant difference in survival.

¶ Patients were stratified based on margin status, tumor diameter (≤3 cm), and nodal status.

§ Local tumor as first site of failure.

Neoadjuvant therapy for pancreatic cancer

Potential benefits of neoadjuvant therapy compared with adjuvant therapy for pancreatic cancer include decreased toxicity, enhanced efficacy, improved compliance, and increased likelihood of an R0 resection (Crane *et al.* 2006b). These benefits have been demonstrated in rectal cancer where a large phase III trial by Sauer *et al.* reported improved local control, sphincter sparing, and toxicity with neoadjuvant versus adjuvant CRT (Sauer *et al.* 2004). For example, in a multivariate analysis of 120 patients with resectable pancreatic cancer, neoadjuvant CRT resulted in less treatment-related toxicity and actually decreased the risk of anastamotic leaks when compared to those patients receiving adjuvant CRT (Lowy *et al.* 1997).

The most extensive experience utilizing preoperative CRT has been reported by M.D. Anderson (Raut *et al.* 2004; Pisters *et al.* 2005). In early neoadjuvant studies, patients were treated with standard fractionated radiation (1.8 Gy daily/50.4 Gy total) and protracted infusional 5-FU. This was converted to a 'rapid-fractionated' radiotherapy course of 3.0 Gy daily for a total dose of 30 Gy followed by an intraoperative boost of 10 Gy (total biologic equivalent dose similar to 50.4 Gy) (Pisters *et al.* 2002; Crane *et al.* 2003). IORT was subsequently abandoned because of toxicity and patients now receive gemcitabine- and cisplatin-based CRT followed by gemcitabine (400 mg/m^2 weekly) prior to resection. Patients who received preoperative gemcitabine-based CRT were more likely to undergo a successful pancreaticoduodenectomy procedure compared with those patients with 5-FU-based CRT (Crane *et al.* 2006b). Pathologic response data was also improved with gemcitabine-based CRT compared to 5-FU-based CRT (Crane *et al.* 2002).

Approximately 25% of patients who start neoadjuvant therapy do not undergo successful resection due to tumor progression or development of a significant medical comorbidity (Raut *et al.* 2004). These patients are spared the morbidity of a pancreaticoduodenectomy procedure which may not have benefited the patient if performed at the time of diagnosis because of the presence of subclinical micrometastatic disease. Patients with positive margins (often retroperitoneal) following surgical resection are more likely to have recurrent disease. Data from M.D. Anderson suggest that patients who received neoadjuvant therapy were less likely to have gross positive margins (R2 = 0%) and local recurrence (10%) compared with patients treated initially with surgery.

Those opposed to neoadjuvant therapy believe that patients could progress locally or systemically while receiving neoadjuvant CRT. Neoadjuvant CRT however offers early systemic treatment as opposed to delaying chemotherapy until after a patient recovers from surgery (6–8 weeks). Other potential negatives of neoadjuvant therapy include overtreatment of patients who may not have needed adjuvant therapy and the inability to accurately stage patients before initiating treatment.

Prior to initiation of neoadjuvant therapy, all patients should be appropriately staged as resectable, borderline resectable, unresectable, or metastatic with high-resolution CT imaging and presented in a multidisciplinary setting to determine the optimal treatment plan (Varadhachary *et al.* 2006). Future clinical studies should evaluate the benefits and potential toxicities of neoadjuvant chemoradiation and/or chemotherapy in patients with resectable pancreatic cancer. The role of intraoperative high-dose and electron beam radiation is currently unclear but may become increasingly important with effective systemic and targeted therapies.

Locally unresectable pancreatic cancer

External beam irradiation with or without chemotherapy

The GITSG trial prospectively randomized 194 patients with unresectable locally advanced pancreatic adenocarcinoma to evaluate whether CRT is superior to RT (Moertel *et al.* 1981). Patients were stratified based on institution, location of primary (head vs. body/tail), grade, surgery (+/– GI or biliary bypass), and ECOG performance status (0 vs. 1 vs. 2–3). The three groups included: (i) RT 60 Gy alone (n = 25); (ii) RT 40 Gy + 5-FU (n = 83); and (iii) RT 60 Gy + 5-FU (n = 86). Patients received 40 Gy (split course) +/– a 20 Gy boost. 5-FU, 500 mg/m^2 IVP was delivered on days 1–3 of each 2000-cGy course. Maintenance weekly 5-FU was given 4 weeks after RT for 2 years or until tumor progression. The median survival for the RT-alone group, 40 Gy/5-FU, and 60 Gy/5-FU was 6, 10, and 10.5 months respectively. For locally advanced non-metastatic pancreatic cancer, this study demonstrated that concurrent 5-FU and radiation is superior to RT alone.

The GITSG and modern trials conclude that the use of external-beam irradiation plus chemotherapy in unresectable pancreatic cancer results in almost a doubling of median survival (overall survival) when compared with surgical bypass or stent placement alone (3–6 months vs. 9–13 months) and an increase in 2-year overall survival from 0–5% to 10–20%. However, 5-year survivors are rare and local control is infrequent.

The Cochrane Collaboration reviewed 50 clinical trials (n = 7043) pertaining to unresectable pancreatic cancer published between 1966 and 2005 (www.cochrane.org). Chemotherapy significantly reduced the 1-year mortality 0.37 (p = 0.00001) when compared with best supportive care. CRT improved 1-year survival (0 vs. 58%, p = 0.001) when compared to best supportive care. However, CRT was associated with more toxicity in the study.

Modern series have implemented gemcitabine with radiation because of its benefit over 5-FU in metastatic disease and for its radiosensitizing properties shown *in vivo* and *in vitro* (Burris *et al.* 1997; Lawrence *et al.* 1999). Currently there is no standard regimen of gemcitabine and radiation. Variations in radiation portal (tumor + margin vs. tumor + regional LN), total dose, and fractionation (30/3 Gy vs. >=50.4/1.8 Gy) are common (McGinn *et al.* 2001). Similarly, gemcitabine frequency and dose is variable (weekly vs. biweekly) (Crane *et al.* 2001). A study by Li *et al.* randomized 34 patients with unresectable, non-metastatic pancreatic cancer to 5-FU vs. gemcitabine-based (weekly) CRT (tumor + regional LN) (Li *et al.* 2003). The response rate (50% vs. 13%) and median survival (14.5 vs. 6.7) were superior in the gemcitabine arm, but the control arm had inferior outcomes compared to historical studies, and toxicity requiring hospitalization was reported in one-third of all patients. The Cancer and Leukemia Group B (CALGB) evaluated gemcitabine given 40 mg/m^2 biweekly with radiation (tumor + regional LN) for patients with unresectable disease (Blackstock *et al.* 2003). A large proportion of patients developed grade 3 or 4 toxicity. The study resulted in good local control but no apparent improvement in survival over standard 5-FU-based CRT. McGinn *et al.* incorporated full-dose weekly gemcitabine (1000 mg/m^2) with dose-escalated radiation (McGinn *et al.* 2001). A total dose of 36 Gy (2.4 Gy daily) delivered to the tumor plus a 1-cm margin was found to be the maximum tolerated dose (MTD). This regimen was expanded to a multi-institutional phase II study in patients with potentially resectable pancreatic cancer (Talamonti *et al.* 2006). In this trial patients received 7 infusions of gemcitabine (1000 mg/m^2) with concurrent radiation (36 Gy in 2.4-Gy fractions) delivered over 9 weeks. Resection was attempted 4–6 weeks later. Nineteen patients (95%) completed therapy without interruption, and one experienced grade 3 gastrointestinal toxicity. Of 20 patients taken to surgery, 17 (85%) underwent resection. Pathologic analysis revealed clear margins in 94% and negative lymph nodes in 65% of specimens. With a median follow-up of 18 months, seven (41%) of the 17 patients with resected disease were alive with no recurrence, three (18%) were alive with distant metastases, and seven (41%) had died. This regimen appears efficacious; however, since a large proportion of patients developed metastatic disease, the next trial incorporates concurrent CRT (30 Gy in 2-Gy fractions) with full-dose gemcitabine and oxaliplatin.

Capecitabine is an oral form of 5-FU which is preferentially metabolized to its active form at the site of the tumor. It has been recently substituted for bolus or infusional 5-FU in patients with resected and unresectable pancreatic cancer. Capecitabine has been shown to have equivalent efficacy to gemcitabine in locally advanced or metastatic pancreatic cancer (Cartwright *et al.* 2002). A phase I trial reported by Crane *et al.* demonstrated the safety of capecitabine with bevacizumab (targeted therapy against VEGF) and radiation in patients with unresectable pancreatic cancer (Crane *et al.* 2006a). Adjustment of capecitabine during treatment was shown to decrease the risk of advanced toxicity. RTOG 0411 evaluated this regimen in a multi-institutional setting and has rapidly reached its targeted accrual (results not yet reported). Additional studies are needed to determine optimal dosing and scheduling of capcitabine (5 vs. 7 days a week) with radiation and how it can be integrated with newer targeted therapies.

Multiple classes of targeted agents including epidermal growth factor receptor (EGFR) inhibitors, inhibitors of vascular endothelial growth factor receptor (VEGF), farnesyl transferase inhibitors, and cyclooxygenase-2 inhibitors have been evaluated in patients with locally advanced and metastatic pancreatic cancer. The combination of gemcitabine and erlotinib was found to be superior to gemcitabine alone in patients with locally advanced or metastatic pancreatic cancer with a significant improvement in survival (1-year 17% vs. 24%). Erlotinib has been shown to be a radiosensitizer *in vivo* (Chinnaiyan *et al.* 2005). A phase I study combining erlotinib (50–150 mg/day), paclitaxel and radiation (50.4 tumor + LN) followed by maintenance erlotinib (150 mg/day) for patients with unresectable or incompletely resected pancreatic cancer was recently reported by Iannitti *et al.* (Iannitti *et al.* 2005). The MTD of erlotinib was 50 mg when combined with paclitaxel, and concurrent radiation. Reported toxicities included diarrhea, dehydration, rash, myelosuppression, and small bowel stricture. The median survival of 13 patients with locally advanced disease was 14 months, and 46% had a partial response. Another study combined capcitabine, gefitinib (250 mg/daily), and radiation (50.4 Gy to tumor + LN) for unresectable pancreatic patients (Czito *et al.* 2006). The study was closed due to 6/10 patients developing a DLT (diarrhea). Additional studies are needed to determine how to safely combine targeted therapies with chemotherapy and radiation.

Role of intraoperative irradiation with or without external beam irradiation

The combination of external-beam irradiation (EBRT) plus intraoperative electron radiotherapy (IOERT) or brachytherapy has resulted in an improvement in local control in IOERT series from Massachusetts General Hospital (Willett *et al.* 2005) and Mayo Clinic (Gunderson *et al.* 1987; Gunderson *et al.* 1995), but this has not translated into an improvement in either median or 5-year survival. The lack of survival improvement was likely related to a high incidence of abdominal failure in both groups. As many as 54% of patients developed liver or peritoneal metastases in the IOERT group (56% in the non-IOERT group). IOERT analyses from MGH and other institutions have also implicated distant intra-abdominal failure as a significant problem. Variations in the dose of IORT, sequence of IORT with EBRT (pre-/post-surgery), patient selection, small numbers, and inconsistent use of chemotherapy complicates the true efficacy of IORT in patients with unresectable pancreatic cancer. In an effort to improve patient selection for IOERT, Garton *et al.* treated patients with full-dose EBRT prior to IOERT (Garton *et al.* 1993). Two months after EBRT, patients received IOERT only if they failed to develop progression of disease (73%). The actual incidence of local control at 1 and 2 years was 86% and 68%, respectively, with a median survival of 14.9 months. Compared to 56 patients treated with EBRT following IOERT, patients receiving neoadjuvant treatment had better outcomes. Patient selection, however, could explain these differences.

An update of the Massachusetts General Hospital series reported on 150 patients who received external-beam radiation before and/or after IOERT (10–20 Gy) with some patients receiving chemotherapy (Willett *et al.* 2005). Most patients underwent a surgical bypass procedure at the time of IOERT. The diameter of the IOERT treatment applicator (surrogate of tumor size) was predictive for long-term survival. Twenty-six patients treated with a small-diameter applicator (5–6 cm) had 2- and 3-year actuarial survival rates of 27% and 17%, respectively. No patients treated with a 9-cm diameter applicator survived beyond 18 months. The authors suggest that innovative protocols combining IOERT with CRT are warranted for small unresectable tumors.

References

Ben-Josef E, Shields AF, Vaishampayan U *et al.* (2004) Intensity-modulated radiotherapy (IMRT) and concurrent capecitabine for pancreatic cancer. *Int J Radiat Oncol Biol Phys* 59(2): 454–9.

Blackstock AW, Tepper JE, Niedwiecki D, Hollis DR, Mayer RJ, Tempero MA. (2003) Cancer and leukemia group B (CALGB) 89805: Phase II chemoradiation trial using gemcitabine in patients with locoregional adenocarcinoma of the pancreas. *Int J Gastrointest Cancer* 34(2–3): 107–16.

Blackstock AW, Mornex F, Partensky C *et al.* (2006) Adjuvant gemcitabine and concurrent radiation for patients with resected pancreatic cancer: A phase II study. *Br J Cancer* 95(3): 260–5.

Burris HA 3rd, Moore MJ, Andersen J *et al.* (1997) Improvements in survival and clinical benefit with gemcitabine as first-line therapy for patients with advanced pancreas cancer: A randomized trial. *J Clin Oncol* 15(6): 2403–13.

Cameron JL, Riall TS, Coleman J, Belcher KA. (2006) One thousand consecutive pancreaticoduodenectomies. *Ann Surg* 244(1): 10–15.

Cartwright TH, Cohn A, Varkey JA *et al.* (2002) Phase II study of oral capecitabine in patients with advanced or metastatic pancreatic cancer. *J Clin Oncol* 20(1): 160–4.

Chinnaiyan P, Huang S, Vallabhaneni G *et al.* (2005) Mechanisms of enhanced radiation response following epidermal growth factor receptor signaling inhibition by erlotinib (tarceva). *Cancer Res* 65(8): 3328–35.

Crane C, Janjan N, Evans D *et al.* (2001) Toxicity and efficacy of concurrent gemcitabine and radiotherapy for locally advanced pancreatic cancer. *Int J Gastrointest Cancer* 29(1): 9–18.

Crane CH, Abbruzzese JL, Evans DB *et al.* (2002) Is the therapeutic index better with gemcitabine-based chemoradiation than with 5-fluorouracil-based chemoradiation in locally advanced pancreatic cancer? *Int J Radiat Oncol Biol Phys* 52(5): 1293–302.

Crane CH, Ellis LM, Abbruzzese JL *et al.* (2006a) Phase I trial evaluating the safety of bevacizumab with concurrent radiotherapy and capecitabine in locally advanced pancreatic cancer. *J Clin Oncol* 24(7): 1145–51.

Crane CH, Varadhachary G, Wolff RA, Pisters PW, Evans DB. (2006b) The argument for pre-operative chemoradiation for localized, radiographically resectable pancreatic cancer. *Best Pract Res Clin Gastroenterol* 20(2): 365–82.

Czito BG, Willett CG, Bendell JC *et al.* (2006) Increased toxicity with gefitinib, capecitabine, and radiation therapy in pancreatic and rectal cancer: Phase I trial results. *J Clin Oncol* 24(4): 656–62.

Disis ML, Cheever MA. (1998) HER-2/neu oncogenic protein: Issues in vaccine development. *Crit Rev Immunol* 18(1–2): 37–45.

Dragovich T, Huberman M, Von Hoff DD*et al.* (2006) Erlotinib plus gemcitabine in patients with unresectable pancreatic cancer and other solid tumors: Phase IB trial. *Cancer Chemother Pharmacol*

Foo ML, Gunderson LL, Nagorney DM *et al.* (1993) Patterns of failure in grossly resected pancreatic ductal adenocarcinoma treated with adjuvant irradiation +/- 5 fluorouracil. *Int J Radiat Oncol Biol Phys* 26(3): 483–9.

Garofalo M, Flannery T, Regine W. (2006) The case for adjuvant chemoradiation for pancreatic cancer. *Best Pract Res Clin Gastroenterol* 20(2): 403–16.

Garton GR, Gunderson LL, Nagorney DM *et al.* (1993) High-dose preoperative external beam and intraoperative irradiation for locally advanced pancreatic cancer. *Int J Radiat Oncol Biol Phys* 27(5): 1153–7.

Gastrointestinal Tumor Study Group. (1987) Further evidence of effective adjuvant combined radiation and chemotherapy following curative resection of pancreatic cancer. gastrointestinal tumor study group. *Cancer* 59(12): 2006–10.

Greten TF, Jaffee EM. (1999) Cancer vaccines. *J Clin Oncol* 17(3): 1047–60.

Gunderson LL, Martin JK, Kvols LK *et al.* (1987) Intraoperative and external beam irradiation +/- 5-FU for locally advanced pancreatic cancer. *Int J Radiat Oncol Biol Phys* 13(3): 319–29.

Gunderson LL, Nagorney DM, Martenson JA *et al.* (1995) External beam plus intraoperative irradiation for gastrointestinal cancers. *World J Surg* 19(2): 191–7.

Iannitti D, Dipetrillo T, Akerman P *et al.* (2005) Erlotinib and chemoradiation followed by maintenance erlotinib for locally advanced pancreatic cancer: A phase I study. *Am J Clin Oncol* 28(6): 570–5.

Kalser MH, Ellenberg SS. (1985) Pancreatic cancer. adjuvant combined radiation and chemotherapy following curative resection. *Arch Surg* 120(8): 899–903.

Klinkenbijl JH, Jeekel J, Sahmoud T *et al.* (1999) Adjuvant radiotherapy and 5-fluorouracil after curative resection of cancer of the pancreas and periampullary region: Phase III trial of the EORTC gastrointestinal tract cancer cooperative group. *Ann Surg* 230(6): 776–82; discussion 782–4.

Koong AC, Le QT, Ho A *et al.* (2004) Phase I study of stereotactic radiosurgery in patients with locally advanced pancreatic cancer. *Int J Radiat Oncol Biol Phys* 58(4): 1017–21.

Koong AC, Christofferson E, Le QT *et al.* (2005) Phase II study to assess the efficacy of conventionally fractionated radiotherapy followed by a stereotactic radiosurgery boost in patients with locally advanced pancreatic cancer. *Int J Radiat Oncol Biol Phys* 63(2): 320–3.

Laheru D, Yeo C, Biedrzycki B *et al.* (2005a) A safety and efficacy trial of lethally irradiated allogeneic pancraetic tumor cells transfected with the GM-CSF gene in combination with adjuvant chemoradiotherapy for the treatment of adenocarcinoma of the pancreas. *Proc AACR/NCI/EORTC*: 204.

Laheru D, Biedrzycki B, Thomas AM, Jaffee EM. (2005b) Development of a cytokine-modified allogeneic whole cell pancreatic cancer vaccine. *Methods Mol Med* 103: 299–327.

Lawrence TS, Eisbruch A, McGinn CJ, Fields MT, Shewach DS. (1999) Radiosensitization by gemcitabine. *Oncology (Williston Park)* 13(10 Suppl 5): 55–60.

Li CP, Chao Y, Chi KH *et al.* (2003) Concurrent chemoradiotherapy treatment of locally advanced pancreatic cancer: Gemcitabine versus 5-fluorouracil, a randomized controlled study. *Int J Radiat Oncol Biol Phys* 57(1): 98–104.

Lowy AM, Lee JE, Pisters PW *et al.* (1997) Prospective, randomized trial of octreotide to prevent pancreatic fistula after pancreaticoduodenectomy for malignant disease. *Ann Surg* 226(5): 632–41.

McGinn CJ, Zalupski MM, Shureiqi I *et al.* (2001) Phase I trial of radiation dose escalation with concurrent weekly full-dose gemcitabine in patients with advanced pancreatic cancer. *J Clin Oncol* 19(22): 4202–8.

Milano MT, Chmura SJ, Garofalo MC *et al.* (2004) Intensity-modulated radiotherapy in treatment of pancreatic and bile duct malignancies: Toxicity and clinical outcome. *Int J Radiat Oncol Biol Phys* 59(2): 445–53.

Moertel CG, Frytak S, Hahn RG *et al.* (1981) Therapy of locally unresectable pancreatic carcinoma: A randomized comparison of high dose (6000 rads) radiation alone, moderate dose radiation (4000 rads + 5-fluorouracil), and high dose radiation + 5-fluorouracil: The gastrointestinal tumor study group. *Cancer* 48(8): 1705–10.

Neoptolemos JP, Dunn JA, Stocken DD *et al.* (2001) Adjuvant chemoradiotherapy and chemotherapy in resectable pancreatic cancer: A randomised controlled trial. *Lancet* 358(9293): 1576–85.

Neoptolemos JP, Stocken DD, Friess H *et al.* (2004) A randomized trial of chemoradiotherapy and chemotherapy after resection of pancreatic cancer. *N Engl J Med* 350(12): 1200–10.

Picozzi VJ, Kozarek RA, Traverso LW. (2003) Interferon-based adjuvant chemoradiation therapy after pancreaticoduodenectomy for pancreatic adenocarcinoma. *Am J Surg* 185(5): 476–80.

Pisters PW, Hudec WA, Lee JE *et al.* (2000) Preoperative chemoradiation for patients with pancreatic cancer: Toxicity of endobiliary stents. *J Clin Oncol* 18(4): 860–7.

Pisters PW, Wolff RA, Janjan NA *et al.* (2002) Preoperative paclitaxel and concurrent rapid-fractionation radiation for resectable pancreatic adenocarcinoma: Toxicities, histologic response rates, and event-free outcome. *J Clin Oncol* 20(10): 2537–44.

Pisters PW, Wolff RA, Crane CH, Evans DB. (2005) Combined-modality treatment for operable pancreatic adenocarcinoma. *Oncology (Williston Park)* 19(3): 393–416.

Raut CP, Evans DB, Crane CH, Pisters PW, Wolff RA. (2004) Neoadjuvant therapy for resectable pancreatic cancer. *Surg Oncol Clin N Am* 13(4): 639–61, ix.

Regine W, Winter K, Abrams R *et al.* (2006) RTOG 9704 a phase III study of adjuvant pre and post chemoradiation (CRT) 5-FU vs. gemcitabine (G) for resected pancreatic adenocarcinoma. *ASCO* Abstract #407.

Sauer R, Becker H, Hohenberger W *et al.* (2004) Preoperative versus postoperative chemoradiotherapy for rectal cancer. *N Engl J Med* 351(17): 1731–40.

Sindelar WF, Kinsella TJ. (1999) Studies of intraoperative radiotherapy in carcinoma of the pancreas. *Ann Oncol* 10 Suppl 4: 226–30.

Talamonti MS, Small W Jr, Mulcahy MF *et al.* (2006) A multi-institutional phase II trial of preoperative full-dose gemcitabine and concurrent radiation for patients with potentially resectable pancreatic carcinoma. *Ann Surg Oncol* 13(2): 150–8.

Varadhachary GR, Tamm EP, Abbruzzese JL *et al.* (2006) Borderline resectable pancreatic cancer: Definitions, management, and role of preoperative therapy. *Ann Surg Oncol* 13(8): 1035–46.

Wang RF, Rosenberg SA. (1999) Human tumor antigens for cancer vaccine development. *Immunol Rev* 170: 85–100.

Willett CG, Del Castillo CF, Shih HA *et al.* (2005) Long-term results of intraoperative electron beam irradiation (IOERT) for patients with unresectable pancreatic cancer. *Ann Surg* 241(2): 295–9.

Wong AA, Delclos ME, Wolff RA *et al.* (2005) Radiation dose considerations in the palliative treatment of locally advanced adenocarcinoma of the pancreas. *Am J Clin Oncol* 28(3): 227–33.

Yeo CJ, Abrams RA, Grochow LB *et al.* (1997) Pancreaticoduodenectomy for pancreatic adenocarcinoma: Postoperative adjuvant chemoradiation improves survival. A prospective, single-institution experience. *Ann Surg* 225(5): 621–33; discussion 633–6.

Novel agents

Manuel Hidalgo

During the last few years, an increasing number of new drugs, many of them targeted to specific alterations in malignant cells, have been tested in pancreatic cancer as well as in other tumors (Von Hoff & Bearss 2002). The rationale to develop these drugs in pancreatic cancer comes from the better understanding of the biologic basis of the disease making possible the identification and validation of some of these targets. In addition, the poor prognosis of patients with pancreatic cancer and the evidence that conventional chemotherapy may have really reached a plateau with regard to improving outcome has also motivated an aggressive evaluation of new drugs in this disease. In the next few paragraphs, we discuss the results of the main clinical studies available thus far with novel agents including matrix metalloproteinase inhibitors, inhibitors of angiogenesis, agents targeted to the Ras oncogene, inhibitors of the EGFR family of membrane receptors, somatostatin analogs, and gene therapy strategies. Table 21.6 summarizes the key features of selected studies conducted with novel drugs in pancreatic cancer.

Matrix metalloproteinase inhibitors

The matrix metalloproteinases (MMPs) are a group of closely related proteases, which are dysregulated in the majority of human neoplasms including pancreatic cancer (Hidalgo & Eckhardt 2001). The increased activity of these enzymes has been related to tumor growth, progression, invasion, generation of blood vessels, and metastasis. Several inhibitors of the MMPs have been developed as anticancer agents and two of them, marimastat and BAY12-9566, have been more extensively studied in pancreatic cancer.

Marimastat is a non-peptidomimetic global inhibitor of the MMP family including MMP1, 2, and 9. In phase I studies in pancreatic cancer, doses from 10 to 25 mg orally twice a day were well tolerated. A large phase II study that enrolled 113 patients, in which 90% of the patients were treated at the 25-mg once a day dose, reported a 30% decline or stabilization in the

Table 21.6 Studies with novel drugs in advanced pancreatic cancer.

Novel agent	Author	Gemcitabine dose/schedule	Novel drug dose/schedule	Phase	Number of patients	Response rate (%)	Median survival (months)	1-year survival (%)
MMPI	Rosemurgy *et al.* (1999)	Ø	Marimastat 5–75 mg oral bid 10–25 mg oral/day	I	64	NR	5.3	21
MMPI	Evans *et al.* (2001)	Ø	Marimastat 10–100 mg oral bid[1]	II	130		3.8	
MMPI	Bramhall *et al.* (2001)	Arm A: 1000 mg/m² weekly × 7; 1 wk rest; day 1, 8, 15 q 4 wks Arm B, C, D: Ø	Arm A: Ø Arm B: Marimastat 5 mg bid Arm C: Marimastat 10 mg bid Arm D: Marimastat 25 mg bid	III	103 104 105 102		5.6 3.7 3.5 4.2	19 14 14 20
MMPI	Bramhall *et al.* (2002)	1000 mg/m² weekly × 7; 1 wk rest; day 1, 8, 15 q 4 wks	Arm A: Marimastat 10 mg bid Arm B: placebo	III	120 119	11 16	5.5 5.5	NR NR
MMPI	Moore *et al.* (2003)	Arm A: 1000 mg/m² weekly × 7; 1 wk rest; day 1, 8, 15 q 4 wks	Arm B: BAY-12-9566 800 mg oral bid	III	139 138		6.59 3.74 $p < 0.001$	
Angiogenesis inhibitor	Kindler *et al.* (2005)	1000 mg/m² day 1, 8, 15 q 4 wks	Bevacizumab 10 mg/kg0iv day 1 and 15	II	52	21	8.8	29
FTI	Cohen *et al.* (2003)	Ø	Tipifarnib 300 mg orally bid	II	20	0	4.8	NR
FTI	Van Cutsem *et al.* (2002)	1000 mg/m² weekly × 7; 1 wk rest; day 1, 8, 15 q 4 wks	Arm A: Tipifarnib 200 mg po bid Arm B: Placebo	III	688		6.4 6.1	27 24
FTI	Lersch *et al.* (2001)	Arm A: 1000 mg/m² weekly × 7; 1 wk rest; day 1, 8, 15 q 4 wks	Arm B: lonafarnib 200 mg po bid	II	30 33	3 6	4.4 3.3	NR
EGFR	Safran *et al.* (2004)	1000 mg/m² weekly × 7; 1 wk rest; day 1, 8, 15 q 4 wks	Trastuzumab 4 mg/Kg loading dose followed by 2 mg/kg weekly dose	II	35	6	7	19
EGFR	Xiong *et al.* (2004)	1000 mg/m² weekly × 7; 1 wk rest; day 1, 8, 15 q 4 wks	Cetuximab 400 mg/m² loading dose followed by 250 mg/m² maintenance dose	II	41	12	7	31.7
EGFR	Moore *et al.* (2005)	1000 mg/m² weekly × 7; 1 wk rest; day 1, 8, 15 q 4 wks	Arm A: Placebo Arm B: Erlotinib 100 mg daily (23 patients received 150 mg)	III	569	NA	5.9 6.4	17 24 ($p = 0.02$)

[1] 90% of the patients received 25-mg dose.

[2] Actuarial estimated.

tumor marker CA19-9 and a median survival of 3.8 months, and 51% of the patients had improvement in symptoms. Twenty-nine per cent of the patients developed arthralgias, the most common toxicity encountered with marimastat (Rosemurgy *et al.* 1999). The efficacy and toxicity of marimastat at doses of 5, 10 and 25 mg twice a day was compared to gemcitabine in a phase III study (Bramhall *et al.* 2001). Patients treated with gemcitabine had a longer progression-free survival of 3.8 months versus 1.9–2 months for the marimastat-treated group ($p = 0.001$). Overall survival was also better for gemcitabine (5.6 months) and significantly worse for patients treated with marimastat at doses of 5 and 10 mg while no statistically significant differences were observed in overall survival with the 25-mg twice a day dose. A subset analysis in this study showed that the benefit of gemcitabine was restricted to patients with advanced disease and that patients with locally advanced tumors benefited from marimastat supporting the hypothesis that these drugs may be more active in the situation of early disease. Finally, the combination of gemcitabine with marimastat was tested against gemcitabine in a randomized phase III study with no improvement in any parameter of outcome in the combined treatment group (Bramhall *et al.* 2002).

The second MMP inhibitor extensively studied in pancreatic cancer is BAY12-9566, a peptidomimetic inhibitor specific for MMP2 and 9. The drug was compared in a phase III study to single-agent gemcitabine (Moore *et al.* 2003). Two hundred and seventy patients of a planned sample of 350 were enrolled after an interim analysis demonstrated that patients treated with gemcitabine had a significantly better time to tumor progression (3.5 vs. 1.6 months, $p < 0.001$) and overall survival (6.59 vs. 3.74, $p < 0.001$). Quality-of-life analysis also favored gemcitabine. In summary, these studies suggest that current MMP inhibitors do not have relevant antitumor activity in patients with advanced pancreatic cancer. Whether or not these drugs or newer-generation analogs would be effective in earlier stages of pancreatic cancer remains to be determined.

Angiogenesis inhibitors

Pancreatic cancer is not an exception to the rule that tumors require the generation of blood vessels to grow, invade and metastasize. The drug of this class of agents that has been tested more exhaustively in pancreatic cancer is bevacizumab, a recombinant humanized monoclonal antibody against the vascular endothelial growth factor (VEGF). Bevacizumab has been studied in combination with gemcitabine in a phase II study (Kindler *et al.* 2005). Patients with advanced or locally advanced pancreatic cancer received gemcitabine 1000 mg/m^2 day 1, 8, and 15 every 28 days and bevacizumab, 10 mg/kg intravenously on day 1 and 15. A total of 52 patients were treated. Eleven patients (21%) had confirmed partial responses and 77% of the patients were alive at 6 months. Median survival was 8.8 months. Pretreatment plasma VEGF levels did not correlate with outcome. Grade 3 and 4 toxicities included hypertension in 19% of the patients, thrombosis in 13%, visceral perforation in 8%, and bleeding in 2%. These results prompted the initiation of a definitive phase III study under the auspices of the Cancer and Leukemia Group B (CALGB 80303). Though the final data have not been presented yet, a press release note informed that the trial did not meet its primary endpoint. While the results of this trial demonstrate that bevacizumab does not have a role in patients with advanced pancreatic cancer, it does not mean that targeting angiogenesis is an ineffective approach to treat this tumor type. Currently, there are a large number of inhibitors of angiogenesis in clinical development that likely will be evaluated in pancreatic cancer as well.

Inhibitors of the oncogene Ras

Mutations in the oncogene Ras are the most frequent genetic abnormality in pancreatic cancer. Because Ras requires farnesylization to be active, a post-translational modification mediated by the enzyme farnesyl-transferase, inhibitors of this enzyme have been developed as potential Ras inhibitors (Adjei 2001). Two of these agents tipifarnib and lonafarnib have been studied in disease-oriented studies in pancreatic cancer. Tipifarnib was tested in a single-agent phase II study in patients with advanced pancreatic cancer administered at a dose of 300 mg orally twice a day (Cohen *et al.* 2003). Twenty patients were treated with no objective responses and a median survival of less than 5 months. Correlative studies conducted in peripheral blood mononuclear cells demonstrated partial inhibition of the target enzyme. In parallel to this study, a randomized phase III study compared the combination of tipifarnib with gemcitabine against gemcitabine plus placebo in patients with advanced pancreatic cancer (Van Cutsem *et al.* 2002). Six hundred and eighty-eight patients were treated and no improvement in outcome was demonstrated in patients treated with the combination as summarized in Table 21.6. Lonafarnib was evaluated in a randomized phase II study in comparison to gemcitabine. The 3-month progression-free survival rate was 23% for patients treated with lonafarnib and 31% with gemcitabine, and the median overall survival was 3.3 months and 4.4 months respectively (Lersch *et al.* 2001). There were two partial responses in patients treated with lonafarnib and one partial response observed in one patient treated with gemcitabine. Overall, lonafarnib was better tolerated than gemcitabine in that study (Lersch *et al.* 2001).

Inhibitors of the EGFR family of receptors

The EGFR family of receptors is formed by four related transmembrane receptors which are composed of a external ligand binding domain, a transmembrane domain, and an intracellular domain with tyrosine kinase (TK) activity. These receptors are frequently dysregulated in cancer and have been associated with the process of tumor growth, invasion and metastasis, exiting considerable interest in developing these drugs for cancer treatment. Pharmacologically, the inhibitors of the EGFR belong to two broad classes of drugs including monoclonal antibodies against the extracellular domain of the receptor and small molecules inhibitors of the intracellular TK domain. The studies conducted in pancreatic cancer have mainly tested the combination of these drugs with gemcitabine (Jimeno & Hidalgo 2005).

Safran and collaborators reported a phase II study of trastuzumab, a monoclonal antibody that targets the Her-2 receptor, in combination with gemcitabine in patients with pancreatic cancer (Safran *et al.* 2004). Up to 21% of pancreatic cancers are Her-2 positive and preclinical studies have shown that inhibition of Her-2 signaling with trastuzumab is associated with antitumor effects in pancreatic cancer models. Patients with Her-2 positive (2 or 3+ as determined by immunohistochemistry) pancreatic cancer received gemcitabine 1000 mg/m^2 weekly for 7 consecutive weeks followed by 1 week of rest and then weekly for 3 weeks every 4 weeks and trastuzumab, 2 mg/kg/week following an initial loading dose of 4 mg/kg. Sixteen per cent of patients screened tested positive for Her-2. A total of 34 patients were enrolled. Two patients (6%) had a partial response and the median survival and 1-year survival were 7 months and 19%. Xiong and collaborators conducted a phase II study of gemcitabine and cetuximab, a monoclonal antibody against the EGFR in EGFR-positive pancreatic cancer patients. Forty-one patients were treated in the study. The overall response rate was 12% with a median survival of 7.1 months and 1-year survival of 31.7% (Xiong *et al.* 2004). Eighty-eight per cent of patients developed rash, which was grade 3 in 12% of patients. As noted in other studies with EGFR inhibitors, longer survival was associated with more severe grade of rash in that trial, with median survival durations of 5.7 months, 8.0 months, and 13.9 months among patients with grade 1, 2, and 3 rash. This strategy has been tested in a phase III study run by the Southwest Oncology Group (SWOG) that enrolled more than 700 patients and whose results will be soon available.

The second clinically relevant classes of agents that inhibit the EGFR are small molecule inhibitors of the receptor TK. There are several of these agents currently in clinical development. Two of these compounds, EKB-569 and erlotinib, have been specifically developed in pancreatic cancer. EKB-569 is an irreversible inhibitor of the EGFR and Her-2 receptors has completed a phase I study in combination with gemcitabine. Erlotinib, a specific and selective inhibitor of the EGFR, has been tested in combination with gemcitabine in a phase III study in patients with locally advanced and advanced pancreatic cancer (Moore *et al.* 2005). The study conducted by the National Cancer Institute of Canada randomized 569 patients with locally advanced (25%) or metastatic (75%) pancreatic adenocarcinoma not preselected for EGFR expression to receive standard-dose gemcitabine in combination with either erlotinib, 100 mg daily, or placebo. The addition of erlotinib to gemcitabine resulted in a statistically significant improvement in survival (HR 0.81; 95% CI 0.67–0.97; $p = 0.025$), with improvement in the median survival from 5.9 months to 6.4 months. The 1-year survival rate improved from 17% to 24% with the addition of erlotinib. The progression-free survival also improved significantly in the gemcitabine/erlotinib group (HR 0.76; $p = 0.003$). The most common side-effects, as expected with erlotinib, were grade 1 and 2 rash and diarrhea. The incidence of serious adverse effects was relatively low and similar in the two groups with the exception of rash, diarrhea, and stomatitis, which were more frequent in the erlotinib group. EGFR levels were tested in 162 tumor samples using immunohistochemistry and were positive in 53%. No clear differences in survival were noted in EGFR-positive patients. As demonstrated with other EGFR inhibitors, the development of drug-induced rash was associated with a better survival. These data led to the regulatory approval of erlotinib for treatment of patients with locally advanced or advanced pancreatic cancer in combination with gemcitabine.

Cox-2 inhibitors

The Cox-2 enzyme is overexpressed in pancreatic cancer and in preclinical studies and pharmacologic inhibition of this enzyme has been associated with antitumor effects in pancreatic cancer likely mediated by an antiangiogenesis and apoptosis inducing mechanism (Maitra *et al.* 2002; Tseng *et al.* 2002).

Other new approaches to systemic disease

In addition to the strategies described in the preceding paragraphs in more detail, there are some other drugs and therapeutic strategies that been used in advanced pancreatic cancer such as gene therapy, immunotherapy, and hormone-based therapies. As discussed in previous sections of this chapter, pancreatic cancer is characterized for lacking multiple genes such as p16, p53 and dpc 4 among others. Hecht *et al.* conducted a phase I/II study of ONYX-015, a E1B-55kD gene-deleted replication-selective adenovirus that preferentially replicates in and kills malignant cells that are p53 defective (Hecht *et al.* 2000). Twenty-one patients with locally advanced adenocarcinoma of the pancreas or with metastatic disease, but minimal or absent liver metastases, underwent eight sessions of ONYX-015 delivered by endoscopic ultrasound (EUS) injection into the primary pancreatic tumor over 8 weeks. The final four treatments were given in combination with gemcitabine 1000 mg/m^2. Two patients had partial regressions of the injected tumor. Local complications were tolerable with the use of oral prophylactic antibiotics and a transgastric injection approach only (Hecht *et al.* 2000).

References

Adjei AA. (2001) Blocking oncogenic Ras signaling for cancer therapy. *J Natl Cancer Inst* 93: 1062–74.

Bramhall SR, Rosemurgy A, Brown PD, Bowry C, Buckels JA. (2001) Marimastat as first-line therapy for patients with unresectable pancreatic cancer: a randomized trial. *J Clin Oncol* 19: 3447–55.

Bramhall SR, Schulz J, Nemunaitis J, Brown PD, Baillet M, Buckels JA. (2002) A double-blind placebo-controlled, randomised study comparing gemcitabine and marimastat with gemcitabine and placebo as first line therapy in patients with advanced pancreatic cancer. *Br J Cancer* 87: 161–7.

Cohen SJ, Ho L, Ranganathan S *et al.* (2003) Phase II and pharmacodynamic study of the farnesyltransferase inhibitor R115777 as initial therapy in patients with metastatic pancreatic adenocarcinoma. *J Clin Oncol* 21: 1301–6.

Evans JD, Stark A, Johnson CD *et al.* (2001) A phase II trial of marimastat in advanced pancreatic cancer. *Br J Cancer* 85: 1865–70.

Hecht J BR, Bedford R, Abbruzzese J, *et al.* (2003) A Phase I/II trial of intratumoral endoscopic ultrasound (EUS) injection of onyx-015 with intravenous gemcitabine in unresectable pancreatic carcinoma. *Clin Cancer Res* 9(2): 555–61.

Hidalgo M, Eckhardt SG. (2001) Development of matrix metalloproteinase inhibitors in cancer therapy. *J Natl Cancer Inst* 93: 178–93.

Jimeno A, Hidalgo M. (2005) Blockade of epidermal growth factor receptor (EGFR) activity. *Crit Rev Oncol Hematol* 53: 179–92.

Kindler HL, Friberg G, Singh DA *et al.* (2005) Phase II trial of bevacizumab plus gemcitabine in patients with advanced pancreatic cancer. *J Clin Oncol* 23: 8033–40.

Lersch CVCE, Amado R, Ehninger G *et al.* (2001) Randomized Phase II study of SCH 66336 and gemcitabine in the treatment of metastatic adenocarcinoma of the pancreas. *Proc Am Soc Clin Oncol.*

Maitra A, Ashfaq R, Gunn CR *et al.* (2002) Cyclooxygenase 2 expression in pancreatic adenocarcinoma and pancreatic intraepithelial neoplasia: an immunohistochemical analysis with automated cellular imaging. *Am J Clin Pathol* 118: 194–201.

Moore MJ, Hamm J, Dancey J *et al.* (2003) Comparison of gemcitabine versus the matrix metalloproteinase inhibitor BAY 12–9566 in patients with advanced or metastatic adenocarcinoma of the pancreas: A Phase III Trial of the National Cancer Institute of Canada Clinical Trials Group. *J Clin Oncol* 21: 3296–302.

Moore MJ, Goldstein D, Hamm J *et al.* (2005) Erlotinib plus gemcitabine compared to gemcitabine alone in patients with advanced pancreatic cancer. A Phase III trial of the National Cancer Institute of Canada Clinical Trials Group (NCICCTG). *J Clin Oncol* 23(16S): 1s. Abstract 1.

Rosemurgy A, Harris J, Langleben A, Casper E, Goode S, Rasmussen H. (1999) Marimastat in patients with advanced pancreatic cancer: a dose-finding study. *Am J Clin Oncol* 22: 247–52.

Safran H, Iannitti D, Ramanathan R *et al.* (2004) Herceptin and gemcitabine for metastatic pancreatic cancers that overexpress HER-2/neu. *Cancer Invest* 22: 706–12.

Tseng WW, Deganutti A, Chen MN, Saxton RE, Liu CD. (2002) Selective cyclooxygenase-2 inhibitor rofecoxib (Vioxx) induces expression of cell cycle arrest genes and slows tumor growth in human pancreatic cancer. *J Gastrointest Surg* 6: 838–43; discussion 844.

Van Cutsem EW *et al.* (2004) Phase III trial comparing gemcitabine plus tipifarnib compared with gemcitabine plus placebo in advanced pancreatic cancer (PC). *J Clin Oncol* 22(8): 1430–8.

Von Hoff DD, Bearss D. (2002) New drugs for patients with pancreatic cancer. *Curr Opin Oncol* 14: 621–7.

Xiong HQ, Rosenberg A, Lobuglio A *et al.* (2004) Cetuximab, a monoclonal antibody targeting the epidermal growth factor receptor, in combination with gemcitabine for advanced pancreatic cancer: a multicenter phase II Trial. *J Clin Oncol* 22: 2610–16.

Prognosis and follow-up

Jeffrey Infante & Wells Messersmith

Introduction

Pancreatic ductal adenocarcinoma remains one of the most lethal human cancers. Despite being the 10th most common cause of incident cancer in men and women, it is the fourth most common cause of death (Jemal *et al.* 2005). As with many solid malignancies in which good early detection strategies do not exist, the overall prognosis remains extremely poor for most patients. At the time of the diagnosis, the most critical determinant of outcome in patients with pancreatic cancer is whether the tumor can be completely resected. Pylorus-preserving pancreaticoduodenectomy, or Whipple procedure, is the standard operation for patients with resectable ductal adenocarcinoma of the head of the pancreas. Surgical resection offers the only chance of a curative treatment paradigm. Unfortunately, approximately 85% of patients present with advanced unresectable disease (DiMagno *et al.* 1999), and are treated palliatively. As would be expected, survival greatly depends on resectability. Though the majority of pancreas cancers are adenocarcinomas, there are multiple histologic variants in which the expected survival is less well defined, including neuroendocrine neoplasms of the pancreas and intraductal papillary mucinous neoplasms (IPMNs).

Resected adenocarcinoma of the pancreas

Survival is significantly better for patients with pancreatic cancers localized to the pancreas and regional lymph nodes, where surgical resection offers the only chance of cure. For patients with resectable ductal adenocarcinoma of the head of the pancreas, the 5-year overall survival rate is approximately 8–20% (Geer & Brennan 1993; Sohn *et al.* 2000; Regine *et al.* 2006; Ries *et al.* 2006). Two large surgical series from Johns Hopkins and from Memorial Sloan-Kettering Cancer Center suggest the median survival is approximately 17 months with an overall survival of approximately 60–65% at 1 year and 17–20% at 5 years (Geer & Brennan 1993; Sohn *et al.* 2000). The SEER (Surveillance Epidemiology and End Results) suggests the 5-year overall survival rate is much worse, 19.6% for those localized to the pancreas only, but 8.2% if there is lymph node involvement (Ries *et al.* 2006). In the Radiation Therapy Oncology Group's recently presented trial RTOG 9704, the 190 patients with resected head of the pancreas tumors randomized to the treatment arm of concurrent 5-FU with radiation

Table 21.7 Prognosis of pancreatic cancer patients as defined by selected clinical trials and case series.

	Author	Study design	Treatment	Median survival	Overall survival
Adenocarcinoma					
Resected	Regine (2006)	Phase III RCT	5-FU/XRT→Gem	19 months	3-year—31%
Locally advanced unresectable	GTSG (1998)	Phase III RCT	5-FU/XRT→SMF	10 months	1-year—41%
Metastatic	Burris (1997)	Phase III RCT	Single agent Gem	6 months	1-year—18%
Neuroendocrine	Kouvaraki (2004)	Retrospective series	5-FU+Strep+Dox	37 months	2-year—74%
IPMNs					
Invasive	Sohn TA (2004)	Retrospective series	Resection	Not Stated	5-year—43%
Non-invasive	Sohn TA (2004)	Retrospective series	Resection	N/A	5-year—77%

RCT, randomized controlled trial; GTSG, Gastrointestinal Tumor Study Group; 5-FU, 5-fluorouracil; XRT, radiation; Gem, gemcitabine; Strep, streptozosin; Dox, doxorubicin.

followed by more gemcitabine experienced a median survival of 18.8 months and a 3-year overall survival of 31% (Regine *et al.* 2006).

Clinicopathologic parameters provide some information about whether a patient will achieve long-term survival. Tumor diameter > 2.5–3.0 cm, positive lymph nodes, positive margins, and poor differentiation are all features that have consistently been associated with a worse prognosis (Geer & Brennan 1993; Sohn *et al.* 2000; Infante *et al.* 2007). The delay in presentation and the systemic nature of this disease is exemplified by the fact that 80–85% of resected patients have positive lymph nodes, and approximately 40% have positive microscopic margins (Infante *et al.* 2007). Some studies suggest that tumors arising from the body and tail of the pancreas have a slightly worse prognosis than those arising from the head of the pancreas since they often present later with an increased size and stage (Sohn *et al.* 2000).

Numerous genetic and epigenetic alterations occur during the development of pancreatic adenocarcinoma. Several studies have investigated whether genetic changes that are important for pancreatic cancer development influence prognosis (Hruban *et al.* 2000). The first molecular marker with prognostic significance was the DNA index (Allison *et al.* 1998). Although DNA index is not used clinically, it indicated that molecular markers could provide information about the malignant behavior of tumors of the pancreas. As the understanding of the molecular and genetic changes that lead to pancreatic neoplasia has grown, so has the hope that molecular markers will be identified that better predict tumor behavior and the response to rational therapies.

An obvious start to the search for such biomarkers is to focus on the genetic changes that are important in the development of pancreas cancer as outlined in the progression model by Hruban *et al.* (Hruban *et al.* 2000). The model correlates somatic genetic changes with the histologic progression from normal pancreatic tissue through the precursor lesions (PanINs 1–3) and eventually into infiltrating adenocarcinoma. Almost all pancreatic adenocarcinomas activate K-ras by mutation (~90%), and inactivate *p16* genetically or epigenetically (>95%), suggesting that if these markers had any prognostic ability it would apply to only a minority of individuals. SMAD4/DPC4 is genetically inactivated in ~55% of pancreatic ductal adenocarcinomas, making this the most common known mode of inactivation of the TGFβ pathway. Protein expression of SMAD4 is a reliable predictor of SMAD4 genetic status and has been used to evaluate the role of SMAD4 inactivation in pancreatic cancer prognosis among patients undergoing pancreatic resection, but results have not been consistent in three studies (Tascilar *et al.* 2001; Biankin *et al.* 2002; Infante *et al.* 2007).

Epigenetic changes that are thought to contribute to pancreatic cancer progression include inactivation of *SPARC, RELN, TFPI-2*, and less commonly, hMLH1 (Ueki *et al.* 2000; Sato *et al.* 2003; Sato *et al.* 2004; Sato *et al.* 2006) and possibly others (Sato & Goggins 2006a,b).

No epigenetic markers have consistently been found to correlate with prognosis. Recently, SPARC expression in the peritumoral fibroblasts of the neighboring stroma was shown to be a strong marker of poor prognosis in patients with pancreas cancer who undergo a Whipple procedure with curative intent (Infante *et al.* 2007). Patients whose pancreatic cancer stroma labeled positive for SPARC had a significantly worse prognosis, with a median survival of 15 months as compared to 30 months for those whose stroma did not express SPARC. Approximately 13% of patients whose stroma expressed SPARC were alive at 4 years as compared to 43% of patients whose stroma lacked SPARC expression. SPARC was the first non-tumor-associated protein shown to correlate with survival in this patient population. The mechanisms by which peritumoral fibroblast SPARC expression portends to a significantly poor patient prognosis are not yet understood.

Despite the great advances in understanding the molecular and genetic changes that lead to neoplasia, no molecular marker has been studied enough to be used in clinical decision making. The sialylated Lewis^a blood group antigen CA19-9 is the only marker that has a role in the management of pancreatic cancer. Perioperative serum levels of CA19-9 have been shown to predict survival in patients with resectable pancreatic adenocarcinoma. It is expected that 10–20% of pancreatic cancers do not shed the marker in the serum, often referred to as non-secretors, and will have undetectable preoperative CA19-9 levels. Preoperative CA19-9 is associated with stage and tumor burden (Ferrone *et al.* 2006). Berger *et al.* suggested that patients who present with resectable adenocarcinoma of the pancreas and are CA19-9 non-secretors do just as well as those with normal CA19-9, and do significantly better than those that present with elevated CA19-9 levels (Berger *et al.* 2004). The use of preoperative a CA19-9 level of elevation as a predictor of outcome has been more difficult since levels are often distorted in the presence of biliary obstruction. A postoperative decrease in CA19-9 levels (Glenn *et al.* 1988; Ferrone *et al.* 2006), and a postoperative value of <200 U/mL are predictors of survival (Ferrone *et al.* 2006).

In summary, resection offers the only curative approach with this disease. Unfortunately, only ~15% of patients are candidates for resection at the time of diagnosis. If patients are able to undergo resection, only around 60% are an R0 resection and the vast majority of patients already have lymph node metastasis. This aggressive biology translates into a very poor 5-year overall survival of 5–25%. A precipitous postoperative decrease in CA19-9 portends to a better survival. Other molecular markers expressed in the tumor or the surrounding stroma appear to have prognostic capacity, but are not yet generalizable to the clinic.

Locally advanced unresectable adenocarcinoma of the pancreas

Due to proximity and the inherent aggressive biology, pancreatic tumors frequently invade adjacent structures such as superior mesenteric and celiac vascular structures, making curative resection impossible. Approximately 30–40% of pancreatic cancer patients present with such locally advanced, non-metastatic disease. In general, treatment efforts in this setting are palliative, except in the rare case where one achieves a significant enough response to allow surgical resection. The true natural history of untreated locally advanced pancreas cancer is hard to define since there are no trials in this subgroup that randomized to an arm of best supportive care. Optimal treatment for locally advanced pancreatic cancer remains controversial, where most practitioners in the United States recommend combined chemotherapy (usually 5-FU based) and radiation (typically 54 Gy in 1.8-Gy fractions), followed by more chemotherapy. Three randomized studies have demonstrated a modest survival benefit of combined modality therapy over chemotherapy or external-beam radiation alone (Moertel *et al.* 1969; Moertel *et al.* 1981; Gastrointestinal Tumor Study Group 1988). The median survival in these trials ranged from 8–11 months with the proportion surviving 1 year anywhere from 25% to 44%. Some oncologists recommend chemotherapy alone for locally advanced disease. In this scenario, gemcitabine is commonly used, based on the randomized trial by Burris *et al.* in which 26% of the study subjects had locally advanced disease (Burris *et al.* 1997). Unfortunately, the results for patients with locally advanced disease were not reported separately from those with metastatic disease.

Metastatic adenocarcinoma of the pancreas

Metastatic pancreas cancer is a uniformly aggressive and fatal disease. The natural history of advanced pancreas cancer is often characterized by increased pain, persistent weight loss, and a progressive decline in performance status. Three trials have randomized patients with metastatic pancreas cancer to chemotherapy versus best supportive care. In these trials the median survival in the untreated arms was 7–17 weeks (Mallinson *et al.* 1980; Frey *et al.* 1981; Palmer *et al.* 1994).

Gemcitabine was the first chemotherapy agent approved by the FDA for the treatment of advanced pancreas cancer. Burris *et al.* published the pivotal trial comparing single-agent gemcitabine to 5-FU (Burris *et al.* 1997). As compared to weekly bolus 5-FU, gemcitabine met its primary endpoint of clinical benefit (improved pain control, analgesic consumption, and performance status). The median survival in the gemcitabine-treated group was 5.6 months, with 18% alive at 1 year. This was marginally but significantly better than the 5-FU arm with a median survival of 4.4 months and 2% alive at 1 year. Gemcitabine has been compared against multiple other cytotoxic chemotherapy agents either alone or in combination, but unfortunately there has been little improvement in prognosis. Recently, a small molecule inhibitor of the epidermal growth factor tyrosine kinase pathway, erlotinib (Tarceva), was approved for the treatment of metastatic pancreas cancer. Despite a marginal improvement in median survival, the proportion of patients alive at 1 year with the combination of gemcitabine with erlotinib was 26% as compared to 20% for those treated with gemcitabine alone (Moore *et al.* 2005).

Neuroendocrine neoplasms of the pancreas

Neoplasms of the endocrine pancreas are rare, accounting for approximately 2% of all pancreatic tumors. Although outcomes are typically better than adenocarcinomas of the pancreas, prognosis is heterogeneous and largely dependent on histologic classification. Multiple classifications exist, but the World Health Organization (WHO) separates these tumors in to functioning or non-functioning neoplasms of benign behavior, neoplasms of uncertain behavior, well-differentiated carcinomas, and poorly differentiated carcinomas/small-cell carcinomas. Tumors that are thought to have 'benign' behavior are characteristically confined to the pancreas, without perineural or perivascular invasion, <2 cm in diameter, <2 mitotic figures per 10× high-power field, and <2% Ki-67-positive cells.

Clinically, all patients with disease localized to the pancreas should be approached surgically along a curative paradigm. Independent of the surgical procedure (pancreaticoduodenectomy, distal pancreatectomy, or tumor enucleation), margin status appears to be the most important prognostic surgical feature (Phan *et al.* 1998). In the Johns Hopkins retrospective surgical series, the 5-year survival rate was 91% for those with benign tumors as compared to 49% for those with malignant tumors. A second smaller surgical series from UCLA found the 5-year survival of malignant neuroendocrine tumors to be 77% (Kazanjian *et al.* 2006). Whether non-functional tumors have an inherently worse biology remains controversial since most present later in their natural history with increased size and stage (Kent *et al.* 1981; White *et al.* 1994; Hochwald *et al.* 2002).

Similar to metastatic adenocarcinoma, metastatic neuroendocrine carcinomas of the pancreas are incurable and treated on a palliative paradigm. However, response rates to chemotherapy are improved (approximately 15–40%) and prognosis is markedly better (Kouvaraki *et al.* 2004; Kulke *et al.* 2006). In one series of 84 patients treated with 5-FU, doxorubicin and streptozosin, the median overall survival was 37 months and 2-year survival was 74% (Kouvaraki *et al.* 2004). The presence of >75% involvement of the liver significantly reduced these survival estimates.

Cystic neoplasms of the pancreas

Cystic neoplasms of the pancreas are rare, and comprise only 1% of pancreatic cancers. The most common cystic neoplasm is an IPMN, but others include mucinous cystic neoplasms, serous cystadenomas, papillary cystic tumors, and cystic islet cell tumors. The WHO characterizes IPMNs as intraductal mucin-producing neoplasms with tall, columnar, mucin-containing epithelium with or without papillary projections. This definition now includes a portion of tumors previously termed papillary carcinoma, ductectatic mucinous cystadenomas, and villous adenomas. IPMNs have clear malignant potential and seem to follow an adenoma–carcinoma sequence of progression from an IPMN adenoma, to borderline IPMN with dysplasia, to IPMN with CIS (carcinoma *in situ*), and finally to invasive carcinoma. The natural history is unclear, but time of progression of an adenoma to invasive carcinoma appears to take at least 5 years (Sohn *et al.* 2004).

Following resection, IPMNs that are classified as non-invasive (which includes 'adenoma', 'borderline', and 'CIS') have a significantly better prognosis as compared to those IPMNs that are associated with invasive cancer. In one retrospective study from Johns Hopkins, 136 patients underwent pancreatic resection of an IPMN between 1987 and 2003 (Sohn *et al.* 2004). The 5-year overall survival for those IPMNs with invasive cancer appears to be 36–43% (Chari *et al.* 2002; Sohn *et al.* 2004). If nodes are involved and/or the residual margins are positive, patients do much worse and survival mimics patients with invasive ductal adenocarcinoma.

The 5-year overall survival was 77% for those with non-invasive IPMNs. As in another study, this favorable prognosis was independent of the degree of epithelial dysplasia (Chari *et al.* 2002; Sohn *et al.* 2004). Although this is an overall good prognosis, it reaffirms the real possibility of the development of an invasive cancer in the pancreatic remnant despite clear surgical margins (Chari *et al.* 2002). Postoperative surveillance is critical in this subgroup. The prognostic significance of main duct versus branch duct variants of IPMNs remain controversial.

Follow-up and surveillance

Most patients that are able to achieve an R0 resection for adenocarcinoma of the pancreas will undergo adjuvant therapy with either chemotherapy or combined chemotherapy with radiation. Following completion of adjuvant therapy, patients tend to be followed closely since disease will eventually recur in approximately 75% of the patients and they will ultimately succumb to their disease. The National Comprehensive Cancer Network recommends surveillance every 3–6 months for 2 years and then annually with a history and physical examination and CA19-9. CT scans of the chest, abdomen and pelvis are often included, despite minimal evidence to support their use. Currently there is no evidence to support a role for PET scans with surveillance.

For patients with non-invasive IPMNs that underwent a full pancreatectomy, no surveillance is necessary. For patients with non-invasive IPMNs that undergo a partial pancreatectomy, the value of surveillance is debated since the possibility of recurrence in the pancreatic remnant is only approximately 8% (Chari *et al.* 2002). For patients with invasive IPMNs, some experts recommend imaging surveillance since recurrence rates are higher and if the recurrence occurs in the remnant, a repeat surgical procedure may be curative. There are no consensus recommendations regarding IPMNs.

Conclusions

In summary, the vast majority of pancreatic neoplasms are adenocarcinomas and prognosis remains grim. Most patients present with advanced unresectable disease. Of the 15% that are able to undergo surgical resection, less than 25% are alive and free of disease at 5 years. Average survival in locally advanced, unresectable disease is estimated to be between 8–11 months. For those with distant metastasis, the median survival is approximately 6 months.

Similar to adenocarcinomas, surgical resection offers the only chance at cure for neuroendocrine neoplasms of the pancreas. However, survival is markedly improved, especially if clear margins are obtained. Metastatic neuroendocrine tumors are also more responsive to chemotherapy and the median survival has reached close to 3 years in some studies.

IPMNs clearly have malignant potential and surgical resection is the treatment of choice. Non-invasive IPMNs have a low risk of recurrence in the pancreatic remnant. Invasive IPMNs have a high rate of recurrence, either locally or distant. The median overall survival following resection is only marginally better than that of typical adenocarcinoma of the pancreas.

References

Allison DC, Piantadosi S, Hruban RH *et al.* (1998) DNA content and other factors associated with ten-year survival after resection of pancreatic carcinoma. *J Surg Oncol* 67: 151–9.

Berger AC, Meszoely IM, Ross EA, Watson JC, Hoffman JP. (2004) Undetectable preoperative levels of serum CA 19–9 correlate with improved survival for patients with resectable pancreatic adenocarcinoma. *Ann Surg Oncol* 11: 644–9.

Biankin AV, Morey AL, Lee CS *et al.* (2002) DPC4/Smad4 expression and outcome in pancreatic ductal adenocarcinoma. *J Clin Oncol* 20: 4531–42.

Burris HA 3rd, Moore MJ, Andersen J *et al.* (1997) Improvements in survival and clinical benefit with gemcitabine as first- line therapy for patients with advanced pancreas cancer: a randomized trial. *J Clin Oncol* 15: 2403–13.

Chari ST, Yadav D, Smyrk TC *et al.* (2002) Study of recurrence after surgical resection of intraductal papillary mucinous neoplasm of the pancreas. *Gastroenterology* 123: 1500–7.

Dimagno EP, Reber HA, Tempero MA. (1999) AGA technical review on the epidemiology, diagnosis, and treatment of pancreatic ductal adenocarcinoma. American Gastroenterological Association. *Gastroenterology* 117: 1464–84.

Ferrone CR, Finkelstein DM, Thayer SP, Muzikansky A, Castillo CF-D, Warshaw AL. (2006) Perioperative CA19–9 levels can predict stage and survival in patients with resectable pancreatic adenocarcinoma. *J Clin Oncol* 24: 2897–902.

Frey C, Twomey P, Keehn R, Elliott D, Higgins G. (1981) Randomized study of 5-FU and CCNU in pancreatic cancer: report of the Veterans Administration Surgical Adjuvant Cancer Chemotherapy Study Group. *Cancer* 47: 27–31.

Gastrointestinal Tumor Study Group (1988) Treatment of locally unresectable carcinoma of the pancreas: comparison of combined-modality therapy (chemotherapy plus radiotherapy) to chemotherapy alone. Gastrointestinal Tumor Study Group. *J Natl Cancer Inst* 80: 751–5.

Geer RJ, Brennan MF. (1993) Prognostic indicators for survival after resection of pancreatic adenocarcinoma. *Am J Surg* 165: 68–72; discussion 72–3.

Glenn J, Steinberg WM, Kurtzman SH, Steinberg SM, Sindelar WF. (1988) Evaluation of the utility of a radioimmunoassay for serum CA 19-9 levels in patients before and after treatment of carcinoma of the pancreas. *J Clin Oncol* 6: 462–8.

Hochwald SN, Zee S, Conlon KC *et al.* (2002) Prognostic factors in pancreatic endocrine neoplasms: an analysis of 136 cases with a proposal for low-grade and intermediate-grade groups. *J Clin Oncol* 20: 2633–42.

Hruban RH, Goggins M, Parsons J, Kern SE. (2000) Progression model for pancreatic cancer. *Clin Cancer Res* 6: 2969–72.

Infante JR, Matsubayashi H, Sato N *et al.* (2007) Peritumoral fibroblast SPARC expression and patient outcome with resectable pancreatic adenocarcinoma. *J Clin Oncol* 25(3): 319–25.

Jemal A, Murray T, Ward E *et al.* (2005) Cancer statistics, 2005. *CA Cancer J Clin* 55: 10–30.

Kazanjian KK, Reber HA, Hines OJ. (2006) Resection of pancreatic neuroendocrine tumors: results of 70 cases. *Arch Surg* 141: 765–70.

Kent RB 3rd, Van Heerden JA, Weiland LH. (1981) Nonfunctioning islet cell tumors. *Ann Surg* 193: 185–90.

Kouvaraki MA, Ajani JA, Hoff P, Wolff R, Evans DB, Lozano R, Yao JC. (2004) Fluorouracil, doxorubicin, and streptozocin in the treatment of patients with locally advanced and metastatic pancreatic endocrine carcinomas. *J Clin Oncol* 22: 4762–71.

Kulke MH, Stuart K, Enzinger PC *et al.* (2006) Phase II Study of temozolomide and thalidomide in patients with metastatic neuroendocrine tumors. *J Clin Oncol* 24: 401–6.

Mallinson CN, Rake MO, Cocking JB *et al.* (1980) Chemotherapy in pancreatic cancer: results of a controlled, prospective, randomised, multicentre trial. *Br Med J* 281: 1589–91.

Moertel CG, Childs DS Jr, Reitemeier RJ, Colby MY Jr, Holbrook MA. (1969) Combined 5-fluorouracil and supervoltage radiation therapy of locally unresectable gastrointestinal cancer. *Lancet* 2: 865–7.

Moertel CG, Frytak S, Hahn RG *et al.* (1981) Therapy of locally unresectable pancreatic carcinoma: a randomized comparison of high dose (6000 rads) radiation alone, moderate dose radiation (4000 rads + 5-fluorouracil), and high dose radiation + 5-fluorouracil: The Gastrointestinal Tumor Study Group. *Cancer* 48: 1705–10.

Moore MJ, Goldstein D, Hamm J *et al.* (2005) Erlotinib plus gemcitabine compared to gemcitabine alone in patients with advanced pancreatic cancer. A phase III trial of the National Cancer Institute of Canada Clinical Trials Group [NCIC-CTG]. *J Clin Oncol (Meeting Abstracts)* 23: 1.

Palmer KR, Kerr M, Knowles G, Cull A, Carter DC, Leonard RC. (1994) Chemotherapy prolongs survival in inoperable pancreatic carcinoma. *Br J Surg* 81: 882–5.

Phan GQ, Yeo CJ, Hruban RH, Lillemoe KD, Pitt HA, Cameron JL. (1998) Surgical experience with pancreatic and peripancreatic neuroendocrine tumors: review of 125 patients. *J Gastrointest Surg* 2: 472–82.

Regine WF, Winter KW, Abrams R *et al.* (2006) RTOG 9704 a phase III study of adjuvant pre and post chemoradiation (CRT) 5-FU vs. gemcitabine (G) for resected pancreatic adenocarcinoma. *J Clin Oncol (Meeting Abstracts)* 24: 4007.

Ries LAG, Harkins D., Krapcho M *et al.*, eds. (2006) *Seer Cancer Statistics Review, 1975–2003*. National Cancer Institute. Bethesda, MD. http://seer.cancer.gov/csr/1975_2003/ [based on November 2005 seer data submission, posted to the seer web site 2006].

Sato N, Goggins M (2006a). Epigenetic alterations in intraductal papillary mucinous neoplasms of the pancreas. *J Hepatobiliary Pancreat Surg* 13(4): 280–5.

Sato N, Goggins M (2006b). The role of epigenetic alterations in pancreatic cancer. *J Hepatobiliary Pancreat Surg* 13(4): 286–95.

Sato N, Fukushima N, Maehara N *et al.* (2003) SPARC/osteonectin is a frequent target for aberrant methylation in pancreatic adenocarcinoma and a mediator of tumor-stromal interactions. *Oncogene* 22: 5021–30.

Sato N, Parker AR, Fukushima N *et al.* (2004) Epigenetic inactivation of TFPI-2 as a common mechanism associated with growth and invasion of pancreatic ductal adenocarcinoma. 24: 850.

Sato N, Fukushima N, Chang R, Matsubayashi H, Goggins M (2006) Differential and epigenetic gene expression profiling identifies frequent disruption of the RELN pathway in pancreatic cancers. *Gastroenterology* 130: 548.

Sohn TA, Yeo CJ, Cameron JL *et al.* (2000) Resected adenocarcinoma of the pancreas-616 patients: results, outcomes, and prognostic indicators. *J Gastrointest Surg* 4: 567–79.

Sohn TA, Yeo CJ, Cameron JL, Hruban RH, Fukushima N, Campbell KA, Lillemoe KD. (2004) Intraductal papillary mucinous neoplasms of the pancreas: an updated experience. *Ann Surg* 239: 788–97; discussion 797–9.

Tascilar M, Skinner HG, Rosty C *et al.* (2001) The SMAD4 protein and prognosis of pancreatic ductal adenocarcinoma. *Clin Cancer Res* 7: 4115–21.

Ueki T, Toyota M, Sohn T *et al.* (2000) Hypermethylation of multiple genes in pancreatic adenocarcinoma. *Cancer Res* 60: 1835–9.

White TJ, Edney JA, Thompson JS, Karrer FW, Moor BJ. (1994) Is there a prognostic difference between functional and non-functional islet cell tumors? *Am J Surg* 168: 627–9; discussion 629–30.

22 Cholangiocarcinoma

Edited by Ravi S. Chari

Diagnosis

Overview

Ravi S. Chari

Making a definitive diagnosis of cholangiocarcinoma is difficult. However, since resection offers the only chance for cure, if cholangiocarcinoma is clinically suspected, the resection should not be delayed by the absence of a tissue diagnosis. To determine resectability, all of the available clinical and radiologic data are needed. Currently there is no system that stratifies patients into subgroups based on their potential for resection. The current American Joint Commission on Cancer Staging system (Table 22.1) is based on pathologic data and can convey information pertaining to the patient's prognosis. This staging system, however, does not predict the likelihood of resection for stage I–III patients (Burke *et al.* 1998; Jarnagin *et al.* 2001). The Bismuth–Corlette system (Table 22.2) can reliably stratify patients based on the location and extent of the tumor in the biliary tree (Bismuth *et al.* 1992). Although this system is useful for description of the tumors, it also is not predictive for resectability or survival.

References

Bismuth H, Nakache R, Diamond T. (1992) Management strategies in resection for hilar cholangiocarcinoma. *Ann Surg* 215(1): 31–8.

Burke EC, Jarnagin WR, Hochwald SN, Pisters PW, Fong Y, Blumgart LH. (1998) Hilar cholangiocarcinoma: patterns of spread, the importance of hepatic resection for curative operation, and a presurgical clinical staging system. *Ann Surg* 228(3): 385–94.

Jarnagin WR, Fong Y, DeMatteo RP *et al.* (2001) Staging, resectability, and outcome in 225 patients with hilar cholangiocarcinoma. *Ann Surg* 234(4): 507–17.

Gastrointestinal Oncology: A Critical Multidisciplinary Team Approach. Edited by J. Jankowski, R. Sampliner, D. Kerr, and Y. Fong.

History

T. Markley Earl, Burnett S. Kelly & Ravi S. Chari

Cholangiocarcinomas are rare malignant tumors arising from the epithelium of the bile ducts. Biliary tract malignancies have traditionally included tumors arising from the gallbladder, extrahepatic biliary tree and ampulla of Vater while intrahepatic malignancies were classified as primary liver tumors. More recently, tumors identified as arising from biliary epithelium exclusive of the gallbladder and ampulla have been termed cholangiocarcinomas and further subdivided into intra- and extrahepatic tumors. Intrahepatic tumors originate from either small intrahepatic ductules or large intrahepatic ducts near the hilum. The extrahepatic ducts are divided into perihilar (including the confluence of the left and right ducts) and distal segments with the transition occurring where the common bile duct lies posterior to the duodenum. Perihilar tumors are further sub classified according to the Bismuth–Corlette system depending on the pattern of involvement of the hepatic ducts (Table 22.2). The hepatic duct bifurcation is the most frequently involved site with approximately 60% of cholangiocarcinomas found in this region. These tumors often involve major hilar vascular structures making resection difficult; however, optimal treatment is duct resection with or without accompanying hepatectomy. Distal tumors are the second most common and are usually treated with pancreaticoduodenectomy. Purely intrahepatic tumors occur most rarely and are treated with hepatic resection. Surgical resection with negative margins remains the mainstay of treatment and is the most important factor for long-term survival; however this is not possible in the majority of patients.

Symptoms

The initial symptoms of biliary tract cancers are usually caused by obstruction of the biliary drainage system often resulting in painless jaundice. Common symptoms include pruritus (66%), abdominal pain (30–50%), weight loss (30–50%) and fever (up to 20%). These symptoms tend to occur earlier in tumors of the

Table 22.1 Current American Joint Commission on cancer staging system for cholangiocarcinoma.

Stage 0	Tis	N0	M0
Stage I	T1	N0	M0
Stage II	T2	N0	M0
Stage III	T1 or T2	N1 or N2	M0
Stage IVA	T3	Any N	M0
Stage IVB	Any T	Any N	M1
Tis	Carcinoma *in situ*		
T1	Tumor invades the subepithelial connective tissue		
T2	Tumor invades perifibromuscular connective tissue		
T3	Tumor invades adjacent organs		
N0	No regional lymph node metastases		
N1	Metastasis to hepatoduodenal ligament lymph nodes		
N2	Metastasis to peripancreatic, periduodenal, periportal, celiac, and/or superior mesenteric artery lymph nodes		
M0	No distant metastasis		
M1	Distant metastasis		

Table 22.2 The Bismuth–Corlette classification scheme of biliary strictures.

Type I	Tumor involves the common hepatic duct
Type II	Tumor involves the bifurcation of the common hepatic duct
Type IIIa	Tumor involves the right hepatic duct
Type IIIb	Tumor involves the left hepatic duct
Type IV	Tumor involves both the right and left hepatic ducts

extrahepatic biliary tree and develop later in more proximal disease. Pain, fatigue, weight loss and malaise are often associated with advanced disease. The pain is often described as a constant dull ache in the right upper quadrant and is more common in cancer of the gallbladder. Cholangitis is an unusual presentation but is suggested by the presence of fever, chills, right upper quadrant pain and jaundice with or without the presence of hemodynamic compromise. The diagnosis of cholangiocarcinoma in patients with a history of primary sclerosing cholangitis (PSC) can be problematic, but is often suggested by a declining performance status and increasing cholestasis. Other symptoms due to biliary obstruction include dark urine and acholic stools.

Risk factors

Primary sclerosing cholangitis

Despite the rarity of these tumors, several risk factors for cholangiocarcinoma are known. The majority of these are associated with biliary stasis, infection or exposure to carcinogens. Perhaps the most significant association of cholangiocarcinoma is to primary sclerosing cholangitis. Lifetime risks of cholangiocarcinoma ranging from 10 to in excess of 30% have been reported. A strong association exists between primary sclerosing cholangitis and chronic ulcerative colitis. Between 60 and 80% of patients with primary sclerosing cholangitis will have concurrent ulcerative colitis and total proctocolectomy does not diminish the risk of developing the condition. The time to diagnosis of cholangiocarcinoma ranges from 1 to 25 years, although one-third of these will be found within 2 years following the diagnosis of primary sclerosing cholangitis and the duration of disease does not appear to alter the risk.

Differentiation of benign biliary strictures that characterize this disease from cholangiocarcinoma remains a difficult clinical problem. Patients with primary sclerosing cholangitis who develop cholangiocarcinoma will typically do so in the fifth decade of life, 20 years earlier than those who develop the disease in the absence of primary sclerosing cholangitis. Approximately 10% of patients undergoing liver transplantation for primary sclerosing cholangitis are found to have cholangiocarcinoma in the hepatectomy specimen. Because of the increased utilization of liver transplantation for patients with sclerosing cholangitis and subsequent decrease in mortality due to hepatic failure, cholangiocarcinoma has become the leading cause of death in patients with this disease.

Biliary infestations

The association between the liver fluke *Opisthorchis viverrini* and cholangiocarcinoma has been recognized for some time and the relationship of *Clonorchis sinensis* remains highly probable. Infection with these parasites results in a 25- to 50-fold increase in the risk of bile duct cancer. Infestation is endemic to southeast Asia with *O. viverrini* occurring predominantly in Thailand, Laos and northern Malaysia, and *C. sinensis* predominant in China, Korea, Taiwan and Vietnam. A 1994 report from the World Health Organization estimates the global number of liver fluke infestations at 17 million. Infestation occurs when humans or other animals ingest raw fish containing the infective cysts of the fluke (metacercariae). Following consumption, the infective metacercariae excyst in the duodenum and move up the bile tree and develop into adults in the intrahepatic bile ducts. The adult flukes lay eggs that are excreted in the host feces. The eggs are ingested by snails of the *Bithynia* species where they hatch and mature into cercariae. The freely swimming cercariae leave the snail and find cyprinoid fish where they develop into metacercariae in the muscle and connective tissue.

Early pathologic consequences of liver fluke infection consist of acute inflammation of the second-order bile ducts and periportal connective tissue along with death of hepatocytes and biliary epithelial cells. As the flukes develop into adults they induce hyperplasia of the bile duct epithelium, adenoma formation and granulomatous reaction with subsequent scarring. Chronic inflammation with resultant hyperplasia of the bile duct epithelium, increased formation of endogenous carcinogen, activation of drug-metabolizing enzymes and increased nitric oxide production likely act in concert during the development of cholangiocarcinoma.

Choledochal cyst

An increased incidence of cholangiocarcinoma has been noted in patients with choledochal cysts. The incidence of cholangiocarcinoma in patients with cystic abnormalities of the bile ducts has been found to range from 2.5% to 28%. Most patients with biliary cystic disease have been found to have an abnormally high entry of the pancreatic duct into the common bile duct, a finding associated with gallbladder cancer. Several studies have suggested that this anomaly results in reflux of exocrine pancreatic secretions into the bile duct leading to inflammation and possible malignant transformation of the biliary epithelium. Resection of the extrahepatic biliary tree lowers the risk of cholangiocarcinoma in all but those patients with intrahepatic or combined intra- and extrahepatic cystic disease.

Hepatolithiasis

Hepatolithiasis is rare in Europe and North America but is relatively common in several parts of Asia and is associated with an increase risk of cholangiocarcinoma. Malignant transformation seems to be associated with chronic inflammation due to bile stasis and recurrent bacteria infections that characterize the disease. Viral hepatitis and liver cirrhosis regardless of etiology has been suggested as risk factors for cholangiocarcinoma. Hepatitis C virus (HCV) RNA has been detected in cholangiocarcinoma tissue supporting the potentially proneoplastic role of HCV in biliary tract epithelium.

Other

Chronic exposure to ionizing radiation has been associated with increased incidence of cholangiocarcinoma. Thorotrast, a suspension containing the radioactive compound thorium dioxide, was a commonly used contrast medium in the early part of the last century and has been linked to bile duct cancer. Following injection, the drug distributes to the liver, spleen, and lymph nodes where it undergoes decay by alpha particle emission with a half-life of over 400 years. A number of other carcinogens have been implicated in cholangiocarcinoma including dioxin, asbestos, and dietary nitrosamines.

At least two genetic disorders are associated with an increased risk of cholangiocarcinoma: Lynch syndrome II and a rare inherited disorder called multiple biliary papillomatosis. An association between hepatitis C and cholangiocarcinoma was initially suggested in 1991, and a more recent prospective case–control study from Japan has reported that the risk of developing cholangiocarcinoma in patients with cirrhosis related to HCV is 3.5% over 10 years. An association between hepatitis B and cholangiocarcinoma has also been suggested but it is less compelling.

Summary

Despite the known risk factors, several with marked increase in risk, many cases of cholangiocarcinoma occur in patients without risk factors. Clinical suspicion in patients with compatible clinical history remains the key to prompt diagnosis.

References

Ahrendt SA, Nakeeb A, Pitt HA. (2001) Liver tumors: cholangiocarcinoma. *Clin Liver Dis* 5(1): 191–218.

De Groen PC, Gores GJ, LaRusso NF, Gunderson LL, Nagorney DM. (1999) Biliary tract cancers. *N Engl J Med* 341(18): 1368–78.

Patel T. (2006) Cholangiocarcinoma. *Nat Clin Pract Gastroenterol Hepatol* 3(1): 33–42.

Shaib YH, El-Serag HB, Davila JA, Morgan R, McGlynn KA. (2005) Risk factors of intrahepatic cholangiocarcinoma in the united states: a case-control study. *Gastroenterology* 128(3): 620–6.

Watanapa P, Watanapa WB. (2002) Liver fluke-associated cholangiocarcinoma. *Br J Surg* 89(8): 962–70.

Clinical

T. Markley Earl, Burnett S. Kelly & Ravi S. Chari

The clinical presentation of cholangiocarcinoma varies depending upon the site of tumor origin. Approximately 90% of patients with perihilar and distal tumors present with jaundice while those with intrahepatic tumors tend to present with abdominal pain and subsequently have a liver mass identified on imaging studies. Fever is an uncommon symptom regardless of tumor location, but is slightly more common in patients with perihilar tumors. Cholangitis is rare at the time of diagnosis but can develop after biliary tract manipulation. Stigmata of tumor-related cachexia such as temporal wasting may be present in patients presenting with advanced disease. Other physical signs include hepatomegaly and a palpable gallbladder or mass, depending on location of the tumor.

Laboratory abnormalities can be divided into those as a result of biliary obstruction and those due to the secretion of abnormal products by the tumor. Biliary obstruction and resultant cholestasis results in elevation of the total bilirubin with a significant proportion being conjugated (direct) due to intact hepatic function. Alkaline phosphatase and γ-glutamyltransferase are also elevated in the presence of biliary tract obstruction. Levels of transaminases are often normal or only mildly elevated. Longstanding obstruction of the common hepatic or bile duct can lead to deficiency of fat-soluble vitamins and subsequent increase in the prothrombin time or international normalized ratio (INR).

Several tumor markers may be secreted into the bile or blood; most are non-specific but may be of diagnostic value in patients with cholangiocarcinoma. The majority of studies in this area have focused on identifying cholangiocarcinoma in patients with primary sclerosing cholangitis due to the increased incidence in this population and the difficulty in differentiating benign and malignant lesions on cholangiography.

Serum levels of cancer antigen (CA) 19-9 are widely used, particularly for detecting cholangiocarcinoma in patients with primary sclerosing cholangitis (PSC). However, the accuracy of serum CA19-9 is variable. In one study of 333 patients with PSC, of whom 13% were diagnosed with cholangiocarcinoma, a level of >180 U/mL had a sensitivity of 67% and a specificity of 98%. In another report of 218 patients with PSC, a level of >129 U/mL was 79% sensitive and 99% specific for the diagnosis of cholangiocarcinoma. In this study the positive predictive value was only 57%.

The optimal value for CA19-9 that best discriminates between benign or malignant disease is difficult to ascertain and is influenced by the presence of cholangitis and cholestasis. A value of >7 U/mL was found to be 73% sensitive and 63% specific for malignant disease in patients without either cholangitis or cholestasis. In contrast, using the same value in the presence of either condition reduced specificity to 42%. Increasing the cutoff value to >300 U/mL increased specificity to 87% but reduced sensitivity to 41%. Serum CA19-9 levels should therefore be re-evaluated following resolution of cholangitis or cholestasis.

Serum levels of carcinoembryonic antigen (CEA) are neither sufficiently sensitive nor specific to diagnose cholangiocarcinoma. Biliary levels have been evaluated, and a fivefold increase has been reported in patients with cholangiocarcinoma compared to those with benign strictures. However, this finding has not been consistent across studies. The use of CEA in combination with CA19-9 (King's College formula) has been utilized with varying results, including one study indicating a sensitivity less than that of CA19-9 alone. Numerous other markers including CA 125 and IL-6 have been investigated; however none have proven significant utility in the diagnosis of cholangiocarcinoma. Further genomic and proteomic analyses may yield novel markers capable of reliably detecting biliary tract malignancies.

References

Bjornsson E, Kilander A, Olsson R. (1999) CA19-9 and CEA are unreliable markers for cholangiocarcinoma in patients with primary sclerosing cholangitis. *Liver* 19(6): 501–8.

De Groen PC, Gores GJ, LaRusso NF, Gunderson LL, Nagorney DM. (1999) Biliary tract cancers. *N Engl J Med* 341(18): 1368–78.

Kim HJ, Kim MH, Lim BC *et al.* (1999) A new strategy for the application of CA19-9 in the differentiation of pancreaticobiliary cancer: analysis using a receiver operating characteristic curve. *Am J Gastroenterol* 94(7): 1941–6.

Levy C, Lymp J, Angulo P, Gores GJ, Larusso N, Lindor KD. (2005) The value of serum CA19-9 in predicting cholangiocarcinomas in patients with primary sclerosing cholangitis. *Dig Dis Sci* 50(9): 1734–40.

Siqueira E, Schoen RE, Silverman W *et al.* (2002) Detecting cholangiocarcinoma in patients with primary sclerosing cholangitis. *Gastrointest Endosc* 56(1): 40–7.

Histopathology

Elizabeth I. Johnston & Mary Kay Washington

Macroscopy

Cholangiocarcinoma is the second most frequent primary hepatic malignancy following hepatocellular carcinoma (HCC), and comprises 10–15% of hepatobiliary neoplasms (Lazaridis *et al.* 2005). On gross examination, intrahepatic cholangiocarcinomas are gray-white to tan masses arising in a non-cirrhotic liver. The edges may be infiltrative or nodular and well-defined, and small tumor satellite lesions may be distributed throughout the liver. Large lesions may show central necrosis and occasionally hemorrhage. Most cholangiocarcinomas are firm due to a prominent desmoplastic stroma, and may be gritty from the presence of dystrophic calcifications. Intraductal growth of the tumor may be seen as papillary excrescences within dilated ducts. Extrahepatic hilar cholangiocarcinomas often show a periductal growth pattern and appear firm, tan-white and ill-defined. These lesions are difficult to distinguish from scar in the hepatic hilum. Additionally, the liver is frequently bile stained as a result of biliary obstruction (Colombari *et al.* 1995).

Histopathology

The majority of cholangiocarcinomas are mucin-producing adenocarcinomas. The most common histologic pattern consists of small, tubular glands and duct-like structures comprised of low columnar or cuboidal cells with clear to eosinophilic cytoplasm and round to oval, basally-located nuclei. Rare intracytoplasmic lumen formation is observed. Mucin can be seen in the glandular lumina and/or in the cytoplasm. A desmoplastic stroma is characteristically present. The fibrosis may occasionally be the predominant feature, with only a few tumor cells visible. Dystrophic calcification is often seen in these primarily desmoplastic tumors. Perineural and lymphovascular invasion is readily identified. Cholangiocarcinomas often show growth within portal tracts, either by spread within portal vein branches or within the intrahepatic bile ducts. Although cholestasis may be prominent in adjacent liver, bile production is not a feature of cholangiocarcinoma.

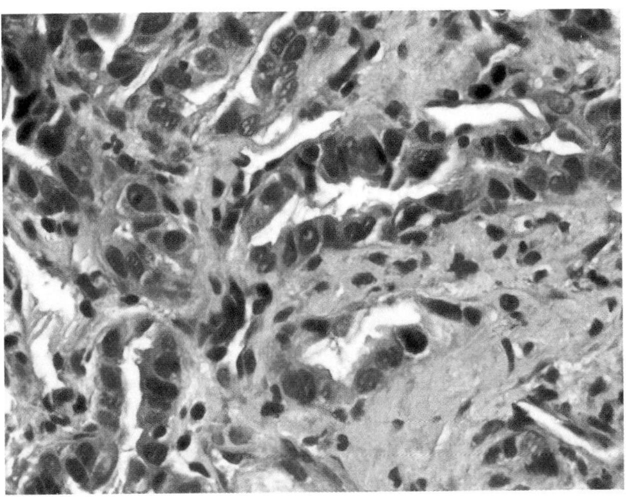

Fig. 22.1 Moderately differentiated cholangiocarcinoma demonstrating glandular formation, moderate pleomorphism, nuclear enlargement, nuclear membrane irregularity, and prominent nucleoli, surrounded by desmoplastic stroma (H&E, 40×).

A large portion of cases may appear moderately to poorly differentiated. The glands may be smaller, or cells may appear in small clusters without lumen formation. A larger degree of cellular and nuclear variation in size and shape may be seen (Fig. 22.1). Prominent nucleoli and frequent mitoses are present. Mucin production may be scant, but is often demonstrable by use of special stains for mucin.

A minority of cholangiocarcinomas demonstrate varying patterns, including mucinous (colloid), cholangiolocellular, signet-ring cell, squamous, sarcomatoid, clear cell, papillary, mucoepidermoid, and lymphoepithelioma-like. Intraductal cholangiocarcinomas are rarely seen and histologically resemble villous adenomas; high-grade dysplasia is generally required to make the diagnosis (Nakajima *et al.* 1988; Colombari *et al.* 1995).

Immunohistochemistry

Cholangiocarcinoma is positive for epithelial markers such as cytokeratin 7 (CK7) and CK19, variably positive for CK20, and shows cytoplasmic and/or membranous staining for polyclonal CEA. Cholangiocarcinoma is uniformly negative for HepPar-1 and AFP (Lau *et al.* 2002).

Molecular biology

Considerable progress has been made in understanding the molecular pathogenesis of cholangiocarcinoma. Molecular alterations lead to increased growth and proliferation, avoidance of apoptosis, tumor invasion and metastasis. K-ras and p53 mutations are found in the majority of sporadic cholangiocarcinomas as well as those arising in primary sclerosing cholangitis. Other molecular alterations include e-cadherin, α-catenin, β-catenin, matrix metalloproteinase (MMP), p16, p21, bcl-2, HGF/c-met, EDG/c-erbB-2, and COX-2. Comparative genomic hybridization studies show distinctive features of genetic alterations in intrahepatic cholangiocarcinoma compared to hepatocellular carcinoma, with intrahepatic cholangiocarcinoma showing changes similar to pancreatic and colorectal carcinomas, in the form of gains of 5p, 7p, 13q, and 20q (Koo *et al.* 2001).

Biliary brushing cytology

Endoscopic techniques are becoming more sophisticated and cytologic sampling of the extrahepatic biliary tree is being increasingly utilized for diagnosis of biliary disease. Biliary tract brushing cytology is recognized as the superior method over bile duct washings or direct bile sampling. Most studies demonstrate a sensitivity rate for detection of carcinoma ranging from 30% to 88% and a specificity rate of nearly 100% (Selvaggi *et al.* 2004). The low sensitivity rate may be partly attributed to the diagnostic challenge posed by biliary tract cytology, even for the experienced pathologist; reactive cholangiocytes may be nearly impossible to differentiate from dysplastic cells. Key morphologic criteria for malignancy include a background of dysplastic cells singly and in clusters, with marked nuclear overlap and crowding, high nuclear to cytoplasmic ratio, irregular nuclear membranes, coarse chromatin, and prominent nucleoli. The pathologist may be reluctant to diagnose carcinoma in the absence of many of the above features; therefore, while there are essentially no false positive diagnoses, a negative result does not reliably exclude malignancy.

Differential diagnosis

The most difficult differential consideration in diagnosing cholangiocarcinoma is metastatic adenocarcinoma, particularly pancreatic, breast, and lung. Immunohistochemical stains are of limited use in this situation, and the distinction may be impossible in a needle biopsy specimen. The diagnosis therefore depends on the clinical exclusion of a primary site elsewhere. Immunohistochemistry may be useful in distinguishing cholangiocarcinoma from metastatic colorectal carcinoma, however. Cholangiocarcinomas are generally positive for CK7 and negative for CK20, while colorectal metastases show the opposite immunoreactivity (CK7–/C20+).

HCC occasionally has a pseudoglandular architecture that is difficult to distinguish from the trabecular pattern of cholangiocarcinoma. Cholangiocarcinoma generally has a more abundant desmoplastic stroma. Immunohistochemistry is useful in this setting; polyclonal carcinoembryonic antigen (CEA) will show a cytoplasmic and/or membranous pattern in cholangiocarcinoma, rather than the canalicular pattern seen in HCC. In addition, α-fetoprotein (AFP) and HepPar-1 are almost always positive in HCC and negative in cholangiocarcinoma.

Electron microscopy, although seldom indicated, demonstrates the features of adenocarcinoma in cholangiocarcinoma, such as microvilli and true lumen formation.

Occasionally bile duct adenoma or an atypical proliferation of bile ducts may be difficult to distinguish from a well-differentiated cholangiocarcinoma. A careful examination of low-power architecture and high-power cytologic features is helpful in this setting.

Epithelioid hemangioendothelioma (EH) is another primary liver tumor that may show single cells and clusters of cells with intracytoplasmic vacuoles and moderate anisocytosis. Immunophenotyping easily distinguishes this tumor from cholangiocarcinoma; EH shows expression of CD34, factor VIII-related antigen, and other endothelial cell markers, which are absent in cholangiocarcinoma.

Combined hepatocellular/cholangiocarcinoma

There are rare cases of malignant epithelial tumors in the liver that show features of both cholangiocarcinoma and hepatocellular carcinoma, and they are designated 'combined hepatocellular-cholangiocarcinoma' in the WHO classification. Studies have resulted in several classification schemes for these tumors. One scheme divides combined HCC-CCC into three categories: 'double cancer' (areas of HCC and CCC are present separately); 'combined type' (both components are present adjacent to each other and mixed together as one mass); and 'mixed type' (both components are intimately mixed). Another scheme put forth by Goodman seems to be more reliable, and also uses three divisions: collision type (separate areas of HCC and CCC)), transitional type (intermixed patterns), and fibrolamellar carcinoma type (inclusion of this type is controversial). There are several proposed pathways of histogenesis of these combined tumors. They may arise independently, and thus be designated a 'double cancer'. One may arise first and subsequently be 'transformed' into the other. Finally, the cancer may arise from progenitor cells with the ability to differentiate into either hepatocytes or cholangiocytes (Tickoo *et al.* 2002).

Combined HCC-CCC has been reported to share the same associations as hepatocellular carcinoma, including cirrhosis, hepatitis B and C, and elevated AFP levels. Recently, use of *in situ* hybridization for albumin mRNA has been shown to be a sensitive and specific marker for hepatocellular differentiation, and is demonstrated in the cholangiocarcinoma 'glandular' areas of combined tumors. These tumors also show varying positivity for cytokeratins 7 and 19 (biliary), CK 8 and 18 (hepatocyte), polyclonal CEA, and AFP, additionally supporting divergent differentiation.

The prognosis of combined HCC-CCC is poor; tumors disseminate widely through spread to regional lymph nodes and distant organs. In one study, the median survival rates for resectable tumors was 26 months and only 6.5 months for unresectable disease (Tickoo *et al.* 2002). The metastases tend to maintain the mixed pattern or occasionally exhibit only hepatocellular differentiation.

References

Colombari R, Tsui WM. (1995) Biliary tumors of the liver. *Semin Liver Dis* 15(4): 402–13.

Koo SH, Ihm CH, Kwon KC, Park JW, Kim JM, Kong G. (2001) Genetic alterations in hepatocellular carcinoma and intrahepatic cholangiocarcinoma. *Cancer Genet Cytogenet* 130(1): 22–8.

Lau SK, Prakash S, Geller SA, Alsabeh R. (2002) Comparative immunohistochemical profile of hepatocellular carcinoma, cholangiocarcinoma, and metastatic adenocarcinoma. *Hum Pathol* 33(12): 1175–81.

Lazaridis KN, Gores GJ. (2005) Cholangiocarcinoma. *Gastroenterology* 128(6): 1655–67.

Nakajima T, Kondo Y, Miyazaki M, Okui K. (1988) A histopathologic study of 102 cases of intrahepatic cholangiocarcinoma: Histologic classification and modes of spreading. *Hum Pathol* 19(10): 1228–34.

Selvaggi SM. (2004) Biliary brushing cytology. *Cytopathology* 15(2): 74–9.

Tickoo SK, Zee SY, Obiekwe S *et al.* (2002) Combined hepatocellular-cholangiocarcinoma: a histopathologic, immunohistochemical, and in situ hybridization study. *Am J Surg Pathol* 26(8): 989–97.

Imaging and staging

Christopher D. Anderson, T. Markley Earl, Stephen J. Meranze & Ravi S. Chari

There is no single staging system for cholangiocarcinoma that preoperatively stratifies patients into subgroups based on their potential for resection and survival. The current American Joint Commission on Cancer Staging system (Table 22.1) is based on pathologic data and can convey information pertaining to the patient's prognosis. This staging system, however, cannot predict the likelihood of resection for stage 1–3 patients (Burke *et al.* 1998; Jarnagin *et al.* 2001). Similarly, the Bismuth–Corlette system can reliably stratify patients based on the location and extent of the tumor in the biliary tree (Bismuth *et al.* 1992). Although this system is useful for description of the tumors, it is not predictive for resectability or survival. Jarnagin and colleagues have proposed a clinical tumor staging system which accounts for local tumor extent and correlates with resectability and patient survival (Jarnagin *et al.* 2001). There are also multicenter reviews under way to develop a better staging system.

Because margin-negative resection is the only chance for long-term survival in patients with cholangiocarcinoma, all imaging studies should be aimed at assessing respectability (Anderson *et al.* 2004). Four basic determinations need to be made: (i) extent of tumor within the biliary tree; (ii) vascular invasion; (iii) hepatic lobar atrophy; and (iv) metastatic disease.

Table 22.3 Radiologic criteria that suggest unresectability.

Bilateral hepatic duct involvement up to secondary radicals
Bilateral hepatic artery involvement
Encasement of the portal vein proximal to its bifurcation
Atrophy of one hepatic lobe with contralateral portal vein encasement
Atrophy of one hepatic lobe with contralateral biliary radical involvement
Distant metastasis

Radiographic findings that suggest unresectability of perihilar tumors include bilateral hepatic duct involvement up to secondary radicals, encasement or occlusion of the main portal vein, lobar atrophy with encasement of the contralateral portal vein branch, involvement of bilateral hepatic arteries, or atrophy of one liver lobe with contralateral secondary biliary radical involvement (Burke *et al.* 1998; Jarnagin *et al.* 2001; Chari *et al.* 2003; Anderson *et al.* 2004). Our criteria for unresectability are summarized in Table 22.3. However, some authors have reported an overestimation of tumor extent as the most common mistake from the current imaging modalities (Otto *et al.* 2004). Multiple reviews have demonstrated that involvement of the main portal vein is the only independent predictor of unresectability (Burke *et al.* 1998; Jarnagin *et al.* 2001). In addition, the presence of hepatic lobar atrophy, ipsilateral branch portal vein involvement and ipsilateral secondary ductal radical involvement are predictors of the need of hepatectomy in order to achieve a margin-negative resection (Burke *et al.* 1998; Jarnagin *et al.* 2001).

Ultrasound

Most jaundiced patients will undergo transabdominal ultrasound (US) as a first-line imaging modality. US is operator dependent, but is a sensitive method for visualizing the bile ducts, confirming ductal dilatation, ruling out choledocholithiasis, and defining the level of the obstruction (Saini 1997; Sharma & Ahuja 1999). Centers with expertise in duplex US have demonstrated this method as an accurate predictor of vascular involvement and resectability. Hann and collegues demonstrated in a small series of patients that duplex US is equivalent to CT portography and angiography for detecting lobar atrophy, the level of biliary obstruction, hepatic parenchymal involvement, and venous invasion (Hann *et al.* 1997). However, this level of expertise is not widely available and US in the staging of cholangiocarcinoma most importantly can demonstrate ductal dilation and suggest the level of obstruction.

Magnetic resonance cholangiopancreatography

Magnetic resonance cholangiopancreatography (MRCP) has become the preferred investigation for suspected hilar tumors at most major centers. This method provides more information than invasive cholangiography and avoids the risks associated with biliary intubation. MRCP has the capability to evaluate the entire biliary tree, while also identifying any intrahepatic mass lesions. In one study of 126 patients with suspected biliary obstruction, MRCP detected 12 of 14 malignant obstructions, and had a positive predictive value of 86%, and a negative predictive value of 98% (Guibaud *et al.* 1995). In a second series comparing MRCP with endoscopic retrograde cholangiography (ERC) in 40 patients with malignant perihilar obstruction, both techniques detected 100% of biliary obstructions, but MRCP was superior in definition of the anatomical extent of tumor (Yeh *et al.* 2000). MRCP also provides information regarding the hilar vascular structures, nodal status, distant metastasis, and lobar atrophy (Guthrie *et al.* 1996; Lee *et al.* 2003; Schwartz *et al.* 1998).

Computed tomography

In centers without MRCP expertise, contrasted computed tomography (CT) and invasive cholangiography compliment each other in the evaluation of hilar tumors. In addition, CT may compliment MRCP in the evaluation of the tumor's relationship to surrounding structures. CT is sensitive for the detection of intrahepatic bile duct tumors, the level of biliary obstruction, and the presence of lobar atrophy. In addition, CT permits visualization of the pertinent nodal basins (Chen *et al.* 2002). Performance of a triple-phase helical CT will detect essentially all cholangiocarcinomas greater than 1 cm (Tillich *et al.* 1998; Valls *et al.* 2000). At least one study has suggested that the relationship of the tumor to the vessels and surrounding organs is more easily evaluated using CT than MRCP (Zhang *et al.* 1999). However, CT alone may only be able to establish resectability in approximately 60% of patients (Zhang *et al.* 1999). Although there are currently no studies specifically evaluating CT angiography (CTA) in the staging of cholangiocarcinoma, this modality is considered the most sensitive imaging technique for the detection of hepatic lesions (Kim *et al.* 2002). This modality is important for the diagnosis of peripheral (intrahepatic) cholangiocarcinoma, and our current practice is to obtain a CTA to assess hepatic arterial and portal venous involvement for hilar tumors. This modality replaces invasive arteriograms and compliments MRCP in the assessment of patients for resectability.

Although not required in patients deemed resectable by CT (or CTA) and MRCP, invasive cholangiography may provide additional diagnostic data (FNA, or brush cytology). It is also utilized by centers who perform preoperative biliary drainage (discussed later). It can be performed via ERC or percutaneous transhepatic cholangiography (PTC). The choice of modality depends in part upon the level of expertise available at each center. For hilar tumors, ERC is preferred in patients with PSC since the marked stricturing of the intrahepatic biliary tree makes a percutaneous approach difficult. Conversely, PTC provides information about the intrahepatic ducts more reliably and is the preferred study in most centers for patients without PSC (Pitt *et al.* 1995a; Pitt *et al.* 1995b). In patients deemed unresectable, PTC and ERC are the primary modes of palliative therapy.

PET and endoscopic ultrasound

Positron emission tomography (PET) can reliably detect cholangiocarcinomas as small as 1 cm (Delbeke *et al.* 1998; Kluge *et al.* 2001; Anderson *et al.* 2003). PET may demonstrate distant metastatic disease not detected by other radiologic studies, in 30% of patients (Anderson *et al.* 2003). In addition, PET may be useful for detecting primary cholangiocarcinoma in patients with PSC (Kluge *et al.* 2001; Anderson *et al.* 2003). Although the cost effectiveness of PET use for cholangiocarcinoma staging has yet to be evaluated, this modality can be a useful tool when a nuclear radiologist with extensive experience with PET is available.

Endoscopic ultrasound (EUS) is routinely used in the evaluation of distal common bile duct cholangiocarcinomas. However, the role of EUS in hilar tumors is evolving. EUS-guided fine needle aspiration has been demonstrated to be very effective for obtaining tissue diagnosis of hilar tumors (Fritscher-Ravens *et al.* 2004; Meara *et al.* 2006). The usefulness of routine EUS for the staging of hilar tumors has yet to be fully evaluated. At least one early study demonstrated an overall accuracy of 84% and 55–75% respectively for T and N stages when compared to pathologic staging (Tio *et al.* 1991).

References

Anderson CA, Rice M, Pinson CW, Chapman WC, Chari RS, Delbeke D. (2004) FDG PET imaging in the evaluation of gallbladder carcinoma and cholangiocarcinoma. *J Gastrointest Surg* 8: 90–7.

Anderson CD, Pinson CW, Berlin J, Chari RS. (2004) Diagnosis and treatment of cholangiocarcinoma. *Oncologist* 9: 43–57.

Bismuth H, Nakache R, Diamond T. (1992) Management strategies in resection for hilar cholangiocarcinoma. *Ann Surg* 215: 31–8.

Burke EC, Jarnagin WR, Hochwald SN, Pisters PW, Fong Y, Blumgart LH. (1998) Hilar cholangiocarcinoma: patterns of spread, the importance of hepatic resection for curative operation, and a presurgical clinical staging system. *Ann Surg* 228: 385–94.

Callery MP, Strasberg SM, Doherty GM, Soper NJ, Norton JA. (1997) Staging laparoscopy with laparoscopic ultrasonography: optimizing resectability in hepatobiliary and pancreatic malignancy. *J Am Coll Surg* 185: 33–9.

Chari RS, Anderson CA, Saverese DMF. (2003) Treatment of cholangiocarcinoma I. In: Rose BD,ed. *UpToDate*. UpToDate, Wellesley, MA.

Chen CY, Shiesh SC, Tsao HC, Lin XZ. (2002) The assessment of biliary CA 125, CA19-9 and CEA in diagnosing cholangiocarcinoma—the influence of sampling time and hepatolithiasis. *Hepatogastroenterology* 49: 616–20.

Conner S, Barron E, Wigmore SJ, Madhavan KK, Parks RW, Garden OJ. (2005) The utility of laparoscopic assessment in the preoperative staging of suspected hilar cholangiocarcinoma. *J Gastrointest Surg* 9: 476–80.

Corvera CU, Weber SM, Jarnagin WR. (2002) Role of laparoscopy in the evaluation of biliary tract cancer. *Surg Oncol Clin N Am* 11: 877–91.

Delbeke D, Martin WH, Sandler MP *et al.* (1998) Evaluation of benign vs malignant hepatic lesions with positron emission tomography. *Arch Surg* 133: 510–15.

Fritscher-Ravens A, Broering DC, Knoefel WT *et al.* (2004) EUS-guided fine-needle aspiration of suspected hilar cholangiocarcinoma in potentially operable patients with negative brush cytology. *Am J Gastroenterol* 99: 45–51.

Guibaud L, Bret PM, Reinhold C, Atri M, Barkun AN. (1995) Bile duct obstruction and choledocholithiasis: diagnosis with MR cholangiography. *Radiology* 197: 109–15.

Guthrie JA, Ward J, Robinson PJ. (1996) Hilar cholangiocarcinomas: T2-weighted spin-echo and gadolinium-enhanced FLASH MR imaging. *Radiology* 201: 347–51.

Hann LE, Greatrex KV, Bach AM, Fong Y, Blumgart LH. (1997) Cholangiocarcinoma at the hepatic hilus: sonographic findings. *AJR Am J Roentgenol* 168: 985–9.

Jarnagin WR, Fong Y, DeMatteo RP *et al.* (2001) Staging, resectability, and outcome in 225 patients with hilar cholangiocarcinoma. *Ann Surg* 234: 507–17.

Kim HC, Kim TK, Sung KB *et al.* (2002) CT during hepatic arteriography and portography: an illustrative review. *Radiographics* 22: 1041–51.

Kluge R, Schmidt F, Caca K *et al.* (2001) Positron emission tomography with [(18)F]fluoro-2-deoxy-D-glucose for diagnosis and staging of bile duct cancer. *Hepatology* 33: 1029–35.

Lee MG, Park KB, Shin YM *et al.* (2003) Preoperative evaluation of hilar cholangiocarcinoma with contrast-enhanced three-dimensional fast imaging with steady-state precession magnetic resonance angiography: comparison with intraarterial digital subtraction angiography. *World J Surg* 27: 278–83.

Meara RS, Jhala D, Eloubeidi MA *et al.* (2006) Endoscopic ultrasound-guided FNA biopsy of bile duct and gallbladder: analysis of 53 cases. *Cytopathology* 17: 42–9.

Otto G, Romaneehsen B, Bittinger F *et al.* (2004) Preoperative imaging of hilar cholangiocarcinoma: surgical evaluation of standard practises. *Z Gastroenterol* 42: 9–14.

Pitt HA, Nakeeb A, Abrams RA *et al.* (1995a) Perihilar cholangiocarcinoma. Postoperative radiotherapy does not improve survival. *Ann Surg* 221: 788–97.

Pitt HA, Dooley WC, Yeo CJ, Cameron JL. (1995b) Malignancies of the biliary tree. *Curr Probl Surg* 32: 1–90.

Saini S. (1997) Imaging of the hepatobiliary tract. *N Engl J Med* 336: 1889–94.

Schwartz LH, Coakley FV, Sun Y, Blumgart LH, Fong Y, Panicek DM. (1998) Neoplastic pancreaticobiliary duct obstruction: evaluation with breath-hold MR cholangiopancreatography. *AJR Am J Roentgenol* 170: 1491–5.

Sharma MP, Ahuja V. (1999) Aetiological spectrum of obstructive jaundice and diagnostic ability of ultrasonography: a clinician's perspective. *Trop Gastroenterol* 20: 167–9.

Tillich M, Mischinger HJ, Preisegger KH, Rabl H, Szolar DH. (1998) Multiphasic helical CT in diagnosis and staging of hilar cholangiocarcinoma. *AJR Am J Roentgenol* 171: 651–8.

Tio TL, Cheng J, Wijers OB, Sars PR, Tytgat GN. (1991) Endosonographic TNM staging of extrahepatic bile duct cancer: comparison with pathological staging. *Gastroenterology* 100: 1351–61.

Valls C, Guma A, Puig I *et al.* (2000) Intrahepatic peripheral cholangiocarcinoma: CT evaluation. *Abdom Imaging* 25: 490–6.

Weber SM, DeMatteo RP, Fong Y, Blumgart LH, Jarnagin WR. (2002) Staging laparoscopy in patients with extrahepatic biliary carcinoma. Analysis of 100 patients. *Ann Surg* 235: 392–9.

Yeh TS, Jan YY, Tseng JH *et al.* (2000) Malignant perihilar biliary obstruction: magnetic resonance cholangiopancreatographic findings. *Am J Gastroenterol* 95: 432–40.

Zhang Y, Uchida M, Abe T, Nishimura H, Hayabuchi N, Nakashima Y. (1999) Intrahepatic peripheral cholangiocarcinoma: comparison of dynamic CT and dynamic MRI. *J Comput Assist Tomogr* 23: 670–7.

Treatment

Overview

Ravi S. Chari

The only durable chance for cure in patients with cholangiocarcinoma is surgical resection. Our approach to suspected hilar cholangiocarcinoma is to perform radiologic staging as described in the previous section. This includes triple phase CT, and PET; very frequently, ERC with biliary drainage has already been performed by the time the patient is referred, and often patients are sent with worsening jaundice or cholangitis as a result of the biliary intervention. We frequently see the bilirubin rise for 2 to 3 weeks after the drainage procedure, and most often this is as a result of cholangitis that accompanies it.

Patient selection and timing are critical factors to operative success. The postoperative course has two significant considerations: postoperative liver failure and high physiologic toll on the patient. The most significant complication after resection is liver failure; however, poor preoperative performance status will also predict poor outcome. While preoperative biliary drainage has been associated with an increased risk of cholangitis and longer postoperative hospital stay in patients with obstructive jaundice who then undergo resection, cholestasis, biliary cirrhosis, and liver dysfunction develop rapidly in the face of unrelieved biliary obstruction. Liver dysfunction is one of the main factors that increase postoperative morbidity and mortality following surgical resection, and thus biliary drainage in high-risk patients should be performed following preoperative radiologic staging. Similarly, many patients present with significant compromise in their performance status, such that major operative intervention should not be considered, simply based on their inability to survive. Thus, we also perform non-operative biliary drainage in those whom operative intervention is deemed not immediately safe (Figure 22.2). Definitive operative intervention is then usually deferred until the serum

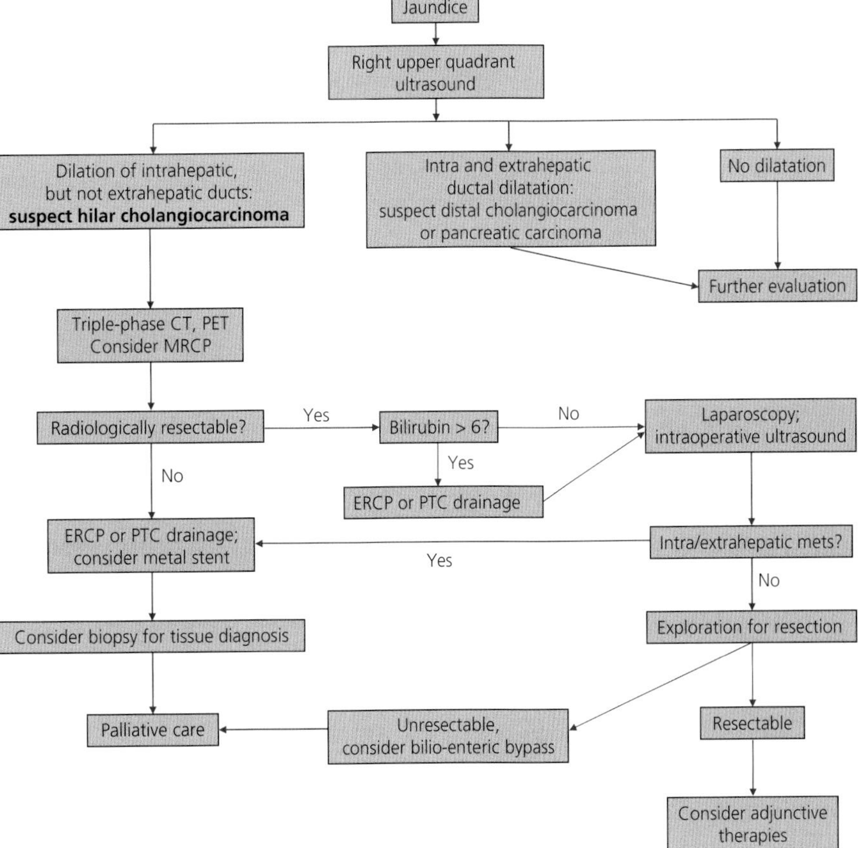

Fig. 22.2 Flow chart depicting the work-up and treatment of a patient with suspected hilar cholangiocarcinoma. Ultrasound demonstrating dilation of intrahepatic bile ducts without extrahepatic dilatation suggests a hilar neoplasm. CT angiogram offers the best detail of the involved vasculature, lymph node basins, and any intrahepatic lesions. PET can detect unsuspected distant or intrahepatic metastases in up to 30% of patients with cholangiocarcinoma. MRCP offers good resolution of both the intrahepatic and extrahepatic biliary tree, but should be substituted with PTC or ERCP in patients that will require preoperative or palliative biliary drainage. Laparoscopy will detect intra-abdominal metastases in up to 30% of patients. Not all patients undergoing exploration for resection will be resectable, and when patients are found to be unresectable at exploration, operative biliary–enteric bypass should be considered (From Anderson CD, Pinson CW, Berlin J, Chari RS. (2004) Diagnosis and treatment of cholangiocarcinoma. *The Oncologist* 9(1): 43–57.

bilirubin is less than 3 mg/dL. Nevertheless, in those patients who are potentially resectable, laparoscopic staging can be accomplished shortly after the drainage procedure in the face of increased bilirubin. If extrahepatic disease or nonresectable tumor is found, curative resection is not possible, and alternative management strategies can be considered at this point.

Reference

Anderson CD, Pinson CW, Berlin J, Chari RS. (2004) Diagnosis and treatment of cholangiocarcinoma. *Oncologist* 9(1): 43–57.

Surgery

Christopher D. Anderson & Ravi S. Chari

Preoperative selection

Patients who are resectable by the radiologic criteria discussed earlier should be physically and nutritionally fit to undergo a major liver resection. All patients should have adequate liver function, and operative planning should ensure adequate remnant liver volume. Liver dysfunction is one of the main contributors to postoperative morbidity and mortality following hepatic resection. In the setting of cholangiocarcinoma requiring hepatic resection, preoperative biliary drainage in patients with severe elevation of serum bilirubin has been associated with increased survival (Su *et al.* 1996a; Strasberg 1998; Yi *et al.* 2004; Zhang *et al.* 2006). We advocate preoperative biliary drainage in patients with a serum bilirubin level greater than 6–10 mg/dL and thus would perform invasive cholangiography in this group of patients.

A significant number of patients deemed radiologically resectable will have peritoneal implants or N2 lymph node (peripancreatic, paraduodenal, celiac, superior mesenteric, posterior pancreaticoduodenal) involvement which is not easily detected on preoperative imaging studies; endoscopic ultrasound can clarify involvement. Diagnostic laparoscopy will help identify as many as 42% of these patients before committing them to a laparotomy (Callery *et al.* 1997; Corvera *et al.* 2002; Weber *et al.* 2002; Connor *et al.* 2005). In addition, laparoscopy offers the opportunity for intraoperative hepatic ultrasound which may be useful for the detection of occult intrahepatic metastases. While not routine at most centers, laparoscopy should be considered when planning resections on patients with cholangiocarcinoma.

Resection

The primary goal of operation in patients with hilar cholangiocarcinoma is the achievement of a microscopically negative resection margin as this is the patient's only chance for long-term survival. A recent report demonstrated no 5-year survivors following extrahepatic bilary resection alone, and no difference in survival between unresectable patients and those resected with a microscopically positive margin (Jarnagin & Shoup 2004). At a minimum, this requires resection of the extrahepatic biliary tree and a subhilar lymphadenectomy. The recent literature demonstrates that the addition of an en bloc partial hepatectomy is required in most cases to achieve margin-negative resections (Klempnauer *et al.* 1997; Burke *et al.* 1998; Nimura *et al.* 2000; Chari *et al.* 2003; Anderson *et al.* 2004; Jarnagin & Shoup 2004). Indeed, the rate of margin-negative resections has consistently been reported above 75% when partial hepatectomy is added to the biliary resection (Tsao *et al.* 2000; Nakeeb *et al.* 2002; Hemming *et al.* 2005). In addition, many authors advocate routinely including caudate lobectomy to all resections to increase the margin-negative rate (Tsao *et al.* 2000). These aggressive strides to achieve margin-negative resections have increased 5-year survival to above 50% in some series (Burke *et al.* 1998; Nakeeb *et al.* 2002). However, the perioperative mortality rates accompanying these more extensive resections are slightly higher than those accompanying local excision only (8–10% vs. 2–4%) (Cameron *et al.* 1990; Hadjis *et al.* 1990; Pichlmayr *et al.* 1996; Su *et al.* 1996; Lillemoe & Cameron 2000; Nimura *et al.* 2000; Nakeeb *et al.* 2002; Hemming *et al.* 2005).

Portal vein embolization

To increase the margin-negative resection rate when extensive hepatic resection is required, the use of preoperative portal vein embolization (PVE) has been advocated (Hemming *et al.* 2003; Nimura *et al.* 2000). The rationale for the use of PVE is to induce compensatory hypertrophy of the future remnant liver and thus minimize postoperative liver dysfunction (Nagino *et al.* 1995). By allowing a larger volume resection to be carried out safely, PVE may allow negative resection margins to be obtained in patients who would otherwise be unresectable because of concerns of insufficient postoperative residual liver volume (Hemming *et al.* 2003; Abdalla *et al.* 2002). In one recent study, patients who underwent preoperative unilateral PVE or whose tumor had caused unilateral PVE had significantly lower operative mortality (Hemming *et al.* 2005).

Lymph node status

In addition to margin status, regional lymph node involvement may correlate with postoperative survival (Klempnauer *et al.* 1997). In one review, patients without nodal involvement had 3- and 5-year survivals of 55% and 30% respectively, while patients with regional lymph node involvement had survivals of 32% and 14.7% respectively (Kitagawa *et al.* 2001). However, a recent report demonstrated no decreased survival in patients with isolated hepatoduodenal lymph node involvement (Jarnagin & Shoup 2004). To this end, many authors do not consider the presence of hepatoduodenal lymph node involvement a contraindication to resection. However, there are currently no data to support a more extensive lymph node resection.

Liver transplantation

Liver transplantation for cholangiocarcinoma is controversial, and most centers have abandoned this as an indication for liver transplantation (Goldstein *et al.* 1993; Jeyarajah & Klintmalm 1998; Meyer *et al.* 2000). However, some reports of success have been published (Iwatsuki *et al.* 1998), and radical multiabdominal organ 'cluster' transplants for selected patients with cholangiocarcinoma have been reported (Alessiani *et al.* 1995). A review of 207 patients who underwent liver transplantation for cholangiocarcinoma reports 1-, 2- and 5-year survivals as 72, 48, and 23% respectively, but over 50% of patients had recurrence within 2 years (Meyer *et al.* 2000). A second review with a 30% 3-year survival reported that small tumor size and a single tumor focus are positive prognostic indicators (Shimoda *et al.* 2001).

Despite these discouraging reports, trials in highly selected patients using specific neoadjuvant protocols have shown encouraging results Rea *et al.* have reported 28 patients with unresectable, stage I and II hilar cholangiocarcinoma in patients with PSC. All patients had a negative staging laparotomy and underwent neoadjuvant therapy with external-beam irradiation, systemic 5-FU, brachytherapy with ^{192}Ir plus oral capecitabine prior to liver transplantation. The actuarial post transplantation 5-year survival was 82%. A follow-up study comparing aggressive neoadjuvant chemoradiation and liver transplantation versus resection showed better 5-year survival and less recurrence in the transplantation group (Rea *et al.* 2005). While this study has been criticized due to the lack of intention to treat analysis in the transplantation group and non-equivalent cohorts, these results are promising and would support further study of liver transplantation in patients with node negative disease. Other centers are currently enrolling patients in clinical trials to further evaluate liver transplantation for patients with cholangiocarcinoma. In addition, these results support the formation of more aggressive clinical trials of neoadjuvant therapy prior to resection.

Surgical palliation

Between 50 and 90% of patients with cholangiocarcinoma are not candidates for curative resection (Vauthey & Blumgart 1994; Chari *et al.* 2003). The goal of care in patients who are unresectable should be focused on first on quality of life and relief of symptoms (pain, pruritus, jaundice) and second on extending survival. Currently recommended palliative measures for patients with unresectable cholangiocarcinoma have recently been reviewed (Anderson *et al.* 2004). It is worth mentioning here that biliary–enteric bypass has traditionally been the primary method of palliation for patients with unresectable cholangiocarcinomas and biliary obstruction. The indications for operative drainage have narrowed due to equivalent palliative results of stenting procedures with a decrease in morbidity. However, patients found to be unresectable at the time of exploration remain ideal candidates for biliary–enteric bypass. There seems to be no obvious advantage of bilateral ductal bypass, and unilateral intrahepatic ductal bypass has been shown to provide adequate palliation (Baer *et al.* 1994). Complex biliary enteric bypass procedures should remain in the armamentarium of hepatobiliary surgeons who treat cholangiocarcinoma.

References

Abdalla EK, Barnett CC, Doherty D, Curley SA, Vauthey JN. (2002) Extended hepatectomy in patients with hepatobiliary malignancies with and without preoperative portal vein embolization. *Arch Surg* 137(6): 675–80.

Alessiani M, Tzakis A, Todo S, Demetris AJ, Fung JJ, Starzl TE. (1995) Assessment of five-year experience with abdominal organ cluster transplantation. *J Am Coll Surg* 180(1): 1–9.

Anderson CD, Pinson CW, Berlin J, Chari RS. (2004) Diagnosis and treatment of cholangiocarcinoma. *Oncologist* 9(1): 43–57.

Baer HU, Rhyner M, Stain SC *et al.* (1994) The effect of communication between the right and left liver on the outcome of surgical drainage for jaundice due to malignant obstruction at the hilus of the liver. *HPB Surg* 8(1): 27–31.

Burke EC, Jarnagin WR, Hochwald SN, Pisters PW, Fong Y, Blumgart LH. (1998) Hilar cholangiocarcinoma: patterns of spread, the importance of hepatic resection for curative operation, and a presurgical clinical staging system. *Ann Surg* 228(3): 385–94.

Callery MP, Strasberg SM, Doherty GM, Soper NJ, Norton JA. (1997) Staging laparoscopy with laparoscopic ultrasonography: optimizing resectability in hepatobiliary and pancreatic malignancy. *J Am Coll Surg* 185(1): 33–9.

Cameron JL, Pitt HA, Zinner MJ, Kaufman SL, Coleman, J. (1990) Management of proximal cholangiocarcinomas by surgical resection and radiotherapy. *Am J Surg* 159(1): 91–7.

Chari RS, Anderson CA, Saverese, DMF. (2003) Treatment of cholangiocarcinoma I. In: Rose BD, ed. *UpToDate.* UpToDate, Wellesley, MA.

Connor S, Barron E, Wigmore SJ, Madhavan KK, Parks RW, Garden OJ. (2005) The utility of laparoscopic assessment in the preoperative staging of suspected hilar cholangiocarcinoma. *J Gastrointest Surg* 9(4): 476–80.

Corvera CU, Weber SM, Jarnagin WR. (2002) Role of laparoscopy in the evaluation of biliary tract cancer. *Surg Oncol Clin N Am* 11(4): 877–91.

Goldstein RM, Stone M, Tillery GW *et al.* (1993) Is liver transplantation indicated for cholangiocarcinoma? *Am J Surg* 166(6): 768–71.

Hadjis NS, Blenkharn JI, Alexander N, Benjamin IS, Blumgart LH. (1990) Outcome of radical surgery in hilar cholangiocarcinoma. *Surgery* 107(6): 597–604.

Hemming AW, Reed AI, Fujita S, Foley DP, Howard RJ. (2005) Surgical management of hilar cholangiocarcinoma. *Ann Surg* 241(5): 693–9.

Hemming AW, Reed AI, Howard RJ *et al.* (2003) Preoperative portal vein embolization for extended hepatectomy. *Ann Surg* 237(5): 686–93.

Iwatsuki S, Todo S, Marsh JW *et al.* (1998) Treatment of hilar cholangiocarcinoma (Klatskin tumors) with hepatic resection or transplantation. *J Am Coll Surg* 187(4): 358–64.

Jarnagin WR, Shoup M. (2004) Surgical management of cholangiocarcinoma. *Semin Liver Dis* 24(2): 189–99.

Jeyarajah DR, Klintmalm GB. (1998) Is liver transplantation indicated for cholangiocarcinoma? *J Hepatobiliary Pancreat Surg* 5(1): 48–51.

Kitagawa Y, Nagino M, Kamiya J *et al.* (2001) Lymph node metastasis from hilar cholangiocarcinoma: audit of 110 patients who underwent regional and paraaortic node dissection. *Ann Surg* 233(3): 385–92.

Klempnauer J, Ridder GJ, von Wasielewski R, Werner M, Weimann A, Pichlmayr R. (1997) Resectional surgery of hilar cholangiocarcinoma: a multivariate analysis of prognostic factors. *J Clin Oncol* 15(3): 947–54.

Lillemoe KD, Cameron JL. (2000) Surgery for hilar cholangiocarcinoma: the Johns Hopkins approach. *J Hepatobiliary Pancreat Surg* 7(2): 115–21.

Meyer CG, Penn I, James L. (2000) Liver transplantation for cholangiocarcinoma: results in 207 patients. *Transplantation* 69(8): 1633–7.

Nagino M, Nimura Y, Kamiya J *et al.* (1995) Right or left trisegment portal vein embolization before hepatic trisegmentectomy for hilar bile duct carcinoma. *Surgery* 117(6): 677–81.

Nakeeb A, Tran KQ, Black MJ *et al.* (2002) Improved survival in resected biliary malignancies. *Surgery* 132(4): 555–63.

Nimura Y, Kamiya J, Kondo S *et al.* (2000) Aggressive preoperative management and extended surgery for hilar cholangiocarcinoma: Nagoya experience. *J Hepatobiliary Pancreat Surg* 7(2): 155–62.

Pichlmayr R, Weimann A, Klempnauer J *et al.* (1996) Surgical treatment in proximal bile duct cancer. A single-center experience. *Ann Surg* 224(5): 628–38.

Rea DJ, Heimbach JK, Rosen CB *et al.* (2005) Liver transplantation with neoadjuvant chemoradiation is more effective than resection for hilar cholangiocarcinoma. *Ann Surg* 242(3): 451–8.

Shimoda M, Farmer DG, Colquhoun SD *et al.* (2001) Liver transplantation for cholangiocellular carcinoma: analysis of a single-center experience and review of the literature. *Liver Transpl* 7 (12): 1023–33.

Strasberg SM. (1998) Resection of hilar cholangiocarcinoma. *HPB Surg* 10(6): 415–18.

Su CH, Tsay SH, Wu CC *et al.* (1996) Factors influencing postoperative morbidity, mortality, and survival after resection for hilar cholangiocarcinoma. *Ann Surg* 223(4): 384–94.

Tsao JI, Nimura Y, Kamiya J *et al.* (2000) Management of hilar cholangiocarcinoma: comparison of an American and a Japanese experience. *Ann Surg* 232(2): 166–74.

Vauthey JN, Blumgart LH. (1994) Recent advances in the management of cholangiocarcinomas. *Semin Liver Dis* 14(2): 109–14.

Weber SM, DeMatteo RP, Fong Y, Blumgart LH, Jarnagin WR. (2002) Staging laparoscopy in patients with extrahepatic biliary carcinoma. Analysis of 100 patients. *Ann Surg* 235(3): 392–9.

Yi B, Zhang BH, Zhang YJ *et al.* (2004) Surgical procedure and prognosis of hilar cholangiocarcinoma. *Hepatobiliary Pancreat Dis Int* 3(3): 453–7.

Zhang BH, Cheng QB, Luo XJ *et al.* (2006) Surgical therapy for hilar cholangiocarcinoma: analysis of 198 cases. *Hepatobiliary Pancreat Dis Int* 5(2): 278–82.

Chemotherapy

Laura A. Williams & Jordan Berlin

Adjuvant

Because the efficacy of chemotherapy for biliary tract cancer in the advanced setting has been difficult to demonstrate, data in the adjuvant setting are limited. Most reports use 5-FU alone or in combination with other agents such as methotrexate, leucovorin, platinums, or interferon-α without any improvement in survival over surgery alone (Anderson *et al.* 2004). There has been one phase III trial which included both pancreas and biliary tract cancers (Takada *et al.* 2002). Patients were randomized to receive either surgery alone or mitomycin C in combination with infusional 5-FU following resection. Five hundred and eight patients were randomized, including 148 patients with gallbladder cancer. Although a statistically significant difference in survival was not demonstrated for the group overall, in the 112 patients with gallbladder cancer who were evaluated, there was a statistically significant improvement in 5-year survival rate for the chemotherapy group (26%) compared with the control group (14%), $p = 0.0367$. However, upon stratification for 'curative' versus 'non-curative' resection, the benefit appeared to be limited to those patients deemed to have a 'non-curative' resection. It is unclear at this time if there is any benefit to adjuvant therapy, particularly newer regimens that have not yet been tested in this setting.

Treatment of advanced disease

Traditional chemotherapy

Several chemotherapy agents have been evaluated in biliary tract cancer patients with limited efficacy. As with all GI malignancies, 5-FU has been evaluated in numerous combinations for this disease. Single-arm trials have examined 5-FU in combination with leucovorin, platinums, anthracyclines, and interferon in various permutations yielding median survival times ranging from 5–14 months and response rates of 10–40% (Patt *et al.* 1996; Sanz-Altamira *et al.* 1998; Patt *et al.* 2001; Malik & Aziz 2003). Phase III trials are rare and patient numbers are small. However, one such trial evaluated the use of 5-FU and leucovorin chemotherapy (sometimes with etoposide) versus best supportive care (Glimelius *et al.* 1996). This trial randomly assigned both biliary tract and pancreas cancer patients together. In this study, chemotherapy provided a longer survival time (6 months) when compared to best supportive care (2.5 months). Although these survival times remained the same for the biliary tract cancer patients when evaluated separately, only 37 biliary tract cancer patients were enrolled on the trial. Perhaps more importantly, though, in this trial quality of life scores and quality-adjusted survival time were better for the patients treated with chemotherapy.

There may be other agents that would better combine with 5-FU than etoposide. For example, the combination of 5-FU, leucovorin and oxaliplatin (FOLFOX 3) was examined in a small study of 16 patients with advanced biliary tract adenocarcinoma and demonstrated an impressive disease control rate of 56% with a median survival time of 9.5 months (Nehls *et al.* 2002).

In previous phase II trials, response rates of 8–60% have been observed for single-agent gemcitabine with stable disease in 28–85% of patients (Scheithauer 2002). Overall survival ranged from 6.3–16 months. Therefore, attempts to improve upon these preliminary results with combination therapy have been made.

Gemcitabine in combination with 5-FU was reported in a two-part sequential phase II study with 18 patients treated with gemcitabine alone and 22 patients treated with gemcitabine, 5-FU and leucovorin (Gebbia *et al.* 2001). In the single-agent gemcitabine group, time to progression was 3.4 months with a median overall survival of 8 months and 22% of patients alive at 1 year. The combination arm yielded a 4.1 month time to progression with a median overall survival of 11 months and 36% alive at one year. Other studies of the combination of gemcitabine with 5-FU or capecitabine have shown response rates in the 10–30% range with overall survival from 6–14 months (Jacobson *et al.* 2003; Hsu *et al.* 2004; Alberts *et al.* 2005; Cho *et al.* 2005; Knox *et al.* 2005).

Gemcitabine has been combined with platinum agents as well. Patients with advanced biliary tract adenocarcinoma were treated in a phase II study of gemcitabine 1000 mg/m^2 as a 10 mg/m^2/min infusion on day 1, followed by oxaliplatin 100 mg/m^2 as a 2-h infusion on day 2 every 2 weeks (GEMOX) (Andre *et al.* 2004). 'Group A,' defined as patients with an ECOG performance status of 0–2, bilirubin <2.5× normal, and no prior chemotherapy achieved an objective response rate of 36%, stable disease in 26% and a median overall survival of 15.4 months. These results were updated at the 2006 American Society of Clinical Oncology meeting, now observing a median overall survival of 8.25 months (Andre *et al.* 2006). Approximately 10% of patients experienced grade 3 or 4 hematologic toxicity. Non-hematologic toxicities included pain, ALT elevation, fatigue, infection, nausea, vomiting, diarrhea and sensory neuropathy, all reported to have <10% incidence. Gemcitabine in combination with cisplatin in phase II studies have demonstrated response rates ranging from 27.5% to 48% with overall survival ranging from 7–11 months (Table 22.4).

The efficacy of chemotherapy in biliary tract cancer was recently evaluated in a pooled analysis of 88 trials presented by Eckel (Eckel *et al.* 2006). Overall response rates ranged from 0–83% with a pooled response rate of 23.3%. The median progression-free survival was 4.1 months with a median overall survival of 8.0 months. The addition of platinum analogs increased the response rate of 5-FU from 17% to 27% and increased the response rate of gemcitabine from 22% to 42%. Whenever combining chemotherapy agents, the additional side-effects also have to be taken into account.

Table 22.4 Response to chemotherapy for biliary tract adenocarcinoma. RR, response rate; OS, overall survival.

Reference	Chemotherapy	No. Patients	RR	OS (months)
Malik (2003)	5-FU/LV	30	7%	14.8
Patt (1996)	5-FU/IFN	35	34%	12
Patt (2001)	5-FU/IFN/cisplatin/ doxorubicin	41	21.1%	14
Nehls (2002)	FOLFOX3	16	19%	9.5
Nehls (2004)	CapeOx	56	29%	NR
Ducreux (2005)	HD 5-FU	29	7.1%	5
Ducreux (2005)	5-FU/cisplatin	29	19%	8
Penz (2001)	Gemcitabine	32	22%	11.5
Arroyo (2001)	Gemcitabine	39	36%	6.5
Tsavaris (2004)	Gemcitabine	30	30%	14
Gelibter (2005)	Gemcitabine FDR	40	15%	10
Jacobson (2003)	Gemcitabine/5-FU	42	9.5%	6.8
Hsu (2004)	Gemcitabine/5-FU	28	21.4%	4.7
Alberts (2005)	Gemcitabine/5-FU	42	9.5%	9.7
Knox (2005)	Gemcitabine/capecitabine	45	31%	14
Cho (2005)	Gemcitabine/capecitabine	44	32%	14
Thongprasert (2005)	Gemcitabine/cisplatin	40	27.5%	9
Reyes-Vidal (2004)	Gemcitabine/cisplatin	42	48%	7
Kim (2006)	Gemcitabine/cisplatin	29	34.5%	11
Andre (2006)	GEMOX	70	NR	8.25

Targeted therapy

Because of the insufficiency of traditional chemotherapy in biliary tract cancers, alternate strategies are sought. EGFR (also called HER-1) expression is increased in the majority of bile duct cancers along with its ligand TGF-α (Lee *et al.* 1995). Additionally, HER-2, which can dimerize with EGFR, is also overexpressed in 24–65% of biliary cancers (Lee & Pirdas 1995; Ogo *et al.* 2006; Thomas *et al.* 2006). In response to EGF stimulation, cholangiocarcinoma cell lines showed sustained EGFR activation due to defective receptor internalization (Yoon *et al.* 2004). However, treatment with EGFR kinase inhibitors attenuated the EGF stimulated growth in these cells. Forty-two patients with either unresectable or metastatic biliary cancers were treated with erlotinib 150 mg/day (Philip *et al.* 2006); 57% of patients had received prior chemotherapy for their disease. The estimated overall confirmed response rate was 8% with an additional 43% achieving stabilization of disease; 11% of first-line patients and 21% of second-line patients were progression free at 24 weeks. Median overall survival was 7.5 months. The investigational agent, NVP-AEE788, inhibits both the EGFR and ErbB-2. *In vitro* data suggested even greater growth inhibition of biliary tract cancer cell lines with this agent compared to erlotinib (Wiedmann *et al.* 2006). Lapatinib is also an inhibitor of both EGFR and HER-2. Unfortunately, a clinical study presented at the 2006 American Society of Clinical Oncology meeting failed to demonstrate any activity in biliary tract cancer (gallbladder and bile duct) (Ramanathan *et al.* 2006).

Summary

Traditional chemotherapy, most notably gemcitabine or 5-FU alone or in combination with a platinum agent, demonstrates modest efficacy in terms of response rate and improved median survival and additionally shows an improvement in quality of life when compared with supportive care alone. Agents targeting the EGF receptor have shown promise, but further research regarding the underlying pathogenesis of biliary tract cancer will be necessary to best utilize these and other therapies.

References

Alberts SR, Al-Khatib H, Mahoney MR et *al.* (2005) Gemcitabine, 5-fluorouracil, and leucovorin in advanced biliary tract and gallbladder carcinoma: a North Central Cancer Treatment Group phase II trial. *Cancer* 103(1): 111–18.

Anderson CD, Pinson CW, Berlin J, Chari RS. (2004) Diagnosis and treatment of cholangiocarcinoma. *Oncologist* 9(1): 43–57.

Andre T, Tournigand C, Rosmorduc O et *al.* (2004) Gemcitabine combined with oxaliplatin (GEMOX) in advanced biliary tract adenocarcinoma: a GERCOR study. *Ann Oncol* 15(9): 1339–43.

Andre T, Reyes-Vidal JM, Fartoux P et *al.* (2006) An international multicenter phase II trial of gemcitabine and oxaliplatin (GEMOX) in patients with advanced biliary tract cancer. *J Clin Oncol* ASCO Annual Meeting Proceedings 24(18S): 211s, abstract 4135.

Arroyo G, Gallardo J, Rubio B et *al.* (2001) Gemcitabine in advanced biliary tract cancer (ABTC). Experience from Chile and Argentina in phase II trials. *Proc Am Soc Clin Oncol* 20(1 of 2): 157a, abstract 626.

Cho JY, Paik YH, Lee SJ et *al.* (2005) Capecitabine combined with gemcitabine (CapGem) as first-line treatment in patients with advanced/ metastatic biliary tract carcinoma. *Cancer* 104(12): 2753–8.

Ducreux M, VanCutsem E, VanLaethem JL et *al.* (2005) A randomized phase II trial of weekly high-dose 5-fluorouracil with and without folinic acid and cisplatin in patients with advanced biliary tract carcinoma: results of the 40955 EORTC trial. *Eur J Cancer* 41(3): 398–403.

Eckel F, Schmid RM. (2006) Chemotherapy in advanced biliary tract carcinoma: a comprehensive analysis. *J Clin Oncol* 2006 ASCO Annual Meeting Proceedings Part I 24(18S): 626s, number 14036.

Gebbia V, Giuliani F, Maiello E et *al.* (2001) Treatment of inoperable and/or metastatic biliary tree carcinomas with single-agent gemcitabine or in combination with levofolinic acid and infusion fluorouracil: results of a multicenter phase II study. *J Clin Oncol* 19(20): 4089–91.

Gelibter A, Malaguti P, DiCosimo S et *al.* (2005) Fixed dose-rate gemcitabine infusion as first-line treatment for advanced-stage carcinoma of the pancreas and biliary tree. *Cancer* 104(6): 1237–45.

Glimelius B, Hoffman K, Sjoden PO *et al.* (1996) Chemotherapy improves survival and quality of life in advanced pancreatic and biliary cancer. *Ann Oncol* 7(6): 593–600.

Hsu C, Shen YC, Yang CH et *al.* (2004) Weekly gemcitabine plus 24-h infusion of high-dose 5-fluorouracil/leucovorin for locally advanced or metastatic carcinoma of the biliary tract. *Br J Cancer* 90(9): 1715–19.

Jacobson SD, Alberts SR, Mahoney MR et *al.* (2003) Phase II trial of gemcitabine, 5-fluorouracil, and leucovorin in patients with unresectable or metastatic biliary and gallbladder carcinoma: A North Central Cancer Treatment Group (NCCTG) study. *J Clin Oncol* ASCO Annual Meeting Proceedings 22(2): 275, abstract 1102.

Kim ST, Park JO, Lee J et *al.* (2006) A phase II study of gemcitabine and cisplatin in advanced biliary tract cancer. *Cancer* 106(6): 1339–46.

Kim YW, Huh SH, Park YK et *al.* (2001) Expression of the c-erb-B2 and p53 protein in gallbladder carcinomas. *Oncol Rep* 8(5) 1127–32.

Knox JJ, Hedley D, Oza A et *al.* (2005) Combining gemcitabine and capecitabine in patients with advanced biliary cancer: a phase II trial. *J Clin Oncol* 23(10): 2332–8.

Lee CS, Pirdas A. (1995) Epidermal growth factor receptor immunoreactivity in gallbladder and extrahepatic biliary tract tumors. *Pathol Res Pract* 191(11): 1087–91.

Malik IA, Aziz Z. (2003) Prospective evaluation of efficacy and toxicity of 5-FU and folinic acid (Mayo Clinic regimen) in patients with advanced cancer of the gallbladder. *Am J Clin Oncol* 26(2): 124–6.

Nehls O, Klump B, Arenau HT et *al.* (2002) Oxaliplatin, fluorouracil and leucovorin for advanced biliary system adenocarcinomas: a prospective phase II trial. *Br J Cancer* 87(7): 702–4.

Nehls O, Oettle H, Hartmann JT et *al.* (2004) A multicenter phase II study of capecitabine plus oxaliplatin (CapOx) in advanced biliary system adenocarcinomas. *ASCO Annual Meeting Proc* 22: 335, abstract 4091.

Ogo Y, Nio Y, Yano S et *al.* (2006) Immunohistochemical expression of HER-1 and HER-2 in extrahepatic biliary carcinoma. *Anticancer Res* 26(1B): 763–70.

Patt YZ, Jones DV, Hoque A et *al.* (1996) Phase II trial of intravenous fluorouracil and subcutaneous interferon alfa-2b for biliary tract cancer. *J Clin Oncol* 14(8): 2311–15.

Patt YZ, Hassan MM, Lozano RD et *al.* (2001) Phase II trial of cisplatin, interferon α-2b, doxorubicin, and 5-fluorouracil for biliary tract cancer. *Clin Can Res* 7(11): 3375–80.

Penz M, Kornek GV, Raderer M et *al.* (2001) Phase II trial of two-weekly gemcitabine in patients with advanced biliary tract cancer. *Ann Oncol* 12(3): 183–6.

Philip PA, Mahoney MR, Allmer C et *al.* (2006) Phase II study of erlotinib in patients with advanced biliary cancer. *J Clin Oncol* 24(19): 3069–74.

Ramanathan RK, Belani CP, Singh DA et *al.* (2006) Phase II study of lapatinib, a dual inhibitor of epidermal growth factor receptor (EGFR) tyrosine kinase 1 and 2 (Her2/Neu) in patients with advanced biliary tree cancer or hepatocellular cancer. A California Consortium Trial. *J Clin Oncol* 2006 ASCO Annual Meeting Proceedings 24(18S Part I): 181s, abstract 4010.

Reyes-Vidal JM, Gallardo J, Yanez E et *al.* (2004) Gemcitabine and cisplatin in the treatment of patients with unresectable or metastatic gallbladder cancer: results of the phase II GOCCHI study 2000–13. ASCO GI Cancers Symposium, abstract 87. www.asco.org/portal/site/ASCO/menuitem.34d60f5624ba07fd506fe310ee37a01d/?vgnextoid=76f8201eb61a7010VgnVCM100000ed730ad1RCRD&vmview=abst_detail_view&confID=27&abstractID=203

Sanz-Altamira PM, Ferrante K, Jenkins RL et *al.* (1998) A phase II trial of 5-fluorouracil, leucovorin, and carboplatin in patients with unresectable biliary tree carcinoma. *Cancer* 82(12): 2321–5.

Scheithauer W. (2002) Review of gemcitabine in biliary tract carcinoma. *Sem Oncol* 29(6 Suppl 20): 40–5.

Takada T, Amano H, Yasuda H et *al.* (2002) Is postoperative adjuvant chemotherapy useful for gallbladder carcinoma? *Cancer* 95(8): 1685–95.

Thomas MB, Kawamoto T, Tarco E et *al.* (2006) Amplification of erbB2 (HER-2/neu) gene expression in gallbladder and in bile duct cancer. 2006 ASCO GI Cancers Symposium, abstract 217. www.asco.org/portal/site/ASCO/menuitem.34d60f5624ba07fd506fe310ee37a01d/?vgnextoid=76f8201eb61a7010VgnVCM100000ed730ad1RCRD&vmview=abst_detail_view&confID=41&abstractID=293

Thongprasert S, Napapan S, Charoentum C, Moonprakan S. (2005) Phase II study of gemcitabine and cisplatin as first line chemotherapy in inoperable biliary tract carcinoma. *Ann Oncol* 16(2): 279–81.

Tsavaris N, Kosmas C, Panagiotis G et *al.* (2004) Weekly gemcitabine for the treatment of biliary tract and gallbladder cancer. *Invest New Drugs* 22(2): 193–8.

Wiedmann M, Feisthammel J, Bluthner T et *al.* (2006) Novel targeted approaches to treating biliary tract cancer: the dual epidermal growth factor receptor and ErbB-2 tyrosine kinase inhibitor NVP-AEE788 is more efficient than the epidermal growth factor receptor inhibitors gefitinib and erlotinib. *Anti-Cancer Drugs* 17(7): 783–95.

Yoon JH, Gwak GY, Lee HS et *al.* (2004) Enhanced epidermal growth factor receptor activation in human cholangiocarcinoma cells. *J Hepatol* 41(5): 808–14.

Role of radiation therapy

Jayamarx Jayaraman & A. Bapsi Chakravarthy

The role of radiation in cholangiocarcinoma remains controversial. There are no large randomized studies to guide treatment. Given the rarity of the disease, this is unlikely to ever happen. We are, therefore, limited to develop treatment guidelines based on patterns of failure data as well as non-randomized, single-institution studies which compare results to historical controls. The majority of single-institution studies are retrospective in nature and have included a heterogeneous patient population who have been treated with a wide variety of doses and schedules of radiation over a long period of time, with or without chemotherapy, making interpretation of the data even more difficult.

Resectable disease

Preoperative chemoradiation

Although neoadjuvant chemoradiation has been used successfully in many sites of the gastrointestinal tract (Bosset *et al.* 1997; Sauer *et al.* 2004), very few studies have used this approach for the treatment of cholangiocarcinomas. Preoperative therapy has several theoretical advantages including the early initiation of both systemic and local treatments in a disease which has a high risk for both. By postponing surgery until completion of chemoradiation, patients with disease that quickly spreads may be spared the morbidity of surgery.

In a retrospective analysis, 9 patients (5 hilar, 4 distal) treated with preoperative chemoradiation consisting of continuous-infusion 5-FU and radiation had a higher rate of margin-negative resections (100%) compared to those treated with surgery alone (54%) (McMasters *et al.* 1997). In another retrospective analysis of 22 patients treated with neoadjuvant continuous infusion 5-FU and radiation, 4 of 14 (29%) patients showed a clinical response while 2 of 14 had a complete response (Deodato *et al.* 2006).

A phase I study from Duke University treated patients with resectable or locally advanced pancreatic and biliary cancer with neoadjuvant eniluracil/5-FU and radiation (4500 cGy followed by 540 cGy by reduced fields). One of the patients achieved a pathologic complete response. Four of 13 patients underwent margin-negative resections. The study concluded neoadjuvant concurrent chemoradiation is effective and well tolerated (Czito *et al.* 2006). Patients who underwent low-dose neoadjuvant radiation of 10.5 Gy (3 fractions of 3.5 Gy) were found to have no wound implantation compared to a 20% rate of wound implants in those who underwent surgery alone (Gerhards *et al.* 2000). In general, preoperative chemoradiation is seldom used outside of a clinical trial.

Adjuvant chemoradiation

Proximal/hilar cholangiocarcinomas

As the patterns of recurrence following resection of hilar cholangiocarcinomas is predominantly local–regional, postoperative radiation has been used to help decrease the risk of local recurrence. Patients with local–regional recurrence often suffer from symptoms of obstructive jaundice, pain, pruritus, fever and sepsis. Therefore, local control remains an important goal in the treatment of proximal/hilar cholangiocarcinomas.

Several single institutional retrospective analyses show an improvement in median survival with the addition of radiation to surgery. Investigators from the University of Amsterdam found that in 112 patients who underwent resection for hilar cholangiocarcinoma, median survival was improved for the patients who received adjuvant radiotherapy (24 vs. 8 months) (Gerhards *et al.* 2003) (Table 22.5).

In contrast to the above, other studies suggest that there is no benefit to the addition of radiation (Ben-David *et al.* 2006). Japanese investigators who retrospectively analysed 69 patients following surgery for cholangiocarcinoma found no benefit to the addition of radiation (Sagawa *et al.* 2005). In a prospective study from Johns Hopkins, patients who underwent curative resection the addition of radiation (external beam with/without intraluminal brachytherapy) did not improve median survival, which was 20 months (Pitt *et al.* 1995). In a retrospective analysis from the same institution, there was no significant improvement in 5-year survival with the use of adjuvant radiation (Cameron *et al.* 1990) (Table 22.5).

Distal cholangiocarcinomas

Distal cholangiocarcinomas are similar to pancreatic cancers. They are located at the head of the pancreas and resection requires a pancreaticoduodenectomy. They generally have a better prognosis than proximal tumors as they are more likely to be resectable and often present earlier with symptoms of obstructive jaundice. However, their proximity to the small bowel makes delivery of large doses of radiation difficult.

Investigators from Johns Hopkins described 34 patients with distal common bile duct cholangiocarcinoma treated with pancreaticoduodenectomy, followed by adjuvant concurrent chemoradiation. This group experienced longer median survival (36.9 months) than historical controls from the same institution treated with surgery alone (22 months) (Hughes *et al.* 2005).

Unresectable disease

Many studies have examined the role of primary radiation with or without chemotherapy for unresectable disease (Table 22.6). In a retrospective study from China 75 patients with unresectable or node-positive intrahepatic cholangiocarcinoma were evaluated. Thirty-eight patients received external-beam radiotherapy (median total dose 50 Gy, range 30–60 Gy, at 2 Gy/fraction, 5 times a week). One-year survival was improved in the patients who received external-beam radiotherapy compared with patients treated with surgery alone (36.1% vs. 19%). Patients with lymph node metastases (treated with hepatectomy and external-beam radiotherapy) experienced a longer median

Table 22.5 Resectable disease.

Author	Number of patients	RT	Dose (Gy)	Chemotherapy	Median survival (months)
Gerhards *et al.* (2003)	71	Yes	46	No	24
			42 + 10*		
	20	No		No	8
Hughes *et al.* (2005)	34	Yes	40–54	5-FU	36.9
	30	No		No	22
Sagawa *et al.* (2005)	39	Yes	37.5	No	23
			37.2 + 36.9*		
	30	No		No	20
Pitt *et al.* (1995)	23	Yes	46 ± 13†	No	14
			51‡		
	27	No		No	15

* Intraluminal brachytherapy dose.

† Resectable (EBRT ± iridium).

‡ Unresectable.

Table 22.6 Unresectable disease.

Author	Number of patients	RT	Dose (Gy)	Chemotherapy	Median survival (months)
Brunner *et al.* (2004)	25	Yes	45–50.4 ± 10*	5-FU or gemcitabine	16.5
	39	No		No	9.3
Grove *et al.* (1991)	19	Yes	12.6–64	No	12.2
	9	No		No	2.2

* High dose rate iridium-192.

survival (468 days) than those who did not receive external-beam radiotherapy (211 days) (Zeng *et al.* 2006).

A retrospective study from Germany analyzed 98 patients with unresectable biliary carcinoma. All patients underwent palliative biliary stent placement. Twenty-five patients were treated with chemoradiation therapy consisting of 45–50.4 Gy using three-dimensional conformal radiotherapy. Concurrent chemotherapy (5-FU or gemcitabine) was also given. Patients treated with chemoradiation had a longer median survival than patients treated with stenting alone (16.5 months vs. 9.3 months) (Brunner *et al.* 2004).

Newer radiation therapy techniques

Despite the use of external-beam radiation with chemotherapy, most patients will have local recurrence and obstruction of the biliary tree resulting in jaundice, pruritus and sepsis. Doses of 50–54 Gy in 1.8–2-Gy fractions are utilized due to the sensitivity of the adjacent small bowel to higher doses of radiation. These doses, however, are insufficient to eradicate gross disease and therefore techniques that involve dose escalation including 3D conformal therapy, intensity-modulated radiation therapy, and radiosurgery have all been tried for this disease.

Conventional CT-based radiation planning allows the physician to outline more precisely the tumor and normal tissue with better visualization than was possible using conventional X-ray simulators. Recent improvements in computerized treatment planning now allow not only better visualization of the target and avoidance structures, but also allow the computer to design the optimum fields and blocks. More precise delivery of dose to the target while sparing surrounding normal tissue is now possible with the use of computer-aided planning (intensity-modulated radiation therapy)(Ben-Josef *et al.* 2005; Milano *et al.* 2004).

Finally, radiosurgery, a technique that uses multiple fields to cone down on the tumor, can be used to treat the tumor while sparing surrounding normal tissue. German investigators reported a case study of a patient diagnosed with unresectable Klatskin's tumor who was treated with stereotactic radiotherapy using a body frame (Becker *et al.* 2005).

More recently 4D treatment planning software is being developed which takes into account not only CT-guided anatomic detail and precision planning abilities but also respiratory motion. A few centers are now able to treat using machines that use respiratory gating to track the tumor during respiration. Whether such sophisticated treatment systems will result in better survival remains to be seen. They do, however, allow for much higher doses to be delivered safely.

Intraluminal brachytherapy

Another way to increase the dose to the tumor while sparing normal tissue is the use of intraluminal brachytherapy. Although there have been no randomized trials, several series have shown that when brachytherapy is combined with external beam it enhances the survival. Brachytherapy can be given with low or high dose rate applicators. Low dose rate brachytherapy using iridium-192 is the most popular. This is placed through a percutaneous transhepatic biliary stent and remains in place for approximately 2 days. The patient remains hospitalized in a special lead-shielded hospital room so as not to expose others to radiation. Due to the rapid dose fall-off, doses of 20–30 Gy can be safely delivered to the area 0.5–1 cm from the radioactive source. This treatment is often combined with external-beam radiation using doses of 45–50.4 Gy (in 25 to 28 fractions).

Some studies have found that the addition of an intraluminal boost provides good local control and improved quality of life for patients (Takamura *et al.* 2003). In a study from the Mayo Clinic, 24 patients with extrahepatic bile duct carcinoma were treated with external-beam irradiation (median dose was 50.4 Gy delivered in 1.8-Gy/day fractions) and low dose rate brachytherapy using iridium-192 (20 Gy). Nine patients also received 5-FU. Median survival was 12.8 months with a 2-year survival of 18.8% and 5-year survival rate of 14.1%. The study concluded that survival can be improved by adding intraluminal brachytherapy to external-beam irradiation (Foo *et al.* 1997).

High-dose-rate (HDR) brachytherapy

With the advent of the high dose rate applicator, the equivalent biologic dose can be given in a much shorter period of time with no risk of radiation exposure to healthcare staff. As the patient is treated within minutes in a shielded area in the radiation oncology suite, special hospital beds with lead shielding are no longer required. Investigators from Japan described 31 patients with unresectable extrahepatic bile duct carcinoma who received external-beam radiation alone, or external beam with high dose rate brachytherapy boost. This study concluded that HDR intraluminal brachytherapy is well tolerated and improved time to tumor recurrence (Shin *et al.* 2003). Another study analysed 30 patients with bile duct carcinomas (palliative resection or inoperable) who were treated with external-beam radiation (30–45 Gy) and intraluminal high dose rate brachytherapy (20–45 Gy). The study concluded that combination of 40 Gy of external-beam radiation and 20 Gy of brachytherapy is well tolerated (Fritz *et al.* 1994).

Intraoperative radiotherapy (IORT)

Intraoperative brachytherapy is a method that utilizes a single dose of external-beam radiation to the tumor bed at the time of surgery. Low-energy photons or electrons are typically used. Normal structures can be physically moved out of the way. Very few centers have the shielded operating rooms that are required for this type of radiation delivery. In a retrospective analysis of 47 patients diagnosed with stage IVA Klatskin's tumor who had microscopic residual noted at surgery, 19 patients underwent resection alone and the remaining 28 patients received adjuvant radiotherapy (external beam and IORT, external beam alone, and IORT alone). The local regional control was better in patients who received adjuvant radiation. The investigators recommended IORT in combination with external-beam radiation (Todoroki *et al.* 2000).

Charged particle radiotherapy

Charged particles such as protons and helium ions have also been utilized. These particles are able to deliver a very high dose to a very small volume. There are only a handful of treatment centers that have particle accelerators. Patients with microscopic residual disease had an improved median survival with the addition of conventional radiation therapy ($p = 0.01$) but this was even higher with the use of charged particle therapy ($p = 0.0005$). Patients with gross residual disease had a smaller but still statistically significant improvement in survival following adjuvant radiation using conventional therapy ($p = 0.05$) which was statistically more significant with the use of charged particle therapy ($p = 0.04$). Median survival for the entire group treated with surgery alone, adjuvant radiotherapy, and charged particles were 6.5, 11, and 14 months respectively and 16, 16, and 23 months for those who were treated with curative intent (Schoenthaler *et al.* 1994).

Neoadjuvant chemoradiation followed by liver transplant

Given the poor prognosis of this disease, investigators have evaluated novel treatment approaches including neoadjuvant chemoradiation followed by liver transplant. In a study from the Mayo Clinic the survival of patients with hilar cholangiocarcinoma who underwent neoadjuvant therapy followed by liver transplantation was improved compared to patients who underwent resection alone (Rea *et al.* 2005). See also the section on surgery in this chapter.

Treatment recommendations

Given the paucity of randomized data, no definitive conclusions can be drawn but we recommend the use of adjuvant chemoradiation using external-beam radiation for patients with *high risk features* such as positive lymph nodes or positive margins. Chemotherapy consists of continuous infusion 5-FU based on its demonstrated radiosensitizing potential in other sites of the gastrointestinal tract (O'Connell *et al.* 1994). The radiation dose we recommend would be 50.4 Gy to the surgical bed and surrounding lymph nodes.

In locally advanced disease and/or unresectable disease we consider the use of chemoradiation using external-beam doses of 50.4–54 Gy, 1.8 Gy/fraction with concurrent continuous-infusion 5-FU. Patients with a good performance status and appropriate tumor geometry can be considered for brachytherapy boost using high dose rate intraluminal brachytherapy 500 cGy to 0.5-cm depth.

References

Becker G, Momm F, Schwacha H *et al.* (2005) Klatskin tumor treated by inter-disciplinary therapies including stereotactic radiotherapy: a case report. *World J Gastroenterol* 11(31): 4923–6.

Ben-David MA, Griffith KA, Abu-Isa E *et al.* (2006) External-beam radiotherapy for localized extrahepatic cholangiocarcinoma. *International Journal of Radiation Oncology Biology Physics* 66(3): 772–9.

Ben-Josef E, Normolle D, Ensminger WD *et al.* (2005) Phase II trial of high-dose conformal radiation therapy with concurrent hepatic artery floxuridine for unresectable intrahepatic malignancies. *J Clin Oncol* 23(34): 8739–47.

Bosset JF, Gignoux M, Triboulet JP *et al.* (1997) Chemoradiotherapy followed by surgery compared with surgery alone in squamous-cell cancer of the esophagus. *N Engl J Med* 337: 161–7.

Brunner TB, Schwab D, Meyer T, Sauer R. (2004) Chemoradiation may prolong survival of patients with non-bulky unresectable extrahepatic biliary carcinomaa retrospective analysis. *Strahlenther Onkol* 180(12): 751–7.

Cameron JL, Pitt HA, Zinner MJ, Kaufman SL, Coleman J. (1990) Management of proximal cholangiocarcinomas by surgical resection and radiotherapy. *Am J Surg* 159(1): 91–8.

Czito BG, Hong TJ, Cohen DP *et al.* (2006) A phase I study of eniluracil/5-FU in combination with radiation therapy for potentially resectable and/or unresectable cancer of the pancreas and distal biliary tract. *Cancer Invest* 24(1): 9–17.

Czito BG, Hurwitz HI, Clough RW *et al.* (2005) Adjuvant external-beam radiotherapy with concurrent chemotherapy after resection of primary gallbladder carcinoma: a 23-year experience. *Int J Radiat Oncol Biol Phys* 62(4): 1030–4.

De Groen PC, Gores GJ, Larusso NF, Gunderson LL, Nagorney DM. (1999) Biliary tract cancers. *N Engl J Med* 341(18): 1368–78.

Deodato F, Clemente G, Mattiucci GC *et al.* (2006) Chemoradiation and brachytherapy in biliary tract carcinoma: Long-term results. *Int J Radiat Oncol Biol Phys* 64(2): 483–8.

Foo ML, Gunderson LL, Bender CE, Buskirk SJ. (1997) External radiation therapy and transcatheter iridium in the treatment of extrahepatic bile duct carcinoma. *Int J Radiat Oncol Biol Phys* 39(4): 929–35.

Fritz P, Brambs HJ, Schraube P, Freund U, Berns C, Wannenmacher M. (1994) Combined external beam radiotherapy and intraluminal high dose rate brachytherapy on bile duct carcinomas. *Int J Radiat Oncol Biol Phys* 29(4): 855–61.

Gerhards MF, Gonzalez DG, Ten Hoopen-Neumann H, Van Gulik TM, De Wit LT, Gouma DJ. (2000) Prevention of implantation metastases after resection of proximal bile duct tumours with pre-operative low dose radiation therapy. *Eur J Surg Oncol* 26(5): 480–5.

Gerhards MF, Van Gulik TM, Gonzalez Gonzalez D, Rauws EA, Gouma DJ. (2003) Results of postoperative radiotherapy for resectable hilar cholangiocarcinoma. *World J Surg* 27(2): 173–9.

Grove MK, Hermann RE, Vogt DP, Broughan TA. (1991) Role of radiation after operative palliation in cancer of the proximal bile ducts. *Am J Surg* 161(4): 454–8.

Hughes M, Frassica D, Yeo C, Riall T, Laheru D, Abrams R. (2005) Adjuvant concurrent chemoradiation for adenocarcinoma of the distal common bile duct. *Int J Radiat Oncol Biol Phys* 63(S1):S14, abstract 24.

McMasters KM, Tuttle TM, Leach SD *et al.* (1997) Neoadjuvant chemoradiation for extrahepatic cholangiocarcinoma. *Am J Surg* 174(6): 605–9.

Milano MT, Chmura SJ, Garofalo MC *et al.* (2004) Intensity-modulated radiotherapy in treatment of pancreatic and bile duct malignancies: toxicity and clinical outcome. *Int J Radiat Oncol Biol Phys* 59(2): 445–53.

O'Connell MJ, Martenson JA, Wieand HS *et al.* (1994) Improving adjuvant therapy for rectal cancer by combining protracted-infusion fluorouracil with radiation therapy after curative surgery. *N Engl J Med* 331(8): 502–7.

Pitt HA, Nakeeb A, Abrams RA *et al.* (1995) Perihilar cholangiocarcinoma. Postoperative radiotherapy does not improve survival. *Ann Surg* 221(6): 788–98.

Rea DJ, Heimbach JK, Rosen CB *et al.* (2005) Liver transplantation with neoadjuvant chemoradiation is more effective than resection for hilar cholangiocarcinoma. *Ann Surg* 242(3): 451–61.

Sagawa N, Kondo S, Morikawa T, Okushiba S, Katoh H. (2005) Effectiveness of radiation therapy after surgery for hilar cholangiocarcinoma. *Surg Today* 35(7): 548–52.

Sauer R, Becker H, Hohenberger W *et al.* (2004) Preoperative versus postoperative chemoradiotherapy for rectal cancer. *N Engl J Med* 351(17): 1731–40.

Schoenthaler R, Phillips TL, Castro J, Efird JT, Better A, Way LW. (1994) Carcinoma of the extrahepatic bile ducts. The University of California at San Francisco experience. *Ann Surg* 219(3): 267–74.

Shin HS, Seong J, Kim WC *et al.* (2003) Combination of external beam irradiation and high-dose-rate intraluminal brachytherapy for inoperable carcinoma of the extrahepatic bile ducts. *Int J Radiat Oncol Biol Phys* 57(1): 105–12.

Takamura A, Saito H, Kamada T *et al.* (2003) Intraluminal low-dose-rate 192Ir brachytherapy combined with external beam radiotherapy and biliary stenting for unresectable extrahepatic bile duct carcinoma. *Int J Radiat Oncol Biol Phys* 57(5): 1357–65.

Todoroki T, Ohara K, Kawamoto T *et al.* (2000) Benefits of adjuvant radiotherapy after radical resection of locally advanced main hepatic duct carcinoma. *Int J Radiat Oncol Biol Phys* 46(3): 581–7.

Zeng ZC, Tang ZY, Fan J *et al.* (2006) Consideration of the role of radiotherapy for unresectable intrahepatic cholangiocarcinoma: a retrospective analysis of 75 patients. *Cancer J* 12(2): 113–22.

Ablation

Christopher D. Anderson & Ravi S. Chari

There are few long-term studies regarding the use of ablation therapies in the treatment of liver neoplasms. The majority of studies evaluating hepatic ablative therapies group numerous types of liver tumors together; thus there are few reports from which information specific for cholangiocarcinoma may be obtained. Ablative therapies are not equivalent to resection and should not be thought of as a less invasive substitute therapy. There are no data evaluating the long-term outcomes of ablation and resection remains the only potential curative therapy. Radiofrequency ablation (RFA) and photodynamic therapy (PDT) are the most commonly employed techniques for cholangiocarcinoma. In general, RFA has been used for unresectable intrahepatic cholangiocarcinoma or intrahepatic metastases. In addition, newer techniques such as endoscopic PDT have shown promise for both palliation and adjuvant therapy of cholangiocarcinoma.

Radiofrequency ablation (RFA)

RFA uses a high-frequency alternating current delivered directly into the tumor via an electrode. This produces heat via friction from the movement of ions within the tissue. Tissue necrosis occurs as local tissue temperature increases (Curley 2001). The amount of tissue destroyed using RFA is dependent on the impedence of the tissue in question and the square of the distance from the electrode (Buscarini *et al.* 2005). Thus rapid cooling of tissues or proximity to large blood vessels (which may act as a heat sink) limits the tissue coagulation potential (Lencioni *et al.* 2004). RFA requires imaging assistance and can be performed percutaneously, laparoscopically, or at laparotomy. Experience with these techniques varies widely among institutions. While the majority of RFA ablations for liver tumors can be safely carried out percutaneously, many authors advocate performing these procedures via laparotomy or laparoscopy whereby the use of intraoperative ultrasound increases the detection of occult metastases (Wood *et al.* 2000).

RFA has been used extensively for liver tumors. Reports on its specific use for cholangiocarcinoma are limited to case reports and/or portions of larger series of hepatic tumors. However, many reports on the use of RFA for hepatocellular carcinoma and metastatic colorectal carcinoma exist in the literature. Extrapolating from the available metastatic colorectal cancer data, RFA would seem most useful in patients who are not resectable, or who have recurrent disease. The available data would suggest 3-year survivals between 33 and 52% following RFA, although this is not cholangiocarcinoma specific (Solbiati *et al.* 2001; Oshowo *et al.* 2003; Lencioni *et al.* 2004). Information regarding disease-free survival and/or 5-year survival is extremely limited. RFA is best utilized for smaller-sized tumors (<3 cm diameter), and has local recurrences reported between 3 and 39% (Curley *et al.* 1999; Siperstein *et al.* 2000; Solbiati *et al.* 2001; Higgins & Berger 2006). RFA for the treatment of unresectable cholangiocarcinoma is only possible for intrahepatic tumors or hepatic metastasis from perihilar or distal (periampullary) tumors.

Endoscopic photodynamic therapy (PDT)

Although not widely available, PDT is emerging as an important palliative option for patients with unresectable cholangiocarcinoma. PDT employs a porphyrin photosensitizer which localizes to the mitochondria of tumor cells 24–48 hours following intravenous administration. Direct illumination of the tumor bed with a specific wavelength results in activation of the photoagent and induction of cell death, primarily through apoptosis, microvascular damage, and an antitumor immune response (Berr 2004; Harrod-Kim 2006). PDT has been shown to regress carcinomas of the skin, lungs, pharynx, esophagus, and stomach. The tumoricidal tissue penetration achieved is a depth of 4 mm and hence it is regarded as a palliative option (Berr 2004).

In one study, 39 patients with cholangiocarcinoma were randomized to treatment with either biliary stenting plus PDT or stenting alone (Ortner *et al.* 2003). Patients receiving PDT had higher median survival (493 days vs. 98 days), better quality of life scores, and better stabilization of Karnofsky performance status than did the stenting group (Ortner *et al.* 2003). A more recent study has verified these results (Zoepf *et al.* 2005). PDT is now being studied as a form of neoadjuvant therapy as a means of improving the likelihood of achieving a margin-negative resection (Berr *et al.* 2000; Wiedmann *et al.* 2003).

Summary

Ablative technologies continue to evolve and newer modalities may be developed in the future. RFA is restricted to intrahepatic cholangiocarcinoma, while PDT is limited to large duct involvement. Currently, PDT and RFA can be considered useful neoadjuvant, adjuvant and palliative measures in patients with cholangiocarcinoma.

References

Berr F. (2004) Photodynamic therapy for cholangiocarcinoma. *Semin Liver Dis* 24(2): 177–87.

Berr F, Tannapfel A, Lamesch P *et al.* (2000) Neoadjuvant photodynamic therapy before curative resection of proximal bile duct carcinoma. *J Hepatol* 32(2): 352–7.

Buscarini E, Savoia A, Brambilla G *et al.* (2005) Radiofrequency thermal ablation of liver tumors. *Eur.Radiol* 15(5): 884–94.

Curley SA, Izzo F, Delrio P *et al.* (1999) Radiofrequency ablation of unresectable primary and metastatic hepatic malignancies: results in 123 patients. *Ann Surg* 230(1): 1–8.

Curley SA. (2001) Radiofrequency ablation of malignant liver tumors. *Oncologist* 6(1): 14–23.

Harrod-Kim P. (2006) Tumor ablation with photodynamic therapy: introduction to mechanism and clinical applications. *J Vasc Interv Radiol* 17(9): 1441–8.

Higgins H, Berger DL. (2006) RFA for liver tumors: does it really work? *Oncologist* 11(7): 801–8.

Lencioni R, Crocetti L, Cioni D, Della PC, Bartolozzi C. (2004) Percutaneous radiofrequency ablation of hepatic colorectal metastases: technique, indications, results, and new promises. *Invest Radiol* 39(11): 689–97.

Ortner ME, Caca K, Berr F *et al.* (2003) Successful photodynamic therapy for nonresectable cholangiocarcinoma: a randomized prospective study. *Gastroenterology* 125(5): 1355–63.

Oshowo A, Gillams A, Harrison E, Lees WR, Taylor I. (2003) Comparison of resection and radiofrequency ablation for treatment of solitary colorectal liver metastases. *Br J Surg* 90(10): 1240–3.

Siperstein A, Garland A, Engle K *et al.* (2000) Local recurrence after laparoscopic radiofrequency thermal ablation of hepatic tumors. *Ann Surg Oncol* 7(2): 106–13.

Solbiati L, Ierace T, Tonolini M, Osti V, Cova L. (2001) Radiofrequency thermal ablation of hepatic metastases. *Eur J Ultrasound* 13(2): 149–58.

Wiedmann M, Caca K, Berr F *et al.* (2003) Neoadjuvant photodynamic therapy as a new approach to treating hilar cholangiocarcinoma: a phase II pilot study. *Cancer* 97(11): 2783–90.

Wood TF, Rose DM, Chung M, Allegra DP, Foshag LJ, Bilchik AJ. (2000) Radiofrequency ablation of 231 unresectable hepatic tumors: indications, limitations, and complications. *Ann Surg Oncol* 7(8): 593–600.

Zoepf T, Jakobs R, Arnold JC, Apel D, Riemann JF. (2005) Palliation of nonresectable bile duct cancer: improved survival after photodynamic therapy. *Am J Gastroenterol* 100(11): 2426–30.

Prognosis and follow-up

Christopher D. Anderson & Ravi S. Chari

Overall, the diagnosis of cholangiocarcinoma carries an extremely poor prognosis. The overall 5-year survival for patients with cholangiocarcinoma is between 5 and 10%. This is in part related to the late presentation of most patients and the inability of margin-negative resection to be achieved. The vast majority of patients with unresectable disease die between 6 months and 1 year following diagnosis (Carriaga & Henson 1995; Burke *et al.* 1998). Death usually occurs from liver failure or infectious complications accompanying the advancing biliary obstruction. Patients who are explored for potentially curative resections have reported 5-year survival rates from 8 to 44% (Hadjis *et al.* 1990; Bismuth *et al.* 1992; Nagorney *et al.* 1993; Washburn *et al.* 1995; Pichlmayr *et al.* 1996b; Su *et al.* 1996; Nagino *et al.* 1998; Nimura *et al.* 1998; Lillemoe & Cameron 2000; Nimura *et al.* 2000; Saldinger & Blumgart 2000; Jarnagin *et al.* 2001; Nakeeb *et al.* 2002; Nakagohri *et al.* 2003). In studies that compared outcomes after a histologically negative margin with those after a positive margin, the 5-year survival rates were greater when a negative margin was obtained, 19–47% versus 0–12% (Hadjis *et al.* 1990; Pichlmayr *et al.* 1996; Su *et al.* 1996; Lillemoe & Cameron 2000; Jarnagin *et al.* 2001; Nakeeb *et al.* 2002). For patients with distal cholangiocarcinoma, the achievement of a margin-negative resection via a pancreaticoduodenectomy results in a 21–54% 5-year survival (Nagorney *et al.* 1993; Fong *et al.* 1996; Wade *et al.* 1997). There are less data regarding the specific prognosis of intrahepatic cholangiocarcinoma. However, at least one report shows a 60% 3-year survival following R0 resection (Nagorney *et al.* 1993). Regardless of the location of the tumor, the prognosis of cholangiocarcinoma depends on the achievement of a R0 resection. There is no demonstrated survival advantage of chemotherapy or radiation therapy; however these modalities remain important considerations for quality of life. There may be a slight survival advantage from ablative therapies in patients who are unresectable. Further studies are needed.

Follow-up for patients after resection of cholangiocarcinoma should be focused on the early detection of recurrent or metastatic disease. Tumor markers such as CA19-9 should be checked yearly if they were elevated preoperatively. In addition to physical exam and routine laboratory tests (serum bilirubin, alkaline phosphatase, and transaminases), it has been our practice to follow patients with axial imaging (CT or MRI) at 4-month intervals for the first year postoperatively and then every 6 months for two years. We then recommend it yearly thereafter for at least 3 years. Locoregional disease is the pattern of recurrence in cholangiocarcinoma. PET imaging is useful in patients suspected for having recurrence, but should not be a scheduled screening exam (Anderson *et al.* 2004).

References

Anderson CA, Rice MH, Pinson CW, Chapman WC, Chari RS, Delbeke D. (2004) Fluorodeoxyglucose PET imaging in the evaluation of gallbladder carcinoma and cholangiocarcinoma. *J Gastrointest Surg* 8(1): 90–7.

Bismuth H, Nakache R, Diamond T. (1992) Management strategies in resection for hilar cholangiocarcinoma. *Ann Surg* 215(1): 31–8.

Burke EC, Jarnagin WR, Hochwald SN, Pisters PW, Fong Y, Blumgart LH. (1998) Hilar cholangiocarcinoma: patterns of spread, the importance of hepatic resection for curative operation, and a presurgical clinical staging system. *Ann Surg* 228(3): 385–94.

Carriaga MT, Henson DE. (1995) Liver, gallbladder, extrahepatic bile ducts, and pancreas. *Cancer* 75(1 Suppl): 171–90.

Fong Y, Blumgart LH, Lin E, Fortner JG, Brennan MF. (1996) Outcome of treatment for distal bile duct cancer. *Br J Surg* 83(12): 1712–15.

Hadjis NS, Blenkharn JI, Alexander N, Benjamin IS, Blumgart LH. (1990) Outcome of radical surgery in hilar cholangiocarcinoma. *Surgery* 107(6): 597–604.

Jarnagin WR, Fong Y, DeMatteo RP *et al.* (2001) Staging, resectability, and outcome in 225 patients with hilar cholangiocarcinoma. *Ann Surg* 234(4): 507–17.

Lillemoe KD, Cameron JL. (2000) Surgery for hilar cholangiocarcinoma: the Johns Hopkins approach. *J Hepatobiliary Pancreat Surg* 7(2): 115–21.

Nagino M, Nimura Y, Kamiya J *et al.* (1998) Segmental liver resections for hilar cholangiocarcinoma. *Hepatogastroenterology* 45(19): 7–13.

Nagorney DM, Donohue JH, Farnell MB, Schleck CD, Ilstrup DM. (1993) Outcomes after curative resections of cholangiocarcinoma. *Arch Surg* 128(8): 871–7.

Nakagohri T, Asano T, Kinoshita H, Kenmochi T, Urashima T, Miura F, Ochiai T. (2003) Aggressive surgical resection for hilar-invasive and peripheral intrahepatic cholangiocarcinoma. *World J Surg* 27(3): 289–93.

Nakeeb A, Tran KQ, Black MJ *et al.* (2002) Improved survival in resected biliary malignancies. *Surgery* 132(4): 555–63.

Nimura Y, Kamiya J, Nagino M *et al.* (1998) Aggressive surgical treatment of hilar cholangiocarcinoma. *J Hepatobiliary Pancreat Surg* 5(1): 52–61.

Nimura Y, Kamiya J, Kondo S *et al.* (2000) Aggressive preoperative management and extended surgery for hilar cholangiocarcinoma: Nagoya experience. *J Hepatobiliary Pancreat Surg* 7(2): 155–62.

Pichlmayr R, Weimann A, Klempnauer J *et al.* (1996) Surgical treatment in proximal bile duct cancer. A single-center experience. *Ann Surg* 224(5): 628–38.

Saldinger PF, Blumgart LH. (2000) Resection of hilar cholangiocarcinoma–a European and United States experience. *J Hepatobiliary Pancreat Surg* 7(2): 111–14.

Su CH, Tsay SH, Wu CC *et al.* (1996) Factors influencing postoperative morbidity, mortality, and survival after resection for hilar cholangiocarcinoma. *Ann Surg* 223(4): 384–94.

Wade TP, Prasad CN, Virgo KS, Johnson FE. (1997) Experience with distal bile duct cancers in U.S. Veterans Affairs hospitals: 1987–1991. *J Surg Oncol* 64(3): 242–5.

Washburn WK, Lewis WD, Jenkins RL. (1995) Aggressive surgical resection for cholangiocarcinoma. *Arch Surg* 130(3): 270–6.

23 Neuroendocrine Tumors

Edited by Ursula Plöckinger

History and histopathology

Guido Rindi & Cesare Bordi

History

The endocrine tumors of the gastrointestinal tract, also defined as neuroendocrine tumors (NET), originate from or, if you prefer, are made of cells with a phenotype largely overlapping that of cells belonging to the so-called diffuse endocrine system (DES) of the gut and are comprehensively defined as 'entero-endocrine' cells.

The identification of endocrine tumors and enteroendocrine cells largely coincides, and dates back to the 19th century when histology and histochemistry were initially established as novel branches of medical science. As early as the second half of the 19th and early 20th centuries 'different' cells of the gastric and intestinal mucosa were identified (Heidenhain 1870). The staining of these cells was obtained thanks to the interaction with chromium salt and for this reason were named as enterochromaffin cells (Ciaccio 1907). At about the same time secretin was discovered by Bayliss and Starling in 1902 and the gut was identified as the source of bloodborne agents, 'hormones', capable of eliciting physiologic effects at distance (Bayliss & Starling 1902). This was the observation that established endocrinology as a novel branch of medicine.

Other similar epithelial cells in different organs of the human body were subsequently described because of their failure to take up conventional stains (Feyrter 1938). These cells were named 'clear cells' and included those with intrinsic silver-reducing capacity (chromaffin cells) previously described by Masson (Gosset & Masson 1914). Given their wide distribution, these cells were grouped in the so-called 'diffuse endocrine system' (DES), a complex network of cells with not entirely clarified regulatory function (Feyrter 1938). It was hypothesized that these cells have local, 'paracrine', function via the production and secretion of peptides or amines (Feyrter 1953). This unitarian theory was refreshed about 40 years ago, in 1966, when Sir A. G. E. Pearse identified a group of cells containing amines and/or with the property of taking up amine precursors which are then transformed into amines by intracellular decarboxylation (Pearse 1966). These cells were grouped in the APUD system (amine uptake and decarboxylation) which also comprised, together with several other cell types, the argentaffin, 5-hydroxytryptamine-storing cell (Erspamer & Asero 1952) of the gastrointestinal tract. The APUD concept reinforced the local regulatory role proposed for DES cells and introduced the idea that the disperse endocrine cells were actually a neuron-like element with a neuroectodermal derivation. Although the neural crest origin was subsequently proven only for the nerve elements of the gut plexuses (Le Douarin & Teillet 1973) and not for endocrine cells (Andrew *et al.* 1983), this theory reinforced the unitarian concept of common functional properties of enteroendocrine cells. The subsequent identification of several peptide/amine hormones and the recognition that DES cells are the source of such substances made possible the development of the current classification in specific cell types according to the cell main hormonal product (Rindi *et al.* 2004).

In parallel with the development of the concept of a gut diffuse endocrine network, a non-conventional, epithelial tumor with slow-growing attitude was identified and defined as 'karzinoide' (carcinoid, i.e. carcinoma-like) by Oberendorfer (Öberendorfer 1907). Two previous reports also described ileal 'carcinomas' with features potentially consistent with a carcinoid diagnosis, one of which had liver metastases in association with a typical functional syndrome (Lubarsch 1888; Ransom 1890). The argentaffin properties of some of these tumors were described and their relationship with the enterochromaffin cells was subsequently established (Gosset & Masson 1914). The production of serotonin was later demonstrated in carcinoid tumor extracts (Ratzenhofer & Lembeck 1954).

Gastrointestinal Oncology: A Critical Multidisciplinary Team Approach.
Edited by J. Jankowski, R. Sampliner, D. Kerr, and Y. Fong.

Tumor histogenesis

Since the discovery of secretin by Bayliss and Starling many hormones have been identified in the gut so that the gastroenteropancreatic tract is recognized as the largest endocrine organ of the whole human body. As many as 15 highly specialized epithelial cells of endodermal origin makes the diffuse endocrine system of the gut. Gut endocrine cells constitute a complex regulatory network exerting local control on secretion, absorption, motility, mucosal cell proliferation/differentiation and possibly immune barrier. This is realized by the synthesis and release of multiple active molecules, including peptide hormones and biogenic amines specific for each individual cell type.

Endocrine cells share several antigens with neural cells. These molecules are defined as neuroendocrine (NE) markers. Specific histochemical techniques were firstly developed and include silver impregnation methods like the Masson–Fontana stain for argentaffinity (i.e. the ability of endocrine cells to take up and reduce silver ions in the absence of reducing agents), or the Grimelius' stain for argyrophilia (i.e. the ability of endocrine cells to take up and reduce silver ions in the presence of reducing agents). Nowadays immunohistochemistry makes easier and more effective the detection of cytosol NE markers like NSE and PGP 9.5 and of granular NE markers of large-dense-core vesicles (LDCV), like chromogranin A and related fragments, or of small synaptic-like vesicles (SSV), like synaptophysin. Such NE markers are defined 'general markers' since they identify an endocrine phenotype common to most endocrine cells of the gut. The specific cell subtyping can be obtained by the identification of the cell-specific hormonal product(s) (specific markers) at immunohistochemistry and/or by the assessment of LDCV morphology at electron microscopy.

Gut endocrine cells are a plastic cell population capable of adapting to different physiologic and pathologic stimuli (Rindi *et al.* 2004). Indeed, endocrine cells appear to differentiate in the gut via tissue-specific pathways, which may be disrupted and investigated by genetic manipulation in mice. In particular genetic evidences indicate that endocrine-committed cells may be sensitive to physiologic stimuli as well as transforming agents. It is therefore likely that, in humans too, immature, endocrine-committed cells may transform giving origin to gut endocrine tumors.

Histopathology

Premalignant presentations

Proliferative changes of gut endocrine cells include both hyperplastic and dysplastic lesions. Premalignant presentations or true preneoplastic lesions, i.e. lesions with a defined potential for tumor development, are by definition only the dysplastic lesions. Although hyperplastic growth was identified at all sites of the gut, dysplastic lesions have been defined and classified only for the histamine-producing, enterochromaffin-like (ECL) cells of the stomach (Solcia *et al.* 1998). Dysplastic 'precarcinoid' growth is limited to the mucosa, is below 500 μm in size and is composed of some way atypical ECL cells with reduced reactivity to silver stain. Four types of dysplastic lesions are recognized: (i) the enlarging micronodule (size above 150 μm); (ii) the fusing micronodule; (iii) the microinvasive lesion; and (iv) the nodule with newly formed stroma. Usually dysplastic changes associate with mixed patterns of ECL cell hyperplasia. Very recently the proliferative changes of gastrin-producing (G) cells were described and classified in the duodenum of MEN1 patients using the same approach as defined for gastric ECL cells (Anlauf *et al.* 2005). An 'enlarged nodule' of gastrin-positive cells with solid architecture and size 90–210 μm was identified as a potential dysplastic, precursor lesion for duodenal gastrinoma.

Neoplastic lesions

According to the anatomical and functional heterogeneity of the cells of origin, gut endocrine tumors represent a heterogeneous group of neoplasms with remarkable clinicopathologic differences. The novel WHO classifications are recommended to better define and diagnose gut endocrine tumors (Solcia *et al.* 2000; Hamilton & Aaltonen 2000; DeLellis *et al.* 2004). Pure NE tumors are classified on an anatomical basis (stomach, duodenum and upper jejunum; ileum; appendix; colon and rectum), cell type (e.g. gastrin-producing G-cell tumors) and status of differentiation for the large majority of tumor cells. Two broad classes are defined as (i) well-differentiated tumors/carcinomas and (ii) poorly differentiated endocrine carcinomas.

In well-differentiated endocrine neoplasms three categories are defined at diagnosis as: (i) 'benign behavior' tumors, or tumors with potentially benign course; (ii) 'uncertain-behavior' tumors, or tumors with potentially low-grade malignant course; and (iii) 'carcinomas', with low-grade malignant course. Well-differentiated tumors/carcinomas are composed of tumor cells closely resembling their normal counterparts and may associate with unregulated hormone secretion.

Conversely, poorly differentiated endocrine carcinomas are invariably high-grade malignant, are virtually never associated with a hormone-related clinical syndrome and display an abortive endocrine phenotype being more commonly reputed to derive from endocrine-committed, multipotent cells rather than from differentiated endocrine cells. Histopathologic criteria of differentiation are provided.

Well-differentiated tumors/carcinomas

In general, well-differentiated tumors are characterized by a 'so called' organoid/endocrine architecture with solid islets, trabecular, glandular, acinar or mixed patterns (Fig. 23.1) (Soga & Tazawa 1971). As a rule no necrosis is observed. The stroma is normally delicate and extremely rich in microvasculature, or,

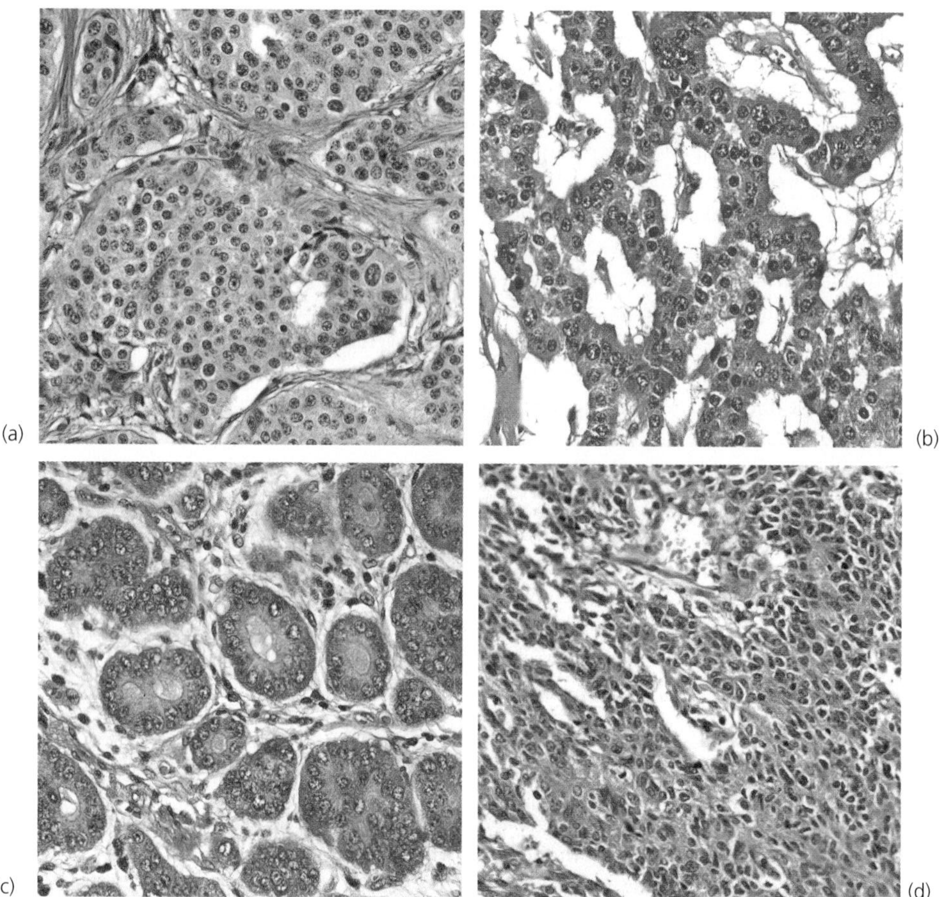

Fig. 23.1 Histology of endocrine tumors according to Soga and Tazawa (1971). (a) Well differentiated endocrine carcinoma of the ileum displaying a structure characterized by solid islets, a pattern originally defined 'type A' as it is composed of 'nodular solid nests'. The tumor cells show low atypia, no mitosis, and no necrosis; this pattern is typically observed in tumors mainly composed of serotonin-producing enterochromaffin (EC) cells, as in this case. H&E, ×200 original magnification. (b) Well-differentiated endocrine tumor of the pancreas, not associated with any hyperfunctional syndrome (non-functioning), showing a mainly trabecular structure with large spaces, often with evident vessel. This pattern was originally defined as 'type B' since it is composed of 'trabecular or ribbon-like structure forming a frequent anastomosing pattern'. These features are typically seen when tumors are formed by glucagon-producing A cells, as in this case. Tumor cells display mild atypia; H&E, ×200 original magnification. (c) Well-differentiated EC cell endocrine carcinoma of the ileum displaying a characteristic glandular structure, also defined as 'type C' since it is composed of 'tubular, acinar or rosette-like structures'. No significant cell atypia is observed. This carcinoma is actually of 'mixed type' as it shows a predominantly solid islet structure (see a) in other fields. H&E, ×200 original magnification. (d) Poorly differentiated endocrine carcinoma of the colon with a prevalent solid sheet structure, severe cell atypia and mitoses. This pattern is also defined as 'type D', since it is 'of lower atypical differentiation'. Other areas of this carcinoma show extensive necrosis. H&E, ×180 original magnification.

in some instances, may be abundant and fibrous, often displaying deposition of amorphous hyaline material, amyloid. Round calcium deposits, also defined as psammoma bodies, are observed only rarely and typically within the acinar structure of somatostatin-producing D-cell tumors of the duodenum. Tumor cells display bland features, are rather monomorph in shape, with abundant, variably eosinophilic cytoplasm, regular round nuclei and overall low cytologic atypia. As a rule, a very low number of typical mitoses (if any) is observed and, accordingly, the proliferation index as assessed by Ki-67 is rather low.

In some instances, namely in well-differentiated endocrine carcinomas, histologic aspects demonstrating a less organoid, more solid structure, moderate cytologic atypia with occasional mitoses, moderately higher Ki-67 index and/or punctate necrosis may suggest a higher grade of histologic malignancy. No grading system is defined by the WHO classifications however, despite several independent investigations suggesting its value (Capella *et al.* 1995; Rindi *et al.* 1999; Hochwald *et al.* 2002; Van Eeden *et al.* 2002). Recently a comprehensive working scheme was proposed and awaits confirmation of its potential efficiency on study series (Rindi *et al.* 2006).

The functional differentiation status is normally assessed by immunohistochemistry for general and specific endocrine markers. In pathology practice a widely used general NE marker panel comprises the vesicular markers chromogranin A and synaptophysin. Cytosol markers like neuron-specific enolase (NSE) and protein gene product 9.5 (PGP 9.5) may be used only to meet specific diagnostic demands, namely when possible technical artifacts require multiple NE antigen targeting, or if requested by the clinician. It is expected that almost all well-differentiated tumor cells express uniformly and intensely all the above-mentioned markers.

Immunohistochemistry for hormones (specific markers) may readily identify specific tumor cell types. Typically not all tumor cells exhibit positive immunoreactivity for specific hormonal markers given the multiple cell-type components often observed (Solcia *et al.* 1998). Hormone immunohistochemistry is helpful for diagnostic purposes and allows the cell type definition as requested by the WHO classifications (Hamilton & Aaltonen 2000; Solcia *et al.* 2000; DeLellis *et al.* 2004).

Poorly differentiated carcinomas

As a rule, poorly differentiated carcinomas display a prevalent solid structure with large cell islands or sheets with abundant necrosis, often central, and variably abundant fibrous stroma at periphery. These features are overall defined as 'geographical chart' architecture. Within the cancer islands, tumor cells may be detached with a loose phenotype and single cell necrosis; the stroma is usually scant and poor in microvasculature. Cancer cells display an epithelial feature, are round/polygonal in shape, of small to medium size with severe cellular atypia, abundant mitoses frequently atypical and high Ki-67 proliferation index. A poorly differentiated carcinoma with large, pleomorphic cells has also been reported (Crafa *et al.* 2003).

The functional differentiation status when investigated with the minimal immunohistochemical panel mentioned above and including chromogranin A and synaptophysin, show abundant and diffuse positive staining for synaptophysin in most cancer cells while, by converse, chromogranin A is usually scant or absent. This latter feature reflects the rare occurrence of well-developed LDCV granules as assessed by ultrastructural investigation (Solcia *et al.* 1998). The absence of chromogranin A is consistent with the 'on/off' switch function of chromogranin A gene in mammalian cells (Kim *et al.* 2001). Accordingly, no or only scant hormone immunoreactivity is detected. Cytosol markers like NSE and PGP9.5 are intensely expressed in the large majority of cancer cells. The use of histochemistry for mucins (PAS or PAS–Alcian blue stains) and of an extended immunohistochemical panel for non-granular NE markers including NSE, PGP9.5 and the neural adhesion molecule CD56 N-CAM, may be of help for difficult diagnoses.

Predictors of malignancy

The clinical behavior of gut endocrine tumors span from a benign/low-grade malignant in well-differentiated tumors/carcinomas, to highly malignant in poorly differentiated carcinomas. The histologic criteria are sufficient to reach a diagnosis of poorly differentiated carcinoma and such diagnosis implies a poor clinical outcome given the aggressive behavior of such endocrine cancer type. By converse, in the WHO classification the definition of well-differentiated carcinoma requires the evidence of malignancy at diagnosis, i.e. the presence of synchronous metastasis and/or deep wall invasion (Solcia *et al.* 2000; Hamilton & Aaltonen 2000; DeLellis *et al.* 2004). In the absence of such evidence the behavior of well-differentiated tumors is difficult to foresee. The identification of defined predictors of malignancy with proven prognostic impact may help allocating specific cases in the category of 'benign' or 'uncertain behavior'. These predictors of malignancy, and when numerical their relative cut-offs, differ in tumors at different anatomical sites (Solcia *et al.* 2000; Hamilton & Aaltonen 2000; DeLellis *et al.* 2004).

Several clinicopathologic parameters have been investigated and are considered as helpful in assessing a malignant potential in the absence of actual malignancy. Such parameters include: tumor size (larger tumors are more aggressive); invasion of nearby tissue (pancreas or appendix) or wall invasion beyond the submucosa; angioinvasion and invasion of perineural spaces; solid structure; necrosis; overt cell atypia; ploidy status (aneuploidy correlates with poor prognosis); more than two mitoses in 10 microscopic high power fields (HPF); Ki-67 index of more than 2% or of more than 100 in 10 HPF; loss of chromogranin A immunoreactivity, argyrophilia or hormone expression; and nuclear *p53* protein accumulation. Some of these variables proved effective in retrospective studies and especially in gastric and pancreatic tumors. However consistent data are missing for mid- and lower-gut tumors. The recent proposal for a TNM staging and grading of foregut endocrine tumors includes part of the above evidence (Rindi *et al.* 2006) and will be of help for a more rationale patient stratification and a more effective and standardized management.

Acknowledgements

This work was in part supported by grants from the Italian Ministry of the University and Scientific Research (MIUR-2005069205) and the University of Parma.

References

Andrew A, Kramer B, Rawdon BB. (1983) Gut and pancreatic amine precursor uptake and decarboxylation cells are not neural crest derivatives. *Gastroenterology* 84: 429–31.

Anlauf M, Perren A, Meyer CL *et al.* (2005) Precursor lesions in patients with multiple endocrine neoplasia type 1-associated duodenal gastrinomas. *Gastroenterology* 128: 1187–98.

Bayliss WM, Starling EH. (1902) On the causation of the so-called peripheral reflex secretion of the pancreas. *Proc R Soc Lond B Biol Sci* 69: 352–3.

Capella C, Heitz PU, Hofler H, Solcia E, Kloppel G. (1995) Revised classification of neuroendocrine tumours of the lung, pancreas and gut. *Virchows Arch* 425: 547–60.

Ciaccio C. (1907) Sopra speciali cellule granulose della mucosa intestinale. *Arch Ital Anat Embriol* 6: 482.

Crafa P, Milione M, Azzoni C, Pilato FP, Pizzi S, Bordi C. (2003) Pleomorph poorly differentiated endocrine carcinoma of the rectum. *Virchows Arch* 442: 605–10.

Delellis RA, Lloyd RV, Heitz PU, Eng C, eds. (2004) *World Health Organization Classification of Tumours Pathology and Genetics of Tumours of Endocrine Organs.* Lyon, IARC Press.

Erspamer V, Asero B. (1952) Identification of enteramine, the specific hormone of the enetrochromaffin cell system, as 5-hydroxytryptamine. *Nature* 169: 800–1.

Feyrter F. (1938) Über diffuse endokrine epitheliale Organe. *Liepzig Zentr Inn Mediz* 29: 545–71.

Feyrter F. (1953) *Über die Peripheren Endockrinen (Parakrinen) Druesen des Menschen.* Maudrich W, Wien, Düsseldorf.

Gosset A, Masson P. (1914) Tumeurs endocrine de l'appendice. *Presse Medicale* 25: 237.

Hamilton SR, Aaltonen LA, eds. (2000) *World Health Organization Classification of Tumours, Pathology and Genetics of Tumours of the Digestive System.* IARC Press, Lyon.

Heidenhain R. (1870) Unterschunger über den Bau der Labdrüser. *Ark Mikrosk Anat* 6: 368–406.

Hochwald SN, Zee S, Conlon KC, Colleoni R, Louie O, Brennan MF, Klimstra DS. (2002) Prognostic factors in pancreatic endocrine neoplasms: an analysis of 136 cases with a proposal for low-grade and intermediate-grade groups. *J Clin Oncol* 20: 2633–42.

Kim T, Tao-Cheng, J-H, Eiden LE, Loh PY. (2001) Chromogranin A, an 'On/Off' switch controlling dense-core secretory granule biogenesis. *Cell* 106: 499–509.

Le Douarin NM, Teillet MA. (1973) The migration of neural crest cells to the wall of the digestive tract in avian embryo. *J Embryol Exp Morphol* 30: 31–48.

Lubarsch O. (1888) Uber den primaren Krebs des Ileum nebst Bemerkungen uber das gleichzeitige Vorkommen von Krebs und Tuberkulose. *Virchows Arch* 3: 280–317.

Öberendorfer S. (1907) Karzinoide tumoren des Dünndarms. *Frankfurter Zeischrift Pathologie* 1: 426–32.

Pearse AGE. (1966) Common cytochemical properties of cells producing polypeptide hormones, with particular reference to calcitonin and C-cells. *Vet Records* 79: 303–13.

Ransom WB. (1890) A case of primary carcinoma of the ileum. *Lancet* 2: 1020–3.

Ratzenhofer M, Lembeck F. (1954) [5-Hydroxytryptamine in carcinoids of the gastrointestinal system.]. *Z Krebsforsch* 60: 169–95.

Rindi G, Azzoni C, La Rosa S *et al.* (1999) ECL cell tumor and poorly differentiated endocrine carcinoma of the stomach: prognostic evaluation by pathological analysis. *Gastroenterology* 116: 532–42.

Rindi G, Leiter AB, Kopin AS, Bordi C, Solcia E. (2004) The 'normal' endocrine cell of the gut: changing concepts and new evidences. *Ann N Y Acad Sci* 1014: 1–12.

Rindi G, Kloppel G, Alhman H *et al.* (2006) TNM staging of foregut (neuro)endocrine tumors: a consensus proposal including a grading system. *Virchows Arch* 449: 395–401.

Soga J, Tazawa K. (1971) Pathologic analysis of carcinoids; histologic reevaluation of 62 cases. *Cancer* 28: 990–8.

Solcia E, Capella C, Fiocca R, Sessa F, Larosa S, Rindi G. (1998) Disorders of the endocrine system. In: Ming SC, ed. *Pathology of the Gastrointestinal Tract,* 2nd edn. Williams and Wilkins, Philadelphia.

Solcia E, Klöppel G, Sobin LH. (2000) *Histological Typing of Endocrine Tumours.* Springer-Verlag, New York.

Van Eeden S, Quaedvlieg PF, Taal BG, Offerhaus GJ, Lamers CB, Van Velthuysen ML. (2002) Classification of low-grade neuroendocrine tumors of midgut and unknown origin. *Hum Pathol* 33: 1126–32.

Diagnosis, staging, prognosis and follow-up

Gastric neuroendocrine tumors

Gianfranco Delle Fave

Introduction

Gastric endocrine tumors are rare neoplasms occurring in 1–2 cases/1,000,000 persons/year, and account for 8.7% of all gastrointestinal neuroendocrine tumors. Their reported frequency has increased over the last 50 years, and is similar with respect to gender, incidence being 1.2 and 1.8/1,000,000 persons/year in white males and females, respectively (Modlin *et al.* 2004). It is questionable whether the increased incidence has any significance or whether it is just the result of the increased number of endoscopic procedures performed.

Differently from endocrine tumors occuring in other organs, gastric tumors are still widely known as 'carcinoids'. Thus, in the present chapter, all gastric endocrine tumors will be referred to as 'gastric carcinoids'.

The most frequently used classification of gastric carcinoids is based on their clinical features. From this viewpoint, according to the presence of a background gastric pathology, three different types of gastric carcinoids can be distinguished. They are different in both clinical and pathologic features, which reflect differences in diagnostic approach and clinical management (Table 23.1).

Type I gastric carcinoid

The definition of type I gastric carcinoid is based on the definite demonstration of a peculiar background gastric pathology, which is atrophic body gastritis (ABG). ABG is characterized by atrophy of the gastric body mucosa, defined as loss of the relative glands which are replaced by intestinal metaplasia or by fibrosis, hypergastrinemia and hypo-/achlorhydria. Gastric carcinoids develop in 1–5% of patients with achlorhydric ABG (Annibale *et al.* 2001a; Burkitt & Pritchard 2006) and consequent hypergastrinemia; they represent the most common type of gastric carcinoid, accounting for 70–80% of all cases. They are localized in the gastric fundus/body, are usually small (<1–2 cm), often multiple, and more frequently diagnosed in females aged >50 years. Not associated with the typical carcinoid syndrome, type I gastric carcinoids are usually included in the

Table 23.1 Classification and general features of gastric carcinoids.

	Background pathology	Circulating gastrin	Intragastric pH	Macroscopic	Metastases	Histologic pattern/WHO classification
Type I	ABG	↑↑	↑↑	Frequently intramucosal Single/multiple Flat/polypoid <2 cm	Exceptional	Usually benign, rarely low-grade malignant No cell atypia Ki-67 <2% WDET
Type II	MEN1/ZES	↑↑	↓↓	Frequently intramucosal Usually multiple Polypoid <2 cm	Up to 30%	Usually benign or low-grade malignant Possible invasion and loss of differentiation Rare cell atypia Ki-67 usually <2% WDET > WDEC > PDEC
Type III	Sporadic	↔	↔	Single Polypoid Often ulcerated, >1–2 cm	50–100%	Frequent invasion Frequent cell atypia Ki-67 >2% Usually WDEC or PDEC Less commonly WDET

'non-functioning' group of neuroendocrine tumors. The patients are usually asymptomatic, and the diagnosis is often accidental during gastroscopy performed for dyspepsia or anemia—either iron deficient or pernicious—which represent the most frequent manifestations of ABG. The only known risk factor for the subsequent development of carcinoid in patients with ABG is a previous finding of ECL cell dysplasia, which carries a 26-fold increased risk (Annibale *et al.* 2001a). From a histologic viewpoint, the majority of ABG patients show a micronodular pattern of hyperplasia which represents the result of longstanding hypergastrinemia, and not the epiphenomenon of mucosal atrophy, due to the growth of ECL cells in oxyntic glands after loss of parietal and chief elements. Chronic hypergastrinemia has a proliferative effect on gastric ECL cells which can contribute to the development of carcinoid tumors; in patients with ECL carcinoid and ABG, after antrectomy the volume fraction of ECL cells is significantly reduced, thus confirming the importance of the specific stimulus of antral G cells removed by antrectomy.

Histologically, type I carcinoids are limited to the mucosa and often submucosa, showing a mixed architectural pattern characterized by areas of both Soga type A (solid) and Soga type B (trabecular) fields. The neighboring endocrine cells are hyperplastic and dysplastic, so that often in a single microscopic field, many of the steps of the hyperplasia–dysplasia–neoplasia sequence are present. The antral G cells are hyperplastic. The relatively benign behavior of these lesions is confirmed by the absence (or very low number) of mitoses and the low Ki-67 index, which is usually <30 × 10 HPF (Rindi *et al.* 1999). Thus, these tumors correspond to well-differentiated endocrine tumors (WDETs) in the WHO classification; however, occasional angio- or regional lymph-node invasion and exceptional distant metastases have been reported (Delle Fave *et al.* 2005).

Type II gastric carcinoid

Type II gastric carcinoids may develop in the course of ZES and are usually associated with multiple endocrine neoplasia (MEN1). They represent 5% of all gastric carcinoids. It has been observed that patients with MEN1/ZES have a 20–30% risk of developing type II gastric carcinoid, in contrast to patients with sporadic ZES (non-MEN1-associated) who develop gastric carcinoid in 0–1% of cases. Based on these observations, type II carcinoids in MEN1/ZES may be considered as a part of the MEN1 syndrome, rather than a simple consequence of chronic hypergastrinemia. Furthermore, although they usually develop in the gastric fundus/body, they have been rarely observed also in the gastric antrum, suggesting that factors other than hypergastrinemia may be involved in the development of tumors. Among these factors, genetic defects of the MEN1 gene seem to be directly responsible for the development of the tumor.

Sporadic ZES is, of course, the best model for investigating the ECL cell response to hypergastrinemia alone because it allows the separation of hypergastrinemia from the genetic MEN1 background. It has been observed that in sporadic ZES patients, an important increase in endocrine cell volume in acid-secreting mucosa is sustained by only ECL cell increase. Recently, 106 patients with sporadic ZES have been investigated, and ECL cell changes have been detected in most of them. In this large cohort of patients, it was observed that 99% of them had ECL hyperplasia and abnormal a-human chorionic gonadotropin (a-hCG) staining, and that the changes were advanced in 50% of cases. A long-term follow-up observation confirmed that the risk of developing gastric carcinoids is low in sporadic ZES patients (at least 100 times less than in patients with MEN1/ZES) for at least 15–20 years (Peghini *et al.* 2002).

These observations confirm that hypergastrinemia per se can only initiate the ECL cell modifications, but other elements, such as the inherited loss of heterozygosity (LOH) on 11q13 in MEN1 (or the environmental gastric changes of ABG in type I tumors), are required as 'transforming factors' responsible for the neoplastic transformation.

Type II carcinoids are usually small (<1–2 cm) and often multiple. The histologic patterns of type II carcinoids are similar to those in type I except for the absence of the surrounding mucosal atrophy. Therefore, type II carcinoids are usually classified as WDETs, which may be extended to the submucosa, and which usually have a good prognosis. However, regional lymph nodes have been reported to be involved in up to 30% of patients, and some authors have described an association with malignant neuroendocrine gastric carcinoma. Therefore a type II gastric carcinoid can be also referred to as a well-differentiated endocrine carcinoma (WDEC) if the gastric tumor invades as far as the muscularis propria, presents with angioinvasion, or is associated with metastases. Poorly differentiated endocrine carcinomas (PDECs) have also occasionally been associated with MEN1 but are more likely to be sporadic and are therefore better described in the section on type III gastric carcinoids.

Type III gastric carcinoid

Also called 'sporadic,' due to the absence of any specific gastric pathology, type III gastric carcinoids account for the remaining 15–20% of tumors. They usually are single and large (>2 cm), and grow from the gastric body/fundus in the context of a normal (non-atrophic) surrounding mucosa and in the absence of circulating hypergastrinemia. They are more frequent in males aged >50 years and can show typical carcinoid features (WDET), but in particular when exceeding 2 cm, nuclear atypia, high mitosis rate and high Mib1-Ki-67 values are observed (Rindi *et al.* 1999). Liver or lymph-node metastases are frequent, and they are strictly related to tumor size, although metastases have also been described in tumors measuring a few millimetres in size. Therefore many sporadic gastric carcinoids are classified as WDECs or more aggressive PDECs which may either derive from dedifferentiation of WDECs or appear *de novo* within the stomach (Delle Fave *et al.* 2005) (Table 23.1). There are two histologic patterns in this last group. The best known is the small cell carcinoma; the other, called large cell neuroendocrine carcinoma, is rare, and presents cells with abundant cytoplasm organized in an organoid, trabecular, nest, rosette-like pattern; nuclei are vesicular and nucleoli are prominent. Both of these variants need immunohistochemical examination with cytosolic non-granular markers (synaptophisin, PGP 9.5, NSE, CD 56/N-CAM) to verify their endocrine origin, because the granular markers—chromogranin-A in particular—are negative.

Genetic factors and molecular pathology of gastric carcinoids

The molecular bases of the pathogenesis of gastric carcinoids are unclear, and most data come from studies which include gastric 'endocrine tumors' without any details on the background pathology and the grade of differentiation. As the pathological features, growth factors, genetic background, prognosis and treatment of the various types of gastric endocrine tumors are different, this issue raises particular concern.

Available molecular and genetic data are not sufficient to define which patients with known background pathologies (ABG or MEN1/ZES) are at higher risk of developing gastric carcinoids, which patients with type II and III gastric carcinoid present a higher risk of metastatic disease, or what the origin of gastric PDEC (i.e. from ECL cells, other endocrine cells, or exocrine cells) is.

The best genetic model for investigating the developement of gastric carcinoid is offered by type II lesions occuring in patients with MEN1. Debelenko *et al.* demonstrated that the MEN1-typical LOH at 11q13 is present in 75% of MEN1/ZES-related gastric carcinoids, and is associated with the deletion of the MEN1 locus in every individual patient (Debelenko *et al.* 1997). Therefore, type II gastric carcinoids occuring in MEN1/ZES are a specific tumor type due to menin inactivation, and not only an epiphenomenon due to hypergastrinemia.

This view is supported by the clinical observation that patients with sporadic ZES rarely develop gastric carcinoids compared with patients with MEN1/ZES, suggesting that the genetic factor plays a major role in the development of these tumors.

On the other hand, it has been reported that normalization of gastrin levels following surgical excision of the gastrinoma is able to induce regression of gastric carcinoids in MEN1/ZES, thus suggesting a necessary, yet not sufficient role for gastrin.

The actual prevalence of type-II gastric carcinoids is also difficult to assess, as these tumors are often small and intramucosal, and the probability of detecting them is related directly to the number of biopsies taken during gastroscopy. A similar problem applies to type I lesions. This makes it possible but difficult to detect molecular or genetic factors that predict the risk of developing gastric carcinoids in patients with MEN1/ZES.

With respect to type I gastric carcinoids, a first important point regards the actual neoplastic nature of these lesions. D'Adda *et al.* have investigated 16 type I gastric carcinoids and revealed that all but two were monoclonal as assessed by the pattern of X-chromosome inactivation (D'Adda *et al.* 1999). Therefore, despite their indolent behaviour, type I gastric carcinoids are true neoplasms.

If type I gastric carcinoids are tumors, one would expect some genetic changes to be causitive of the initiation and mainteinance of their growth. Furthermore, as the prevalence of carcinoid lesions in patients with ABG and hypergastrinemia is relatively low (Annibale *et al.* 2001a), some undescribed factors other than gastrin are likely to contribute to carcinogenesis. Indeed, several genetic or molecular abnormalities have been reported in these neoplasms, with findings suggesting a similar mechanism to the one reported for type II lesions.

LOH analysis has revealed allelic losses in the 11q13 region in 50% of type I gastric carcinoids, suggesting similar mechanisms of carcinogenesis for type I and type II carcinoids. Furthermore, the expression of the pancreatitis-associated protein RegI-α, has been found to be increased in patients with hypergastrinemia, and its missense mutations in patients with both type I and type II gastric carcinoids (Higham *et al.* 1999). It has been speculated that Reg might act as a negative regulator of ECL growth, whose loss of function could contribute to the development of carcinoids.

A role for the anti-apoptotic protein BCL-2 has also been proposed. It has been demonstrated that the protein is expressed by human ECL cells independent of the circulating gastrin levels, with higher BCL-2 immunoreactivity found in patients with ABG. It was hypothesized that the anti-apoptotic activity of BCL-2 may contribute to the development of carcinoid tumors by extending the exposure of hyperplastic ECL cells to other unknown factors.

The expression of p21 and p27 has also been recently investigated in a series of gastric WDETs (Doganavsargil *et al.* 2006). All cases expressed p27, while p21 expression was more frequent in patients with gastric atrophy (i.e. type-I carcinoids). As expected, Ki-67 scores were very low. Interpretation of these results is troublesome, as again this series is heterogeneous, but it is inferred that loss of p27 expression suggests more aggressive behavior.

While for gastrin-dependent (type I and II) lesions, there is evidence for a role of both endocrine and genetic factors in the development of the neoplastic lesions, type III carcinoids should arise due to genetic/molecular abnormalities only, most of which are presently unknown. The histopathologic features, and the aggressive clinical behavior of these tumors suggest a fundamental difference from both type I and II lesions. However, genetic changes at 11q13 have been reported in 25% to 62% of type III gastric carcinoids, thus suggesting that some common events may be shared by all gastric carcinoids.

Indeed, Pizzi *et al.* compared sporadic gastric WDEC to PDEC by analysing a wide series of genetic alterations and reported a similar profile in the two groups. Except for LOH at TP53, nuclear expression of p53 and loss of FHIT expression were all rare events in WDEC compared to PDEC (Pizzi *et al.* 2003). Similar findings were reported by others, with overexpression of p53 reported in 58%, and its mutation in 73% of gastric endocrine carcinomas, compared to 0% for typical gastric carcinoids. These latter results illustrate a clear molecular difference between those gastric endocrine tumors defined as 'carcinoid' or 'benign' or 'WDET', or types I and II, and most of the sporadic gastric endocrine neoplasms (type III) designed are WDEC or PDEC. It has also been speculated that these second and more aggressive phenotypes may arise from endocrine components of adenocarcinoma, with which they share molecular and clinical features, such as the altered p53 function. More recently, the expression of AgNOR has also been found to be suggestive of a more aggressive behavior, with higher scores found in type III cases (Giuffre *et al.* 2006). AgNOR scores are also correlated with Ki-67 scores. Therefore, a role for AgNOR as a possible tool able to predict a more aggressive phenotype has been suggested.

Factors affecting the progression of gastric carcinoids, and accounting for the different metastatic ability of different subtypes, have not been specifically investigated (Delle Fave *et al.* 2005). A recent report described that up to 4.6% of MEN1/ZES patients develop metastases from gastric carcinoids. Even if given the possibility of metastases due to other concomitant endocrine tumors, a definite figure is difficult to obtain. In this context, the recently suggested ability of gastrin to upregulate the expression of MMP9, which has been linked with ECM invasion, seems of interest. It was also demonstrated that menin can inhibit this effect of hypergastrinemia, which results in *in vivo* overexpression of MMP9 in patients with type II gastric carcinoid.

Beta-microseminoprotein has also been proposed as a marker of progression in gastric carcinoids, as it was found to stain in all patients evaluated with type III or metastatic gastric carcinoids.

Diagnostic approach to patients with gastric endocrine tumors

Due to their peculiar heterogeneity in terms of biologic and clinical features, which reflect different prognosis, a multidisciplinary approach is required to obtain an optimal management of this disease.

The diagnosis of gastric carcinoids is usually an accidental finding in the course of upper endoscopy. Once the carcinoids have been found, the initial approach to the patient should be based on the investigation of the possible presence of background pathology (ABG, MEN1/ZES), in order to properly classify the tumor (Fig. 23.2). For this, an accurate pathologic evaluation of the tumor tissue and of the gastric mucosa is mandatory. Upper endoscopy with an extensive bioptic sampling of the gastric body mucosa is required to investigate the presence of ABG. If ABG has been ruled out, a detailed clinical and family history may be helpful toward understanding if the carcinoid is a manifestation of a MEN1 syndrome. An adequate biochemical assessment should be performed to complete the patient evaluation, and should include the following.

Fasting gastrin levels

Elevated gastrin levels usually occur in patients with type I carcinoids in the context of achlorhydric ABG, as well as in type II tumors associated with hypersecretive MEN1/ZES. It may be difficult to discriminate between these opposite conditions, based on fasting gastrin levels only. In fact, two-thirds of

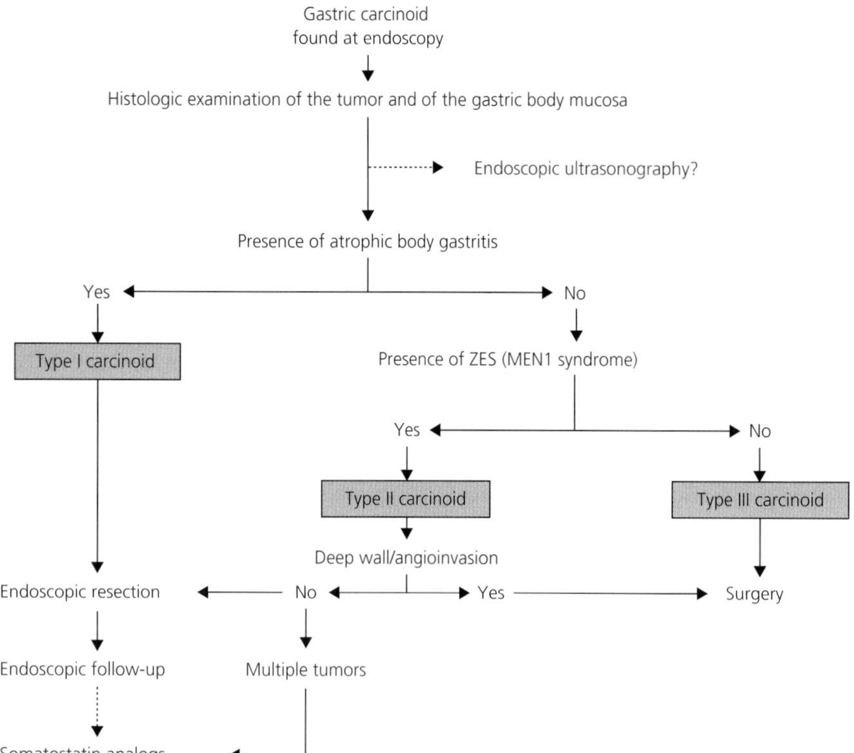

Fig. 23.2 Diagnostic algorithm for gastric neuroendocrine tumors.

gastrinoma patients have fasting gastrin levels <10-fold normal that overlap with gastrin levels seen in other more common conditions, such as ABG, or simple *Helicobacter pylori* infection. In these patients, gastrin provocative tests are needed to establish the diagnosis. On the contrary, abnormal gastrin levels are not expected in type III carcinoids.

Gastrin provocative tests

In suspected type II carcinoids as a manifestation of MEN1 syndrome, provocative tests may help diagnose ZES. Whereas numerous gastrin provocative tests have been proposed, only the secretin and calcium tests are considered useful for the investigation of the presence of ZES. The secretin test is a crucial element in the diagnosis of this pathology. The criterion with the highest sensitivity and specificity is an increase of gastrin ≥120 pg/mL after the secretin injection (Berna *et al.* 2006). A positive gastrin provocative test may discriminate between hypergastrinemia related to achloridric ABG and acid hypersecretion related to ZES.

Chromogranin A (CgA)

Circulating CgA is the most accurate non-specific tumor marker for diagnosis and follow-up of neuroendocrine tumors, including gastrinomas with ZES. However, it is well known that CgA may rise also in several conditions other than NETs, such as long-term use of proton pump inhibitors, primary parathyroid hyperplasia, thyroid C-cell hyperplasia, non-neuroendocrine cancers, and in patients with ABG.

Additional biomarkers for the evaluation of ABG are represented by *H. pylori* antibodies, and serum pepsinogen I, which, together with gastrin levels, have been proposed as a useful biochemical panel for the initial evaluation of patients with suspected ABG. The majority of these patients, in fact, show evidence of *H. pylori* infection, and have low levels of serum pepsinogen I, together with hypergastrinemia (Annibale *et al.* 2001b; Väänänen *et al.* 2003).

In addition, gastric juice pH assessment, by the evaluation of basal and pentagastrin-stimulated gastric acid secretions, may be useful to confirm achloridria in ABG, or, on the contrary, to demonstrate gastric acid hypersecretion in ZES patients (Table 23.1).

Endoscopic ultrasonography has been proposed as an additional diagnostic tool able to determine the depth of invasion of submucosal tumors, and to stage the disease by excluding the presence of perigastric lymph node. However, although promising, the role of EUS in gastric carcinoids is still not definitively standardized.

Management of patients with gastric endocrine tumors

After the type of carcinoid has been defined, the patient should be evaluated by a team made up of gastroenterologists, pathologists, oncologists, and surgeons, in order to determine the modality of treatment and follow-up.

Type I carcinoids are generally considered slow-growing tumors with low aggressive behavior. Although up to 50% of these tumors may present with microscopic invasion of lymphatics, angioinvasion and the development of distant metastases are very unusual events which have been reported in less than 2% of cases (Table 23.1). This indolent behavior is also confirmed by the low risk of deep wall invasion, occurring in 0–10% of cases, and by the high long-term survival rate, which has been reported to be 100%, suggesting that the presence of this tumor does not have much impact on patient life (Rindi *et al.* 1999).

The treatment of type I gastric carcinoids has been poorly investigated, with conflicting conclusions often based on case reports or small case series. Indeed, while some authors have suggested that endoscopic resection of the tumor is sufficient, others consider a more aggressive surgical approach advisable, especially in the case of multiple tumors and/or in the presence of recurrence of the disease during follow-up. Antrectomy has been suggested due to the possibility of removing the source of gastrin production and thus the stimulus to ECL cell proliferation. More aggressive surgery—including subtotal or total gastrectomy—has been also suggested. Recently, technical progress in endoscopy has led to the possibility of endoscopic mucosal resection which has been used in gastric tumors, including carcinoids. An additional option for treatment of type I gastric carcinoid is the somatostatin analog octreotide, on account of its ability to control hypergastrinemia and related ECL cell growth. There have been reports of tumor regression in patients with type I carcinoid. Furthermore, together with α-interferon, somatostatin analog determined the disappearance of liver metastases in two patients with type I gastric carcinoid previously treated by gastrectomy. However, due to their indolent course, an appropriate surveillance endoscopic follow-up based on gastroscopy with multiple gastric biopsy, and a conservative approach with endoscopic resection and, eventually, somatostatin analogs, seems appropriate in type I gastric carcinoids (Fig. 23.2).

The diagnosis of type II carcinoids is usually made by gastroscopy and is performed as part of routine management of patients with MEN1 and ZES. Lympho- and angioinvasion are frequently observed in these patients; however, distant metastases occur in approximately 10–20% of patients (Table 23.1). Although most type II carcinoid tumors are not invasive, aggressive cases have been described. It has in fact recently been reported that in patients with longstanding ZES/MEN1 the gastric carcinoid tumors may be aggressive and metastasize to the liver. The management of type II gastric carcinoid has to be approached in the context of the MEN1 syndrome which is present in these patients. If the tumor is amenable to endoscopic resection, polypectomy should be performed in order to obtain a full histologic evaluation and to plan future follow-up. However, type II carcinoids are often multiple and thus not suitable for complete endoscopic resection. In these cases, the somatostatin analog octreotide has been demonstrated to be effective at reducing tumor growth. As with type I carcinoids, gastric surgery should be performed only in highly selected patients, particularly if the histologic examination shows the features of PDEC (Fig. 23.2).

The therapeutic approach to type III gastric carcinoid is usually based on surgical tumor resection, and the patients should be managed similarly to those with gastric adenocarcinoma. The risk of metastases and the prognosis also depend on the histologic features of the tumor which affect tumor growth. In fact, metastases are found in 50–70% of well-differentiated tumors and in up to 100% of poorly differentiated tumors (Table 23.1). This aggressive tumor behavior is confirmed by the high risk of tumor-related death, which occurs in 25–30% and 75–87% at a median interval from diagnosis of 28 and 7 months in patients with well-differentiated and poorly differentiated tumors, respectively (Rindi *et al.* 1999). Somatostatin analogs are not indicated for treatment of such tumors.

Acknowledgement

Work supported by grants from Italian Ministry of University (PRIN 2005 prot. 2005069205_005) and from University of Roma 'La Sapienza' (prot. C26A058912).

References

Annibale B, Azzoni C, Corleto VD *et al.* (2001a) Atrophic body gastritis patients with enterochromaffin-like cell dysplasia are at increased risk for the development of type I gastric carcinoid. *Eur J Gastroenterol Hepatol* 13: 1449–56.

Annibale B, Negrini R, Caruana P *et al.* (2001b) Two-thirds of atrophic body gastritis patients have evidence of Helicobacter pylori infection. *Helicobacter* 6: 225–33.

Berna MJ, Hoffmann KM, Long SH, Serrano J, Gibril F, Jensen RT. (2006) Serum gastrin in Zollinger–Ellison Syndrome: II. Prospective study of gastrin provocative testing in 293 patients from the National Institutes of Health and comparison with 537 cases from the literature. evaluation of diagnostic criteria, proposal of new criteria, and correlations with clinical and tumoral features. *Medicine (Baltimore)* 85: 331–64.

Burkitt MD, Pritchard DM. (2006) Review article: pathogenesis and management of gastric carcinoid tumors. *Aliment Pharmacol Ther* 24: 1305–20.

D'Adda T, Candidus S, Denk H *et al.* (1999) Gastric neuroendocrine neoplasms: tumor clonality and malignancy-associated large X-chromosomal deletions. *J Pathol* 189: 394–401.

Debelenko LV, Emmert-Buck MR, Zhuang Z *et al.* (1997) The multiple endocrine neoplasia type I gene locus is involved in the pathogenesis of type II gastric carcinoids, *Gastroenterology* 113: 773–81.

Delle Fave G, Capurso G, Milione M, Panzuto F. (2005) Endocrine tumors of the stomach. *Best Pract Res Clin Gastroenterol* 19: 659–73.

Doganavsargil B, Sarsik B, Kirdok FS, Musoglu A, Tuncyurek M. (2006) p21 and p27 immunoexpression in gastric well differentiated endocrine tumors (ECL-cell carcinoids). *World J Gastroenterol* 12: 6280–84.

Giuffre G, Mormandi F, Barresi V, Bordi C, Tuccari G, Barresi G. (2006) Quantità of AgNORs in gastric endocrine carcinoid tumors as a potential prognostic tool. *Eur J Histochem* 50: 45–50.
Higham AD, Bishop LA, Dimaline R *et al.* (1999) Mutations of RegIalpha are associated with enterochromaffin-like cell tumor development in patients with hypergastrinemia. *Gastroenterology* 116: 1489–91.
Modlin IM, Lye KD, Kidd M. (2004) A 50-year analysis of 562 gastric carcinoids: small tumor or larger problem? *Am J Gastroenterol* 99: 23–32.
Peghini PL, Annibale B, Azzoni C *et al.* (2002) Effect of chronic hypergastrinemia on human enterochromaffin-like cells: insights from patients with sporadic gastrinomas. *Gastroenterology* 123: 68–85.
Pizzi, Azzoni C, Bassi D *et al.* (2003) Genetic alterations in poorly differentiated endocrine carcinomas of the gastrointestinal tract. *Cancer* 98: 1273–82.
Rindi G, Azzoni C, La Rosa S *et al.* (1999) ECL cell tumor and poorly differentiated endocrine carcinoma of the stomach: prognostic evaluation by pathological analysis. *Gastroenterology* 116: 532–42.
Väänänen H, Vauhkonen M, Helske T *et al.* (2003) Non-endoscopic diagnosis of atrophic gastritis with a blood test. *Eur J Gastroenterol Hepatol* 15: 885–91.

Gastrinoma

Frédérique Maire & Philippe Ruszniewski

Definition

Gastrinomas are gastrin-secreting tumors, that result in the Zollinger–Ellison syndrome (ZES) by gastric acid hypersecretion. Gastrin, released from the tumor into the circulation, exerts trophic effects on parietal cells and histamine-producing enterochromaffin-like (ECL) cells, which result in hyperchlorhydria and gastric mucosal thickening.

A subset of endocrine tumors with immunohistochemical expression of gastrin but without evidence of Zollinger–Ellison syndrome should be designated as functionally inactive endocrine tumors expressing gastrin, but not as gastrinomas.

Localization

The majority of gastrinomas arise in the duodenum or in the pancreas. The recent increasing occurrence of duodenal lesions (mostly first part of the duodenum) is due to improved imaging modalities, and particularly the wide use of endoscopic ultrasonography, perioperative transillumination and duodenotomy. Increasing evidence suggests that lymph node primary gastrinomas exist (5% of gastrinomas). Unusual sites of gastrinomas have been reported including liver, biliary tract, gallbladder, ovary, jejunum, or kidney.

Gastrinomas can occur in either the sporadic form or in association with MEN1 in up to 25% (Modlin *et al.* 2006). Sporadic duodenal gastrinomas are located in the submucosa and are most often less than 1 cm in diameter. Sporadic pancreatic gastrinomas usually have a diameter of 2 cm or more. They have been reported more frequently in the head of the pancreas but have been described in all parts of the organ. MEN1-related gastrinomas are usually small, located in the duodenum and frequently multifocal.

Epidemiology

Pancreatic endocrine tumors are rare with an incidence of about 1 in 100,000 (Modlin *et al.* 2006). Gastrinomas represent 15% of all pancreatic endocrine tumors and are the second most frequently occurring functional pancreatic endocrine tumors. The incidence of gastrinomas has been reported at about 0.5–3 patients per year per million inhabitants (Modlin *et al.* 2006).

The male to female ratio is 1.5 : 2.1. Gastrinomas are usually diagnosed between the ages of 50 and 70 years.

Clinical presentation

The diagnosis of gastrinomas is considered in patients with unusual peptic ulcer disease (associated neither with *H. pylori* infection, nor with use of anti-inflammatory drugs) and/or complicated peptic ulcer disease, that is refractory to conventional treatment (Table 23.2). Ulceration of the upper gastrointestinal mucosa develops in more than 90% of patients. Occasionally the distal duodenum and/or jejunum can also be involved.

Esophageal involvement occurs in 10–60% of patients, and includes heartburn and dysphagia due to gastroesophageal reflux and its complications.

Diarrhea develops in 50–65% of patients and can either precede, accompany or follow the peptic ulcer disease. Diarrhea results from the large volume of gastric acid produced. In addition, acid inactivation of the pancreatic enzymes and acid damage to enterocytes also contribute to it. The resolution of diarrhea when patients take antisecretory medications is very suggestive of ZES syndrome (Mignon *et al.* 1995).

Table 23.2 Schematic presentation of clinical situations suggesting a diagnosis of ZES. From Mignon *et al.* (1995).

Duodenal ulcer + acid hypersecretion
Duodenal ulcer without *Helicobacter pylori* infection
Duodenal ulcer resistant to adequate medical therapy
Postoperative recurrent ulcer
Severe esophagitis related to gastroesophageal reflux
Duodenal ulcer + chronic diarrhea
Unexplained chronic diarrhea
Duodenal ulcer + primary hyperparathyroidism
Duodenal ulcer + raised serum gastrin
Metastatic liver +/– duodenal ulcer and without primary adenocarcinoma
Member of kindred with MEN1 or ZES

Cushing's syndrome in relation to an ectopic production of ACTH has been reported in 5% of patients with ZES.

In a recent review, the delay between the onset of the symptoms and the time of diagnosis was 5.2 years (Norton *et al.* 2006).

Positive diagnosis

The diagnosis of ZES is based on the finding of elevated fasting serum gastrin associated with gastric acid hypersecretion. A reliable test is the measurement of gastric acid secretion through a nasogastric tube. Proton pump inhibitors (PPIs) have to be interrupted at least 5 days before testing. Gastric analysis through a nasogastric tube traditionally has been considered as the gold standard in the diagnosis of ZES, but it has fallen out of favor with clinicians as a result of time-consuming procedure (more than 1 hour to perform) and of significant patient discomfort. Recently, a rapid simple endoscopic technique whereby a single 15-minute sample of gastric juice can be collected under direct endoscopic visualization has been proposed, with an excellent agreement for determination of acid ouput and acid concentration between conventional and endoscopic techniques (Oh *et al.* 2006)

The diagnostic criteria for ZES are as follows : basal acid output (BAO) ≥ 15 mmol/h is suggestive of ZES diagnosis but can overlap with other situations. Threshold value of 100% specificity is obtained only for BAO ≥ 38 mmol/h (Mignon *et al.* 1995).

Elevated fasting serum gastrin is suggestive of ZES, but can be observed in other conditions, like *H. pylori* infection, antral G-cell hyperplasia/hyperfunction, atrophic gastritis or use of PPIs. Very high fasting serum gastrin levels >100-fold normal (5–9% of ZES patients) are specific of ZES. Normal fasting serum gastrin values have been reported in less than 3% of patients with ZES (Berna *et al.* 2006). Two-thirds of ZES patients have fasting serum gastrin values <10-fold normal, not specific of ZES. In these two latter situations, gastrin provocative tests are needed to establish the diagnosis. A secretin infusion (2U/kg intravenously in 2 min) induces a marked increase in both serum gastrin and acid output (≥18 mmol/h) in 90% of ZES patients (Mignon *et al.*1995). An increase of serum gastrin >200 pg/mL is diagnostic of ZES (Tomassetti *et al.* 2005). Recently, a large prospective study proposed new diagnostic criteria (Berna *et al.* 2006). An increase from fasting gastrin to post-secretin gastrin ≥120 pg/mL has the highest sensitivity (94%) and specificity (100%) for diagnosis. The authors suggest that secretin stimulation should be used as the first-line provocative test because of its greater sensitivity and simplicity and lack of side-effects. The calcium test should be considered in patients with a strong clinical suspicion of ZES but a negative secretin test. There is agreement in the literature that calcium and meal tests are less useful than secretin for detecting ZES.

Staging

Accurate localization of the primary gastrinoma and tumor staging are required as the first step of the management of these patients.

Localization of the primary tumor

Transabdominal abdominal ultrasound (US) remains poor in detecting small pancreatic and extrapancreatic gastrinomas.

Computed tomography (CT) with bolus of contrast administration can achieve sensitivities ranging from 82% to 92%. Small size of non-metastatic gastrinomas limits the performance of CT with a 30% tumor detection rate for lesions measuring 1–3 cm.

Magnetic resonance imaging (MRI), using T1-weighed fat suppression images, has a good sensitivity for endocrine tumors, and is considered as the most sensitive technique for demonstrating liver metastases (Tomassetti *et al.* 2005).

Endoscopic ultrasonography (EUS) provides excellent sensitivity (90%) in the detection of small pancreatic tumors (Table 23.3). Characteristic EUS features of endocrine lesions include an homogenous hypoechoic pattern with or without calcifications and peripheral rim enhancement (Fig. 23.3) (O'Toole *et al.* 1999). Occasionally these tumors may be hyperechoeic or rarely cystic. A normal pancreatic EUS examination is a strong argument for an extrapancreatic tumor location. Exploration for duodenal gastrinomas, which are frequently small submucosal lesions, requires an approach with a hyperinflated water balloon and interchangeable 10- and 12-MHz frequencies (Fig. 23.3). The sensitivity of EUS is only 40–60% for duodenal tumor detection (Norton *et al.* 2004). Combination of EUS with standard axial endoscopy is also recommended to increase tumor localization. In addition, cytologic or histologic confirmation of small pancreatic endocrine tumors can be performed

Table 23.3 Endoscopic ultrasonography for the localization of gastrinomas, from Norton *et al.* (2004). Restricted to analyses with at least five patients with gastrinoma.

Author (year)	Number of patients	% EUS localization
Palazzo (1992)	15	60%
Rosch (1992)	7	86%
Ruszniewski (1995)	22	28% DUO; 75% PAN; 62% LN
Cadiot (1996)	21	57% DUO (33% EUS/24%ENDO)
Zimmer (1996)	12	63% DUO; 89% PAN
Proye (1998)	15	28% DUO; 85% (PAN + LN)
De Angelis (1999)	8	38% DUO; 80% LN
Anderson (2000)	18	100% PAN
Mirallie (2002)	26	46% DUO; 75% PAN; 57% LN

DU, duodenal; PAN, pancreatic; ENDO, endoscopic results; LN, lymph node; EUS, endoscopic ultrasound.

(a) 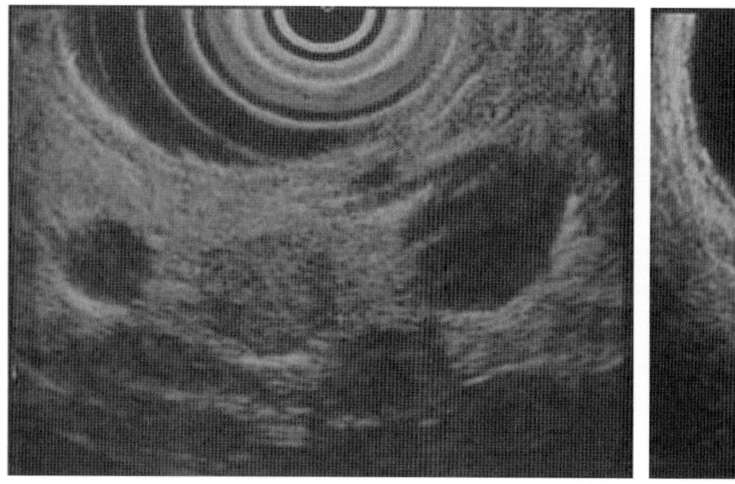

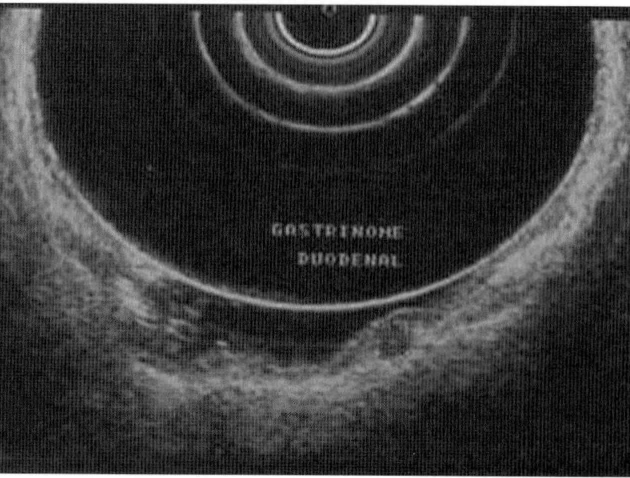

(b)

Fig. 23.3 Endoscopic ultrasonography. Left, diagnosis of a pancreatic endocrine tumor. Right, diagnosis of a small duodenal gastrinoma.

safely using EUS-guided fine needle aspiration biopsy, but in practice is rarely necessary. A careful search for lymph node involvement in patients with endocrine tumors of the duodenopancreatic area is also mandatory. Characteristic features predictive of malignant lymph node involvement including large, well demarcated nodes with a hypo- or isoechoic homogeneous pattern with peripheral rim enhancement have been previously documented. A complete examination requires an evaluation of peripancreatic, mesenteric, pyloric, celiac and hepatic root lymph node chains.

Somatostatin receptor scintigraphy (SRS) has been shown to be of value in patients with gastrinomas. SRS is more sensitive in both localizing the primary and identifying liver metastases than conventional methods such as US, CT and MRI. However, because the sensitivity of SRS correlates with the size of gastrinoma, only 30% of gastrinomas <1 cm in diameter can be visualized by this technique. Interestingly, combination of EUS and SRS increased sensitivities for detection of isolated duodenal gastrinomas and peripancreatic lymph nodes to 88% and 91%, respectively.

In practice, SRS and CT scan with contrast are recommended as a routine preoperative imaging, prior to EUS (Fig. 23.4).

Gastrin receptor scintigraphy (GRS) is a new imaging method recently developed for the detection of endocrine tumors, as gastrin-binding CCK2 receptors are expressed on these tumors. In a recent study, the overall tumor-detection rate was 74% for GRS and 82% for SRS. GRS performed better than SRS in 22% of patients, equivalent images were obtained in 30% and SRS performed better in 40% (Gotthardt *et al.* 2006).

Functional studies, measuring hormonal gradients by transhepatic portal venous sampling, have been proposed. A modification of the hormonal gradient during angiography has been developed using secretin injected selectively in each artery that feeds the pancreas and the duodenum, and hepatic venous samplings are collected and assayed for gastrin gradients. The sensitivity and the specificity of this test are greater than 90%, but it is invasive and requires considerable expertise. It has thus been largely supplanted by the combination of SRS, EUS and preoperative explorations.

If a primary gastrinoma cannot be identified by conventional techniques (10–20% of patients), operative techniques such as duodenal transillumination, operative ultrasound and/or duodenotomy will accurately localize close to 100% of tumors in specialized centers.

TNM staging

In 2006, the European Neuroendocrine Tumor Society (ENETS) proposed a consensus in TNM staging of foregut endocrine tumors (Table 23.4) (Rindi *et al.* 2006). TNM staging has been validated as predictive of survival in patients with gastrinomas (Ellison *et al.* 2006).

Prognosis

With the development of effective gastric antisecretory drugs, first with H2 antagonists in the 1970s and later PPIs, the prognostic of patients with gastrinomas radically changed. Complications related to acid hypersecretion are now well controlled by medical treatment and an increasing proportion of patients are dying from the malignant nature of the gastrinoma. The overall 5-year survival for all gastrinomas is between 60 and 70% (Roy *et al.* 2001). One-third of patients already have metastases at initial presentation. Approximately 25% of patients with Zollinger–Ellison syndrome follow an aggressive course, with development of liver metastases and an overall 10-year survival of 30% (Roy *et al.* 2001). The remaining 75% have a very indolent growth.

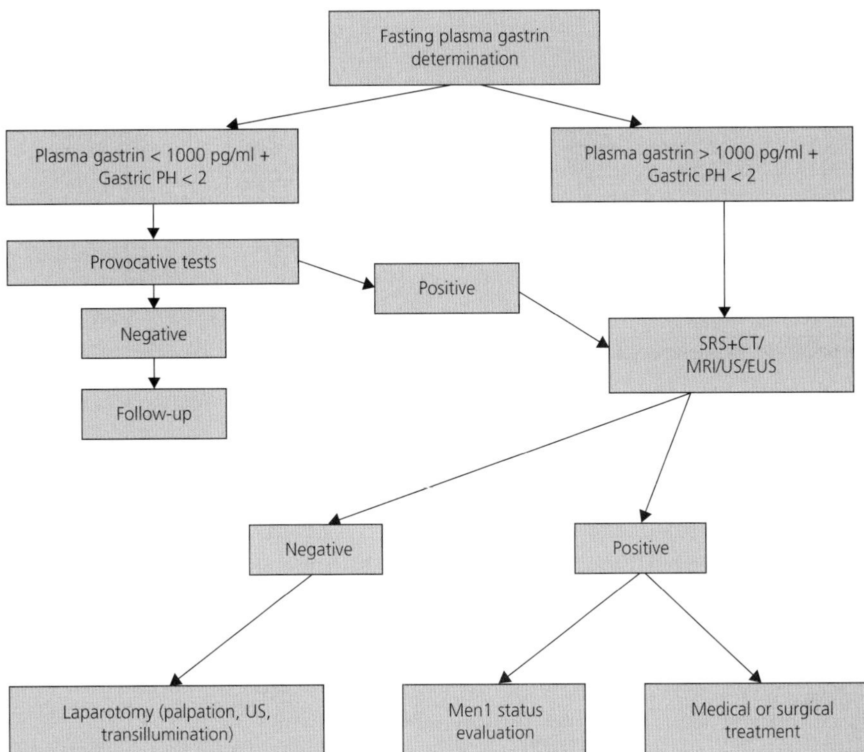

Fig. 23.4 Diagnostic algorithm for Zollinger–Ellison syndrome, from Tomassetti *et al.* (2005). SRS, somatostatin receptor scintigraphy; CT, computed tomography; MRI, magnetic resonance imaging; US, ultrasonography; EUS, endoscopic ultrasonography.

Table 23.4 Proposal for a TNM classification and disease staging for endocrine tumors of the pancreas. From Rindi *et al.* (2006).

T: primary tumor

TX	Primary tumor cannot be assessed
T0	No evidence of primary tumor
T1	Tumor limited to the pancreas and size <2 cm
T2	Tumor limited to the pancreas and size 2–4 cm
T3	Tumor limited to the pancreas and size >4 cm or invading duodenum or bile duct
T4	Tumor invading adjacent organs (stomach, spleen, colon, adrenal gland) or the wall of large vessels (celiac axis or superior mesenteric artery)

For any T, add (m) for multiple tumors

N: regional lymph nodes

NX	Regional lymph node cannot be assessed
N0	No regional lymph node metastasis
N1	Regional lymph node metastasis

M: distant metastases

MX	Distant metastasis cannot be assessed
M0	No distant metastases
M1*	Distant metastasis

Disease stages

Stage I	T1	N0	M0
Stage IIa	T2	N0	M0
Stage IIb	T3	N0	M0
Stage IIIa	T4	N0	M0
Stage IIIb	Any T	N1	M0
Stage IV	Any T	Any N	M1

[a] M1: presence of any single or multiple metastases at any distant anatomical site (including non-regional nodes).

Prognostic factors

The factors associated with a poor prognosis include the presence of liver metastases, the extent of liver metastases, the development of bone metastases or ectopic Cushing's syndrome, a large primary tumor (>3 cm), female gender, sporadic tumor and pancreatic location of the primary tumor (rather than duodenal) (Yu *et al.* 1999). The presence of liver metastases is the most important determinant of survival.

Effect of a surgical approach

The possibility of altering the natural history of gastrinomas by surgery is supported by several studies. A first study in 1994 showed that surgery decreased the rate of development of liver metastases; however, the follow-up duration and number of patients were not sufficient to demonstrate an effect on survival (Fraker *et al.* 1994). Two recent studies showed that surgical approach leads to long-term survival in these patients. One reported the following of 33 patients with pancreatic endocrine tumor (including 13 gastrinomas). The 5-, 10-, and actuarial 25-year survival rates for patients with malignant tumors were 81%, 72%, and 36%, respectively. The survival rate was significantly related to the patients'age at time of initial operation (better in patients younger than 50 years) and the presence or development of metastases (Fendrich *et al.* 2006). The other study by Norton *et al.* (2006), including 195 patients with ZES, demonstrated that surgery increases survival by significantly decreasing the development of advanced disease and increasing disease-related survival (Fig. 23.5). Fifteen-year disease-related survival was 98% and 74% for operated and unoperated patients, repectively.

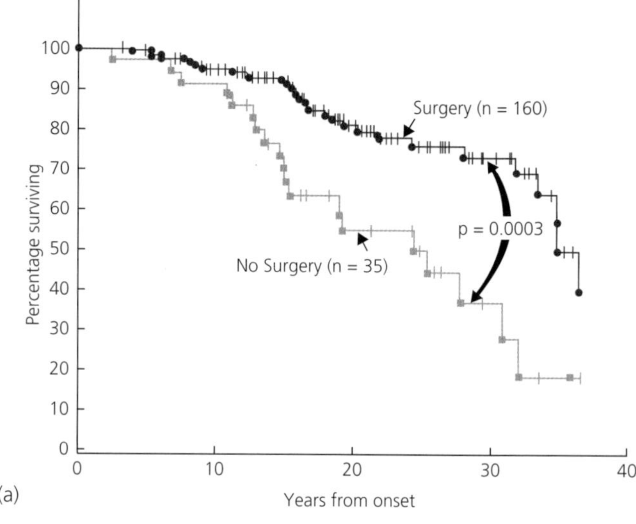

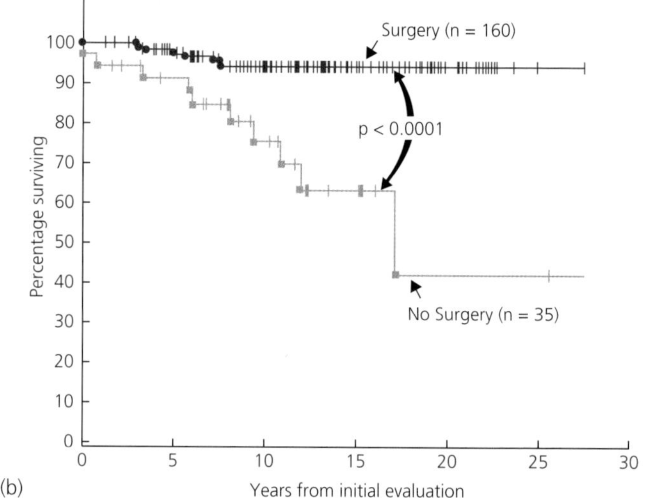

Fig. 23.5 Total survival and liver metastasis-free survival in 195 patients with gastrinomas, from Norton *et al.* (2006). Total survival from onset of ZES (a) and liver metastases free from initial evaluation (b) are shown for the 160 surgical and 35 non-surgical patients.

Follow-up

The two main therapeutic objectives in patients with gastrinomas are the control of gastric acid hypersecretion and the control of neoplasia growth.

IPPs has proven to be safe and effective in controlling acid hypersecretion. While efficacy is suggested by resolution of diarrhea and endoscopic healing of mucosal lesions, formal gastric secretory analysis has the best predictive value. A reliable criterion for the control of hypersecretion is the reduction of the BAO below 10 mEq/h within the hour prior to the next dose of antisecretory medication. In patients with previous partial gastrectomy or severe peptic esophagitis, the BAO before the next scheduled dose should be below 5 and 1 mEq/h, respectively.

Antisecretory drugs are known to increase plasma gastrin levels to within 2–4 times the baseline. There have been concerns that prolonged large doses of PPIs might lead to the development of enterochromaffin-like (ECL) cell hyperplasia due to the trophic effect of PPI-induced hypergastronemia. Currently, PPIs have not been found to increase the risk of gastric carcinoids in humans treated for non-ZES-related peptic conditions. In contrast, long-term hypergastrinemia in patients with ZES-associated MEN1 has been associated with gastric carcinoid tumors, whereas gastric carcinoids in sporadic ZES are very rare. Thus, while high gastrin levels appear to be a necessary condition for ECL cell proliferation, other factors are required for the initiation of ECL cell replication.

In conclusion, treatment efficacy should be monitored annually in patients with gastrinomas with careful clinical appraisal and endoscopic and gastric analysis. Endoscopic surveillance should also be employed yearly for ZES patients with MEN1 (and probably less frequently in sporadic cases) to screen for ECL carcinoids and to propose their resection once they reach a significant size.

References

Berna MJ, Hoffmann KM, Long SH, Serrano J, Gibril F, Jensen RT. (2006) Serum gastrin in Zollinger–Ellison syndrome: II. Prospective study of gastrin provocative testing in 293 patients from the National Institutes of Health and comparison with 537 cases from the literature. Evaluation of diagnostic criteria, proposal of new criteria, and correlations with clinical and tumoral features. *Medicine (Baltimore)* 85: 331–64.

Ellison EC, Sparks J, Verducci JS *et al.* (2006) 50-year appraisal of gastrinoma: recommendations for staging and treatment. *J Am Coll Surg* 202: 897–905.

Fendrich V, Langer P, Celik I *et al.* (2006) An aggressive surgical approach leads to long-term survival in patients with pancreatic endocrine tumors. *Ann Surg* 244: 845–51.

Fraker DL, Norton JA, Alexander HR, Venzon DJ, Jensen RT. (1994) Surgery in Zollinger–Ellison syndrome alters the natural history of gastrinoma. *Ann Surg* 220: 320–30.

Gotthardt M, Behe MP, Grass J *et al.* (2006) Added value of gastrin receptor scintigraphy in comparison to somatostatin receptor scintigraphy in patients with carcinoids and other neuroendocrine tumors. *Endocr Relat Cancer* 13: 1203–11.

Mignon M, Jais P, Cadiot G, Ben Yedder D, Vatier J. (1995) Clinical features and advances in biological criteria for Zollinger–Ellison syndrome. In: Mignon M, Jensen RT, eds. *Endocrine Tumors of the Pancreas. Recent Advances in Research and Management*, vol. 23, pp. 223–39. Krager, Basel.

Modlin MI, Zikusoka M, Kidd M, Latich I, Eick G, Romanyshyn J. (2006) The history and epidemiology of neuroendocrine tumors. In: Caplin M, Kvols L, eds. *Handbook of neuroendorine tumors. Their current and future management*, pp. 7–36. Bioscientifica.

Norton JA, Jensen RT. (2004) Resolved and unresolved controversies in the surgical management of patients with Zollinger–Ellison syndrome. *Ann Surg* 240: 757–73.

Norton JA, Fraker DL, Alexander HR *et al.* (2006) Surgery increases survival in patients with gastrinoma. *Ann Surg* 244: 410–9.

Oh DS, Wang HS, Ohning, GV, Pisegna JR. (2006) Validation of a new endoscopic technique to assess acid output in Zollinger–Ellison syndrome. *Clin Gastroenterol Hepatol* 4: 1467–73.

O'Toole D, Palazzo L, Ruszniewski P. (1999) Role of endoscopic ultrasonography in endocrine tumors of the duodenopancreatic region. In: Mignon M, Colombel JF, eds. *Recent Advances in the Pathophysiology and Management of Inflammatory Bowel Diseases and Digestive Endocrine Tumors*, pp. 229–40. John Libbey Eurotext, Paris.

Rindi G, Kloppel G, Alhman H *et al.* (2006) TNM staging of foregut (neuro)endocrine tumors: a consensus proposal including a grading system. *Virchows Arch* 449: 395–401.

Roy PK, Venzon DJ, Feigenbaum KM *et al.* (2001) Gastric secretion in Zollinger–Ellison syndrome. Correlation with clinical expression, tumor extent and role in diagnosis–a prospective NIH study of 235 patients and a review of 984 cases in the literature. *Medicine (Baltimore)* 80: 189–222.

Tomassetti P, Campana D, Piscitelli L *et al.* (2005) Treatment of Zollinger–Ellison syndrome. *World J Gastroenterol* 11: 5423–32.

Yu F, Venzon DJ, Serrano J *et al.* (1999) Prospective study of the clinical course, prognostic factors and survival in patients with longstanding Zollinger–Ellison syndrome. *J Clin Oncol* 17: 615–30.

Insulinoma

Wouter W. de Herder

Diagnosis

Symptoms and clinical signs

Insulinomas generally present with signs and symptoms of hypoglycemia caused by inappropriate insulin secretion. Hypoglycemic symptoms can be grouped into those resulting from neuroglycopenia (commonly including headache, diplopia, blurred vision, confusion, dizziness, abnormal behavior, lethargy, amnesia; whereas rarely, hypoglycemia may result in seizures and coma); and those resulting from the activated autonomic nervous system (including sweating, weakness, hunger, tremor, nausea, feelings of warmth, anxiety, and palpitations).

Clinical tests

The diagnosis of insulinoma can be absolutely established using the following six strict criteria:

1 documented blood glucose levels ≤2.2 mmol/L (≤40 mg/dL)

2 concomitant insulin levels ≥6 μU/L (≥36 pmol/L; ≥3 μU/L by ICMA).

3 C-peptide levels ≥200 pmol/L

4 proinsulin levels ≥5 pmol/L

5 β-hydroxybutyrate levels ≤2.7 mmol/L

6 absence of sulfonylurea (metabolites) in the plasma and/or urine.

Further controlled testing includes the 72-hour fast, which is the gold standard for establishing the diagnosis of insulinoma. When the patient develops symptoms and the blood glucose levels are ≤2.2 mmol/L (≤40 mg/dL), blood is also drawn for C-peptide, proinsulin and insulin. Failure of appropriate insulin suppression in the presence of hypoglycemia substantiates an autonomously secreting insulinoma.

Histopathology

The WHO classifies functioning endocrine tumors of the pancreas, like insulinomas, into three categories:

1 well-differentiated endocrine tumors, with benign or uncertain behavior at the time of diagnosis

2 well-differentiated endocrine carcinomas with low-grade malignant behavior

3 poorly differentiated endocrine carcinomas, with high-grade malignant behavior.

Most insulinomas are classified as WHO 1.

Imaging and staging

Insulinomas are usually solitary and intrapancreatic in location. They are characteristically small, with approximately two-thirds

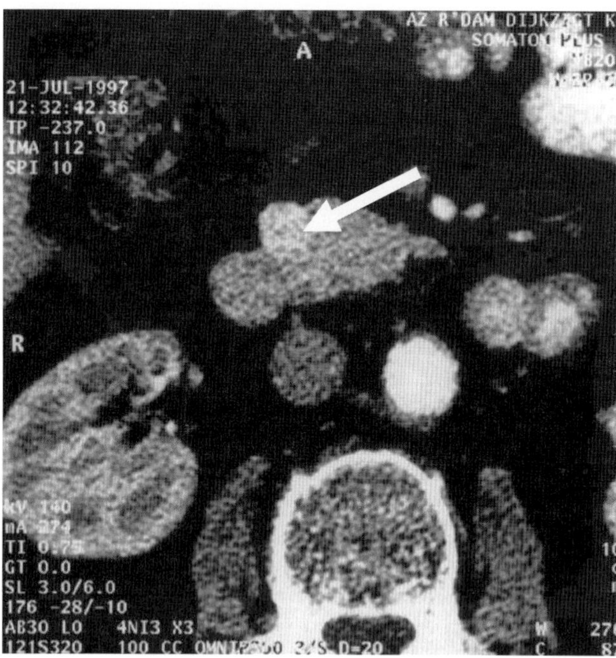

Fig. 23.6 Abdominal CT in the transverse plane showing a hypervascular tumor (insulinoma) in the pancreatic body (arrow).

being ≤2 cm at presentation. The three most useful imaging modalities are gadolinium-enhanced dynamic MRI, three-phase computed tomography (CT), and endoscopic ultrasound. Other imaging modalities which can be applied for the visualization or localization of insulinomas are: transabdominal ultrasound, selective celiac and mesenteric arteriography, venography and venous sampling, ^{111}In-pentetreotide scintigraphy, PET with ^{11}C-5-hydroxytryptophan (5-HTP), ^{11}C-l-DOPA, ^{18}F-DOPA, or ^{67}Ga-DOTA-DPhe^{1}-Tyr^{3}-octreotide (^{67}Ga-DOTATOC) and intraoperative ultrasound, or laparoscopic intraoperative ultrasound. Insulinomas are staged according to the recently developed TNM classification and disease staging for endocrine tumors of the pancreas.

Treatment

Surgical management

At operation, the entire pancreas is explored. Tumor enucleation is preferred. Central or distal pancreatectomy are safe and effective alternatives. In specific cases laparoscopic surgery seems feasible.

Medical management

Medical management is reserved only for patients who are unable or unwilling to undergo surgical treatment, for preoperative control of blood glucose levels, or for unresectable metastatic disease.

Dietary management is designed to prevent prolonged periods of fasting. Diazoxide is the most effective drug for controlling hypoglycemia. However, it has side-effects. Somatostatin analogs like octreotide and lanreotide can be useful in preventing hypoglycemia in those patients with somatostatin receptor subtype 2-(^{111}In-pentetreotide scintigraphy) positive tumors, but can worsen hypoglycemia in those patients with tumors that do not express this receptor subtype.

Malignant insulinomas account for only about 5–10% of all insulinomas. The median disease-free survival after curative resection is 5 years, but recurrence occurs in more than 60% at a median interval of 2.5–3 years. Median survival with recurrent tumor is less than 2 years. Palliative resection may prolong median survival. When surgical options to address malignancy have been exhausted, other debulking procedures like: radiofrequency thermoablation, cryotherapy, hepatic artery embolization and chemoembolization, and peptide receptor radionuclide therapy have been utilized yielding temporary palliation. Systemic chemotherapeutic options include combinations of adriamycin or doxorubicin and streptozocin, which can result in a significant tumor regression rate, and remission from hypoglycemic symptoms can be extended for up to 1.5 years.

References

de Herder WW. (2004) Insulinoma. *Neuroendocrinology* 80 (Suppl 1): 20–22.

Grant CS. (2005) Insulinoma. *Best Pract Res Clin Gastroenterol* 19: 783–98.

Rindi G, Kloppel G, Alhman H *et al.* (2006) TNM staging of foregut (neuro)endocrine tumors: a consensus proposal including a grading system. *Virchows Arch* 449: 395–401.

Service FJ. (1995) Hypoglycemic disorders. *N Engl J Med* 332: 1144–52.

Service FJ. (1997) Insulinoma and other islet-cell tumors. *Cancer Treat Res* 89: 335–46.

Service FJ, Dale AJ, Elveback LR, Jiang NS. (1976) Insulinoma: clinical and diagnostic features of 60 consecutive cases. *Mayo Clin Proc* 51: 417–29.

Stabile BE. (1997) Islet cell tumors. *Gastroenterologist* 5: 213–32.

Non-functioning endocrine tumors of the pancreas

Dimitrios Papadogias & Gregory Kaltsas

Introduction

Non-functioning endocrine tumors of the pancreas are neoplasms of neuroendocrine differentiation that are mainly defined by their histopathologic classification. Neuroendocrine cells are characterized by the expression of vesicular proteins such as chromogranin A and/or synaptophysin, and/or non-specific cytosolic markers, such as neuron-specific enolase (NSE) (Solcia *et al.* 2000). The absence of any distinct clinical symptoms suggestive of a hypersecretory state denotes the 'non-functioning' status of these tumors. However, non-functioning tumors may well exhibit immunohistochemical positivity for several hormones, neuropeptides and/or neurotransmitters (Oberg *et al.* 2004; Ramage *et al.* 2005). In addition, with prolonged follow-up non-functioning pancreatic endocrine tumors can occasionally evolve into functioning tumors following the synthesis and secretion of various biologic active substances (Oberg *et al.* 2004; Kaltsas *et al.* 2004a).

Classification and epidemiology

The WHO classifies non-functioning pancreatic endocrine tumors according to a uniform classification scheme for endocrine tumors that is aimed at predicting biologic behavior (Solcia *et al.* 2000). This system is independent of the site of the primary and is based on a combination of the classical gross and microscopic structural criteria and the incorporation of the Ki-67 proliferative index (or the conventional mitotic index) (Solcia *et al.* 2000; Kaltsas *et al.* 2004a; Oberg *et al.* 2004). According to this system non-functioning pancreatic endocrine tumors are classified as: (i) well-differentiated endocrine tumors, with benign or uncertain behavior at the time of diagnosis; (ii) well-differentiated endocrine carcinomas, with low-grade malignant behavior; and (iii) poorly differentiated endocrine carcinomas, with high-grade malignant behavior (Table 23.5). The majority of pancreatic endocrine tumors, between 60 and 100%, are classified as well-differentiated endocrine carcinomas; such tumors are slowly growing and can exhibit phases of standstill and/or even phases of regression (Mignon 2000; Kaltsas *et al.* 2004a). Poorly differentiated pancreatic endocrine carcinomas behave very aggressively, similarly to small cell carcinomas (Oberg *et al.* 2004).

Although epidemiologic series have shown that pancreatic endocrine tumors account for 3–10% of all pancreatic tumors, autopsy series have revealed a much higher incidence of approximately 1.6–10% cases per year (Mignon 2000; Barakat *et al.* 2004). Tumors identified at autopsy are usually less than 1 cm in size, and most probably represent benign microadenomas without any clinical significance and/or hormonal hypersecretion (Barakat *et al.* 2004). It is thought that pancreatic endocrine tumors that are clinically important develop with an incidence of 3.5–4/10^6/year (Mignon 2000; Barakat *et al.* 2004). With the application of newer and more sensitive imaging modalities, the number of incidentally identified clinically significant non-functioning pancreatic endocrine tumors has increased (Kaltsas *et al.* 2004b; Oberg *et al.* 2004). Thus, although in earlier series the percentage of these tumors was estimated to be between 18 and 66% of all pancreatic endocrine tumors, more recent studies have shown that the majority of pancreatic endocrine tumors are non-functioning (Barakat *et al.* 2004; Oberg *et al.* 2004). The peak incidence of these tumors is during the fifth decade of life, with equal distribution between the sexes (Ramage *et al.* 2005).

Diagnosis and staging

The diagnosis of non-functioning pancreatic endocrine tumors is usually made late when the disease has already progressed. This is due to the lack of the characteristic clinical presentation of a secretory syndrome, and the fact that the majority of these tumors are well differentiated and therefore slow growing (Kaltsas *et al.* 2004a; Oberg *et al.* 2004). Thus, patients harboring such tumors may run a prolonged course with maintenance of a good performance status besides extensive tumor load. Occasionally patients with pancreatic endocrine tumors have been misdiagnosed as suffering from pancreatic adenocarcinomas; in such cases, the unexpected prolonged survival and the good performance status of the patients directs to the correct diagnosis (Kaltsas *et al.* 2004a). The diagnosis is based on the combination of non-specific clinical features with the aid of more specific biologic and imaging modalities and final histologic confirmation.

Table 23.5 Current applicable criteria for the classification and prognosis of endocrine pancreatic tumors.

Biologic behavior	WHO classification	Metastases	Invasion	Histologic differentiation	Tumor size (cm)	Angioinvasion	Ki-67 (%)
Benign (low risk)	Group 1	–	–	Well-differentiated	≤1 cm	–	<2
Benign or low-grade malignant (intermediate risk)	Group 1	–	–	Well-differentiated	>2 cm	±	<2
Low-grade malignant	Group 2	+	+	Well-differentiated	Usually > 3 cm	+	>2
? Intermediate*	? Group 2–3	+	+	Intermediate	Any size	+	2–20
High-grade malignant	Group 3	+	+	Poorly differentiated	Any size	+	>20

* Within this group the biologic behavior of tumors expressing lower proliferative index (PI) may be different to those with higher PI.

Clinical presentation

Pancreatic endocrine tumors can synthesize and store substances that are common to all endocrine tumors (chromogranins), and occasionally cell specific hormones, neuroamines and/or other compounds of neuroendocrine differentiation (Oberg *et al.* 2004; Ramage *et al.* 2005). Their clinical silence is due to either absence of a secretory product or the secretion of substances into the bloodstream in concentrations that are not capable of exerting a biologic effect. Alternatively the absence of symptoms could be the result of inactive hormonal production, cosecretion of peptide inhibitors such as somatostatin or downregulation of peripheral receptors (Oberg *et al.* 2004). Many patients with pancreatic endocrine tumors have elevated levels of peptides not known to cause any specific clinical syndrome such as chromogranins, pancreatic polypeptide (PP), neurotensin, ghrelin, and hCG subunits (Oberg & Eriksson 2005). Although tumors derived from PP cells are clinically silent, there are rare exceptions of PPomas associated with diarrhea, diabetes mellitus, and weight loss (Mignon 2000).

Due to the lack of symptoms related to hormonal hypersecretion, non-functioning pancreatic endocrine tumors are diagnosed late in the course of the disease. As these tumors arise from the pancreatic islet cells, early lesions may not occlude the pancreatic ducts and may remain asymptomatic for many years (Kaltsas *et al.* 2004a). However, when patients harboring such tumors come to medical attention they have large-sized tumors (primary lesion greater than 5 cm), and a significant number, between 60 to 80%, have already developed synchronous liver metastases (Barakat *et al.* 2004; Oberg *et al.* 2004). Primary tumors are mostly localized at the head of the pancreas, followed by the body and tail. Clinical signs and symptoms develop due to the extensive tumor mass, local invasion and compression of nearby structures, and/or the development of distant metastases (Oberg *et al.* 2004). Common presenting symptoms are abdominal pain (35–80%), followed by weight loss (20–35%), and anorexia and nausea (45%). Less commonly, patients may present with intra-abdominal hemorrhage (4–20%), jaundice (17–50%) and/or a palpable mass (7–40%) (Kaltsas *et al.* 2004a; Oberg *et al.* 2004). Although the great majority of pancreatic endocrine tumors are sporadic they can also occur in the context of familial (hereditary) syndromes. In these cases, tumors can be multiple and appear at different stages during the course of the disease (Brandi *et al.* 2001; Ramage *et al.* 2005). The following hereditary syndromes are associated with non-functioning pancreatic endocrine tumors.

Multiple endocrine neoplasia type 1 (MEN1)

MEN1 is a hereditary tumor syndrome that is inherited with the autosomal trait and occurs with high penetrance. The main manifestations of the disease are primary hyperparathyroidism (90–100%), pituitary adenomas (40–50%) and pancreatic endocrine tumors (30–75%) (Brandi *et al.* 2001). Non-functioning pancreatic endocrine tumors occur besides functional tumors; a prevalence of approximately 55% for non-functioning pancreatic endocrine tumors has been encountered in MEN1 patients. These tumors occur at an earlier age, are usually multiple, vary in size from small microadenomas to large-sized tumors, and exhibit a more benign course than sporadic tumors. Their malignant potential is related to the size of the tumor and these tumors are currently the leading cause of disease-specific mortality in patients with MEN1 (Brandi *et al.* 2001). However, only a small number of patients (5–8%) with non-functioning pancreatic endocrine tumors have MEN1 syndrome (Kaltsas *et al.* 2004).

Von Hippel-Lindau disease (VHL)

VHL is an autosomal dominant disease with almost complete penetrance, characterized by the development of several types of neoplasia (Kaltsas *et al.* 2004a; Ramage *et al.* 2005). Hemangioblastomas of the central nervous system, retinal angiomas, renal cell carcinomas and pheochromocytomas are the most common lesions. Non-functioning pancreatic endocrine tumors are part of the syndrome in up to 16% of patients; they frequently coexist with pheochromocytomas and may even precede the manifestation of other lesions (Kaltsas *et al.* 2004a).

Tuberous sclerosis

An association of non-functioning pancreatic endocrine tumors with tuberous sclerosis has also been suggested (Kaltsas *et al.* 2004a).

Biochemical confirmation

Chromogranins are cosecreted with peptidic hormones and amines present in secretory granules and their function is not entirely known (Oberg *et al.* 2004). The most representative is chromogranin A, which is stored in the majority of well-differentiated endocrine tumors (irrespective of their functional status); its release into the circulation can be used as a general marker for the biochemical confirmation of the endocrine nature of the tumor (Oberg *et al.* 2004; Ramage *et al.* 2005). Chromogranin A is used as a tumor marker for non-functioning pancreatic endocrine tumors and can also be of prognostic significance as its concentration probably correlates with the tumor mass (Oberg *et al.* 2004). Non-functioning pancreatic endocrine tumors may secrete hormones and/or neurotransmitters, with serum concentrations clearly above the normal range (e.g. so-called 'silent' tumors), although they are insufficient to induce a hypersecretory syndrome (Kaltsas *et al.* 2004a). The clinical impact of silent tumors compared to non-secreting, non-functioning tumors is still unknown and extensive screening for secreted hormones is not routinely performed (Oberg *et al.* 2004). Occasionally, symptoms suggestive of a secretory syndrome may develop in patients with non-functioning pancreatic endocrine tumors. In such cases, measurement of the relevant hormone or neuroamine is mandatory (Kaltsas *et al.* 2004a; Oberg *et al.* 2004). Basal and meal-stimulated PP measurement may be useful for early detection of pancreatic involvement in MEN1, as it may substantiate the presence of a tumor in 75% of those tested (Oberg *et al.* 2004; Ramage *et al.* 2005).

Functional and radiologic (morphologic) confirmation

Functional imaging: somatostatin-receptor scintigraphy (SRS)

Neuroendocrine tumors express somatostatin receptors and this has led to the development of radiolabeled somatostatin analogs for diagnostic imaging (Kaltsas *et al.* 2005; Ramage *et al.* 2005). There are five somatostatin receptor (SSTR) subtypes, of which subtype 2 and 5 are more widely distributed in pancreatic endocrine tumors (Kaltsas *et al.* 2005). With the exception of insulinomas (approximately 50% express SSTR subtype 2), SRS plays a central role in locating and assessing the primary tumor and metastases in pancreatic endocrine tumors (Oberg *et al.* 2004). In particular, SRS exerts a 90% and 80% sensitivity and specificity for all pancreatic endocrine tumors respectively; in addition, it can also detect lesions expressing SSTRs elsewhere (Kaltsas *et al.* 2005; Ramage *et al.* 2005). Therefore, SRS currently presents the most important modality for localization of the primary and determination of the extent of the disease. Whole-body imaging allows for detection of distant metastases and thus influences therapeutic decisions; the method should always include SPECT and pictures should be taken at 24 and 48 hours (Kaltsas *et al.* 2005; Ramage *et al.* 2005). Positron emission tomography (PET) is a functional imaging technique which reflects tumor metabolism; short-lived positron-emitting isotopes such as ^{18}F ($t_{1/2}$ 2h) and ^{11}C (20 min) are used to label substances of interest (Oberg *et al.* 2004). ^{18}F-deoxyglucose (FDG-PET) is being used as an imaging procedure in common cancer, reflecting increased metabolism of glucose in tumors; however, the majority of well-differentiated pancreatic endocrine tumors do not show increased uptake of FDG (Oberg *et al.* 2004). A specific tracer, the serotonin precursor 5-hydroxytryptophan (5-HTP), has been labeled with ^{11}C and shows increased uptake in neuroendocrine tumors revealing lesions not obvious with the use of other modalities (Kaltsas *et al.* 2004b; Oberg *et al.* 2004). However, this technique is of limited use in non-functioning pancreatic endocrine tumors which are usually large and easily identifiable. Positron emission tomography (PET) and/or PET CT, using Ga-DOTATOC to visualize somatostatin receptors presents a promising new tool although sufficient data are still lacking (Kaltsas *et al.* 2005).

Radiologic confirmation

Following initial staging using SRS further morphologic imaging is required to delineate the exact anatomical location of the primary tumor and/or the extent of metastatic disease. Ultrasonography combined with CT and/or MRI, based on local availability and expertise, are the imaging modalities of choice (Fig. 23.7).

Ultrasonography

With ultrasonography the majority of lesions appear hypoechoic, while larger lesions are more heterogeneous (Kaltsas *et al.* 2005). Endoscopic Ultrasonography (EUS), when available, can be used to obtain an early histologic confirmation and may also be of prognostic significance. This technique is particularly useful when cases of familial syndromes are suspected as it can identify small and multiple lesions that may elude detection by conventional techniques (Kaltsas *et al.* 2005; Oberg & Eriksson 2005). In addition, it offers the possibility of obtaining early tissue diagnosis.

Computed tomography and magnetic resonance imaging

Non-contrast-enhanced CT images display iso- or hypodense lesions compared to the adjacent pancreatic parenchyma and can also reveal areas of calcification and hemorrhage. Following contrast enhancement, the hypervascularity of endocrine

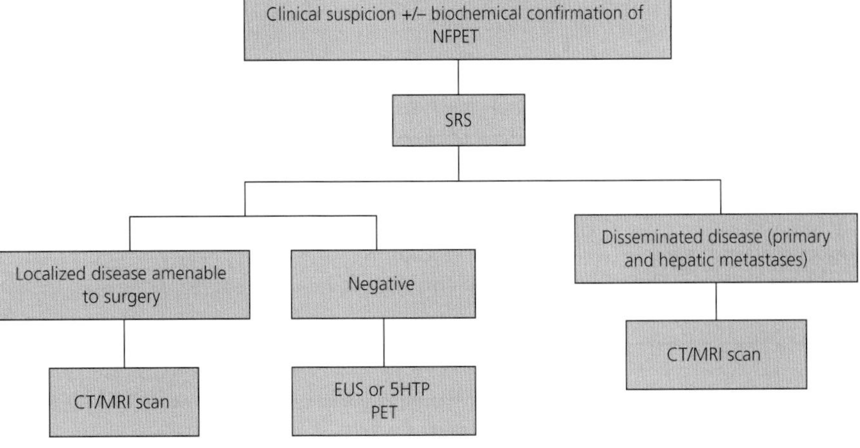

Fig. 23.7 Imaging algorithm for the diagnosis, staging and follow-up of non-functioning pancreatic endocrine tumors (NFPETs). SRS, somatostatin receptor scintigraphy; CT, computed tomography; MRI, magnetic resonance imaging; EUS, endoscopic ultrasonography; PET, positron emission tomography.

tumors becomes prominent and distinguishes them from other pancreatic lesions (Kaltsas *et al.* 2005). Images should be obtained with multidetector CT (2.5-mm section thickness), at the peak arterial phase of contrast enhancement and reconstructed at 1.25-mm thickness (Kaltsas *et al.* 2005). MRI displays hypointense or hyperintense lesions compared to the adjacent pancreatic parenchyma on T1- or T2-weighted images, respectively. Fat-saturated T1-weighted images during the injection of the contrast medium gadolinium reveal the hypervascularity of endocrine tumors; the hyperintensity is best depicted on fat-suppressed T2-weighted images (Kaltsas *et al.* 2005). MRI with a hepatocyte-specific contrast agent may depict small (<1 cm) liver metastases and thus influence decision-making with respect to surgical therapy. To differentiate the hypervascular pancreatic neuroendocrine tumor from hypovascular pancreatic adenocarcinoma, contrast-enhanced techniques (multidetector CT or MRI) are useful. In addition, T2-weighted MR images differentiate the hyperintense neuroendocrine pancreatic tumor from the frequently hypointense adenocarcinoma (Kaltsas *et al.* 2005). Other helpful signs for distinguishing pancreatic endocrine tumors from the more aggressive adenocarcinomas are the mean larger volume, the occasionally cystic component, and the lack of infiltration of peripancreatic fat and vessels in the former group of tumors (Kaltsas *et al.* 2005).

In patients with a high index of clinical suspicion but negative non-invasive imaging studies (US, CT and/or MRI), further diagnostic investigations may include contrast-enhanced US (sensitivity and specificity 94% and 96%, respectively), EUS with biopsies (sensitivity 82–86%) and/or PET imaging using 5-HTP (Kaltsas *et al.* 2005; Oberg & Eriksson 2005). For follow-up, the technique that best visualizes the individual tumor should be used. However, with progressive disease and before therapeutic decisions, a thorough staging (SRS, US and CT/MRI) may be required.

Pathology and genetics

The pathologic report should include detailed description of the macroscopic, microscopic and immunohistochemical features of the tumor, in order to support the diagnosis of an endocrine tumor and allow for its correct classification according to current WHO criteria (Table 23.5). In addition, markers that have been shown to predict the biologic behavior of the tumor should also be included as they can direct therapeutic decisions and intensity of follow-up (Table 23.6). Germline DNA testing is mandatory when familial syndromes are suspected as they can identify asymptomatic carriers and/or exclude, under particular circumstances, non-affected members from prolonged and extensive follow-up.

Histopathology

The majority of non-functioning pancreatic endocrine tumors are well-differentiated tumors without any distinctive histopathologic features. Fine needle aspiration cytology, it may be useful in establishing the correct pre- or intraoperative diagnosis when it is not feasible to obtain a tissue specimen. Although preoperative histology is not required it is an important mean in establishing a preoperative and definitive diagnosis (Ramage *et al.* 2005). An adequate biopsy should be obtained with enough tissue to define tumor features and the biopsy should be repeated if the clinical course changes (Oberg *et al.* 2004). In order to demonstrate the endocrine nature of the neoplastic cells, the immunohistochemical detection of chromogranin A and synaptophysin is necessary and sufficient in most cases. To exclude tumors which may be confused with endocrine lesions, expression of vimentin; nuclear localization of beta-catenin for solid-pseudopapillary tumors; and expression of trypsin for acinar cell carcinoma are useful (Solcia *et al.* 2000). A pathology report of practical clinical use should be able to distinguish between well and poorly differentiated neoplasms and well-differentiated endocrine tumors (benign lesions) from tumors of uncertain behavior and carcinomas (La Rosa *et al.* 1996; Solcia *et al.* 2000). To achieve this, several parameters should be assessed including tumor size, invasion of nearby tissues, number of mitoses and the presence of necrosis (Table 23.6). Evaluation of the mitotic index and the proliferation Ki-67 index are mandatory. While hormones/neurotransmitters like pancreatic polypeptide (40–50%), glucagons (30%), insulin (50%), somatostatin, calcitonin, parathyroid hormone-related peptide (PTHrP) and serotonin may be expressed by non-

Table 23.6 Clinical and histomorphologic features for prognosis and staging non-functioning endocrine pancreatic tumors.

Macroscopic evaluation	Microscopic evaluation	Immunohistochemistry
Tumor size	Mitotic index (number of mitoses in 10 HPF)	Chromogranin A expression
Lymph node metastases	Angioinvasion	Synaptophysin expression
Extrapancreatic invasion	Perineural invasion	Ki-67 index (expressed in% of cells positive)
Distant metastases		

HPF, high power field. Localized disease: High mitotic index and/or proliferative index (% Ki-67), angiinvasion and perineural invasion and more prominent synaptophysin from chromogranin staining characterize 'increased risk tumors'. Presence and number of hepatic metastasis, extrahepatic metastases, high Ki-67% PI consist worse prognostic features.

functioning pancreatic endocrine tumors, their immunohistochemical determination is not necessary for diagnosis and/or tumor subtyping (Oberg *et al.* 2004). However, in the presence of any symptoms suggestive of a secretory syndrome a repeated biopsy performing immunohistochemical determination of the relevant hormone, neuroamine and/or neurotransmitter should be performed (Oberg *et al.* 2004; Oberg & Eriksson 2005).

Genetics

Germline DNA testing for hereditary tumor syndromes is only recommended in specific situations. These include a family history or clinical findings suggesting MEN1 or von Hippel-Lindau disease (VHL), the presence of multiple tumors or the demonstration of precursor lesions, such as evidence of hyperplastic features or microadenomas in the peritumoral pancreatic tissue (Kaltsas *et al.* 2004a). Mutational analysis should be performed to test for menin or VHL mutations. However, MEN1 germline mutation tests may fail to detect 10–20% of those mutations. In such instances 11q13 haplotype testing about the MEN1 locus or genetic linkage can identify MEN1 carriers (Brandi *et al.* 2001). It is important to search thoroughly for MEN1 and other hereditary syndromes in all patients with non-functioning endocrine tumors by obtaining a detailed family history, clinical examination and appropriate investigations when required (Ramage *et al.* 2005).

Prognosis

Most endocrine pancreatic tumors are large well-differentiated (WHO group 2) endocrine carcinomas (Table 23.5) and a significant number of them (up to 80%) have already developed synchronous metastases at the time of diagnosis (Kaltsas *et al.* 2004a; Oberg *et al.* 2005). Prognosis depends on the presence of liver and bone metastases and histopathologic classification; overall 5-year survival ranges between 30% and 63%, with a median survival from the time of diagnosis of 72 months. Actuarial 5- and 10-year survival rates after diagnosis of liver metastases were 46% and 38%, respectively, although aggressive treatment may increase 5-year survival to 63% or 82% (La Rosa *et al.* 1996; Kaltsas *et al.* 2004a; Oberg *et al.* 2004; Ramage *et al.* 2005). The initial number and size of liver metastases, the rapid progression of liver metastases (more than 25% volume increase within 6–12 months), and the development of bone metastases confer a poor prognosis (Kaltsas *et al.* 2004a). Histopathologic staging, including tumor differentiation, tumor size, proliferation marker and angioinvasion, correlates with survival (Tables 23.5 & 23.6). All patients with low-risk tumors were alive after 47 months, 10% of those with intermediate risk tumors had died after 94 months, while 35% of patients with low-grade malignant tumors died after a period of 42 months (La Rossa *et al.* 1996). A considerable number of patients with MEN1 will be found to harbor non-functioning pancreatic endocrine tumors that are probably the leading cause of mortality due to metastatic spread (Brandi *et al.* 2001). There is still controversy around the role of surgical treatment for asymptomatic patients as a mean to diminish malignant dissemination and therefore affect prognosis (Brandi *et al.* 2001).

Follow-up

Follow-up aims to evaluate the results of surgical therapy and/or provide indications for additional treatment. Follow-up investigations should be adjusted according to the type of the tumor (well vs poorly differentiated tumors) and the stage of the disease. Follow-up is based on clinical (symptoms/signs of disease progression, performance status of the patient), biochemical (chromogranin A measurement) and radiologic (morphologic and when necessary functional) assessment. The results of follow-up investigations are used to clarify whether further therapy is required or when this is applied is effective.

Benign or borderline malignant non-functioning pancreatic endocrine tumors

Follow-up includes clinical, laboratory (measurement of chromogranin A) and radiologic examinations. The follow-up intervals should be regular following the initial diagnosis and therapeutic interventions in order to document residual and/or progressive disease. Although complete resection of benign non-functioning pancreatic endocrine tumors is considered to be curative and further follow-up will probably not be necessary, there is still limited experience following the introduction of the WHO classification into clinical practice (Table 23.5). It is probably more reasonable to advocate regular follow-up (every 12 months employing limited resources such as chromogranin A measurements and a single imaging modality) even in patients with favorable prognostic factors. Patients with pancreatic lesions of uncertain behavior (Table 23.5) who have undergone radical surgery cannot be considered cured. Therefore, long-term follow-up every 12 months using ultrasonography and/or MRI/CT scans and biochemical markers (chromogranin A) is suggested. Although limited data derived from prospective studies exist, SRS could be performed 6 months after surgery and/or in the presence of clinical and/or biochemical suspicion of tumor recurrence with negative conventional imaging (Oberg *et al.* 2004; Ramage *et al.* 2005).

Malignant non-functioning pancreatic endocrine tumors

Patients with radically resected malignant tumors should be followed up regularly, every 6 months with biochemical markers (chromogranin A), ultrasonography and/or MRI/CT scans to detect early recurrences (Oberg *et al.* 2004; Ramage *et al.* 2005). The natural history of pancreatic endocrine tumors varies, with some developing recurrences even after periods of prolonged follow-up (Mignon 2000). Recurrences can be either local, locoregional and/or distant; further treatment will be planned according to the site of recurrence and bulk of the disease. Occasionally tumor progression may be rapid, with evidence of disseminated disease in contrast to the histopathologic markers used to predict the biologic behavior of the tumor; in such cases, a further tissue diagnosis may be required to exclude tumor dedifferentiation (Oberg *et al.* 2004; Oberg & Eriksson 2005). This is substantiated further when there is disconcordance between serum markers (decreasing concentrations of serum chromogranin) and radiologic findings (evidence of tumor progression). A more strict follow-up should be advocated for poorly differentiated carcinomas in which radical resection was achieved as early relapse is usually the case (Kaltsas *et al.* 2004a).

Advanced malignant non-functioning pancreatic NET

In patients with rapid tumor growth, and proliferation index greater than 20%, follow-up should be performed more often, every 3 months. Initial follow-up investigations should include clinical, biochemical markers, ultrasonography and/or CT or MRI scans (Oberg *et al.* 2004).

Follow-up of patients with hereditary syndromes

The majority of information for the follow-up of these patients is derived from patients with MEN1. Regular imaging is required, every 6–12 months, to document substantial alterations in the size of the lesions. Although several groups advocate that no intervention should be performed unless a particular tumor is more than 3 cm in size or is growing, others favor earlier intervention if the lesions are more than 1–2 cm in size (Brandi *et al.* 2001). Metastatic disease is likely to be present in a substantial fraction of patients receiving the earliest surgery even in the absence of positive imaging results (Brandi *et al.* 2001). In such cases sensitive techniques such as EUS or PET imaging using 5-HTP may be of value.

Follow-up also influences therapeutic decisions. Therapeutic schemes should be monitored closely and terminated as soon there is disease progression. If no further therapeutic modalities are available, monitoring the disease should be kept at a minimum.

Summary

Non-functioning pancreatic endocrine tumors are the most common endocrine tumors of the pancreas. As the majority of these tumors are well differentiated endocrine carcinomas not associated with any distinct secretory syndrome, they are of large size at presentation and associated with synchronous, mainly hepatic metastases. As clinical presentation is non-specific the general biochemical endocrine marker chromogranin A is of value in directing towards endocrine differentiation of these tumors. The documentation of somatostatin receptors in these tumors with the use of somatostatin receptor scintigraphy facilitates the diagnosis further and helps staging the disease. CT and/or MRI are used for the exact anatomic delineation of the lesions and for further follow-up. In cases where the clinical and/or biochemical suspicion is high but imaging modalities have failed to identify any lesion, EUS and/or PET using specific tracers can be of value. The endocrine nature of the tumor is based on the documentation of specific markers of neuroendocrine differentiation on histology. The incorporation of several microscopic and immunohistochemical features is used to predict the biologic behavior of the tumor and overall prognosis. In the case of multiple tumors and relevant family history, search for a familial tumoral syndrome should be undertaken and genetic screening may be required. Although the prognosis of these tumors is relatively good in the absence of metastases, patients should remain on regular follow-up using a number of biochemical and imaging investigations to document response to treatment and any evidence of disease progression. Follow-up schemes are currently evolving and the intensity and means of follow-up are based on the characteristics of the tumor, extent of the disease and local facilities and expertise.

References

Barakat MT, Meeran K, Bloom SR. (2004) Neuroendocrine tumors. *Endocrin Rel Cancer* 11(1): 1–18.

Brandi ML, Cagel RF, Angeli A *et al.* (2001) Guidelines for diagnosis and therapy of MEN type 1 and type 2. *J Clin Endocrinol Metab* 186: 5658–71.

Kaltsas GA, Besser GM, Grossman AB. (2004a) The diagnosis and medical management of advanced neuroendocrine tumors. *Endocrin Rev* 25: 458–511.

Kaltsas GA, Rockall A, Papadogias D, Reznek R, Grossman AB. (2004b) Recent advances in radiological and radionuclide imaging and therapy of neuroendocrine tumors. *Eur J Endocrinol* 151(1): 15–27.

Kaltsas GA, Papadogias D, Makras P, Grossman AB. (2005) Treatment of advanced newoendocrine tumors with radiolabelled somatostatin analogues. *Endo Rel Cancer* 12(4): 683–99.

La Rosa S, Sessa F, Capella C *et al.* (1996) Prognostic criteria for non-functioning pancreatic endocrine tumors *Virchows Arch* 429(6): 323–33.

Mignon M. (2000) Natural history of neuroendocrine enetropancreatic tumors. *Digestion* 62 (Suppl 1): 51–8.

Oberg K, Eriksson B. (2005) Endocrine tumors of the pancreas. *Best Pract Res Clin Gastroenterol* 19(5): 753–81.

Oberg K, Astrup L, Eriksson B *et al.* (2004) Guidelines for the management of gastroenteropancreatic neuroendocrine tumours (including bronchopulmonary and thymic neoplasms). Part II-specific NE tumour types. *Acta Oncol* 443(7): 626–36.

Ramage JK, Davies AHG, Ardill J *et al.* (2005) Guidelines for the management of gastroenteropancreatic neuroendocrine tumours. *Gut* 54: 1–16.

Solcia E, Kloppel G, Sobin LH. (2000) Histological typing of endocrine tumors. In: *World Health Organization: International Histological Classification of Tumors*, 2nd edn. Springer, Berlin.

Rare functioning pancreatic endocrine tumors

Dermot O'Toole

Introduction

Pancreatic endocrine tumors (PETs) represent a heterogeneous group of tumors depending on their functional status and histologic differentiation. Functioning tumors are defined when clinical symptoms are related to peptide or hormone overproduction. Indeed, non-functioning PETs are reported with increasing frequency (Plockinger & Wiedenmann 2004). The most common functioning tumors of the pancreas include insulinomas and gastrinomas (dealt with elsewhere). This section will deal with a group of rare functioning tumors of the pancreas (RFTs) which by definition are less easy to categorize due to the relatively few data which include small series and numerous case reports. It is also important to adequately define RFTs as tumors whose secreted peptides/hormones are responsible for specific clinical symptoms. Tumors secreting pancreatic polypeptide, human chorionic gonadotrophin subunits, calcitonin, neurotensin or other peptides do not usually produce specific symptoms and should be considered as non-functioning tumors. It is also important to note that several of these RFTs may have extrapancreatic localizations such as VIPomas (10%), somatostatinoma (~50%), GRFoma (70%) and adrenocorticotropic-secreting tumors (ACTHoma) (85%) (Jensen 1999).

The section includes specific headings related to general and specific aspects pertaining to diagnostics and therapeutics in RFTs and in addition specific syndromes (such as VIPoma, glucagonoma).

Epidemiology

The incidence of clinically detected PETs has been reported to be 4–12 per million inhabitants, which is much lower than that reported from autopsy series (about 1%) (Eriksson *et al.* 1990; Modlin *et al.* 2003). When all functioning PETs are considered, insulinomas are the most common (17% incidence), followed by gastrinoma (15%). Rare functioning tumors are by definition far less common, accounting for approximately 10% of PETs, and include VIPoma (2%), glucagonoma (1%), carcinoid (1%) and somatostatinoma (1%). In addition, even rarer tumors secreting adrenocorticotropic hormones (ACTHoma), growth hormone (GRFomas), calcitonin-producing tumors, and parathyroid hormone-related peptide tumors are described, and while the incidence is extremely low clinical awareness is required (Verner & Morrison 1958; Mallinson *et al.* 1974; Ganda *et al.* 1977; Vinik & Moattari 1989; Gorden *et al.* 1989; Kimura *et al.* 1991; Wermers *et al.* 1996; Soga 1998; Soga & Yakuwa 1999; Chastain 2001; Nikou *et al.* 2005).

Clinicopathologic features

Similar to insulinomas and gastrinomas, the majority of RFTs are well-differentiated tumors (Solcia *et al.* 2000). They most frequently present at a malignant stage and the majority are classified as WHO group 2; liver metastases are common (Long *et al.* 1981; Gorden *et al.* 1989; Wermers *et al.* 1996; Smith *et al.* 1998; Nikou *et al.* 2005). Precise survival rates specific to RFTs are impossible to ascertain as data, logically, included functioning tumors as a whole. Bearing this in mind, 5-year survival rates are reported to be 60–100% for localized disease, 40% for regional disease, and 29% for distant metastases; the rate is reported to be close to 80% for all stages (Eriksson *et al.* 1990; Eriksson & Oberg 1993; Modlin *et al.* 2003). The average age at diagnosis of RFTs is 50–55 years and they have an equal sex distribution (Wermers *et al.* 1996; Smith *et al.* 1998; Nikou *et al.* 2005). These tumors can be associated with the multiple endocrine neoplasia type 1 syndrome (MEN1; an autosomal dominantly-inherited predisposition to develop multiple tumors on the endocrine system—most frequently involving the parathyroids, pituitary and pancreas). Overall 15–30% of patients with PETs will have MEN1. Clinical awareness of the possibility of MEN1 is important due to the possibility of the development of multiple tumors occurring either synchronously or metachronously (Skogseid *et al.* 1991). The incidence of MEN1 in patients with RFTs is not known but figures suggested in recent studies indicated a rate of about 2% for VIPomas and glucagonomas (Levy-Bohbot *et al.* 2004; Gibril *et al.* 2004). The incidence of MEN1 in somatostatinomas and GRFomas may be higher. Even in the absence of MEN1, patients with malignant functioning tumors may present with mixed syndromes, or the tumors may change clinically over time.

Diagnostic procedures

Pathology

A pathologic diagnosis is mandatory in all cases and is easily obtained on tumor biopsy performed either in cases of hepatic metastases (e.g, ultrasound-guided biopsy) or of the primary tumor (preferably using EUS-FNA if locally-advanced, or at surgery). Pathologic diagnosis of RFTs is performed using conventional hematoxylin–eosin staining, immunohistochemical staining with chromogranin, and synaptophysin (Fig. 23.8) (Solcia *et al.* 2000). Immunohistochemistry using specific antibodies depending on the clinical situation may also be applied. Important adjuncts in distinguishing well from poorly differentiated tumors include determination of mitotic index by counting 10 HPF, and calculation of Ki-67 index by immunohistochemistry is mandatory (Solcia *et al.* 2000).

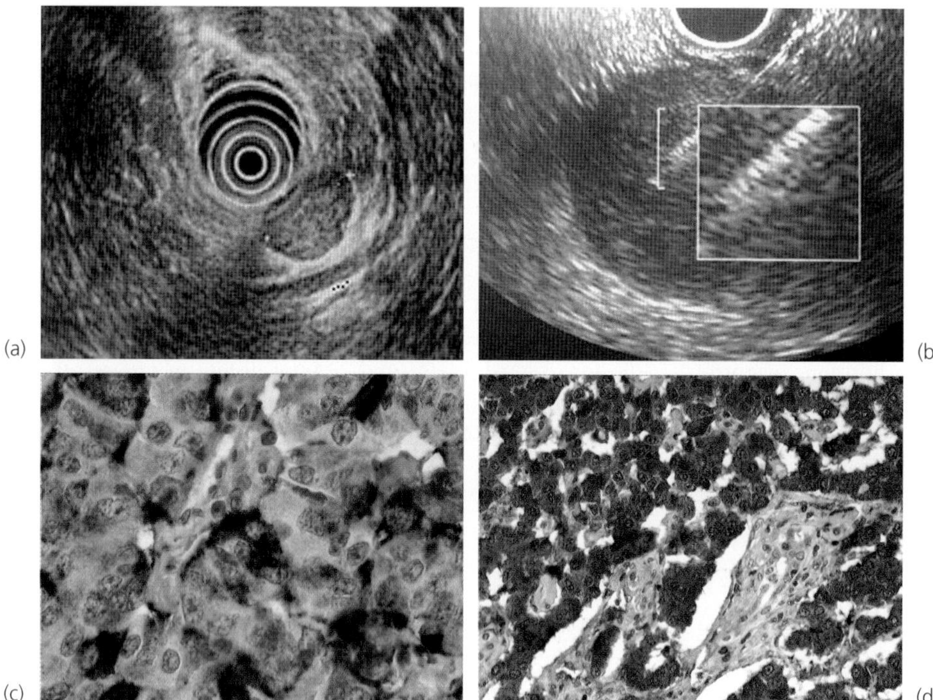

Fig. 23.8 Example of a well-differentiated endocrine tumor of the pancreatic body. (a) At radial echoendoscopy, the tumor is homogeneous and hypoechoic with well-circumscribed borders and posterior reinforcement. (b) EUS-FNA is demonstrated with the 22-gauge needle perfectly centered in the lesion permitting histologic analysis; immunohistochemistry is thus possible showing cordonal sheets of regular cells staining for chromogranin A (c) and synamptophysin (d).

Biology

The diagnosis for the majority of RFTs is prompted by clinical suspicion (e.g. chronic diarrhea with electrolyte disturbance in patients with VIPoma or the association of the typical migratory skin rash and diabetes in cases of glucagonoma). Biologic tests should include specific markers depending on clinical symptoms (VIP, glucagon, somatostatin, GRF, ACTH) and in addition, general markers (chromogranin A and pancreatic polypeptide) should be performed as for other functioning and non-functioning PETs (Smith *et al.* 1998; Long *et al.* 1981; Guillausseau *et al.* 1982; Capella *et al.* 1983; Nikou *et al.* 2005). Genetic testing for MEN1 should be performed in case of suspected familial predisposition to MEN1 or if the presence of other associated endocrinopathies (e.g. elevated serum calcium or PTH suggesting hyperparathyroidism and prolactinoma, respectively).

Imaging

The standard imaging procedures for RFTs, like other PETs, include EUS, contrast-enhanced helical CT or MRI of the abdomen (for both primary tumor and detection of metastases) in combination with SRS. Image-fusion data, combining CT and SRS (SPECT), appears promising (Gabriel *et al.* 2005) in helping to accurately locate tumoral residues and in planning surgery (Fig. 23.9). EUS is a proven method in detecting most PETs and can be combined with EUS-FNA with microbiopsy (Anderson *et al.* 2000; Gines *et al.* 2002) (Fig. 23.8). The majority of RFTs are positive using SRS (Fig. 23.9) and this should be used routinely in the investigation of both primary and metastatic disease (Lebtahi *et al.* 1999; Kwekkeboom *et al.* 2000; Lebtahi *et al.* 2002) prior to treatment planning especially surgery. ^{68}Gallium-labeled somatostatin analog PET has been recently found to detect even small tumors and should prove a promising technique in the future (Hofmann *et al.* 2001; Kowalski *et al.* 2003). Standard PET with ^{18}-F-glucose is not efficient in detecting well-differentiated tumors, whether functioning or not, but may have some value in the detection of aggressive poorly differentiated PETs (Eriksson *et al.* 2005). Recently, data using PET with 5-HTP or L-DOPA has also shown promising results and may be an option for detection of small well differentiated tumors (Hoegerle *et al.* 2001; Eriksson *et al.* 2005; Orlefors *et al.* 2005).

Treatment

Medical

Control of symptoms

As in patients with insulinomas and gastrinomas, beginning specific medical therapy to control the frequent debilitating symptoms in relation to hormone/peptide overproduction is urgent. Fortunately, both somatostatin analogs and interferon have been shown to be effective in the control of symptoms in functioning PETs (Plockinger *et al.* 2004) and this also includes RFTs (Gorden *et al.* 1989; Wermers *et al.* 1996; Nikou *et al.* 2005). In fact about 80–90% of patients with VIPoma and

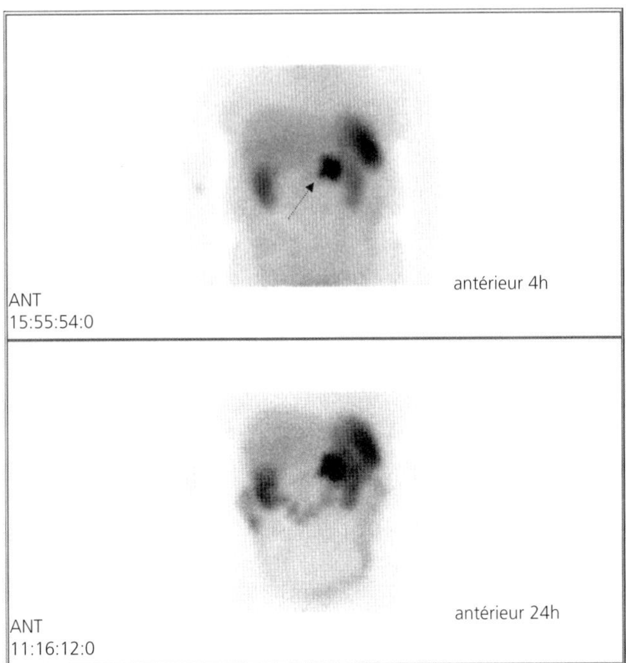

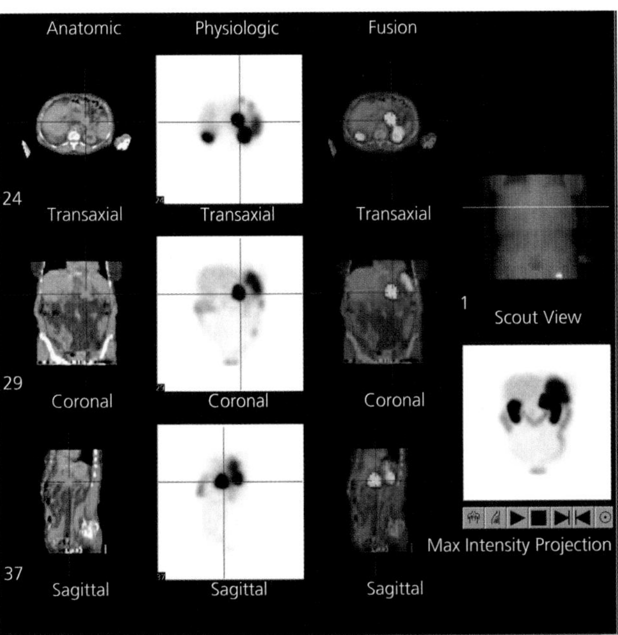

Fig. 23.9 (a) Planar views (anterior and posterior) of standard somatostatin receptor scintigraphy demonstrating intense uptake in a VIPoma of the pancreatic body/tail at 4 and 24 hrs. (b) Combined SPECT/CT fusion allows for both scintigraphic and CT localization of the tumor.

glucagonoma improve very promptly, overcoming diarrhea and skin rash, and 60–80% have a reduction in VIP and glucagon levels. Symptomatic relief is not always related to reduction in circulating hormone levels, indicating that somatostatin analogs have direct effects on the peripheral target organ. Escape from symptomatic control can be seen quite frequently but an increase in the dose of somatostatin analogs can help temporarily. In the control of symptoms, somatostatin analog therapy should be initiated with short-acting substances (octreotide 100 μg subcutaneously × 2–3) for 1–2 days with titration according to clinical response, then the patient can be transferred to slow-release Lanreotide-SR® i.m., Lanreotide autogel® s.c. or Sandostatin–LAR® i.m. (every 4 weeks) (Oberg *et al.* 2004).

Specific antitumor therapy

The antitumor efficacy of somatostatin analogs appears less pronounced according to recent data, with objective tumor responses of <10% (Aparicio *et al.* 2001; Faiss *et al.* 2003; Welin *et al.* 2004; Arnold *et al.* 2005); however, disease stabilization of up to 40% has been reported and these agents may be of value in subgroups of patients with slowly progressive well-differentiated tumors expressing sst_2 receptor subtypes (i.e. a positive SRS) (Faiss *et al.* 2003; Arnold *et al.* 2005). Likewise, interferon may be indicated in metastatic low proliferating tumors and can be effective in VIPomas not responding to somatostatin analogs (Oberg *et al.* 1985) but this requires confirmation in a controlled manner (Faiss *et al.* 2003; Arnold *et al.* 2005). Use of bispecific or multispecific ligands recognizing several sst subtypes may have more pronounced effects as antioncogenics (O'Toole *et al.* 2006).

Systemic chemotherapy is indicated in patients with metastatic and progressive RFTs using combinations of streptozotcin and 5-FU and or doxorubicin with current objective response rates in the order of 35% (Kouvaraki *et al.* 2004; Delaunoit *et al.* 2004). This is considerably lower than the 69% reported by Moertel *et al.*in 1992 (Moertel *et al.* 1992) which is probably explained by the crude methods employed to measure tumor response at that time. Currently trials are under way examining newer cytotoxic candidates such as agents directed at the rich vascular network in PETs (antiangiogenics, e.g. VEGF inhibitors) or internal kinases integral in proliferation pathways (e.g. sunitinib, a multitarget kinase inhibitor) (Yao *et al.* 2005; Kulke *et al.* 2005). Another exciting area in the treatment of digestive endocrine tumors relates to the development of peptide receptor radionuclide therapy (PRRT). This has been made possible due to development of chelators suitable for radiometal labeling allowing for coupling of modified somatostatin analogs with trivalent metal ions (indium, gallium, yttrium, lutetium, etc.), thus allowing for further potential in diagnostic and therapeutic applications. Limited experience is available concerning PRRT in the treatment of RFTs; however, its efficacy in other advanced PETs with positive SRS has been demonstrated (Waldherr *et al.* 2002; Kwekkeboom *et al.* 2005). This therapeutic option should be considered for patients with advanced disease in whom other treatment options have failed; indeed, use of PRRT as first line therapy may be justified in certain cases and further trials are required to correctly place PRRT in treatment algorithms of PETs.

Surgical and cytoablative therapies

Surgery

Indications for surgery depend on clinical symptoms, tumor size and location, malignancy and metastatic spread. Curative surgery is always recommended whenever feasible after careful symptomatic control of the clinical syndrome (Wermers *et al.* 1992); the latter may be achieved by medical or locoregional treatments. Curative surgery can also be aimed for in patients with metastatic disease, including 'localized' metastatic disease to the liver (Akerstrom 1996). The type of surgery depends on the location of the primary tumor: pancreaticoduodenal resection (Whipple's operation), distal pancreatic resection, tumor enucleation, or enucleation in combination with resection (Kianmanesh *et al.* 2005a). If malignancy is suspected, adequate lymph node clearance is mandatory.

In case of surgery for liver metastases, complete resection (R0) of metastases should always be considered both in functioning and non-functioning tumors. Liver surgery includes metastasis enucleation, segmental resection(s), hemihepatectomy or extended hemihepatectomy (Ahlman *et al.* 2000). Intraoperative US should be performed for detection of all liver metastases. Prior to performing liver surgery, metastatic disease should be confined to the liver. The presence of liver metastases is the major prognostic indicator in patients with PETs and surgical resection appears to strongly favor clinical outcome as defined in multiple series (Kianmanesh *et al.* 2005b). Liver surgery can be performed concomitantly with surgery to the primary tumor or on a separate occasion. In patients with RFTs specific measures to avoid hormonal crisis are required during surgery (notably perioperative somatostatin analog infusion) and specified anesthetic considerations (Wermers *et al.* 1992). Palliative surgery (to primary or metastases) may also be performed following multidisciplinary discussions and includes palliative or debulking resections (resection of >90% of tumor burden) to control symptoms related to hormonal hypersecretion (Guillausseau *et al.* 1982; Smith *et al.* 1998; Wermers *et al.* 1992; Nikou *et al.* 2005). Bilateral adrenalectomy should be considered in selected cases with ACTH secretion resulting in Cushing syndrome (Maton *et al.* 1986; Yu *et al.* 1999). The exact role of liver transplantation in patients with RTFs has not been defined; however, it may be indicated for a small number of patients without extrahepatic metastases (Ahlman *et al.* 2004), in whom life-threatening hormonal symptoms persist despite maximal medical therapy and where standard surgery is not feasible.

Cytoablative methods

Selective embolization alone or in combination with intra-arterial chemotherapy (chemoembolization using streptozotocine, doxorubicin, mitomycin C etc.) is an established procedure effective in controlling symptoms and controlling tumor progression in functioning digestive endocrine tumors including PETs (O'Toole *et al.* 2003). Symptomatic responses of about 60% are reported with an approximately 40–50% tumor response (Ruszniewski *et al.* 1993; Clouse *et al.* 1994; Ruszniewski & Malka 2000; Roche *et al.* 2003; Gupta *et al.* 2005). It has not been established whether chemoembolization is more efficient than embolization alone. In experienced centers the mortality rate is low; however, significant morbidity may occur (hepatic or renal failure). The post-embolization syndrome is frequent, with fever (sometimes prolonged), right upper quadrant pain, nausea, elevation of liver enzymes and a decrease in albumin and PK (O'Toole *et al.* 2003). Adequate analgesia and hydration are recommended during and following treatment and prophylaxis with somatostatin analogs is always indicated when embolizing functioning tumors. Contraindications to chemoembolization are complete portal vein thrombosis, hepatic insufficiency and a previous pancreaticoduodenectomy, which may expose the patient to severe complications (notably sepsis).

Other local ablative methods which may be used alone or in combination with surgery include radiofrequency ablation (RFA), cryotherapy and laser therapy (Cozzi *et al.* 1995; Shapiro *et al.* 1998; Wessels & Schell 2001; Hellman *et al.* 2002; Berber *et al.* 2002; Dick *et al.* 2003; Mensel *et al.* 2005). Local ablative methods are usually reserved to treat limited disease (<8–10 metastases of <4–5 cm in diameter).

Multiple endocrine neoplasia type 1 (Wermer's syndrome)

Multiple endocrine neoplasia type 1 (MEN1) is an autosomal dominant inherited predisposition to the development of multiple adenomas or tumors of diverse endocrine tissue. The disorder results from a mutation in the tumor suppressor gene *menin* located at 11q13 (Chandrasekharappa *et al.* 1997). This affection has a high penetrance and phenotypic manifestations include adenomas of the parathyroids and pituitary as well as pancreatic and duodenal endocrine tumors (most frequently gastrinomas), adrenal tumors, ECLomas of the gastric fundus (as part of the Zollinger–Ellison syndrome) and thymic or bronchial tumors. Genetic mutations observed in patients with MEN1 are quite dispersed along the coding sequence and no genotype/phenotype correlation exists (Chandrasekharappa *et al.* 1997; Lemmens *et al.* 1997). The syndrome is diagnosed in the fourth or fifth decades, but biochemical evidence of lesions associated with MEN1 may be observed as early as in adolescence. Overall, gastrinomas have the most frequent association with MEN1 (25%) and other functioning pancreatic tumors more rarely found to exist as part of this inherited predisposition: insulinomas (5–8%) and RFTs (as discussed above). MEN1 should be suspected if there is a family or personal history of endocrinopathies, recurrent peptic ulcer disease, a history of renal colic (or nephrolithiases or hypercalcemia) or pancreatic endocrine tumor syndromes. In patients with gastrinomas the association with parathyroid adenomas is frequent and requires parathormone and ionized calcium measurements as well as ultrasound of the parathyroids; 25% of all MEN1/ZES patients lack a family history of MEN1, supporting the need to genetically screen all ZES patients for MEN1. In other endocrine tumors of the pancreas or duodenum where the incidence of MEN1 is lower, genetic testing should be performed in the event of a family history of MEN1, suspicious clinical or laboratory data for MEN1 are found or multiple tumors are present raising the possibility of MEN1.

Identification of patients with MEN1 is extremely important as the prognosis and therapy is altered in its presence. In patients with MEN1-associated gastrinomas the pancreas and duodenum usually harbor multiple tumors, invariably of small size, and curative resection is impossible in the absence of a total pancreaticoduodenectomy—the latter is not justified in the majority of cases. Some groups adopt an monitoring system reserving limited resection once tumors exceed 2 cm in order to avoid metastatic spread (Norton & Jensen 2004; Thomas-Marques *et al.* 2006). Surgery may be obviously required to control symptoms in patients presenting with other functional pancreatic tumors such as insulinoma, VIPoma etc. In addition, the incidence of malignant non-functioning pancreatic tumors in patients with MEN1 has been reported to reach about 50% in a recent series (Thomas-Marques *et al.* 2006) and appear to be aggressive with a recently reported 10-year survival of 62% versus 86% for functional tumors (Levy-Bohbot *et al.* 2004).

Standardized screening enables the detection of asymptomatic tumor disease at a mean of 25 years and this is in contrast to non-screened patients in whom 75% present with morbidity related to their endocrine tumors and a significant number have malignant transformation (Skogseid *et al.* 1996). The role of EUS in screening and guiding treatment in asymptomatic MEN1-associated GEP has been recently reported by two groups (Gauger *et al.* 2003; Thomas-Marques *et al.* 2006). The recent series by the French GTE (Groupe des tumeurs endocrines) reported on a prospective screening programme using EUS as a screening method in non-functioning asymptomatic MEN1 patients (half had minor biochemical abnormalities) (Thomas-Marques *et al.* 2006). No comparison with other imaging methods was made. Twenty-eight tumors (55%) were detected in 51 patients at a median age of 39 years (range: 16–71). The median size and number of tumors per patient were 6 mm (range 6–60 mm) and 3 (range 1–9), respectively. Interestingly, tumors were ≥10 mm for 37% of patients and ≥20 mm in 14% (Thomas-Marques *et al.* 2006). This study also analysed the rate of tumor progression as defined by a significant increase in tumor size (increase of at least 10 mm) or number (>50% increase in total number) at follow-up EUS in 16 patients with initially abnormal EUS findings. Tumors remained stable at a median of 50 months (range 12–70 months) in 63% of patients; however, 37% presented an increase in number or size of lesions (Thomas-Marques *et al.* 2006). New pancreatic lesions were also observed in three patients who had undergone surgery and were monitored by EUS. Follow-up EUS in patients with normal findings at initial examination was limited to three patients—two developed small lesions at screening EUS at 12, 24 and 48 months and five other patients had normal CT. On the basis of a metastatic risk estimated at 18% for tumors >20 mm, this group as well as the NIH, propose surgery for tumors exceeding 20 mm (Thomas-Marques *et al.* 2006; Norton & Jensen 2004). For the French GTE the proposed EUS screening schedule is as follows: first follow-up EUS at 5 years if normal screening EUS, at 3 years if tumors <10 mm, and at 1 or 2 years when initial tumors are larger (Thomas-Marques *et al.* 2006). The age at which EUS is to be performed has not been clearly established and the GTE proposes EUS in all adults at diagnosis of MEN1 and in children with suspicion of pancreatic or duodenal involvement (symptoms or positive non-invasive imaging) (Thomas-Marques *et al.* 2006).

VIPoma or Vermer–Morrison syndrome

The secretion of vasoactive intestinal hormone (VIP) stimulates enterocytic intestinal secretion of water and electrolytes. Water and electrolyte loss may be massive and two-thirds of patients have more than 3 L of stools/day (Rambaud *et al.* 1986). The basis of treatment includes the correction of dehydration and electrolyte disturbances by the administration of i.v. perfusions with electrolytes as required, combined with somatostatin analogs (Gordon *et al.* 1989; Matuchansky & Rambaud 1995; Eriksson & Oberg 1999; Park *et al.* 1996). Thereafter, a search for the primary tumor as well as eventual metastases (approximately 60%; Matuchansky & Rambaud 1995; Park *et al.* 1996) can be performed prior to proposing a surgical resection. Somatostatin and its analogs decrease the liberation of VIP (and eventually other peptides which are cosecreted by the tumor) but also have a direct effect by inhibiting enterocyte secretion of water and electrolytes (Ruskone *et al.* 1982). VIP levels decrease in 89% of patients treated with somatostatin analogs but levels only normalize in about 33% (Gordon *et al.* 1989). These agents are also effective in abolishing or improving the debilitating diarrhea (85% response rate) encountered in these patients (Gordon *et al.* 1989; Nikou *et al.* 2005). The effects of somatostatin analogs are prolonged in approximately half of patients but require increase doses in a quarter and the remainder experience early escape. Theses agents are well tolerated and use of a prolonged release formulation can be recommended following dose adjustments with immediate preparations (Oberg *et al.* 2004). In patients who experience resistance or escape (tachyphalaxis), changing one analog for another may prove beneficial; addition of rescue immediate-release formulations may also prove efficacious (Oberg *et al.* 2004). Interferon-alpha has also been employed in this clinical situation but with inconsistent results (Oberg *et al.* 1985; Cellier *et al.* 2000).

Glucagonoma

The glucagonoma syndrome includes the association of necrolytic migratory erythema, weight loss (often severe) and diabetes. Other clinical manifestations include thromboses, chelitis and glossitis, anemia, and neuropsychiatric symptoms (Mallinson *et al.* 1974; Guillausseau & Guillausseau-Scholer 1995; Wermers *et al.* 1996; Frankton & Bloom 1996). These symptoms and signs are in relation either directly or indirectly to excessive secretion of glucagon. Low serum amino acid concentrations, which appear at least partially responsible for the generation of the skin rash, results from protein hypercatabolism due to increased gluconeogenesis induced by glucagon hypersecretion. In more than 80% of cases, the tumor is metastatic at the time of diagnosis (Mallinson *et al.* 1974; Guillausseau & Guillausseau-Scholer 1995; Wermers *et al.* 1996; Frankton & Bloom 1996) and chances of a surgical cure are low. Symptomatic treatment is essential and relies on correction of metabolic disorders (nutrition, insulin therapy, and preventative measures against thrombosis etc.) associated with the administration of somatostatin analogs (Guillausseau & Guillausseau-Scholer 1995; Wermers *et al.* 1996; Frankton & Bloom 1996); ablative and/or cytoreductive strategies may be required to control symptoms. Specific antitumor therapy (chemotherapy, chemoembolization) can thereafter be discussed. In a series of 43 patients treated with the somatostatin analog octreotide, skin rashes improved in 27 (63%), and glucagon levels decreased or normalized in 36 (84%) and 4 (9%) cases, respectively (Guillausseau & Guillausseau-Scholer 1995). The median dose used was 300 μg/day. Somatostatin analogs appear less effective in correcting the cachexia and diabetes (Frankton & Bloom 1996). Escape or resistance to treatment occurred in one third of patients within 6 months, required dose increases (Guillausseau & Guillausseau-Scholer 1995).

Other functioning tumors

Other types of functioning tumors are exceptionally rare and include somatostatinoms and tumors secreting the following hormones: ACTH (ACTHomas), GRF (GRFomas), PTH (PTHomas) and serotonin (pancreatic 'carcinoids'). Somatostatinomas are usually localized to the pancreas or duodenum (65%) and may be associated with MEN1. Duodenal tumors may be associated with neurofibromatosis. Specificities regarding symptomatic control in these scarce tumors are largely poorly analysed due to their rarity; however, somatostatin analogs may be effective (except for somatostatinomas). Surgery and other antitumoral strategies applying to more frequent PETs should also be applied to these more frequent variants. In patients with ACTH-secreting tumors, bilateral adrenalectomy should be considered prior to treatment of the primary tumor as hypertensive crises in these patients are often difficult to control and may be life-threatening. Patients with sporadic gastrinomas and ectopic ACTH secretion had a poorer natural history compared to those without Cushing syndrome (Yu *et al.* 1999).

References

Ahlman H, Wangberg B, Jansson S *et al.* (2000) Interventional treatment of gastrointestinal neuroendocrine tumors. *Digestion* 62 (Suppl 1): 59.

Ahlman H, Friman S, Cahlin C *et al.* (2004) Liver transplantation for treatment of metastatic neuroendocrine tumors. *Ann N Y Acad Sci* 1014: 265.

Akerstrom G. (1996) Management of carcinoid tumors of the stomach, duodenum, and pancreas. *World J Surg* 20(2): 173.

Anderson MA, Carpenter S, Thompson NW, Nostrant TT, Elta GH, Scheiman JM. (2000) Endoscopic ultrasound is highly accurate and directs management in patients with neuroendocrine tumors of the pancreas. *Am J Gastroenterol* 95(9): 2271.

Aparicio T, Ducreux M, Baudin E *et al.* (2001) Antitumor activity of somatostatin analogues in progressive metastatic neuroendocrine tumors. *Eur J Cancer* 37(8): 1014.

Arnold R, Rinke A, Klose KJ *et al.* (2005) Octreotide versus octreotide plus interferon-alpha in endocrine gastroenteropancreatic tumors: a randomized trial. *Clin Gastroenterol Hepatol* 3(8): 761.

Berber E, Flesher N, Siperstein AE. (2002) Laparoscopic radiofrequency ablation of neuroendocrine liver metastases. *World J Surg* 26(8): 985.

Capella C, Polak JM, Buffa R *et al.* (1983) Morphologic patterns and diagnostic criteria of VIP-producing endocrine tumors. A histologic, histochemical, ultrastructural, and biochemical study of 32 cases. *Cancer* 52(10): 1860.

Cellier C, Yaghi C, Cuillerier E *et al.* (2000) Metastatic jejunal VIPoma: beneficial effect of combination therapy with interferon-alpha and 5-fluorouracil. *Am J Gastroenterol* 95(1): 289.

Chandrasekharappa SC, Guru SC, Manickam P *et al.* (1997) Positional cloning of the gene for multiple endocrine neoplasia-type 1. *Science* 276(5311): 404.

Chastain MA. (2001) The glucagonoma syndrome: a review of its features and discussion of new perspectives. *Am J Med Sci* 321(5): 306.

Clouse ME, Perry L, Stuart K, Stokes KR. (1994) Hepatic arterial chemoembolization for metastatic neuroendocrine tumors. *Digestion* 55 (Suppl 3): 92.

Cozzi PJ, Englund R, Morris DL. (1995) Cryotherapy treatment of patients with hepatic metastases from neuroendocrine tumors. *Cancer* 76(3): 501.

Delaunoit T, Ducreux M, Boige V *et al.* (2004) The doxorubicin-streptozotocin combination for the treatment of advanced well-differentiated pancreatic endocrine carcinoma; a judicious option? *Eur J Cancer* 40(4): 515.

Dick EA, Joarder R, de Jode M *et al.* (2003) MR-guided laser thermal ablation of primary and secondary liver tumors. *Clin Radiol* 58(2): 112.

Eriksson B, Oberg K. (1993) An update of the medical treatment of malignant endocrine pancreatic tumors. *Acta Oncol* 32(2): 203.

Eriksson B, Oberg K. (1999) Summing up 15 years of somatostatin analog therapy in neuroendocrine tumors: future outlook. *Ann Oncol* 10 (Suppl 2): S31.

Eriksson B, Arnberg H, Lindgren PG *et al.* (1990) Neuroendocrine pancreatic tumors: clinical presentation, biochemical and histopathological findings in 84 patients. *J Intern Med* 228(2): 103.

Eriksson B, Orlefors H, Oberg K, Sundin A, Bergstrom M, Langstrom B. (2005) Developments in PET for the detection of endocrine tumors. *Best Pract Res Clin Endocrinol Metab* 19(2): 311.

Faiss S, Pape UF, Bohmig M *et al.* (2003) Prospective, randomized, multicenter trial on the antiproliferative effect of lanreotide, interferon alfa, and their combination for therapy of metastatic neuroendocrine gastroenteropancreatic tumors–the International Lanreotide and Interferon Alfa Study Group. *J Clin Oncol* 21(14): 2689.

Frankton S, Bloom SR. (1996) Glucagonomas. *Baillière's Clin Gastroenterol* 10: 697–705.

Gabriel M, Hausler F, Bale R *et al.* (2005) Image fusion analysis of (99m)Tc-HYNIC-Tyr(3)-octreotide SPECT and diagnostic CT using an immobilisation device with external markers in patients with endocrine tumors. *Eur J Nucl Med Mol Imaging* 32(12): 1440.

Ganda OP, Weir GC, Soeldner JS *et al.* (1977) 'Somatostatinoma': a somatostatin-containing tumor of the endocrine pancreas. *N Engl J Med* 296(17): 963.

Gauger PG, Scheiman JM, Wamsteker EJ, Richards ML, Doherty GM, Thompson NW. (2003) Role of endoscopic ultrasonography in screening and treatment of pancreatic endocrine tumors in asymptomatic patients with multiple endocrine neoplasia type 1. *Br J Surg* 90(6): 748.

Gibril F, Schumann M, Pace A, Jensen RT. (2004) Multiple endocrine neoplasia type 1 and Zollinger–Ellison syndrome: a prospective study of 107 cases and comparison with 1009 cases from the literature. *Medicine (Baltimore)* 83(1): 43.

Gines A, Vazquez-Sequeiros E, Soria MT, Clain JE, Wiersema MJ. (2002) Usefulness of EUS-guided fine needle aspiration (EUS-FNA) in the diagnosis of functioning neuroendocrine tumors. *Gastrointest Endosc* 56(2): 291.

Gorden P, Comi RJ, Maton PN, Go VL. (1989) NIH conference. Somatostatin and somatostatin analogue (SMS 201–995) in treatment of hormone-secreting tumors of the pituitary and gastrointestinal tract and non-neoplastic diseases of the gut. *Ann Intern Med* 110(1): 35.

Guillausseau PJ, Guillausseau C, Villet R *et al.* (1982) [Glucagonomas. Clinical, biological, anatomopathological and therapeutic aspects (general review of 130 cases]. *Gastroenterol Clin Biol* 6(12): 1029.

Guillausseau PJ, Guillausseau-Scholer C. (1995) Glucagonomas : clinical presentation, diagnosis, and advances in management. In: Mignon MJR, ed. *Endocrine Tumors of the Pancreas. Recent Advances in Research and Management*, p. 183. *Front Gastrointest Res*, vol 23. Karger, Basel.

Gupta S, Johnson MM, Murthy R *et al.* (2005) Hepatic arterial embolization and chemoembolization for the treatment of patients with metastatic neuroendocrine tumors: variables affecting response rates and survival. *Cancer* 104(8): 1590–602.

Hellman P, Ladjevardi S, Skogseid B, Akerstrom G, Elvin A. (2002) Radiofrequency tissue ablation using cooled tip for liver metastases of endocrine tumors. *World J Surg* 26(8): 1052.

Hoegerle S, Altehoefer C, Ghanem N *et al.* (2001) Whole-body 18F dopa PET for detection of gastrointestinal carcinoid tumors. *Radiology* 220(2): 373.

Hofmann M, Maecke H, Borner R *et al.* (2001) Biokinetics and imaging with the somatostatin receptor PET radioligand (68)Ga-DOTATOC. preliminary data. *Eur J Nucl Med* 28(12): 1751.

Jensen R. (1999) Nautural history of digestive endocrine tumors. In: Mignon M, ed. *Recent Advances in the Pathophysiology and Management of Inflammatory Bowel Disease and Digestive Endocrine Tumors*, p. 192. John Libbey Eurotext, Paris.

Kianmanesh R, O'Toole D, Sauvanet A, Ruszniewski P, Belghiti J. (2005a) [Surgical treatment of gastric, enteric, and pancreatic endocrine tumors Part 1. Treatment of primary endocrine tumors]. *J Chir (Paris)* 142(3): 132.

Kianmanesh R, O'Toole D, Sauvanet A, Ruszniewski P, Belghiti J. (2005b) [Surgical treatment of gastric, enteric pancreatic endocrine tumors. Part 2. treatment of hepatic metastases]. *J Chir (Paris)* 142(4): 208.

Kimura W, Kuroda A, Morioka Y. (1991) Clinical pathology of endocrine tumors of the pancreas. Analysis of autopsy cases. *Dig Dis Sci* 36(7): 933.

Kouvaraki MA, Ajani JA, Hoff P *et al.* (2004) Fluorouracil, doxorubicin, and streptozocin in the treatment of patients with locally advanced and metastatic pancreatic endocrine carcinomas. *J Clin Oncol* 22(23): 4762.

Kowalski J, Henze M, Schuhmacher J, Macke HR, Hofmann M, Haberkorn U. (2003) Evaluation of positron emission tomography imaging using [68Ga]-DOTA-D Phe(1)-Tyr(3)-Octreotide in comparison to [111In]-DTPAOC SPECT. First results in patients with neuroendocrine tumors. *Mol Imaging Biol* 5(1): 42.

Kulke M, Lenz HJ, Meropol NJ *et al.* (2005) A phase 2 study to evaluate the efficacy and safety of SU11248 in patients (pts) with unresectable neuroendocrine tumors (NETs). *J Clin Oncol* A4008.

Kwekkeboom D, Krenning EP, de Jong M. (2000) Peptide receptor imaging and therapy. *J Nucl Med* 41(10): 1704.

Kwekkeboom DJ, Teunissen JJ, Bakker WH *et al.* (2005) Radiolabeled somatostatin analog [^{177}Lu-DOTA0,Tyr3]octreotate in patients with endocrine gastroenteropancreatic tumors. *J Clin Oncol* 23(12): 2754.

Lebtahi R, Cadiot G, Sarda L *et al.* (1997) Clinical impact of somatostatin receptor scintigraphy in the management of patients with neuroendocrine gastroenteropancreatic tumors. *J Nucl Med* 38(6): 853.

Lebtahi R, Le Cloirec J, Houzard C *et al.* (2002) Detection of neuroendocrine tumors: 99mTc-P829 scintigraphy compared with 111In-pentetreotide scintigraphy. *J Nucl Med* 43(7): 889.

Lemmens I, Van de Ven WJ, Kas K *et al.* (1997) Identification of the multiple endocrine neoplasia type 1 (MEN-1) gene. The European Consortium on MEN-1. *Hum Mol Genet* 6(7): 1177.

Levy-Bohbot N, Merle C, Goudet P *et al.* (2004) Prevalence, characteristics and prognosis of MEN 1-associated glucagonomas, VIPomas, and somatostatinomas: study from the GTE (Groupe des Tumeurs Endocrines) registry. *Gastroenterol Clin Biol* 28(11): 1075.

Long RG, Bryant MG, Mitchell SJ, Adrian TE, Polak JM, Bloom SR. (1981) Clinicopathological study of pancreatic and ganglioneuroblastoma tumors secreting vasoactive intestinal polypeptide (vipomas). *Br Med J (Clin Res Ed)* 282(6278): 1767.

Mallinson CN, Bloom SR, Warin AP, Salmon PR, Cox B. (1974) A glucagonoma syndrome. *Lancet* 2(7871): 1.

Maton PN, Gardner JD, Jensen RT. (1986) Cushing's syndrome in patients with the Zollinger–Ellison syndrome. *N Engl J Med* 315(1): 1.

Matuchansky C, Rambaud JC. (1995) VIPomas and endocrine cholera: clinical presentation, diagnosis, and advances in management. In: Mignon MJRT, ed. *Endocrine tumors of the pancreas. Recent advances in research and management*, p 166. *Front Gastrointest Res*, vol 23. Karger, Basel.

Mensel B, Weigel C, Heidecke CD, Stier A, Hosten N. (2005) [Laser-induced thermotherapy (LITT) of tumors of the liver in central location: results and complications]. *Rofo* 177(9): 1267.

Modlin IM, Lye KD, Kidd M. (2003) A 5-decade analysis of 13,715 carcinoid tumors. *Cancer* 97(4): 934.

Moertel CG, Lefkopoulo M, Lipsitz S, Hahn RG, Klaassen D. (1992) Streptozocin-doxorubicin, streptozocin-fluorouracil or chlorozotocin in the treatment of advanced islet-cell carcinoma. *N Engl J Med* 326(8): 519.

Nikou GC, Toubanakis C, Nikolaou P *et al.* (2005) VIPomas: an update in diagnosis and management in a series of 11 patients. *Hepatogastroenterology* 52(64): 1259.

Norton JA, Jensen RT. (2004) Resolved and unresolved controversies in the surgical management of patients with Zollinger–Ellison syndrome. *Ann Surg* 240(5): 757.

Oberg K, Alm G, Lindstrom H, Lundqvist G. (1985) Successful treatment of therapy-resistant pancreatic cholera with human leucocyte interferon. *Lancet* 1(8431): 725.

Oberg K, Kvols L, Caplin M *et al.* (2004) Consensus report on the use of somatostatin analogs for the management of neuroendocrine tumors of the gastroenteropancreatic system. *Ann Oncol* 15(6): 966.

Orlefors H, Sundin A, Garske U *et al.* (2005) Whole-body (11)C-5-hydroxytryptophan positron emission tomography as a universal imaging technique for neuroendocrine tumors: comparison with somatostatin receptor scintigraphy and computed tomography. *J Clin Endocrinol Metab* 90(6): 3392.

O'Toole D, Maire F, Ruszniewski P. (2003) Ablative therapies for liver metastases of digestive endocrine tumors. *Endocr Relat Cancer* 10(4): 463.

O'Toole D, Saveanu A, Couvelard A *et al.* (2006) The analysis of quantitative expression of somatostatin and dopamine receptors in gastro-entero-pancreatic tumors opens new therapeutic strategies. *Eur J Endocrinol*, in press.

Park SK, O'Dorisio MS, O'Dorisio TM. (1996) Vasoactive intestinal polypeptide-secreting tumors: biology and therapy. *Baillieres Clin Gastroenterol* 10(4): 673.

Plockinger U, Wiedenmann B. (2004) Diagnosis of non-functioning neuro-endocrine gastro-enteropancreatic tumors. *Neuroendocrinology* 80 (Suppl 1): 35.

Plockinger U, Rindi G, Arnold R *et al.* (2004) Guidelines for the diagnosis and treatment of neuroendocrine gastrointestinal tumors. A consensus statement on behalf of the European Neuroendocrine Tumor Society (ENETS). *Neuroendocrinology* 80(6): 394.

Rambaud JC, Hautefeuille M, Ruskone A, Jacquenod P. (1986) Diarrhoea due to circulating agents. *Clin Gastroenterol* 15(3): 603.

Roche A, Girish BV, de Baere T *et al.* (2003) Trans-catheter arterial chemoembolization as first-line treatment for hepatic metastases from endocrine tumors. *Eur Radiol* 13(1): 136.

Ruskone A, Rene E, Chayvialle JA *et al.* (1982) Effect of somatostatin on diarrhea and on small intestinal water and electrolyte transport in a patient with pancreatic cholera. *Dig Dis Sci* 27(5): 459.

Ruszniewski P, Malka D. (2000) Hepatic arterial chemoembolization in the management of advanced digestive endocrine tumors. *Digestion* 62 (Suppl 1): 79.

Ruszniewski P, Rougier P, Roche A *et al.* (1993) Hepatic arterial chemoembolization in patients with liver metastases of endocrine tumors. A prospective phase II study in 24 patients. *Cancer* 71(8): 2624.

Shapiro RS, Shafir M, Sung M, Warner R, Glajchen N. (1998) Cryotherapy of metastatic carcinoid tumors. *Abdom Imaging* 23(3): 314.

Skogseid B, Eriksson B, Lundqvist G *et al.* (1991) Multiple endocrine neoplasia type 1: a 10-year prospective screening study in four kindreds. *J Clin Endocrinol Metab* 73(2): 281.

Skogseid B, Oberg K, Eriksson B *et al.* (1996) Surgery for asymptomatic pancreatic lesion in multiple endocrine neoplasia type I. *World J Surg* 20(7): 872.

Smith SL, Branton SA, Avino AJ *et al.* (1998) Vasoactive intestinal polypeptide secreting islet cell tumors: a 15-year experience and review of the literature. *Surgery* 124(6): 1050.

Soga J. (1998) Statistical evaluation of 2001 carcinoid cases with metastases, collected from literature: a comparative study between ordinary carcinoids and atypical varieties. *J Exp Clin Cancer Res* 17(1): 3.

Soga J, Yakuwa Y. (1999) Somatostatinoma/inhibitory syndrome: a statistical evaluation of 173 reported cases as compared to other pancreatic endocrinomas. *J Exp Clin Cancer Res* 18(1): 13.

Solcia E, Klöppel G, Sobin LH. (2000) Histological typing of endocrine tumors. In: Solcia E, Klöppel G, Sobin LH, eds. *Histological Typing of Endocrine Tumors (International Classification of Tumors)*. Springer, Berlin.

Thomas-Marques L, Murat A, Delemer B *et al.* (2006) Prospective endoscopic ultrasonographic evaluation of the frequency of nonfunctioning pancreaticoduodenal endocrine tumors in patients with multiple endocrine neoplasia type 1. *Am J Gastroenterol* 101(2): 266.

Verner JV, Morrison AB. (1958) Islet cell tumor and a syndrome of refractory watery diarrhea and hypokalemia. *Am J Med* 25(3): 374.

Vinik AI, Moattari AR. (1989) Treatment of endocrine tumors of the pancreas. *Endocrinol Metab Clin North Am* 18(2): 483.

Waldherr C, Pless M, Maecke HR *et al.* (2002) Tumor response and clinical benefit in neuroendocrine tumors after 7.4 GBq (90)Y-DOTATOC. *J Nucl Med* 43(5): 610.

Welin SV, Janson ET, Sundin A *et al.* (2004) High-dose treatment with a long-acting somatostatin analogue in patients with advanced midgut carcinoid tumors. *Eur J Endocrinol* 151(1): 107.

Wermers RA, Fatourechi V, Kvols LK. (1996) Clinical spectrum of hyperglucagonemia associated with malignant neuroendocrine tumors. *Mayo Clin Proc* 71(11): 1030.

Wessels FJ, Schell SR. (2001) Radiofrequency ablation treatment of refractory carcinoid hepatic metastases. *J Surg Res* 95(1): 8.

Yao C, Ng C, Hoff PM *et al.* (2005) Improved progression free survival (PFS), and rapid, sustained decrease in tumor perfusion among patients with advanced carcinoid treated with bevacizumab. *J Clin Oncol* A4007.

Yu F, Venzon DJ, Serrano J *et al.* (1999) Prospective study of the clinical course, prognostic factors, causes of death, and survival in patients with long-standing Zollinger–Ellison syndrome. *J Clin Oncol* 17(2): 615.

Midgut and appendiceal tumors

Barbro Eriksson

Introduction

Neuroendocrine tumors of the gastrointestinal tract have traditionally been called 'carcinoids'. The most common carcinoid is nowadays the small intestinal carcinoid. Although most midgut carcinoids are non-functioning, those that have metastasized to the liver can give rise to the carcinoid syndrome caused by an excess production of amines and peptides. The carcinoid syndrome consists of diarrhea, flush, and carcinoid heart disease. Carcinoid heart disease mainly involves tricuspid and pulmonary valves. Measurements of urinary 5-HIAA and plasma chromogranin A establish biochemical diagnosis. Staging, which is important for the therapeutic decision, is best achieved by performing somatostatin receptor scintigraphy. Survival depends on the stage at diagnosis and the proliferation index and in patients with liver metastases at diagnosis 10-year survival rates have been <30%.

Neuroendocrine (NE) tumors of the gastrointestinal tract, previously called 'carcinoids', are rare tumors. They originate from the enterochromaffin Kulschitzky cells of the intestine and have the capacity to produce various amines and peptides. Traditionally, these tumors were classified according to embryonic origin into foregut (stomach, duodenum, and pancreas), midgut (small bowel, appendix, cecum, and proximal colon) and hindgut carcinoids (distal colon and rectum) (Williams & Sandler 1963). However, a new revised WHO classification has introduced the general terms neuroendocrine tumor and neuroendocrine carcinoma of different organs (Capella *et al.* 1994). Based on a combination of microscopic structural criteria and immunohistochemistry using the proliferation index (PI) Ki-67 or mitotic index, benign tumors are distinguished from those with uncertain behavior and those which are high-grade malignant.

Diagnosis

Epidemiology

The most recent studies indicate an overall incidence of midgut carcinoids of 0.2–2 per year (Hemminki & Li 2001; Modlin *et al.* 2003). However, autopsy studies revealed a much higher incidence, indicating the subclinical behavior of most of these tumors (Berge & Linell 1976). The incidence of the carcinoid syndrome has been reported to be between 0.5/100.000 and 0.7/100,000 (Berge & Linell 1976; Hemminki & Li 2001; Modlin *et al.* 2003).

Hence, the incidence of endocrine midgut tumors is much higher than those in the foregut and hindgut region. Tumors of the lower jejunum and ileum account for 23–28% of all gastrointestinal endocrine tumors (Kulke & Mayer 1999; Modlin *et al.* 2003). Midgut endocrine tumors occur in an equal proportion in males and females, with an age peak in the sixth and seventh decades (Modlin *et al.* 2003). Midgut tumors have been reported to be multicentric in 26–30% and associated with other non-carcinoid malignancies (adenocarcinoma of the gastrointestinal tract, breast cancer, and others) in 15–29% (Modlin *et al.* 2003). These frequent NET develop quite preferentially in the terminal ileum and ocassionally in the immediately adjacent cecum, including the cecal valve.

The incidence rate of appendiceal endocrine tumors has been reported to be 0.075 new cases per 100,000 per year (Modlin *et al.* 2003). Interestingly, appendiceal carcinoids from being the most common carcinoids now constitute 19% of all gastrointestinal tumors and hence are less frequent than small intestinal carcinoids (Modlin *et al.* 2003). They appear at an earlier age, most commonly in the fourth and fifth decades of life, and are more often seen in women.

NE midgut tumors are seldom part of a familiar genetic disorder. However, a familiar clustering of midgut carcinoids (in two to three generations) appears to exist although the genetic background has not yet been elucidated (Kaltsas *et al.* 2004b).

Clinical presentation

Endocrine midgut tumors can be divided according to their clinical behavior into functioning and non-functioning tumors; the latter constitute about 90% of the tumors (Capella *et al.* 1994). The functioning tumors are responsible for the carcinoid syndrome. Most endocrine midgut tumors are well differentiated and slow growing, whereas a minority have a more aggressive course (Kaltsas *et al.* 2004b).

Carcinoid tumors less than 1 cm in diameter that are confined to the mucosa and submucosa generally do not cause any symptoms and are discovered while searching for a primary tumor in patients newly diagnosed with liver metastases or incidentally during colonoscopy. At the time of diagnosis, midgut carcinoid tumors are commonly larger than 2 cm and have invaded the muscularis propria and also metastasized to regional lymph nodes. Typical symptoms include intermittent abdominal discomfort misinterpreted as irritable bowel disease, sometimes for many years. Peritumoral fibrosis can lead to intestinal obstruction by adhesions of intestinal loops or luminal stricture (Marshall & Bodnarchuk 1993). Furthermore, fibrosis around mesenteric metastases causes fixation of the ileal mesentery to the retroperitoneum, with fibrous bands obstructing the small intestine and transverse colon. This desmoplastic reaction may culminate in hydronephrosis or small bowel ischemia (Sakai *et al.* 2000). The patients may then complain of feeding-related abdominal pain, obstipation of diarrhea, a palpable abdominal mass, or weight loss.

Appendiceal carcinoids are typically detected incidentally during appendectomy. They can contribute to the development of appendicitis by obstructing the lumen.

The carcinoid syndrome

The enterochromaffin cells and carcinoid tumors have the capacity to produce amines, such as 5-hydroxytryptamine (serotonin). In the liver, serotonin is metabolized to 5-hydroxyindoleacetic acid (5-HIAA) (Kema *et al.* 2000). In patients with liver metastases or extrahepatic metastases (retroperitoneum, ovaries), excess serotonin will enter the systemic circulation.

The carcinoid syndrome was first described by Thorson *et al.*in 1954 and includes symptoms of flush, diarrhea, carcinoid heart disease, and bronchoconstriction (Thorsson 1954). It is almost exclusively associated with midgut carcinoids. The diarrhea is believed to be caused by the excess production of serotonin or other factors (Oberg *et al.* 1987; von der Ohe *et al.*

1993), whereas the flush may be mediated by vasoactive substances such as tachy- and bradykinins (Norheim *et al.* 1987b).

Diarrhea, occurring in up to 80% of patients, can be hormonal caused by serotonin or possibly other substances, but other mechanisms can also produce diarrhea. Short bowel syndrome following bowel resection to remove primary tumor or metastases may lead to considerable malabsorption of fat, bile acids and bacterial overgrowth.

Flushing occurs in up to 90% of patients and is usually provoked by spicy food, alcohol, and physical and psychologic stress, and is often worse in the morning. The typical midgut flush is diffuse and erythematous, commonly affecting the face, neck and upper chest, and of short duration, lasting from 1 to 5 minutes. Patients with a later stage of malignant carcinoid demonstrate a more violaceous flush, which affects the same areas of the body often lasting a little longer.

Carcinoid heart disease develops in 40–45% of patients (Zuetenhorst *et al.* 2003) and was described as the cause of death of one-third of patients (Norheim *et al.* 1987a). It is characterized by plaque-like, fibrous endocardial thickening that principally involves the right side of the heart, causing retraction and fixation of the leaflets of the tricuspid and pulmonary valves as well as diminished right ventricular function (Simula *et al.* 2002). Tricuspid regurgitation is a nearly universal finding. These valvular lesions will eventually lead to right-sided heart failure. The pathogenesis of the fibrosis in the right side of the heart has not been established. Several studies have shown that U-5-HIAA and tachykinins are higher in those patients with carcinoid heart disease than in those without it (Norheim *et al.* 1987a). Serotonin and tachykinins are probably involved but other factors are most likely involved as well, such as members of the TGF-β-family and a downstream mediator of TGF- β activities, connective tissue growth factor (CTGF), participating in matrix formation and collagen deposition (Waltenberger *et al.* 1993).

The causative agent for bronchial constriction is not known, but both tachykinins and bradykinins have been suggested as mediators. These agents can constrict smooth muscle in the respiratory tract and also cause local edema in the airways (Hua *et al.* 1984; Gardner *et al.* 1967).

Carcinoid crisis is a severe exacerbation of symptoms often provoked by anesthesia or invasive procedures, such as surgery, if the patients are not on continuous somatostatin analog treatment. The clinical picture includes severe flushing, hypo- or hypertension, diarrhea, severe bronchospasm and cardiac arrythmias.

Diagnostic procedures

Biochemical diagnosis

A clinical constellation of symptoms should lead to confirmation of the diagnosis using biochemical tests.

Patients with NE tumors of the midgut have increased serotonin production, and elevated serotonin levels can be measured directly in the plasma or indirectly via the serotonin metabolite, 5-HIAA, in the urine (Feldman & O'Dorisio 1986). Elevated 24-hour urinary 5-HIAA levels have a sensitivity of 73% and a specificity of 100% in predicting the presence of a carcinoid tumor in the midgut area (Feldman & O'Dorisio 1986; Ardill & Erikkson 2003). Collection of urine should be performed during diet restriction (bananas, chocolate, tea, coffee, walnuts, and spicy food should be avoided). Usually the mean of two 24-hour collections is estimated.

Plasma chromogranin A is increased in 87% of patients with midgut carcinoids (Janson *et al.* 1997). It also appears to correlate with tumor burden and can therefore be used to predict prognosis, particularly in classic midgut carcinoid tumors (Janson *et al.* 1997). This relationship is attested by a postresection study in which the presence of ileal lymph node metastases was associated with chromogranin A elevation in all 25 patients, whereas only three had elevation of 5-HIAA (Eriksson & Oberg 1991). Often elevation of chromogranin A can precede radiologic evidence of a recurrence in different types of NE tumors.

If chromogranin A and urinary 5-HIAA are normal but a midgut carcinoid is strongly suspected, a provocative test with pentagastrin measuring the tachykinin, neuropeptide K (NPK), can be performed (Modlin & Tang 1997).

False positive elevation of chromogranin A can be seen in renal impairment, liver failure, atrophic gastritis, and inflammatory bowel disease (Granberg *et al.* 1999).

Imaging

Topographic localization of the primary tumor and metastases should be undertaken before a therapeutic strategy can be established. Care should be taken to consider features special to carcinoids, such as multicentricity, associated neoplasms, peritoneal and cardiac manifestations.

Many radiologic techniques have been used to localize and image carcinoid tumors; however, the utility is dependent of tumor size and location. In most patients with a metastasized midgut carcinoid, transabdominal US is often the initial imaging procedure disclosing the presence of liver metastases (Andersson *et al.* 1987). The sensitivity has been rather poor but with new contrast media this has improved and it may also be used to guide percutaneous coarse-needle biopsies for histopathologic diagnosis. Additionally, contrast-enhanced CT or MRI can be performed, which complement each other (Ricke *et al.* 2001; Bader *et al.* 2001; Kaltsas *et al.* 2004a). The sensitivity of these methods has improved during the last few years; for example three-phase high-resolution CT, and CT/MRI can also visualize desmoplastic reactions in the mesentery. In the detection of liver metastases, MRI is considered to be superior to CT (Bader *et al.* 2001). However, none of these methods are particularly sensitive in the detection of small primary tumors.

Midgut carcinoid tumors express large numbers of high-affinity somatostatin receptors in 80–90% of patients, a phenomenon that can be exploited for scintigraphic imaging (Reubi 2003; de Herder *et al.* 2003). ^{111}In-labeled DTPA-d-Phe-10-(octreotide) (Octreoscan®) was developed for scintigraphy because it shares the receptor-binding profile of octreotide, rendering it an ideal radiopharmaceutical for imaging of

SSTR2- and SSTR5-positive tumors (Krenning *et al.* 1993; Kwekkeboom & Krenning 1996). It is now used routinely to stage carcinoid tumors and can detect both primary tumors and metatstatic lesions in lung, breast, and bone, not apparent by conventional radiologic imaging techniques. It is a non-invasive whole-body examination, which is performed over 2 days, and provides staging of the disease and should be the initial imaging procedure. Several studies have shown that performing Octreoscan alters the management of NE tumor patients in up to 40% of cases (Termanini *et al.* 1997). There are some limitations to the method with regard to the spatial resolution (<1 cm) and negativity in lesions lacking the expression of SSTR2 and 5. Additional CT/MR should be performed for exact anatomic localization and estimation of size of lesions.

Colonoscopy can identify primary tumors in the distal ileum, at the iliocecal valve or in the right-sided colon. Barium enema and enteroclysis of the small intestine, both established methods for detection of small primaries, are rarely indicated (Taal *et al.* 1996). Instead, new methods such as caspsule endoscopy or double balloon enteroscopy are promising but their utility has not yet been elucidated.

Other imaging techniques that have been used include ^{123}I- or ^{131}I-meta-iodobenzylguanidin (MIBG)-scintigraphy, based on the presence of catecholamine transporters in the tumors; however, the sensitivity in midgut carcinoids varies between 60 and 85% (Taal *et al.* 1996). Promising new whole-body techniques are PET with specific tracers for neuroendocrine tumors, ^{18}F-DOPA and ^{11}C-5-hydroxytryptophan (Orlefors *et al.* 1998; Hoegerle *et al.* 2001). These tracers were developed based on the amine precursor uptake and decarboxylation (APUD) properties of NE tumors. Both methods have been shown to be superior to Octreoscan for the detection of small primaries and lymph node metastases (Orlefors *et al.* 1998; Hoegerle *et al.* 2001). Whereas ^{11}C-5-HTP appears to be a universal tracer for NE tumors (lung, pancreas, midgut, hindgut) with more than 90% sensitivity (Orlefors *et al.* 1998), ^{18}F-DOPA is excellent for detection of classical midgut carcinoids (>90% sensitivity) (Koopmans *et al.* 2006) but not as sensitive for visualization of 'non-carcinoid' tumors (<25%) (Montravers *et al.* 2006).

Recently, PET tracers based on the presence of somatostatin receptors in NE tumors have come into use, mainly ^{68}Ga-DOTATOC, in several centers (Hofmann *et al.* 2001). ^{68}Ga-DOTATOC-PET has already been shown to be more sensitive than Octreoscan (Hofmann *et al.* 2001), detecting 30% more lesions. Another advantage of using this PET tracer is the fact that no cyclotron is required, which should make the procedure less expensive and more accessible and the examination can be performed in 1 day. Furthermore, this method should allow quantification of the density of somatostatin receptors, which could help to optimize treatment with radiolabeled somatostatin analogs.

Echocardiography is mandatory in patients with the carcinoid syndrome to confirm or exclude carcinoid heart disease (Lundin *et al.* 1990). Conventional bone scan can be performed in the few cases where Octreoscan fails to visualize skeletal metastases. MRI and plain X-ray can be performed to determine the extent of bone involvement and risk of fractures.

Histopathology

To establish the diagnosis of a midgut carcinoid tumor, the growth pattern of the tumor can be looked at. However, the most important immunohistochemical marker for these tumors is a positive staining for chromogranin A (Lloyd & Wilson 1983). Previously more laborious silver stainings indicating argyrophilic and argentaffin properties of the midgut tumors were used, but nowadays in clinical practice, staining for chromogranin A is a routine procedure. In cases of unknown primary, identification of enterochromaffin cells can be achieved by staining for serotonin.

Staging

As mentioned above, there is a revised WHO classification for NE tumors based on combining microscopic structural criteria and immunohistochemistry with the proliferation marker Ki-67. For midgut and appendiceal carcinoids the clinicopathologic staging according to WHO is the following (Solcia 2000).

Midgut and appendiceal carcinoids: clinicopathologic staging

1 Well-differentiated endocrine tumor (carcinoid): Benign behavior: confined to the mucosa-submucosa, non-angioinvasive, <1 cm in size
- 1.1 Serotonin-producing tumor
- 1.2 Enteroglucagon-producing tumor

2 Uncertain behavior: non-functioning, confined to mucosa-submucosa, >1 cm in size, or angioinvasive
- 2.1 Serotonin-producing tumor
- 2.2 Enteroglucagon-producing tumor

3 Well-differentiated endocrine carcinoma (malignant carcinoid), low-grade malignant, deeply invasive (muscularis propria or beyond), or with metastases
- 3.1 Serotonin-producing tumor with or without carcinoid syndrome
- 3.2 Enteroglucagon-producing carcinoma

4 Poorly differentiated endocrine carcinoma (small-cell carcinoma), high-grade malignant

5 Mixed exocrine-endocrine carcinoma—moderate to high-grade malignant

Endocrine tumors of the appendix: clinicopathologic staging

1 Well-differentiated endocrine tumor (carcinoid), benign behavior, non-funtioning, confined to appendiceal wall, non-angioinvasive
- 1.1 Serotonin-producing tumor
- 1.2 Enteroglucagon-producing tumor—uncertain behavior, non-functioning, confined to subserosa, >2 cm in size, or angioinvasive tumor

2 Well-differentiated endocrine carcinoma (malignant carcinoid), low-grade malignant, invading the mesoappendix or beyond, and/or with metastases
- 2.1 Serotonin-producing endocrine tumor with or without carcinoid syndrome

3 Mixed exocrine-endocrine carcinoma

4 Low-grade, malignant, goblet cell carcinoid

The new imaging techniques have greatly facilitated a more exact staging of NE tumors. A tumor/nodes/metastases (TNM) classification is under way to supplement the European Neuroendocrine Tumor Society (ENETS) revised guidelines for midgut carcinoid tumors. After validation, this TNM classification will hopefully provide a powerful prognostic tool that can also allow more reliable comparisons between different clinical studies.

Prognosis

The prognosis of endocrine tumors of the distal small intestine is rather different from that of tumors originating in the duodenum, stomach and rectum, since they frequently metastasize to regional lymph nodes and later to the liver (Strodel *et al.* 1983; Burke *et al.* 1997). The 10-year survival rate is approximately 60% if liver metastases are absent, and 15–25% in the presence of liver metastases at diagnosis (McDermott *et al.* 1994; Quaedvlieg *et al.* 2001). Hence, the stage of the disease at presentation affects the survival. Also tumor grade is of importance, since patients with slow-growing well-differentiated tumors with low Ki-67 live longer than those with a high Ki-67.

In a relatively recently published retrospective study, removal of the primary could make the prognosis more favorable (Hellman *et al.* 2002).

Patients with appendiceal carcinoids have a more favorable prognosis. Tumors <2 cm in size, confined to the appendiceal wall and not angioinvasive are cured by appendectomy (Thompson *et al.* 1985; Moertel *et al.* 1987; MacGillivray *et al.* 1992). Invasion of the mesoappendix, a size of >2 cm and angioinvasion indicate an uncertain malignant behavior as does the location of the tumor at the base of the appendix with involvement of the surgical margin or cecum (Solcia 2000). Five-year survival of patients with appendiceal carcinoid is 95% for localized disease, 83% for those with regional disease and 34% for those with distant metastases (Thompson *et al.* 1985; Moertel *et al.* 1987; MacGillivray *et al.* 1992).

The new TNM classification and grading system will as mentioned be an important prognostic tool.

Follow-up during/after treatment

Patients with liver metastases

Ultrasonography or MR/CT and biochemical markers, including those initially elevated every 3 months. Diagnosis of bone metastases (if clinical signs are present) by Octreoscan and/or bone scan and MR.

Patients without liver metastases

Long-term follow-up because of the possibility of late recurrences. If curative surgery has been performed, Octreoscan or PET should be done after 6 months. Plasma chromogranin A will signal early recurrence.

References

Andersson T, Eriksson B, Hemmingsson A, Lindgren PG, Oberg K. (1987) *Acta Radiol* 28: 535–9.

Ardill JE, Erikkson B. (2003) *Endocr Relat Cancer* 10: 459–62.

Bader TR, Semelka RC, Chiu VC, Armao DM, Woosley JT. (2001) *J Magn Reson Imaging* 14: 261–9.

Berge T, Linell F. (1976) *Acta Pathol Microbiol Scand [A]* 84: 322–30.

Burke AP, Thomas RM, Elsayed AM, Sobin LH. (1997) *Cancer* 79: 1086–93.

Capella C, Heitz PU, Hofler H, Solcia E, Kloppel G. (1994) *Digestion* 55 (Suppl 3): 11–23.

de Herder WW, Hofland LJ, van der Lely AJ, Lamberts SW. (2003) *Endocr Relat Cancer* 10: 451–8.

Eriksson B, Oberg K. (1991) *Acta Oncol* 30: 477–83.

Feldman JM, O'Dorisio TM. (1986) *Am J Med* 81: 41–8.

Gardner B, Dollinger M, Silen W, Back N, O'Reilly S. (1967) *Surgery* 61: 846–52.

Granberg D, Stridsberg M, Seensalu R *et al.* (1999) *J Clin Endocrinol Metab* 84: 2712–7.

Hellman P, Lundstrom T, Ohrvall U *et al.* (2002) *World J Surg* 26: 991–7.

Hemminki K, Li X. (2001) *Cancer* 92: 2204–10.

Hoegerle S, Altehoefer C, Ghanem N *et al.* (2001) *Radiology* 220: 373–80.

Hofmann M, Maecke H, Borner R *et al.* (2001) *Eur J Nucl Med* 28: 1751–7.

Hua X, Lundberg JM, Theodorsson-Norheim E, Brodin E. (1984) *Naunyn Schmiedebergs Arch Pharmacol* 328: 196–201.

Janson ET, Holmberg L, Stridsberg M *et al.* (1997) *Ann Oncol* 8: 685–90.

Kaltsas G, Rockall A, Papadogias D, Reznek R, Grossman AB. (2004a) *Eur J Endocrinol* 151: 15–27.

Kaltsas GA, Besser GM, Grossman AB. (2004b) *Endocr Rev* 25: 458–511.

Kema IP, de Vries EG, Muskiet FA. (2000) *J Chromatogr B Biomed Sci Appl* 747: 33–48.

Koopmans KP, de Vries EG, Kema IP *et al.* (2006) *Lancet Oncol* 7: 728–34.

Krenning EP, Kwekkeboom DJ, Bakker WH *et al.* (1993) *Eur J Nucl Med* 20: 716–31.

Kulke MH, Mayer RJ. (1999) *N Engl J Med* 340: 858–68.

Kwekkeboom DJ, Krenning EP. (1996) *World J Surg* 20: 157–61.

Lloyd RV, Wilson BS. (1983) *Science* 222: 628–30.

Lundin L, Landelius J, Andren B, Oberg K. (1990) *Br Heart J* 64: 190–4.

MacGillivray DC, Heaton RB, Rushin JM, Cruess DF. (1992) *Surgery* 111: 466–71.

Marshall JB, Bodnarchuk G. (1993) *J Clin Gastroenterol* 16: 123–9.

McDermott EW, Guduric B, Brennan MF. (1994) *Br J Surg* 81: 1007–9.

Modlin IM, Lye KD, Kidd M. (2003) *Cancer* 97: 934–59.

Modlin IM, Tang LH. (1997) *Gastroenterology* 112: 583–90.

Moertel CG, Weiland LH, Nagorney DM, Dockerty MB. (1987) *N Engl J Med* 317: 1699–701.

Montravers F, Grahek D, Kerrou K *et al.* (2006) *J Nucl Med* 47: 1455–62.

Norheim I, Oberg K, Theodorsson-Norheim E *et al.* (1987a) *Ann Surg* 206: 115–25.

Norheim I, Wilander E, Oberg K *et al.* (1987b) *Eur J Cancer Clin Oncol* 23: 689–95.

Oberg K, Theodorsson-Norheim E, Norheim I. (1987) *Scand J Gastroenterol* 22: 1041–8.
Orlefors H, Sundin A, Ahlstrom H *et al.* (1998) *J Clin Oncol* 16: 2534–41.
Quaedvlieg PF, Visser O, Lamers CB, Janssen-Heijen ML, Taal BG. (2001) *Ann Oncol* 12: 1295–300.
Reubi JC. (2003) *Endocr Rev* 24: 389–427.
Ricke J, Klose KJ, Mignon M, Oberg K, Wiedenmann B. (2001) *Eur J Radiol* 37: 8–17.
Sakai D, Murakami M, Kawazoe K, Tsutsumi Y. (2000) *Pathol Int* 50: 404–11.
Simula DV, Edwards WD, Tazelaar HD, Connolly HM, Schaff HV. (2002) *Mayo Clin Proc* 77: 139–47.
Solcia EKG, Sobin LH (in collaboration with 9 pathologists from 4 countries). (2000) *Histological Typing of Endocrine Tumors. WHO International Histological Classification of Tumors*, 2nd edn. Springer, Berlin.
Strodel WE, Talpos G, Eckhauser F, Thompson N. (1983) *Arch Surg* 118: 391–7.
Taal BG, Hoefnagel CA, Valdes Olmos RA, Boot H. (1996) *Eur J Cancer* 32A: 1924–32.
Termanini B, Gibril F, Reynolds JC *et al.* (1997) *Gastroenterology* 112: 335–47.
Thompson GB, van Heerden JA, Martin JK Jr *et al.* (1985) *Surgery* 98: 1054–63.
Thorsson ABG, Waldenstrom J (1954) *Ann Heart J* 47: 795–817.
Waltenberger J, Lundin L, Oberg K *et al.* (1993) *Am J Pathol* 142: 71–8.
Williams ED, Sandler M. (1963) *Lancet* 1: 238–9.
von der Ohe MR, Camilleri M, Kvols LK, Thomforde GM. (1993) *N Engl J Med* 329: 1073–8.
Zuetenhorst JM, Bonfrer JM, Korse CM, Bakker R, van Tinteren H, Taal BG. (2003) *Cancer* 97: 1609–15.

Neuroendocrine tumors of the colon and rectum

Christoph J. Auernhammer

The historical term 'carcinoid' was introduced by Oberndorfer (1907). Williams and Sandler (1963) classified neuroendocrine tumors according to their embryologic site into foregut (bronchopulmonary, stomach, duodenum, pancreas), midgut (jejunum, ileum, appendix, coecum, ascending colon) and hindgut tumors (transverse and descending colon, sigmoid, rectum). The current WHO classification (2000) of neuroendocrine tumors uses a site-specific nomenclature (neuroendocrine tumor of the stomach, duodenum, pancreas, jejunum, ileum, appendix, cecum, colon, rectum) and abandoned the term 'carcinoid' by introducing a histopathologic differentiation (well-differentiated neuroendocrine tumor, well-differentiated neuroendocrine carcinoma, poorly differentiated neuroendocrine carcinoma). This classification adresses the specific tumor entities and their clinical and prognostic characteristics. Neuroendocrine tumors of the colon and rectum (hindgut tumors) will be discussed in this section, focussing on their epidemiology, clinical presentation and diagnosis, staging, prognosis, therapeutic strategies and follow-up.

Epidemiology

In a large series of 13,715 neuroendocrine tumors 24.5% occurred in the trachebronchopulmonary system and 66.9% in the gastrointestinal system. The general incidence of all neuroendocrine tumors increased from 8.5 per 10^6 in the year 1973 to 38.4 per 10^6 in the year 1997. In all neuroendocrine tumors of the gastrointestinal tract, the most common sites are small intestine 41.8–44.7%, rectum 19.6–24.1%, appendix 16.7–24.1%, colon (without rectum and appendix) 7.8–10.6%. In an epidemiologic database of 522,630 colorectal cancers, 96% were adenocarcinomas and 2% were neuroendocrine tumors.

Colon

The incidence of neuroendocrine tumors of the colon is 1.0–2.0 per 10^6 and has remained constant over the last five decades. The incidence of neuroendocrine tumors of the colon does not show any significant racial differences and no gender disparities. The average age at diagnosis is 70 years.

Neuroendocrine tumors of the colon (without rectum and appendix) are most common in the cecum at approximately 50%. Rarer locations are the sigmoid and rectosigmoid junction, ascending colon, hepatic flexure, transverse colon, splenic flexure and descending colon. Thus hindgut colonic neuroendocrine tumors (transverse and descending colon, sigmoid) are rare tumor entities.

Rectum

The incidence of neuroendocrine tumors of the rectum increased constantly from 0.4 per 10^6 in the year 1973 to 4.2 per 10^6 in the year 1997. Within all neuroendocrine tumors of the gastrointestinal tract, the percentage of neuroendocrine tumors of the rectum increased from 8.1% (1973–1979) to 15.7% (1980–1989) and 25.4% (1990–1997). This increase is probably due to increased frequency of endoscopy and increased awareness in histologic diagnosis and reporting. The incidence of neuroendocrine tumors of the rectum is two- to threefold higher in black than in white patients and three- to fourfold higher in Asian than in non-Asian patients. The incidence of neuroendocrine tumors of the rectum does not show any significant gender disparities. The average age at diagnosis is 46–52 years. Currently rectal neuroendocrine tumors are the third most common gastrointestinal neuroendocrine tumor.

Histopathology, staging and grading

The minimum requirement for the histopathologic work-up of a neuroendocrine tumor is to perform an immunhistochemical staining against synaptophysin and chromogranin A.

Neuron-specific enolase and PGP 9.5 can be used as additional general markers for neuroendocrine tumors. While typical midgut carcinoids and neuroendocrine tumors of the proximal colon stain positive against serotonin, neuroendocrine tumors of the rectum generally stain negative against serotonin. Neuroendocrine tumors of the proximal colon are (serotonin-positive) EC cell tumors. In contrast, neuroendocrine tumors of the rectum are well-differentiated L-cell tumors which produce glucagon-like immunoreactants (e.g. glycentin, glucagon-29, glucagon-37), pancreatic polypeptide (PP) and pancreatic-polypeptide–like peptide PYY. The majority (70–80%) of rectal carcinoids shows positive immunhistochemical staining for prostate acid phoshatase, in contrast to only 15% of neuroendocrine tumors of other gastrointestinal sites.

The current WHO classification of neuroendocrine tumors differentiates between well-differentiated endocrine tumors of benign or uncertain behavior (WHO grade I), well-differentiated endocrine carcinomas—low-grade malignant (WHO grade II)) and poorly differentiated endocrine carcinomas—high-grade malignant (WHO grade III). This WHO classification has been very recently accomplished by an ENETS proposal for a TNM classification and a histologic grading system for midgut and hindgut neuroendocrine tumors. The use of this TNM classification (Table 23.7), staging system (Table 23.8), and grading system (Table 23.9) is highly recommended in clinical practice. According to the WHO classification and ENETs grading system, mitotic indexing and determination of the proliferation index Ki-67 by use of the MIB1 antibody are essentially required procedures in the grading process. The ENETS proposal reflects an effort to establish a clinicopathologic report system with high prognostic impact. Therapeutic strategies must be adjusted according to staging and grading in each individual tumor patient.

Rare histopathologic findings are multiple neuroendocrine tumors of the rectum, composite adenoma/adenocarcinoma and carcinoid tumors, or poorly differentiated rectal neuroendocine carcinomas with a high proliferation index Ki-67 > 20% (grading G3).

Table 23.7 TNM classification for neuroendocrine tumors of colon and rectum—a working proposal (excerpted from Rindi *et al.* 2007 with permission from Springer).

T: primary tumor	
TX	primary tumor cannot be assessed
T0	No evidence of primary tumor
T1	Tumor invades mucosa or submucosa
	T1a size <1 cm
	T1b size 1–2 cm
T2	Tumor invades muscularis propria or size >2 cm
T3	Tumor invades subserosa/pericolic/perirectal fat
T4	Tumor directly invades other organs/structures and/or perforates visceral peritoneum
For any T add (m) for multiple tumors	
N: regional lymph nodes	
NX	Regional lymph node status cannot be assessed
N0	No regional lymph node metastasis
N1	Regional lymph node metastasis
M: distant metastases	
MX	Distant metastasis cannot be assessed
M0	No distant metastasis
M1	Distant metastasis

Stage at diagnosis and prognostic markers

Colon

Neuroendocrine tumors of the colon are often diagnosed at a late stage. The incidence of metastasis according to *primary tumor size* is estimated for neuroendocrine tumors of the colon to be 18% for tumors <1 cm and 55% for tumors >2 cm. At diagnosis, 85–90% of all neuroendocrine tumors of the colon are >2 cm and show metastasis in more than 50% of cases (regional 21.9% and distant 32.5%). Accordingly, 5-year cancer-specific survival rates of all stages are 69.5%; this is composed of 5-year cancer-specific survival rates of 94.1% for local stage, 72.5% for regional stage and 27.8% for distant stage.

Table 23.8 Disease staging for neuroendocrine tumors of colon and rectum—a working proposal (excerpted from Rindi *et al.* 2007 with permission from Springer).

Disease stages	T-primary tumor	N-regional nodes	M-distant metastasis
Stage IA	T1a	N0	M0
Stage IB	T1b	N0	M0
Stage IIA	T2	N0	M0
Stage IIB	T3	N0	M
Stage IIIA	T4	N0	M0
Stage IIIB	Any T	N1	M0
Stage IV	Any T	Any N	M1

Table 23.9 Grading for neuroendocrine tumors of colon and rectum—a working proposal (excerpted from Rindi *et al.* 2007 with permission from Springer). Mitotic counts should be assessed in at least 40 high-power fields (HPF) and mitotic counts per 10 HPF should be reported. Ki-67 proliferation index should be assessed by use of the MIB1 antibody and the percentage of positive tumor cells from 2000 analysed tumor cells should be reported.

Grade	Mitotic count (10 HPF)	Ki-67 index (%)
G1	<2	<2
G2	2–20	3–20
G3	>20	>20

Rectum

Neuroendocrine tumors of the rectum are often diagnosed at a local stage (88.2%) and show metastasis in less than 15% of cases (regional 5.0% and distant 6.8%). Accordingly, 5-year cancer-specific survival rates of all stages are 87.5–88.1%; this is composed of cancer-specific 5-year survival rates of 94.9–98.9% for local stage, 53.7% for regional stage and 14.6% for distant stage. Colorectal carcinoids without metastasis have a better prognosis than adenocarcinomas. However, the survival rates of patients with regional or distant metastasized colorectal neuroendocrine carcinomas are comparable and not preferable to those with adenocarcinomas at the same stage.

The typical rectum carcinoid is a solitary well-differentiated neuroendocrine tumor with low proliferation index Ki-67 <2% (grading G1). The incidence of metastasis according to *primary tumor size* is estimated for typical neuroendocrine tumors of the rectum to be 1–3% (up to 7% in single series) for tumors <10 mm, 5–15% (up to 40% in single series) for tumors 10–20 mm and 60–80% for tumors >20 mm. Risk factors for lymph node metastasis are tumor size >10 mm and lymphatic invasion; risk factors for distant metastasis are tumor size >20 mm and venous invasion. Neuroendocrine tumors of the rectum may show an even stronger continous size-dependent risk of metastasis. In several large series of rectum carcinoids (largest series n = 777), metastasis rates were calculated as 1.3–3.7% for tumors <5 mm, 9.7–13.2% for tumors 5–10 mm, 27.6% for tumors 10–20 mm and 53.6–56.7% for tumors >20 mm. The median tumor size in tumors without metastasis versus with metastasis was 8.4 mm versus 14.9 mm. Besides primary tumor size, other important prognostic risk factors are *atypical endoscopic features (central depression, ulceration), depth of invasion (mucosa/submucosa vs muscularis propria or deeper), mitotic rate (Ki-67 < 2%, Ki-67 2–20%, KI-67 > 20%), lymphatic invasion, venous invasion.*

In contrast to typical carcinoids of the rectum, poorly differentiated neuroendocrine carcinomas of the colon and rectum with a high proliferation index Ki-67 > 20% (grading G3) are rare tumors. These high-grade carcinomas can be small-cell carcinomas as well as large-cell carcinomas. Median survival in this rare tumor entity is only 10–15 months and the 2- and 3-year survival rates are only 26% and 13%, respectively.

Clinical presentation and diagnosis

Colon

Hindgut neuroendocrine tumors of the colon are normally diagnosed at a late stage. Clinical symptoms may include abdominal discomfort, change in bowel habit, lower GI bleeding, abdominal pain in the upper right quadrant, weight loss, fatigue, cachexia. Tumor lesions may also be diagnosed incidentally during a routine abdominal ultrasound or colonoscopy. The tumor often presents like an adenocarcionoma of the colon with hepatic metastasis or an abdominal mass lesion of the colon. The histopathology will revise the diagnosis to neuroendocrine carcinoma of the colon.

Staging includes colonoscopy, abdominal ultrasound and CT/MRI of the abdomen. In general, liver metastases of neuroendocrine carcinomas are hypervascularized. Neuroendocrine liver metastasis can appear in abdominal ultrasound as echo-rich or echo-poor lesions; larger lesions often appear as echo-rich lesions with a centrally echo-poor region (probably according to central necrosis). Power Doppler imaging demonstrates hypervascular lesions in 66% of all cases (metastasis of other origin are hypovascular in 80% of all cases). In ultrasound, especially small neuroendocrine liver metastasis might show similarities to hemangiomas. Contrast-enhanced ultrasound demonstrates arterial phase enhancement in approximately 90% of all cases (metastasis of other origin demonstrates arterial phase enhancement in only approximately 20% of all cases). For the assessment of liver metastasis also triphasic CT scan with an hepatic arterial phase is essentially required. In the arterial phase hypervascularization of the metastasis is shown, while in the portal–venous phase neuroendocrine metastasis are often isointense and therefore may be missed. MRI of the liver with gadolinium and liver-specific contrast agents has a higher sensitivity for the staging of liver metastasis than CT. For the value of nuclear imaging techniques and serum tumor markers see the next paragraph.

Rectum

Approximately 50% of all patients with rectal neuroendocrine tumors are asymptomatic and many neuroendocrine tumors of the rectum will be diagnosed as small tumors <1 cm during routine endoscopy. At diagnosis, 66–75% of all rectal neuroendocrine tumors are <1 cm and 84–96% are <2 cm. Symptoms that may occur mostly in larger tumors are anal bleeding, abdominal pain, anorectal discomfort, change in bowel habits, constipation. The tumor is normally not obstructive to the rectum. The tumor lesions can be located up to 20 cm of the anorectal line, but the majority (75%) are located within 8 cm of the anorectal line.

At *endoscopy* tumors appear as small, round, mobile, submucosal tumors with intact mucosa and smooth yellowish surface (Fig. 23.10a). Atypical endoscopic features (central depression or ulceration) are risk factors for metastasis and thus negative prognostic factors. *Routine endoscopy biopsies* are recommended; however, they may be inconclusive due to the submucosal tumor location. The tumors derive from endocrine cells in the depth of the epithelial glands but then regularly invade the submucosa in the large majority of cases. *Endoscopic-ultrasound fine-needle aspiration (EUS-FNA)* may provide cytology with a high diagnostic yield of 95% in rectal tumors.

EUS is highly recommended in order to diagnose tumor size, to stage tumor invasion (mucosa and submucosa, muscularis propria or deeper) and to evaluate perirectal lymph node

(a)
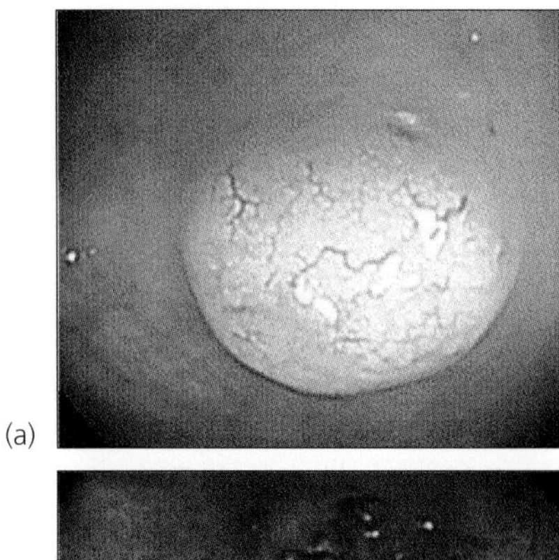

(c)
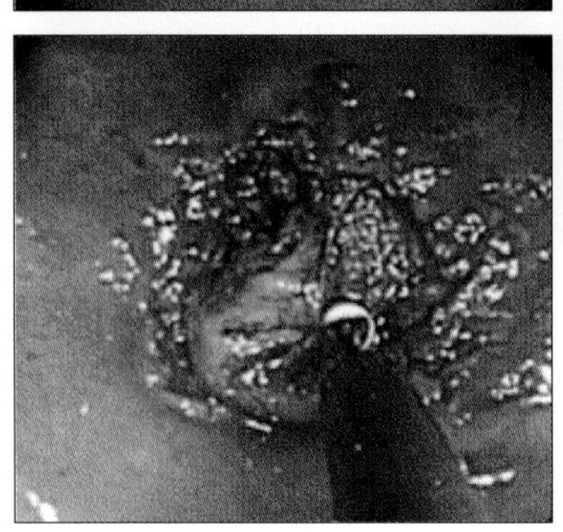

(b)
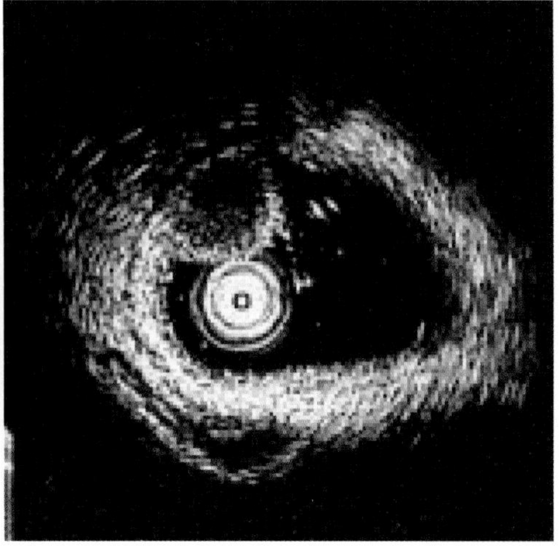

Fig. 23.10 Typical rectal neuroendocrine tumor confined to the submucosa. (a) Endoscopic appearance. Small submucosal tumor with intact mucosa. (b) Endoscopic ultrasound. Rectal neuroendocrine tumor seen as a hypoechoic homogenous mass confined to the submucosa. (c) Endoscopic submucosal dissection of a yellowish tumor. (Figures reprinted from Chen PJ, Hsieh TY, Chao YC. (2007) Clinical challenges and images in GI. *Gastroenterology* 132: 853–4 with permission from Elsevier.)

involvement. The diagnostic value of EUS in staging adenocarcinomas of the rectum has been intensively evaluated and exhibits an accuracy of 80–95% in staging local tumor invasion (T stage) and an accuracy of 70–75% in predicting perirectal lymph node involvement (N stage). In comparison CT and MRI of the pelvis exhibit accuracies of 65–75% and 75–85% in staging local tumor invasion (T stage) and accuracies of 55–65% and 60–65% in predicting perirectal lymph node involvement (N stage) in rectal adenocarcinomas. The diagnostic values of EUS, CT and MRI in staging neuroendocrine tumors of the rectum are probably of similar value but need to be studied more extensively. All methods have only limited value in predicting perirectal lymph node involvement and therefore additional parameters have to be considered for therapeutic decision-making. The majority (75%) of all rectal neuroendocrine tumors are confined to the submucosa, while approximately 20% invade the muscularis propria or deeper. The typical rectal carcinoid appears in EUS as a homogenous hypoechoic mass of the submucosa (Fig. 23.10b). Tumor invasion beyond the submucosa with invasion of the muscularis propria is a negative prognostic sign. Rectal neuroendocrine tumors <1 cm in diameter have a low risk (3%) of metastasis and rectal neuroendocrine tumors of 1–2 cm in diameter have an intermediate risk (10–15%) of metastasis. Local staging with EUS is required to evaluate the extent of rectal wall invasion and perirectal lymph node metastasis. CT/MRI of the pelvis/abdomen are additive methods to adress these questions and in addition can be used to exclude rare hepatic metastasis at this stage. Rectal neuroendocrine tumors >2 cm in diameter often show invasion of the muscularis propria and have a high risk (60%) of regional and distant metastasis. Local staging with endoscopic ultrasound (EUS) and CT/MRI of the pelvis is recommended as well as distant staging with abdominal ultrasound, CT/MRI of the abdomen/liver and chest X-ray/CT of the thorax.

Despite its high diagnostic sensitivity and standard application in neuroendocrine tumors of foregut and midgut origin, the value of 111In-DTPAOC (Octreoscan) SPECT in hindgut neuroendocrine tumors (distal colon and rectum) is discussed controversially in the literature and has not been systematically evaluated in larger studies. In comparison to traditional ^{111}In-DTPAOC (Octreoscan) SPECT, there is a significantly higher sensitivity of ^{99}mTc-EDDA/HYNIC-octreotate SPECT and especially ^{68}Ga-DOTATOC-PET/CT for the detection of somatostatin receptor positive neuroendocrine tumors. For somatostatin receptor-negative neuroendocrine tumors MIBG-scintigraphy is an option. In addition, the ^{18}F-dopa-PET/CT shows high diagnostic sensitivity for somatostatin receptor-negative neuroendocrine tumors and might be also useful in hindgut carcinoids. With regard to hindgut neuroendocrine tumors, no sufficient data on the role of these new promising imaging techniques are available and no recommendations can be given; their use is still investigational. *FDG-PET/CT is not indicated in the majority of neuroendocrine tumors*, as it demonstrates a relatively poor sensitivity in low-grade (G1) and intermediate-grade (G2) neuroendocrine tumors. In contrast, poorly differentiated (high-grade, G3) neuroendocrine carcinomas are a rare indication for FDG-PET/CT in neuroendocrine tumors. *Bone scintigraphy* can be used to assess bone metastasis; however, MRI of the spine and newer PET/CT techniques demonstrate higher sensitivities.

Serum tumor marker chromogranin A is highly recommended as general marker in neuroendocrine tumors, including tumors from the colon and rectum. In contrast, measurement of *5-HIAA in urine and serotonin in serum is neither useful nor indicated in patients with neuroendocrine tumors of the rectum without a carcinoid syndrome.* Most rectal neuroendocrine tumors are not functionally active and the incidence of serotonin-producing EC-cell tumors with carcinoid syndrome in this tumor entity is only 0.2–0.7%. *Serum prostate acid phosphatase* levels may be increased (as 70–80% of rectal carcinoids show positive immunhistochemical staining for prostate acid phosphatase), but its clinical value as a serum tumor marker has not been systematically evaluated.

Therapy

For the indications and results of cytoreductive therapeutic strategies such as surgery of hepatic metastasis and radiofrequency ablation (RFA), debulking surgery, biotherapy, chemotherapy, transarterial hepatic embolization (TAE), selective intra-arterial hepatic radiotherapy (SIRT), peptide receptor radiation therapy (PRRT) with 90yttrium- and ^{177}lutetium-labeled somatostatin analogs, and targeted therapy with tyrosin kinase inhibitors (TKI)/agiogenesis inhibitors in colorectal neuroendocrine carcinomas with distant metastasis (stage M1), please refer to the appropriate chapters in this textbook.

Colon

Most neuroendocrine tumors of the colon are in an advanced stage at diagnosis with tumor size >2 cm and invasion of the muscularis propria. Extended surgery following oncologic surgical rules with hemicolectomy and lymph node dissection should be applied. Aggressive surgery of liver metastasis has been shown to result in an improved survival in several retrospective series of well- and intermediate-differentiated neuroendocrine carcinomas of foregut and midgut origin. Although there are no sufficient data for hindgut neuroendocine carcinomas, a similar approach is recommended.

Rectum

Rectal neuroendocrine tumors <1 cm in diameter are mostly confined to the submucosa and have a low risk of metastasis. These typical tumors (stage IA; T1a, N0, M0) can be locally resected by endoscopic or transanal resection techniques. Cure can be assumed if local excision is complete with histologically clear margins and the tumor is a highly differentiated (low-grade G1) tumor. No further follow-up is required in these cases. Standard polypectomy may not result in complete resection of the submucosal tumor. The following local resection techniques are considered adequate.

1 Endoscopic mucosal resection (EMR). EMR involves the following three steps: submucosal fluid injection to elevate the lesion from the muscularis propria, aspiration of the lesion with a suction cap, and resection with an electrosurgical snare.

2 Endoscopic submucosal dissection (ESD). ESD involves the following three steps: submucosal fluid injection to elevate the lesion from the muscularis propria, 2-mm deep mucosal incision with special cutting knives, and submucosal dissection with an electrosurgical snare or a special cutting knife.

3 Conventional transanal resection allows only resection of lesions located in the distal rectum with a maximum 5–10 cm from the anal verge, while transanal endoscopic microsurgery (TEM) can be performed at any location in the extraperitoneal rectum (e.g. up to 20 cm on the posterior wall, 15 cm laterally and 12 cm on the anterior wall). These different techniques can be used based on local availability and expertise.

Rectal neuroendocrine tumors 1–2 cm in diameter have an intermediate risk of regional metastasis. Provided there is no evidence of invasion of the muscularis muscosae and no evidence of regional lymph node metastasis, tumors of 1–2 cm size (stage IB; T1b, N0, M0) also qualify for local endoscopic resection/transanal surgery. Endoscopic appearance and histologic grading should be further parameters to consider. In these larger tumors >1 cm, ESD and TEM in particular can provide a high rate of *en bloc* resection.

Rectal neuroendocrine tumors >2 cm in diameter often show invasion of the muscularis propria and have a high risk of regional and distant metastasis. Extended surgery with anterior rectal resection or abdominoperineal resection with mesorectal excision and lymph node dissection is recommended in these tumors of size >2 cm (stage IIA; T2, N0, M0), or invasion of the muscularis propria (stage IIA; T2, N0, M0), invasion of the subserosa/perirectal fat (stage IIB; T3, N0, M0), invasion of adjacent organs/structures (stage IIIA; T4, N0, M0), and in all tumors with known regional lymph node involvement (stage IIIB; any T, N1, M0). Some authors favor local excision by transanal surgery also for selected tumors with size >2 cm (stage IIA; T2, N0, M0) or invasion of the muscularis propria (stage IIA; T2, N0, M0). This approach is based on evidence that provided complete local resection of the tumor has been successfully performed, aggressive surgery provides no advantage for the overall survival of theses patients. However, staging of perirectal lymph node involvement with EUS and MRI has only limited sensitivity of approximately 75%. Therefore, extended surgery in these cases should be considered. The value of extended surgery has not been demonstrated in rectal neuroendocrine tumors with diffuse distant metastasis (stage IV; any T, any N, M1). However, the more aggressive approach with surgery of hepatic metastasis in neuroendocrine tumors needs also to be discussed in this tumor entity in the future.

A flowchart of the therapeutic strategy for neuroendocrine tumors of the rectum is shown in Fig. 23.11.

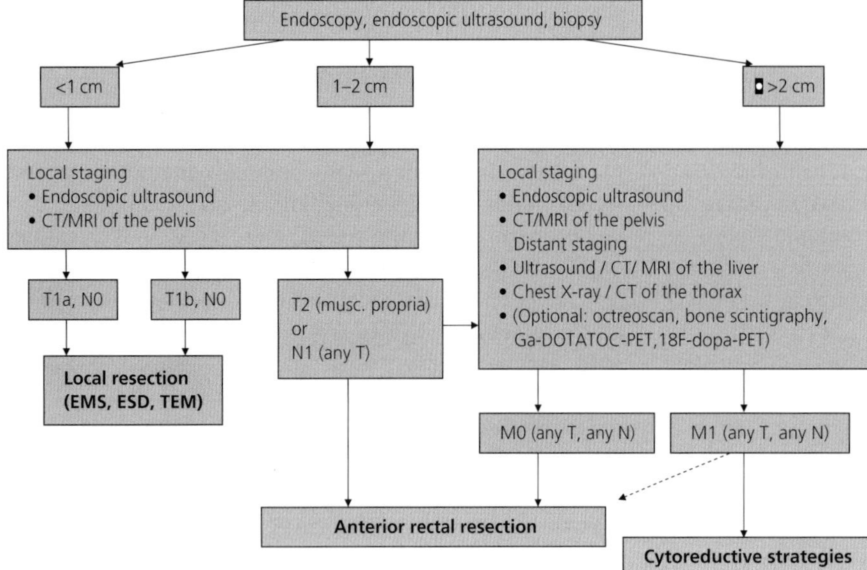

Fig. 23.11 Flow-chart of the therapeutic strategy for neuroendocrine tumors of the rectum (modified from Vogelsang & Siewert 2005).

Synchronous and metachronous second neoplasias

In tumor registers, approximately 13% of all patients with rectal carcinoids show associated synchronous or metachronous non-carcinoid neoplasms. Synchronous malignancies can be diagnosed in 8% of all patients with colorectal carcinoid tumors, while the cumulative 20-year risk of a metachronous cancer is estimated at 22.6%. Thus the overall risk over 20 years exceeds 30%. The *synchronous non-carcinoid secondary malignancies observed in patients with colorectal carcinoids* are mostly due to a significantly increased risk ratio (observed cancers/expected cancers) of cancers of the gastrointestinal tract: colorectal cancer (relative risk 7.7), cancers of the small bowel (relative risk 38.7) and cancers of the esophagus/stomach (relative risk 2.4). In absolute numbers, *colorectal adenocarcinomas are the most common secondary carcinoma in patients with colorectal carcinoids.* In a large series of 2086 patients with colorectal carcinoids, there were observed 126 secondary colorectal cancers. The *metachronous non-carcinoid secondary malignancies that can be observed in patients with a colorectal carcinoid in their history* are mostly due to a significantly increased ratio (observed cancers/expected cancers) of the following non-GI tract cancers: lung cancer (relative risk 2.5), prostate cancer (relative risk 2.0). and urinary tract cancer (relative risk 2.0). No statistically significant increased risk was observed for gynecologic and breast cancer.

Recommendations

In every patient diagnosed with a colorectal neuroendocrine tumor, associated secondary non-carcinoid cancers should be excluded by total colonoscopy, gastroduodenoscopy, (small bowel examination if there are suggestive symptoms), chest X-ray, prostate examination and urine analysis. Regular follow-up and surveillance at appropriate intervals is recommended. For repeat colonoscopy, an interval of 1 year after diagnosis and afterwards regular intervals of 3–5 years have been suggested.

Follow-up

There exist no data or general recommendations on the follow-up of patients with colorectal neuroendocrine tumors. The follow-up strategy depends on the postsurgical situation (R0 or R1) and on prognostic risk factors (stage, histopathologic grading, clinical aggressiveness) of the tumor. In general, visits every 3–4 months within the first year and every 4–6 months in the subsequent years seem appropriate for the majority of all well-differentiated (G1) and intermediate-differentiated (G2) tumors, but may be insufficient for poorly differentiated G3 tumors with high proliferation index. Visits include appropriate imaging studies (CT/MRI) and appropriate serum tumor markers (chromogranin A). ^{111}In-DTPAOC (Octreoscan) SPECT is only recommended at annual intervals.

In the R0 situation of typical rectal carcinoids (tumor size <1 cm confined to the submucosa [T1a, N0, M0]; proliferation index Ki-67 < 2% [grade G1]) a local endoscopy after 4–6 months seems suitable. In the R0 situation of tumors with larger tumor size (tumor size >2 cm or invasion beyond the submucosa into muscularis propria [T2 ,N0, M0]) or intermediate grading (Ki-67 2–20% [grade G2]) an early follow-up in 3–4 months with local endoscopy and CT/MRI of abdomen/pelvis is recommended. Additional follow-ups at individually adjusted appropriate intervals seems feasible.

References

Bhutani MS. (2007) Recent developments in the role of endoscopic ultrasonography in diseases of the colon and rectum. *Curr Opin Gastroenterol* 23: 67–73.

Konishi T, Watanabe T, Lishimoto J, Kotake K, Muto T, Nagawa H. (2007) Prognosis and risk factors of metastasis in colorectal carcinoids: results of a nationwide registry over 15 years. *Gut* 56: 863–8.

Modlin IM, Lye KD, Kidd M. (2003) A 5-decade analysis of 13,715 carcinoid tumors. *Cancer* 97: 934–59.

Plockinger U, Rindi G, Arnold R *et al.*; European Neuroendocrine Tumour Society. (2004) Guidelines for the diagnosis and treatment of neuroendocrine gastrointestinal tumours. A consensus statement on behalf of the European Neuroendocrine Tumour Society (ENETS). *Neuroendocrinology* 80: 394–424.

Rindi G, Kloppel G, Couvelard A *et al.* (2007) TNM staging of midgut and hindgut (neuro) endocrine tumors: a consensus proposal including a grading system. *Virchows Arch* [Epub ahead of print]

Soga J. (1997) Carcinoids of the rectum: an evaluation of 1271 reported cases. *Surg Today* 27: 112–19.

Soga J. (2005) Early-stage carcinoids of the gastrointestinal tract. An analysis of 1914 reported cases. *Cancer* 103: 1587–95.

Tichansky DS, Cagir B, Borrazzo E *et al.* (2002) Risk of secondary cancers in patients with colorectal carcinoids. *Dis Colon Rectum* 45: 91–7.

Vogelsang H, Siewert JR. (2005) Endocrine tumors of the hindgut. *Best Prac Res Clin Gastroenterol* 19: 739–51.

Wang AY, Ahmad NA. (2006) Rectal carcinoids. *Curr Opin Gastroenterol* 22: 529–35.

Imaging of gastroenteropancreatic neuroendocrine tumors

Anders Sundin

Introduction

Most gasteroenteropancreatic neuroendocrine tumors (NETs) are well differentiated and slow growing, but this group of neoplasms also comprise less common dedifferentiated tumors with an aggressive behavior. NETs may produce hormones, according to the cell of origin, or they may be non-functional. In case of hormonal overproduction, symptoms may be very severe even when the tumor is small. Depending on the tumor's anatomic localization, site-specific symptoms may arise. A midgut carcinoid (MGC) may for example lead to gastrointestinal obstruction and/or ischemia because of a mesenteric metastasis with a surrounding desmoplastic reaction and kinking of the bowel and encasement of the superior mesenteric artery and vein. Symptoms from a NET can be vague and in patients with MGC there may be a delay in the diagnosis for 2–3 years. Also, NETs may be found incidentally when the patient undergoes surgery for abdominal disease of other origin, for example as with appendical carcinoids. These differences in tumor growth, hormonal function and localization are reflected in the tumor's clinical presentation. Consequently, the need for diagnostic procedures and the choice of methods depend on the individual patient's tumor status at clinical presentation and must be considered accordingly. The various imaging aspects to be considered in the choice of methods, or combination of modalities, are related to diagnosis of the primary tumor, evaluation of the local extent of the lesion and its relation to adjacent anatomical structures, staging of the tumor concerning regional and distant metastases and evaluation of tumor somatostatin receptor density. After surgery and start of medical treatment, imaging is needed for therapy monitoring and detection of recurrent disease, respectively. The imaging work-up may involve EUS, conventional radiologic techniques for morphologic diagnosis such as CT, MRI and US and functional techniques including SRS with SPECT and PET.

Imaging methods

Computed tomography

CT is available in most departments as one of the most frequently employed methods for tumor imaging including NETs. Current CT scanners are spiral or helical CT scanners. The patient is positioned on a couch or 'table' and is moved continuously through the gantry of the scanner during rotation of the X-ray tube which thereby, relative to the patient, describes a spiral movement. In multidetector CT (MDCT) or multichannel CT (MCCT) helical scanners, several parallel detector rows are utilized to acquire multiple transaxial images per tube rotation. The recent generations of CT scanners, equipped with at least 64 detector rows and with a tube rotation time of 0.3–0.5 s, are able to produce hundreds or more of 1-mm or sub-mm transaxial images per tube rotation and allow examination of the abdomen and thorax during one breath-hold. Incremental CT scanning, in which the patient couch is moved stepwise through the gantry while producing one image at each table position and per tube rotation, will still be in use for some years to come. In comparison with MDCT, incremental CT has considerable limitations with regard to image quality and appropriate use of intravenous contrast media.

CT of the neck and thorax is generally performed using standard examination protocols whereas the technique for CT of the abdomen is usually adapted according to tumor type and application (e.g. detection of primary tumor, staging, therapy monitoring).

Two hours before CT of the abdomen about 800 mL of a very dilute iodine contrast material, or tap water, is routinely administered for opacification of the bowel.

When CT of the pancreas and abdominal CT angiography is performed, the patient drinks about 400 mL of water starting 15 minutes before the examination. Before CT of the pancreas an anticholinergic drug is often administered intravenously. In this manner the duodenum is filled with water, the bowel movements are temporarily inhibited and the pancreas is therefore better delineated and tumors in the duodenum may easier be depicted.

With modern MDCT scanners, 1-mm or sub-mm transaxial images are regularly reconstructed and are used to create 2–3-mm multiplanar reformats (MPRs) in the coronal and sagittal plane. Also, volume reconstruction technique (VRT) may be applied to produce 3D images and maximum intensity projections (MIPs) may be reconstructed to better appreciate vascular anatomy and pathology. For the image reading in the transaxial plane the thin sections may be utilized but generally a slice thickness of 2–5 mm is used.

For CT of the liver and pancreas, triple-phase examination is recommended and includes scanning before (native phase) and during intravenous contrast enhancement in the late arterial (portal venous inflow) phase and in the venous (portal–venous) phase. The reason for performing a triple-phase examination is the variation in vascularity of NET liver metastases and EPTs. Some are well vascularized and are best depicted in the late arterial contrast enhancement phase and other, less vascularized lesions, are better delineated in the venous phase. This variation in lesion vascularity is seen between different patients and in the liver of the same patient and may also vary over time due to tumor growth and as an effect of treatment. Some metastases are diagnosed only at CT performed before contrast enhancement. Medical therapy may initiate fatty infiltration of the liver with a decrease of the attenuation in normal liver parenchyma. In this situation, liver metastases previously best delineated during intravenous contrast enhancement may at follow-up be diagnosed in the native phase only. The effect of treatment may also change the enhancement pattern of the liver metastases accordingly. The risk of misinterpreting so-called 'spared areas' or 'skip lesions', i.e. areas of normal parenchyma in a fatty infiltrated liver, to represent metastases is also reduced by using triple-phase CT examination. The same holds true for focal fatty infiltration in the liver.

The depiction of well-vascularized liver metastases in the late arterial contrast enhancement phase depends on the intravenous influx of iodine. A high injection rate (>3 mL/s) by use of a power injector and/or a high iodine concentration (≥300 mgI/mL) is therefore recommended to optimize the image quality. By contrast, the diagnosis of poorly vascularized liver metastases in the venous contrast enhancement phase relies on sufficient enhancement of the normal liver parenchyma. Therefore the administered volume of the contrast medium is best based on the patient's body weight (1.5–2 mL/kg of contrast media; approximately 300 mgI/mL). The amount of contrast medium should always be considered in relation to the patient's renal function which may be impaired especially in the diabetic and older patient and as a result of chemotherapy. The cardiovascular status of the patient affects the timing of the scanning in relation to the contrast medium administration. Most modern CT scanners are, however, equipped with computer software to allow monitoring of the aortic enhancement during contrast administration in order to determine the optimum time point for examination start.

For preoperative evaluation, CT of the abdomen performed in the late arterial phase usually allows evaluation of the larger arteries in relation to the tumor lesions. Abdominal CT angiography (early arterial contrast enhancement phase) is therefore generally not mandatory in the initial work-up but should be added in case of any interpretation difficulties with regard to vascular anatomy or encasement.

The rest of the abdomen, below the liver, can be examined in the venous phase only, corresponding to approximately 60–90 s after start of contrast injection.

CT of the neck and thorax is generally performed when both arteries and veins are opacified by the contrast medium. This corresponds to approximately 30 and 40 s after start of contrast injection at 3 mL/s for the neck and thorax, respectively.

Magnetic resonance imaging

The development of MRI technique over the last few years has increased the spatial resolution, and faster acquisitions allow examination during one breath-hold which decreases or eliminates respiratory image artefacts and facilitates the use of intravenous contrast media. The addition of fat-suppressed sequences may also increase the tissue contrast.

For MRI of the liver and pancreas, dynamic scanning during intravenous contrast enhancement every 30 seconds to include the early and late arterial and the venous phases is recommended. MRI of the pancreas regularly includes magnetic resonance cholangiopancreatography (MRCP) to visualize the pancreatic duct and duct obstruction.

Except for the conventional extracellular gadolinium (Gd)-based MRI contrast media, with a pharmacokinetical pattern similar to that of iodine contrast media for CT, several new preparations are available for contrast-enhanced MRI.

Other gadolinium chelates (Gd-DTPA, Gd-EOB-DTPA) immediately after injection act as extracellular contrast agents but are only to a limited extent eliminated with glomerular filtration. Instead they accumulate in the hepatocytes for a relatively long time period following injection (a quarter of an hour to 2 hours depending on the chelate), and opacify the normal liver parenchyma, thereby making tumor tissue appear hypointense. Mn-DPDP is a manganese-based hepatocyte specific contrast agent which, between 15 minutes and 4 hours after injection, has a strong paramagnetic effect and causes an increased signal in the normal liver parenchyma. Mn-DPDP may also be used for MRI of the pancreas.

Superparamagnetic iron oxide (SPIO) particles are composed of iron oxide crystals coated with dextran or carboxydextran and are taken up by the Kupffer cells but are not retained in tumor tissue. The particles induce strong relaxation effects in the normal liver parenchyma which turns hypointense, while tumors appear hyperintense relative to the liver parenchyma.

Ultrasound

Abdominal ultrasound and CT are complementary radiologic methods to diagnose liver metastases, lymph node metastases, mesenteric metastases and other intra-abdominal and retroperitoneal lesions. Free fluid in the abdomen and pleural spaces may also be detected. US is operator sensitive and an optimal examination technique is essential. The possibility of using different transducers with appropriate ultrasound frequencies is important. The deeper portions of the abdomen, especially in obese patients, require the better penetration of a low-frequency transducer than more superficial areas where high-frequency transducers are generally preferred because of their better spatial resolution.

The recent developments in US have increased the spatial resolution and the introduction of intravenous contrast media has facilitated tumor characterization and detection of liver metastases but this has also been shown for EPTs. By dynamic scanning during intravenous contrast enhancement the temporal and spatial enhancement pattern in the tumor may be evaluated in the arterial, venous and late phase. Using intravenously contrast-enhanced US, liver metastases as small as 3 mm may be detected and previously equivocal tumor findings at unenhanced US or at CT may be characterized.

In our department US and CT are used every second time for therapy monitoring of abdominal NET disease. Exceptions are patients with tumors that are not depicted by one of the methods and obese patients in whom US is a less appropriate choice of imaging method. This procedure also reduces the radiation dose to these patients who are generally monitored over many years of therapy. US-guided tissue biopsies may safely and rapidly be performed whereas CT-guided procedures are more complicated and time consuming. This is also true for US-guided radiofrequency ablation (RFA) of liver metastases.

Endoscopic ultrasound is one of the most important and powerful imaging techniques to localize EPTs in patients presenting with symptoms and/or biochemical evidence of a functioning tumor. EUS is operator dependent and the results vary also with the localization of the tumor with lower sensitivity for tumors in the pancreatic tail and the duodenal wall. High-frequency transducers are utilized and tumors with merely a few mm diameters may be detected. The technique also allows fine needle aspiration (FNA) for cytology.

Peroperative or intraoperative US is used during laparotomy and laparascopic surgery to localize EPTs and increases the sensitivity compared to intraoperative palpation alone. Peroperative US can also delineate the relationship of the tumor to the pancreatic duct. The sensitivity for detecting liver metastases also increases when the transducer can be positioned on the liver surface. A liver resection, because of metastases, may also be combined with an intraoperative US-guided RFA.

Somatostatin receptor scintigraphy

SRS is an established functional technique for NET imaging. It is based on targeting of somatostatin receptors on the tumor cells, generally by using the somatostatin analog octreotide which is labeled with ^{111}In. ^{111}In-DTPA-octreotide is available as a commercial product (OctreoScan®). SRS generally employs both planar imaging of the whole body and SPECT of the abdomen and, when indicated, also of the thorax. The transaxial SPECT images are generally reformatted in the coronal (Fig. 23.12) and sagittal plane.

Besides being a sensitive imaging method for tumor detection and staging, SRS can predict a beneficial effect of somatostatin analog therapy on hormonal hypersecretion and provide a tool to select appropriate patients for peptide receptor radionuclide therapy. In order to estimate the tumor somatostatin receptor density the tumor-to-liver uptake ratio can be used as an approximate measure.

Recent SPECT cameras are equipped with a diagnostic-quality CT scanner to correct the images for attenuation and to supply an anatomical map for morphologic correlation of the SPECT findings. The use of SPECT-CT hybrid systems improves the accuracy of SRS by allowing better definition of the extent of the disease, differentiation of physiologic uptake from tumor and diagnosing additional lesions.

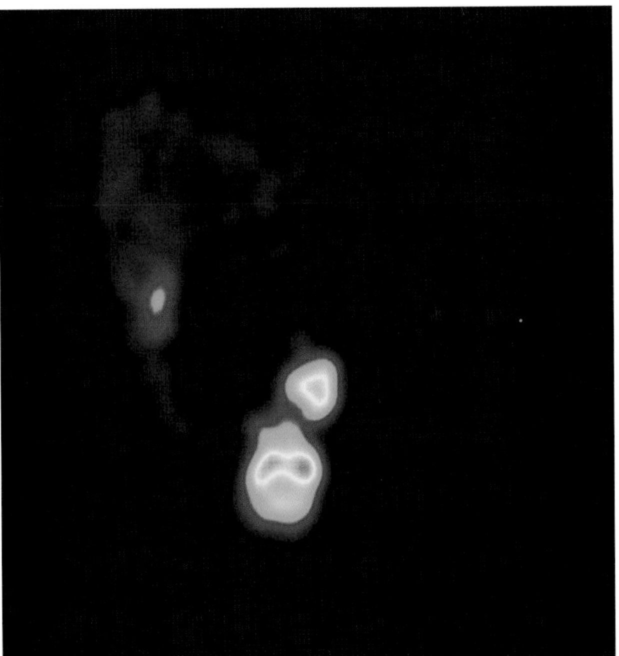

Fig. 23.12 ^{111}In-octreotide SPECT, coronal reformatted image, showing a very high tracer accumulation in a mesenteric metastasis from a midgut carcinoid.

Positron emission tomography

PET is a technique by which various aspects of biologic function may be imaged (e.g. metabolism, receptor density, enzyme function, and blood flow). The molecules utilized for PET are labeled with a positron emitter which typically has a short half-life (^{15}O $t_{1/2} = 2$ min, ^{11}C $t_{1/2} = 20$ min, ^{18}F $t_{1/2} = 110$ min). The PET camera resembles a CT scanner with a patient couch and a gantry which holds tens of thousands of detectors. PET using ^{18}F-labeled deoxyglucose (FDG) has during recent years evolved as a powerful functional technique for tumor imaging. After injection of FDG, allowing about 1 hour for tumor accumulation and elimination from normal tissues, the patient is positioned in the PET camera. A positron is emitted, collides with an electron and both are annihilated and converted to two antiparallel high-energy 511 keV photons which reach the detectors in the gantry and the line of decay is registered. At each bed position the lines of decay from about a 15-cm axial section of the body are registered by the detectors and are reconstructed to transaxial images representing radioactivity concentration. With a PET/CT camera, in which a CT scanner also has been fitted into the PET gantry, a CT examination can be performed in the same imaging session. The CT examination is used to correct the PET images for attenuation and provides an anatomical map for correlation of the PET findings.

FDG is, however, not useful for NET imaging except for dedifferentiated tumors and cancers with neuroendocrine differentiation. For PET of NETs other tracers have therefore been synthesized such as ^{18}F-L-DOPA, ^{68}Ga-octreotide and ^{11}C-5-hydroxy tryptophane (5-HTP). ^{18}F-L-DOPA and 5-HTP are amine precursors which are taken up by the tumor cells and by decarboxylation are converted to the corresponding amines (dopamine and serotonine). For somatostatin receptor imaging by PET ^{68}Ga-octreotide is used.

Angiography

Abdominal angiography and venous sampling is currently not often used in the radiologic work-up in NET patients, and in our center angiography is performed only in connection with intra-arterial embolization of liver metastases.

Imaging of NETs and image findings

Neuroendocrine gastric tumors

Type I and small (<1 cm) type II tumors rarely require imaging procedures besides endoscopy. With larger and growing tumors EUS can detect invasion of the wall and visualize lymph nodes, and EUS-guided FNA may confirm metastasis. If this is the case abdominal CT or MRI (depending on local availability and expertise) and SRS is recommended. For type III tumors preoperative imaging generally includes EUS. In case of a well-differentiated tumor, staging may be performed by whole-body CT and SRS and with poorly differentiated tumors by whole-body CT. In the latter tumors FDG-PET may also be considered.

Duodenal neuroendocrine tumors

EUS can detect tumor invasion of the wall and visualize lymph nodes and EUS-guided FNA may confirm metastasis. In case of a functional tumor, further imaging employs abdominal CT or MRI and SRS,whereas for non-functional tumors SRS cannot generally be recommended.

Endocrine pancreatic tumors (EPT)

The radiologic work up should localize the primary tumor, determine the position of the tumor in relation to the pancreatic duct and bile duct, evaluate possible vascular encasement and stage the disease with respect to regional and distant metastases. Disseminated disease often involves the liver but metastases may be found in a variety of locations e.g. in distant lymph nodes and bone.

The radiologic diagnosis in patients presenting with symptoms and/or biochemistry consistent with a *functioning EPT* is often a challenge, since the tumors often are small, especially insulinomas or gastrinomas, and may be multiple (MEN1). Therefore several methods are often required to locate the tumor including EUS, CT, MRI, US, and SRS. Depending on the local availability and expertise, especially regarding EUS and MRI, the sequence of imaging modalities used to localize the primary tumor varies. Some centers advocate EUS early in this sequence because of the high sensitivity in detecting EPTs, ranging approximately 70–95% (Anderson *et al.* 2000; Fidler & Johnson 2001) but with generally lower sensitivity for tumors in the tail of the pancreas and for extrapancreatic EPTs.

The initial imaging method is, however, generally CT or MRI. Often one of these methods is sufficient to detect the disease; for example about half of the gastrinomas are malignant and have metastasized in a vast majority of these cases at the time of clinical presentation (Fig. 23.13). The reported sensitivity for CT to detect an EPT is 70–100% (Ichikawa *et al.* 2000; Fidler & Johnson 2001) but only 50% for gastrinoma (Fidler & Johnson 2001). For MRI the sensitivity ranges from 70 to 95% (Ichikawa *et al.* 2000; Thoeni *et al.* 2000). If one or the other method of CT and/or MRI is negative, EUS is then often utilized as the next imaging modality.

For localization of EPTs, SRS may also be performed; it has a reported sensitivity of 60–95% (Fidler & Johnson 2001). The sensitivity of SRS for insulinoma is lower, approximately 50–60% (de Herder *et al.* 2005) and EUS is therefore preferred to SRS in the imaging sequence for these tumors.

Some departments with an expertise in contrast-enhanced US utilize this method, which, in a recent study, showed a sensitivity of 94% for EPT localization (Rickes *et al.* 2006). Before the surgical decision, morphologic imaging by CT or MRI is

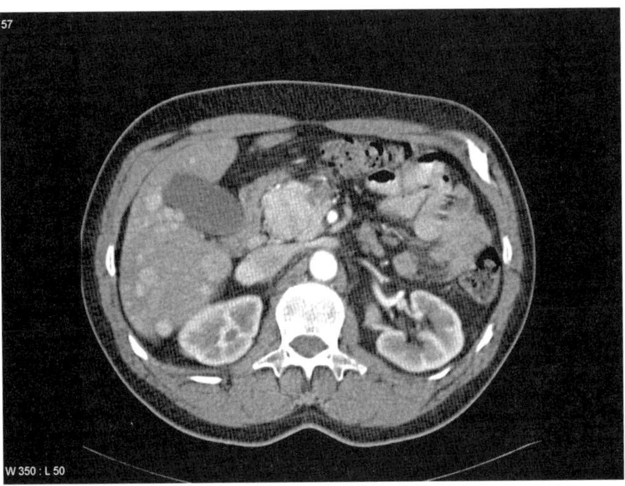

Fig. 23.13 CT in the arterial contrast enhancement phase of a gastrinoma in the pancreatic head and multiple well-vascularized liver metastases.

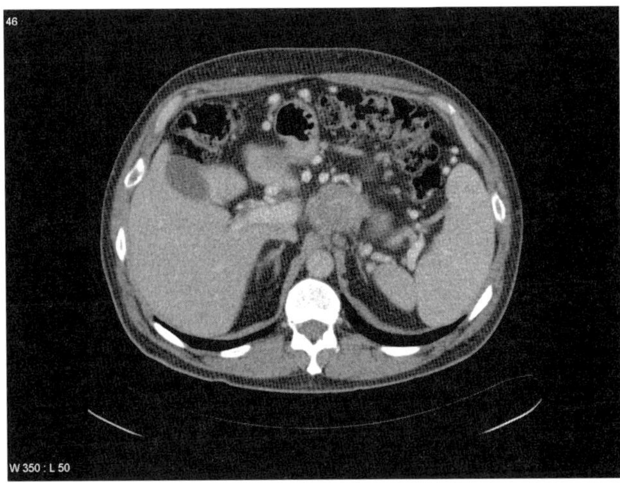

Fig. 23.14 CT in the venous contrast enhancement phase of an endocrine pancreatic tumor in the pancreatic body causing encasement of the spleenic vein with development of collateral veins.

needed to evaluate vascular encasement and to stage the disease. Functional imaging by SRS is, with the exception for cases of benign insulinomas, generally recommended for tumor staging and for evaluation of somatostatin receptor status.

The *non-functioning EPTs* are generally larger than the functioning tumors at the time of clinical presentation and may in many cases also have metastasized. Radiologic imaging by CT or MRI is therefore generally sufficient together with SRS for evaluation non-abdominal metastases and/or of somatostatin receptor status. For dedifferentiated EPTs and endocrine pancreatic cancers FDG-PET may instead be considered.

EPT imaging findings

A small functioning EPT is rarely diagnosed in the non-enhanced CT examination but it may help to identify calcifications in an underlying tumor. At MRI the tumor generally shows a low signal in T1-weighted sequences and mostly a high signal in T2, although the latter may vary. At CT and MRI, insulinomas and gastrinomas typically show a marked contrast enhancement in the late arterial phase (portal venous inflow phase) and by contrast-enhanced US a 'vascular blush' in the tumor may be seen during the arterial phase. EPTs are rather frequently also identified in the venous contrast enhancement phase in which the tumor sometimes may be even better seen than in the late arterial phase. Approximately 25% of gastrinomas are located outside the pancreas and are found in the duodenum, the stomach and the hepatoduodenal ligament.

Other less frequently occurring hormone-producing EPTs (e.g. glucagonoma, VIPoma) tend to be larger and often metastases are present at the time of diagnosis. These tumors may be confused with ductal pancreatic cancers but the pattern of vascular compromise is somewhat different with EPTs more often encasing the superior mesenteric vein and the portal vein. The non-functioning EPTs are generally not as well vascularized as the functioning tumors.

Even with fairly large EPTs and vascular encasement, often a narrow layer of fat is left between the superior mesenteric artery and the tumor. Tumor extending into the superior mesenteric vein and the portal vein is only rarely seen and biliary obstruction is atypical. Especially with larger tumors, occlusion of the splenic vein is fairly common and is accompanied by development of tortuous collateral veins around the stomach and in the mesentery (Fig. 23.14).

PET with ^{11}C-L-DOPA, ^{18}F-L-DOPA, ^{11}C-5-HTP and ^{68}Ga-octreotid has been performed in small groups of patients with EPTs with promising results. For the individual patient PET has a great impact when no other method has been able to localize the tumor. However, further comparative studies in larger groups of patients are needed to establish the role of PET imaging in EPT patients.

Midgut carcinoids and appendiceal carcinoids

The symptoms of MGC are frequently considered non-specific and the diagnosis is therefore often delayed. Therefore, the diagnosis is often established when the tumor has already metastasized. Consequently, imaging in most of these patient is mainly concentrated on tumor staging, describing the extent of metastases, vessel encasement by mesenteric metastases and assessing the liver involvement. This imaging work-up generally comprises CT of the abdomen and thorax but, depending on the local availability and expertise, MRI may instead be preferred. SRS is performed for functional imaging and staging of the disease and to evaluate the somatostatin receptor status (Fig. 23.12) as a means for the therapeutic decision. SRS has shown a very high sensitivity for carcinoid tumors which are visualized in approximately 60–95% of patients (Modlin *et al.* 2006).

MGC imaging findings

MGCs typically metastasize to the mesentery and to the liver. Retroperitoneal lymph node metastases are also common, typically located near the aorta and inferior vena cava (Fig. 23.15), and retrocrural lymph node metastases are sometimes present. Lymph node metastases are also frequently located ventrally in the lower thorax adjacent to the heart. More seldom thoracic metastases are found (e.g. in mediastinal lymph nodes). Sometimes peritoneal carcinomatosis is seen and metastases to bone, subcutis, brain, breast and pancreas.

The CT and MRI image of a *mesenteric carcinoid metastasis* is often characteristic. It is typically located near a loop of bowel, frequently in or near the right iliac fossa, indicating the site of the primary tumor. They can often be seen to induce an intense desmoplastic reaction, causing contraction and adherence of the adjacent bowel loop, with kinking which may result in partial or complete intestinal obstruction. This is reflected in the CT and MRI image as a central rounded soft tissue mass, typically with one or several calcifications, surrounded by radiating streaks in the mesenteric fat resembling spokes in a wheel (Fig. 23.16). Mesenteric metastases may also be found more centrally near the mesenteric root. Encasement of the superior mesenteric artery and vein is common and is important to evaluate before surgical resection of the mesenteric metastases and the primary tumor which is generally performed in these patients to prevent future intestinal complications of the disease. A sign of intestinal ischemia is thickening of the bowel wall. The extent of involvement of the superior mesenteric artery, and whether this is rather peripheral or more centrally located, is best evaluated by abdominal CT angiography but the late arterial contrast enhancement phase is generally sufficient (Fig. 23.17). The corresponding assessment in this regard for the superior mesenteric vein is best performed in the venous phase (Fig. 23.18).

Metastases to the peritoneum are frequently found in the form of mesenteric lymph nodes. Peritoneal carcinosis may be seen as an irregular sponge-like band-formed opacity, typically near the anterior abdominal wall, or in the form of multiple disseminated discrete lesions. These can sometimes be located on the liver surface and mimic liver metastases (Fig. 23.19).

PET with ^{11}C-L-DOPA, ^{18}F-L-DOPA, ^{11}C-5-HTP and ^{68}Ga-octreotide has been performed in small groups of MGC patients with promising results. As in cases of occult EPT, PET has also a great impact in the individual MGC patient when no other method has been able to localize the tumor. However, larger

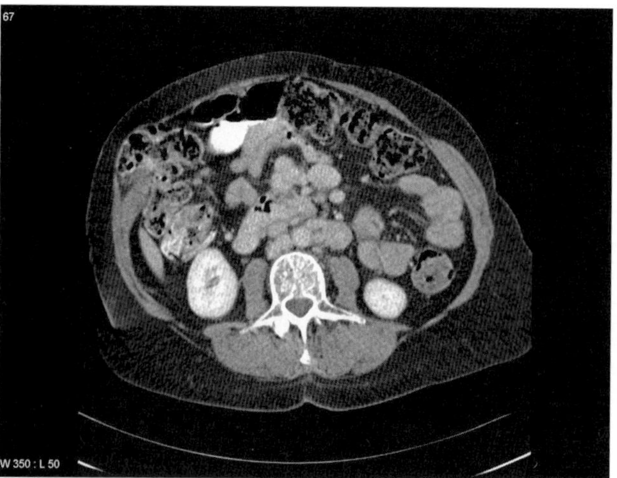

Fig. 23.15 CT of midgut carcinoid metastases to the mesentery and around the aorta and inferior vena cava.

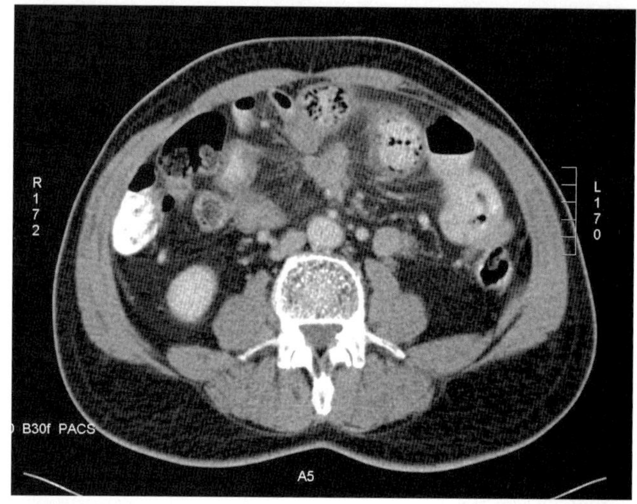

(a)

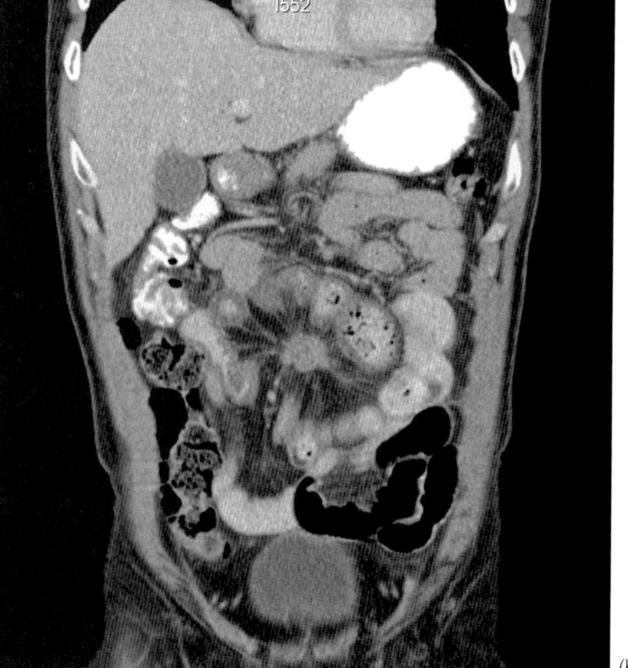

(b)

Fig. 23.16 CT of a mesenteric metastasis from a midgut carcinoid with a pronounced desmoplastic reaction and 'spoke wheel pattern'. (a) Transaxial image; (b) coronal reformatted image.

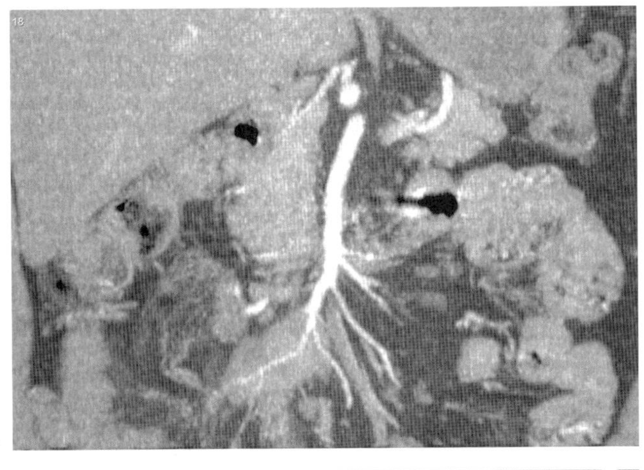

(a)

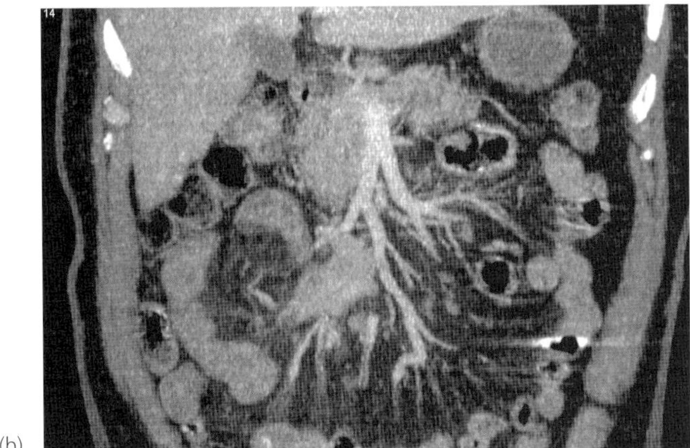

(b)

Fig. 23.17 CT coronal maximum intensity projection (MIP). (a) The arterial contrast enhancement phase showing encasement of the superior mesenteric artery by a mesenteric metastasis from a midgut carcinoid. (b) The venous contrast enhancement phase showing occlusion of the superior mesenteric vein.

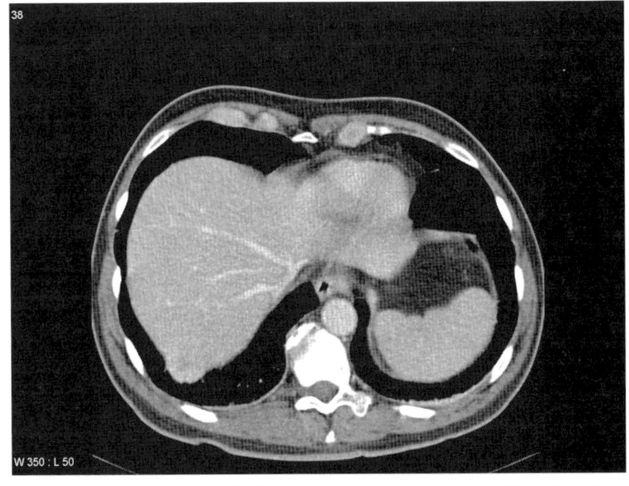

(a)

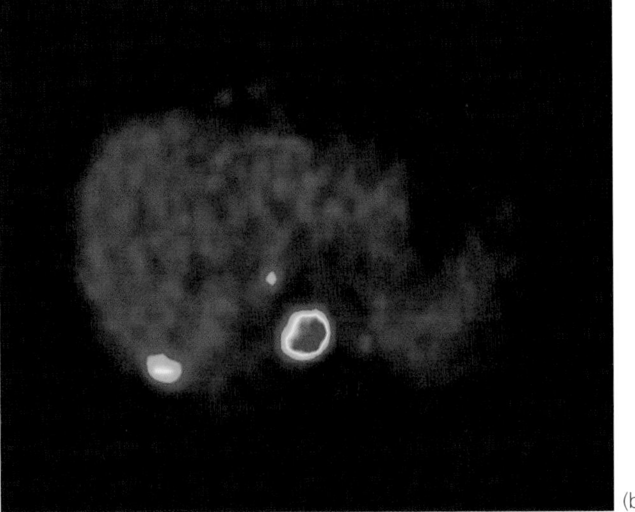

(b)

Fig. 23.18 (a) CT of a subdiaphragmal peritoneal metastasis on the posterior liver surface. (b) ^{11}C-5-HTP-PET showing the peritoneal metastasis and in addition a previously undiagnosed peritoneal metastasis and a bone metastasis in a vertebral body.

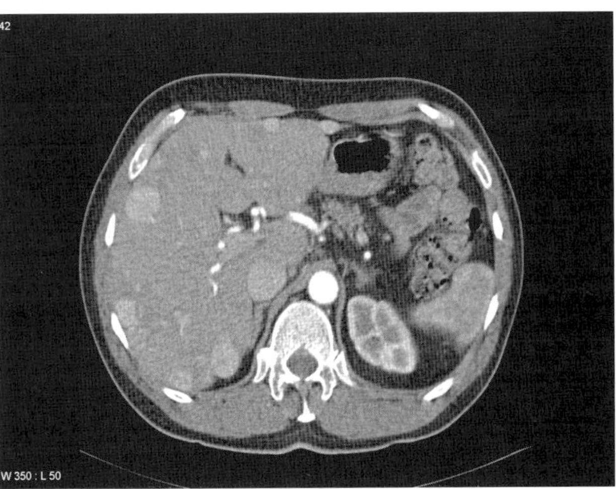

Fig. 23.19 CT in the arterial contrast enhancement phase showing several well-vascularized liver metastases from an endocrine pancreatic tumor.

groups of patients are needed in comparative studies to establish the role of PET with various tracers in MGC patients.

Appendical carcinoids are in the vast majority of patients an incidental finding in a surgically removed appendix or are discovered at surgery initiated because of symptoms of appendicitis. These patients are subject to radiologic imaging following surgery with CT and SRS of the abdomen when the tumor exceeds 2 cm and with CT and SRS of the abdomen and thorax after the finding of a goblet-cell carcinoid of any size.

Rectal and colonic carcinoids

A completely resected small (<1 cm) tumor rarely requires imaging procedures besides endoscopy to detect possible additional lesions in the colon. In patients with larger tumors and with invasion of the bowel wall, staging is generally performed by CT and SRS of the abdomen and chest. In case of a poorly differentiated tumor and a negative SRS, FDG-PET may be performed.

When a rectal tumor is considered for resection, preoperative evaluation is performed by MRI or transrectal EUS, depending on local availability and expertise.

NET liver metastases

NET liver metastases are generally described as well vascularized. This may, however, vary between patients and within the liver of the same patient. The visibility of the lesions may also vary depending on the effect of therapy on the normal liver parenchyma and on the metastases. Therefore triple-phase scanning with CT or dynamic examination with MRI during intravenous contrast enhancement is required to appropriately evaluate NET liver metastases.

The primary imaging work-up generally includes CT or MRI and SRS. If the primary tumor is unknown, both abdomen and thorax are included. Before liver resection with curative intent, which may be performed in combination with RFA, imaging generally includes MRI and SRS and, if available, contrast-enhanced US may be added. For therapy monitoring during medical therapy, CT in combination with US is usually sufficient but depending on the local availability and expertise MRI may be preferred instead. The sensitivity for detecting liver metastases in general is approximately 50–75% for CT and about 70–90% for MRI (Lencioni *et al.* 2004). In a recent review, the sensitivity for contrast-enhanced US was 87% and for intraoperative US 98% (Hohmann *et al.* 2004). In a study comparing CT, MRI and SRS for detection of NET liver metastases, the respective sensitivity was 79%, 95% and 49% (Dromain *et al.* 2005) and another study on CT and SRS reported a sensitivity of 100% and 90%, respectively.

NET imaging findings

At CT, well vascularized NET liver metastases appear in the portal venous inflow (late arterial) contrast enhancement phase as high-attenuation lesions relative to the low-attenuation non-enhanced liver parenchyma (Fig. 23.20). The poorly

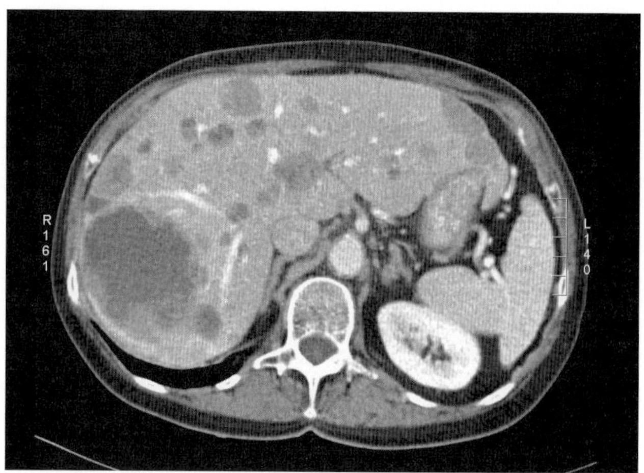

Fig. 23.20 CT in the venous contrast enhancement phase showing several poorly vascularized liver metastases from a midgut carcinoid. Extensive necrosis is seen in the large metastasis in the posterior aspect of the right liver lobe.

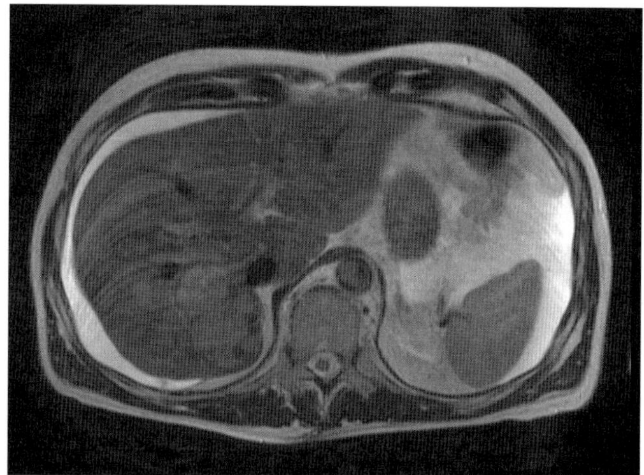

(a)

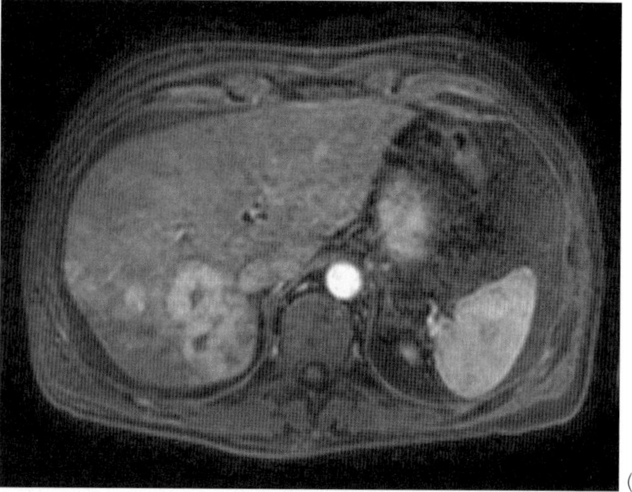

(b)

Fig. 23.21 (a) MRI T2-weighted sequence. (b) Gadolinium contrast-enhanced MRI in the arterial phases showing liver metastases from a midgut carcinoid in the posterior aspect of the right liver lobe.

vascularized lesions are best depicted in the venous contrast enhancement-phase as low-attenuating areas relative to the contrast-enhanced liver parenchyma (Fig. 23.21). Peripheral contrast enhancement and central necroses are often seen, the latter especially in the larger metastases (Fig. 23.21). Larger metastases are fairly often visible in the native images but most lesions are isoattenuating with the native liver and only possible to delineate during contrast enhancement. Occasional calcifications, indicating an underlying metastasis, are best seen in the native images.

At MRI, metastases from NETs to the liver often show low signal intensity in T1-weighted images and high signal intensity in T2-weighted images. Fat-suppressed T2-weighted sequences may increase the lesion to liver contrast. During dynamic imaging following intravenous contrast enhancement using conventional Gd contrast media, the pattern is similar to that of CT with well-vascularized lesions enhancing in the arterial phase and the poorly vascularized lesions being best depicted in the venous phase.

PET with ^{68}Ga-octreotide, ^{18}F-L-DOPA and ^{11}C-5-HTP have shown promising visualization of NET liver metastases in small groups of patients but as previously stated, comparative studies in larger groups of patients are needed to better define the role for PET imaging in this respect.

Future prospects

By replacing older equipment with MDCT scanners, the high axial resolution of these scanners will provide the means to regularly view images in the axial, coronal and sagittal planes and the high examination speed will make it possible to optimize contrast media technique. This will probably increase lesion detectability and facilitate the preoperative anatomical interpretation. Contrast-enhanced US will probably continue to expand and is likely to influence the future imaging work-up in NET patients. Similarly to PET-CT, the escalating use of hybrid SPECT-CT is expected to increase the sensitivity of SRS. However, the better spatial resolution of PET (about 0.5 cm) compared to SPECT (approximately 1–1.5 cm) will favor the replacement of SRS by ^{68}Ga-octreotide-PET. The ongoing expansion of PET-CT for tumor imaging and the research on new PET tracers for NET imaging may in a near future have an impact also on PET-CT imaging of NET patients.

References

Anderson MA, Carpenter S, Thompson NW, Nostrant TT, Elta GH, Scheiman JM. (2000) Endoscopic ultrasound is highly accurate and directs management in patients with neuroendocrine tumors of the pancreas. *Am J Gastroenterol* 95: 2271–7.

de Herder WW, Kwekkeboom DJ, Valkema R *et al.* (2005) Neuroendocrine tumors and somatostatin: imaging techniques. *J Endocrinol Invest* 28 (11 Suppl): 132–6.

Dromain C, de Baere T, Lumbroso J *et al.* (2005) Detection of liver metastases from endocrine tumors: a prospective comparison of somatostatin receptor scintigraphy, computed tomography, and magnetic resonance imaging. *J Clin Oncol* 23: 70–8.

Fidler JL, Johnson CD. (2001) Imaging of neuroendocrine tumors of the pancreas. *Int J Gastrointest Cancer* 30: 73–85.

Hohmann J, Albrecht T, Oldenburg A, Skrok J, Wolf KJ. (2004) Liver metastases in cancer: detection with contrast-enhanced ultrasonography. *Abdom Imaging* 29: 669–81.

Ichikawa T, Peterson MS, Federle MP *et al.* (2000) Islet cell tumor of the pancreas: biphasic CT versus MR imaging in tumor detection. *Radiology* 216: 163–71.

Lencioni R, Cioni D, Crocetti L, Della Pina C, Bartolozzi C. (2004) Magnetic resonance imaging of liver tumors. *J Hepatol* 40: 162–71.

Modlin IM, Latich I, Zikusoka M, Kidd M, Eick G, Chan AK. (2006) Gastrointestinal carcinoids: the evolution of diagnostic strategies. *J Clin Gastroenterol* 40: 572–82.

Rickes S, Monkemuller K, Malfertheiner P. (2006) Contrast-enhanced ultrasound in the diagnosis of pancreatic tumors. *JOP* 7: 584–92.

Thoeni RF, Mueller-Lisse UG, Chan R, Do NK, Shyn PB. (2000) Detection of small, functional islet cell tumors in the pancreas: selection of MR imaging sequences for optimal sensitivity. *Radiology* 214: 483–90.

Treatment

Overview

Rudolf Arnold & Anja Rinke

Special features of neuroendocrine tumors that influence therapeutic decisions

Neuroendocrine tumors are rare compared to other epithelial tumor entities. They are characterized by a number of specific features which have to be recognized if treatment of patients with these tumors is intended.

- Tumors can be benign, but are mostly malignant.
- They grow, in general, slowly compared with the more aggressively proliferating adenocarcinomas of the gastrointestinal tract.
- Neuroendocrine tumors are mostly functionally inactive; however, some are functionally active and lead to well-known, sometimes dramatic clinical syndromes as a consequence of excess hormone release by the tumor cells.
- The quality of life of patients with non-functioning tumors is frequently uncompromised, even in those with diffuse metastatic spread.
- Some malignant tumors never develop metastases and only the primary grows.
- Others develop lymph node metastases, others metastases into lymph nodes and the liver, others develop additional metastases into the bone, skin, brain and elsewhere.
- Some patients reveal few (low tumor load), others many metastases (high tumor load).

• Although the histology is very similar in most tumors despite a different origin of the primary (foregut, midgut, hindgut), tumor biology may differ considerably.
• Histologic differentiation of the tumors can change with time: after years of very slow progression of a highly differentiated tumor, growth can explode as a result of tumor dedifferentiation; obviously, this would also modify therapeutic strategy.
• Neuroendocrine tumors can arise solitarily and as part of genetic syndromes such as MEN1 syndrome, von Hippel–Lindau syndrome and others.

It is, therefore, easy to understand that treatment strategies have to be adjusted to these differences in origin (foregut, midgut, hindgut), in biology, growth pattern and, most importantly, according to the quality of lifeof an individual patient (Arnold 2005).

Modalities and limitations of treatment

The currently available treatment options and possible indications for treatment are summarized in Figs 23.22 & 23.23. They should recognize the specific features of neuroendocrine tumors. Contrary to the more frequently occurring adenocarcinomas, most treatment schedules are not based on proper prospective and controlled studies.

Surgery

Curative surgery is the major goal in neuroendocrine tumors. Surgical removal of an insulinoma, gastrinoma, appendiceal carcinoid and other resectable functioning and non-functioning tumors or endoscopic polypectomoy of a small gastric or rectal carcinoid is the major option. However, it is questionable whether or not in the presence of metastases removal of the primary is mandatory with respect to prevention of disease progression, long-term survival and quality of life. Surgeons favor removing an asymptomatic primary midgut tumor even in the presence of liver metastases to avoid later obstruction of the bowel by the growing primary or to prevent later developing desmoplastic reaction with the consequence of impaired bowel function. Some studies suggest a survival benefit of patients if a primary located in the midgut is removed. However, this assumption is not based on prospective studies. Similar considerations are true for the removal of a primary pancreatic tumor in the presence of metastases. A further unsettled problem is multiple pancreatic tumors in the presence of MEN1. Should they all be removed surgically if they are functionally inactive? It is easy to identify and remove an insulinoma in a patient with MEN1, but it may be difficult to identify such a single functionally active tumor within a pancreas containing multiple non-functioning tumors (Chamberlain *et al.* 2000; Akerström *et al.* 2001).

All patients? Patients with MEN1 and multiple tumors?
Slowly growing tumors? Patients with low tumor load?
Patients with high tumor load?
Rapidly growing tumors? Symptomatic patients?
Asymptomatic patients? Patients with stable disease?
Highly differentiated tumors? Poorly differentiated tumors?

Fig. 23.22 The therapeutic dilemma: whom to treat?

Curative surgery Palliative surgery
Chemotherapy Biotherapy
Peptide receptor radionuclide therapy Chemoembolization
Ablative therapy
Transplantation Endoscopic treatment

Fig. 23.23 How to treat? The therapeutic alternatives.

Biotherapy

Octreotide, its long-acting analogs and interferon-alpha are accepted major milestones in managing symptoms from neuroendocrine tumors such as watery diarrhea in VIPoma, flush and diarrhea in carcinoid syndrome, migratory erythema and anorexia in glucagonoma syndrome. However, although an antiproliferative effect of octreotide and its analogs has been suggested by several prospective studies, there are currently no placebo-controlled prospective studies available that support the hypothesis. Such studies would be highly desirable since not all tumors seem to respond to octreotide and its long-acting analogs and the costs of this treatment are expensive. Interferon-alpha is an alternative option to octreotide and is able to reduce symptoms in patients with functioning neuroendocrine tumors and to inhibit tumor growth. Side-effects are more prominent and available studies concerning growth inhibition are not placebo-controlled (Öberg & Ericsson 1991; Ducreux *et al.* 2000; Garland *et al.* 2003; Faiss *et al.* 2003; Arnold *et al.* 2005).

Chemotherapy

Neuroendocrine tumors are, in general, less sensitive to chemotherapy than other epithelial tumors. There are two exceptions: rapidly growing, mostly poorly differentiated tumors with a high Ki-67 index in histology which respond to etoposide plus cisplatin; and highly differentiated neuroendocrine tumors of pancreatic origin responding to streptozotocin-containing combinations. In contrast, other foregut tumors such as malignant neuroendocrine tumors of the stomach and duodenum, and all midgut and hindgut tumors are more or less resistant to chemotherapy. Even within pancreatic tumors, only some, mostly malignant insulinomas and VIP-producing tumors, do respond to a protocol with streptozotocin plus doxorubicin or 5-fluorouracil. Other pancreatic tumors with a comparable histology respond rarely; some do respond, some not. At a very recent ASCO meeting the combination of temozolomide, an oral dacarbacin, together with the tyrosine kinase inhibitor bevacizumab has also been shown to be active in malignant pancreatic but not in malignant intestinal neuroendocrine tumors (carcinoids). The reason why gastrointestinal neuroendocrine tumors in contrast to tumors of pancreatic origin are less sensitive to these chemotherapeutic regimens is unknown, as is the reason why only some and not all pancreatic tumors respond despite identical histology (Moertel *et al.* 1992; Arnold 2005).

Ablative therapy

Locoregional strategies like chemoembolization with vascular occlusion inducing ischemia in liver metastases which are mostly highly vascularized or regional destruction with either percutaneous alcohol injection, cryoablation or radiofrequency ablation have been shown to effectively reduce tumor tissue. Excellent tumor response rates have been achieved with chemoembolization and other local ablative procedures for liver metastases. However, whether or not this is followed by a survival advantage has not been demonstrated clearly since no comparative studies have been performed (Ruszniewski *et al.* 1993; Arnold 2005).

Peptide receptor radionucleide therapy

Peptide receptor radionucleide therapy is undoubtedly the most spectacular progress within the available therapeutic strategies. It is based on the presence of high numbers of somatostatin receptors, mainly subtype sst^2, on the surface of tumor cells. An increasing number of patients with metastatic disease have been successfully treated with this approach and ^{90}yttrium and ^{177}lutetium-labeled somatostatin analogs are currently under investigation. Serious toxic side-effects especially to the bone marrow, kidney and liver which occurred frequently at the beginning could be avoided in more recent studies by appropriate dosimetry, kidney protection using coadministration of amino acid solutions and by paying careful attention to pretherapeutic kidney and bone marrow function. Unfortunately, protocols which describe how peptide receptor radionucleide therapy should be offered to individual patients and the respective results are published from few institutions only, and are therefore difficult to compare with institutions not publishing their protocols and results. There is, currently, no agreement concerning indications for treatment. Should peptide receptor radionucleide therapy be offered to patients at diagnosis, i.e. as first-line therapy, or after failure of biotherapy, to patients with low or high tumor load, to slowly or more rapidly growing tumors? Do patients respond to treatment irrespective of the origin of the primary (foregut, midgut, hindgut)? What should be done in patients who do not respond to this regimen? Such questions need to be answered to offer the physicians caring for an individual patient the best arguments for adequate therapeutic decision-making (Valkema *et al.* 2006).

Extrahepatic metastases

Metastases outside the liver do not necessarily respond to systemic treatment with chemotherapy, biotherapy or peptide receptor radionucleide therapy as shown for liver and lymph node metastases. Bone metastases in particular are frequently less sensitive to these treatment schedules. Patients with bone involvement respond favorably to biphosphonate treatment. Brain metastases merit radiosurgery, and metastases elsewhere should be removed surgically if possible.

Definition of response

Response to antiproliferative treatment is defined by WHO criteria as progression, stable disease, partial response and complete response. However, this definition does not contain a time frame. Since most malignant epithelial tumors are growing rapidly such a time frame is not necessary in the clinical setting. The spontaneous tumor growth of neuroendocrine tumors is very slow in many patients. Within a time interval of 3 months many tumors and of 6 months some tumors do not fulfil the criterion of a 25% increase or decrease in volume. A WHO compatible response may be observed in this example after 3–9 months or even longer. Therefore, true response to a specific antiproliferative treatment can only be supposed if the spontaneous tumor growth prior to treatment in a specific patient is documented. The spontaneous growth characteristics should be investigated with imaging procedures before treatment in every patient. Otherwise, an apparent response to treatment as stabilization of tumor growth can just mirror spontaneous tumor behavior and not an influence of treatment. This demand is not fulfilled by many studies and even in recent studies spontaneous tumor growth has not been reported. Therefore, if studies describe stable disease in response to treatment, this can only be judged as antiproliferative response if tumor progress occurred prior to treatment. Of course, every tumor documented by imaging procedures must have grown to reach its documented size as otherwise it would not exist. However, growth of neuroendocrine tumors is not necessarily linear and phases of growth may be followed by phases of growth arrest or slowing down of growth (Arnold 2005).

Treatment of neuroendocrine tumors according to the site of the primary

Tables 23.10–23.12 summarize current standards of the treatment of neuroendocrine tumors according to the site of the primary. Fig. 23.24 presents a proposal as to how patients with metastatic disease should be treated according to individual tumor growth. In this proposal curative or palliative surgery will be offered to every patient. Subsequent treatment depends on the extent of tumor progression. Patients with stable disease, i.e. tumors that do not progress for a period of 3–6 months should not be treated with any of the available antiproliferative

Table 23.10 Treatment of gastric carcinoids.

Tumor type	Endoscopy	Surgery	Biotherapy	Chemotherapy	Ablative therapy	Radioligand therapy
Carcinoid of the stomach						
Type 1						
Solitary <2 cm	Yes	Ø	Ø	Ø	Ø	Ø
Solitary >2 cm	Ø	Yes	Ø	Ø	Ø	Ø
Multiple <2 cm	Yes	Ø	Ø	Ø	Ø	Ø
Type 2						
Solitary <2 cm	Yes	Ø	Ø	Ø	Ø	Ø
Solitary >2 cm	no	Yes	Ø	Ø	Ø	Ø
Multiple	Yes	Ø	Ø	Ø	Ø	Ø
Type 3						
<2 cm	?	Yes	Ø	Ø	Ø	Ø
>2 cm	Ø	Yes	Ø	Ø	Ø	Ø
Regional metastases	Ø	Yes	Ø	Ø	Ø	Ø
Liver metastases	Ø	Yes*	Ø	?†	?†	?†

* Low tumor load.
† Efficacy not established.
Ø Not indicated.

Table 23.11 Treatment of pancreatic and duodenal tumors.

Tumor type	Endoscopy	Surgery	Biotherapy	Chemotherapy	Ablative therapy	Radioligand therapy
NET pancreas						
<2 cm	Ø	Yes	Ø	Ø	Ø	Ø
>2 cm	Ø	Ye	Ø	Ø	Ø	Ø
Regional metastases	Ø	Yes	Ø	Ø	Ø	Ø
Liver metastases	Ø	Yes*	Yes†	Yes‡	Yes§	Yes
Multiple tumors (MEN1)	Ø	?§	Ø	Ø	Ø	Ø
NET duodenum						
<2 cm	Yes	Yes	Ø	Ø	Ø	Ø
>2 cm	Ø	Yes	Ø	Ø	Ø	Ø
Regional metastases	Ø	Yes	Ø	Ø	Ø	Ø
Liver metastases	Ø	Yes*	Yes†	Yes‡	Yes§	Yes
Multiple tumors (MEN1)	Ø	?	Ø	Ø	Ø	Ø

* Low tumor load.
† Efficacy unpredictable, no placebo controlled studies available.
‡ Effective in malignant insulinoma and VIPoma, efficacy unpredictable in non-functioning tumors.
§ No controlled studies available.
Ø Not indicated.

strategies until further tumor progression. Patients with very slowly growing tumors are candidates for biotherapy since this treatment option is easy to perform and can be self-administered. The author of this report prefers long-acting somatostatin analogs as the first option due to the lack of severe side-effects, thus providing an unimpaired life quality as compared to interferon-alpha. In patients with further tumor growth interferon-alpha can be added since some studies suggest an additive antiproliferative effect although prospective controlled studies do not support this concept. In patients with metastatic disease who do not respond to biotherapy, chemotherapy in the case of a pancreatic tumor, chemoembolization, ablative strategies and radioligand therapy are alternative options equal in rank. However, no studies are available demonstrating the superiority of one of these treatment options. Chemotherapy has not been shown to be effective in midgut and hindgut tumors. Liver transplantation should be considered for patients with liver metastases only after surgical removal of the primary and exclu-

Table 23.12 Treatment of midgut and hindgut tumors.

Tumor type	Endoscopy	Surgery	Biotherapy	Chemotherapy	Ablative therapy	Radioligand therapy
NET midgut						
<2 cm	Ø	Yes	Ø	Ø	Ø	Ø
>2 cm	Ø	Yes	Ø	Ø	Ø	Ø
Regional metastases	Ø	Yes	Ø	Ø	Ø	Ø
Liver metastases	Ø	Yes*	Yes**	Ø	Yes***	Yes***
NET hindgut						
Colon						
<2 cm	Ø	Yes	Ø	Ø	Ø	Ø
>2 cm	Ø	Yes	Ø	Ø	Ø	Ø
Regional metastases	Ø	Yes	Ø	Ø	Ø	Ø
Liver metastases	Ø	Yes*	?†	Ø	Yes‡	Yes‡
Rectum						
<2 cm	Yes	Ø	Ø	Ø	Ø	Ø
>2 cm	Ø	Yes	Ø	Ø	Ø	Ø
Regional metastases	Ø	Yes	Ø	Ø	Ø	Ø
Liver metastases	Ø	Yes*	?†	Ø	Yes‡	Yes‡

* Low tumor load.
† Efficacy unpredictable.
‡ Efficacy possible, no controlled studies available.
Ø Not indicated.

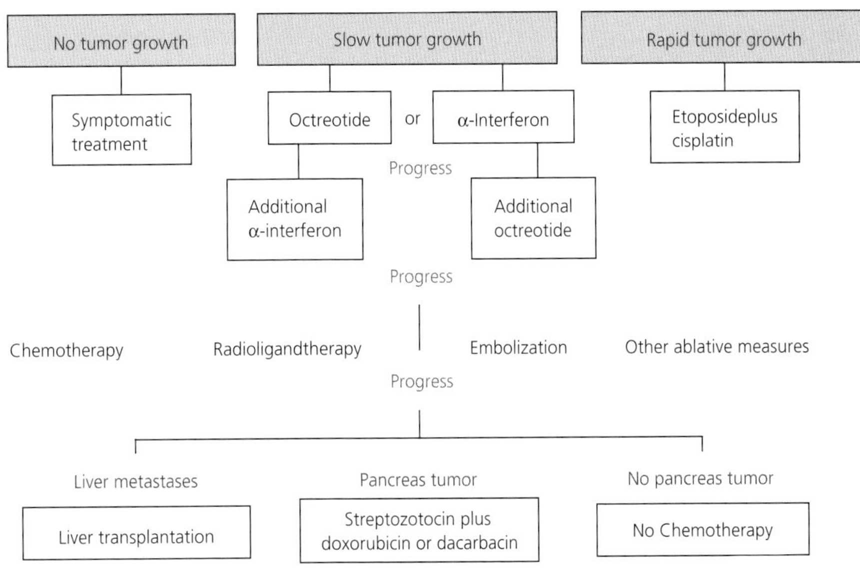

Fig. 23.24 Therapeutic options for neuroendocrine tumors.

sion of extrahepatic tumor spread by the available imaging methods. In patients with rapidly progressing tumors and those with poorly differentiated tumors chemotherapy with cisplatin and etoposide is the primary treatment option.

References

Arnold R, ed. (2005) Endocrine tumours of the gastrointestinal tract: Part I and II. In: BEST Practice and Research. *Clin Gastroenterol* 19(5).

Arnold R, Rinke A, Klose K-J *et al.* (2005) Octreotide versus octreotide plus interferon-alpha in endocrine gastroenteropancreatic tumors: a randomized trial. *Clin Gastroenterol Hepatol* 3: 761–71.

Akerström G, Hellman P, Öhrvall U. (2001) Midgut and hindgut carcinoid tumors. In: Doherty GM, Skögseid B, eds. *Surgical Endocrinology*, pp. 447–59. Lippincott Williams & Wilkins, Philadelphia.

Chamberlain RS, Canes D, Brown KT *et al.* (2000) Hepatic neuroendocrine metastases: Does intervention alter outcomes? *J Am Coll Surg* 190(4): 432–45.

Ducreux M, Ruszniewski P, Chayvialle JA *et al.* (2000) The antitumoral effect of the long-acting somatostatin analog lanreotide in neuroendocrine tumors. *Am J Gastroenterol* 95(11): 3276–81.

Faiss S, Pape UR, Bohmig M *et al.* (2003) Prospective, randomized, multicenter trial on the antiproliferative effect of lanreotide, interferon alfa, and combination on gastroenteropancreatic tumors—the international lanreotide and interferon alfa study group. *J Clin Oncol* 21(14): 2689–96.

Garland J, Buscombe JR, Bouvier C *et al.* (2003) Sandostatin LAR (long-acting octreotide acetate) for malignant carcinoid syndrome: a 3-year experience. *Aliment Pharmacol Ther* 17: 437–44.

Moertel CG, Lefkopoulo M, Lipsitz S, Hahn RG, Klaassen D. (1992) Streptozocin-doxorubicin, streptozocin-fluorouracil or chlorozotocin in the treatment of advanced islet-cell carcinoma. *N Engl J Med* 326: 519–23.

Oberg K, Eriksson B. (1991) The role of interferons in the management of carcinoid tumours. *Br J Haematol* 79(Suppl 1): 74–7.

Ruszniewski P, Rougier P, Roche A *et al.* (1993) Hepatic arterial chemoembolization in patients with liver metastases of endocrine tumors. *Cancer* 71: 2624–30.

Valkema R, Pauwels S, Kvols LK *et al.* (2006) Survival and response after peptide receptor radionuclide therapy with [90Y-DOTAO,Tyr3] octreotide in patients with advanced gastroenteropancreatic neuroendocrine tumors. *Semin Nucl Med* 36: 147–56.

Surgery: pancreatic tumors

Göran Åkerström & Per Hellman

Introduction

Among the endocrine pancreatic tumors (EPTs), insulinoma and gastrinoma may cause severe, potentially life-threatening hormonal symptoms despite inconspicuous size, but can be surgically removed due to increased efficiency of pre- and intra-operative localization diagnosis. Other entities, glucagonoma, VIPoma, and non-functioning endocrine pancreatic tumors are often large and metastasizing, but may require all efforts of surgical debulking to alleviate hormonal symptoms, and/or have favorable survival. Prospective screening is recommended in MEN1 for detection of EPTs and early surgery before metastases have developed. A great challenge is to develop surgery for efficient removal of primary tumors and metastases, and to undertake operation with minimal morbidity and mortality. Proliferation and genetic markers can help foresee prognosis and select patients for surgery, and possibly avoid higher-grade malignant lesions, such as poorly differentiated neuroendocrine carcinoma (with higher Ki-67 proliferation index), which may be more efficiently managed with chemotherapy.

Insulinomas

Insulinomas account for approximately 25% of EPTs and are most prevalent of the functioning tumors. They occur most frequently at an age of around 40–60 years. The majority is sporadic, but 5–10% may be familial and associated with the hereditary MEN1 syndrome, and may then affect also younger individuals. MEN1 patients typically have multiple tumors, which may be synchronous or develop asynchronously, whereas sporadic lesions tend to be solitary.

Patients with insulinoma suffer from more or less severe hypoglycemia, with symptoms of neuroglycopenia and of catecholamine excess during early morning or afternoon fasting or in association with exercise. Since symptoms are often puzzling and misinterpreted, the diagnosis may be delayed for years. Crucial for early diagnosis is to liberally determine serum glucose in patients with unclear attacks of neurologic or psychiatric symptoms, or with bizarre behavior, seizures, or coma. Many patients have become obese, being accustomed to frequent nightly meals to avoid hypoglycemia and this may occasionally complicate surgery. Diagnosis is settled by demonstration of hypoglycemia (serum glucose concentrations <45 mg/dL) during a supervised fasting test together with inappropriately high serum insulin, and this should imply any detectable insulin during the fasting hypoglycemia. Insulin/glucose quotients, which we used to rely on, have proven less relevant, since 20% of patients may have normal or only slightly elevated insulin values. Before the patient is accepted for surgery it is crucial to show corresponding rise in C-peptide to help exclude factitia, implying self-administration of insulin or peroral antidiabetic medication, which indeed is claimed to be more common than insulinoma, and where surgery of course should be avoided. Oral sulfonylurea antidiabetics should also be excluded by plasma measurement. The ratio of proinsulin to total immunoreactive insulin values is usually <20% in normal individuals, but tends to be higher (>30%) in patients with insulinoma. Unusually high proinsulin/insulin ratio >50% is often seen with malignant insulinoma, but can occur also with 25% of benign insulinoma.

Indications for surgery

Hypoglycemia due to insulinoma is not well controlled by medical treatment, and surgery should with few exceptions be recommended. Operation is generally possible also in elderly individuals, who may be offered considerable relief of sometimes severe or incapacitating symptoms or even threatening mental disability. Some patients may have been thought to have developing dementia and will generally become lucid after successful surgery. When diagnosis is obtained surgery should not be postponed since patients with severe hypoglycemic attacks may risk permanent cerebral damage. Some institutions recommend a preoperative treatment period with diazoxide or somatostatin analog to evaluate response and tolerance if surgery should fail. We do not recommend this since somatostatin analog treatment is rarely efficient and diazoxide may have severe side-effects, with fluid retention and edema, that may complicate surgery.

Localization diagnosis

Insulinomas are unusual among endocrine pancreatic tumors since 90% are benign and single, and therefore generally available for surgical removal. However, most insulinomas are small, with size from 6 mm to commonly around 1–1.5 cm; 90% have been smaller than 2 cm. Ectopic extrapancreatic tumors have been rare, less than 1%, and have occurred in the proximity of the pancreas, generally in the duodenal wall. Insulinomas have been uniformly distributed between the head, body and tail of the pancreas. Malignant insulinomas are rare, accounting for 5–10% of cases, and should be suspected in patients with unusually large tumors (>4 cm in diameter). The malignant diagnosis requires histologic demonstration of local invasion in surrounding tissue or the presence of metastases. Multiple insulinomas may be encountered in 8–17% of cases, most often in MEN1 patients, but also without apparent association with this syndrome.

Because most insulinomas may be safely visualized at surgery by an experienced surgeon it has sometimes been claimed that localization diagnosis may not be necessary. However, with improvement of methods preoperative localization has become increasingly important to ensure successful outcome, also since we have learned that diffuse β-cell nesidioblastosis may occasionally be encountered in adults with hyperinsulinemic hypoglycemia. Accurate preoperative localization correlates with higher probability of cure. *Spiral CT* with i.v. contrast enhancement (or occasionally *MRI*) is routinely performed to provide anatomy and rule out presence of liver metastases, but also to detect the unusual larger tumors that could indicate malignancy. The i.v. contrast at CT may cause a tumor blush due to increased vascularity; otherwise these investigations have low sensitivity for detection of the smallest insulinomas. In contrast to other EPTs less than 50% of insulinomas are visualized by octreoscan because of inconsistent expression of somatostatin receptors.

During recent years *endoscopic ultrasound (EUS)* has appeared as the most efficient method for preoperative localization of the smaller insulinomas, with reported near 90% sensitivity and has replaced many other procedures (Anderson *et al.* 2000). An image of the pancreas is generated through the duodenal and stomach walls by an endoscope that should pass to the third portion of the duodenum to visualize also the uncinate process. Insulinomas in the pancreatic body and tail are imaged by scanning through the posterior wall of the stomach. False-positive findings may be accessory spleens or lymph glands within the pancreas, and some isoechoic (6%) or pedunculated tumors may fail visualization. EUS can reveal important relations to the pancreatic duct, and some equipment may be used for tumor biopsy.

An increasingly applied localization method is the *selective arterial stimulation (SAS) test*, with calcium gluconate injection into arteries supplying the pancreas, and concomitant hepatic vein sampling for insulin, which can regionalize an insulinoma to the head, body or tail of the pancreas (Doppman *et al.* 1995). The test is performed with an initial angiogram that may visualize the typical tumor blush of the insulinoma, and is of greatest value in reoperative cases, but is also used before primary operation when other localization studies are negative. When the test demonstrates insulin secretion from multiple areas of the pancreas, multiple insulinoma (MEN1 patients) or nesidioblastosis should be suspected.

Intraoperative ultrasound (IOUS) has been the greatest breakthrough in localization of occult insulinomas and is now generally considered mandatory for insulinoma operation together with complete pancreatic exploration and palpation at surgery (Fig. 23.25). The IOUS will efficiently detect typically hypoechogenic insulinomas and can identify tumors a few mm in size. It can demonstrate the surgical anatomy and guide safest approach to avoid injuries of the pancreatic duct during tumor removal, and can also reveal tumor bilobation that has to be appreciated at enucleation. The investigation is highly operator dependent and should be done by an experienced investigator.

Surgical treatment

Exposure of the pancreas is generally achieved via bilateral subcostal incision with a fixed upper abdominal retractor. The head of the pancreas is mobilized to the aorta by a Kocher manoeuvre, and the ventral and dorsal surfaces of the pancreatic head are dissected, with the uncinate process carefully freed from the portomesenteric vein. The distal pancreas is explored via the lesser sac, with incision of the retroperitoneum at the lower pancreatic border, allowing blunt dissection of the pancreatic body and tail to the mesenteric vein. The entire pancreas is palpated bidigitally and scanned with IOUS from the anterior and posterior surfaces (Fig. 23.25). An insulinoma often appears as a brownish-red mass possible to palpate between fingers as a firm discrete mass (Fig. 23.26). Tumors deep within the pancreatic head and in the uncinate process are difficult to palpate, especially in patients with previous pancreatitis. Combination of IOUS and palpation increases sensitivity of insulinoma detection to nearly 100%, but requires complete surgical exploration. Tumors in the proximal pancreas are generally enucleated with incision of the parenchyma parallel to the pancreatic duct, and with blunt dissection of the tumor and careful ligation of vessels and duct tributaries. Some pancreatic head tumors adjacent to the pancreatic duct (or bile duct) may be safer enucleated towards a catheter introduced by ERCP or duodenotomy. Rare large tumors with suspicion of malignancy require pancreaticoduodenectomy. Also pancreatic tail tumors may be safely enucleated if located on either edge of the pancreatic body or tail, or on the ventral or dorsal surface at distance from the duct. Resection is chosen for distal tumors close to the duct to minimize the risk of pancreatic effusion, or if a plane between the tumor capsule and the pancreatic parenchyma is not easily found. Distal pancreatic resection can be made spleen-preserving with benign tumors, if the splenic vein is not located

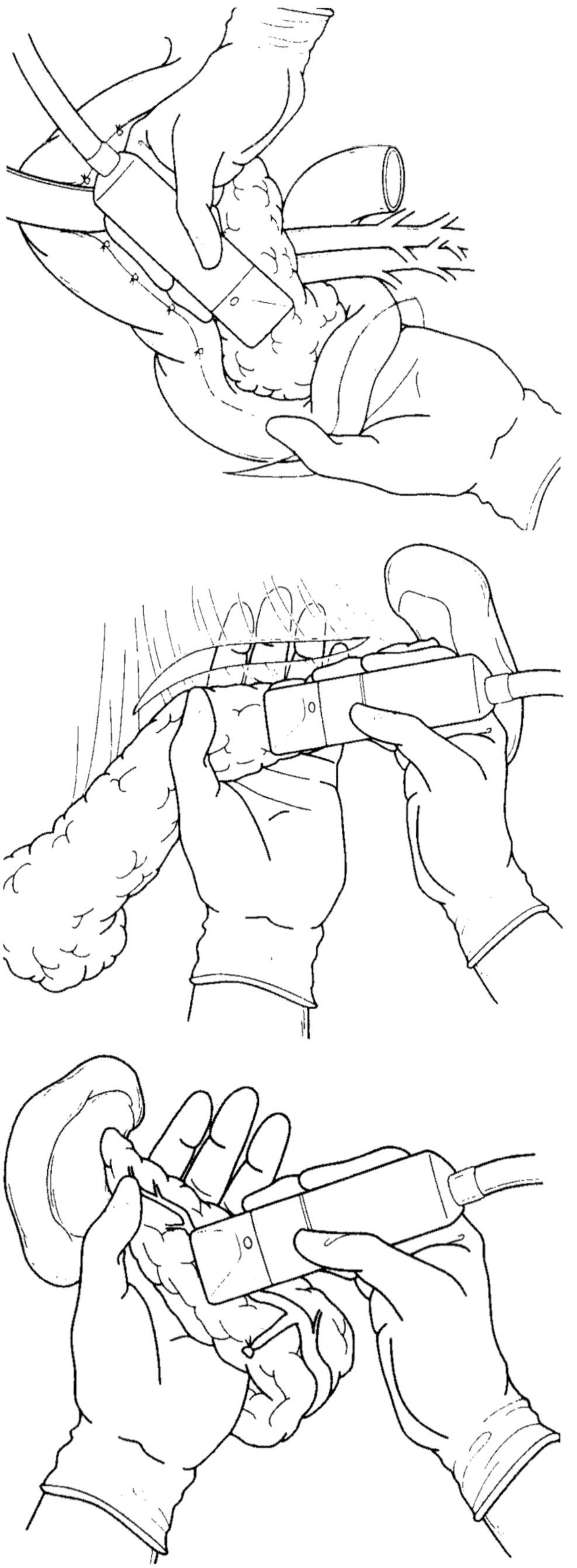

(a)

(b)

(c)

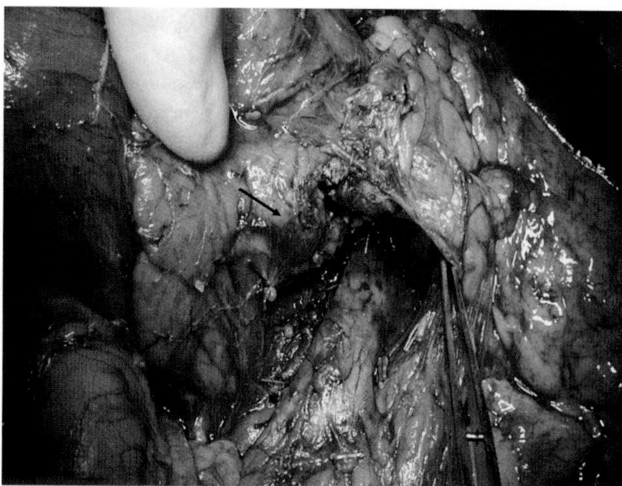

Fig. 23.26 Pancreatic head insulinoma possible to enucleate after release of attachments to mesenteric vein and with pancreatic duct proven to be at distance by IOUS. From Åkerström G, Hellman P. (2007) Neuroendocrine tumors. *Best Practice Research Clinical Endocrinology and Metabolism* 21(1): 87–109, with permission.

within the distal pancreatic parenchyma, but this is avoided with large or malignancy suspect insulinoma, since the splenic hilum is often a first site of metastases. Rapid intraoperative insulin assay has been applied to verify successful insulinoma excision, but generally this is done by frozen section analysis.

Complications due to postoperative pancreatic effusion are expected in 10–20%, with risk for formation of pseudocyst, abscess and chronic fistula formation. This is prevented by cautious operative technique and liberal prolonged closed suction drainage, with especial caution after tumor enucleation in the pancreatic head. Enucleation cavities should not be closed by suture.

Blind distal pancreatic resection should not be undertaken if an insulinoma is not found, because 50% of occult insulinomas are located in the pancreatic head or uncinate process. In such case the abdomen should be closed, and the patient subjected to further investigation to verify the biochemical diagnosis and once again exclude factitious insulin administration. More extensive localization procedures are applied before reoperation, including the SAS intraarterial stimulation test.

Fig. 23.25 Intraoperative ultrasound (IOUS) scanning (a) of the pancreatic head after extensive Kocher mobilization, (b) of the body and tail after mobilization along the inferior and superior border, and (c) of the posterior surface after medial reflection of the tail and spleen. IOUS scanning with a 7.5–10-MHz probe can identify nearly 100% of insulinomas, which typically appear sonolucent and hypoechogen. Scanning with a 5-MHz probe may reveal occult liver metastases. From Lowney J, Doherty GM (2001). In: Doherty GM, Skogseid B, eds. *Surgical Endocrinology*. Lippincott Williams & Wilkins, Philadelphia, with permission.

Laparoscopic surgery

Recently laparoscopic removal of insulinoma has been applied in many centers, and can be associated with increased patient comfort and reduced hospital stay. The operation is facilitated by laparoscopic ultrasonography, but may be complicated especially for pancreatic head tumors by higher risk of pancreatic effusion (20–40%). Distal pancreatic resection has been most often performed laparoscopically, enucleation from the pancreatic head has been considered more difficult, but may sometimes be safer with a preoperatively introduced pancreatic duct catheter. The laparoscopic surgery should be selected for preoperatively well visualized tumors, and should be performed only by expert laparoscopists.

Adult nesidioblastosis

Although representing a controversial issue, symptomatic hypoglycemia has been reported in adult individuals without insulinoma, but with diffuse beta-cell proliferation due to islet hypertrophy or nesidioblastosis (Service *et al.* 2005). The condition has been named adult nesidioblastosis, and the patients have been claimed to have typically postprandial, rather than fasting-provoked hyperinsulinemic hypoglycemia, with diagnosis confirmed by a meal test causing hypoglycemia and inappropriate insulin and C-peptide levels. The diagnosis can be supported if the SAS test shows insulin secretion from multiple areas of the pancreas and MEN1 is excluded, and the test may be used to direct gradient-guided subtotal pancreatic resection. Nesidioblastosis has also been reported in patients previously subjected to gastric bypass surgery for extreme obesity. In patients with nesidioblastosis reversal of hypoglycemia has been reported after 60–90% distal pancreatic resection, but cure has not been universal, and apparently sometimes less efficient in females. Some patients have been long-term palliated by medical treatment with calcium blockers. A preoperative treatment period with diazoxide has been suggested to help determine the extent of the required pancreatic resection, with more extensive (85%) resection recommended in patients refractory to the drug. We still await further studies that will clarify this syndrome and the role for surgery versus medical treatment.

Malignant insulinomas

Malignant insulinomas account for 5–10% of patients with endogenous hypoglycemia. Hypoglycemia may be severe in some patients, who may need continuous glucose infusion and cannot undergo a fasting test. High proinsulin/insulin ratio (>50%) may indicate malignant insulinoma, but occurs also with benign tumors. The malignant insulinoma is generally large, >4 cm, with an average size of ~6 cm depicted from older series. The diagnosis of malignancy requires demonstration of local invasion or metastases, with local infiltration as the only manifestation of malignancy in ~5%. Aggressive attempts of resection should be considered in patients with malignant insulinoma and even palliative debulking may yield survival benefit. If malignancy is suspected distal resection should include the spleen and peripancreatic lymph nodes. However, many patients with malignant insulinomas appear with spread metastases in the liver, lungs and lymph nodes, and are scarcely available for tumor reduction, with survival strongly dependent on response to chemotherapy. Some patients have larger, apparently dedifferentiated malignant insulinoma, with slight insulin hypersecretion and less severe hypoglycemia. These patients in particular can be helped by surgical removal of the large pancreatic tumor and in absence of spread metastases can experience long-term survival or cure. Ten-year survival of ~30% has been reported in patients with malignant insulinoma.

Gastrinoma: Zollinger–Ellison syndrome

Gastrinomas account for ~20% of functioning EPTs. The majority are sporadic, but as many as 30% occur as a part of the MEN1 syndrome, and even without a family history all Zollinger–Ellison syndrome (ZES) patients should be carefully evaluated for the syndrome. Gastrinomas and ZES constitute a rare cause of peptic ulcer disease with typically recurrent, atypical, multiple and complicated ulcers, very often with concomitant diarrhea, and/or esophagitis, and in 20% only diarrhea. Gastrin levels are often markedly increased, together with raised basal acid output with low gastric pH. Serum gastrin >1000 pg/mL and gastric pH < 2 is diagnostic of ZES. In patients with lower gastrin a secretin test may be required, which is diagnostic if there is paradoxal rise in gastrin, 200 pg/mL over baseline, but 15% of ZES patients have negative test. The important differential diagnosis is atrophic gastritis, where patients have high gastrin without gastric acid and high gastric pH, and pH > 3 excludes ZES.

Pancreatic gastrinomas have generally been large, malignant tumors, with high incidence of metastases at an early stage (lymph node metastases ~45% and liver metastases ~60%) and often rather rapid progression. Low cure rate was reported after attempts of surgical excision of gastrinoma until in 1989–1990, when duodenal gastrinomas were recognized as the most common gastrinomas, and subsequently found to constitute the primary tumor in 60–70% of sporadic ZES, and 90% of MEN1-associated ZES (Thompson *et al.* 1989; Pipeleers-Marichal *et al.* 1990). MEN1 ZES patients have often had multiple duodenal tumors (Fig. 23.27). The duodenal gastrinomas have been revealed as typically very tiny submucosal tumors, often smaller than 0.5 cm, being most frequently located in the first and second portion of the duodenum, but possible to find in the entire duodenum to the Treitz ligament. These tumors have great tendency to lymph node metastases (~45%), but liver metastases have generally been late and occurred in a minority of patients (~10%), and this has been considered to provide an obvious possibility for successful surgical removal that could prevent or delay development of liver metastases. The duodenal

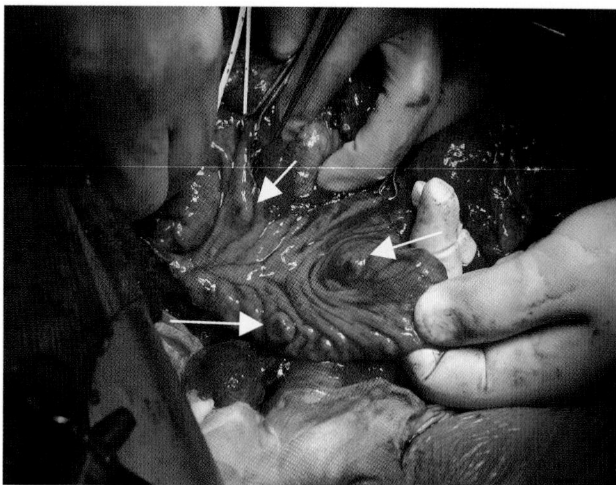

Fig. 23.27 Multiple duodenal gastrinomas in MEN1 patient. From Åkerström G, Hellman P. (2007) Neuroendocrine tumors. *Best Practice Research Clinical Endocrinology and Metabolism* 21(1): 87–109, with permission.

tumor entity may have represented the primary tumor in patients with 'primary lymph node gastrinoma', diagnosed in up to 10% of patients with ZES, where the primary tumor may have been minimal and remained undetected.

Indications for surgery

All sporadic ZES patients should be considered for surgery, unless there is spread or unresectable liver metastases, and the operation should routinely include exploration of the duodenum and pancreas. Surgery is liberally undertaken also in absence of positive localization diagnosis, since especially these patients may have resectable duodenal gastrinomas. Prior to surgery the patients routinely receive treatment with high-dose proton pump inhibitor and often also somatostatin analog to minimize risk of ulcer complications.

Localization diagnosis

Sporadic pancreatic gastrinomas causing ZES have been solitary and generally large (>1 cm in diameter—substantiating that gastrin is an ectopic hormone for pancreatic tumors), and have occurred with nearly equal frequency in the entire pancreas. The small duodenal gastrinomas are rarely detected by preoperative localization studies. Spiral CT with i.v. contrast (or MRI) is routinely performed in ZES patients to visualize lymph node and liver metastases prior to surgery. However, small duodenal tumors are not detectable, and instead larger lymph node metastases around the pancreatic head are easily mistaken to represent the primary tumor. Octreoscan has special affinity for gastrinoma, and can often (~90%) reveal lymph node and liver metastases, and occasional larger primary tumors, and 5-HTP-PET investigation has appeared even more sensitive. EUS can detect pancreatic and few larger duodenal gastrinomas, and often lymph gland metastases, but will rarely visualize the smallest duodenal tumors. The selective arterial stimulation test (the SAS, Imamura test) was originally developed with injection of pentagastrin for visualization of gastrinoma, and may provide tumor regionalization, and demonstrate presence or absence of liver metastases (Imamura & Takahashi 1993). The SAS test can be applied if other localization studies are negative, and is otherwise undertaken prior to reoperation.

Surgical treatment

The surgical cure rate in ZES patients increased markedly after 1990, when it was appreciated that the majority of gastrinomas occur in the duodenum (Norton *et al.* 1999). In operation for gastrinoma the pancreas is explored and investigated with IOUS as depicted for insulinoma, and the duodenum is freed to the Treitz ligament. The duodenal gastrinomas may be visualized by longitudinal duodenotomy at surgery with inversion of the lumen for careful palpation of the mucosa. The smallest duodenal submucosal tumors, sometimes only 1–2 mm in size, can be identified by palpation as tiny nodules under the mucosa. The small duodenal gastrinomas can be removed by mucosal dissection, whereas larger tumors (>5 mm) require full-thickness duodenal wall excision. Pancreatic gastrinomas have often been possible to enucleate. Lymph node metastases on the pancreatic surface, originating from an undiscovered duodenal gastrinoma, may have close attachment to the pancreatic capsule and should not be mistaken to represent pancreatic tumors. Pancreaticoduodenectomy is required for large gastrinomas in the pancreatic head and occasional larger, invasive duodenal tumors. Surgery in patients with gastrinoma should invariably include clearance of lymph node metastases around the pancreas and duodenum, and along the hepatic–celiac and mesenteric artery (important location with primary tumor in distal duodenum), and should aim to identify and remove also resectable liver metastases.

If a gastrinoma is not found at exploration the liver is palpated and investigated by IOUS for a rare primary hepatic gastrinoma. The distal duodenum and proximal jejunum should also be explored and the ovaries in a female patient.

Prognosis

All gastrinomas are potentially malignant. Survival has been favorable in patients with duodenal gastrinomas also with presence of lymph node metastases. Removal of regional metastases possibly limits further spread, and few (~10%) patients with duodenal gastrinomas have developed liver metastases (Norton *et al.* 1999). Adverse prognostic factors have been primary tumor of pancreatic origin or large duodenal tumors, presence of liver or bone metastases, and very high serum gastrin. The small duodenal gastrinomas often have remarkably slow progression with ~90% 10-year survival, whereas pancreatic gastrinomas have more rapid progression with only 60% 10-year survival.

Glucagonomas

Glucagonomas are uncommon, representing ~10% of functioning EPT, and are most frequent around 50 years of age. The patients have mild diabetes, hypoaminoacidemia, and a typical intensely pruritic skin rash, necrolytic migrating erythema, which often starts in the groin and migrates to extremities. In addition they have tendency for deep venous thrombosis and thrombophlebitis, and may at advanced stages develop cachexia. Diagnosis is based on demonstration of raised plasma glucagon and is often delayed. Marked palliation and preparation for operation is achieved by parenteral nutritional and by treatment with somatostatin analog, which tends to heal the skin lesion. Antithrombotic medication should also be given, because of the high risk for thrombosis and pulmonary embolism during surgery. The glucagonomas are generally located in the pancreatic body or tail and are often large, between 4 and 15 cm in diameter. The tumors are malignant in ~80% and often present with regional lymph gland metastases in the splenic hilum. Patients should be treated with pancreatic resection or subtotal pancreatectomy dependent on tumor location, together with clearance of regional lymph node metastases, and therefore with splenectomy as part of the procedure. IOUS can help detect occult liver metastases that can be resected or ablated. Tumor progression is often slow despite presence of metastases, and during a long disease course the patients may require sequential excision of lymph node or liver metastases, with 5 years or more between recurrent lesions. A 10-year survival of ~50% has been reported.

Vipomas

Tumors secreting vasoactive intestinal peptide (VIP) cause the WDHA (watery diarrhea, hypokalemia, achlorhydria) syndrome characterized by severe secretory diarrhea with volumes exceeding 3L/day, hypokalemic acidosis and dehydration. Due to vasodilatory effect of VIP patients may exhibit flush, and some patients have hypercalcemia. Correct diagnosis is obtained by demonstration of raised VIP values. Intensive treatment with somatostatin analog and intravenous fluid and electrolyte resuscitation is often urgently required before operation due to risk for severe dehydration. The tumors are generally large and located within the pancreatic tail, 50% of patients have metastases at presentation. Treatment is surgical excision, and debulking surgery should be considered in patients with metastases, consisting of pancreatectomy and resection or ablation of liver metastases and even resection of lung metastases if present. Routine cholecystectomy may facilitate treatment with long-acting somatostatin analog. A 10-year survival of ~40% is reported.

Somatostatinoma

Somatostatinomas occur in the duodenum or in the pancreas. The duodenal somatostatinomas are more common in patients with von Recklinghausen disease, and may occasionally have concomitant pheochromocytoma. These tumors are usually small and diagnosed because of bleeding or ampullary obstruction with jaundice. The pancreatic somatostatinomas may be associated with the somatostatinoma syndrome consisting of diabetes mellitus, cholelithiasis and steatorrhea, but may also lack typical symptoms. The patients may require local resection or pancreaticoduodenectomy together with regional lymph node clearance.

Corticotropin-producing tumors

EPTs may secrete ACTH or CRH causing a severe ectopic Cushing syndrome. Most of these tumors have metastases and rapid disease progression, some have concomitant production of gastrin and may have suffer from a ZES. Ketoconazole treatment is usually inefficient and patients may suffer from severe hypokalemia and require bilateral adrenalectomy. Debulking surgery of the pancreatic tumor or metastases is rarely efficient treatment.

Non-functioning endocrine pancreatic tumors

The non-functioning EPTs are not related to any clinical syndrome of hormone excess (Hellman *et al.* 2000; Kouvaraki *et al.* 2005). They may have no hormone secretion, due to absence of secretory granulae, or release amounts insufficient to cause clinical symptoms. The majority have increased serum values of chromogranin A, common are also raised values of pancreatic polypeptide (PP) revealed in 50–70%, fewer have low values of insulin/proinsulin, glucagon or calcitonin without symptoms. The non-functioning tumors have increased in frequency and now constitute 30–50% of EPT. They account for 3–5% of pancreatic tumors, but are important to recognize because of markedly better survival prospects than patients with adenocarcinoma. The non-functioning EPTs are most often diagnosed at the age of ~50–60 years, but also occur in younger individuals, where they may be discovered as unusually large tumors without the typical malignant cachexia of pancreatic carcinoma (Fig. 23.28).

Diagnosis of the non-functioning tumors can be made by demonstrating hypervascularization of primary tumor and metastases on contrast-enhanced CT, and positive octreoscan, raised serum levels of chromogranin A or serum PP, or by ultrasound-guided fine or semifine needle biopsy stained with chromogranin A or synaptophysin. EUS may also be used for biopsy.

The non-functioning endocrine pancreatic tumors most commonly (60%) occupy the pancreatic head, but may occur in the entire pancreas. They may cause jaundice or discomfort

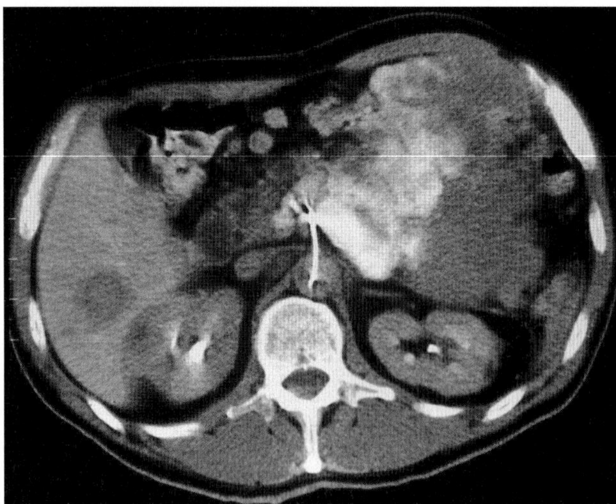

(a)

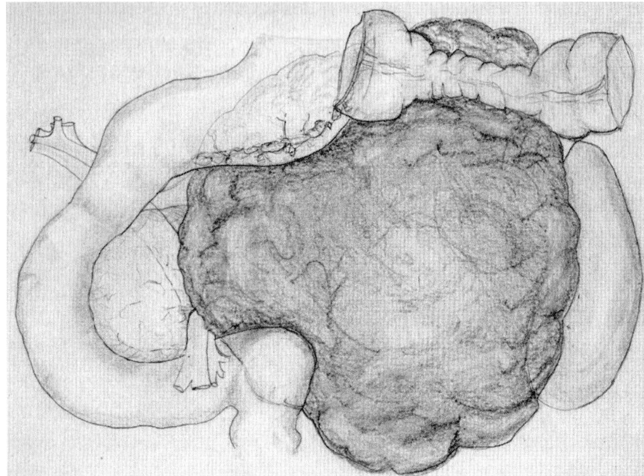

(b)

Fig. 23.28 (a) CT image and (b) drawing of non-functioning pancreatic head tumor with growth in transverse colon. The celiac–hepatic artery, mesenteric artery, and portomesenteric vein could be dissected from the tumor capsule. From Hellman *et al.* (2000) *World J Surg* 24: 1353–7, with permission.

due to local extension or pain due to pancreatitis, though jaundice may be absent also with conspicuously large pancreatic head tumors. Although growth is typically slow compared to adenocarcinomas, the progress is variable, some are indolent with growth only of the primary lesion, whereas others progress rapidly with lymph node and liver metastases. High Ki-67 proliferation index (>5%) and high frequency of chromosomal rearrangements have been associated with more rapid progression. Generally extra-abdominal spread from endocrine pancreatic tumors occurs late.

Even when survival is extended the pancreatic tumors *per se* may be the cause of morbidity. The tumors tend to grow into surrounding structures, the ventricle, the duodenum, or the transverse colon, and may then be associated with obstruction or bleeding. With continuous growth in the pancreatic head and body, the mesenteric vein is often invaded and occluded, causing portal hypertension and increased tendency to gastrointestinal bleeding, and eventually mesenteric thrombosis and intestinal ischemia. Also the celiac, the hepatic, and the mesenteric artery may be involved.

Surgical treatment

Surgery is indicated for removal of the primary tumor to reduce risk for the mesenteric vein involvement or gastric outlet obstruction, and to facilitate efficient chemotherapy, and may be undertaken also in presence of low-volume liver metastases (Hellman *et al.* 2000; Kouvaraki *et al.* 2005). Also the largest EPTs can often be removed by extended pancreaticoduodenectomy or subtotal pancreatectomy, even in presence of portal hypertension, sometimes with use of vein graft (from internal jugular or saphenous vein) to restore patency of the mesenteric vein (Hellman *et al.* 2000; Kouvaraki *et al.* 2005). Involvement of the mesentericoceliac arterial axis has been claimed to contraindicate surgery, but in our experience the central axis arteries may often be dissected free, or they may be graft substituted. Extensive dissection around the mesenteric artery may cause severe diarrhea due to denervation of intestinal plexa, and significantly impair the patients' general condition.

Prognosis

Presence and extent of liver metastases is the main determinant of survival. The rate of metastases varies from 62 to 92%. Results of surgery for large non-functioning tumors have reported 5-year survival of 65%, and 10-year survival of ~50% or more with extensive removal of metastases. Survival advantage has been evident in absence of liver metastases or if such metastases have been resected. Merely palliative surgery with remaining tumor has resulted in poor survival. The operative mortality of the aggressive surgery has varied from 0 to 15%; the risks have been associated mainly with complications due to mesenteric vein or artery occlusion. Peroperative morbidity has varied between 6 and 39%, pancreatic effusion and abscess formation has been a problem in many series, but generally resolved with efficient drainage.

Endocrine pancreatic tumors associated with MEN1

Pancreatico-duodenal endocrinopathy involvement occurs clinically in around 50% of MEN1 patients (Åkerström *et al.* 2002). Non-functioning EPTs secreting PP are the most prevalent tumors, occurring in nearly all patients, often also coincident with the functioning tumors. Gastrinoma and ZES have been the most common functioning tumors, encountered in nearly 50% of MEN1 patients; insulinoma has occurred in 20%, glucagonoma and VIPoma in <5%. Insulinoma has been the most frequent functioning tumor in teenagers. The MEN1 syndrome has been diagnosed in 30% of ZES patients, but only in 5–10% of patients with insulinoma. Raised hormone values are often seen without presence of hormonal syndrome; most common are raised serum values of PP, gastrin and chromogranin A.

Malignant pancreatic tumors are the most common cause of disease-related death in MEN1 kindreds, and screening for the endocrinopathy coupled to early intervention once a tumor is identified has appeared justified from the disease history. The MEN1 pancreas typically harbors numerous microadenomas, but during a patient's lifetime only few will grow to clinically relevant tumors. Disease progress is often slow with the MEN1 tumors, larger tumors are likely to become aggressive and metastasizing, though also the small gastrinomas spread early to regional lymph nodes. In the absence of distant metastases surgery is invariably recommended for MEN1 insulinomas and rare VIPomas or glucagonomas, but has been controversial with MEN1 ZES because long-term cure is rarely achieved. However, follow-up studies of MEN1 kindreds have indicated that ZES appears as a late feature of the disease with metastases already present in 30–50% of patients. Surgical removal of gastrinoma and lymph gland metastases appear to decrease risk for development of liver metastases, and since this is a negative prognostic factor we and others propose surgery also for ZES patients for malignancy prevention and to facilitate medical treatment. Non-functioning EPT can often be diagnosed earlier by screening with biochemical markers consisting of pancreatic hormones (especially PP is sensitive), and chromogranin A. We suggest MEN1 patients be subjected to pancreatic exploration even in absence of hormone excess syndrome, when these markers are unequivocally raised and EUS or any other radiologic investigation (spiral CT or 5-HTP PET) indicate presence of a tumor of ~1 cm or larger (Åkerström *et al.* 2002; Hellman *et al.* 2005). Others have required larger tumor size of 2 or 3 cm for tumor removal, which in our opinion implies higher risk for already developed metastases. Our active prophylactic pancreatic surgery in MEN1 recommends operation in relatively young patients subjected to the screening program, since age may also be important for tumor progression.

Surgical treatment

MEN1 patients are most often subjected to 80% distal pancreatic resection combined with enucleation of tumors in the pancreatic head, with the aim of minimize the risk of developing diabetes (Fig. 23.29) (Åkerström *et al.* 2002). Tumors smaller than ~5 mm in the pancreatic head may be difficult to enucleate and may be left for observation. Duodenotomy is done in patients with raised gastrin or ZES to identify and remove duodenal gastrinomas, which may often be multiple (Fig. 23.27). Pancreaticoduodenectomy may occasionally be required in MEN1 patients with bulky tumors of any entity in the pancreatic head or duodenum, and has also been proposed for efficient eradication of MEN1 ZES. However, we do not propose routine pancreaticoduodenectomy for MEN1 ZES patients since many have concomitant non-functioning tail tumors, and this procedure will also cause difficulties treating recurrent tumors of any entity. Moreover, after pancreaticoduodenectomy liver metastases cannot be treated with embolization because of risk of ascending infection via the hepaticojejunostomy. Reoperation may be required in MEN1 patients with enucleation or resection of new tumors, and has in our experience been uneventful. Lymph gland or liver metastases may occasionally require surgery. Total pancreatectomy may be needed for very large malignant tumors, but has only occasionally been performed in our MEN1 patients. Liberal pancreatic surgery in MEN1 patients has to be performed with minimal morbidity and virtually absent mortality, achieved by cautious dissection and adequate drainage of enucleated areas, resection surfaces, or anastomoses.

The active surgical strategy in MEN1 has appeared to reduce the risk of metastases or death from pancreatic malignancy in MEN1 patients, but requires longer follow-up and randomized evaluation.

References

Åkerström G, Hessman O, Skogseid B. (2002) Timing and extent of surgery in symptomatic and asymptomatic neuroendocrine tumors of the pancreas in MEN 1. *Langenbeck's Arch Surg* 386: 558–69.

Anderson MA, Carpenter S, Thompson NW *et al.* (2000) Endoscopic ultrasound is highly accurate and directs management in patients with neuroendocrine tumors of the pancreas. *Am J Gastroenterol* 95: 2271–7.

Doppman JL, Chang R, Fraker DL *et al.* (1995) Localization of insulinomas to regions of the pancreas by intra-arterial stimulation with calcium. *Ann Intern Med* 123: 269–73.

Hellman P, Andersson M, Rastad J *et al.* (2000) Surgical strategy for large or malignant endocrine pancreatic tumours. *World J Surg* 24: 1353–60.

Hellman P, Hennings J, Åkerström G, Skogseid B. (2005) Endoscopic ultrasonography for evaluation of pancreatic tumours in multiple endocrine neoplasia type 1. *Br J Surg* 92: 1508–12.

Imamura M, Takahashi K. (1993) Use of selective arterial secretin injection test to guide surgery in patients with Zollinger–Ellison syndrome. *World J Surg* 17: 433–8.

Kouvaraki MA, Solorzano CC, Shapiro SE *et al.* (2005) Surgical treatment of non-functioning pancreatic islet cell tumors. *J Surg Oncol* 89: 170–85.

Norton JA, Fraker DL, Alexander HR. (1999) Surgery to cure the Zollinger–Ellison syndrome. *N Engl J Med* 341: 635–44.

Pipeleers-Marichal M, Somer G, Willems G *et al.* (1990) Gastrinomas in the duodenums of patients with multiple endocrine neoplasia type 1 and the Zollinger–Ellison syndrome. *N Engl J Med* 322: 723–7.

Service GJ, Thompson GB, Service FJ *et al.* (2005) Hyperinsulinemic hypoglycemia with nesidioblastosis after gastric-bypass surgery. *N Engl J Med* 353: 249–53.

Thompson NW, Vinik AI, Eckhauser FE. (1989) Microgastrinomas of the duodenum. A cause of failed operation for the Zollinger–Ellison syndrome. *Ann Surg* 209: 396–404.

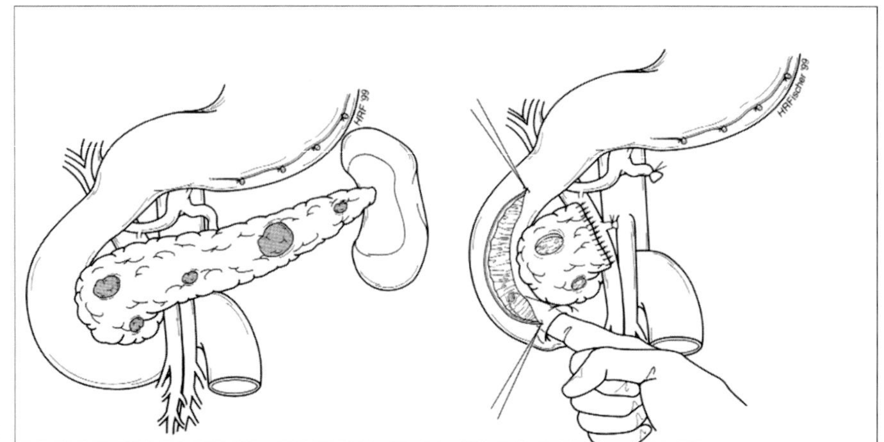

(a)

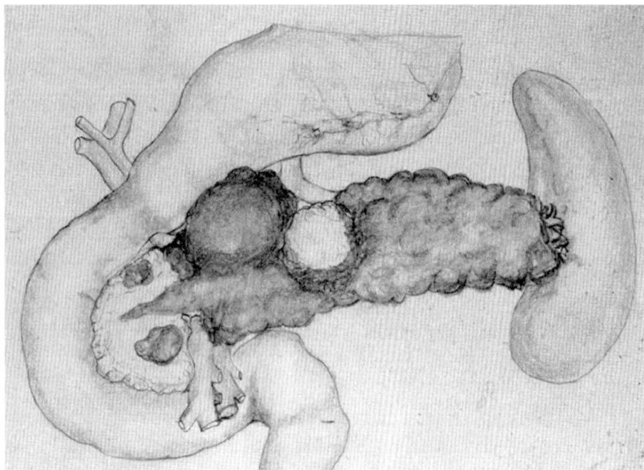

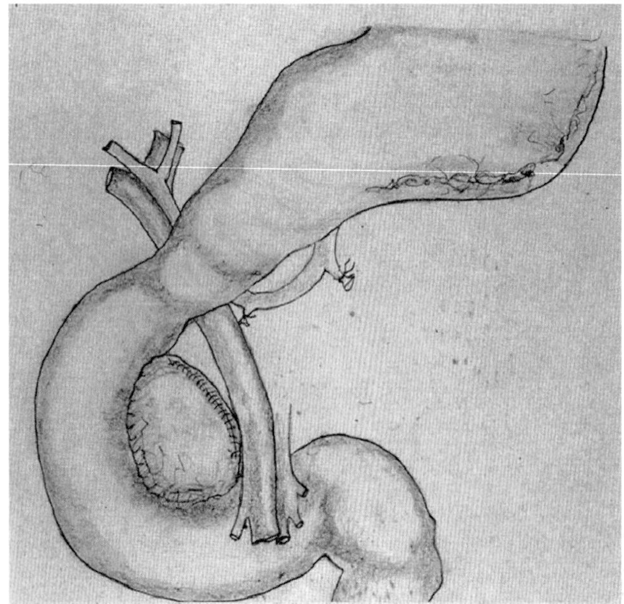

(b)

Fig. 23.29 (a) The commonly applied (80%) subtotal distal pancreatectomy in MEN1 patients (N Thompson procedure), combined with enucleation of tumors in the pancreatic head. Duodenotomy (right) is undertaken in patients with raised serum-gastrin. (b) Drawing of non-functioning pancreatic tumor of the pancreatic body and tail in 25-year-old male patient with MEN1 and raised serum PP, glucagon and chromogranin A values. The tumor was removed by distal pancreatic resection with dissection of tumor extension and two separate tumors in the pancreatic head, with a small part of the pancreatic head remaining (right) without development of diabetes. From Skogseid B *et al.* (2001). In: Doherty GM, Skogseid B, eds. *Surgical Endocrinology*. Lippincott Williams & Wilkins, Philadelphia, with permission.

Surgery: midgut tumors

Matthias Rothmund

General

Midgut neuroendocrine tumors (midgut NETs) most often originate from the terminal ileum but may be located within the jejunum and the duodenum as well. The primary tumor usually is small (a few millimeters in diameter) and located within the submucosa and may be visible at surgery only as a tiny submucosal nodule with localized fibrosis and thickening of the intestinal wall (Akerstrom *et al.* 2005) (Fig. 23.30). One-third of the patients have multiple primary tumors in the adjacent intestine (Fig. 23.31). Some authors suggest lymphatic dissemination as a possible explanation for this feature (Akerstrom *et al.* 2005). Mesenteric lymph node metastases occur frequently even with the smallest tumors, and tend to be markedly larger than the primary tumor or tumors.

Intestinal obstruction is almost never caused by the tumor itself but develops because of distinct mesenteric fibrosis ('desmoplastic reaction') leading to shrinkage of the mesenteric root, kinking of the adjacent small bowel and fibrotic banding that may result in intestinal obstruction. Chronic intestinal ischemia is a consequence of the combination of vascular sclerosis and constriction due to vessel encasement by the mesenteric tumor in line with the desmoplastic reaction and hormone-release (Ohrvall *et al.* 2000) (Fig. 23.32).

Surgical intervention has to be considered as one of the corner stones in the multidisciplinary treatment of these tumors, even in patients with non-resectable peritoneal or lymphatic metastases.

In cases of limited non-metastatic disease surgery represents the most important and only potential curative therapy. The extent of surgery is dependent on localization, size and entity of the tumor.

Even in the case of metastatic spread to the liver, palliative resection of the primary tumor together with the attaining lymph nodes has to be performed to prevent further involvement of the mesenteric root with subsequent irresectability.

Surgery can alleviate symptoms in nearly 80% of patients with advanced disease (Makridis *et al.* 1997) and leads to prolongation of 5-year survival rate (Hellman *et al.* 2002b). Hence, even when cure cannot be achieved due to metastatic spread to the liver or gross involvement of mesenteric lymph nodes, incomplete resection ('tumor debulking') may be indicated to facilitate medical therapy and improve quality of life.

Repeated surgery may be needed in case of recurrent symptoms due to progression after primary surgery. Reoperation can be very difficult because of harsh fibrosis and regrowth of tumor. Fistulation, intestinal devascularization or short bowel syndrome are possible complications thereafter. Therefore, surgery for midgut NET can be challenging and referral to institutions with special experience is strongly recommended.

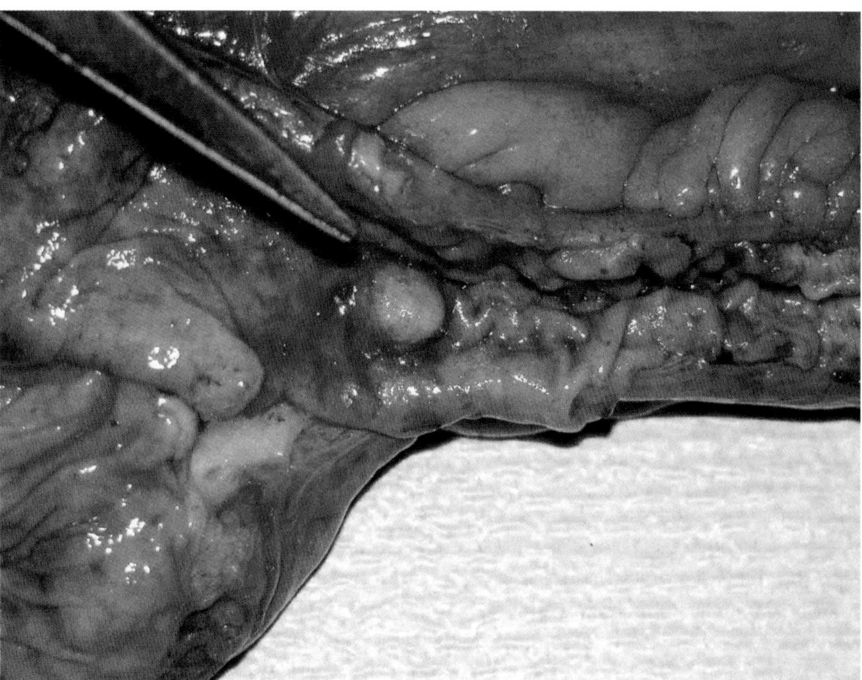

Fig. 23.30 Primary midgut NET within the terminal ileum close to the ileocecal valve presenting as a small, hard, flat, submucous and fibrotic knot with a size of 1 cm.

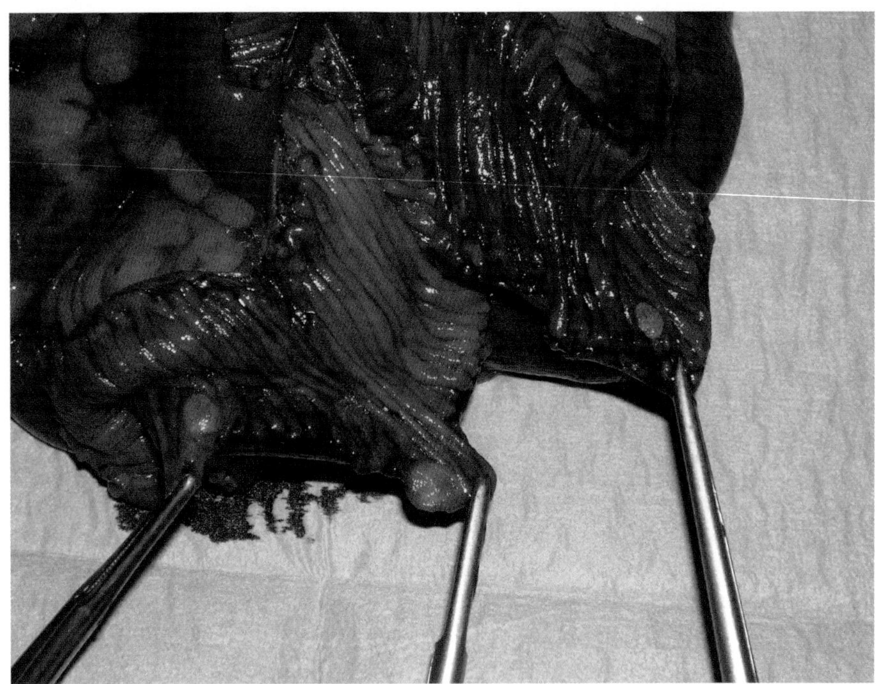

Fig. 23.31 Multicentric midgut NET within the terminal ileum.

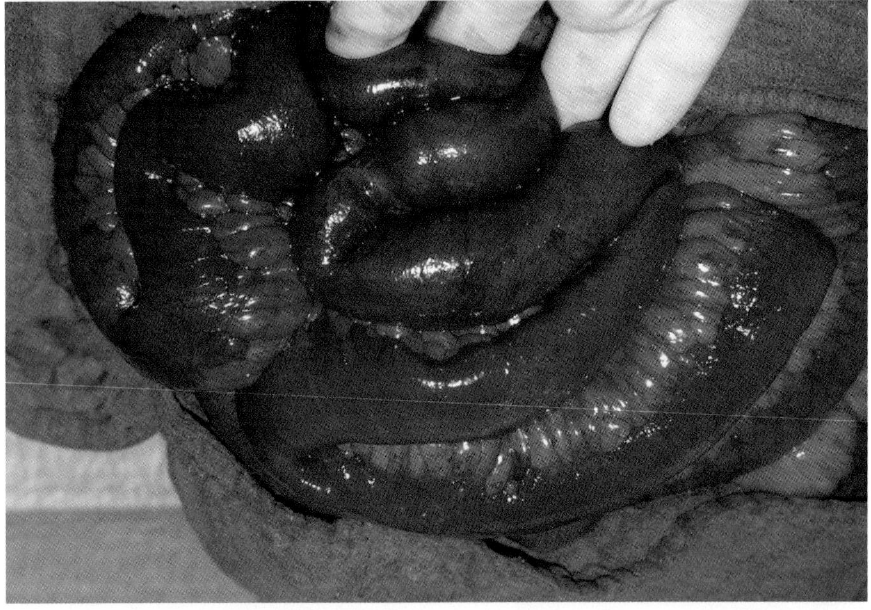

Fig. 23.32 Small bowel ischemia due to entrapment of appertaining vessels by a conglomerate of mesenteric lymph nodes.

Symptoms and diagnostic procedures

Midgut NET tend to grow slowly. Many patients endure periods of unspecific episodic abdominal discomfort, mostly cramps or pain, before the disease becomes overt (Akerstrom *et al.* 2005). Abdominal symptoms may increase until bowel obstruction or intestinal ischemia develops causing chronic pain, vomiting etc., and the patient requires surgery. Gastrointestinal bleeding may be another, though rare, initial manifestation of NET. Metastatic spread to extra-abdominal sites such as the skeleton (spine, ribs and skull), the lungs, central nervous system, mediastinal and peripheral lymph nodes, ovaries, breast, and skin may occur and an enlarged neck lymph node may be the earliest sign of the disease.

Symptoms always imply an advanced tumor stage and represent complications of lymph node metastases in the mesentery, or metastases in the liver ('carcinoid syndrome') or at distant sites.

Nearly half of the tumors will be detected during emergency surgery for obstruction or signs of 'appendicitis', without preoperative knowledge of the underlying illness (Akerstrom *et al.* 2005). Diagnosis may be confirmed after detection of liver metastases. With metastatic spread to the liver, symptoms according to serotonine release may develop and are summarized as the 'carcinoid syndrome'.

Monoamine oxidases in the liver can detoxify serotonine from primaries and mesenteric metastases, and therefore the carcinoid syndrome tends to develop only if the patient has a large amount of liver metastases. The carcinoid syndrome, with flush, diarrhea, right-sided heart valve fibrosis, and bronchial obstruction, occurs in approximately 20% of patients with midgut NET of the ileum or jejunum (Akerstrom *et al.* 2005).

Frequency of lymph node metastases at presentation of a midgut NET is directly associated with tumor size and dependent on tumor localization (Fig. 23.33). Depth of tumor invasion and multilocular disease promote the occurrence of lymph node metastases. Lymph nodes will be affected in approximately 44% if tumor size is below 1 cm. If tumor size exceeds 2 cm, lymphatic metastases will be detectable in approximately 82% (Memon & Nelson 1997).

The extent of lymphatic and liver metastases at the time of diagnosis represents the most reliable prognostic factor. Five-year survival drops from 73% in patients with a limited disease to approximately 50% in patients with liver metastases (Modlin *et al.* 2003).

Midgut NET can be diagnosed by demonstration of raised levels of the serotonine metabolite 5-hydroxy-indoleacetic acid (5-HIAA) in 24-hour urinary samples. The increase in this metabolite is specific for midgut NET, but appears only in advanced disease states, and generally indicates the presence of liver metastases (Akerstrom *et al.* 2005). Alternatively, plasma chromogranin A can be measured as a sensitive but somewhat unspecific parameter for diagnosis and disease progression. Chromogranin A reflects the tumor burden and is commonly used to follow results of treatment, although false increases may occur (Akerstrom *et al.* 2005).

Dynamic CT with contrast enhancement can efficiently demonstrate mesenteric metastases and retroperitoneal tumor extension. A mesenteric tumor with radiating densities is considered pathognomonic for mesenteric metastases of midgut NET (Akerstrom *et al.* 2005). CT can reveal relations between

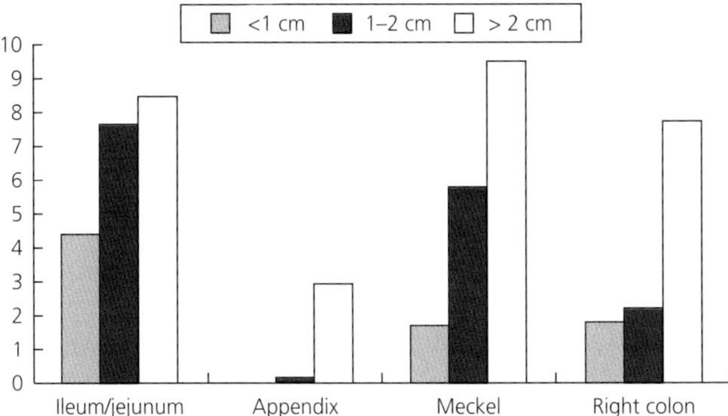

Fig. 23.33 Risk for mesenteric lymph node metastases depending on size and location of the midgut NET as indicator of tumor aggressiveness.

mesenteric metastases and the mesenteric arteries and veins. In advanced cases with intestinal ischemia dilated peripheral mesenteric veins and edematous loops of intestine may be visible. CT with images before and after intravenous contrast administration and in arterial and venous phases is often used to visualize liver metastases, but has rather low sensitivity for small lesions. MRI can sometimes demonstrate liver metastases more efficiently. Percutaneous ultrasound is used to guide fine or semi-fine needle biopsy for histologic diagnosis of liver or mesenteric metastases (Akerstrom *et al.* 2005).

Octeotide scan has a sensitivity of more than 90% and is routinely used to determine metastatic spread, especially to extra-abdominal sites. The investigation can visualize bone metastases better than bone scan, which may fail to identify osteolytic lesions. PET with the serotonin precursor 5-hydroxytryptophan labeled with ^{11}C (5HTP-PET) can identify midgut NET with a high sensitivity, and is used to monitor treatment effects (Akerstrom *et al.* 2005).

Perioperative management and informed consent

If a midgut NET is already diagnosed, the patient's consent form has to include possible extension of surgical resection to unexpected liver and lymph node metastases and resection of parts of the intestine threatened by desmoplastic reaction of the tumor. The patient must be informed that the disease might be much more extended than expected preoperatively. At the same time, the possibility of incomplete resection ('tumor debulking') instead of complete removal if involvement of large parts of the intestine is present has to be explained.

Anesthesiology plays an important role in the treatment of patients with NET. Patients with NET can have perioperative flush, diarrhea or bronchial obstruction due to hormone secretion. Electrolyte imbalance should be carefully adjusted.

Careful premedication to combat anxiety is mandatory because stress can trigger episodes of flush. Additional prophylaxis against the effects of the mediators by H1 and H2 receptor blockage and methysergide is necessary.

Any manipulation of neuroendocrine tumors carries the possibility of provoking a carcinoid crisis. This is a reaction to the release of different substances such as serotonin, callikrein, bradykinin, histamine or tachykinin. These substances are known to cause partly antidromic effects on the blood pressure and pulse, leading to unpredictable interactions. The most frequent feature is the development of life-threatening hypotension and bronchial spasm that are typically difficult to adjourn.

Somatostatin or octreotide should be given perioperatively as a prophylaxis against the carcinoid crisis (intravenously, starting 24 hours ahead of surgery: octreotide at a dose of 50–200 μg/h) (Oberg *et al.* 2004).

For emergency surgery in therapy-naïve patients with functional NETs, a 500–1000 μg i.v. bolus of octreotide or 500 μg s.c. should be given 1–2 h before surgery (Oberg *et al.* 2004).

The recommended intraoperative use of octreotide for carcinoid crisis with hypotension is bolus i.v. doses of 500–1000 μg, with treatment repetition at 5-min intervals until control of symptoms is achieved. Alternatively, following an i.v. bolus dose, continuous i.v. infusion of octreotide at a dose of 50–200 μg/h may be given. In any patient who has required supplemental dosing during a procedure, the postoperative dose would be 50–200 μg/h for 24 h, followed by resumption of the preoperative treatment schedule (Oberg *et al.* 2004).

Somatostatin or its analogs are able to inhibit peptide release out of cells from the GEP system. Instability of circulation that occurs despite that is difficult to treat and differentiate from other circumstances such as hypovolemia. If hypotension occurs, substitution of i.v. liquids should be accompanied by i.v. bolus as described above. Sympathomimetics are prohibited, because of their ability of peptide release by α-receptors.

Patients have to be monitored at an intensive care unit after surgery.

To minimize the perioperative risk in patients with NET one should consider the guidelines shown in Table 23.13.

Surgery

Primary midgut NETs tend to be deposited to the right side of the mesenteric artery and typically are located at the most distal part of the ileum. The primary tumor usually presents as a small, hard, flat, submucous and fibrotic nodule with a median size of 0.5–1 cm and a grayish to whitish color (Fig. 23.30). If this tumor cannot be moved against the underlying tissue, this has to be interpreted as a sign of invasion of the muscularis propria.

Characteristically the primary tumor is surrounded by fairly extensive areas of fibrosis eventually accompanied by gross lymph node involvement or liver metastases.

Within surgery, mobilization of the right hemicolon and dissection of adhesions should be the initial step. Freeing the mesenteric root will help to identify the mesenteric vessels. Without careful dissection of the mesenteric root wedge resection in the fibrotic and contracted mesentery may easily compromise the main mesenteric artery and devascularize a major part of the small intestine with creation of a short bowel syndrome (Makridis *et al.* 1997; Ohrvall *et al.* 2000). The tumor may appear to be non-resectable because of intestinal entrapment or mesenteric metastases encasing major intestinal blood vessels. In these cases, dividing the mesenteric lymph node conglomerate even with cutting through the tumor mass may allow separation from the vessels, thus preserving important arcades along the intestine. This may permit a more limited intestinal resection and reduce the risk of creating a short bowel syndrome. Intestinal bypass should be avoided wherever possible, mainly because intestinal ischemia may develop in disengaged intestinal segments. Bypass procedures should only be selected when extensive tumor growth or fibrosis inhibit appropriate dissection (Ohrvall *et al.* 2000).

Because of frequent lymphatic involvement even in the case of a small tumor, extended resection together with the relevant lymph nodes is essential (Fig. 23.34).

When the primary lesion and regional metastases are removed by wedge resection of the mesentery, lymph node metastases should be cleared as effectively as possible by dissection around the mesenteric artery, aiming to preserve the vascular supply and to limit intestinal resection.

The goal of any surgical intervention is to remove the primary tumor together with the affected lymph nodes as completely as possible. At the same time, the main intestinal vascular supply and important peripheral collaterals have to be preserved to maintain as much small intestine as possible. This procedure is also indicated in the presence of liver metastases.

Table 23.13 Nine rules for dealing with midgut NET.

1 Midgut NET tend to grow slowly
2 Midgut NET have better prognosis than carcinomas at the same locations; in individual cases progress is not predictable
3 Aggressiveness and prognosis are dependent on the location (e.g. appendix vs. ileum)
4 The carcinoid syndome is a marker of advanced, almost always metastatic disease
5 Hepatic and lymphatic metastases represent no contraindication towards surgical intervention
6 Surgery at early disease stage is the only available cure
7 Even repeated palliative surgery is indicated wherever possible for debulking, to treat intestinal obstruction or cardiac valve involvement
8 Primary tumors should be removed wherever possible, even in cases of metastastic spread to the liver
9 Any intervention has to be performed under application of octreotide or somatostatin to prevent carcinoid crisis

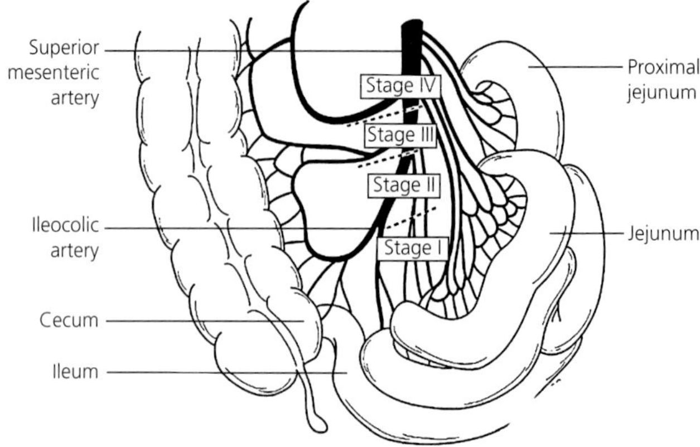

Fig. 23.34 Stages of midgut NET mesenteric metastases. Stage I : lymph node(s) involving the mesentery close to the intestine. Stage II: metastases involving arterial branches close to the mesenteric artery. Stage III: Metastases extend along the superior mesenteric artery (without encircling). Stage IV: Metastases extend retroperitoneally, behind or above the pancreas, or grow around the mesenteric artery and involve the origin of proximal jejunal arteries on the left side of the superior mesenteric artery (modified according to Akerstrom *et al.* 2005 and Ohrvall 2000).

Long-acting somatostatin analogs may increase quality of life and life expectancy in patients with liver metastases and help to control the carcinoid syndrome, but abdominal complications will become of increasing concern and appear to be a principal cause of death (Makridis *et al.* 1997; Akerstrom *et al.* 2005). The possibility of preventing or delaying these complications represents the indication for abdominal surgery even in patients with advanced disease. If a grossly radical tumor removal is achieved, the patients may remain symptom free for extended periods.

In patients with advanced local disease or liver metastases, simultaneous cholecystectomy should be performed to avoid gall = bladder necrosis if embolization of liver metastases becomes necessary. Liver resection should be performed if removal of approximately 90% of metastases is feasible without danger to the patient.

Careful examination of the whole intestine has to be performed to discover possible multicentric NETs or simultaneous neoplasms (detectable in 8–29%) (Modlin *et al.* 2003).

Surgery can be extremely challenging and boundaries are set in terms of large resections of small intestine. Careful dissection may help to preserve enough bowel to prevent short bowel syndrome.

Reoperation

Reoperation is recommended if the primary tumor and bulking of mesenteric metastases have not been removed during initial surgery, since any remaining mesenteric tumor is likely to cause future abdominal complications (Akerstrom *et al.* 2005).

Midgut NETs progress slowly, but recurrence with liver metastases is likely to occur in more than 80% of patients with long-term follow-up (Akerstrom *et al.* 2005).

During periods of medical treatment, mesenteric tumor and fibrosis may progress and increase vascular and intestinal entrapment. Many patients will develop episodes of feeding-related abdominal pain and diarrhea resulting in malnutrition and malaise. These symptoms are probably attributable to renewed tumor growth and impending intestinal ischemia and have to be recognized as indications of threatening complications. Reoperation should be considered before complications necessitate emergency surgery which is difficult or impossible to manage in these patients.

Results of surgery and prognosis

Usually NETs of the midgut are rather slow growing. Patients tend to have long survival times; the median survival for patients with midgut NET is approximately 9 years from the time of diagnosis (Makridis *et al.* 1997). Median survival in patients with carcinoid syndrome and liver metastases is approximately 7 years and in advanced carcinoid heart disease up to 4 years (Makridis *et al.* 1997). If synchronous or metachronous gastrointestinal adenocarcinomas develop, prognosis will be limited by the adenocarcinoma.

The benefit of surgery mainly consists of favorable and long-lasting relief of abdominal symptoms. Hellman *et al.* (2002b) reported a median survival of 12.4 years and a 5-year survival of 91% in patients without liver metastases in a series of 300 patients after resection of mesenteric metastases. Significant symptom alleviation and long disease-free survival have been repeatedly reported as a result of liver surgery in patients with the carcinoid syndrome (Hellman *et al.* 2002a; Akerstrom *et al.* 2005), although randomized evaluation is missing. Sustained symptom palliation and reduction of tumor markers are achieved especially after removal of large (>10 cm) dominant lesions, or if 90% of the tumor volume can be excised. Five-year survival of 70% or more has been reported after grossly radical liver surgery, and symptom palliation has been obtained also with non-curative resections (Akerstrom *et al.* 2005). The risk of liver failure can be reduced by two-stage liver resection combined with portal embolization to trigger liver regeneration. Indications have been widened by the possibility of combining liver resection with RFA. Virtually every patient will present with new metastases after liver resection or ablative therapy, but often with slow progression.

NET of the appendix and within a Meckel's diverticulum

Appendiceal NETs are the most prevalent NETs found at autopsy studies. Tumors are most often discovered by coincidence at operation for appendicitis (incidence: 1/200 appendectomies) (Memon & Nelson 1997). Women are more often affected than men. Patients are generally younger than those with other NETs; the mean age at tumor discovery is 41 years (Memon & Nelson 1997). Children may be affected; the prevalence is even higher in children than in adults. It is possible that most of the tumors never reach clinical significance or undergo spontaneous involution. In a series of 40 children with appendiceal NET incidentally found at appendectomy, no recurrence could be found in a median follow-up of 18 years (Parkes *et al.* 1993). The reason for the benign characteristics of appendiceal NETs still remains unclear, but a different origin has been discussed: appendiceal NETs seem to originate from specialized subepthelial neuroendocrine cells in contrast to other NETs, which originate from neuroendocrine epithelial cells.

Characteristically tumors are located at the tip of the appendix (up to 70%) and are small in size (up to 90% <1 cm) leading to a favorable prognosis for these tumors. Tumors smaller than 1 cm almost never metastasize, and tumors between 1 and 2 cm metastasize in up to 1%. The occurrence of metastases rises up to 85% when tumor size exceeds 2 cm (Stinner & Rothmund 2005).

Because of their benign character simple appendectomy represents the treatment of choice if tumor size is smaller than 1 cm. Right hemicolectomy should be performed if tumor size exceeds 2 cm. Tumors between 1 and 2 cm in diameter may be treated either by appendectomy or right hemicolectomy. The latter should be preferred if the tumor is localized close to the appendiceal basis or if histologically unfavorable signs of malignancy occur (like infiltration of the mesoappendix, serosa or high mitotic rate within the tumor).

The adenocarcinoid of the appendix is a special form of appendiceal NET. It is an infrequent tumor with histologic features of both adenocarcinoma and carcinoid tumor. Although its malignant potential remains unclear, adenocarcinoids seem to be biologically more aggressive than conventional appendiceal NETs. In the case of an appendiceal adenocarcinoid simple appendectomy is only appropriate if tumor size is less than 1 cm, there is no tumor extension beyond the appendical adventitia, there are fewer than 2 mitoses per 10 high-power fields found in histological slides, and there are free surgical margins.

Otherwise, right hemicolectomy seems to be indicated. The risk for developing colorectal adenocarcinoma seems to be extremely high in patients treated for appendiceal adenocarcinoid and warrants close follow-up with colonoscopic screening (Bucher *et al.* 2005).

NETs within a Meckel's diverticulum are extremely rare. Morphology is similar to NET of the appendix, but the incidence of lymph node metastases is higher. The risk of metastases is 6.3% with a diameter of 5 mm, 26.3% when tumor size is between 6 and 10 mm, and 58% when tumor size is between 1 and 2 cm. Therefore, NETs within a Meckel's diverticulum have to be treated by radical resection of the appertaining lymphatic tissue similar to NET of the small bowel.

References

Akerstrom G, Hellman P, Hessman O, Osmak L. (2005) Management of midgut carcinoids. *J Surg Oncol* 89(3): 161–9.

Bucher P, Gervaz P, Ris F, Oulhaci W, Egger JF, Morel P. (2005) Surgical treatment of appendiceal adenocarcinoid (goblet cell carcinoid). *World J Surg* 29(11): 1436–9.

Hellman P, Ladjevardi S, Skogseid B, Akerstrom G, Elvin A. (2002a) Radiofrequency tissue ablation using cooled tip for liver metastases of endocrine tumors. *World J Surg* 26(8): 1052–6.

Hellman P, Lundstrom T, Ohrvall U *et al.* (2002b) Effect of surgery on the outcome of midgut carcinoid disease with lymph node and liver metastases. *World J Surg* 26(8): 991–7.

Makridis C, Ekbom A, Bring J *et al.* (1997) Survival and daily physical activity in patients treated for advanced midgut carcinoid tumors. *Surgery* 122(6): 1075–82.

Memon MA, Nelson H. (1997) Gastrointestinal carcinoid tumors: current management strategies. *Dis Colon Rectum* 40(9): 1101–18.

Modlin IM, Lye KD, Kidd M. (2003) A 5-decade analysis of 13,715 carcinoid tumors. *Cancer* 97(4): 934–59.

Oberg K, Kvols L, Caplin M *et al.* (2004) Consensus report on the use of somatostatin analogs for the management of neuroendocrine tumors of the gastroenteropancreatic system. *Ann Oncol* 15(6): 966–73.

Ohrvall U, Eriksson B, Juhlin C *et al.* (2000) Method for dissection of mesenteric metastases in mid-gut carcinoid tumors. *World J Surg* 24(11): 1402–8.

Parkes SE, Muir KR, Al SM *et al.* (1993) Carcinoid tumours of the appendix in children 1957–1986: incidence, treatment and outcome. *Br J Surg* 80(4): 502–4.

Stinner B, Rothmund M. (2005) Neuroendocrine tumours (carcinoids) of the appendix. *Best Pract Res Clin Gastroenterol* 19(5): 729–38.

Surgery: liver metastases

Håkan Ahlman & Michael Olausson

Neuroendocrine tumors of the gastrointestinal tract (carcinoids and endocrine pancreatic tumors, EPTs) are rare diseases with an incidence of 1–2 per 100,000 population (Modlin & Sandor 1997). In the presence of liver metastases these patients may suffer from disabling symptoms due to hormone overproduction. Patients with localized disease can be resected for cure but also patients with liver metastases can undergo potentially curative tumor resection. However, long-term follow-up of the latter cases indicates frequent recurrence of tumor (Norton 1994; Chamberlain *et al.* 2000; Sarmiento & Que 2003; Sutcliffe *et al.* 2004). By close biochemical monitoring of tumor markers combined with newer techniques for tumor visualization, such as octreotide scintigraphy, spiral CT and MR, and PET using precursors of biogenic amines, these recurrences can be diagnosed at an early stage so that repeat surgical procedures can be performed (Olausson *et al.* 2007).

If all tumor can be resected the duration and quality of life for these patients can be greatly enhanced (Pederzoli *et al.* 1999; Chamberlain *et al.* 2000; Norton *et al.* 2003). Even in patients not suitable for curative liver surgery, debulking (or cytoreductive surgery) can be considered if the main tumor burden can be safely excised (Sarmiento & Que 2003). The aim of this type of treatment is palliation of hormonal symptoms and pain. Active surgical treatment was recommended early for well-differentiated NE tumors, since many of these have relatively slow growth (McEntee *et al.* 1990; Carty *et al.* 1992; Norton 1994; Que *et al.* 1995). More extensive surgery of NE tumor disease can today be performed with low mortality and morbidity and liver surgery can safely be combined with advanced gastrointestinal procedures (Chen *et al.* 1998; Chung *et al.* 2001; Norton *et al.* 2003).

The surgical treatment can also cause relief of secondary symptoms, such as biliary or bowel obstruction, bleeding and mass effects. Since patients with advanced disease often have different types of metastatic spread, they are best managed by a multidisciplinary team. In one large series half of the patients had extrahepatic metastases and more than 80% bilobar liver metastases. Accordingly, some were only medically treated, while the others had interventional treatment by hepatic arterial embolization (HAE) or resection. With this selection bias the interventionally treated groups had a survival advantage after 3 years of follow-up, even more pronounced after 5 years. Both HAE and resection provided good palliation of both hormonal and pain symptoms (Chamberlain *et al.* 2000).

Preoperative considerations

Prior to all interventional treatment of NE tumors, the tumor type and hormone production must be assessed. Patients with *midgut carcinoids* are pretreated with long-acting somatostatin analogs, such as octreotide, to prevent carcinoid crises during intervention. In case of a crisis reaction (severe facial flushing, bronchoconstriction, and hypotension) adrenergic drugs should be avoided, since carcinoid tumor cells may express adrenoceptors and a vicious circle with excessive release of serotonin and tachykinins can be initiated. Instead, the surgical manipulation should be interrupted, volume substituted according to hemodynamic parameters and i.v. doses of octreotide and cortisone given. Spinal anesthesia with markedly reduced arterial blood pressure may elicit carcinoid crises due to compensatory release of catecholamines from the adrenals, in turn activating serotonin release from the tumor. For postoperative pain epidural analgesia is preferred (Ahlman *et al.* 1988). Of particular importance is awareness of significant carcinoid heart disease, since these patients can develop right-sided heart failure with increased central venous pressure and risk back-bleeding from hepatic veins during liver surgery. Valve replacement prior to hepatic resection may be indicated for patients at risk (Westberg *et al.* 2001; Sarmiento & Que 2003). *Foregut carcinoids* with excess production of histamine can cause an 'atypical carcinoid syndrome' (generalized flushing, bronchoconstriction, hypotension, lacrimation, and cutaneous edema); HAE in these patients can be contraindicated due to uncontrollable release reactions. Correct diagnosis relies on analysis of the main histamine metabolite methylimidazole acetic acid (MelmAA) in urine. Patients with histamine-producing tumors are optimally pretreated with a combination of somatostatin analogs, blockade of histamine (H_1 and H_2) receptors and cortisone. Histamine-liberating agents, such as morphine and tubocurarine, should be avoided (Ahlman *et al.* 1992). For patients with *glucagonoma*, or *VIPoma*, preoperative treatment with octreotide is usually sufficient. Skin lesions (necrolytic migrating erythema) associated with infection, sometimes seen in glucagonoma patients, can heal rapidly with somatostatin analogs, antibiotics, and amino acid supplementation prior to surgery. During this period, low-dose heparin is recommended due to increased risk of thrombosis associated with glucagonoma. Patients with *gastrinoma* maintain their medication with proton pump inhibitors for a period after removal of the tumor, since they have elevated gastric acid secretion due to hypertrophy of the gastric mucosa. Patients with large *insulinomas* may require hypertonic glucose after tumor removal and close glucose monitoring is necessary.

Interventional treatment of liver metastases

Curative and palliative treatment of liver metastases can be demanding and often involves several treatment modalities. If liver transplantation is planned as a second step, then it is important to resect all extrahepatic tumor. There is no general agreement when to start the palliative surgical treatment; for example gastrinomas metastatic to the liver show most variable growth rates in individual patients, which influences the decision-making (Sutliff *et al.* 1997).

The surgical treatment for liver metastases can be divided into three modalities:

- liver resection
- regional or local procedures
- liver transplantation.

Liver resection

Anatomical liver resection can be performed for lesions situated within any of the eight liver segments (each supplied by branches of the hepatic arteries and portal vein) draining into an hepatic duct (Fig. 23.35). For curative resection a good clearance margin is required, but for NE tumors resected for palliation this margin can be narrowed and local tumor deposits removed by atypical resections. The extension of tumor is assessed by inspection, palpation, and intraoperative ultrasound. The latter technique reveals the relation between the tumor and the portal/hepatic veins, which is of special importance for ablative procedures.

The liver is sagitally divided by the three major hepatic veins, which delineate the type resections: *left hepatectomy* (removal of segments II–III), *right hepatectomy* (removal of segments V–VIII), and *trisegmentectomy* (removal of the three central segments, sometimes also the caudate lobe, segment I). Resection of the individual segments requires identification and subsequent ligation of the portal pedicle. This can be difficult for segments VII–VIII resulting in impaired venous drainage from the residing lower segments. This type of resection is rarely

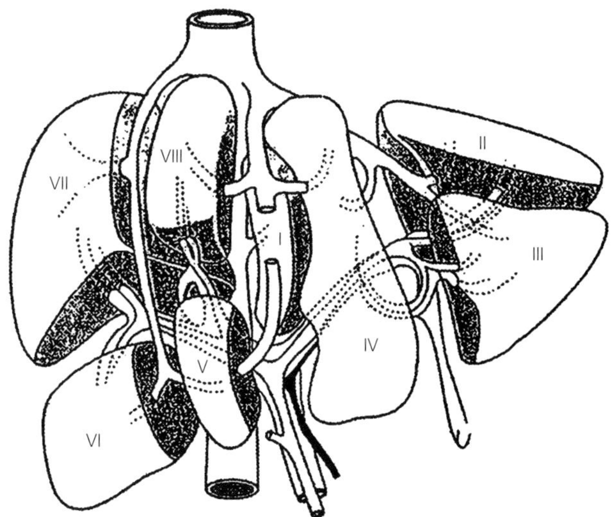

Fig. 23.35 Surgical anatomy of the liver. I–VIII, Liver segments I–VIII.

performed. Superficial liver metastases can safely be removed by wedge excisions.

A transverse subcostal incision is used, but the patient should be scrubbed up to the sternal notch in case the vena cava needs to be controlled above the diaphragm. For all resections, the liver should be fully mobilized by division of the major ligaments. The inferior vena cava can be controlled by a sling below the liver.

Left hepatectomy. The left and middle hepatic veins have their junction at variable levels, which means that they cannot always be controlled separately outside the liver. Division of the liver parenchyma can be performed by several techniques, for example the finger fracture technique or by the harmonic scalpel/ultrasonic surgical aspirator, which destroys liver cells leaving the biliary and vascular structures intact for ligation. To minimize bleeding from the raw surface a superficial argon beam coagulator is often used.

Right hepatectomy. The most common variant in arterial anatomy is replacement of the right hepatic artery by a branch of the superior mesenteric artery. For right-sided tumors preoperative angiography, or MR angiography, is therefore valuable. For right hepatectomy the right hepatic vein can be controlled outside the liver. It is important to have control of the free edge of the lesser omentum to prevent bleeding; occlusion can be applied by the so-called Pringle's maneuver. The safe duration of total hepatic ischemia at normothermia may exceed 1 h, but can be shorter with hepatic dysfunction. The shortest possible clamping (often intermittent) should be used, since it is associated with intestinal congestion and accumulation of metabolites.

Extended right lobe resection. In some cases extended right lobe resections, leaving only the two left liver segments, can be performed. A residual liver less than 20–25% may lead to hepatic failure. To reduce mortality and morbidity preoperative portal embolization of the tumor-carrying right lobe can be performed, which over 2–3 weeks induces hypertrophy of the intact left liver. Thereafter the planned resection can be safely performed (Farges & Belghiti 1999).

Metastasectomy of multiple deposits usually requires clamping of inflow vessels, incision by diathermy and blunt dissection, followed by ligation of vessels and bile leaks. To obtain optimal cytoreduction the principles of anatomical resection, wedge resection, and metastasectomy are often combined.

For postoperative management epidural, or patient-controlled analgesia, is used. After major liver surgery hypoglycemia and hypoalbuminemia should be avoided. Clotting should be monitored and fresh plasma used when necessary. As with all elective surgical interventions, the operative mortality must be kept low. Prophylactic use of antibiotics has markedly reduced infectious complications.

Results of liver surgery

Over the last decade very active surgery has become increasingly more common as primary treatment for well-differentiated endocrine carcinomas (WDECs) and their metastases (Table 23.14). Curative liver surgery (no gross residual tumor) should be considered for all patients with resectable disease, since this is the only long-term effective strategy (Norton *et al.* 2003). Palliative (cytoreductive) liver surgery can be considered for patients with slow tumor growth and severe hormonal symptoms. Palliative liver resections are generally performed in patients in whom more than 90% of the tumor volume can be safely excised (Sarmiento & Que 2003). Preoperative HAE can occasionally be used to shrink tumors, especially since patients with large tumor bulk have worse prognosis when treated by surgery alone (Sutcliffe *et al.* 2004).

Table 23.14 Five-year survival after surgery for liver metastases of NE tumors.

Carty *et al.* (1992)	n = 17	79%
Söreide *et al.* (1992)	n = 75	70%
Ahlman *et al.* (1996)	n = 14	100%*
Chen *et al.* (1998)	n = 15	73%
Chamberlain *et al.* (2000)	n = 34	76%
Pascher *et al.* (2000)	n = 25	76%
Nave *et al.* (2001)	n = 31	47%
Sarmiento *et al.* (2000)	n = 170	61%

* Patients selected for R0 resection.

In series of patients with NE tumors 20 years ago, the liver resection rate with curative intent was about 10% (Galland & Blumgart 1986; Hughes & Sugarbaker 1987). This was partly ascribed to the fact that many tumors had diffuse spread within the liver at clinical presentation. In our own prospective series of 64 consecutive patients with the midgut carcinoid syndrome and liver metastases, 14 patients (22%) with unilateral liver disease underwent intentionally curative liver surgery and normalized their tumor markers, i.e. plasma chromogranin A and urinary 5-HIAA (Wängberg *et al.* 1996). The survival in this group of patients after 5 years (100%) compared favorably with those treated with HAE (63%) or bio- or chemotherapy (0%) after resection of the primary. These findings emphasize the importance of patient selection. In other series as many as 40–50% of patients with NE tumors underwent liver resection, when both palliative and curative procedures were considered (Carty *et al.* 1992; Que *et al.* 1995; Dousset *et al.* 1996; Chamberlain *et al.* 2000; Sarmiento & Que 2003). Recently, in a small consecutive series curative liver resection was performed in 50% of the patients (Norton *et al.* 2003). In the reported series at centers of expertise, the mortality was low (<6%) and the complication rate below 30% (Fig. 23.36).

Even with so-called curative resections the tumor may recur. It is therefore of importance to have these patients under surveillance using biochemical tumor markers (general markers like chromogranin A and tumor-specific amines/peptide hormones) in combination with octreotide scintigraphy plus SPECT and spiral CT/MRI in order to early detect subclinical disease and perform repeat surgery. This strategy has been

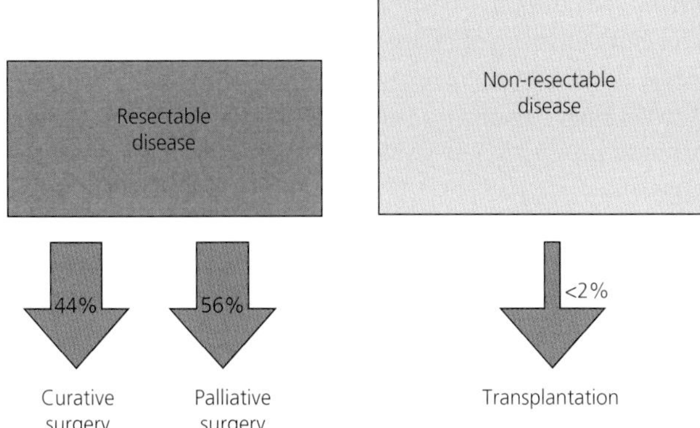

Fig. 23.36 Flow chart for surgical treatment of NE liver metastases. At centers of expertise the liver resection rate for both curative and palliative procedures is high (40–50%; see text). In the large Mayo series (n = 170) 44% of resected patients had intentionally curative procedures and 56% had palliative procedures, but still the non-resectable cases dominate. In the non-resectable group a small proportion of patients can be considered for transplantation (<2%).

successful in patients with WDEC treated by transplantation; in our experience scintigraphy was superior to biochemical markers in case of somatostatin receptor-positive tumors (Olausson *et al.* 2007).

Twenty years ago Norton *et al.* (1986) reported the outcome of aggressive surgery in selected patients with advanced gastrinoma. They all underwent major liver resections combined with other debulking procedures at tumor progression and chemotherapy. On a short-term basis good symptomatic relief and markedly reduced tumor markers were seen; out of 42 consecutive patients with EPT treated over a 10-year period at the NIH, 17 were resected and 25 were inoperable and only medically treated (Carty *et al.* 1992). There was a 5-year survival advantage in the surgically treated group (79%) versus the medically treated (28%) in this selected series. There was no operative mortality, but the tumor disease recurred in all surgically treated patients within 8 years. On the other hand, such delay of tumor growth with a long medication-free interval, also observed for midgut carcinoids, is a major therapeutic advantage in itself (Wängberg *et al.* 1996). Very similar 5-year survival rates for surgically treated patients with NE tumors and liver metastases were reported from MSKCC (Chamberlain *et al.* 2000), Chicago (Yao *et al.* 2001), and Hannover (Nave *et al.* 2001) (see Table 23.14). Surgery with curative intent was the best prognostic factor; others related to size of the liver tumors, site of the primary and prior resection of the primary tumor. Mc Entee *et al.* (1990) from the Mayo Clinic reported encouraging results 15 years ago in 37 patients (carcinoids or EPTs) treated with liver resection. This series included 17 curative resections; 9 patients with hormonal symptoms were all completely relieved. Twenty patients underwent palliative resections; 16 patients had hormonal symptoms and half of them obtained symptom control. In a later report from the same center 74 patients with metastatic NE tumors had undergone liver resection; the 4-year survival was 73%, even though nearly two-thirds of the procedures were palliative (Que *et al.* 1995). In a recent review Sarmiento & Que (2003) stated that patients with reasonable performance status, whose primary tumor was controlled and whose extrahepatic metastases were limited, were all assessed for liver surgery. Forty-four per cent of their patients had undergone R0 resection with low mortality (<1.2%) and morbidity (15%), but the recurrence rate at 5 years was 84%. Control of symptoms was achieved in 93% after debulking with a median duration of 45 months. The 5- and 10-year survival rates were 61% and 35%, respectively (Table 23.14). Thus, data from several major centers all support active intervention of NE liver metastases, even though the role of palliative surgery for enhanced survival is still not proven in randomized studies (Fig. 23.36).

Regional or local procedures

Regional hyperthermia

At advanced stage of histamine-producing tumors, ischemic liver treatment is potentially dangerous due to uncontrollable release of tumor products. In individual patients with the foregut carcinoid syndrome we have used heat-stable cytotoxic drugs (melphalan plus cisplatin) delivered by regional hyperthermic liver perfusion. During perfusion the venous effluent from the liver with vasoactive substances was shunted from the systemic circulation avoiding adverse effects. Cytostatic perfusion of the isolated liver with simultaneous filtration of portal vein blood and maintained systemic circulation were made possible by a special perfusion catheter inserted in the cava. The surgical technique involves isolation of the hepatic artery, portal vein, and cava inferior and superior to the liver together with a temporary portocaval shunt (allowing maintained blood flow rates in both the hepatic artery and portal system) (Scherstén *et al.* 1991). Repeat hyperthermic perfusion can be difficult to perform due to intense fibrotic reaction of the vessels used for perfusion.

Local ablation

In elderly patients, or patients with progressive tumors after previous treatment, percutaneous *alcohol injections* into isolated liver lesions have been attempted to destroy tumor tissue. Tumor volume is estimated ultrasonographically and the lesions injected with equal volumes of absolute alcohol. During injection the lesions develop high echogenicity. With repeat injections marked symptom palliation related to reduced tumor markers and proven tumor regression can be achieved. The tumor can also be destroyed by *cryosurgical techniques* or by *interstitial laser*. The freeze damage is caused by intra- and extracellular crystal formation, dehydration, and vascular damage. Cryosurgery is less effective close to large vessels ('heat-sink') and should not be used for large tumors due to risk for coagulopathies, respiratory distress syndrome, and acute renal failure. Cryoprobes can be equipped with intraoperative ultrasound and can destroy tumors deep in the liver without damaging the normal overlying parenchyma. In short series good symptomatic relief has been reported (Cozzi *et al.* 1995). Today the most commonly used technique is *radiofrequency ablation*, which causes selective thermocoagulation of lesions up to 3–4 cm in diameter. Tumor adjacent to large vessels can usually be treated, since the vessels are protected by cooling due to bloodstream effects (Bilchik *et al.* 1999; Siperstein *et al.* 2000; Wessels & Schnee 2001). Ultrasound is usually the imaging guidance, but open thermosensitive MR systems for monitoring of coagulative effects are being developed. These ablative techniques can be used in open or laparoscopic surgery, or percutaneously, and are valuable complements to liver resection, such as for recurrent tumors in the residual liver after resection (Fig. 23.37). Multiple lesions can be treated in one single session.

Liver transplantation

Metastases from gastrointestinal NE tumors can be slowly growing and limited to the liver for long periods, which leaves a therapeutic window for orthotopic liver transplantation (OLT) in selected patients. Current data suggest that the primary tumor should be removed by a first operation, so that disease stability can be assessed. Patients with favorable biologic features (WDEC with low proliferation and stable disease) and with no extrahepatic metastases may even be cured by OLT. More difficult to predict are the patients with non-resectable disease limited to the liver, who do not respond to previous interventional treatment, or patients with life-threatening hormone production (e.g. histamine or insulin) occasionally transplanted for palliation (Rosado & Gores 2003). An upper age limit of 55 years has been suggested. Some centers will not accept tumor mass exceeding 50% of liver volume (Schweizer *et al.* 1993), although no strict studies on NE tumor volume and outcome of transplantation are available. Poorly differentiated endocrine carcinomas (PDECs) very seldom present at a stage when they are resectable. Due to poor prognosis transplantation is contraindicated for these highly proliferative tumors.

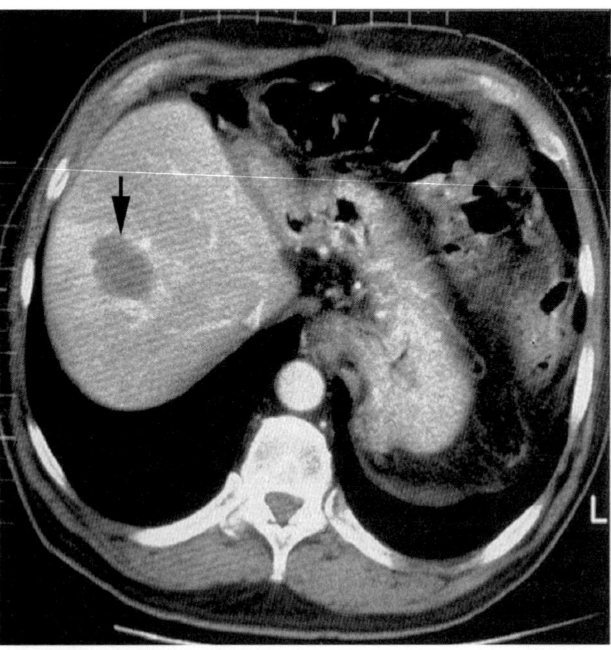

Fig. 23.37 CT scan of an EPT patient previously subjected to 'curative' left hemihepatectomy. Three years later there is recurrence of a centrally located lesion in the residual liver, which was treated with radiofrequency ablation (arrow).

A careful evaluation of the outcome of primary surgery (complete excision of locoregional disease) is important, since growth of residual tumor may accelerate during immunosuppression (Gulanikar *et al.* 1991). Using biochemical markers and imaging procedures residual extrahepatic tumors can be revealed in a high proportion of patients worked up for OLT. It therefore seems reasonable to follow a *two-step strategy* with histology-proven radical resection of the primary carcinoid, or EPT with tail location. If effective chemotherapy is available, it would be desirable before transplantation. EPT with head location can be treated by a Whipple procedure followed by OLT, or by tumor excision and multivisceral transplantation (MVTx) in one setting (Olausson *et al.* 2007).

Results of transplantation

In 1994 Bechstein and Neuhaus reviewed the world literature of 30 patients with different NE tumor types (15 EPT and 15 carcinoids) treated with OLT. The 1-year survival was 52% with transplantation-associated deaths in half of the patients within 8 months. Four years later, much more favorable survival figures were reported. The actuarial 5-year survival from Hannover was 80%; only one out of 12 patients with OLT died of recurrent tumor (Lang *et al.* 1997). Similar figures were indicated for patients with carcinoids in contrast to the rather poor survival of patients with EPTs (8%) in a French multicenter study of 31 patients (Le Treut *et al.* 1997). On the other hand, in an English series carcinoid patients had high recurrence rate and shorter survival probably due to relatively long interval between diagnosis and OLT (Sutcliffe *et al.* 2004). Lehnert in 1998 reviewed the first 103 reported cases in Europe with OLT as treatment of NE tumors with 5-year overall and disease-free survival of 47% and 24%, respectively. Survival seemed to be favorably influenced by young age (<50 years), absence of hilar lymph node metastases, and less extensive upper abdominal surgery. Certain tumor sites (lung and small bowel) and octreotide treatment prior to surgery may be other positive prognostic factors. For MVTx the prognosis for NE tumors widely surpassed other tumor types, such as sarcoma, hepatocellular cancer, or cholangiocarcinoma. Patients with no lymph node metastases, no vascular invasion and only liver metastases had a much lower recurrence rate (Alessiani *et al.* 1995).

Our experience of OLT (n = 10), or MVTx (n = 5), during 1997–2005 as treatment of WDEC tumors included 10 EPTs and 5 carcinoids. All procedures were performed with curative intent and the hepatic tumors had limited proliferation (Ki-67 ≤ 10%). This series differs from previous ones in several aspects; patients up to 60 years and a majority with large tumor burden in the liver (>50%) were included. The patients with MVTx all had higher proliferation than the OLT patients and also had different immunosuppression and may thus represent a negative selection bias. Of the 10 OLT patients only one died of recurrent tumor during a mean observation time of 54 ± 10 months; two of the carcinoid patients have remained tumor-free during 57 and 70 months, respectively. Of the 5 MVTx patients two died of transplantation-associated causes within 2–4 months, one of recurrent tumor after 27 months and two are alive; one with recurrent tumor after 4 years (now observed 66 months) and one is tumor-free after 1 year. With careful tumor monitoring and repeat surgery at tumor recurrence the probability of escaping tumor-related death after OLT in our series was 0.9 after 6 years; 1.0 for carcinoids and 0.8 for EPT, i.e. the initial survival of grafts and patients do not differ from those obtained for benign disease (Florman *et al.* 2002). However, the probability of escaping recurrence after MVTx, or OLT, was about 0.2 after 5 years in our series in agreement with others. To date about 130 OLT for NE tumors have been performed world-wide, but only 8 patients were tumor-free after 5 years.

The best 1-year survival rate for OLT (77%) was reported by van Vilsteren (2006) versus 70% for OLT and MVTx in our series, but it must be borne in mind that short-time survival only reflects slow growth of these tumors. In our series two patients with carcinoid tumors received somatostatin receptor-targeted radiotherapy (^{177}Lu-octreotate, 7.0–7.5 GBq × 4) as completion treatment when they presented with non-resectable disease after OLT; one with marked tumor regression and total symptom control during 4 years, the other with almost complete tumor regression during the first 2 years of observation.

For EPT a cut-off value of 5% for proliferation identifies patients with shorter survival (Pelosi *et al.* 1996), but our series included patients with Ki-67 levels up to 10%. In a study of 19 OLT patients with long follow-up, low Ki-67 levels (<5%) and regular expression of the adhesion molecule E-cadherin were associated with better prognosis, while analysis of p53 expression did not improve prognostic accuracy (Rosenau *et al.* 2002). In conclusion, OLT can offer good relief of symptoms and long disease-free intervals with initial survival of grafts and patients as seen in cirrhosis, but the experience with MVTx is still too limited. Prospective studies to define the best criteria to predict clinical outcome of OLT are still to be defined.

References

Ahlman H, Åhlund L, Dahlström A *et al.* (1988) The use of SMS 201–995 and provocation tests in carcinoid patients in preparation for surgery and hepatic arterial embolisation. *Anesth Analg* 67: 1142–8.

Ahlman H, Wängberg B, Nilsson O *et al.* (1992) Aspects of diagnosis and treatment of the foregut carcinoid syndrome. *Scand J Gastroenterol* 27: 459–71.

Ahlman H, Westberg G, Wängberg B *et al.* (1996) Treatment of liver metastases of carcinoid tumors. *World J Surg* 20: 196–202.

Alessiani M, Tzakis A, Todo S *et al.* (1995) Assessment of 5-year experience with abdominal cluster transplantation. *J Am Coll Surg* 180: 1–9.

Anthuber M, Jauch KW, Briegel J *et al.* (1996) Results of liver transplantation for gastroenteropancreatic tumor metastases. *World J Surg* 20: 73–6.

Arnold JC, O'Grady JG, Bird GL *et al.* (1989) Liver transplantation for primary and secondary hepatic apudomas. *Br J Surg* 76: 248–9.

Bechstein W, Neuhaus P. (1994) Liver transplantation for hepatic metastases of neuroendocrine tumors. *Ann NY Acad Sci* 733: 507–14.

Bilchik AJ, Rose DM, Allegra DP *et al.* (1999) Radiofrequency ablation: a minimally invasive technique with multiple applications. *Cancer J Sci Am* 5: 356–61.

Carty SE, Jensen RT, Norton JA. (1992) Prospective study of aggressive resection of metastatic pancreatic endocrine tumors. *Surgery* 112: 1024–31.

Chamberlain RS, Canes D, Brown KT *et al.* (2000) Hepatic neuroendocrine metastases: does intervention alter outcomes? *J Am Coll Surg* 190: 432–45.

Chen H, Hardacre JM, Uzar A *et al.* (1998) Isolated liver metastases from neuroendocrine tumors: does resection prolong survival? *J Am Coll Surg* 187: 88–92.

Chung MH, Pisegna J, Spirt M *et al.* (2001) Hepatic cytoreduction followed by a novel long-acting somatostatin analog: a paradigm for intractable neuroendocrine tumors. *Surgery* 130: 954–62.

Coppa J, Pulvirenti A, Schiavo M *et al.* (2001) Resection versus transplantation for liver metastases from neuroendocrine tumors. *Transpl Proc* 3: 1537–9.

Cozzi PJ, Englund R, Morris DL. (1995) Cryotherapy treatment of patients with hepatic metastases from neuroendocrine tumors. *Cancer* 76: 501–9.

Dousset B, Saint-Marc O, Pitre J *et al.* (1996) Metastastic endocrine tumors: medical treatment, surgical resection, or liver transplantation. *World J Surg* 20: 908–14.

Farges O, Belghiti J. (1999) Options in the resection of endocrine liver metastases. Mignon M, Colombel JF, eds. *Recent Advances in the Pathophysiology and Management of Inflammatory Bowel Disease and Digestive Endocrine Tumors*, pp. 335–7. J Libbey Eurotext, Paris.

Florman S, Toure B, Kim L *et al.* (2004) Liver transplantation for neuroendocrine tumors. *J Gastrointest* 8: 208–12.

Frilling A, Malago M, Weber F *et al.* (2006) Liver transplantation for patients with metastatic endocrine tumors: single-center experience with 15 patients. *Liver Transpl* 12: 1089–96.

Galland RB, Blumgart LH. (1986) Carcinoid syndrome: surgical management. *Br J Hosp Med* 35: 168–70.

Gulanikar AC, Kotylak G, Bitter-Suermann J. (1991) Does immunosuppression alter the growth of metastatic liver carcinoid after orthotopic liver transplantation? *Transpl Proc* 23: 2197.

Hughes KS, Sugarbaker PH. (1987) Resection of the liver for metastatic solid tumors. In: Rosenberg SA, ed. *Surgical Treatment of Metastatic Cancer*, pp 125–64. Lippincott, Philadelphia.

Lang H, Oldhafer KJ, Weimann A *et al.* (1997). Liver transplantation for metastatic neuroendocrine tumors. *Ann Surg* 225: 347–54.

Le Treut YP, Delpero JR, Dousset B *et al.* (1997) Results of liver transplantation in the treatment of metastatic tumors: A 31-case French multicentric report. *Ann Surg* 225: 355–64.

Lehnert T. (1998) Liver transplantation for metastatic neuroendocrine carcinoma. *Transplantation* 66: 1307–12.

Makowka L, Tzakis AG, Mazzaferro V *et al.* (1989) Transplantation of the liver for metastatic endocrine tumors of the intestine and pancreas. *Surg Gynecol Obstet* 168: 107–11.

Mc Entee GP, Nagorney DM, Kvols LK *et al.* (1990) Cytoreductive hepatic surgery for neuroendocrine tumors. *Surgery* 108: 1091–6.

Modlin IM, Sandor A. (1997) An analysis of 8305 cases of carcinoid tumors. *Cancer* 79: 813–29.

Nave H, Mossinger E, Feist H *et al.* (2001) Surgery as primary treatment in patients with liver metastases from carcinoid tumors: a retrospective unicentric study over 13 years. *Surgery* 129: 170–5.

Norton JA. (1994) Surgical management of carcinoid tumors: Role of debulking and surgery for advanced disease. *Digestion* 55: 98–103.

Norton JA, Sugarbaker PH, Doppman JL *et al.* (1986) Aggressive resection of metastatic disease in selected patients with malignant gastrinoma. *Ann Surg* 203: 352–9.

Norton JA, Warren RS, Kelly MG *et al.* (2003) Aggressive surgery for metastatic liver neuroendocrine tumors. *Surgery* 134: 1057–63.

Olausson M, Friman S, Herlenius G *et al.* (2007) Orthotopic liver or multivisceral transplantation as treatment of metastatic neuroendocrine tumors. *Liver Transplantation* (in press).

Pascher A, Steinmüller T, Radke C *et al.* (2000) Primary and secondary manifestation of neuroendocrine tumors. *Langenbacks Arch Surg* 385: 265–70.

Pederzoli P, Falconi M, Bonora A *et al.* (1999) Cytoreductive surgery in advanced endocrine tumors of the pancreas. *Ital J Gastroenterol Hepatol* 31: 207–12.

Pelosi G, Bresaola E, Bogina G *et al.* (1996) Endocrine tumors of the pancreas: Ki-67 immunoreactivity on paraffin sections is an independent predictor for malignancy. *Hum Pathol* 27: 1124–34.

Que FG, Nagorney DM, Batts KP *et al.* (1995) Hepatic resection for metastatic neuroendocrine carcinomas. *Am J Surg* 169: 36–42.

Ringe B, Lorf T, Dopkens K *et al.* (2001) Treatment of hepatic metastases from gastroenteropancreatic tumors role of liver transplantation. *World J Surg* 25: 697–9.

Rosado B, Gores GJ. (2004) Liver transplantation for neuroendocrine tumors: Progress and uncertainty. *Liver Transpl* 10: 712–13.

Rosenau J, Bahr MJ, von Wasielewski R *et al.* (2002) Ki-67, E-cadherin, and p 53 as prognostic indicators of long-term outcome of liver transplantation for metastatic neuroendocrine tumors. *Transplantation* 73: 386–94.

Routley D, Ramage JK, McPeake J *et al.* (1995) Orthotopic liver transplantation in the treatment of metastatic neuroendocrine tumors of the liver. *Liver Transplant Surg* 1: 118–21.

Sarmiento JM, Que FG. (2003) Hepatic surgery for metastases from neuroendocrine tumors. *Surg Oncol Clin N Am* 12: 231–42.

Scherstén T, Ahlman H, Wängberg B *et al.* (1991) Hyperthermic liver perfusion chemotherapy in the treatment of the foregut carcinoid syndrome. *Lancet* 338: 568–369.

Schweizer RT, Alsina AE, Rosson R *et al.* (1993) Liver transplantation for metastatic neuroendocrine tumors. *Transplant Proc* 25: 1973.

Siperstein A, Garland A, Engle K *et al.* (2000) Laparoscopic radiofrequency ablation of primary and metastatic liver tumors. Technical considerations. *Surg Endosc* 14: 400–5.

Sutliff VE, Doppman JL, Gibril LF *et al.* (1997) Growth of newly diagnosed untreated metastatic gastrinomas and predictors of growth pattern. *J Clin Oncol* 15: 2420–31.

Sutcliffe R, Maquire D, Ramage J *et al.* (2004) Management of neuroendocrine liver metastases. *Am J Surg* 187: 39–46.

Söreide O, Berstad T, Bakka A *et al.* (1992) Surgical treatment as a principle in patients with advanced abdominal carcinoid tumors. *Surgery* 111: 48–54.

Van Vilsteren FGI, Baskin-Bey ES, Nagorney DM *et al.* (2006) Liver transplantation for gastroenteropancreatic neuroendocrine cancers: Defining selection criteria to improve survival. *Liver Transpl* 12: 448–56.

Wängberg B, Westberg G, Tylén U *et al.* (1996) Survival of patients with disseminated midgut carcinoid tumors after aggressive tumor reduction. *World J Surg* 20: 892–9.

Wessels FJ, Schell SR. (2001) Radiofrequency ablation treatment of refractory carcinoid metastases. *J Surg Res* 95: 8–12.

Westberg G, Wängberg B, Ahlman H *et al.* (2001) Prediction of prognosis by echocardiography in patients with the midgut carcinoid syndrome. *Br J Surg* 88: 865–72.

Yao KA, Talamonti MS, Nemcek A *et al.* (2001) Indications and results of liver resection and hepatic chemoembolization for metastatic gastrointestinal neuroendocrine tumors. *Surgery* 130: 677–82.

Ablative therapy

Massimo Falconi & Rossella Bettini

Introduction

Hepatic metastases occur in 25–90% of patients with endocrine tumors of gastrointestinal origin. Although endocrine tumors are generally characterized by a fairly unaggressive biology and slow growth, the presence of liver metastases nonetheless influence overall prognosis and quality of life. The 5-year survival of patients with liver metastases is 40% compared to 75–99% for those without hepatic metastasis. Moreover, the metastatic growth rate appears to correlate with survival.

The extended survival after diagnosis of neuroendocrine neoplasia makes the quality of life an important consideration and is influenced by the tumor mass and hormonal symptoms related to tumor load. In reality, carcinoid syndrome usually occurs only in patients with liver metastases due to the production and release of serotonin directly into the bloodstream.

Therefore, efficacious treatment of hepatic metastases should increase survival if the hepatic tumor is reduced by 90% or more. In the presence of hormonal hypersecretion, symptoms are proportional to tumor bulk, and subsequently any substantial degree of debulking should provide symptomatic improvement due to a reduction in hormonal secretion.

Surgery is the treatment of choice, but it is often unfeasible due to either extensive tumor burden or the presence of metastases that are critically situated within the liver, precluding safe resection. Systemic treatments are frequently insufficient. The effects of somatostatin analogs, useful in the initial control of hormonal symptoms, tend to decrease over time. Chemotherapy is not particularly effective, especially in patients with liver metastases of midgut origin.

Due to the above-mentioned characteristics and the typical presence of metastatic disease often isolated to the liver, the use of locoregional ablative therapies has been favored.

Indications of ablative therapies

The target of ablative techniques is metastatic disease to the liver and its indications include treatment of hepatic metastases in patients who are not candidates for surgery or as an adjunct to surgical resection. Usually the primary tumor site should be already controlled or resection planned at the time of ablative therapy of liver metastases. Ablative therapies can be performed percutaneously or intraoperatively, and in this latter situation, either during open surgery or under laparoscopic guidance.

Ablative techniques render a larger percentage of patients candidates for surgery with radical intent, even if metastases are deep within liver parenchyma or in locations not amenable to conventional surgical excision. Usually small metastases can be effectively ablated with relatively minimal damage to the adjacent parenchyma. Moreover, because of the limited invasiveness of ablative procedures, they can also be used to successfully treat patients with invalidating comorbid diseases, or who have undergone previous liver surgery. Another advantage of percutaneous ablation therapies is the possibility of carrying out subsequent treatment sessions.

Ablative therapies may also be used as 'bridge' procedures or to control hormonal symptoms when the disease is present outside the liver, even though these indications are more controversial. One such application is in single metachronous metastases for which surgical therapy might be postponed for a few months in order to ensure that no other lesions are present. Another possible indication is liver metastases with a different pattern of octreoscan positivity; ablative therapies can be utilized for the treatment of octreoscan-negative lesions, while radio-receptor targeted therapy can be used for other lesions.

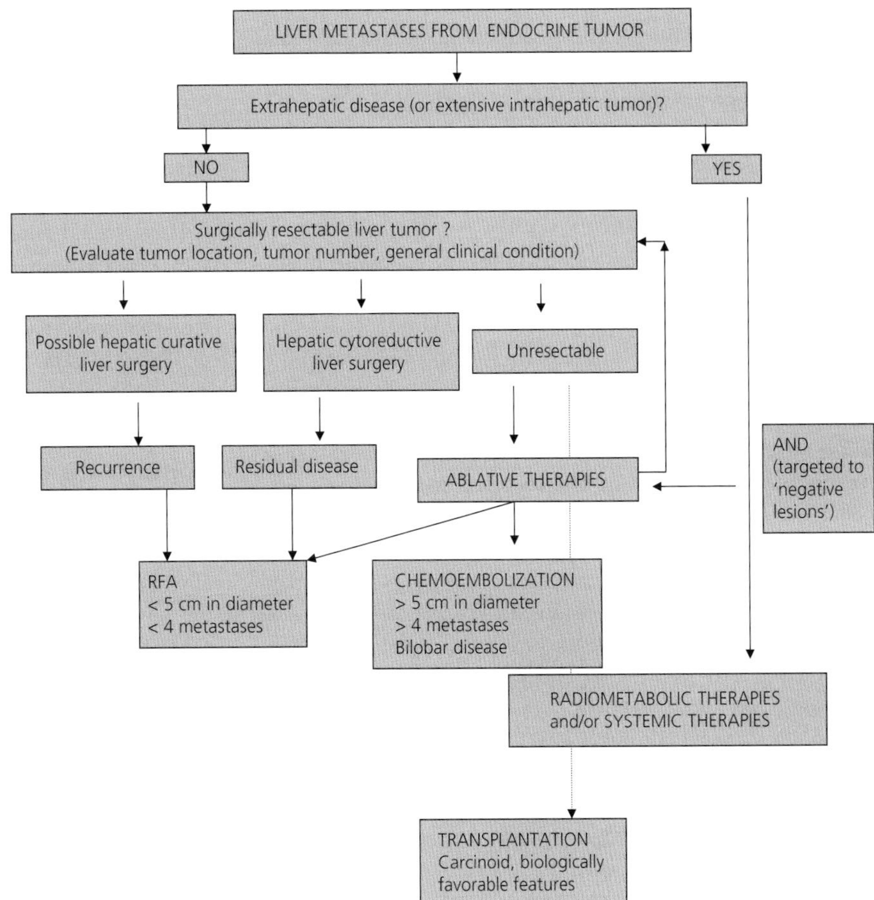

Fig. 23.38 Possible algorithm for the management of hepatic metastases from endocrine tumors with particular attention to the indications of ablative therapies.

Vascular occlusive strategies: hepatic arterial embolization and transarterial chemoembolization

Principles, technique, indications and contraindications

Hepatic metastases of neuroendocrine gastrointestinal tumors derive almost all their blood supply from the hepatic artery, whilst the normal liver has twice the blood supply, 25% provided by the hepatic artery and 75% by the portal vein. Arterial hypervascularization of liver metastases from endocrine tumors prompted previous investigators to develop techniques directed at interrupting the arterial blood supply with the aim of inducing tumor ischemia and necrosis, while portal vein flow protects normal liver parenchyma from infarction.

Initially ischemia was achieved by aggressive techniques such as *surgical ligation of the hepatic artery*. However this method is no longer recommended due to the high mortality rates (up to 20%) and the short-lived clinical response (less than 4 months) caused by rapid revascularization and formation of collateral vessels. Due to advances in percutaneous techniques, selective portal surgical ligation may be used during surgery targeted to the primary tumor, or when a major hepatic resection is planned during a second operation. In this latter case, ischemia is more targeted to causing hypertrophy of the contralateral liver lobe, rather than to control the disease. Transient hepatic ischemia, performed by traction on the hepatic artery with an external vessel loop for a few minutes, is also obsolete.

At present vascular occlusion can be achieved percutaneously with highly selective techniques such as hepatic artery embolization (HAE) which can also be combined with transcatheter arterial chemotherapy (TACE).

Due to frequent vascular abnormalities, the procedure begins in both cases with diagnostic angiography of the celiac axis and the superior mesenteric artery using the Seldinger technique. Care is also taken to assess portal vein patency, since embolization in this situation causes hepatic infarction. Selective catheterization as proximal as possible of the hepatic artery branches in the vascular distribution of the tumor has the advantage of leaving the main segmental arteries open and avoiding rapid collateral development.

In *hepatic artery embolization (HAE)* the procedure consists of the selective injection of embolizing agents, until a marked decrease in blood flow is observed. The use of absorbable gelatine sponge fragments (Gelfoam®), microspheres (Embosphere®) and non-absorbable polyvinyl alcohol (PVA) particles (Ivalon®) has been reported. Iodized oil (Ethiodol® or Lipiodol®) has the advantage of facilitating identification of tumors and following their morphologic evolution.

Transcatheter arterial chemotherapy (TACE) is based on the same interventional radiologic procedure as HAE. Once selective catheterization is obtained the procedure requires the injection of cytotoxic drugs previously emulsified in iodized oil and dissolved in saline and water-soluble iodinated contrast agent. After injection, the embolization is performed distally in hepatic artery to reduce blood flow.

The most commonly administered cytotoxic drugs are doxorubicin (50 mg/m^2) or streptozotocin (1.5 g/m^2). The association of vascular occlusive strategies with cytotoxic agents has been reported to be more efficacious in anoxic cells. Anoxia and reduced vascularization can moreover increase local drug concentrations 10- to 100-fold compared to systemic infusion, while simultaneous embolization prolongs dwelling times of the drug in cancer cells. The response rates of neoplasms to chemotherapy drugs are proportional to the area under the drug concentration time curve.

These procedures can be repeated every 1–3 months, but the optimal timing of sequential cycles is unclear. As for the number of cycles, a minimum of two TACE sessions seems to be required to achieve a maximal tumor response. A high Lipiodol® uptake (>50%) as determined by postoperative CT seems to be predictive of better response.

The development of radionucleotide therapy performed with somatostatin analogs has been a substantial advance during the past 5 years. Recently embolization has been associated with intra-arterial administration of ^{90}Y-DOTA-lanreotide directly to the liver metastasis. In patients with tumors that are primarily restricted to the liver, this therapy can achieve higher intratumoral concentrations and provide more effective treatment of somatostatin receptor-positive liver metastases from neuroendocrine tumors.

Contraindications of hepatic arterial embolization procedures include complete portal vein thrombosis, hepatic insufficiency and previous biliary anastomoses. Diffuse liver involvement in the absence of hepatic insufficiency is not a contraindication.

However if the hepatic involvement is extensive the morbidity rate is significantly higher. Actually this parameter seems to be the most important factor predicting response to both surgical treatment and TACE. Roche reported a response rate to TACE of 3% for liver involvement less than 30%, which decreased to 23% if the involvement was more than 60% ($p = 0.016$).

Complications

Minor side-effects seen in the 'post-embolic syndrome' are common, although mostly transient and self-limiting. It generally lasts 1–3 days, but may continue for a week and although the severity may differ it is seen in 20–80% of patients. The symptoms include abdominal pain (50–60%), fever (30–60%), nausea and vomiting (50–70%) and increased serum transaminases (100%).

Major side-effects are less frequent but are nonetheless clinically relevant, occurring in about 10% of cases, and include renal and liver failure, upper gastrointestinal bleeding due to the occurrence of ischemic peptic ulcer, cholecystitis, hepatic abscess and intestinal ischemia. To prevent or reduce these complications, patients should be pretreated with intravenous hydration and antibiotics, and postoperatively with analgesics and antiemetic therapies. In carcinoid tumors a hormonal crisis should be avoided by administrating intravenous octreotide.

The mortality rate for embolization is about 3–5%.

Results

It is difficult to compare data regarding the results and survival between different reports due to the large variations encountered such as different numbers of cycles, the concomitant use of other medical treatment such as somatostatin analogs or chemotherapy and, for TACE, the use of different cytotoxic agents.

In patients suffering from pancreatic endocrine tumors, Ajani performed sequential hepatic *embolization* with a median number of four procedures and reported a partial response in 60% (12 of 20) of cases with a median survival of 33.7 months (Ajani *et al.* 1988). Schell *et al.* reported symptomatic improvement after hepatic arterial embolization in 64% of patients, with a reduction of tumor burden in 79% of cases (Schell *et al.* 2002). When a low number of repeated procedures were performed, Erikkson *et al.* reported an overall objective response of approximately 50%, even if the median duration of response (12 months) was similar (Eriksson *et al.* 1998).

Whether chemoembolization is preferable to embolization alone is unclear. Following the report by Moertel *et al.*, in which the combination of intravenous chemotherapy after hepatic arterial occlusion was more efficacious in the long term and had a higher regression rate compared to occlusion alone, many investigators favored chemoembolization (Moertel *et al.* 1994). TACE is reported to lead to slightly better biochemical and tumor responses.

Gupta and colleagues have recently published a study in which TACE did not show any therapeutic benefits over HEA in patients with carcinoid tumors. On the contrary, metastases from pancreatic endocrine tumors seem to benefit from addition of intra-arterial chemotherapy to embolization. This unusual result may be explained by the resistance to chemotherapy reported for carcinoid tumors (Gupta *et al.* 2005).

The combination of peripheral hepatic artery embolization with local cytotoxic chemotherapy effectively reduces hormonal symptoms and tumor burden (Table 23.15).

TACE has proven effective in symptom relief in 67–100% of patients suffering from either a carcinoid or islet cell tumor. The amelioration of symptoms in carcinoid syndrome is confirmed by the decrease in urinary 5-HIAA seen in 50–91% of patients with carcinoid disease.

An objective tumor response rate of 33–86% was also confirmed in many series. A recent series by Roche *et al.* confirmed previous reports in 14 patients treated with TACE as first-line option with an objective tumor response of 86% and obtained a 5-year survival of 83% (Roche *et al.* 2003). Whether or not survival is prolonged following TACE has yet to be demonstrated.

Studies that have compared the results of hepatic resection with embolization with or without intra-arterial chemotherapy have demonstrated prolonged survival in the former.

Chamberlain reported a 5-year survival of 76% in those patients treated surgically (including curative and partial resections) and 53% for those treated with hepatic artery embolization. There were no 5-year survivors in those treated medically (Chamberlain *et al.* 2000). Nonetheless a combination of surgery, ablation and TACE can be used to render a larger number of patients with neuroendocrine metastases eligible for aggressive management. Touzios reported a 5-year survival rate of 96% in patients treated with resection and ablation, which decreased to 50% in those treated with TACE and 25% in untreated patients (Touzios *et al.* 2005).

For patients with non-resectable tumors these procedures appear to offer the best hope of controlling multiple masses (more than four lesions) as well as tumors larger than 5 cm in diameter. Moreover they can be used to treat a higher area of liver compared to ablative therapies, independently of the size and location of the tumor(s).

Hepatic radioembolization using microspheres labeled with radioactive isotopes such as yttrium-90 has been described since 1990, although the hepatic artery administration of radioreceptor peptide may be a more attractive approach for the future. In particular, it permits delivering therapeutic irradiation to the liver and differentially to tumors within the liver. Initial data indicate that it is a safe and effective palliative approach, even if more studies are necessary to compare the effectiveness of ^{90}Y-DOTA Lanreotide with that of TACE. Comparative dosing studies with intravenous ^{90}Y-DOTA lanreotide therapy are also needed (McStay *et al.* 2005).

Local ablative techniques

Local ablative therapies are well established for unresectable hepatocellular carcinomas (HCCs) and liver metastases from colorectal carcinoma (CRC), although only a few small series have been published for endocrine hepatic metastases. Due to the above-mentioned characteristics, local ablative techniques are usually reserved for patients with limited or localized disease. They can also be used in residual disease as an adjunct to surgery (Atwell *et al.* 2005).

Percutaneous alcohol injection

Alcohol injection under ultrasound guidance into liver metastases has been used for different tumors, but the experience with endocrine tumors is limited. Ethanol causes dehydration of neoplastic cells and subsequent coagulation necrosis, followed by fibrous reaction and small vessel thrombosis. It is an inexpensive method with limited collateral injury to adjacent liver, and is usually indicated only for single unresectable liver metastases less than 3 cm. It has also been shown to be effective for small HCCs, but is not effective for metastases from CRC.

Table 23.15 Reported data from the literature on the post-TACE results (according to WHO criteria).

References	n	Type of tumor	Drug	Sustained relief (%) (symptomatic pts)	HIAA reduction >50%	Response rate (%)	Mean duration (months)	Progression rate (%)
Therasse *et al.* (1993)	23	Carcinoids	DOX	100	91	35	–	12
Ruszniewski *et al.* (1993)	18	Carcinoids	DOX (50 mg/m²)	73	57	33	21	17
	5	ICC						
Hajarizadeh *et al.* (1992)		Carcinoids	CDDP, MMC, DOX + 5-FU*		–	50	10.6	–
Mavligit *et al.* (1993)	5	ICC	CDDP + vinblastine†	–	–	80	18.5	–
Clouse *et al.* (1994)	20	Carcinoids	DOX (40–80 mg)	100	100	95	8.5	–
		ICC						
Diaco *et al.* (1995)	10	Carcinoids	CDDP, MMC, DOX + 5-FU*	100	60PR	42	10	
					30SD	6		
Ruszniewski & Malka (2000)	8	Carcinoids	STZ (1.5 g/m²)	67	50	53	10.5	26
	7	ICC						
Kress *et al.* (2003)‡	12	Carcinoids	DOX (20–40 mg)	0	66	8PR		19
	8	ICC				54SD		
Roche *et al.* (2003)§	10	Carcinoids	DOX (25–120 mg)	90	75	86	–	14
	4	Unknown				43PR	25PR	
						29MR	14MR	
						14 SD	7SD	

ICC, islet cell carcinoma; CDDP, cisplatin; MMC, mitomycin C; DOX, doxorubicin; STZ, streptozotocin; PR, partial response (>50% reduction); SD, stable disease; MR, minor response (25–50% reduction).

* CDDP; MMC; DOX + 5-FU; CDDP (100 mg); MMC (30 mg); DOX (30 mg) + sequential intra-arterial 5-FU (2 g/day for 5 days).

† CDDP + vinblastine: CDDP (150 mg) + sequential intrarterial vinblastine (10 mg/m²).

‡ >50% of the treated patients had a tumor burden >50%.

§ First-line treatment.

Endocrine tumors, due to their high degree of vascularization, will likely give better results. However the response to percutaneously administered alcohol is varied. There is a scarcity of data pertaining to endocrine tumors. Livraghi *et al.* reported a complete response in all four endocrine hepatic metastases treated with percutaneous alcohol injection (Livraghi *et al.* 1991).

Laser-induced thermal therapy

A novel approach is the local ablation of tumor using thermal coagulation, or laser-induced thermal therapy (LITT). However, there are scarce data using the method in endocrine tumors. Veenendaal *et al.* reported that with the use of simultaneous multiple fibers, LITT or next-generation bipolar RFA can ablate tumors as large as 7 cm in diameter and up to seven lesions during a single session (Veenendaal *et al.* 2006).

Cryosurgery

Principles, technique, indications and contraindications

Cryosurgical ablation was developed 150 years ago for treating breast and cervical cancer. However, recent technical advances in ultrasonography and cryosurgical delivery systems, allowing accurate monitoring of freezing process, have permitted good results in colorectal hepatic metastases. At present it is usually performed during laparotomy and only less than 10% of patients are treated laparoscopically. Consequently it is considerably more expensive than percutaneous techniques.

From a technical point of view, one or more cryoprobes, depending on the tumor size, are inserted into the neoplasm under ultrasonography guidance. Liquid nitrogen circulating in the probes causes freezing and tumoral destruction in an area termed 'the ice ball'. Cell death is caused by a combination of direct freezing, denaturation of cellular proteins, cell membrane rupture, cell dehydration and ischemic hypoxia. Tumoral freezing is monitored by ultrasonography until the 'ice ball' surrounds the tumor with a 1 cm margin of normal tissue. After removal of the cryoprobes, the tract is packed for hemostasis.

Complications

The complication rate of cryotherapy is generally greater (near 20%) than that for radiofrequency ablation. Complications include hemorrhage, pleural effusion, abscess formation, biliary strictures or perforation, small vessel ischemia, arteriovenous fistula formation and thrombocytopenia.

Results

Bilchick *et al.* reported successful results in terms of reducing tumor markers (near 90%) and symptom control with a median duration of 10 months using cryoablation (Bilchik *et al.* 1997). Additionally even if it has replaced been by RFA in most centers, which can also be used more safely in a percutaneous manner, it is an important supplement to surgical resection, allowing regional destruction to lesions not amenable to resection.

One possible advantage of this method over RFA is that it can be used near large vessels, with a very low risk of thrombosis. As previously reported by Bilchick *et al.* in a large study of 308 patients suffering from unresectable primary and secondary tumors, lesions >3 cm may be treated more effectively by cryosurgery than by RFA ablation (Bilchik *et al.* 2000).

Radiofrequency ablation

Principles, technique, indications and contraindications

Although RFA is a fairly new technique, converting RF waves into heat, various studies have demonstrated its effectiveness in the treatment of unresectable hepatocellular carcinomas and hepatic metastases of colon carcinoma.

During RFA a small electrode is placed within the tumor to deliver a high-frequency alternating current in the range of radiofrequency waves (near 460 kHz) into the surrounding tissues, causing molecular vibration which is then converted into frictional heat and subsequent thermal coagulative necrosis.

Lesions that are 2.5 cm in diameter or smaller can be treated with a single cycle, while larger tumors require overlapping ablations. Depending on the techniques, the ideal tumor candidates for RFA are less than 3.5 cm in diameter and are completely surrounded by hepatic parenchyma, 1 cm or more deep to the liver capsule, and 2 cm or more away from large hepatic portal veins.

RFA can be performed either intraoperatively (even at laparoscopy) or percutaneously. A multivariate meta-analysis suggested that the latter was associated with a higher risk of local recurrence. Careful diagnostic laparoscopy allows better evaluation of potential extrahepatic disease. Moreover, when associated with an ultrasonography laparoscopic probe, it allows detection of any additional areas with metastatic disease in the liver parenchyma. In addition, during laparoscopy lesions located near the periphery of the liver may also be treated.

RFA is especially suitable for repeated treatment in patients with local recurrence or new metastases that have developed during follow-up. It is also useful as an adjunct to surgical therapy.

Complications

The complication rate of RFA is 3–7%. Minor complications include sepsis and bile leakage, while major complications comprise abscesses and bleeding. The mortality rate is near zero.

Results

The role and effectiveness of RFA in the treatment of hepatic metastases has been demonstrated by recent case series. Berber *et al.* published the largest series to date of intraoperative laparoscopic RFA performed on 234 hepatic neuroendocrine metastases in 34 patients. Relief of symptoms was achieved in

95% of cases, with significant or complete symptom control in 80% for a mean of 10 months. After treatment, 65% of patients demonstrated a partial or significant decrease in tumor markers. Data from 32 patients showed local recurrence at 3% of the treated metastatic sites, documented between 6 and 12 months after RFA. Overall, 41% of patients showed no progression, with a median survival of 1.6 years after RFA (Berber *et al.* 2002).

In another study by Hellman *et al.*, 43 hepatic metastases in 21 patients were treated with either RFA alone or associated with surgery. The sizes of the hepatic metastases ranged from 2 to 7 cm. Fifteen patients were treated with curative intent, however only four remained free of residual disease at follow-up. The local recurrence rate was 4.6% at 2-year follow-up (Hellman *et al.* 2002).

Conclusions

Published data confirm the value of a multimodal approach in the treatment of endocrine tumors. Given the established success, surgical resection is the gold standard treatment of endocrine hepatic metastases when possible. However locoregional ablative strategies are an effective adjunctive treatment to surgery or medical treatment in metastatic disease.

The most effective management strategy and timing of treatments remains unclear. Moreover, optimal therapy must be tailored for each patient. When local ablative therapies are used early in the course of disease the occurrence of carcinoid syndrome with end stage disease can be postponed.

In case of multiple lesions and bilobar involvement, TACE should be the method of choice since it gives acceptable results in terms of both control of symptoms and tumor response. It can also be combined with systemic treatments to improve the results.

RFA is usually reserved for patients with limited or localized disease, but can also be used in residual disease as adjunct to surgery.

Clinicians still need to carry out more studies to define the role of ablative therapies in the multimodal treatment of endocrine tumors, especially in terms of timing and indications.

References

Ajani JA, Carrasco CH *et al.* (1988) Islet cell tumors metastatic to the liver: effective palliation by sequential hepatic artery embolization. *Ann Intern Med* 108(3): 340–4.

Atwell TD, Charboneau JW *et al.* (2005) Treatment of neuroendocrine cancer metastatic to the liver: the role of ablative techniques. *Cardiovasc Intervent Radiol* 28(4): 409–21.

Berber E, Flesher N, Siperstein AE. (2002) Laparoscopic radiofrequency ablation of neuroendocrine liver metastases. *World J Surg* 26(8): 985–90.

Bilchik AJ, Sarantou T *et al.* (1997) Cryosurgical palliation of metastatic neuroendocrine tumors resistant to conventional therapy. *Surgery* 122(6): 1040–7; discussion 1047–8.

Bilchik AJ, Wood TF *et al.* (2000) Cryosurgical ablation and radiofrequency ablation for unresectable hepatic malignant neoplasms: a proposed algorithm. *Arch Surg* 135(6): 657–62; discussion 662–4.

Chamberlain RS, Canes D, Brown KT *et al.* (2000) Hepatic neuroendocrine metastases: does intervention alter outcomes? *J Am Coll Surg* 190(4): 432–45.

Clouse ME, Perry L, Stuart K, Stokes KR. (1994) Hepatic arterial chemoembolization for metastatic neuroendocrine tumors. *Digestion* 55 (Suppl 3): 92–7.

Diaco DS, Hajarizadeh H *et al.* (1995) Treatment of metastatic carcinoid tumors using multimodality therapy of octreotide acetate, intra-arterial chemotherapy, and hepatic arterial chemoembolization. *Am J Surg* 169(5): 523–8.

Eriksson BK, Larsson EG *et al.* (1998) Liver embolizations of patients with malignant neuroendocrine gastrointestinal tumors. *Cancer* 83(11): 2293–301.

Gupta S, Johnson MM, Murthy R *et al.* (2005) Hepatic arterial embolization and chemoembolization for the treatment of patients with metastatic neuroendocrine tumors: variables affecting response rates and survival. *Cancer* 104(8): 1590–602.

Hajarizadeh H, Ivancev K *et al.* (1992) Effective palliative treatment of metastatic carcinoid tumors with intra-arterial chemotherapy/chemoembolization combined with octreotide acetate. *Am J Surg* 163(5): 479–83.

Hellman P, Ladjevardi S, Skogseid B, Akerstrom G, Elvin A. (2002) Radiofrequency tissue ablation using cooled tip for liver metastases of endocrine tumors. *World J Surg* 26(8): 1052–6.

Kress O, Wagner HJ *et al.* (2003) Transarterial chemoembolization of advanced liver metastases of neuroendocrine tumors—a retrospective single-center analysis. *Digestion* 68(2–3): 94–101.

Livraghi T, Vettori C *et al.* (1991) Liver metastases: results of percutaneous ethanol injection in 14 patients. *Radiology* 179(3): 709–12.

Mavligit GM, Pollock RE *et al.* (1993) Durable hepatic tumor regression after arterial chemoembolization-infusion in patients with islet cell carcinoma of the pancreas metastatic to the liver. *Cancer* 72(2): 375–80.

McStay MK, Maudgil D *et al.* (2005) Large-volume liver metastases from neuroendocrine tumors: hepatic intraarterial 90Y-DOTA-lanreotide as effective palliative therapy. *Radiology* 237(2): 718–26.

Moertel CG, Johnson CM *et al.* (1994) The management of patients with advanced carcinoid tumors and islet cell carcinomas. *Ann Intern Med* 120(4): 302–9.

Roche A, Girish BV, de Baere T *et al.* (2003) Trans-catheter arterial chemoembolization as first-line treatment for hepatic metastases from endocrine tumors. *Eur Radiol* 13(1): 136–40.

Ruszniewski P, Rougier P *et al.* (1993) Hepatic arterial chemoembolization in patients with liver metastases of endocrine tumors. A prospective phase II study in 24 patients. *Cancer* 71(8): 2624–30.

Ruszniewski P, Malka D. (2000) Hepatic arterial chemoembolization in the management of advanced digestive endocrine tumors. *Digestion* 62 (Suppl 1): 79–83.

Schell SR, Camp ER *et al.* (2002) Hepatic artery embolization for control of symptoms, octreotide requirements, and tumor progression in metastatic carcinoid tumors. *J Gastrointest Surg* 6(5): 664–70.

Therasse E, Breittmayer F *et al.* (1993) Transcatheter chemoembolization of progressive carcinoid liver metastasis. *Radiology* 189(2): 541–7.

Touzios JG, Kiely JM *et al.* (2005) Neuroendocrine hepatic metastases: does aggressive management improve survival? *Ann Surg* 241(5): 776–83; discussion 783–5.

Veenendaal LM, Borel Rinkes IH *et al.* (2006) Multipolar radiofrequency ablation of large hepatic metastases of endocrine tumors. *Eur J Gastroenterol Hepatol* 18(1): 89–92.

Radiolabeled somatostatin analogs

Dik J. Kwekkeboom, Jaap J.M. Teunissen, Boen L. Kam, Roelf Valkema, Wouter W. de Herder & Eric P. Krenning

Introduction

Treatment with radiolabeled somatostatin analogs is a promising new tool in the management of patients with inoperable or metastasized endocrine tumors. Symptomatic improvement may occur with all ^{111}In, ^{90}Y, or ^{177}Lu-labeled somatostatin analogs that have been used for peptide receptor radionuclide therapy (PRRT). The results that were obtained with [^{90}Y-DOTA^0,Tyr^3]octreotide and [^{177}Lu-DOTA^0,Tyr^3]octreotate are very encouraging in terms of tumor regression. Also, if kidney-protective agents are used, the side-effects of this therapy are few and mild, and the duration of the therapy response for both radiopharmaceuticals is more than 30 months. Lastly, the patients' self-assessed quality of life increases significantly after treatment with [^{177}Lu-DOTA^0,Tyr^3]octreotate. These data compare favorably with the limited number of alternative treatment approaches. If more widespread use of PRRT can be guaranteed, such therapy might well become the therapy of first choice in patients with metastasized or inoperable GEP tumors.

Endocrine gastroenteropancreatic (GEP) tumors, which comprise functioning and non-functioning endocrine pancreatic tumors and carcinoids, are usually slow growing. When metastasized, treatment with somatostatin analogs results in reduced hormonal overproduction and symptomatic relief in most cases. Treatment with somatostatin analogs is however seldom successful in terms of tumor size reduction (Arnold *et al.* 1993; Janson & Oberg 1993; Ducreux *et al.* 2000).

A new treatment modality for patients with inoperable or metastasized endocrine GEP tumors is the use of radiolabeled somatostatin analogs. The majority of endocrine GEP tumors possess somatostatin receptors and can therefore be visualized using the radiolabeled somatostatin analog [^{111}indium-DTPA^0]octreotide (OctreoScan®). A logical sequence to this tumor visualization *in vivo* was therefore to also try to treat these patients with radiolabeled somatostatin analogs.

Studies with [^{111}In-DTPA^0]octreotide

Because at that time no other chelated somatostatin analogs labeled with beta-emitting radionuclides were available, early studies in the mid- to late 1990s used [^{111}In-DTPA^0]octreotide for PRRT. Initial studies with high dosages of [^{111}In-DTPA^0]octreotide in patients with metastasized neuroendocrine tumors were encouraging with regard to symptom relief, but partial remissions (PRs) were exceptional. Two out of 26 patients with GEP tumors who were treated with high dosages of [^{111}In-DTPA^0]octreotide, and received a total cumulative dose of more than 550 mCi (20 GBq), had a decrease in tumor size of between 25 and 50%, as measured on CT scans (Valkema *et al.* 2002). None, however, had PR (Table 23.16). In another study in 27 patients with GEP tumors, PR was reported in 2 out of 26 patients with measurable disease (Anthony *et al.* 2002) (Table 23.16). Both series had relatively high numbers of patients who were in a poor clinical condition upon study entry. Also,

Table 23.16 Tumor responses in patients with GEP tumors, treated with different radiolabeled somatostatin analogs. Adapted from: Kwekkeboom *et al.* (2005), with permission.

Center (reference)	Ligand	Patient no	Tumor response					
			CR	PR	MR	SD	PD	CR + PR
Rotterdam (Valkema *et al.* 2002)	[^{111}In-DTPA^0]octreotide	26	0	0	5 (19%)	11 (42%)	10 (38%)	0%
New Orleans (Anthony *et al.* 2002)	[^{111}In-DTPA^0]octreotide	26	0	2 (8%)	NA	21 (81%)	3 (12%)	8%
Milan (Bodel *et al.* 2003)	[^{90}Y-DOTA^0,Tyr^3]octreotide	21	0	6 (29%)	NA	11 (52%)	4 (19%)	29%
Basel (Waldherr *et al.* 2001, 2002)	[^{90}Y-DOTA^0,Tyr^3]octreotide	74	3 (4%)	15 (20%)	NA	48 (65%)	8 (11%)	24%
Basel (Waldherr *et al.* 2002)	[^{90}Y-DOTA^0,Tyr^3]octreotide	33	2 (6%)	9 (27%)	NA	19 (57%)	3 (9%)	33%
Rotterdam (Valkema *et al.* 2003)	[^{90}Y-DOTA^0,Tyr^3]octreotide	54	0	4 (7%)	7 (13%)	33 (61%)	10 (19%)	7%
Rotterdam (Kwekkeboom *et al.* 2005)	[^{177}Lu-DOTA^0,Tyr^3]octreotate	131	3 (2%)	32 (26%)	24 (19%)	44 (35%)	22 (18%)	28%

many had progressive disease when entering the study. The most common toxicity in both series was due to bone marrow suppression. Serious side-effects consisted of leukemia and myelodysplastic syndrome (MDS) in three patients who had been treated with total cumulative doses of >2.7 Ci (100 GBq) (and estimated bone marrow radiation doses of more than 3 Gy) (Valkema *et al.* 2002). One of these patients had also been treated with chemotherapy, which may have contributed to or caused this complication. Anthony *et al.* (2002) reported renal insufficiency in one patient which was probably not treatment related, but due to pre-existent retroperitoneal fibrosis. Transient liver toxicity was observed in three patients with widespread liver metastases. Although in both series favorable effects on symptomatology were reported, CT-assessed tumor regression was observed only in rare cases. This is not surprising, since ^{111}In-coupled peptides are not ideal for PRRT because of the small particle range and therefore short tissue penetration.

Studies with [^{90}Y-DOTA^0,Tyr^3]octreotide

The next generation of somatostatin receptor-mediated radionuclide therapy used a modified somatostatin analog, [Tyr^3]octreotide, with a higher affinity for the somatostatin receptor subtype 2, and a different chelator, DOTA instead of DTPA, in order to ensure a more stable binding of the intended beta-emitting radionuclide ^{90}yttrium (^{90}Y). Using this compound (^{90}Y-DOTATOC; OctreoTher®), different phase 1 and phase 2 PRRT trials have been performed.

Otte *et al.* (1999) and Waldherr *et al.* (2001, 2002a) (Basel, Switzerland) reported different phase 1 and phase 2 studies in patients with neuroendocrine GEP tumors. In their first reports, using a dose-escalating scheme of four treatment sessions up to a cumulative dose of 160 mCi (6 GBq)/m^2, and at which time renal protection with amino acid infusion was not performed in half of the patients, renal insufficiency developed in 4/29 patients. The overall response rate in GEP tumor patients who were either treated with 160 mCi (6 GBq)/m^2 (Waldherr *et al.* 2001), or, in a later study, with 200 mCi (7.4 GBq)/m^2 in 4 doses (Waldherr *et al.* 2002a), was 24% (Table 23.16). In a subsequent study, with the same dose of 200 mCi (7.4 GBq)/m^2 administered in two sessions, complete and partial remissions were found in one third of 36 patients (Waldherr *et al.* 2002b) (Table 23.16). It should be emphasized, however, that this was not a randomized trial comparing two dosing schemes.

Chinol *et al.* (Milan, Italy) (Chinol *et al.* 2002), described dosimetric and dose-finding studies with [^{90}Y-DOTA^0,Tyr^3] octreotide with and without the administration of kidney-protecting agents. No major acute reactions were observed up to an administered dose of 150 mCi (5.6 GBq) per cycle. Reversible grade 3 hematologic toxicity was found in 43% of patients injected with 140 mCi (5.2 GBq), which was defined as the maximum tolerated dose per cycle. None of the patients developed acute or delayed kidney failure, although follow-up was short. Partial and complete remissions were reported by the same group in 28% of 87 patients with neuroendocrine tumors (Paganelli *et al.* 2002).

In a more detailed publication from the same group, Bodei *et al.*(2003) report the results of a phase 1 study in 40 patients with somatostatin receptor-positive tumors, of whom 21 had GEP tumors. Cumulative total treatment doses ranged from 160 to 300 mCi (5.9–11.1 GBq), given in two treatment cycles. Six of 21 (29%) patients had tumor regression (Table 23.16). Median duration of the response was 9 months.

Another study with [^{90}Y-DOTA^0,Tyr^3]octreotide is a multicenter phase 1 study which was performed in Rotterdam (the Netherlands), Brussels (Belgium) and Tampa (USA), in which 60 patients received escalating doses up to 400 mCi (14.8 GBq)/m^2 in four cycles or up to 250 mCi (9.3 GBq)/m^2 single dose, without reaching the maximum tolerated single dose (Valkema *et al.* 2003). The cumulative radiation dose to kidneys was limited to 27 Gy. All received amino acids concomitant with [^{90}Y-DOTA^0,Tyr^3]octreotide for kidney protection. Three patients had dose-limiting toxicity: one liver toxicity, one thrombocytopenia grade 4 (<25 × 10^9/L), and one MDS. Four out of 54 (8%) patients who had received their maximum allowed dose had PR, and 7 (13%) had a minor response (MR) (25–50% tumor volume reduction) (Table 23.16). The median time to progression in the 44 patients who had either stable disease (SD), MR, or PR was 30 months.

Bushnell *et al.* (Iowa City, USA) (Bushnell *et al.* 2003) reported a favorable clinical response as determined by a scoring system that included weight, patient-assessed health score, Karnofsky score, and tumor-related symptoms, in 14/21 patients who were treated with a total cumulative dose of 360 mCi [^{90}Y-DOTA^0,Tyr^3]octreotide in three treatment cycles.

Despite differences in protocols used, complete plus partial remissions in most of the different studies with [^{90}Y-DOTA^0,Tyr^3]octreotide are in the same range, in between 10 and 30%, and therefore better than those obtained with [^{111}In-DTPA^0]octreotide.

Studies with [^{177}Lu-DOTA^0,Tyr^3]octreotate

The somatostatin analog [DTPA^0,Tyr^3]octreotate differs from [DTPA^0,Tyr^3]octreotide only in that the C-terminal threoninol is replaced with threonine. Compared with [DTPA^0,Tyr^3] octreotide, it shows an improved binding to somatostatin receptor positive tissues in animal experiments (De Jong *et al.* 1998). Also, its DOTA-coupled counterpart, [DOTA^0, Tyr^3]octreotate, labeled with the beta- and gamma-emitting radionuclide ^{177}lutetium (^{177}Lu), was reported very successful in terms of tumor regression and animal survival in a rat model (Erion *et al.* 1999). Reubi *et al.* (Reubi *et al.* 2000) reported a ninefold increase in affinity for the somatostatin receptor subtype 2 for [DOTA^0,Tyr^3]octreotate when compared with [DOTA^0,Tyr^3]octreotide, and a six- to sevenfold increase in affinity for their yttrium-loaded counterparts.

In a comparison in patients, it was found that the uptake of radioactivity, expressed as percentage of the injected dose of [^{177}Lu-DOTA^0,Tyr^3]octreotate, was comparable to that after [^{111}In-DTPA^0]octreotide for kidneys, spleen and liver, but was three- to fourfold higher for 4 of 5 tumors (Kwekkeboom *et al.* 2001). Therefore, [^{177}Lu-DOTA^0,Tyr^3]octreotate potentially represents an important improvement because of the higher absorbed doses that can be achieved to most tumors with about equal doses to potentially dose-limiting organs and because of the lower tissue penetration range of ^{177}Lu if compared with ^{90}Y, which may be especially important for small tumors.

The first treatment effects of [^{177}Lu-DOTA^0,Tyr^3]octreotate therapy were described in 35 patients with neuroendocrine GEP tumors, who had a follow-up of 3 to 6 months after receiving their final dose (Kwekkeboom *et al.* 2003). Patients were treated with dosages of 100, 150, or 200 mCi (3.7, 5.6, or 7.4 GBq) [^{177}Lu-DOTA^0,Tyr^3]octreotate, up to a final cumulative dose of 600–800 mCi (22.2–29.6 GBq), with treatment intervals of 6–9 weeks.

The effects of the therapy on tumor size were evaluable in 34 patients. Three months after the final administration a complete remission (CR) was found in one patient (3%), PR in 12 (35%), SD in 14 (41%), and progressive disease (PD) in 7 (21%), including three patients who died during the treatment period. The side-effects of treatment with [177Lu-DOTA0,Tyr3] octreotate were few and mostly transient, with mild bone marrow depression as the most common finding.

More recently, an analysis of this treatment in 131 patients with neuroendocrine GEP tumors was reported (Kwekkeboom *et al.* 2005). Fifty-five of the 131 (42%) patients had documented progressive disease within 1 year before the start of the therapy, 37 (28%) had stable disease, and in 39 (30%) information on disease progression was absent. Treatment intervals were 6–10 weeks, except in 4 patients who had persistent thrombocytopenia and in 13 others because of reasons unrelated to the treatment. In 116 patients, the final intended cumulative dose of 600–800 mCi was administered. Ten of the 15 remaining patients died of progressive disease before completing their treatment.

Nausea and vomiting within the first 24 h after the administration were present in 31% and 14% of the administrations, respectively. Mild abdominal pain was noticed by 12% of the patients, especially those with liver enlargement. Increased hair loss was noticed by 64% of the patients; hair regrowth occurred within 3 months after the last administration.

Serious side-effects occurred in 2 patients. One patient in whom in the year preceding the therapy serum creatinine concentrations had risen from 60–70 μmol/L to 90–100 μmol/L, and who had a urinary creatinine clearance of 41 mL/min when entering the study, eventually developed renal insufficiency 1.5 years after receiving her last treatment. A kidney biopsy demonstrated tubular depositions and microangiopathy. Eventually, the patient refrained from hemodialysis and died shortly thereafter. In another patient who had diffuse liver metastases from an endocrine pancreatic tumor which had grown rapidly in the months preceding the therapy, an increase in upper abdominal pain and a deterioriation of liver functions occurred in the days and weeks following the first administration. The patient developed hepatorenal syndrome and died after 5 weeks.

WHO toxicity grade 3 or 4 anemia (Hb 4.0–4.9 or <4.0 mmol/L, respectively), leucocytopenia (WBC 1.0–1.9 or $<1.0 \times 10^9$/L, respectively), or thrombocytopenia (platelets 25.0–49.9 or $<25 \times 10^9$/L, respectively) occurred after 0.4% and 0.0%, 1.3% and 0.0%, and 1.5% and 0.2% of the administrations, respectively. Patients who had been treated with chemotherapy had significantly more frequently thrombocytopenia toxicity grade ≥2, whereas patients older than 70 years of age had a significantly higher frequency of WHO toxicity grade ≥2 leucocytopenia, especially neutropenia. Mean Hb, leucocytes and platelets decreased significantly during treatment, but were not significantly different from pretreatment values 18–24 months after the last therapy. Neither serum creatinine nor creatinine clearance changed significantly.

Tumor size could be evaluated in 125 patients. CR was found in 3 (2%) patients, PR in 32 (26%), MR in 24 (19%), SD in 44 (35%), and PD in 22 (18%) patients, including the 10 patients who died before the intended cumulative dose was reached (Table 23.16) (Figs 23.39 & 23.40). Higher remission rates were positively correlated with high uptake during pretherapy [111In-DTPA0]octreotide scintigraphy and a limited number of liver metastases, whereas PD was significantly more frequent in patients with a low Karnofsky performance score (KPS) and extensive disease (Figs 23.41–23.43).

Median follow-up in the 103 patients who either had SD or tumor regression was 16 months and median time to progression was more than 36 months.

Another study evaluated the quality of life (QoL) in 50 patients with metastatic somatostatin receptor-positive GEP tumors treated with [^{177}Lu-DOTA^0,Tyr^3]octreotate (Teunissen *et al.* 2004). The patients completed the European Organization for the Research and Treatment of Cancer Quality of Life Questionnaire C30 before therapy and at follow-up visit 6 weeks after the last cycle. A significant improvement in the global health status/QoL scale was observed after therapy with [^{177}Lu-DOTA^0,Tyr^3]octreotate. Furthermore, significant improvement was observed in the role, emotional, and social function scales. The symptom scores for fatigue, insomnia, and pain decreased significantly. Patients with proven tumor regression most frequently had an improvement of QoL domains.

Studies with other radiolabeled somatostatin analogs

Chelated lanreotide, another somatostatin analog, labeled with ^{111}In for diagnostic purposes and with ^{90}Y for therapeutic use, has been advocated because of its better binding than

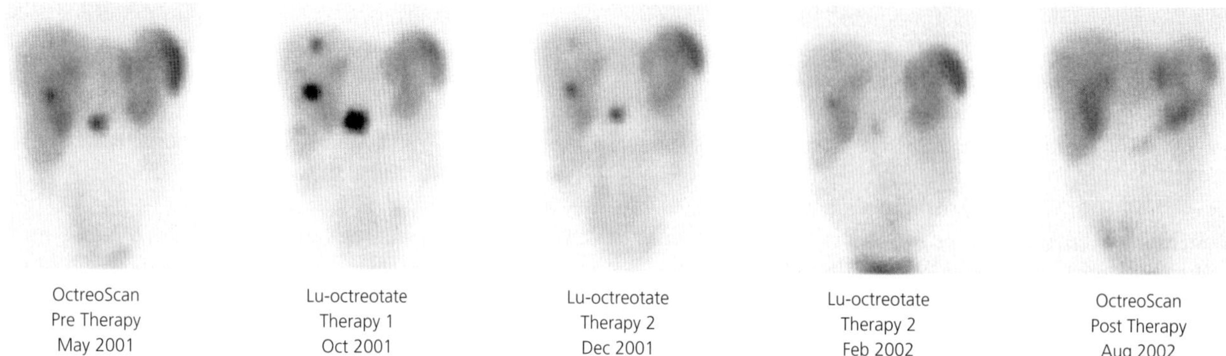

Fig. 23.39 Scintigrams in a patient with a neuroendocrine tumor of the pancreas with liver metastases. Anterior abdominal images. Furthest left and right panels show the scintigrams 24 h after injection of 6 mCi (222 MBq) [^{111}In-DTPA0]octreotide (OctreoScan) before and 6 months after the last therapy with ^{177}Lu-octreotate, respectively. Before therapy, uptake in the pancreatic lesion and one liver lesion is seen; no pathologic uptake on the post-therapy scan (although small spots still visible with SPECT imaging). Middle three panels: scans 3 days after each therapy cycle with 200 mCi (7.2 GBq) ^{177}Lu-octreotate. Notice the more intense uptake on the first post-therapeutic scan compared to the octreoscan. Also notice the decrease in tumor uptake after each subsequent therapy cycle. The patient had PR. Progression was apparent again in July 2003.

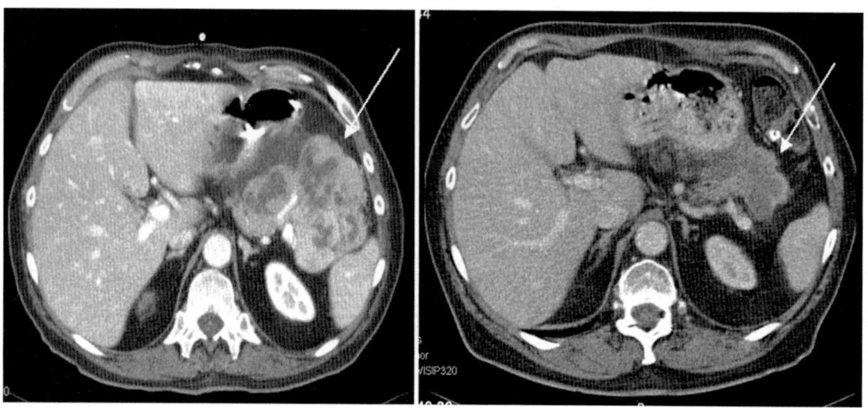

Fig. 23.40 CT scan images in a patient with a non-functioning neuroendocrine tumor of the tail of the pancreas (arrows) before (left) and 6 weeks after the last treatment with ^{177}Lu-octreotate. Before the treatment, the patient had lost more than 15 kg of body weight. At the time of scanning 8 months later (right), he had regained 14 kg. Scaling is identical. Notice the decrease in tumor size and the increase in body circumference.

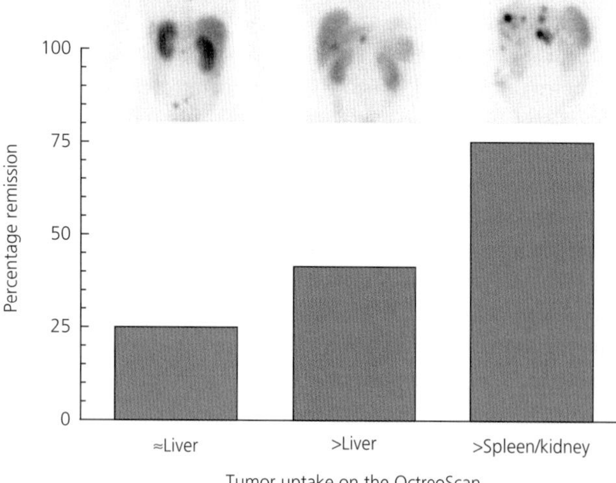

Fig. 23.41 Relationship between the chances of achieving a tumor remission (MR, PR, or CR) after treatment with ^{177}Lu-octreotate and visually scored uptake on the pretherapeutic OctreoScan. Examples of uptake scores are indicated. Data from an analysis of 131 patients with GEP tumors (Kwekkeboom *et al.* 2005).

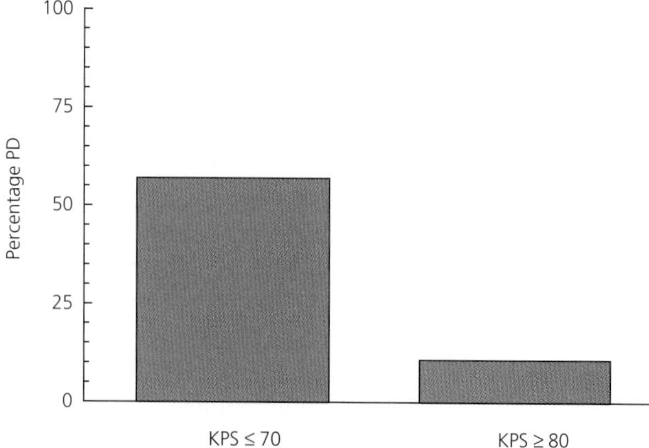

Fig. 23.42 Relationship between the chances of having progressive disease after treatment with ^{177}Lu-octreotate and Karnofsky Performance Score (KPS). Patients in poor clinical condition at the start perform worse. Data from an analysis of 131 patients with GEP tumors (Kwekkeboom *et al.* 2005).

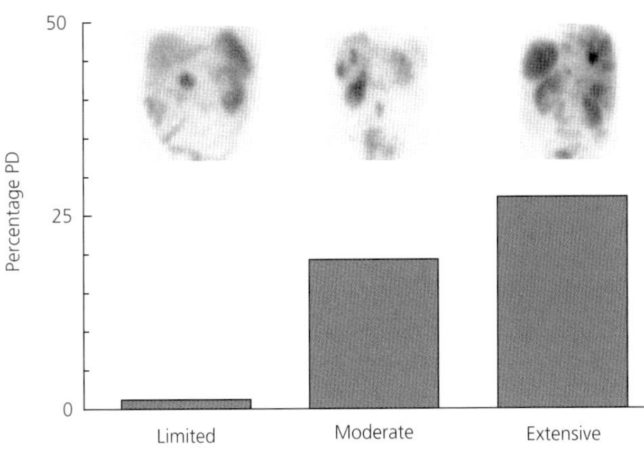

Fig. 23.43 Relationship between the chances of having progressive disease after treatment with ^{177}Lu-octreotate and tumor extent on the OctreoScan at the start. Examples of tumor extent are indicated. Patients with extensive tumor burden perform worse. Data from an analysis of 131 patients with GEP tumors (Kwekkeboom *et al.* 2005).

[^{111}In-DTPA^{0}]octreotide to the somatostatin receptor subtypes 3 and 4 (Virgolini *et al.* 2002). This claim has been questioned (Reubi *et al.* 2000). Although this compound has been used to treat patients with GEP tumors, it shows poorer affinity than radiolabeled [DOTA^{0}, Tyr^{3}]octreotide/octreotate for the somatostatin receptor subtype 2, which is predominantly overexpressed in GEP tumors (Reubi *et al.* 2000).

Comparison of the different treatments

Treatment with radiolabeled somatostatin analogs is a promising new tool in the management of patients with inoperable or metastasized neuroendocrine tumors. The results that were obtained with [^{90}Y-DOTA^{0},Tyr^{3}]octreotide and [^{177}Lu-DOTA^{0},Tyr^{3}]octreotate are very encouraging, although a direct, randomized comparison between the various treatments is lacking. Also, the reported percentages of tumor remission after [^{90}Y-DOTA^{0},Tyr^{3}]octreotide treatment vary. This may have several causes. The administered doses and dosing schemes differ: some studies use dose-escalating schemes, whereas others use fixed doses; also, there are several patient and tumor characteristics that determine treatment outcome, such as amount of uptake on the octreoscan, the estimated total tumor burden, and the extent of liver involvement. Therefore, differences in patient selection may play an important role in determining treatment outcome. Other factors that can have contributed to the different results that were found in the different centers performing trials with the same compounds, may be differences in tumor response criteria, and centralized versus decentralized follow-up CT scoring. Therefore, in order to establish which treatment scheme and which radiolabeled somatostatin analogs or combination of analogs is optimal, randomized trials are needed.

Comparison with chemotherapy

In order to better evaluate the response to PRRT it would have been preferable that a randomized trial were performed comparing PRRT to no further treatment at all. This however, is presently no longer possible, since patients can be treated with PRRT in several medical centers and since the results of such treatment are so impressive that withholding it to half of the patients in an experimental setting cannot be ethically justified. However, Faiss *et al.* (2003) recently reported tumor remissions in 4 out of 80 (5%) GEP tumor patients who had progressive disease at study entry and were treated with somatostatin analogs and/or interferon alpha. By contrast, we found tumor remissions in 47% of our patients who were treated with ^{177}Lu-octreotate, whether or not they had PD at study entry (Kwekkeboom *et al.* 2005). It seems highly unlikely that such a difference could have been caused by patient selection.

Apart from the proportion of patients with a tumor remission, the duration of such a response is another important treatment outcome parameter. Reported response rates for single-agent and combination chemotherapy in patients with endocrine GEP tumors are for instance as high as 40–60% for well-differentiated pancreatic tumors and poorly differentiated tumors from any origin, whereas success rates for midgut tumors rarely exceed 20% in recent studies (Moertel 1983; Moertel *et al.* 1980, 1992; Cheng & Saltz 1999; Van Hazel *et al.* 1983; Bukowski *et al.* 1994; Ritzel *et al.* 1995; Andreyev *et al.* 1995; Neijt *et al.* 1995 ; Ansell *et al.* 2001; for a review see O'Toole *et al.* 2004). High response rates have been reported in older series (Moertel 1983; Moertel *et al.* 1980; Moertel *et al.* 1992), but in these studies the response evaluation also included biochemical responses (changes in serum tumor marker levels) as well as physical examination for the evaluation of hepatomegaly. Indeed, much of the discrepancy between older and more recent studies can be ascribed to differences in response criteria, as is illustrated in a more recent study by Cheng and Saltz (1999) who described that their percentage of patients with an objective response would have increased from 6% to 25% if they had accepted not only measured CT scan changes as response criteria, but also decreases of hepatomegaly assessed with physical examination. Despite the varying percentages of objective responses that have been reported for chemotherapy, the median time to progression in most of the studies is less than 18 months. In this respect, treatment with ^{90}Y-octreotide or ^{177}Lu-octreotate perform considerably better with a median time to progression of more than 30 and more than 36 months, respectively (Valkema *et al.* 2003; Kwekkeboom *et al.* 2005).

When to treat?

With ^{177}Lu-octreotate we treated both patients who had progressive disease at baseline and those who were stable or in whom disease progression was not documented. The reason for this was that for many of these patients waiting for disease progression would have involved a serious deterioriation in their clinical condition.

Tumor remission was positively correlated with a high uptake during [^{111}In-DTPA^{0}]octreotide scintigraphy and a limited number of liver metastases, whereas disease progression was significantly more frequent in patients with a low performance status and a high tumor load (Kwekkeboom *et al.* 2005). This implies that the chances of a successful treatment are better if patients are treated in an early stage of their disease. In contrast to what we reported earlier in a much smaller group of patients (Kwekkeboom *et al.* 2003), the percentage of patients with a remission does not differ significantly between those patients who have disease progression at baseline and those who have not; therefore, to wait for disease progression has no advantage in terms of chances of success. On the other hand, firm conclusions on the effect of our therapy on overall survival cannot be drawn from this or any other study with radiolabeled somatostatin analogs, as randomized trials comparing treatment with radiolabeled analogs to no additional treatment have not been performed.

Options to improve PRRT

From animal experiments it can be inferred that ^{90}Y-labeled somatostatin analogs may be more effective for larger tumors, whereas ^{177}Lu-labeled somatostatin analogs may be more effective for smaller tumors, but their combination may be the most effective (De Jong *et al.* 2002). Therefore, apart from comparisons between radiolabeled octreotate and octreotide, and between somatostatin analogs labeled with ^{90}Y or ^{177}Lu, PRRT with combinations of ^{90}Y- and ^{177}Lu-labeled analogs should also be evaluated.

Future directions to improve this therapy may also include the use of radiosensitizing chemotherapeutical agents. Chemosensitization with 5-fluorouracil (5-FU) in combination with ^{90}Y-labeled antibody radioimmunotherapy is feasible and safe (Wong *et al.* 2003). Also, chemosensitization with 5-FU combined with ^{111}In-DTPA-octreotide treatment resulted in symptomatic response in 71% of patients with neuroendocrine tumors (Kong *et al.* 2005), whereas other studies using only ^{111}In-DTPA-octreotide treatment reported such responses in lower percentages (Valkema *et al.* 2002; Anthony *et al.* 2002). Numerous trials of the effects of combined chemotherapy and (fractionated) external-beam radiotherapy have been performed. In many of these, 5-FU was used. More recent trials used the prodrug of 5-FU, capecitabine, which has the advantage of oral administration. Also with the combination of radiotherapy and capecitabine, an increased efficacy in terms of tumor growth control was reported if compared to radiotherapy as single treatment modality (Rich *et al.* 2004). If capecitabine is used in relatively low doses (1600–2000 mg/m^2/day), grade 3 hematologic or other toxicity is rare (Dunst *et al.* 2002; Rich *et al.* 2004). For these reasons, we recently planned a randomized multicenter trial comparing treatment with ^{177}Lu-octreotate with and without capecitabine in patients with GEP tumors.

Conclusions

Treatment with radiolabeled somatostatin analogs is a promising new tool in the management of patients with inoperable or metastasized neuroendocrine tumors. Symptomatic improvement may occur with all ^{111}In, ^{90}Y, or ^{177}Lu-labeled somatostatin analogs that have been used for PRRT. The results that were obtained with [^{90}Y-DOTA^{0},Tyr^{3}]octreotide and [^{177}Lu-DOTA^{0},Tyr^{3}]octreotate are very encouraging in terms of tumor regression. Also, if kidney protective agents are used, the side-effects of this therapy are few and mild, and the duration of the therapy response for both radiopharmaceuticals is more than 30 months. Lastly, the patients' self-assessed quality of life increases significantly after treatment with [^{177}Lu-DOTA^{0}, Tyr^{3}]octreotate. These data compare favorably with the limited number of alternative treatment approaches. If more widespread use of PRRT can be guaranteed, such therapy might well become the therapy of first choice in patients with metastasized or inoperable GEP tumors.

References

Andreyev HJ, Scott-Mackie P, Cunningham D *et al.* (1995) Phase II study of continuous infusion fluorouracil and interferon alfa-2b in the palliation of malignant neuroendocrine tumors. *J Clin Oncol* 13: 1486–92.

Ansell SM, Pitot HC, Burch PA, Kvols LK, Mahoney MR, Rubin J. (2001) A phase II study of high-dose paclitaxel in patients with advanced neuroendocrine tumors. *Cancer* 91: 1543–8.

Anthony LB, Woltering EA, Espanan GD, Cronin MD, Maloney TJ, McCarthy KE. (2002) Indium-111-pentetreotide prolongs survival in gastroenteropancreatic malignancies. *Semin Nucl Med* 32: 123–32.

Arnold R, Benning R, Neuhaus C *et al.* (1993) Gastroenteropancreatic endocrine tumours: effect of sandostatin on tumour growth. The German Sandostatin Study Group. *Digestion* 1993 54 (Suppl 1): 72–75.

Bodei L, Cremonesi M, Zoboli S *et al.* (2003) Receptor-mediated radionuclide therapy with ^{90}Y-DOTATOC in association with amino acid infusion: a phase I study. *Eur J Nucl Med Mol Imaging* 30: 207–16.

Bukowski RM, Tangen CM, Peterson RF *et al.* (1994) Phase II trial of dimethyltriazenoimidazole carboxamide in patients with metastatic carcinoid. *Cancer* 73: 1505–8.

Bushnell D, O'Dorisio T, Menda Y *et al.* (2003) Evaluating the clinical effectiveness of ^{90}Y-SMT 487 in patients with neuroendocrine tumors. *J Nucl Med* 44: 1556–60.

Cheng PN, Saltz LB. (1999) Failure to confirm major objective antitumor activity for streptozocin and doxorubicin in the treatment of patients with advanced islet cell carcinoma. *Cancer* 86: 944–8.

Chinol M, Bodei L, Cremonesi M, Paganelli G. (2002) Receptor-mediated radiotherapy with Y-DOTA-DPhe-Tyr-octreotide: the experience of the European Institute of Oncology group. *Semin Nucl Med* 32: 141–7.

De Jong M, Breeman WA, Bakker WH *et al.* (1998) Comparison of (111)In-labeled somatostatin analogues for tumor scintigraphy and radionuclide therapy. *Cancer Res* 58: 437–41.

De Jong M, Valkema R, Jamar F *et al.* (2002) Somatostatin receptor-targeted radionuclide therapy of tumors: preclinical and clinical findings. *Semin Nucl Med* 32: 133–40.

Ducreux M, Ruszniewski P, Chayvialle JA *et al.* (2000) The antitumoral effect of the long-acting somatostatin analog lanreotide in neuroendocrine tumors. *Am J Gastroenterol* 95: 3276–81.

Dunst J, Reese T, Sutter T *et al.* (2002) Phase I trial evaluating the concurrent combination of radiotherapy and capecitabine in rectal cancer. *J Clin Oncol* 20: 3983–91.

Erion JL, Bugaj JE, Schmidt MA, Wilhelm RR, Srinivasan A. (1999) High radiotherapeutic efficacy of [Lu-177]-DOTA-Y(3)-octreotate in a rat tumor model. [Abstr] *J Nucl Med* 40: 223P.

Faiss S, Pape UF, Bohmig M *et al.* (2003) Prospective, randomized, multicenter trial on the antiproliferative effect of lanreotide, interferon alfa, and their combination for therapy of metastatic neuroendocrine gastroenteropancreatic tumors—the International Lanreotide and Interferon Alfa Study Group. *J Clin Oncol* 21: 2689–96.

Janson ET, Oberg K. (1993) Long-term management of the carcinoid syndrome. Treatment with octreotide alone and in combination with alpha-interferon. *Acta Oncol* 32: 225–9.

Kong G, Lau E, Ramdave S, Hicks RJ. (2005) High-dose In-111 octreotide therapy in combination with radiosensitizing 5-FU chemotherapy for treatment of SSR-expressing neuroendocrine tumors. [Abstr] *J Nucl Med* 46 (Suppl 2): 151P.

Kwekkeboom DJ, Bakker WH, Kooij PP *et al.* (2001) [^{177}Lu-DOTA0Tyr3]octreotate: comparison with [111In-DTPA0]octreotide in patients. *Eur J Nucl Med* 28: 1319–25.

Kwekkeboom DJ, Bakker WH, Kam BL *et al.* (2003) Treatment of patients with gastro-entero-pancreatic (GEP) tumours with the novel radiolabeled somatostatin analogue [^{177}Lu-DOTA^0,Tyr^3]octreotate. *Eur J Nucl Med Mol Imaging* 30: 417–22.

Kwekkeboom DJ, Teunissen JJ, Bakker WH *et al.* (2005) Treatment with the radiolabeled somatostatin analogue [^{177}Lu-DOTA^0,Tyr^3]octreotate in patients with gastro-entero-pancreatic (GEP) tumors. *J Clin Oncol* 23: 2754–62.

Moertel CG. (1983) Treatment of the carcinoid tumor and the malignant carcinoid syndrome. *J Clin Oncol* 1: 727–40.

Moertel CG, Hanley JA, Johnson LA. (1980) Streptozocin alone compared with streptozocin plus fluorouracil in the treatment of advanced islet-cell carcinoma. *N Engl J Med* 303: 1189–94.

Moertel CG, Lefkopoulo M, Lipsitz S, Hahn RG, Klaassen D. (1992) Streptozocin-doxorubicin, streptozocin-fluorouracil or chlorozotocin in the treatment of advanced islet-cell carcinoma. *N Engl J Med* 326: 519–23.

Neijt JP, Lacave AJ, Splinter TA *et al.* (1995) Mitoxantrone in metastatic apudomas: a phase II study of the EORTC Gastro-Intestinal Cancer Cooperative Group. *Br J Cancer* 71: 106–8.

O'Toole D, Hentic O, Corcos O, Ruszniewski P. (2004) Chemotherapy for gastro-enteropancreatic endocrine tumours. *Neuroendocrinology* 80 (Suppl 1): 79–84.

Otte A, Herrmann R, Heppeler A *et al.* (1999) Yttrium-90 DOTATOC: first clinical results. *Eur J Nucl Med* 26: 1439–47.

Paganelli G, Bodei L, Handkiewicz Junak D *et al.* (2002) 90Y-DOTA-D-Phe1-Tyr3-octreotide in therapy of neuroendocrine malignancies. *Biopolymers* 66: 393–8.

Reubi JC, Schar JC, Waser B *et al.* (2000) Affinity profiles for human somatostatin receptor subtypes SST1-SST5 of somatostatin radiotracers selected for scintigraphic and radiotherapeutic use. *Eur J Nucl Med* 27: 273–82.

Rich TA, Shepard RC, Mosley ST. (2004) Four decades of continuing innovation with fluorouracil: current and future approaches to fluorouracil chemoradiation therapy. *J Clin Oncol* 22: 2214–32.

Ritzel U, Leonhardt U, Stockmann F, Ramadori G. (1995) Treatment of metastasized midgut carcinoids with dacarbazine. *Am J Gastroenterol* 90: 627–31.

Teunissen JJ, Kwekkeboom DJ, Krenning EP. (2004) Quality of life in patients with gastroenteropancreatic tumors treated with [^{177}Lu-DOTA0,Tyr3]octreotate. *J Clin Oncol* 22: 2724–9.

Valkema R, de Jong M, Bakker WH *et al.* (2002) Phase I study of peptide receptor radionuclide therapy with [^{111}In-DTPA^0]Octreotide: the Rotterdam experience. *Semin Nucl Med* 32: 110–22.

Valkema R, Pauwels S, Kvols L *et al.* (2003) Long-term follow-up of a phase 1 study of peptide receptor radionuclide therapy (PRRT) with [90Y-DOTA0,Tyr3]octreotide in patients with somatostatin receptor positive tumours. [Abstr] *Eur J Nucl Med Mol Imaging* 30 (Suppl 2): S232.

Van Hazel GA, Rubin J, Moertel CG. (1983) Treatment of metastatic carcinoid tumor with dactinomycin or dacarbazine. *Cancer Treat Rep* 67: 583–5.

Virgolini I, Britton K, Buscombe J, Moncayo R, Paganelli G, Riva P. (2002) In- and Y-DOTA-lanreotide: results and implications of the MAURITIUS trial. *Semin Nucl Med* 32: 148–55.

Waldherr C, Pless M, Maecke HR, Haldemann A, Mueller-Brand J. (2001) The clinical value of [^{90}Y-DOTA]-D-Phe^1-Tyr^3-octreotide (^{90}Y-DOTATOC) in the treatment of neuroendocrine tumours: a clinical phase II study. *Ann Oncol* 12: 941–5.

Waldherr C, Pless M, Maecke HR *et al.* (2002a) Tumor response and clinical benefit in neuroendocrine tumors after 7.4 GBq (90)Y-DOTATOC. *J Nucl Med* 43: 617–20.

Waldherr C, Schumacher T, Maecke HR *et al.* (2002b) Does tumor response depend on the number of treatment sessions at constant injected dose using 90Yttrium-DOTATOC in neuroendocrine tumors? [Abstr] *Eur J Nucl Med Mol Imaging* 29 (Suppl 1): S100.

Wong JY, Shibata S, Williams LE *et al.* (2003) A phase I trial of 90Y-anti-carcinoembryonic antigen chimeric T84.66 radioimmunotherapy with 5-fluorouracil in patients with metastatic colorectal cancer. *Clin Cancer Res* 9: 5842–52.

Biotherapy and chemotherapy

Ursula Plöckinger

Introduction

Neuroendocrine tumors are classified according to their differentiation, localization and functionality (Table 23.17). The classification and tumor stage have important prognostic implications and influence therapeutic decisions. This section discusses the established indications of biotherapy and chemotherapy in gastrointestinal neuroendocrine tumors of the foregut and midgut, gives some in-depth information on the mechanism and effects of biotherapy and chemotherapy, as well as practical information on indication, dosage and side-effects. Evolving new therapeutic options are discussed later in the chapter (p. 662).

Table 23.17 Criteria for the classification of neuroendocrine tumors.

Localization	Differentiation	Proliferation	Functionality
Stomach	Well-differentiated tumor	Ki-67 </= 2%	Functioning
Duoedenum	Well-differentiated carcinoma	Ki-67 > 2%	Nonfunctioning
Pancreas	Low differentiated carcinoma	Ki-67 > 20%	
Jejunum/ileum			
Colon			
Rectum			

Biotherapy can be used as a symptomatic treatment in patients with functioning neuroendocrine tumors, i.e. in patients with the carcinoid syndrome, watery diarrhea or glucagonoma syndrome. Biotherapy is rarely used for symptomatic treatment of the Zollinger–Ellison syndrome, as proton pump inhibitors are a highly effective and more convenient option in these patients. Symptomatic therapy of insulinomas is rarely necessary, as most of these tumors are benign and thus surgery is curative. In the rare patient with persisting hyperinsulinemia, biotherapy i.e. somatostatin analogs may be an option (see below). To conclude, the objective of symptomatic biotherapy is to reduce signs, symptoms and complications of hormone hypersecretion syndromes in patients with neuroendocrine gastrointestinal tumors, and thus to increase the quality of life and overall survival.

In addition biotherapy has been used as an antiproliferative treatment in slow-growing malignant, well-differentiated (WHO classification) metastasized neuroendocrine carcinomas. While tumor regression is rare, stabilization of tumor growth has been demonstrated. Thus, biotherapy is used with antiproliferative intentions in neuroendocrine tumors of the pancreas and the small bowel.

Most gastroenteropancreatic neuroendocrine tumors are malignant and present with metastatic disease to the lymph nodes and liver, and in later stages with metastases to the bone, brain and other rare locations. Chemotherapy is a palliative option in both slow-growing, well-differentiated or rapidly proliferating, poorly differentiated neuroendocrine tumors. While different treatment regimens have been shown to be effective in well-differentiated pancreatic neuroendocrine carcinomas, chemotherapeutic options for tumors of the small bowel are poor. On the other hand, localization of the primary is not as important for poorly differentiated carcinomas, as these rapidly growing tumors respond to different chemotherapeutic agents, irrespective of the localization of the primary.

In slow-growing, well-differentiated tumors, tumor growth is unpredictable and slow tumor progression may alternate with long intervals of stable disease. Thus, the timing of antiproliferative therapy is not yet clear. As the quality of life is good in most patients with metastasized well-differentiated neuroendocrine tumors, antiproliferative therapy should only be initiated whenever progressive disease has been demonstrated according to standard criteria. On the other hand, poorly differentiated tumors may demonstrate rapid tumor growth and medical treatment should not be withheld.

Biotherapy

Biotherapy is defined as the therapy of hormonal hypersecretion syndromes and/or tumor growth with substances or pharmacologic derivatives thereof, occurring naturally in the body. Despite the widespread therapeutic use of biotherapy in neuroendocrine tumors for more than 20 years, data fulfilling the criteria of evidence-based medicine are rare. The interpretation of study results has to be done with some caveats. Data referring to the therapeutic efficacy of biotherapy only rarely give primary endpoints like mortality or the time to progression. Most studies include a variety of neuroendocrine tumors, the number of patients is low and most studies represent single-center experience. The results of different studies are difficult to compare, as dosage, treatment duration and a variety of different pretreatments were employed. There are only few prospective, randomized multicenter studies in therapy-naïve patients with documented progress before initiation of biotherapy. No placebo group was ever included in these studies. However, despite these drawbacks, there are indications of the benefit of biotherapy on symptoms of hormone hypersecretion, while on the other hand, definite data on the antiproliferative effectiveness and a positive effect on survival are still lacking.

Somatostatin

Endogenous somatostatin (SS) circulates in two biologic active forms, i.e. SS-14 and SS-28. SS binds with high affinity to five G-protein-coupled membrane receptors (sst1–5). Ligand binding inhibits adenylate cyclase activity, reduces calcium influx and negatively influences hormone synthesis and secretion. Physiologically SS regulates hormone secretion from the anterior pituitary, the pancreas, and the gastrointestinal tract. Hence its use in gastrointestinal hypersecretion syndromes has been proposed for the inhibition of autonomous hormone secretion. An inhibitory influence on proliferation may be due to the activation of phosphotyrosine phosphatases and the mitogen-activated protein kinase (MAPK) activity (Lamberts *et al.* 1991). The interference with gene transcription by inhibition of the transcription factor complex activator protein 1 (AP-1) may add to an antiproliferative effect. *In vitro*, high doses of somatostatin analogs (SSA) induce apoptosis in tumor cells, and this could translate into inhibition of tumor growth. Additional antiproliferative effects may be related to the antiangiogenic activity of SS either directly or via inhibition of growth factors like vascular endothelial growth factor, basic fibroblast growth factor and insulin-like growth factor 1 (Dasgupta 2004).

Most neuroendocrine tumors express a high density of somatostatin receptors (Table 23.18). The density of sst is higher in tumor tissue compared to the normal tissue. This allows for specific, tumor tissue-targeted, therapeutic effects and should reduce the number of side-effects i.e. suppression of physiologically secreted hormones. However, sst-subtype expression varies considerably between different tumor types and among tumors of the same type. Even within a given tumor, sst expression is not homogenously distributed (Hofland & Lamberts 2003).

Somatostatin analogs

SSAs were developed to circumvent the short half-life (<3 min) of native SS. The clinically used SSAs preferentially bind to sst2 and sst5 (Table 23.19). [^{111}In] DPTA-octreotide scintigraphy is used for *in vivo* visualization of sst as a diagnostic and staging tool in neuroendocrine tumors. However, results of somatostatin receptor scintigraphy are not closely correlated to the outcome of SSA therapy.

Table 23.18 Somatostatin receptor subtypes mRNA in neuroendocrine tumors.

Tumor	sst1	sst2	sst3	sst4	sst5
Gastrinoma	79%*	93%	36%	61%	93%
Insulinoma	76%	81%	38%	58%	57%
Non-functioning pancreatic tumor	58%	88%	42%	48%	50%
Carcinoid tumor of the gut	76%	80%	43%	68%	77%

* Indicates the percentage of positive tumors for each sst 1–5. mRNA expression may overestimate the number of receptors present, depending on the technique used (PR-PCR, Northern blot, in situ hybridization).

Table 23.19 Binding affinities of somatostatin analogs to somatostatin receptor (sst) subtypes.

sst	SS-14	Octreotide	Lanreotide	Pasireotide
sst1	0.93 ± 0.12	280 ± 80	180 ± 20	9.3 ± 0.1
sst2	0.15 ± 0.02	0.38 ± 0.08	0.54 ± 0.08	1.0 ± 0.1
sst3	0.56 ± 0.17	7.10 ± 1.40	14 ± 9	1.5 ± 0.3
sst4	1.40 ± 0.40	>1000	230 ± 40	>100
sst5	0.29 ± 0.04	6.3 ± 1.0	17 ± 5	0.16 ± 0.1

Binding affinities are given as mean ± SEM IC-50 (nmol/L).

Two different somatostatin analogs, octreotide and lanreotide, are clinically used. For these analogs serum half-life is increased considerably compared to native somatostatin (~2 h). The subcutaneous injectable octreotide has to be given three times daily, while long-acting preparations now available (lanreotide long-lasting [LA] and octreotide long-acting repeatable [LAR]) allow for one intramuscular injection every 2 (lanreotide) to 4 (octreotide LAR) weeks. In the case of lanreotide autogel, an interval up to 6 weeks between injections and the possibility of self-injection, may increase patient comfort and compliance (Table 23.20).

Recently pasireotide has been introduced, an SSA with high affinity for sst1–3 and sst5. It has been shown to be effective in patients who do not respond to the currently available SSA octreotide and lanreotide. However, its use is still restricted to clinical studies.

Octreotide and lanreotide both effectively inhibit autonomous hormone or neurotransmitter secretion by neuroendocrine gastrointestinal tumors. Unfortunately, tachyphylaxis develops after months or even years of treatment in virtually all patients. Tachyphylaxis may be due to desensitization, homologous agonist-induced downregulation in sst numbers on the cell surface, heterologous regulation of SS receptor expression or even SS receptor gene mutations (Hofland & Lamberts 2003). Initially, tachyphylaxis can be reversed by increasing the dose. However, eventually SSA therapy becomes ineffective in all patients.

Indications for SSA therapy

Hormone hypersecretion syndromes

SSAs are indicated in patients with symptoms due to excessive hormone release by a neuroendocrine tumor or its metastases. In patients with the carcinoid syndrome, octreotide LAR is equally potent in the control of flushing and diarrhea if compared to subcutaneous administration. SSAs are indicated in the therapy of the watery diarrhea syndrome, reducing the secretion of vasoactive intestinal peptide, and thus, diarrhea, dehydration and electrolyte imbalance. In patients with insulin hypersecretion, SSAs may reduce the insulin concentration in tumors expressing sufficient sst2 or sst5, i.e. mostly malignant insulinomas. However, as SSAs inhibit glucagon secretion as well, patients have to be observed closely at the beginning of therapy to prevent severe hypoglycemia due to the reduced glucagon-dependent counter-regulation. Thus, diazoxid is the preferred primary therapy for inhibition of insulin secretion, effectively

Table 23.20 Pharmacology of somatostatin analogs.

Drug	Mode of injection	Dosage	Clinical effect
Octreotide	Subcutaneous	3 × 100–300 g/day	Up to 6 h
Octreotide LAR	Intramuscular	10–30 mg/month	Up to 4 weeks
Lanreotide LA	Intramuscular	10–20 mg/14 day	Up to 2 weeks
Lanreotide Autogel	Subcutaneous	60–120 mg/month	Up to 4–6 weeks

reducing the risk of hypoglycemia. SSAs effectively inhibit glucagon secretion in patients with a glucagonoma syndrome; skin lesions improve and catabolism is reduced (Table 23.21).

Antisecretory effect on tumor markers

There is an excellent effect of SSAs on tumor markers (Table 23.22). SSAs induce remission and/or stabilization of tumor markers in approximately 70% of patients (Oberg 1994). The decline of tumor markers, like chromogranin A, is due to the antisecretory effect of SSAs and should not be interpreted as evidence for tumor volume reduction. Unfortunately, the duration of remission is short (median 8 to 12 months), with tachyphylaxis occurring early in the course of therapy.

Antiproliferative therapy

Clinical studies have, so far, given disappointing results with regard to tumor regression. Tumor shrinkage is demonstrated in less than 10% of the patients. However, stabilization of tumor growth, after CT-documented progression prior to treatment, occurs in up to 50% of the patients with neuroendocrine tumors of various locations. Stable disease is observed in 37–45% of the patients with documented tumor progression before SSA therapy (Tables 23.23 & 23.24). The median duration of stabilization was 18–26.5 months (Arnold *et al.* 1996). In a highly selected group of patients with progressive disease, 47% of the patients demonstrated at least stable disease when treated with a high dose of lanreotide (3 × 5 g/day). This was confirmed

Table 23.21 Effects of somatostatin analogs on hypersecretion syndromes

Syndrome	Symptom	Hormone/neurotransmitter	Tumor marker
Carcinoid syndrome	Flush > diarrhea	Serotonin	5-HIAA, CgA
Watery diarrhea syndrome	Diarrhea, dehydration, acidosis	VIP	VIP
Glucagonoma syndrome	Migratory necrolytic erythema	Glucagon	Glucagon
Insulin hypersecretion*	Fasting hypoglycemia	Insulin	Insulin
Zollinger–Ellison syndrome	Peptic ulceration, GERD†	Gastrin	Gastrin

* Benign insulinomas rarely express sufficient sst2 and 5 for SSAs to be effective. Thus, SSAs are only indicated as second-line therapy in malignant insulinomas (see text).

† Gastroesophageal reflux disease.

Table 23.22 Biochemical effect of somatostatin analogs.

n	CR	PR	SD	PD	Author
23	0	9	5	9	Aparicio *et al.* (2001)
39	2	11	15	11	Arnold *et al.* (1996)
13	4	6	3	9	di Bartolomeo *et al.* (1996)
14	0	9			Arnold *et al.* (1993b)
89	6/89 (7%)	35/89 (39%)	23/75 (31%)	29/75 (39%)	

CR, complete response; PR, partial response; SD, stable disease; PD; progressive disease.

Table 23.23 Anti-proliferative effect of somatostatin analogs in patients with progressive disesase.

SSA	Dosage	n	CR	PR	SD	PD	Author
Lanreotide	3000 μg/d	22	0	1	7	14	Faiss *et al.* (2003)
Lanreotide	30 mg/2w	35	0	1	20	14	Aparicio *et al.* (2001)
Octreotide	600–1500 μg/d	52	0	0	19	33	Arnold *et al.* (1996)
Octreotide	1500–3000 μg/d	58	0	2	27	29	di Bartolomeo *et al.* (1996)
Octreotide	600 μg/d	10	0	0	5	5	Arnold *et al.* (1993a)
Lanreotide	15000 μg/d	24	1	1	11	11	Faiss *et al.* (2003)
		201	1 (0.5%)	5 (3%)	89 (44%)	106 (53%)	

CR, complete remission; PR, partial remission; SD, stable disease; PD, progressive disease.

Table 23.24 Anti-proliferative effect of somatostatin analogs in patients without progressive disease.

SSA	Dosage	N	CR	PR	SD	PD	Author
Lanreotide	30 mg/14d	31	–	2 (7%)	25 (81%)	4 (13%)	Wymenga *et al.* (1999)
Lanreotide	30 mg/14d	39	–	4 (10%)	19 (49%)	16 (41%)	Ducreux *et al.* (2000)
Lanreotide	750–12,000 μg/d	19	–	1 (5%)	12 (63%)	6 (32%)	Eriksson *et al.* (1997)
Lanreotide	30 mg/10d	18	–	–	14 (78%)	4 (22%)	Tomassetti *et al.* (1998)
Octreotide	20 mg/28d	16	–	–	14 (88%)	2 (12%)	Tomassetti *et al.* (2000)
Octreotide	20 mg/28d	15	–	1 (7%)	6 (40%)	8 (53%)	Ricci *et al.* (2000)
Octreotide/lanreotide	6000–9000 μg/day	13	–	4 (31%)	1 (8%)	8 (61%)	Anthony *et al.* (1993)
		183	0 (0%)	12 (8%)	91 (60%)	48 (32%)	

CR, complete remission; PR, partial remission; SD, stable disease; PD, progressive disease.

recently in 75% of the patients with advanced midgut carcinoids, with stabilization for 6–24 months. In neuroendocrine tumors of the small intestine, the therapeutic effect of high-dose treatment may be slightly better (stable disease in eight out of ten patients) than with conventional dosage.

Predictors of the clinical outcome of SSA therapy have also been analyzed. A pancreatic primary, with no previous surgical therapy and distant, extrahepatic metastases, indicates a poor response to treatment in multivariate analysis, while age, size of the primary and Ki-67 did not influence the response rate to SSA therapy. Patients achieving a positive response (stabilization) after 6 months of treatment maintain it throughout long-term follow-up and live longer than patients unresponsive to therapy.

Dosage

Therapy with octreotide is usually started with a dose of 300 μg/day s.c. or octreotide LAR 10 mg/4 weeks i.m. or lanreotide LA 30 mg/7–10 days i.m. The dose is then adjusted according to the individual clinical and biochemical response. Octreotide and lanreotide are equally effective in controlling clinical symptoms. After the start of the long-acting formulations, subcutaneous octreotide has to be added for up to 2 months, until steady-state concentrations are achieved. In a rare patient, octreotide s.c. has to be supplemented in addition to the long-acting formulations, due to occasional breakthrough of flush and diarrhea. Subcutaneous octreotide is used in the event of a carcinoid crisis or for prevention of a carcinoid crisis during surgical procedures.

Side-effects of somatostatin analogs

Frequently occurring side-effects like abdominal discomfort, bloating, and steatorrhea, due to the inhibition of pancreatic enzymes, are mostly mild and subside spontaneously within the first weeks of therapy. Persistent steatorrhea can be treated with supplementation of pancreatic enzymes. Cholestasis with subsequent cholecystolithiasis does occur in up to 60% of the patients, due to inhibition of cholecystokinin and production of a lithogenic bile. Prophylactic therapy with chenodeoxycholic acid and ursodeoxycholic acid may be able to prevent the occurrence of gallstone disease in patients on long-term SSA therapy. Due to steatorrhea, malabsorption with reduction of serum vitamin D concentration and subsequently reduced calcium absorption has been observed. In patients on long-term therapy, the vitamin B12 concentration should be monitored. Serum vitamin B12 concentration may decline, possibly due to a direct inhibition of the intrinsic factor secretion at the parietal cell (Plockinger *et al.* 1998). Rarely, a moderate effluvium occurs and is usually reversible when the drug is stopped (Table 23.25).

Table 23.25 Side-effects of somatostatin analogs.

Frequent	Pain and swelling at injection site Loss of appetite, nausea, vomiting Abdominal pain , bloating Diarrhea Gallbladder sludge
Rare	Gallstones Vitamin b12 deficiency Alopecia, allergic skin reaction Bradycardia, pancreatitis
Very rare	Reversible acute hepatitis Reduced glucose tolerance, diabetes mellitus
Laboratory values	Bilirubin, γ-GT increased

In summary, SSAs effectively control symptoms of hypersecretion in patients with neuroendocrine tumors of the gastrointestinal tract. Despite the minor effects on tumor volume reduction observed so far, an antiproliferative effect does occur, with stabilization of the disease for up to 25 months. A possible positive effect on tumor volume regression with high-dose treatment has still to be demonstrated. Survival may be prolonged in those patients responding positively to SSA therapy. In addition, SSAs significantly increase the quality of life in patients with symptoms related to hormone secretion, while side-effects of SSA therapy are limited.

Interferon

Interferon-α 2a, or 2b (IFN) production is a physiologic response to substances such as microbes, tumor cells and antigens. The anti-tumor action of IFN is thought to be due to several, complementary mechanisms. Interferons react with specific cell-surface receptors to activate a cytoplasmatic signal transduction cascade, which, ultimately, induces the transcription of multiple interferon-inducible genes (ISG). ISG probably act as tumor suppressor genes. IFN- α acts on 2′ 5′-A-synthetase and p-68 kinase. Both enzymes induce the degradation of peptide hormone and growth factor mRNA, inhibiting protein synthesis. The induction of 2′ 5′-A-synthetase correlates with clinical efficacy. The antiproliferative effect of IFN is probably due to a blockade of the cell cycle in the transition of G0→G1 (Oberg 1992). This is due to the inhibition of cyclin B expression, resulting in reduced CDC 2 kinase activity and thus inhibition of the cell cycle. Furthermore, induction of apoptosis, as well as increased expression of class I antigens on the tumor cell surface (which marks the cell as a target for cytotoxic T-lymphocytes) may add to the antiproliferative effects. In addition, an antiangiogenic effect has been suggested. An interesting aspect is the observation of an increase in connective tissue paralleled by a reduction in tumor tissue during interferon therapy. Similar changes have been observed in osteosarcoma transplanted to nude mice. This intratumor fibrosis occurs without any change in tumor size (Oberg 1992).

IFN-α has been widely used for the treatment of solid tumors. In neuroendocrine tumors the indications for interferon are comparable to those of SSAs, with carcinoid crisis being the exception. However, there are only few data on the effect of interferon therapy in patients with pancreatic neuroendocrine tumors. Most investigations used recombinant interferon-α 2a or 2b. Human leukocyte interferon can be substituted whenever antibodies develop to recombinant interferon-α 2a.

Indications for interferon-α therapy

Hormone hypersecretion syndromes

Symptomatic remission is seen in 30–70% of patients with carcinoid syndrome, with a better effect of interferon therapy on flushing compared to diarrhea. While the control of symptoms of hypersecretion by interferon is comparable to SSA, its onset of response is delayed.

Antisecretory effects on tumor markers

In neuroendocrine tumors of the gut, a biochemical response is observed in 50% of the patients. Tumor marker remission or stable 5-HIAA concentration occured in 36% and 35% of patients, respectively. Analyzing results of 10 clinical studies with mixed tumor populations (n = 255), a partial remission or stabilization of tumor markers occurs in 44% and 30% of the patients, respectively. These data are comparable to published results of a recent meta-analysis, indicating overall median response rates of biochemical markers in up to 44% of patients (Shah & Caplin 2005).

Antiproliferative therapy

Tumor shrinkage occurs in 10% of patients, whereas stable disease is observed in up to 70%. Progressive disease was seen in 23% of patients. Table 23.26 gives data on a large cohort of patients with evaluable results on tumor mass (n = 274) treated with interferon in 10 studies. In the early studies, the treatment period was too short to evaluate the time to progression. The median survival from the start of therapy for patients with neuroendocrine tumors of the gut was >80 months. IFN-α is preferentially used in patients with metastasizing disease, primarily for control of tumor progression and only secondarily for control of hypersecretion syndromes.

Table 23.26 Antiproliferative effects of interferon therapy.

Interferon	Evaluable patients	CR	PR	SD	PD	Author
IFN	14	–	–	9	5	Doberauer *et al.* (1991)
IFNα	20	–	–	15	5	Tiensuu Janson *et al.* (1992)
IFNα	15	–	3	NI	NI	Dirix *et al.* (1996)
rIFNα	20	–	4	NI	NI	Moertel *et al.* (1989)
rIFNα	12	–	2	9	1	Janson *et al.* (1992)
rIFNα2b	17	–	–	16	NI	Oberg and Eriksson (1989)
rIFNα2b	14	–	–	10	NI	Smith *et al.* (1987)
rIFNα2b	26	–	4	17	NI	Schober *et al.* (1992)
rIFNα2b	25	–	–	16	9	Jacobsen *et al.* (1995)
hIFN/rIFNα	111	–	16	74	21	Oberg & Eriksson (1991)
Total	274		29/274	166/239	41/182	
Percentage			11%	70%	23%	

CR, complete remission; PR, partial remission; SD, stable disease; PD, progressive disease.

Again, the data should be interpreted with caution. Progressive disease, as a prerequisite for study inclusion, was necessary only in a small number of these investigations. Thus, information on spontaneous tumor growth is lacking in most of these studies. Patients with different pretreatment modalities consisting of surgical interventions, embolization therapy and/or chemotherapy have been included. In addition, the dose regimen, the type of IFN- α (rIFN- α 2α, rIFN- α2b, human leukocyte IFN) and treatment time differed considerably between the studies. In these slow-growing tumors, changes might only be obvious after long treatment periods (up to 30 months). No randomized, prospective multicenter studies have been performed and most trials used secondary endpoints like tumor shrinkage or reduction of biochemical markers for evaluation of therapeutic efficacy. Endpoint analysis, i.e. overall survival or time to progression, is given in about one-third of the trials. Overall, results of these investigations delineate a consistent pattern of efficacy for interferon on symptom control.

Dosage

The most effective dose in the treatment of neuroendocrine tumors is 3–10 million IU per day, 3 to 7 days per week. However, the dose tolerated for long-term therapy has to be adjusted individually. Titrating the dose of IFN-α, aiming at a reduction of the leukocyte count to 3×10^9/L reduces the number of side-effects (Oberg 1996). A dose above 12 Mill IU does not result in substantial benefit, but increases toxicity considerably. Pegylated interferon, the long-acting formulation of interferon is available, but not licensed for therapy of neuroendocrine tumors.

Side-effects of interferon therapy

In almost all patients (97%) a 'flu-like' syndrome occurs in the first 5 days. Paracetamol (500–1000 mg) is able to relieve these symptoms. Anorexia, weight loss (59%), and fatigue (51%) may adversely affect well-being. Bone marrow toxicity like anemia, leukocytopenia ($<2.0 \times 10^9$/L) and thrombocytopenia ($<100 \times 10^9$/L) have been observed in 31%, 7% and 18% of patients, respectively, as well as hepatotoxicity (31%). These effects are dose dependent. Autoimmune reactions occur in 20% of patients (Oberg 1994). In a detailed report on autoimmune disorders observed during therapy with INF-α in patients with neuroendocrine tumors of midgut origin, 19% of patients (n = 135) developed autoimmune disorders (3 hyperthyroidism, 10 hypothyroidism, 5 thyroiditis, 4 pernicious anemia and 3 systemic lupus erythematosus) (Table 23.27).

Rare side-effects like depression, mental disturbances and visual impairment may occur. Interferon-neutralizing antibodies can be observed in up to 38% of patients (Oberg 1994). Neutralizing antibodies most frequently occur with recombinant INF-α2a. As neutralizing antibodies may be able to negatively influence the anti-tumor response, measurement of antibodies should be included in the therapeutic regimen. A change from recombinant IFN- α to human leukocyte IFN may bring back anti-tumor efficacy. IFN- α should not be given to patients with pre-existing moderate to severe failure of the liver, kidney or heart. (Table 23.28)

In summary, interferon therapy is primarily given in patients with metastasized neuroendocrine tumors of the gut. The

Table 23.28 Contraindications for interferon.

Heart failure, arrhythmia, myocardial infarction
Epilepsy
Psychiatric disease
Autoimmune disease
Thyroid dysfunction (hyper- or hypothyroidism) insufficiently treated

Table 23.27 Side-effects of interferon.

Side-effects	Occurrence	Therapy
Flu-like symptoms	Frequent	Paracetamol
Myelosuppression	Frequent	Control, dose reduction
Allergic reactions	Occasional	Antiallergic therapy or end of therapy
Hypotension	Rare	Fluids
Weight loss	Rare	End of therapy
Depression, psychiatric disease	Rare	End of therapy
Autoimmune disease: autoimmune thyreoiditis, pneumonitis, diabetes mellitus, systemic lupus erythematodes (sLE), idiopathic thrombocytopenic purpura (ITP)	Rare to very rare	Control, treatment of thyroid dysfunction or diabetes, end of therapy with pneumonitis, sLE, ITP
Visual disturbances	Rare	Control before and during therapy
Transaminases	Very rare	Control, eventually end of therapy
Nephrotic syndrome, kidney failure	Very rare	Control, eventually end of therapy
Hypertriglyceridemia	Very rare	Therapy of hypertriglyeridemia

effect on symptoms of hormone hypersecretion is comparable to SSAs, while the onset of response is delayed compared to SSA. Interferon treatment will not cure the disease; however, it may be able to control tumor growth over extended periods, the smaller the tumor burden, the more so. Thus, interferon should be given rather early in the course of the disease. Side-effects of interferon therapy are more pronounced than with SSA. Individualized doses allow a reasonable quality of life.

Combination therapy: somatostatin analog plus interferon-α

The combination of SSAs and IFN- α was used in an effort to enhance the antiproliferative effect of interferon therapy, to add the positive effect of SSA on hypersecretion syndromes and to reduce the dose of IFN- α and thus the number of IFN-related side-effects.

An early study showed no additional antiproliferative effect with combination therapy. More recent studies demonstrated an increased number of patients with stable disease for tumor volume (57–75%), remission or stabilization of biochemical parameters (77–92%). However, a recent, well-designed prospective multicenter study showed no advantage of combination therapy, neither on biochemical nor antiproliferative results, while the number of side-effects increased (Faiss *et al.* 2003). Thus, if biotherapy with SSA or IFN fails, due to progression of the disease or to tachyphylaxis (SSA), or side-effects are intolerable with IFN-α, the combination of both drugs may be useful in individual patients. The information provided by the recent study on combination therapy, however, does not recommend it is a standard treatment regimen.

In summary, biotherapy is preferentially indicated for the treatment of hormone hypersecretion syndromes in patients with neuroendocrine tumors. Excellent symptomatic relief can be achieved by SSA, IFN- α and other medical treatment strategies. Antiproliferative effects are not convincing, but stabilization of the disease does occur in up to 50% of patients with either SSA or interferon therapy. A combined treatment does not add substantial effect and is not recommended. Side-effects of SSA therapy are minor and quality of life is good with somatostatin analog therapy, while with interferon the drug has to be individually titrated to balance treatment efficacy and side-effects.

Systemic chemotherapy

Chemotherapy is a palliative option in metastasizing neuroendocrine carcinomas. Streptozotocin (STZ), fluorouracil (5-FU), doxorubicin, dacarbazin (DTIC), etoposide and cisplatin have been used. As the response rate to monotherapy has been low, most chemotherapeutic regimens for neuroendocrine tumors rely on combination therapy.

Streptozotocin

STZ is an alkylating nitrosurea compound. It has a glucose moiety, which is supposed to be responsible for the low bone marrow toxicity of the drug, while the nitrosurea component is the actual toxic part. Streptozotocin enters the pancreatic β-cell via the GLUT2 glucose transporter. However, the molecular mechanism of cytotoxicity is still unknown. STZ is effective in the treatment of neuroendocrine tumors of the pancreas. STZ is usually administered intravenously at a dose of 500 mg/m^2/day × 5 days every 6 weeks. It is used in combination with either 5-FU (400 mg/m^2/day × 5 days every 5 weeks) or doxorubicin (50 mg/m^2/day on day 1 and day 22). STZ induces nausea and vomiting in up to 90% of patients, with grade 3 to 4 toxicity in 10%, respectively. Odensatron or other 5HT3-receptor antagonists alleviate these symptoms. STZ is potentially nephrotoxic. Glomerular and tubular dysfunction occur in 20–75% of patients. Nephrotoxicity increases with the duration of drug administration. When protein excretion increases to above 500 mg/24 h or an increase of creatinine above 2 mg/dL occurs, therapy should be interrupted until kidney function falls below this limit. Bone marrow toxicity is low (leukocytopenia or thrombocytopenia in 9% of patients), thus combinations with 5-FU or doxorubicin are possible. Rare side-effects are cardiac arrhythmias, CNS toxicity with mental depression, skin necrosis and diarrhea.

5-Fluorouracil

5-Fluorouracil (5-FU) is a prodrug and needs to be metabolized for antineoplastic action. Its metabolites inhibit thymidilate synthetase, thus blocking DNA synthesis. In addition RNA synthesis is reduced. 5-FU preferentially inhibits proliferating cells, resulting in bone marrow toxicity and gastrointestinal side-effects. Patients with coronary heart disease or cardiomyopathy are at risk for cardiotoxic side-effects. During therapy with 5-FU, the determination of 5-hydroxyindolacetic acid may give false positive results. 5-FU is given as a 4-hour infusion for 5 consecutive days in combination with STZ.

Doxorubicin

Doxorubicin is supposed to interact with DNA base pairs and this may result in steric inhibition of DNA synthesis. Additional antineoplastic actions are possibly due to the formation of free radicals, an effect on tumor cell membranes and the inhibition of topoisomerase II activity. Myelosuppression is a dose-limiting side-effect. Immediate, reversible or irreversible cardiotoxicities (related to the cumulative dose) have been observed. Elderly patients and those with hypertension are at risk. Nausea and vomiting are seen in up to 80% of patients, but antiemetic prophylaxis is effective.

Dacarbazin

Dacarbazin has cytostatic effects and inhibits the cell cycle. Additional effects are a reduction of the DNA synthesis, as well as alkylating effects. Therapy with dacarbazin can induce a rare veno-occlusive syndrome. However, in most patients toxicity is low and the side-effects experienced are mostly nausea and vomiting. Dacarbazin is given as monotherapy (650 mg/m^2 per infusion over 60–90 min).

Cisplatin

Cisplatin is an alkylating agent and thus interferes with DNA replication. Nausea and vomiting occur in up to 75% of patients, myelosuppression is usually mild to moderate, with high-dose therapy (onset after 10 days, nadir between 14 and 23 days and recovery between 21 to 39 days). Nephrotoxicity (acute or chronic renal failure) is possible and the drug should be withdrawn when creatinine is above 1.5 mg/100 mL. A 25% or 50% dose reduction is recommended for creatinine clearance of 46–60 mL/min or 31–45 mL/min, respectively. Adequate hydration prior to cisplatin administration is recommended and serum electrolytes (magnesium included), should be monitored during therapy. Peripheral neuropathy is common and is dose and duration dependent.

Etoposide

Etoposide, a podophyllotoxin derivative, is used in combination with cisplatin for poorly differentiated NET. Cytotoxicity is due to breaks of DNA strands. Etoposide interacts with topisomerase II. The inhibition of the cell cycle during S and G2 phase is cytostatic. Doses less than 400 mg/day can be given as a single dose orally, while higher doses should be divided. In patients with concomitant severe liver and kidney dysfunction dose adjustments are recommended. Side-effects like nausea, vomiting and diarrhea, myelosuppression and alopecia are common. Amenorrhea and ovarian failure occur in up to 38% of patients.

In neuroendocrine tumors of the pancreas overall response rates of 17%, 18–26% and 21% were obtained with monotherapy using STZ, 5-FU and doxorubicin, respectively. Combination therapy for well-differentiated, neuroendocrine tumors of the pancreas, on the other hand, resulted in a median response of 36% (Table 23.29). Median remission lasted 17 months, while median overall survival was almost 2 years (Table 23.29). The combination of STZ and 5-FU (n = 147) resulted in an objective response in 21% of patients, with a median survival time from the start of therapy of less than 8 months. A recent randomized prospective trial (n = 163) failed to confirm the suggested superiority of STZ and doxorubicin over STZ and 5-FU (Sun *et al.* 2005). Objective remission was 16% for both arms, progression-free survival was 4.5 and 5.3 months, respectively. Overall survival was higher with STZ/5FU (24.3 vs 15.7 months, $p < 0.03$, respectively), arguing for the less toxic approach with STZ/5-FU. Other combination schemes like dacarbacin, 5-FU and leucoverin (response rate 27%), dacarbacin, 5-FU and epirubicin (response rate 30%), lomustine and 5-FU (response rate 21%) were comparable. In a recent trial, 84 patients with pancreatic neuroendocrine tumors were treated with STZ, 5-FU and doxorubicin (Kouvaraki *et al.* 2004). This triple combination achieved a response rate of 39% and a median progression free survival of 9.3 months, confirming earlier data in small investigations (Rivera & Ajani 1998; von Schrenck *et al.* 1988).

In contrast, chemotherapy is less effective in neuroendocrine tumors of the gut. An overview over 10 trials (1979–2005) indicates a median response rate of 25% and a median survival of 11 months (Table 23.30). Thus, in well-differentiated neuroendocrine tumors of the gut, chemotherapy is not a preferred option.

More aggressive treatment schemes such as etoposide and cisplatin were ineffective in patients with well-differentiated neuroendocrine tumors. In contrast, in 18 patients with

Table 23.29 Chemotherapy in well-differentiated neuroendocrine tumors of the small bowel.

	n	Response (%)	Median survival	Author
Dox	81	21	11	Engstrom *et al.* (1984)
STZ, 5-FU	80	22	15	Engstrom *et al.* (1984)
STZ, 5-FU	43	33	n.i.	Moertel & Hanley (1979)
STZ, Dox	33	40	11	Frame *et al.* (1988)
STZ, Dox	3	30	5	Pavel *et al.* (2005)
STZ, cyclophosphamide	47	26	n.i.	Moertel & Hanley (1979)
5FU, Dox, DTIC	20	10	5	Di Bartolomeo *et al.* (1995)
5FU, CCNU	16	25	16	Kaltsas *et al.* (2002)
MTX, cyclophosphamide	16	0	n.i.	Moertel *et al.* (1984)
VP16, cisplatin	13	0	n.i.	Moertel *et al.* (1991)
	35	21		

Dox, doxorubicin; n.i., not indicated; STZ, streptoxotocin; 5-FU, 5-fluorouracil; DTIC, dacarbacin; CCNU, lamustine; MTX, methotrexate; VP16, etoposide.

Table 23.30 Results of chemotherapy in neuroendocrine tumors.

Chemotherapy	n	Response (%)	PFS (months)	Median survival	Author
STZ	42	36	17	17	Moertel *et al.* (1980)
DTIC	42	33		19.3	Ramanathan *et al.* (2001)
STZ, 5-FU	42	63	17	26	Moertel *et al.* (1980)
STZ Dox	25	36	22		Eriksson *et al.* (1990)
STZ Dox	16	6	18		Cheng & Saltz (1999)
STZ Dox	3	30		18	Pavel *et al.* (2005)
STZ Dox	36	69	18	26	Moertel *et al.* (1992)
STZ 5-FU	33	45	14	18	Moertel *et al.* (1992)
CLZ 5-FU	44	36	11		Bukowski *et al.* (1992)
STZ 5-FU Dox	10	40		26	von Schrenck *et al.* (1988)
STZ 5-FU Dox	12	55	15	21	Rivera & Ajani (1998)
STZ 5-FU Dox	84	39	18	37	Kouvaraki *et al.* (2004)
5-FU Epi DTIC	15	27	10		Bajetta *et al.* (1998)
5-FU Epi DTIC	32	25	21	38	Bajetta *et al.* (2002)
All	436	39	16.5	25	

STZ, streptozotocin; DTIC, dacarbacin; 5-FU, 5-fluorouracil; CLZ, chlorozotocin; Dox, doxorubicin; Epi, epirubicin.

undifferentiated, anaplastic, neuroendocrine tumors (5 tumors were of midgut/hindgut origin) 67% objective responses were obtained (Moertel *et al.* 1991) with a median duration of remission of less than 8 months.

In interpreting these data it has to be kept in mind that most studies comprise only a small number of patients, and the patients are usually heterogeneous groups with respect to the localization of the tumor, total tumor burden, and pretreatment schemes.

Side-effects of systemic chemotherapy

Frequently occurring side-effects have already been discussed with the substances used. Cardiac arrhythmias, CNS toxicity with mental depression, skin necrosis and diarrhea are rare. The half-life of doxorubicin is prolonged when given in combination with STZ. The doxorubicin dose has therefore to be reduced compared with single-agent treatment. Doxorubicin may aggravate coexistent heart disease not evident at the beginning of therapy.

In summary, combination therapy with STZ, 5-FU, with the possible addition of doxorubicin, are now standard treatment schedules in patients with well-differentiated neuroendocrine tumors of the pancreas. For neuroendocrine tumors of the gut, there is still no convincing evidence for improved survival with chemotherapy and thus other palliative options should be discussed. However, in patients with anaplastic neuroendocrine carcinomas the combination of etoposide and cisplatin yielded a response rate of 67%, making this regimen a rewarding tool in undifferentiated neuroendocrine tumors of the intestine.

Conclusions

In neuroendocrine gastrointestinal tumors, symptomatic biotherapy for functioning tumors is well established, while antiproliferative indications still await the confirmation by prospective, randomized, multicenter trials. Chemotherapy is a well-established option for well-differentiated neuroendocrine carcinomas of the pancreas, while chemotherapeutic regimens have been ineffective in well-differentiated tumors of the small bowel. Poorly differentiated tumors can be treated with cisplatin and etoposide irrespective of the location of the primary. However, new agents like multiligand SSAs, antiangiogenetic substances and multikinase inhibitors may offer new treatment options for these patients.

References

Anthony L, Johnson D, Hande K *et al.* (1993) Somatostatin analogue phase I trials in neuroendocrine neoplasms. *Acta Oncol* 32: 217–23.

Aparicio T, Ducreux M, Baudin E *et al.* (2001) Antitumour activity of somatostatin analogues in progressive metastatic neuroendocrine tumours. *Eur J Cancer* 37: 1014–9.

Arnold R, Benning R, Neuhaus C, Rolwage M, Trautmann ME. (1993a) Gastroenteropancreatic endocrine tumours: effect of sandostatin on tumour growth. The German Sandostatin Study Group. *Digestion* 54 (Suppl 1): 72–5.

Arnold R, Neuhaus C, Benning R *et al.* (1993b) Somatostatin analog sandostatin and inhibition of tumor growth in patients with metastatic endocrine gastroenteropancreatic tumors. *World J Surg* 17: 511–19.

Arnold R, Trautmann ME, Creutzfeldt W *et al.* (1996) Somatostatin analogue octreotide and inhibition of tumour growth in metastatic endocrine gastroenteropancreatic tumours. *Gut* 38: 430–8.

Bajetta E, Rimassa L, Carnaghi C *et al.* (1998) 5-Fluorouracil, dacarbazine, and epirubicin in the treatment of patients with neuroendocrine tumors. *Cancer* 83: 372–8.

Bajetta E, Ferrari L, Procopio G *et al.* (2002) Efficacy of a chemotherapy combination for the treatment of metastatic neuroendocrine tumours. *Ann Oncol* 13: 614–21.

Bukowski RM, Tangen C, Lee R *et al.* (1992) Phase II trial of chlorozotocin and fluorouracil in islet cell carcinoma: a Southwest Oncology Group study. *J Clin Oncol* 10: 1914–8.

Cheng PN, Saltz LB. (1999) Failure to confirm major objective antitumor activity for streptozocin and doxorubicin in the treatment of patients with advanced islet cell carcinoma. *Cancer* 86: 944–8.

Dasgupta P. (2004) Somatostatin analogues: multiple roles in cellular proliferation, neoplasia, and angiogenesis. *Pharmacol Ther* 102: 61–85.

Di Bartolomeo M, Bajetta E, Bochicchio AM *et al.* (1995) A phase II trial of dacarbazine, fluorouracil and epirubicin in patients with neuroendocrine tumours. A study by the Italian Trials in Medical Oncology (ITMO) Group. *Ann Oncol* 6: 77–9.

Di Bartolomeo M, Bajetta E, Buzzoni R *et al.* (1996) Clinical efficacy of octreotide in the treatment of metastatic neuroendocrine tumors. A study by the Italian Trials in Medical Oncology Group. *Cancer* 77: 402–8.

Dirix LY, Vermeulen PB, Fierens H, De Schepper B, Corthouts B, Van Oosterom AT. (1996) Long-term results of continuous treatment with recombinant interferon-alpha in patients with metastatic carcinoid tumors–an antiangiogenic effect? *Anticancer Drugs* 7: 175–81.

Doberauer C, Mengelkoch B, Kloke O, Wandl U, Niederle N. (1991) Treatment of metastatic carcinoid tumors and the carcinoid syndrome with recombinant interferon alpha. *Acta Oncol* 30: 603–5.

Ducreux M, Ruszniewski P, Chayvialle JA *et al.* (2000) The antitumoral effect of the long-acting somatostatin analog lanreotide in neuroendocrine tumors. *Am J Gastroenterol* 95: 3276–81.

Engstrom PF, Lavin PT, Moertel CG, Folsch E, Douglass HO Jr. (1984) Streptozocin plus fluorouracil versus doxorubicin therapy for metastatic carcinoid tumor. *J Clin Oncol* 2: 1255–9.

Eriksson B, Skogseid B, Lundqvist G, Wide L, Wilander E, Oberg K. (1990) Medical treatment and long-term survival in a prospective study of 84 patients with endocrine pancreatic tumors. *Cancer* 65: 1883–90.

Eriksson B, Renstrup J, Imam H, Oberg K. (1997) High-dose treatment with lanreotide of patients with advanced neuroendocrine gastrointestinal tumors: clinical and biological effects. *Ann Oncol* 8: 1041–4.

Faiss S, Pape UF, Bohmig M *et al.* (2003) Prospective, randomized, multicenter trial on the antiproliferative effect of lanreotide, interferon alfa, and their combination for therapy of metastatic neuroendocrine gastroenteropancreatic tumors—the International Lanreotide and Interferon Alfa Study Group. *J Clin Oncol* 21: 2689–96.

Frame J, Kelsen D, Kemeny N *et al.* (1988) A phase II trial of streptozotocin and adriamycin in advanced APUD tumors. *Am J Clin Oncol* 11: 490–5.

Hofland LJ, Lamberts SW. (2003) The pathophysiological consequences of somatostatin receptor internalization and resistance. *Endocr Rev* 24: 28–47.

Jacobsen MB, Hanssen LE, Kolmannskog F, Schrumpf E, Vatn MH, Bergan A. (1995) Interferon-alpha 2b, with or without prior hepatic artery embolization: clinical response and survival in mid-gut carcinoid patients. The Norwegian carcinoid study. *Scand J Gastroenterol* 30: 789–96.

Janson ET, Ronnblom L, Ahlstrom H *et al.* (1992) Treatment with alpha-interferon versus alpha-interferon in combination with streptozocin and doxorubicin in patients with malignant carcinoid tumors: a randomized trial. *Ann Oncol* 3: 635–8.

Kaltsas GA, Mukherjee JJ, Isidori A *et al.* (2002) Treatment of advanced neuroendocrine tumours using combination chemotherapy with lomustine and 5-fluorouracil. *Clin Endocrinol (Oxf)* 57: 169–83.

Kouvaraki MA, Ajani JA, Hoff P *et al.* (2004) Fluorouracil, doxorubicin, and streptozocin in the treatment of patients with locally advanced and metastatic pancreatic endocrine carcinomas. *J Clin Oncol* 22: 4762–71.

Lamberts SW, Krenning EP, Reubi JC. (1991) The role of somatostatin and its analogs in the diagnosis and treatment of tumors. *Endocr Rev* 12: 450–82.

Moertel CG, Hanley JA. (1979) Combination chemotherapy trials in metastatic carcinoid tumor and the malignant carcinoid syndrome. *Cancer Clin Trials* 2: 327–34.

Moertel CG, Hanley JA, Johnson LA. (1980) Streptozocin alone compared with streptozocin plus fluorouracil in the treatment of advanced islet-cell carcinoma. *N Engl J Med* 303: 1189–94.

Moertel CG, O'Connell MJ, Reitemeier RJ, Rubin J. (1984) Evaluation of combined cyclophosphamide and methotrexate therapy in the treatment of metastatic carcinoid tumor and the malignant carcinoid syndrome. *Cancer Treat Rep* 68: 665–7.

Moertel CG, Rubin J, Kvols LK. (1989) Therapy of metastatic carcinoid tumor and the malignant carcinoid syndrome with recombinant leukocyte A interferon. *J Clin Oncol* 7: 865–8.

Moertel CG, Kvols LK, O'Connell MJ, Rubin J. (1991) Treatment of neuroendocrine carcinomas with combined etoposide and cisplatin. Evidence of major therapeutic activity in the anaplastic variants of these neoplasms. *Cancer* 68: 227–32.

Moertel CG, Lefkopoulo M, Lipsitz S, Hahn RG, Klaassen D. (1992) Streptozocin-doxorubicin, streptozocin-fluorouracil or chlorozotocin in the treatment of advanced islet-cell carcinoma. *N Engl J Med* 326: 519–23.

Oberg K. (1992) The action of interferon alpha on human carcinoid tumours. *Semin Cancer Biol* 3: 35–41.

Oberg K. (1994) Endocrine tumors of the gastrointestinal tract: systemic treatment. *Anticancer Drugs* 5: 503–19.

Oberg K. (1996) Neuroendocrine gastrointestinal tumours. *Ann Oncol* 7: 453–63.

Oberg K, Eriksson B. (1989) Medical treatment of neuroendocrine gut and pancreatic tumors. *Acta Oncol* 28: 425–31.

Oberg K, Eriksson B. (1991) The role of interferons in the management of carcinoid tumours. *Br J Haematol* 79 (Suppl 1): 74–7.

Pavel ME, Baum U, Hahn EG, Hensen J. (2005) Doxorubicin and streptozotocin after failed biotherapy of neuroendocrine tumors. *Int J Gastrointest Cancer* 35: 179–85.

Plockinger U, Perez-Canto A, Emde C, Liehr RM, Hopfenmuller W, Quabbe HJ. (1998) Effect of the somatostatin analog octreotide on gastric mucosal function and histology during 3 months of preoperative treatment in patients with acromegaly. *Eur J Endocrinol* 139: 387–94.

Ramanathan RK, Cnaan A, Hahn RG, Carbone PP, Haller DG. (2001) Phase II trial of dacarbazine (DTIC) in advanced pancreatic islet cell carcinoma. Study of the Eastern Cooperative Oncology Group-E6282. *Ann Oncol* 12: 1139–43.

Ricci S, Antonuzzo A, Galli L *et al.* (2000) Long-acting depot lanreotide in the treatment of patients with advanced neuroendocrine tumors. *Am J Clin Oncol* 23: 412–5.

Rivera E, Ajani JA. (1998) Doxorubicin, streptozocin, and 5-fluorouracil chemotherapy for patients with metastatic islet-cell carcinoma. *Am J Clin Oncol* 21: 36–8.

Schober C, Schmoll E, Schmoll HJ *et al.* (1992) Antitumour effect and symptomatic control with interferon alpha 2b in patients with endocrine active tumours. *Eur J Cancer* 28A: 1664–6.

Shah T, Caplin M. (2005) Endocrine tumours of the gastrointestinal tract. Biotherapy for metastatic endocrine tumours. *Best Pract Res Clin Gastroenterol* 19: 617–36.

Smith DB, Scarffe JH, Wagstaff J, Johnston RJ. (1987) Phase II trial of rDNA alfa 2b interferon in patients with malignant carcinoid tumor. *Cancer Treat Rep* 71: 1265–6.

Sun W, Lipsitz S, Catalano P, Mailliard JA, Haller DG. (2005) Phase II/III study of doxorubicin with fluorouracil compared with streptozocin with fluorouracil or dacarbazine in the treatment of advanced carcinoid tumors: Eastern Cooperative Oncology Group Study E1281. *J Clin Oncol* 23: 4897–904.

Tiensuu Janson EM, Ahlstrom H, Andersson T, Oberg KE. (1992) Octreotide and interferon alfa: a new combination for the treatment of malignant carcinoid tumours. *Eur J Cancer* 28A: 1647–50.

Tomassetti P, Migliori M, Gullo L. (1998) Slow-release lanreotide treatment in endocrine gastrointestinal tumors. *Am J Gastroenterol* 93: 1468–71.

Tomassetti P, Migliori M, Corinaldesi R, Gullo L. (2000) Treatment of gastroenteropancreatic neuroendocrine tumours with octreotide LAR. *Aliment Pharmacol Ther* 14: 557–60.

Von Schrenck T, Howard JM, Doppman JL *et al.* (1988) Prospective study of chemotherapy in patients with metastatic gastrinoma. *Gastroenterology* 94: 1326–34.

Wymenga AN, Eriksson B, Salmela PI *et al.* (1999) Efficacy and safety of prolonged-release lanreotide in patients with gastrointestinal neuroendocrine tumors and hormone-related symptoms. *J Clin Oncol* 17: 1111.

Novel agents

Marianne Pavel

Introduction

Cell proliferation and differentiation are regulated by hormones, growth factors and cytokines. These molecules interact with cellular receptors and via a network of intracellular signaling pathways with the nucleus of the cell. In cancer cells key components of these pathways may be altered, overexpressed or mutated, leading to dysregulation of cell signaling, inhibition of cell proliferation and metastasis. The components of these signaling pathways represent potential selective targets for new anticancer therapies. These targets include ligands (e.g. growth factors), cellular receptors, intracellular second messengers and nuclear transcription factors. Neutralization of ligands to prevent their binding to growth factor receptors is one approach exemplified by bevacizumab, a humanized monoclonal antibody targeting circulating vascular endothelial growth factor (VEGF). Another approach is direct inhibition of growth factor receptors either by antibodies directed against the receptor, as has been shown for cetuximab, an antibody against the epidermal growth factor receptor (EGFR) or by inhibiting the kinase activity of receptors by small molecule inhibitors of receptor phosphorylation, as with gefitinib or erlotinib. At the endothelial level PTK/ZK represents another small molecule inhibitor of vascular endothelial growth factor receptor (VEGFR) phosphorylation. Examples for the multispecific inhibition of signaling of cytoplasmic secondary messengers are imatinib, an inhibitor of the kinase activity of bcr-abl, c-kit and platelet derived growth factor receptor (PDGFR), and sunitinib, an inhibitor of RET, c-kit, PDGFR and VEGFR.

Novel therapies have been introduced in the treatment of cancer in recent years. In colon cancer and non-small cell lung cancer (NSCLC) the application of antibodies against circulating growth factors or growth factor receptors represents an established therapy. These antibodies showed significant clinical activity by targeting two major pathways, the EGFR and VEGF signaling pathways in advanced colorectal cancer, especially when combined with chemotherapy. The EGFR tyrosine kinase inhibitor erlotinib showed efficacy in NSCLC after failure of systemic chemotherapy and as first-line therapy.

In the field of neuroendocrine tumors novel drugs have been investigated in clinical trials for the last 2–3 years in a limited number of patients in uncontrolled studies.

Molecular targeted therapies have been of interest for neuroendocrine tumors since the antiproliferative efficacy of standard treatments in patients with metastatic disease is limited, and many tumors express tyrosine kinase receptors, such as PDGFR and VEGFR, and their ligands. While comparative trials to standard treatments are lacking, novel therapies are indicated in the condition of failure to somatostatin analogs, alpha-interferon, systemic chemotherapy, local ablative therapies of liver metastases or peptide receptor radionuclide therapy. Negative somatostatin receptor scintigraphy may be an indication for the earlier use of novel therapies in progressive neuroendocrine tumors, especially of midgut origin.

Novel drugs include angiogenesis inhibitors and molecular targeted therapies. These drugs have been currently under investigation in phase II clinical trials as single or combination therapies with cytotoxic agents (Table 23.31). The expression of potential targets has been investigated in neuroendocrine tumor tissues (Table 23.32). In addition, PDGF, PDGFR-α, PDGFR-β, TGF-α and TGF-β are expressed in neuroendocrine tumor tissue and stroma tissue. Numerous other growth factor receptors, and intracellular second messengers may be other potential targets for growth inhibition of neuroendocrine tumors.

The focus will be on pathways for which inhibitory agents have been currently investigated in phase II clinical trials in neuroendocrine tumor patients. Small patient numbers, the variable tumor course with limited evaluation of tumor growth behavior before initiation of the treatment and different tumor

Table 23.31 Overview of novel agents of phase I and II clinical trials in neuroendocrine tumor patients.

	Authors	Drugs (dose)	Targets	No. of pts.	Design	PD before treatment	Median TTP[1]/TT[2]	Radiologic response (%): EPT/CT	Overall radiologic response (%)	Median progression-free survival
Molecular targeted therapy	Carr *et al.* (2004)	Imatinib (400 mg po bid) + octreotide (n = 21)	c-kit, c-Abl PDGFR	27	Phase II	Yes, in subgroup (n = 14*)	16 wks[2] (12–78+)	N.A.	PR: 3.7 SD: 63/57* PD: 33	24 wks. (38 wks. with octreotide); 1 yr survival: 88%
	Hobday *et al.* (2006)	Gefitinib (250 mg po/d)	EGFR	96	Phase II	Yes	N.A. SD > 4 mo. the TTP prior to study	PR: 10/5 SD: 14/32		8 mo. (CT), 4 mo. (EPT); 6 mo. -PFS: 61% (CT) 31% (EPT)
	Kulke *et al.* (2005)	Sunitinib (50 mg po/d, 4 wks, 2 wks off)	VEGFR PDGFR c-kit	102	Phase II	N.A.	40 wks[1] (CT: 42 wks; EPT: 33 wks)	PR: 13/2 SD: 75/93 PD: 7/0	PR: 9 SD: 82 PD: 4	N.A.
	Yao *et al.* (2006)	RAD001 (5 mg po/d) + octreotide LAR (30 mg q 4 wks.	mTOR VEGF IGF-1	27	Phase II	Yes in subgroup, (n = 17**)	12 wks all at time of evaluation	PR: 18/13 SD: 55/81 PD: 27/6	PR: 15/17.6** SD: 70/59** PD: 15	3 mo.-PFS: 76%; 6 mo.-PFS 65%
Angiogenesis inhibitors	Pavel *et al.* unpubl.	PTK/ZK (1250 mg po./d)	VEGFR-TK	9	Phase I	Yes	9.5 mo[1] (3–18)	1 MR in EPT	PR: 17 SD: 33 PD: 50	6 mo.-PFS 50% 12 mo.-PFS 30%
	Thomas *et al.* (2005)	PTK/ZK 150–1000 mg po.bid	VEGFR-TK	6	Phase I	N.A.	Not specified; 1 patient with EPT > 24 mo.	1 MR (EPT) reported; no details for other patients	N.A.	N.A.
	Kulke *et al.* (2006)	Endostatin (60–90 mg/m^2/d sc.)	Analog of endogenous angiogenesis inhibitor	42	Phase II	No (22 pts. assessable for prior PD: 95% SD > 2 mo.	7.6 mo.[1] (CT), 5.6 mo.[1] (EPT)	N.A.	PR: 0 SD: 80 PD: 20	5.8 mo. (EPT) 7.6 mo. (CT); Overall survival: 17.2 mo. (EPT), 22.6 mo. (CT)
Angiogenesis inhibitors + biotherapy	Yao *et al.* (2005)	Bevacizumab (15 mg/kg) + octreotide vs. PegIFNα-2b 0.5 μg/kg + octreotide	VEGF	22 22	Phase II	N.A.	Not specified	N.A.	Beva./PegIFN PR: 18/0 SD: 77/73 PD: 5/27	18 wks.-PFS: 96% (bevaczumab), 68% (PEG-IFNα-2b)
Angiogenesis inhibitors + chemotherapy	Kulke *et al.* (2006)	Bevacizumab (5 mg/kg iv. q 14 d) + TMZ (150 mg/m^2 po/d 1 wk, 1 wk off)	VEGF	34	Phase II	N.A.	22 wks.[2]	PR: 24/0 SD: 70/92 PD: 6/8	PR: 14 SD: 79 PD: 7	N.A.
	Kulke *et al.* (2006)	Thalidomide (50–400 mg po/d) + TMZ (150 mg/m^2 po/d 1 wk, 1 wk off)	bFGF, VEGF, TNF-a, COX2, EC	29	Phase II	N.A.	7.3 mo.[2] (1–23)	PR + CR: 45/7	CR: 4 PR 21 SD: 68 PD: 7	PFS not reached; 1 yr survival: 79% 2 yr survival: 61%

EPT = endocrine pancreatic tumor, CT = carcinoid tumor, CR = complete response, PR = partial remission, MR = minor remission, PD = progressive disease, SD = stable disease, N.A. = not assessed, EC = endothelial cells, TTP = time to tumor progression, TT = time of treatment, PegIFN = pegylated interferon, PFS = progression free survival, TMZ = temozolomide

Table 23.32 Molecular markers in highly differentiated neuroendocrine carcinomas. Immunohistochemistry expression profiles of endocrine pancreatic tumors (EPT) and carcinoid tumors (CT). Percentages indicate any positive (+) staining and staining graded 2+ or 3+ (Hobday *et al.* 2003).

	EPT (n = 27)		CT (n = 31)	
	Any+	2+ or 3+	any +	2+ or 3+
VEGF	59%	30%	84%	61%
VEGFR-FLK	67%	26%	71%	52%
VEGFR-FLT1	59%	7%	52%	6%
EGFR	22%	19%	100%	77%
HER-2/neu	7%	7%	16%	16%
c-kit	26%	15%	3%	0%
bFGF	26%	11%	16%	0%

VEGF, vascular endothelial growth factor; VEGFR, vascular endothelial growth factor receptor; EGFR, epidermal growth factor receptor; HER2, human epidermal growth factor receptor type 2; c-kit, stem cell factor receptor (CD117); bFGF, basic fibroblast growth factor.

origins limit the significance of these clinical trials and their impact on actual therapeutic strategies.

Molecular targeted therapies

Clinical trials have been conducted in neuroendocrine tumor patients with the tyrosine kinase inhibitors *gefitinib, sunitinib and imatinib*, and the mTOR inhibitor *everolimus*.

Gefitinib

Gefitinib (ZD 1839) is a receptor tyrosine kinase inhibitor of the epidermal growth factor receptor (EGFR). The EGFR is a receptor tyrosine kinase of the ErbB family that is abnormally activated in many epithelial tumors. Two classes of anti-EGFR agents are currently approved for the treatment of patients with cancer: monoclonal antibodies directed against the extracellular domain of the receptor, and low molecular weight ATP-competitive inhibitors of the receptor's tyrosine kinase. EGFR targeting has been demonstrated to be a successful therapy in some epithelial tumors. Anti-EGFR monoclonal antibodies are active in colorectal cancer and NSCLC, the EGFR tyrosine kinase inhibitor erlotinib in NSCLC.

In 96 patients with progressive neuroendocrine tumors (39 with endocrine pancreatic tumors (EPT), 57 with carcinoid tumors) previously treated by other regimens, gefitinib was investigated at a dose of 250 mg p.o. daily. Partial tumor remissions including minor remissions occured in 2 of 40 (5%) patients with carcinoid tumor and 3 of 31 (10%) patients with EPT, stablization of tumor growth in 14% and 32% of patients with EPT and carcinoid tumors, respectively. Progression-free survival at 6 months was 31% for EPT and 61% for carcinoid tumors. Treatment was well tolerated. Fatigue, diarrhea and exanthema grade 3 and 4 occurred in 6, 5 and 3% of patients (Hobday *et al.* 2006). Response was not clearly related to EGFR staining by immunohistochemistry (personal communication, T. Hobday).

From all studies on novel therapies reported so far, this trial seems of greatest significance due to the criteria of tumor progression prior to initiation of gefitinib therapy, thereby allowing to better judge the rate of disease stabilization.

In addition to single EGFR inhibitors other low molecular weight tyrosine kinase inhibitors that target both the EGFR and other members of the EGF family might also be useful novel drugs in the treatment of NET (Table 23.33).

Sunitinib malate

Sunitinib malate is an oral multitargeted tyrosine kinase inhibitor of VEGFR, PDGFR, c-kit, RET and FLT-3 with antiangiogenic and antitumor activities. Efficacy and safety was first studied in patients with GIST following failure of prior imatinib mesylate therapy.

Sunitinib was investigated in 109 patients with advanced unresectable NET (66 with EPT, 43 with carcinoid tumors) at a dose of 50 mg p.o. daily for 4 weeks followed by 2 weeks off treatment. Cycles were repeated every 6 weeks. Median number of cycles was 5, with a range of 1–14. Tumor response rates defined by RECIST criteria in 102 patients were partial response in 9 patients (9%), stable disease in 84 (82%), and progressive disease in 4 (4%). With respect to location of the primary tumor partial tumor remission occured in 13% and 2%, stable disease in 75% and 93% of patients with EPT and carcinoid tumors, respectively. Median time to tumor progression was 40 weeks (33 weeks in EPT, 42 weeks in carcinoids). No data are available on the tumor growth before initiation of sunitinb therapy, thus the percentage of patients who will respond by stable disease is probably overestimated. Side-effects were rare. The most common grade 3 and 4 side-effects included fatigue (25%), neutropenia (16%), thrombocytopenia (8%), hypertension (8%), vomiting (6%), nausea (6%), diarrhea (5%), dehydration (4%), mucosal inflammation (3%), anorexia (3%) and glossodynia (3%). Discontination of the treatment due to side-effects occurred in 7% of patients (Kulke *et al.* 2005).

Imatinib mesylate

Imatinib (STI 571) was the first commercially available small molecule tyrosine kinase inhibitor that blocks the c-kit, c-Abl, and platelet-derived growth factor receptor-β (PDGFR-β) tyrosine kinases and demonstrated remarkable efficacy in chronic myelogenous leukemia (CML) and in gastrointestinal stromal tumors (GIST).

Carcinoid tumors may express PDGF and PDGFR as well as c-kit and might thereby be responsive to imatinib therapy. In 27 previously treated or untreated patients with advanced carcinoid tumors imatinib was used at a dose of 400 mg p.o. bid with concurrent octreotide therapy in 21 patients and prior chemotherapy, hepatic artery embolization, interferon or radiation in 21 patients. Median time of imatinib therapy was 16 weeks (range 12–78).

Table 23.33 Potential novel treatments.

	Drugs	Target	Mechanisms
Growth factor receptor antibodies	Cetuximab, i.v.	EGFR	Receptor antibody
	Trastuzumab, p.o.	HER-2	Receptor antibody
	AMG-479 (Phase I)	IGF-1 R	Receptor antibody
Tyrosine kinase inhibitors	Erlotinib, p.o.	EGFR	TKI
	Lapatinib, p.o.	EGFR, HER2	TKI
	Canertinib (CI-1033), p.o.	EGFR, Her-2, Her-3, Her-4; pan-ErbB inhibitor	TKI
	GW786034, p.o.	VEGFR-1,-2 and -3	
		PDGFR-α and -β, c-kit	TKI
	Zactima (ZD6474), p.o.	VEGFR, EGFR	TKI
	Sorafenib, p.o.	c-Raf-1, B-Raf, VEGFR, PDGFR	TKI
Integrin antagonists	CNTO-95, i.v.	Alpha-v integrin	Human monoclonal antibody
Tubulin-interacting agents	ZD6126, i.v.	Cytoskeleton, microtubules	Microtubule-destabilizer in endothelial cells
	Epothilone B (EPO906), i.v.	Cytoskeleton, microtubules	Microtubule-stabilizer
CDK- inhibitors	R-547, i.v.		
	AT-7519, i.v.	Cyclin-dependent kinases (CDKs) -1, -4 and -2	Selective ATP-competitive CDK inhibitor (inhibitor of cell cycle)
Histone deacetylase inhibitors	SAHA, p.o.		
	MS-275, p.o.		
	Depsipeptide, i.v.	Histone deacetylase (HDAC)	Block angiogenesis and cell cycling
Others	YM-155, i.v.	Survivin	Small molecule inhibitor

TKI, tyrosine kinase inhibitor; MMP, matrix metalloproteinase; VEGFR, vascular endothelial growth factor receptor; EGFR, epidermal growth factor receptor; PDGFR, platelet-derived growth factor receptor; HER2, human epidermal growth factor receptor type 2; IGF-1 R, insulin-like growth factor-1 receptor

One patient (3.7%) with concurrent octreotide therapy developed partial tumor remission and 17 patients (63%) had stable disease. Among 14 patients with progressive disease prior to imatinib, 8 (57%) remained progression free for at least 12 weeks (range 18–52). Median progression-free survival was 24 weeks, and superior in patients with concurrent octreotide compared to imatinib alone (14 vs 38 weeks). Grade 3–4 toxicities included fatigue (26%), diarrhea (11%), fluid retention (11%), nausea (7%), granulocytopenia (7%) and anorexia (4%). The authors suggested the use of imatinib with other agents to improve response rates (Carr *et al.* 2004).

The success of kinase inhibitor therapy might be dependent on the presence of mutations in the target kinase. A lack of antiproliferative activity as known from small cell lung carcinoma (SCLC) patients was associated with absence of c-kit mutations in most of patients. Otherwise mutations may cause acquired resistance to kinase inhibitors as described in CML and GIST.

Everolimus

RAD001 (everolimus) is a mammalian target of rapamycin (mTOR) inhibitor structurally related to rapamycin. The protein kinase mTOR exerts a central control function integrating multiple signaling pathways in response to growth factors and intracellular signaling by nutrients. The mTOR is involved in the regulation of growth-related cellular functions; the best known function is the regulation of translation initiation. Inhibiting mTOR pathway may reduce cell growth and proliferation and impair the metastatic potential of tumor cells. There is an indirect effect on angiogenesis through inhibition of VEGF production by tumor cells. Octreotide is known to inhibit secretion of growth factors from tumor cells, like insulin-like growth factor 1 (IGF-1) and VEGF thereby downregulating autocrine and paracrine growth stimulating effects.

RAD001 (5 mg p.o./day), and the long-acting somatostatin analog octreotide *LAR* (30 mg every 28 days), were given to 32 patients with NET (18 with carcinoid tumors, 13 with EPT). In 27 patients tumor response was assessed by RECIST criteria at week 12. Overall radiologic response rate was 15%. Stable disease was noted in 70% and progressive disease in 15% of patients. With regard to the location of the primary tumor, partial tumor remissions were observed in 2/11 (18%) patients with EPT who were evaluable for tumor response and 2/16 (13%) of carcinoid tumor patients; stable disease occurred in 6/11 (55%) and 13/16 (81%) patients, respectively. Excluding patients with stable disease prior to initiation of RAD001 therapy, results were similar with 10/17 (59%) patients having stable disease and 3/17 (18%) partial tumor remissions.

Chromogranin A decreased by more than 50% in half of patients. Progression-free survival was 76% at 3 months and 65% at 6 months. Treatment was in general well tolerated. The most common toxicity was mild aphthous ulcerations. Side-effects grade 3–4 included fatigue in three patients, and aphthous mucosal ulcers, exanthema, diarrhea and pain in two patients each. Anemia, thrombocytopenia, hyperglycemia and edema developed in one patient each (Yao *et al.* 2006).

Antiangiogenic therapies

Angiogenesis, the formation of new blood vessels from the pre-existing vasculature, is critical for the development and subsequent growth of human tumors and is a prerequisite for the formation of metastases. Various proangiogenic factors, like vascular endothelial growth factor (VEGF), basic fibroblast growth factor (bFGF) and platelet-derived growth factor (PDGF) are released by tumor cells or endothelial cells. VEGF is the most potent endothelial growth factor, mediating its activity through binding to several high-affinity transmembrane endothelial cell receptors, most notably VEGF receptors (VEGFR) types 1 and 2. Binding of VEGF to these receptors leads to intracellular receptor phosphorylation which initiates various intracellular downstream receptor pathways leading to endothelial cell proliferation and migration, and new blood vessel formation whereas binding to VEGFR type 3 leads to lymphangiogenesis.

Neuroendocrine tumors are highly vascular, and express VEGF in up to 90% of tumor tissues investigated. Circulating VEGF levels seem to correlate with tumor progression in neuroendocrine tumor patients.

Antiangiogenic strategies include antibodies against the ligand of the VEGFR, preventing VEGF from binding to its receptor, antibodies against the extracellular domain of the VEGFR, and small molecules interacting with the intracellular domain of the VEGFR thereby inhibiting VEGFR phophorylation and downstream signaling pathways leading to inhibition of endothelial cell differentiation, proliferation and migration. Some of the multispecific tyrosine kinase inhibitors like sunitinib are also angiogenesis inhibitors. Other novel agents like recombinant human endostatin or angiostatin mimic endogeneous angiogenesis inhibitors, whereas matrix metalloproteinase inhibitors inhibit the degradation of the extracellular matrix, one of the first steps in angiogenesis.

In addition, a group of several pharmacologic substances, like thalidomide, squalamine, integrin antagonists, inhibitors of cyclooxygenase-2 block endothelial cells via different mechanisms. There is clinical experience from phase I and II studies with *endostatin*, the anti-VEGF antibody *bevacizumab*, the VEGFR tyrosine kinase inhibitor *PTK/ZK* and *thalidomide* in neuroendocrine tumor patients.

Endostatin

Endostatin is a 20-kd proteolytic fragment of collagen XVIII that has been shown to have antiangiogenic and antitumor activity. Within a multicenter phase II study 42 patients with advanced carcinoid or pancreatic neuroendocrine tumors were treated with recombinant human endostatin administered as a subcutaneous injection bid at a starting dose of 60 mg/m^2/day with dose escalation to 90 mg in those patients who did not achieve the target therapeutic level of 300 ng/mL. None of 40 patients assessable for radiologic response experienced a partial or complete tumor remission by WHO criteria. Stable disease was observed in 32 patients (80%) for a median duration of 10.8 months. However, 11 of 23 patients (48%) assessable for disease progression before study enrolment were reported to have stable disease for at least 6 months prior to study inclusion, and 21 of 22 patients (95%) were reported to have stable disease for at least 2 months prior to study inclusion. Progressive disease occured in 8 patients (20%). Only 6% of 31 patients assessable for chromogranin A response had a more than 50% decrease in baseline serum level and none of the 20 patients assessable for urinary 5-HIAA. The median progression-free survival time was 5.8 months (range 1.9–13.5 months) for patients with EPT and 7.6 months (range 5.3–19.2 months) for patients with carcinoid tumors. Toxicity was low. Most frequent side-effects were usually mild local reactions at injection site (64%), fatigue (30%), abdominal pain (29%) and diarrhea (26%) (Kulke *et al.* 2006a).

Bevacizumab

Bevacizumab, a humanized monoclonal antibody targeting circulating VEGF, is successful in the treatment of colon cancer in combination with standard chemotherapy.

In a first study the combination therapy of bevacizumab and octreotide in highly differentiated neuroendocrine tumors led to a reduction of blood flow and increased vascular permeability at 24 h. In a comparative study of bevacizumab and pegylated interferon-alpha in patients with carcinoid tumors with concurrent octreotide therapy at stable dosage for 2 months at baseline, 4/22 (18%) patients on bevacizumab and 0/22 patients on pegylated interferon-alpha developed partial tumor remissions, whereas stable disease was observed in 17 (77%) patients on bevacizumab and 16 (73%) patients on pegylated interferon-alpha, respectively at week 18. Reduction of 5-HIAA was achieved in 21% on bevacizumab and 43% on pegylated interferon-alpha. Progression-free survival differed at week 18 with 96% for bevacizumab and 68% for pegylated interferon-alpha, however equalled at week 66 after cross-over with combined therapy of both drugs from week 18 (Yao *et al.* 2005).

In a phase II study bevacizumab (5 mg/kg i.v. q 14 days) was used in combination with the alkylating agent temozolomide (TMZ), an oral analog of dacarbazine in patients with advanced neuroendocrine tumors for a median time of 22 weeks. The majority of patients (27/34) had well-differentiated NET, the others moderately to poorly differentiated NET (n = 7). Best confirmed radiologic response to therapy (RECIST) were partial remissions in 24% (4/17) of EPT and none (0/12) of the carcinoid patients while stable disease was observed in 70% (12/17) of patients with EPT and 92% (11/12) of patients with carcinoid tumors. Grade 3–4 toxicities included lymphopenia (62%), thrombocytopenia (21%), leukopenia (6%), vomiting (9%), nausea (6%), fatigue (6%). Hyponatremia, constipation and hypertension were observed in 3% of patients, respectively. Patients received prophylaxis with trimethoprim/sulfamethoxazole and acyclovir due to anticipated adverse events on white blood cells (Kulke *et al.* 2006b).

Vatalanib

Vatalanib [PTK787/ZK 222584 (PTK/ZK)] is an oral multi-VEGF receptor tyrosine kinase inhibitor that blocks tumor angiogenesis and lymphangiogenesis through inhibition of all known VEGF receptor tyrosine kinases. PTK/ZK is currently under investigation in phase II clinical trials in advanced neuroendocrine tumors. Within a preliminary phase I study 9 patients with progressive non-functioning NET including one patient with thyroid carcinoma were treated with escalating doses of i.v. PTK/ZK followed by a maximal oral dose of 1250 mg per day until tumor progression or intolerable toxicity occurred. The patients were pretreated with different regimens (octreotide in 5 patients, alpha-interferon in 5, chemotherapy in 3, ^{90}Y-DOTATOC in 2, irradiation in 2 and chemoembolization in 1). Tumor response was monitored by imaging with CT and MRI of the abdomen, CT of the thorax and FDG-PET. A partial tumor remission occured in one patient with thyroid carcinoma, a stabilization of tumor growth in one patient with EPT, with long-lasting 20% decrease from baseline in the sum of products of perpendicular diameters of all measurable lesions, and stabilization of tumor growth in one patient with thymic neuroendocrine carcinoma (6 months). In another patient with unknown primary tumor there was indication of clinical tumor progression although by imaging stable disease was shown at 3 months. Two other patients out of 6 patients assessable for tumor response had progressive disease at 3 months. The tumor response in the patient with thyroid carcinoma lasted for more than 15 months. The patient with EPT had a benefit for up to 13 months, but was discontinued thereafter due to gastrointestinal bleeding which was not considered to be related to the study drug, because the patient had an invasion of the pancreatic tumor into the small intestine with recurrent gastrointestinal bleeding prior to study enrolment. Tolerability of PTK/ZK was in general good. No other severe toxicities (CTC grade 4) occurred. Two patients stopped oral treatment early for side-effects (dizziness, vomiting and nausea of CTC grade 1–2); another patient was discontinued due to acute hepatitis (CTC grade 3). These patients were not evaluable for tumor response (Pavel *et al.* unpublished data). The most frequent side-effects of p.o. administration of PTK/ZK within this multicenter study of 26 patients with advanced cancer of different origin were dizziness, nausea, vomiting and fatigue. Most adverse events were grade 1 and 2.

Within another phase I study of oral PTK/ZK 6 patients with NET were included. One patient is reported to have developed minor remission of liver lesions and stabilization of the primary tumor in the pancreas. The patient participated in the study for more than 24 months. Initial dose was 750 mg bid; a reduction to 500 mg bid was made because of uncontrolled hypertension and elevated liver enzymes. It is of interest that severe abdominal pain refractory to analgesics subsided with PTK/ZK treatment (Thomas *et al.* 2005). The most common adverse events of PTK/ZK in this study of 43 patients with advanced cancer of different origin were nausea and vomiting usually grade 1 or 2 occurring in 61% and 54% of patients, respectively. These were easily managed with antiemetics. Fatigue was seen in 37%, back pain in 26%, abdominal pain in 23%, and anorexia in 14% of patients. Hypertension was noted in 16%, a grade 3 increase in ALT and AST in 14% of patients.

Thalidomide

Thalidomide, known for its teratogenic potential, is a drug with many pharmacologic properties, including inhibition of angiogenesis and inflammation. Thalidomide apparently interferes with VEGF and basic fibroblast growth factor (bFGF) pathways and the extracellular matrix thereby inhibiting angiogenesis. Bioactivation is required for exertion of its antiangiogenic effects. The drug is currently under investigation for the treatment of several diseases, ranging from inflammatory diseases to cancer. In NET thalidomide (50–400 mg p.o. daily) was applied with the oral chemotherapeutic drug temozolomide (150 mg/m^2 p.o. daily for 1 week followed by 1 week off drug) in a phase II trial in 29 patients (11 EPT, 15 carcinoid tumors, 3 pheochromocytoma). The overall radiologic response rate of 28 assessable patients was 25% (6 PR, 1 CR). Stable disease occured in 19 patients (68%) and progressive disease in 2 (7%). Five of 11 patients (45%) with EPT responded by partial or complete tumor remission, the other responders had metastatic carcinoid and metastatic pheochromocytoma. Median time of tumor response was 13.5 months (range 2–31 months). Of 20 patients with elevated chromogranin A levels at baseline eight (40%) experienced decreases of chromogranin A of more than 50%. The median follow-up time was 26 months (range 3–31). The overall 1 and 2 year survival rates were 79% and 61%. Toxicity was high. Withdrawal of treatment was frequent with 55% of patients stopping therapy after a median time of 8.4 months. The most frequent side-effects usually attributed to thalidomide included fatigue (83%), vomiting (41%), neuropathy (38%), exanthema (38%) and constipation (45%). Mild mood changes and dizziness developed in 31% and 37% of patients, respectively. Lymphopenia grade 3 to 4 was observed in 69% of patients, infections in 37% with 10% of patients having opportunistic infections (Kulke *et al.* 2006c).

Summary and future directions

Molecular targeted therapies and angiogenesis inhibitiors represent a promising approach to antiproliferative therapy of NET. Partial tumor remissions represent a rare event in carcinoid tumors with 0–8%, and occur in 10–18% of patients with

EPT using these novel agents. Percentages of patients with stable disease were high with 55–93%. To our current knowledge stabilization of tumor growth represents a favorable response and may improve survival rates. However tumor growth prior to initiation of these therapies was not documented in the vast majority of the studies. The rates of disease stabilization were lower with gefitinib while this agent was used only in progressive neuroendocrine tumors. Time to tumor progression represents a prognostic marker in neuroendocrine tumors according to well-conducted randomized clinical trials with biotherapy. Considering the naturally indolent growth of neuroendocrine tumors, efficacy from small Phase II studies without this information on spontaneous tumor growth is difficult to assess, and future studies are warranted. The rate of partial tumor remissions may be increased when novel agents are combined with chemotherapy, especially in endocrine pancreatic tumors. Side-effects are minimal with few exceptions when compared to conventional chemotherapeutic agents. However, as with any novel treatment, caution is required with regard to long-term side-effects.

Current ongoing studies (PTK/ZK, sunitinib, RAD001) will further evaluate the efficacy of these novel agents in progressive neuroendocrine tumors after failure of standard therapies.

Larger randomized trials may be necessary to establish the potential clinical benefit of these novel agents and should take into consideration surrogate endpoints of biologic activity.

These future studies should also focus on patients with exposure to fewer prior regimens and novel drugs in combination therapy with biotherapy or chemotherapy. Inhibition of an intracellular signaling pathway can be overcome by tumor cells by directing growth signals through other pathways. The use of novel agents targeting multispecific growth factor signaling in combination with cytotoxic agents or biotherapy seems therefore more promising. Additional novel drugs that have been investigated in other solid tumors in recent or ongoing clinical trials, like integrin antagonists, tubulin-interacting agents, histone deacetylase inhibitors and cyclin-dependent kinase inhibitors might also be attractive therapeutic options in neuroendocrine tumors (Table 23.33). However, it has to be clarified how far these potential targets are relevant for tumor growth and growth control in neuroendocrine tumors.

The greatest challenge will be to determine which patient groups and anticancer drugs are more appropriate for combination therapy with these agents. Assessment of the target gene, mutational status, and target protein expression might be helpful.

The success of kinase inhibitor therapy might be dependent on the presence of mutations in the target kinase. Mutational activation of kinases may indicate which patients are likely to respond to targeted therapies as has been shown for gefitinib in NSCLC patients with EGFR mutations. Examining the number of gene copies of the target may be another useful predictor of efficacy as has been demonstrated for erlotinib in advanced NSCLC with high EGFR gene copy number. In addition, other challenges have to be addressed in the development of effective drugs across different neuroendocrine tumor types to realise an individualized molecular therapy leading to improved patient selection for treatment with novel agents.

The successful integration of targeted agents into clinical routine will depend on the verification of sufficient predictive markers, allowing their economically reasonable usage.

References

Carr K, Yao J, Rashid A *et al.* (2004) A phase II trial of imatinib in patients with advanced carcinoid tumor. In: *2004 ASCO Annual Meeting Proceedings* 22 (Suppl 14S), abstr 4124.

Hobday TJ, Rubin J, Goldberg R, Erlichman C, Lloyd R. (2003) Molecular markers in metastatic gastrointestinal neuroendocrine tumors. In: *2003 ASCO Annual Meeting Proceedings* 22, abstr 1078.

Hobday TJ, Holen K, Donehower R *et al.* (2006) A phase II trial of gefitinib in patients (pts) with progressive metastatic neuroendocrine tumors (NET): A Phase II Consortium (P2C) study. In: *2006 ASCO Annual Meeting Proceedings* 24 (Suppl 18S), abstr 4043.

Kulke MH, Lenz HJ, Meropol NJ *et al.* (2005) Results of a phase II study with sunitinib malate (SU11248) in patients with advanced neuroendocrine tumours (NETs). *Eur J Cancer* Suppl 3(2), abstr 718. Elsevier, Oxford.

Kulke M, Bergsland E, Ryan D *et al.* (2006a) Phase II study of recombinant human endostatin in patients with advanced neuroendocrine tumors. *J Clin Oncol* 24(22): 3555–61.

Kulke M, Stuart K, Earle C *et al.* (2006b) A phase II study of temozolomide and bevacizumab in patients with advanced neuroendocrine tumors. In: *2006 ASCO Annual Meeting Proceedings* 24 (Suppl 18S), abstr 4044.

Kulke MH, Stuart K, Enzinger PC *et al.* (2006c) Phase II study of temozolomide and thalidomide in patients with metastatic neuroendocrine tumors. *J Clin Oncol* 24(3): 401–6.

Thomas AL, Morgan B, Horsfield MA *et al.* (2005) Phase I study of the safety, tolerability, pharmacokinetics, and pharmacodynamics of PTK787/ZK 222584 administered twice daily in patients with advanced cancer. *J Clin Oncol* 23(18): 4162–71.

Yao J, Ng C, Hoff PM *et al.* (2005) Improved progression free survival (PFS), and rapid, sustained decrease in tumor perfusion among patients with advanced carcinoid treated with bevacizumab. *2005 ASCO Annual Meeting Proceedings* 23 (Suppl 16S), abstr 4007.

Yao J, Phan A, Chang D *et al.* (2006) Phase II study of RAD001 (everolimus) and depot octreotide (sandostatin LAR) in patients with advanced low grade neuroendocrine carcinoma (LGNET). *2006 ASCO Annual Meeting Proceedings* 24 (Suppl 18S), abstr 4042.

24 Rare Tumors of the Liver

Shantanu Bhattacharjya, Zahir Soonawalla, Rachel R. Phillips & Peter J. Friend

Introduction

The expansion of and improvements in medical imaging over the last few decades have resulted in an increase in the number of incidentally discovered liver tumors. Though the majority of these tumors are benign, the finding raises concern, and the diagnostic difficulties in elucidating the nature of such lesions forms a significant proportion of the work of a tertiary hepatobiliary multidisciplinary team (MDT). Many of these patients undergo surgery due to diagnostic uncertainty, and a large database review found that 5% of liver resections had benign histology. The vast majority of benign liver lesions do not require resection, and it is therefore important to be able to achieve a reliable diagnosis of such lesions.

The management of any tumor depends upon knowledge of the biology of the tumor and its response to the various therapeutic approaches that are available. Many of the rare tumors of hepatobiliary origin are sufficiently uncommon that there are very few published data regarding the biological behavior or response to therapy, and it is not, therefore, possible to offer an evidence-based treatment for many of the tumors in this group. In general, surgical resection is considered to be the treatment of choice for most malignant tumors in which complete tumor clearance can be accomplished without excessive mortality. It should be stressed that the decision to proceed to surgery must be preceded by a careful assessment of the risks of intervention balanced against the likelihood of useful survival or quality of life benefit. Other treatments, including ablative therapies, are used largely on the basis of experience gained in the treatment of commoner liver tumors.

The first section in this chapter addresses the general principles involved in reaching a diagnosis and recommending therapy and is followed by a more specific discussion of selected individual tumor types. More common benign lesions have been included in this chapter, as they form an important differential diagnosis and are frequently referred to a hepatobiliary MDT.

General principles in the approach to a rare hepatobiliary tumor

Classification of primary tumors of the liver

The liver is composed of cells derived from ectoderm, mesoderm and endoderm. Tumors can develop from any of these elements, either in isolation or in combination. The current classification of primary liver tumors is based on a revised classification of liver tumors by an expert group of histopathologists originally sponsored by the World Health Organization and thereafter by the Armed Forces Institute of Pathology (Ishak 1995; Ishak *et al.* 2003) (Table 24.1). The knowledge of the distribution of these tumors is based on data derived from cancer registries worldwide. These are published in the series of *Cancer Incidence in Five Continents.* However the quality of the data is critically dependant on accurate registration of the various cancers and is yet to be achieved in many parts of the world.

Rare primary hepatobiliary tumors can also be classified as lesions specific to childhood and those that occur at any age. Tumors specific to childhood may be benign conditions, including mesenchymal hamartomas, infantile hemangioendothelioma, hepatic hemangioblastomas and mature teratomas. Malignant tumors of childhood include hepatoblastoma, embryonal sarcoma, rhabdomyosarcoma and germ cell tumors. The incidence of hepatic tumors in childhood is in the region of 0.5–2.5 per million population (Emre & McKenna 2004). Malignant tumors predominate among pediatric liver tumors; hepatoblastomas, hepatocellular carcinomas and other sarcomas comprise 43%, 23% and 6% respectively. There is a male

Gastrointestinal Oncology: A Critical Multidisciplinary Team Approach.
Edited by J. Jankowski, R. Sampliner, D. Kerr, and Y. Fong.
 ISBN: 978-1-4501-2783-7

Table 24.1 An abbreviated classification of primary tumors of the liver.

	Benign	Malignant
Epithelial		
Hepatocellular	Nodular regenerative hyperplasia Focal nodular hyperplasia Hepatocellular adenoma	Hepatocellular carcinoma Fibrolamellar variant Hepatoblastoma
Cholangiocellular	Bile duct adenoma Bile duct cystadenoma Biliary papillomatosis	Cholangiocarcinoma Bile duct cystadenocarcinoma Mixed (cholangiohepatoma)
Non-epithelial		
Blood vessel	Hemangioma Hemangioendothelioma	Hemangiosarcoma Epithelioid hemangioendothelioma
Adipose tissue	Angiomyolipoma	
Mesenchymal	Hemartoma Teratoma	Embryonal sarcoma Rhabdomyosarcoma
Others		Lymphoma Germ cell tumors Carcinoid
Tumor-like lesions	Cysts Hepatic peliosis Inflammatory pseudotumor	

preponderance of 1.8 : 1 for all malignant pediatric liver tumors. The benign tumors include hemangiomas and hemangioendotheliomas (13%), mesenchymal hamartomas (6%), hepatic adenomas (2%), focal nodular hyperplasia (2%), and other benign conditions (5%) (Weinberg & Finegold 1983, 1986).

Benign focal liver masses are present in approximately 9% of adult patients in the developed world. The incidence of individual rare malignant liver tumors in adults is difficult to estimate due to the sporadic nature of these cases.

The etiology of rare hepatobiliary tumors

Many factors have been linked with the development of hepatoblastomas in childhood. These include Beckwith–Wiedemann syndrome, hemihypertrophy, familial adenomatous polyposis, Gardner's syndrome, glycogen storage disease type 1, trisomy 18, fetal alcohol syndrome, prematurity and low birth weight, maternal exposure to oral contraceptives, gonadotrophins, metals, petroleum products and pigments as well as paternal exposure to certain metals (Geiser *et al.* 1970; Sotelo-Avila *et al.* 1980; Koufos *et al.* 1985; Scrable *et al.* 1987; Little *et al.* 1988; Koufos *et al.* 1989; Rainier *et al.* 1995; Simms *et al.* 1995). Amongst tumors that are not specific to childhood, the use of oral contraceptives has been linked to the development of liver cell adenoma and focal nodular hyperplasia (Rabe *et al.* 1994; Benhamou 1997; Heinemann *et al.* 1998; Caballes & Caballes 1999; Ye *et al.* 1999) while exposure to vinyl chloride and thorotrast (previously radiological contrast material) have been linked to the development of angiosarcomas (Simonato *et al.* 1991; Boffetta *et al.* 2003; Lewis & Rempala 2003).

Presentation

The majority of benign primary liver tumors are detected as incidental lesions on imaging. Some come to light following resection of a lesion that was thought to be of a different tumor type. Also, a number of lesions are identified and characterized only at post mortem examination. Malignant liver tumors are usually detected following investigation of a patient presenting either with an upper abdominal mass or with constitutional symptoms. In contrast, rare tumors of the biliary system are usually detected following presentation either as an asymptomatic mass or obstructive jaundice. Much less commonly, a benign lesion may present with intrahepatic or intraperitoneal hemorrhage (e.g. hepatic adenoma) or a high output failure associated with massive arteriovenous shunting (e.g. hemangioendothelioma).

Investigation

Blood tests

Abnormalities in the full blood count (for example a normocytic normochromic anemia with thrombocytosis) are often seen in patients with malignant liver tumors but are of little diagnostic value. On standard biochemical screening, liver function tests are usually normal unless the patient presents with obstructive jaundice. When elevated, α-fetoprotein as well as β-HCG have diagnostic value, as these are secreted by the large majority of hepatoblastomas (and are also useful in follow-up surveillance). Other markers that may be useful include vitamin B12 binding protein and transcobalamin I which are elevated in cases of fibrolamellar hepatocellular carcinoma.

Imaging

Rare liver tumors should be considered in the diagnostic work-up and management of patients presenting either with an incidental hepatic mass or in the differential diagnosis of a patient with known malignancy. The vast majority of liver tumors in the West are secondary and investigations must also be directed to the primary sites must commonly associated with liver maligancy (particularly the gastrointestinal tract). Patient evaluation includes assessment of the most likely underlying pathologic diagnosis, the precise site and volume of disease, its solitary or multifocal nature, any degree of associated vascular invasion or biliary obstruction as well as the presence and extent of any extrahepatic disease.

There is a range of imaging modalities available to facilitate accurate assessment of the liver. Many techniques provide complementary information and the rational use of ultrasound (US), computed tomography (CT) and magnetic resonance (MR) allows optimal assessment and subsequent management in this complex patient group. CT and MR are both excellent modalities for liver imaging. CT enables accurate staging of malignant tumors as well as assessment of any extrahepatic disease. MR can accurately characterise most hepatic pathologies and is the modality of choice in many centres for evaluation of focal and diffuse hepatic parenchymal abnormalities (Powers *et al.* 1994; Hagspiel *et al.* 1995; Levy *et al.* 2002) (Fig. 24.1).

Imaging not only enables detection and characterization of hepatic lesions but also helps guide the most appropriate therapeutic option and monitors response to treatment.

Ultrasound

Ultrasound is often the first imaging modality in the detection of focal or diffuse hepatic parenchymal disorders. It allows accurate assessment of the size and multiplicity of lesions, an indication of their vascularity and evaluation of any biliary obstruction. It is a fast, cheap, non-invasive, readily available investigation that does not involve ionizing radiation. Extra-abdominal disease requires evaluation with CT. The main pitfall of this technique is that it is operator dependent, lacks discriminatory ability and not necessarily reproducible. The addition of intravenous contrast agents concomitantly with US has gained widespread acceptance in the evaluation of focal liver lesions, and has helped increase both the sensitivity and specificity of this test.

Computed tomography

Multislice spiral CT is often the first-line investigation to assess the extent of extrahepatic disease involvement. It can often provide accurate determination of the nature of a focal hepatic abnormality and has the benefit of enabling a rapid evaluation of the whole body. Multiphasic enhanced imaging allows the detection and characterization of most primary and secondary liver neoplasms and demonstrates any complications such as biliary obstruction or vascular invasion. Sequential enhanced sequences often allow assessment of tumor morphology and perfusion and prediction of its likely pathologic nature.

Magnetic resonance imaging

MR is a powerful tool in the evaluation of primary liver neoplasms. Accurate assessment of tumor extent and tissue characterization requires meticulous attention to technical detail and frequently enables an accurate diagnosis. Knowledge of clinical findings and a clear understanding of the segmental anatomy of the liver assist interpretation. The use of advanced techniques in liver MR such as fat suppression, chemical shift imaging and multiphasic dynamic acquisitions following administration of intravenous contrast are of importance in disease detection, pathologic diagnosis and pretreatment assessment. Gadolinium chelate, a non-specific paramagnetic contrast agent, remains the most widely used MR contrast agent. Liver-specific contrast agents, such as mangafodipir trisodium, are selectively taken up by hepatocytes but not by metastatic deposits. Reticuloendothelial system-specific agents, such as

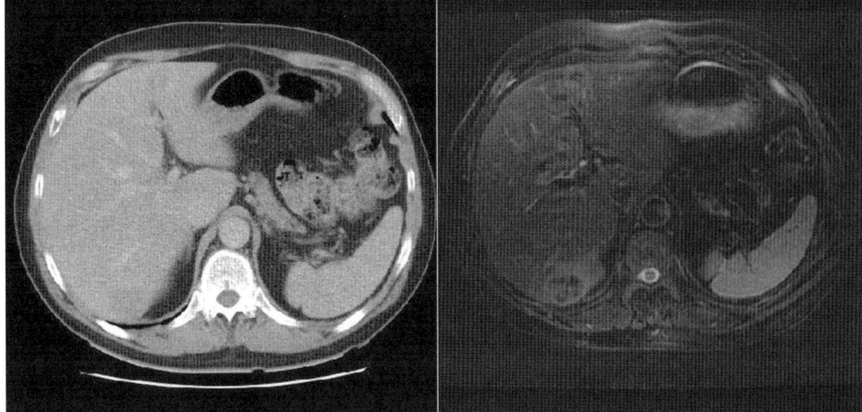

Fig. 24.1 Comparison between conspicuity of lesion on (a) CT and (b) MR in a patient with known metastatic colorectal carcinoma. There are lesions present in both lobes of the liver, more easily appreciated on the MR study (axial T2W with fat suppression).

superparamagnetic iron oxide particles, are selectively captured by the reticuloendothelial (Kuppfer) cells in the liver. Both the above agents increase the signal difference between liver metastases and normal liver parenchyma, thereby improving the detection of focal liver deposits.

Imaging algorithm

If all hepatic parenchymal lesions are to be detected and characterized accurately, it is imperative that attention is given to the precise image acquisition technique, whether on CT or MR. The algorithm shown in Box 24.1 may be of value to narrow the differential diagnosis in adults found to have a hepatic parenchymal lesion.

Biopsy

The role of diagnostic biopsy remains controversial. The argument in favour is the substantial benefit of reaching a definite histologic diagnosis in many cases (the sample is not always satisfactory for diagnostic purposes) (Schnater *et al.* 2005) whilst the arguments against include the risk of peritoneal seeding, bleeding and the fact that with small multifocal lesions, a biopsy is quite likely not to yield a diagnosis (Pelloni & Gertsch 2000; Jones *et al.* 2005). The risk of peritoneal seeding following percutaneous biopsy is probably underestimated and indeed, in the case of rare liver tumors, unknown. The only guide therefore is an estimate based on the incidence of this problem with other tumor types such as hepatocellular cancers and colorectal metastases (Kim *et al.* 2000; Pelloni & Gertsch 2000; Takamori *et al.* 2000; Kosugi *et al.* 2004; Jones *et al.* 2005; Liu *et al.* 2007). Both percutaneous core-biopsy and fine-needle aspiration cytology are useful. Fine-needle aspiration may provide a diagnosis for metastatic tumors, but is unlikely to do so for most rare primary liver tumors. Core biopsy is preferred to reliably obtain a benign diagnosis or identify an unusual malignant tumor.

It is reasonable to offer surgery without a preoperative biopsy for operable lesions whose nature can be unequivocally diagnosed clinically, radiologically and biochemically, or where surgery is the first line of treatment and relatively straightforward. Where this is not possible (the lesion is inoperable or the lesion appears malignant and the tumor type is uncertain or there is a definite role for neoadjuvant therapy), a biopsy is indicated.

Treatment

The majority of benign solid lesions with the exception of liver cell adenomas in adults do not need surgery. Liver cell adenomas have a tendency to grow, a risk of rupture and a potential to turn malignant. There is also often some diagnostic uncertainty in differentiating them from well-differentiated hepatocellular carcinomas, and resection is usually advised. Surgery is the first treatment for operable malignant primary tumors in the liver. For more advanced disease there may be a role for neoadjuvant chemotherapy which may render surgery possible.

The approach to management of rare hepatobiliary tumors is based on the same principles as the management of the com-

Box 24.1 Diagnostic imaging algorithm.

Patient with an incidental hepatic mass or known primary malignancy

Elevated AFP, consider
- Hepatocellular carcinoma
- Hepatoblastoma

CT to assess extrahepatic disease and assess site, size of lesion, evidence of dystrophic calcification, biliary obstruction or vascular invasion

Intra-lesional calcification, consider
- Adenoma
- Hepatocellular carcinoma (particularly fibrolamellar)
- Inflammatory pseudotumor
- Epithelioid hemangioendothelioma
- Undifferentiated embryonal sarcoma
- Infantile hemangioendothelioma
- Intrahepatic cholangiocarcinoma
- Liver metastasis (particularly from colorectal adenocarcinoma)

Regional lymphadenopathy, consider
- Hepatocellular carcinoma
- Biliary cystadenocarcinoma

Vascular invasion, consider
- Hepatocellular carcinoma
- Hepatoblastoma
- Epithelioid hemangioendothelioma

Vascular encasement, consider
- Intrahepatic cholangiocarcinoma

MR to characterize the mass, assess multiplicity and determine surgical resectability

Isointense on unenhanced imaging, consider
- Adenoma
- Focal nodular hyperplasia

Intra-lesional fat, consider
- Adenoma (10%)
- Hepatocellular carcinoma

Intra-lesional hemorrhage, consider
- Adenoma
- Hepatocellular carcinoma
- Hepatoblastoma
- Angiosarcoma
- Infantile hemangioendothelioma
- Undifferentiated embryonal sarcoma
- Intrahepatic cholangiocarcinoma

Presence of central scar, consider
- Focal nodular hyperplasia (scar of increased signal on T2W)
- Fibrolamellar hepatocellular carcinoma (scar of decreased signal on T2W)
- Giant hemangioma

moner primary and secondary tumors of the liver. Cure is only achieved by surgical resection but the risk of surgery must be balanced against the likelihood of cure. Major resectional surgery may be supplemented or replaced by various techniques of local ablation, including radiofrequency ablation, cryotherapy, ethanol injection and high intensity focused ultrasound (HIFU) (Geyik *et al.* 2006; Hanajiri *et al.* 2006; Wu 2006).

The process of assessment for surgery addresses whether the tumor is amenable to resection—whether an operation is likely to remove all viable tumor—and whether the patient is likely to survive and benefit from the procedure. Thus accurate preoperative staging by cross-sectional imaging is essential—to assess both the operability of local disease and the presence of disease distant to the local site. Two major factors determining the morbidity and mortality of liver resection are the health and the volume of the remaining liver parenchyma. Thus an extended lobectomy (removing up to 75% of the liver mass) is associated with a mortality more than double that of a less extensive resection (up to 60% of liver mass).

Liver resection is based on the vascular anatomy of the liver—the precise distribution of the major divisions of the portal vein, hepatic arteries and hepatic veins. The most accurate determination of the local anatomy of the tumor can be made preoperatively by a combination of CT and MR scanning. The most sensitive and accurate determination of the location of the tumor(s) in relation to major blood vessels and the presence of subsidiary tumors within the liver is made by intraoperative ultrasound (Hagspiel *et al.* 1995; Yu & Zhong 1999).

The surgical management of multiple tumors within the liver may require a number of smaller resections of liver parenchyma—as 'non-anatomical' or segmental resections. Ablative techniques, particularly radiofrequency ablation, may be used in such cases, either alone or in conjunction with formal resection and can be delivered under either radiologic guidance (percutaneous) or laparoscopic vision.

Individual tumor types

Benign tumors of childhood

Benign hepatic tumors account for less than 35% of all pediatric liver tumors. The large proportion of these include hemangiomas or vascular malformations followed by mesenchymal hamartomas, adenomas and focal nodular hyperplasia.

Mesenchymal hamartoma

These are rare solitary tumor-like hepatic malformations that usually occur in children under 2 years of age. They account for about 6% of all liver tumors in the pediatric age group and have occasionally been reported in adults. An increased incidence in association with tuberous sclerosis has also been reported.

The clinical presentation is one of progressive abdominal distension in an otherwise asymptomatic infant. They are commoner in males (male to female ratio 2 : 1) and in the right lobe of the liver, and appear as large cystic masses that are not encapsulated and bulge into the adjacent liver parenchyma. Both solid and cystic areas are present, but hemorrhage and necrosis are usually absent.

The lesion probably represents a prenatal abnormality of ductal plate development and is related to polycystic disease, congenital hepatic fibrosis and biliary hamartoma (Dehner *et al.* 1975; Cooper *et al.* 1989). Macroscopically these are large smooth and soft fluctuant tumors that contain multiple cystic spaces filled with a fluid or semisolid gelatinous material. On microscopy there is an irregular mesenchyme with bland characteristics and variable biliary and vascular structures, while portal tracts are absent. The gelatinous stroma contains serous fluid and pseudolymphatic spaces. Extramedullary hematopoiesis is frequently present. A consistent 19q13.4 breakpoint has been identified on cytogenetic analysis (Mascarello & Krous 1992).

Biochemical liver function tests are normal and ultrasound, CT and MRI have characteristic appearances. MR findings depend on whether it is predominantly cystic or predominantly mesenchymal. On T1W images, if cystic, there is varying signal depending on the protein concentration within the cyst locules with marked T2W hyperintensity and internal septations. If mesenchymal, there is low signal on T1W and T2W due to fibrosis.

These lesions are considered to be benign (but there are anecdotal reports of possible malignant transformation). The usual indication for surgical resection is a pressure effect from a large tumor on adjacent structures including adjacent normal liver tissue. The prognosis following resection is excellent.

Hemangioendothelioma

Infantile hemangioendothelioma (type I) in combination with hemangiomas, are the commonest benign liver tumor in the pediatric population accounting for about 18% of all pediatric liver tumors (Davenport *et al.* 1995). Nearly all cases are diagnosed during the first 6 months of life. Females outnumber males in a ratio of 2 : 1.

Most children present with progressive abdominal distension, spontaneous hemorrhage being present occasionally. The natural history is of gradual enlargement during the first 6 months of life. Cutaneous hemangiomas may be present as well and suggest the diagnosis. High-output cardiac failure due to massive vascular flow within the tumor is a common presentation of these tumors. Neonates presenting with cardiac failure often have coexisting congenital heart disease that may delay diagnosis. There may be bruising and petechial hemorrhage from thrombocytopenia (Kasabach Merritt syndrome) or disseminated intravascular coagulation.

The tumor is usually multinodular or diffuse, though solitary tumors have been described. Macroscopically they appear red-brown, spongy with variable degrees of scarring. Microscopically they are subdivided into two types, though both may coexist. Type I lesions have numerous intercommunicating vascular channels lined by a single layer of endothelial cells. Large cavernous spaces may form and hemorrhage and infarction are common features. Extramedullary hematopoiesis is frequent and small bile ducts are present throughout (Ishak *et al.* 1984).

A diagnosis can usually be reached by imaging. On MR the mass is multinodular with heterogeneous signal on T1W due to hemorrhage, necrosis and fibrosis and appears hyperintense on T2W, similar to adult hemangioma. Biopsy can be dangerous.

The majority of lesions regress spontaneously after the first year of life and therefore an expectant policy can be adopted in asymptomatic children. Histologically the lesions are very cellular but are not known to have malignant potential.

For those patients presenting with refractory cardiac failure, management with radiologic embolization or surgical ligation of the hepatic arterial inflow to the tumor may be beneficial. Medical options also include steroid therapy, radiotherapy and chemotherapy with cyclophosphamide. Of these, radiotherapy is reserved for resistant cases as there is a potential for developing a second malignancy in the radiated site. Surgical resection is indicated in patients presenting with major hemorrhage. Transfusion of blood or blood products may be necessary for children with DIC.

Epitheloid hemangioendotheliomas (type II) on the other hand are rare in children but occur more commonly in young women. They are are considered to be low-grade malignant lesions and are slow growing, associated with prolonged survival even in the absence of definitive therapy (Lauffer *et al.* 1996; Makhlouf *et al.* 1999). In children these tumors may exhibit a more aggressive pattern of behavior. Microscopically type II hemangioendotheliomas are characterized by nuclear atypia, multilayering and papillary projections of the endothelial cell lining. They may form solid masses that have mitoses. On CT or MR, there is an evolving pattern with multiple nodules initially that coalesce into large masses. There is often compensatory hypertrophy of the uninvolved portions of the liver. Sequential enhanced imaging demonstrates marked enhancement on the arterial phase of scanning which then becomes isointense to the remainder of the liver.

Liver resection is not always possible and in selected cases liver transplantation can be considered, though recurrence after transplantion continues to remain a problem. More recently, successful treatment with interferon alfa has been recorded. In a recent review most patients presented with multifocal tumor that involved both lobes of the liver. Lung, peritoneum, lymph nodes, and bone were the most common sites of extrahepatic involvement at the time of diagnosis. The most common management was liver transplantation (44.8% of patients), followed by no treatment (24.8% of patients), chemotherapy or radiotherapy (21% of patients), and liver resection (9.4% of patients). The 1-year and 5-year patient survival rates were 96% and 54.5%, respectively, after transplantation; 39.3% and 4.5%, respectively, after no treatment, 73.3% and 30%, respectively, after chemotherapy or radiotherapy; and 100% and 75%, respectively, after liver resection (Mehrabi *et al.* 2006). Liver resection, where possible, is the treatment of choice, followed by transplantation, with chemo- or radiotherapy being reserved for cases where there is evidence of extrahepatic disease.

Hepatic hemangioblastomas

These usually occur as a component of von Hippel–Lindau (VHL) syndrome, which is an inherited multisystem disorder characterized by abnormal growth of blood vessels. While blood vessels normally arborize like trees, in people with VHL little collections of capillaries occur referred to as angiomas or hemangioblastomas. Growths may develop in the retina, certain areas of the brain, the spinal cord, the adrenal glands and other parts of the body (Rojiani *et al.* 1991).

The gene for VHL disease is found on chromosome 3, and is inherited in a dominant fashion. The VHL gene is a tumor suppressor gene and its role in a normal cell is to stop uncontrolled growth and proliferation. If the gene is lost or mutated, then its inhibitory effect on cell growth is lost or diminished, which, in combination with defects in other regulatory proteins, can lead to cancerous growth. Like other tumor suppressor genes, VHL seems to act as a 'gatekeeper' to the multistep process of tumorigenesis.

Hemangioblastomas are well-circumscribed lesions that microscopically appear very cellular. Distant metastases are uncommon. Associations of this tumor type with renal cell carcinoma and phaeochromocytomas are well described. VHL is classified as:

type 1 (angiomatosis without pheochromocytoma)
type 2 (angiomatosis with pheochromocytoma)
type 2A (with renal cell carcinoma)
type 2B (without renal cell carcinoma)
type 2C (only pheochromocytoma and no angiomatosis or renal cell carcinoma).

Imaging is usually diagnostic when all the components of the syndrome are present. Complete resection should be performed where possible and is usually curative.

Mature teratomas

There are relatively few cases of teratoma of the liver that have been reported largely in children and occasionally in adults. Most hepatic teratomas are tridermal with components derived from all three germ layers and appear as partially cystic multilobular tumors. Teratomas can coexist with hepatoblastomas and may be associated with chromosomal abnormalities including trisomy 13. The decision regarding treatment has to be based on the individual case as much about the behavior of these lesions is unknown.

Other benign neoplasms

Hemangiomas

Hemangioma is the commonest benign liver tumor. The reported frequency of these lesions based on autopsy series and ultrasounds ranges from 0.4 to 20%. Hemangiomas can present at any age with a female to male ratio of 3:1 (Gandolfi *et al.* 1991). These lesions appear to have different stages in their development that have been described by various synonyms including cavernous and sclerosing hemangiomas as well as solitary fibrous nodule. Small capillary hemangiomas are commoner than their cavernous counterparts. Cavernous hemangiomas may be associated with focal nodular hyperplasia. Cavernous hemangiomas are considered to be vascular malformations that enlarge by ectasia rather than by hyperplasia. They are likely to be congenital in origin and have no potential for malignant transformation. They are often solitary but multiple lesions may be present in up to 40% patients. They are equally distributed between the right and left lobes of the liver. If the lesions are >5 cm in diameter, they are designated as giant hemangiomas (Belli *et al.* 1992).

Macroscopically these appear as well-circumscribed reddish-purple hypervascular lesions that are surrounded by a fibrous capsule. Microscopically there are large blood-filled spaces lined by endothelium and separated by incomplete fibrous septa. Small hemangiomas may become entirely fibrous and stains such as van Gieson-elastic may be needed to identify thick-walled vessels buried in a hyaline mass.

Hemangiomas are usually found incidentally and the large majority require no further treatment once a diagnosis has been made. Large lesions may become symptomatic because of pressure effects, hemorrhage or thrombosis. Clinically these may present as a non-tender upper abdominal mass. Hemangiomas larger than 5 cm in diameter are referred to as giant hemangiomas. Liver function tests are usually normal. Occasionally there may be associated thrombocytopenia (Kasabach–Merritt syndrome).

The appropriate use of two or three complimentary imaging investigations confirms the diagnosis in most cases. On ultrasound the lesions may appear as well-circumscribed hyperechoic lesions with faint acoustic enhancement. Larger lesions may have mixed echogenicity. CT has characteristic appearances of a hypodense mass with lobulated borders in non-contrast scans. Calcification secondary to fibrosis or thrombosis may be seen in up to 10% cases. On contrast enhancement, these lesions show peripheral nodular enhancement in the early post-contrast phase followed by a centripetal pattern of enhancement in the delayed phase.

More recently MR has emerged as a highly accurate technique for diagnosing and characterizing hemangiomas with 73–100% sensivity and 83–97% specificity. MR shows a well-defined mass with a heterogeneous appearance due to areas of thrombosis, fibrosis or hemorrhage. On T1W images, these lesions are of decreased signal relative to normal liver and on T2W images they are heterogenous and markedly hyperintense relative to normal liver. The enhancement pattern is typically of peripheral enhancement with subsequent infilling of the mass over several minutes, the very prolonged and delayed enhancement due to the lack of intratumoral shunting (Fig. 24.2). The enhancement pattern allows distinction from focal nodular hyperplasia (which also has a central scar) and hypervascular metastases.

Labelled red cell scintigraphy using planar and SPECT imaging is highly specific for diagnosing liver hemangiomas, but is rarely required in clinical practice.

Liver biopsy is usually contraindicated because of the low diagnostic yield and particularly the risk of hemorrhage. However it may sometimes be required for hemangiomas with a large fibrous component that is difficult to characterize.

Most hemangiomas tend to remain stable or involute. The role of sex hormones in causing enlargement during pregnancy or recurrence as a result of steroid medication remains disputed. Nearly all hemangiomas can be safely observed once the diagnosis has been established. The risk of spontaneous rupture of a liver hemangioma is very low, regardless of their size. Active intervention is indicated in cases where symptoms are attributed to the hemangioma or, sometimes, where there is doubt as to the diagnosis. The hemangioma can then be either anatomically resected or enucleated, with anatomical resection being generally preferred where safe. Rarely the lesions may reach a size so as to obstruct hepatic outflow and cause a Budd–Chiari syndrome. A number of other therapeutic procedures have been used in cases of large unresectable symptomatic hemangiomata; these include liver transplantation and also external-beam radiotherapy.

Focal nodular hyperplasia

Focal nodular hyperplasia (FNH) is a non-neoplastic tumor-like condition and is the second most common benign hepatic lesion (after hemangioma). The exact incidence is difficult to define, though in autopsy series an incidence of 0.31% has been reported in adults. These lesions can appear at all ages, are commoner in women in their third and fourth decades, and an apparently increasing incidence may simply be a reflection of improvements in imaging technology. This lesion is generally considered to be a developmental vascular malformation of the liver. An abnormally large feeding vessel is believed to induce changes in sinusoidal pressure and stimulate a hyperplastic response (Wanless *et al.* 1985).

FNH usually presents as a well-defined nodular mass that arises in an otherwise normal liver. Lesions can be superficial, deep or pedunculated, vary in colour from tan to yellow and often have a characteristic dimpled external surface. The majority of lesions are <5 cm in diameter. Microscopically these lesions are composed of cords of hepatocytes subdivided by thin

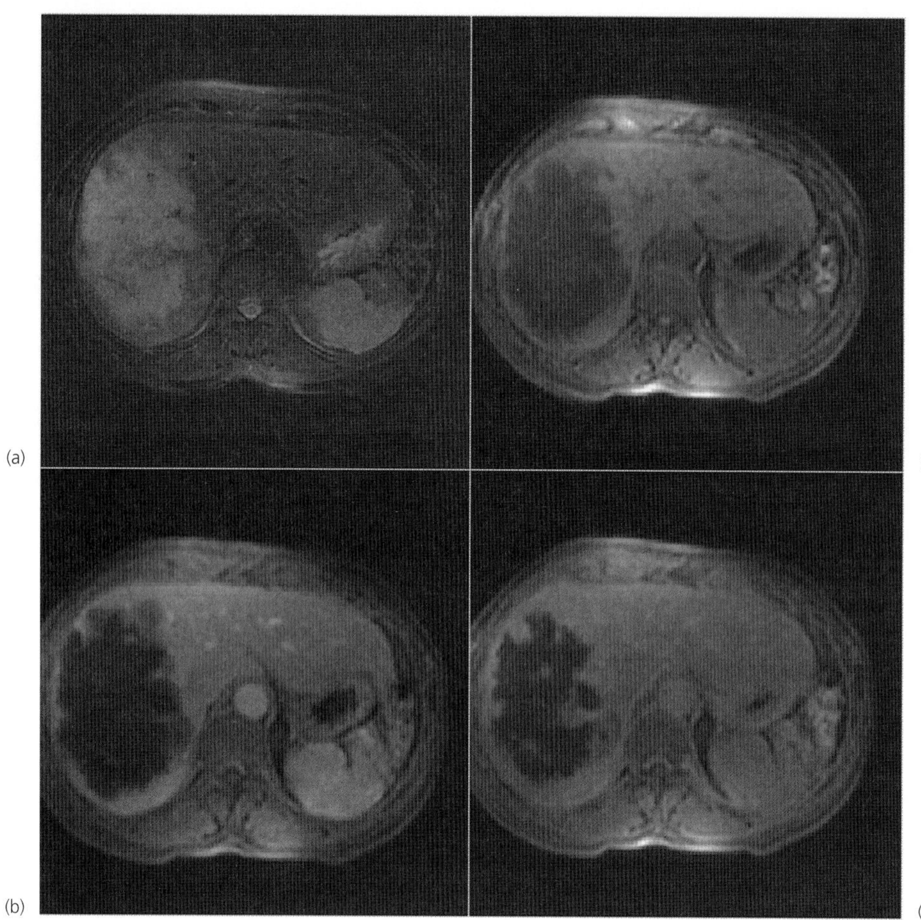

Fig. 24.2 Focal nodular hyperplasia with multiformatted axial MR sequences demonstrating high signal central scar on (a) axial fat suppressed T2W and (b) inversion recovery sequence. The lesion is homogeneous with a central hypointense scar on T1W imaging (c) with marked enhancement post gadolinium and delayed enhancement of the central scar (d).

fibrous septa radiating from a central scar. In 15% of lesions the central scar is not found. Portal tracts and central veins are absent but foci of biliary ductular elements may be present among hepatocytes.

The majority of the patients are asymptomatic and the lesions are usually incidental findings. Symptoms do occur in up to 10% of patients and include vague upper abdominal pain and pressure symptoms. Abdominal examination is usually entirely normal. Very rarely these lesions may bleed, infarct or rupture and therefore present as an acute abdomen. The natural history of these lesions is poorly understood. Increase in size or spontaneous regression appear to occur occasionally.

In most instances FNH can be diagnosed by a combination of imaging studies. Ultrasound lacks specificity but demonstrates a well-defined mass of variable echogenicity. The characteristic central scar is visible in only about 20% cases. Colour Doppler and contrast ultrasound may be able to demonstrate hypervascularity and pulsatile flow in a spoked wheel pattern radiating from the central scar. CT appearances of FNH are variable. On plain scans these appear as homogeneous iso- or hypodense lesions (relative to the normal liver parenchyma). The pathognomonic central scar is frequently absent. On contrast enhancement, these lesions show an immediate transient enhancement after contrast injection. The central scar is best seen as a hypoattenuating area with hyperattenuation of the central feeding vessels. In the portal phase these lesions become isointense. On MR, focal nodular hyperplasia is a homogeneous lesion with a central scar and on T1W images is isointense or occasionally hypointense to normal liver. On T2W images it is usually isointense, or occasionally hyperintense to normal liver. The central scar is hypo- or isointense on T1W and hyperintense on T2W. There is marked enhancement post gadolinium due to its excellent vascularity with delayed enhancement of the central scar (Weimann *et al.* 1997) (Fig. 24.3).

Once the diagnosis of FNH has been made, the vast majority of cases can be simply reassured and observed. The decision to treat is based on a lack of diagnostic certainty or the presence of symptoms. Resection in symptomatic patients alleviates symptoms of vague abdominal pains and or pressure in about 95% of patients. There is a 6% risk that a malignant tumor will be found in patients with an undetermined presumed benign lesion. Surgical excision is therefore preferred for lesions in which the diagnosis is equivocal even after biopsy, and where it can be performed with minimal risk.

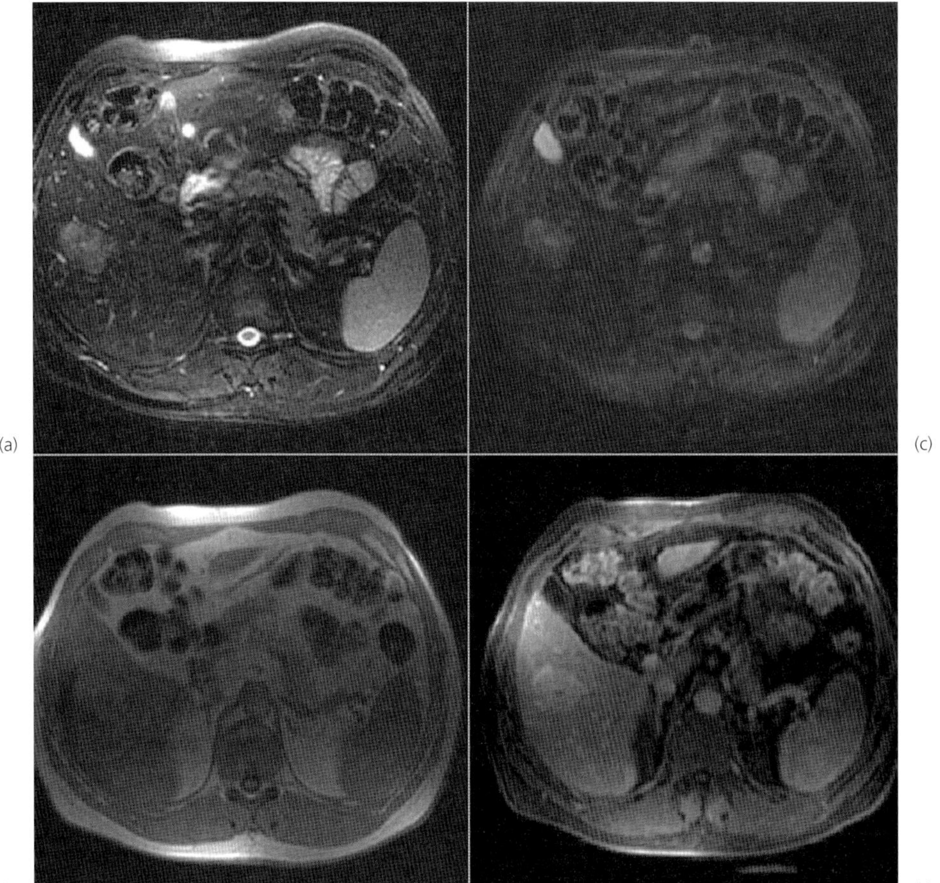

Fig. 24.3 Giant haemangioma. MR demonstrates a well defined lobulated mass with minor internal heterogeneity which is markedly hyperintense on (a) axial fat suppressed T2W image and hypointense on (b) unenhanced T1W image. Following intravenous Gadolinium there is prompt peripheral enhancement on immediate imaging (c) and subsequent infilling of the mass on delayed imaging (d).

Hepatic adenomas

Hepatic adenomas are benign tumors (though some are premalignant) that occur predominantly in young women in the reproductive age group. There is an estimated annual incidence of 3–4 per 100,000 women who are long-term oral contraceptive pill (OCP) users, but only 1 per million population in non-OCP users and women who have used OCPs for less than 2 years. The female to male ratio is reported to be 11 : 1 (Benhamou 1997; Heinemann *et al.* 1998; Mamada *et al.* 2001; Rabe *et al.* 1994).

The development of liver cell adenoma in women taking oral contraceptive steroids relates to dose, duration of usage and increasing age (>30 years) (Rooks *et al.* 1979; Heinemann *et al.* 1998). Of the two common contraceptive steroids, mestranol and ethinyl oestradiol, it was believed that liver cell adenomas were associated more with the former. However, the observed difference is more likely to be due to lower overall doses of the latter. Low-dose oral contraceptives that are used currently seem to carry little risk of tumor development. There is no evidence that the progestogen component of combined medications carries any risk and no association with smoking or alcohol. Other less frequent etiologic agents include clomiphene, danazol, carbamazepine, norethisterone, glycogen storage disease types I, III, IV, familial diabetes mellitus, familial adenomatosis polyposis, Klinefelter syndrome, Hurler's disease and severe combined immune deficiency.

Hepatic adenomas are usually solitary lesions that can achieve considerable size and may sometimes be pedunculated. Macroscopically adenomas have a soft smooth surface and a fleshy appearance with colour ranging from white to brown. Large blood vessels are prominent on the surface of these lesions. The lesions themselves are not encapsulated but develop a pseudocapsule of compressed adjacent liver. Microscopically these are composed of two to three cell thick plates of hepatocytes containing increased deposits of glycogen and fat. These tumors lack the lobular architecture of normal liver and contain no bile ducts. Multiple adenomas are reported to occur in 10–30% of patients (Caballes & Caballes 1999). The presence of more than 10 adenomas in one patient is (arbitrarily) defined as hepatic adenomatosis.

When symptomatic, upper abdominal pain or constitutional symptoms are the usual clinical presentation. Rarely patients may present with massive hemorrhage following intraperitoneal rupture of an adenoma. Liver function tests may be abnormal if the lesion is associated with significant necrosis. In the absence of malignant change these lesions are nearly always associated with a normal αFP.

On ultrasound a hepatic adenoma appears as a well-differentiated hyperechoic lesion. CT appearances are likewise non-specific with appearences of well-demarcated hypodense lesions that may occasionally appear hyperdense because of hemorrhage or necrosis. MR appearances are variable and sometimes these lesions can be difficult to distinguish from hepatocellular cancer. On MRI, adenomas are very similar to the surrounding liver parenchyma on T1W and T2W images. On T1W they may contain areas of high signal due to fatty infiltration or hemorrhage. On T2W, they are heterogeneous with a hypointense rim containing large feeding vessels. They show prompt arterial phase enhancement and become isointense on delayed phases post contrast. Core biopsies are able to diagnose hepatic adenomas, but it can be difficult to differentiate from well-differentiated hepatocellular carcinoma.

Patients with liver cell adenomas are at risk of significant complications including rupture or malignant transformation (Foster & Berman 1994). While this risk is greater in patients who continue to use OCPs or become pregnant, stopping the oral contraceptives does not eliminate this risk. Therefore surgical excision is usually advised, unless their size and number precludes safe resection. Surgical excision should be undertaken in male patients, patients over the age of 50, and those with tumors greater than 5 cm, as there is an increased risk of the tumors being malignant. Bulky lesions causing a mass effect should also be removed. The natural history and biologic behavior of these lesions are poorly understood but elective liver resection for this condition has a less than 1% mortality and low morbidity. Recurrence following resection has not been reported. Patients who present with rupture require emergency intervention. Radiologic embolization can achieve control of hemorrhage in many cases, allowing a more planned approach to liver resection.

Leiomyomatous lesions of the liver

These represent a collection of benign tumors that arise from the mesodermal cell elements within the liver and include leiomyomas, fibromas, fatty tumors amidst a variety of rare tumor types. Hepatic leiomyomas are rare and have mainly been reported in immunodeficient patients. Histologically these have varied appearances, either being composed of monomorphic spindle cells or having a polymorphic appearance with a myxoid stroma and combination of smooth muscle and angiomatous elements. Fibromas are rare and can grow to a considerable size and can have a pedunculated appearance. Focal fatty tumors or fatty nodules composed of either hepatocytes or nodular remanants of non-hepatocyte tissue. Other lipomatous lesions that have been reported in the liver include lipomas and angiomyolipomas (that can occur together with similar renal lesions) that can grow to a considerable size.

A diagnosis can usually be achieved by cross-sectional imaging with ultrasound, CT and MR, occasionally supplemented with a biopsy.

These tumors have a slow indolent course and a benign behavior and usually present as a mass or due to symptoms secondary to pressure effects. Surgical resection when possible may be necessary for symptom control.

Tumor-like lesions in association with acquired immunodeficiency syndrome (AIDS)

This is an interesting group of hepatic conditions that occur in the setting of AIDS but are rare and very unusual in the immunocompetent host. It includes visceral Kaposi's sarcoma, bacillary angiomatosis that has rickettsia like organisms, non-Hodgkin's and Hodgkin's lymphoma, and spindle cell sarcomas in children (Pollock *et al.* 2003). Of these the presence of visceral Kaposi lesions is associated with a poorer prognosis.

Kaposi's sarcoma involves the liver in up to a fifth of autopsied AIDS patients. Primary presentation with hepatic Kaposi's is rare as the liver is usually affected as part of cutaneous and disseminated visceral disease. Macroscopically these appear as 5–10 mm diameter dark red blebs. On cut section. interlacing bands of spindle cells radiate out from the portal triad along the bile ducts. The typical lesion is characterized by bland spindle-shaped cells that arise around bile ducts and form a mesh that contains erythrocytes. Early lesions may be difficult to diagnose as they consist of irregular thin-walled dilated vessels that separate the collagen fibers of capsular and portal connective tissue. Clues to the diagnosis include the diffuse presence of plasma cells, infrequent and normal mitoses, and clusters of intracytoplasmic eosinophillic inclusions which resemble erythrocytes but are smaller. These sarcomas are associated with human herpesvirus 8 infection.

Lymphomas in HIV-infected people are nearly always high-grade B cell in origin and in comparison to non-HIV infected individuals have greater extranodal disease. Typically these lesions develop when the CD4+ lymphocyte counts are less than $100/mm^3$. With improved survival it is expected that the incidence of these lymphomas will rise perhaps to a third of those who survive more than 3 years with AIDS. The liver is involved in over a quarter of AIDS patients with lymphomas, and the liver may be the primary site in these patients. The pathogenesis of these tumors is complicated and associations between the tumors and Epstein–Barr virus and human herpesvirus 8 have been described as well.

Management of Kaposi's sarcoma should be carried out in conjunction with an expert in HIV as definite guidelines do not exist. Factors that need to be considered include the presence of symptoms, effectiveness of antiretroviral therapy, biologic behavior of the lesion and the CD4+ T cell counts (which have a direct relationship with outcome). The various treatment options are outlined in Table 24.2.

Surgery is reserved for rare cases where the tumor becomes symptomatic because of either pressure symptoms or the presence of obstructive jaundice. For the rest, treatment is largely medical. The treatment of HIV-related hepatic lymphoma

Table 24.2 Management of AIDS associated hepatic Kaposi's sarcoma.

Observation and optimization of antiretroviral therapy
Single or limited number of lesions that are symptomatic
Radiation
Intralesional vinblastine
Cryotherapy
Extensive disease
Initial therapy
Interferon-α (if CD4+ T cells < 150/μL)
Liposomal danorubicin
Subsequent therapy
Liposomal doxorubicin
Paclitaxel
Combination chemotherapy with low dose doxorubicin, bleomycin and vinblastine
Radiotherapy

includes combination of highly active antiretroviral therapy and conventional chemotherapy.

Inflammatory pseudotumors

This tumor-like lesion was first recognized in the lungs and thereafter in liver, spleen, pancreas, abdomen, pelvis and orbit. Synonyms include pseudolymphoma, histiocytoma and plasma cell granuloma. Most patients are young with a striking male preponderance.

The etiology and pathogenesis of this condition is poorly understood. Patients often present with symptoms including abdominal pain, fever and weight loss, but jaundice is an uncommon presentation. The lesions occur more commonly in the right lobe of the liver and preponderance in male infants and young adults have been observed.

The histologic picture is dominated by lymphocytic infiltrates with plasma cells, foamy macrophages, lymphoid follicles and giant cells, in a background of spindle cells and marked fibrosis.

Imaging usually reveals a hypovascular lesion. MR appearances are variable, usually mass-like with heterogeneous signal intensity or periportal soft tissue infiltration with a variable enhancement pattern usually hypointense relative to muscle on T1W and hyperintense on T2W. These tumors enhance heterogeneously following contrast.

The biologic behavior of these lesions is not known. Most lesions reported so far have been resected, as they have not been diagnosed before surgery. If the diagnosis is made by biopsy, the lesion can be treated conservatively, and spontaneous regression and response to steroids have been described.

Bile duct adenoma

Bile duct adenomas, also known as benign cholangiomas and cholangioadenomas, are benign intrahepatic epithelial tumors made up of a maze of small bile ducts that are lined by a single layer of cuboidal epithelium that may secrete mucin. They express the same immunophenotype as interlobular bile ducts, but do not communicate with them nor do they have the presence of any bile. It is believed that the tumor is a hamartoma that possibly arises from peribiliary glands. The lesions themselves measure between a few mm to 2 cm in size. They are well circumscribed, non-encapsulated and usually subcapsular. They have a fibrous stroma and may be cellular or hyalinized. The tumor is usually identified as an incidental nodule, often at the time of surgery. The main importance of these lesions is that macroscopically they can be mistaken for liver metastases.

These lesions are benign and require no further treatment once a diagnosis has been established.

Bile duct cystadenoma

Biliary cystadenomas are rare, benign but potentially malignant, multilocular, cystic neoplasms of the biliary ductal system. They usually arise in the liver (80–85%), less frequently in the extrahepatic bile ducts, and rarely in the gallbladder, accounting for less than 5% of cystic neoplasms of the liver. These are rare lesions that are similar in appearance to cystadenomas seen in the pancreas and ovary. They are found more commonly in the liver parenchyma than in the bile duct walls. They are defined as benign cystic tumors lined by mucus-secreting epithelium which may include goblet cells and typically show papillary infoldings. The cells may express carcinoembryonic antigen (Ishak & Rabin 1975).

Two variants have been described—the commoner mucinous and the rarer serous types. The tumors are typically multilocular and macroscopically surrounded by a well-defined fibrous capsule. They are lined by a layer of columnar or cuboidal cells. A basement membrane separates the lining epithelium from the underlying stroma which may be relatively acellular and hyaline, or highly cellular and compacted (mesenchymal).

Mucinous cystadenomas usually occur in middle-aged women and the majority are over 30 years. Approximately 50% present in the right lobe of the liver, 40% in the left lobe and the remainder are bilobar in distribution. Similar cysts may present simultaneously in the pancreas. Serous cystadenomas are rarer (5%) and also have a potential for malignant transformation. The cysts vary in size from a few mm to more than 30 cm in diameter. Symptoms if present are related to size and pressure effects. The premalignant nature or potential for malignant transformation and the tendency to recur, particularly when treated with techniques other than complete excision, are of great concern with these tumors. Furthermore, variable clinical presentation and laboratory and imaging data that are non-specific, preclude reliable differentiation between cystadenoma and cystadenocarcinoma.

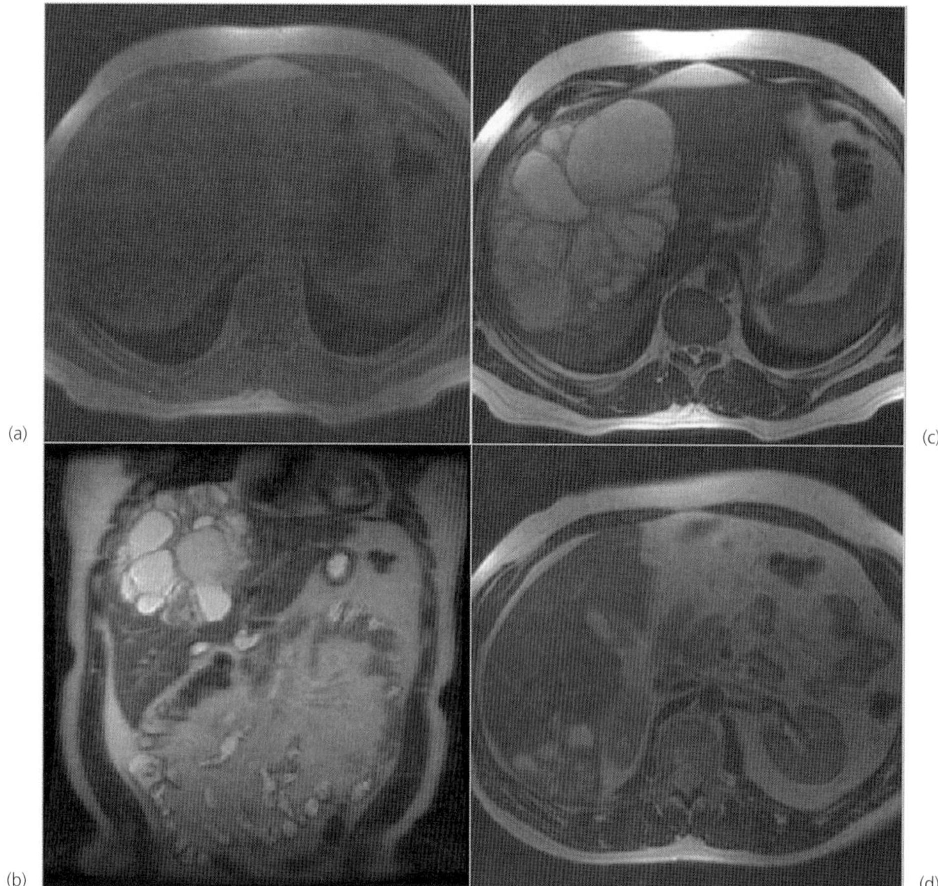

Fig. 24.4 Primary hepatic carcinoid appears as a hypointense mass on T1W imaging (a), a complex multiseptated cystic lesion on T2W in (b) axial and (c) coronal plane and may be multifocal (d).

Of the various hepatic cystic lesions, specific attention should be paid to liver hydatid disease, especially in countries with a high incidence of the disease. They appear morphologically similar to cystadenomas on imaging and can only be differentiated from the latter by serologic tests. Anti-echinococcus granulosis and anti-amebic serologic tests, estimation of CA19-9, CEA and AFP levels, general evaluation of liver and renal function as well as abdominal US, CT and MRI should be performed. Liver function tests may be normal or elevated in cases of intrahepatic or extrahepatic biliary duct compression.

Although they do not rule out cystadenoma when normal, serum CA19-9 levels are believed to be a valuable marker in the diagnosis and monitoring in the postoperative follow-up since they are reported to return to normal after complete resection. Immunoreactivity to CA19-9 is lost when cystadenoma is transformed to cystadenocarcinoma. Measurement of cyst fluid CA19-9 and CEA levels allows differentiation of cystadenomas and cystadenocarcinomas from other hepatic cystic lesions, but is not useful in differentiating between the two (Horsmans *et al.* 1996; Kim 2006; Park *et al.* 2006).

On sonography and CT hepatobiliary cystadenomas exhibit relatively typical findings as a multicystic, space-occupying lesion with septation and papillary mucosal nodes; hence the diagnosis can be made preoperatively in most cases. For differential diagnosis, the malignant form, hepatobiliary cystadenocarcinoma, has to be considered which in the absence of pathognomonic signs of malignancy such as vascular or parietal involvement can only be distinguished from the benign form by histology.

MRI in combination with MRCP is a valuable tool for the diagnosis and differentiation of cystadenoma from other cystic liver lesions. On T1-weighted images, MRI reveals a fluid-containing, multilocular, septated mass with homogenous low signal intensity, the wall and septa of which become enhanced after administration of Gd-DTPA. On T2-weighted images the fluid collections within the tumor demonstrate variable, homogenous high signal intensity while a low-signal-intensity rim represents the wall of the mass. Variable signal intensities on T1- and T2-weighted images depend on the presence of solid components, hemorrhage, and protein content. On T1-weighted images, the signal intensity may change from hypointense to hyperintense while septations may be obscured, and only mild enhancement of the cyst wall is noted after Gd-DTPA administration, as protein concentration and viscosity of the cyst fluid increase. In contrast, on T2-weighted images, signal intensity of the cyst fluid may decrease. Similar changes of the typical MRI appearance of cystadenoma may be caused by internal hemorrhage. MRI can also disclose dilated intrahepatic or extrahepatic bile ducts or demonstrate the relationship of the lesion to vascular structures, and thu, is helpful in planning the surgical procedure.

A preoperative assumption that the lesion is benign based on US, CT or MR findings is not safe and therefore not recommended. The presence of irregular thickness of the wall, mural nodules or papillary projections indicates the possibility of malignancy. Papillary projections in the cyst if seen on contrast-enhanced CT are characteristic of malignant neoplasm. Hypervascularity of mural nodules on CT during arteriography may also indicate malignancy. Septation without nodularity suggests the diagnosis of cystadenoma whereas septation with mural or septal nodules, papillary infoldings, discrete solid masses, and thick, coarse calcifications is suggestive of cystadenocarcinoma. Changes in appearance of the cyst wall may also suggest malignant transformation. Despite these features, however, imaging criteria to differentiate between biliary cystadenoma and cystadenocarcinoma are not reliable.

Complete surgical resection is the treatment of choice for all multiloculated cystic hepatic lesions. If a cystadenoma is suspected or has been diagnosed, surgery is indicated even in asymptomatic patients, since cystadenoma and cystadenocarcinoma cannot be reliably differentiated on the basis of radiologic criteria (Kim 2006). Techniques other than complete excision for treatment of cystic hepatic lesions should not be performed in cystadenomas because they may result in continued tumor growth, recurrence or late malignant transformation of the tumor. Benign biliary cystadenomas are believed to transform to cystadenocarcinomas even decades after partial resection although few of these lesions have been reported. Non-radical therapeutic techniques such as aspiration, fenestration, internal drainage, intratumoral sclerosant application or partial resection of cystadenomas is disappointing since the recurrence rate is extremely high, ranging from 90% to 100% compared to 0–10% after radical resection.

When detected incidentally during surgery for other clinical indications, a complete surgical resection of the tumor should be performed after appropriate staging. Although incidental finding of a cystadenoma after open or laparoscopic fenestration of a hepatic cyst requires complete resection, complete enucleation of the cyst with strict follow-up could be considered as a definitive treatment, with additional surgical intervention only in case of a recurrence or suspicion of malignancy. In cases of communication of an intrahepatic cystadenoma with the biliary tract, biliary fistulae should be confirmed with cholangiography, and if identified, resection of the tumor should be supplemented with suture closure of the fistula.

Biliary papillomatosis

This is a rare condition commoner in middle-aged males (male : female 2 : 1). It is characterized by the presence of multiple papillomas in the intra- and extrahepatic biliary tree. Involvement of the gallbladder and the main pancreatic duct has been reported as well. The lumen of these structures contains soft friable papillary excrescences that are composed of mucus-secreting columnar epithelial cells supported by thin fibrovascular stalks.

The condition is progressive and presents with episodes of hemobilia, obstructive jaundice and sepsis. Temporary treatment measures include curettage and experimental therapies such as photodynamic therapy. Patients usually die from complications of sepsis. Malignant transformation remains a possibility. Liver transplantation is the only potential cure for this condition.

Malignant tumors

Tumors of childhood

Liver cancers comprise about 5% of abdominal solid tumors and 1.1% of all childhood maligancies in the pediatric population. The overall incidence of liver cancer in the age group 0–4 years is in the order of 5 per million population and 1 per million population in other age groups. Hepatoblastoma is the commonest malignant pediatric liver tumor followed by hepatocellular carcinoma and sarcoma.

Hepatoblastoma

Hepatoblastomas comprise 46–64% of malignant liver neoplasms in children. The male to female ratio is about 1.8 : 1. The median age at diagnosis is 18 months though sporadic cases in adults have been reported. Most cases occur before the age of 2½ to 3 years. Congenital hepatoblastomas are rare (Daniel & Kifle 1989; Kaczynski *et al.* 1996; Emre & McKenna 2004).

These tumors may occur in siblings and are associated with Beckwith–Wiedemann syndrome, hemihypertrophy, familial adenomatous polyposis, Gardner's syndrome, glycogen storage disease type 1, trisomy 18, fetal alcohol syndrome, prematurity and low birth weight, maternal exposure to oral contraceptives, gonadotrophins, metals, petroleum products and pigments as well as paternal exposure to certain metals. There is no reported association with chronic liver disease of viral etiology.

Hepatoblastomas present as an abdominal mass (71%), associated with weight loss (24%), anorexia (22%), pain (18%), vomiting (13%), or jaundice (7%).

Five histologic subtypes have been based on light microscopy findings and include fetal, embryonal, mixed mesenchymal, macrotubular, and anaplastic or small cell. The tumor cells appear smaller than normal hepatocytes. Extramedullary hematopoiesis is evident and may be related to the production of cytokines by the tumor. The importance of subtype is in prognostication, with the worst prognosis being the anaplastic or small cell type followed by the embryonal, macrotubular, fetal and mixed mesenchymal variants.

Patients usually have anemia with thrombocytosis and the large majority have elevated α-fetoprotein levels.

On a plain abdominal X-ray these will often show a mass effect; however, this modality has little diagnostic utility. Ultrasound is usually the first imaging modality that is able to differentiate this from renal or adrenal tumors and can also assess blood flow in the tumor. However cross-sectional imaging with CT or MRI is essential to stage the extent of the disease accurately and plan therapy. MR appearances vary with histologic classification; on T1W, the tumor is hypointense to normal liver with focal high-signal areas due to hemorrhage and on T2W, it returns an increased signal. Fibrous septations within the tumor appear as hypointense bands.

An image-guided percutaneous or open biopsy is essential to differentiate the lesion from other tumors such as the malignant germ cell tumor. This is particularly important when neoadjuvant chemotherapy is being contemplated. Although this does impart an increased risk of peritoneal seeding; this is offset by the chemoresponsiveness of these tumors (Schnater *et al.* 2005).

There are various staging classifications. The clinical staging system is based on preoperative assessment and the location of the tumor. The left and right lobes of the liver are divided into lateral and medial and anterior and posterior sectors respectively. The staging system divides patients into four groups depending on the sector(s) involved and vascular involvement. The TNM system stages patients on the basis of tumor size, presence of vascular or lymph node involvement and distant metastasis.

The first clinical decision is whether to initiate neoadjuvant chemotherapy or proceed with surgical resection. While extensive tumors can be downstaged with chemotherapy, thereby facilitating resection, there is no evidence of survival benefit from using neoadjuvant therapy for early, localized tumors that are suitable for resection. One advantage of performing the resection without prior chemotherapy is to reduce the overall need for chemotherapy and minimize the toxic effects of the drugs. However, most patients do not present with resectable disease and therefore require preoperative chemotherapy and a prior liver biopsy. The criteria of inoperability include multifocal and central tumors with significant vascular involvement following chemotherapy. In selected cases there may be a role for liver transplantation. Responsiveness to chemotherapy may be an important prognostic indicator for survival post transplantation. Results following transplantation after chemotherapy to unresectable liver tumors suggest that graft and patient survival rates at 1 year, 3 years and 5 years are in the order of 91%, 91%, and 82% respectively (Reyes *et al.* 2000; Cillo *et al.* 2003).

The 3-year overall survival rates of children with hepatoblastomas has improved from 25% to 80% over the past two decades and can be attributed to progress of chemotherapy regimens. A variety of chemotherapy regimens based on the drugs cisplatin, carboplatinum, doxorubicin, vincristine, adriamycin and actinomycin D have been used. Introduction of cisplatin in the early 1980s was associated with sustained improvement in disease-free survival (Davies *et al.* 2004; Suita *et al.* 2004; Towu *et al.* 2004).

The first chemotherapy regimen that was evaluated in a trial (SIOPEL-1) was using the PLADO regimen (combination cisplatin and adriamycin) preoperatively. 5 years event free and overall survival figures were 66% and 75% respectively (Otte *et al.* 2004). Subsequent studies confirmed that this regimen outperformed earlier regimens albeit at the cost of slightly higher cardiotoxicity. In 1998 following an earlier pilot study (SIOPEL-2) a further study (SIOPEL-3) has been initiated after stratifying the patients into low-risk and high-risk groups based on the presence or absence of vascular invasion, extrahepatic disease and/or metastases. While the results of SIOPEL-3 are awaited, results of SIOPEL-2 suggest that cisplatin alone is effective in low-risk group tumors with a 90% response rate and 91% 3-year overall survival (Perilongo *et al.* 2004). For higher-risk groups no difference in overall survival have been seen between the stratified regimen and the previously used PLADO regimen (Ninane *et al.* 1991).

An overall survival of 60–70% is achievable with non-stage IV hepatoblastoma except for the small cell variant in which the prognosis is poorer (Sasaki *et al.* 2002).

Embryonal sarcoma

Embryonal sarcomas also known as malignant mesenchymoma or undifferentiated sarcoma are very rare primary hepatic tumors in children. The age at diagnosis is between 5 and 15 years.

These tumors are typically diagnosed after 6 years of age with a decline in incidence after 10 years of age. In children, there is a slight male predominance (1.0 : 0.65). In 1978 the reported median survival time was less than 1 year. A recent review of published cases suggests a better outlook with curative surgery with a 5-year survuival of 80% (Weitz *et al.* 2007).

There are no specific clinical features. Tumor-related symptoms might be regarded as abdominal mass with or without upper abdominal pain or swelling. Fever is probably related to the hemorrhage and necrosis found in the majority of these tumors. Jaundice is usually absent. Rupture into the tumor or free rupture into the peritoneal cavity due to rapid growth is not uncommon. Laboratory studies are non-specific, and the α-fetoprotein is not increased.

Radiographs of the abdomen are usually normal. The lesion can be detected by ultrasound, CT and MRI. On CT imaging these tumors appear as hypodense lesions with a pseudocapsule. On MR the tumor is predominantly hypointense relative to the liver on T1W with areas of high signal corresponding to recent hemorrhage. The signal intensity on T2W reflects the cystic or solid nature of the tumor, and if cystic, is markedly hyperintense. Internal debris and septations may be seen on T2W. MRI localizes the lesion more accurately than the other methods, with good resectability correlation. It also can detect vascular invasion, biliary obstruction and hilar adenopathies.

UES of the liver is a neoplasm with primitive mesenchymal phenotype. Tumor size often exceeds 10 cm and can be as large as 30 cm. Macroscopic examination shows a single, well-demarcated, soft, globular mass that frequently has cystic, gelatinous, hemorrhagic and necrotic foci. Microscopic examination reveals a pseudocapsule surrounding a neoplasm, composed predominately of spindle, oval, or stellate cells with ill-defined cell borders. The tumor cells are embedded in an abundant myxoid stroma that contains many thin-walled veins. Bile duct-like structures occasionally appear hyperplastic or reactive, although they, too, may show degenerative changes. Immunohistochemical studies have indicated variable immunoreactivity with antibodies to desmin, muscle-specific actin, and cytokeratin, but not myoglobin. Vimentin and the 'histiocytic' determinants (alpha-1-antitrypsin and alpha-1-antichymotrypsin) are the only consistent immunohistochemical markers expressed by this tumor. However, it is known that the latter two markers are not specific for histiocytes, but are expressed in a range of tissue types including epithelium.

Available treatments include surgery, hepatic arterial ligation, hepatic transplantation, and combinations of surgery and/or chemotherapy and radiation therapy. Radical resection of the tumor is the optimal treatment of choice.

The prognosis for these tumors has been poor until recently and the majority of patients died of tumor recurrence or metastasis within 2 years. The major impediments in achieving long-term, disease-free intervals are local recurrence in the upper abdomen and distant metastases. Recent researchers have shown that pre- and/or postoperative systemic chemotherapy (with cisplatin, andriamycin, cyclophosphamide) and/or radiotherapy, when necessary, can remarkably improve patient's survival. Because the tumor does not produce any characteristic serum markers to permit monitoring of subclinical recurrences, a second-look laparotomy on completion of chemotherapy should be considered. Once there is an evidence of recurrence, resection of the tumor wherever feasible should be performed.

The prognosis is poor and most patients relapse with recurrent disease.

Rhabdomyosarcomas

These are rare highly malignant sarcoma-like lesions. Histologically these are high-grade round cell neoplasms that have abundant cytoplasm with filamentous inclusions. The cells are frequently positive for vimentin and other epithelial antigens. There may be an associated genetic abnormality in chromosome 22.

Rhabdomyosarcomas have no characteristic imaging features, but the diagnosis may be suspected if there are widespread CNS metastases in the presence of a liver mass. These tumors tend to be chemo- and radioresistant. The treatment of choice is surgery if this is feasible.

The prognosis is poor and recurrence and disease progression is usually the rule. Resectional surgery may offer short-term palliation with recurrence and metastases being common.

Germ cell tumors

These are extremely rare tumors and may present as teratomas, choriocarcinomas or yolk sac tumors. In childhood these usually respond to neoadjuvant chemotherapy followed by surgical resection. There have been no studies of adequate size to elucidate the biologic behavior of these lesions.

Other rare malignant neoplasms

Angiosarcomas

Angiosarcomas are rare vascular neoplasms that can occur in the liver in any age group. About 25 cases of this are diagnosed per year in the USA and 1–2 cases per year in the UK. There is a reported association with exposure to arsenic and vinyl chloride-containing compounds as well as exposure to thorotrast, a radiologic contrast agent which is no longer used. Other rare causes include androgenic and anabolic steroids, stilbesterol, oral contraceptives, phenelzine and von Recklinghausen's disease.

The tumor itself is composed of masses of anaplastic spindle cells with sparsely scattered poorly formed vascular channels that are lined by endothelial cells. The tumors tend to be multiple rather than solitary. These are not associated with cirrhosis but can have associated non-cirrhotic periportal and perisinusoidal fibrosis. In a few cases factor VII-related antigen has been demonstrated, suggesting a possible origin from endothelial cells. These tumors tend to be infiltrative. Extramedullary hemopoiesis may be present rarely.

Angiosarcomas usually appear either in children (where some consider these to be a variant of hemangioendothelioma) or later, in the sixth or seventh decades of life. These lesions are locally aggressive and usually present with either an abdominal mass or constitutional symptoms.

There are no specific biochemical changes. Occasionally DIC may be detected.

On dynamic CT these tumors appear as infiltrating enhancing masses that have a centripetal enhancement pattern. If related to thorotrast exposure, high-attenuation thorium deposition may be seen in a reticular pattern in the liver and/or lymph nodes. On MR these lesions appear as a hypointense mass relative to the liver on T1W imaging and is hyperintense on T2W imaging. Peripheral rim enhancement is present after the administration of intravenous gadolinium and persists in the delayed phase images.

The prognosis of these tumors is dismal. Most patients die within 6 months of diagnosis with either liver failure, hypovolemic shock secondary to intra-abdominal hemorrhage or due to disseminated metastasis, particularly to the lung.

Surgical excision is the only effective therapeutic option though the large majority of tumors are inoperable at presentation. This tumor is neither radio- nor chemosensitive and therefore, these modalities do not have a role in the management of this condition.

Leiomyosarcoma

There are a few isolated reports of primary leiomyosarcomas of the liver. These have to be differentiated from metastatic sarcoma that may present as late as 15 years after successful treatment of the primary. These lesions may be related to mesenchymal elements in the inferior vena cava or portal vein. Clinically they present as a mass with or without constitutional symptoms. Imaging appearances may vary and the lesions may appear solid or cystic on imaging depending on their morphology and contents.The natural history of these lesions is to progress slowly and eventually cause liver failure or (rarely) rupture causing intraperitoneal hemorrhage. These tumors like their counterparts elsewhere are relatively chemo- and radiotherapy resistant. Surgical resection where possible is the treatment of choice.

Hepatic carcinoids

Primary hepatic carcinoid tumors are extremely rare. The vast majority of carcinoid tumors of the liver are metastatic either from the gastrointestinal tract or from the bronchus. These tumors have a protracted indolent course and therefore have a more favourable prognosis compared to other primary tumors of the liver. If hepatic carcinoid tumors are functional (secreting), because of direct secretion into the systemic circulation, avoiding the hepatic first-pass effect, these patients are likely to present with the carcinoid syndrome with cutaneous flushing, diarrhea, asthma and cardiac disease including dyspnea on exertion and abnormalities of the pulmonary and tricuspid valves leading to their incompetence. The estimated annual incidence is about 1 per million population.

These tumors arise from cells derived from the neuroectoderm. These are variably referred to as APUD or enterochromaffin cells. In the case of metastatic carcinoid disease, the commonest site for the primary is the appendix, followed by the small bowel, colon and stomach. Clinically these tumors present with an abdominal mass and the carcinoid syndrome.

The presence of functioning carcinoids can be detected by measuring urinary 5-HIAA and serum levels of various markers based on the presentation of the patient. The list of potential markers for GEP-NETs is long. Aside from the hormones of secretory tumors, the most important markers are chromogranin A (CgA), neuron-specific enolase (NSE, gamma-gamma dimer) and synaptophysin (P38). Other markers include synaptobrevin (VAMP-1), synapsin (1A, 1B, 2A, 2B), SV2, protein P65, protein S-100, protein gene product (PGP) 9.5, intermediate filaments (cytokeratins, vimentin, neurofilaments), protein 7B2, chromogranin B (secretogranin I), chromogranin C (secretogranin II), pancreastatin, vasostatin, cytochrome b561, leu-7 (HNK-1), calcitonin, human chorionic gonadotropin-alpha (HCG-α), human chorionic gonadotropin-beta (HCG-), thyroid function tests (TFTs), parathyroid hormone (PTH), calcium, prolactin, α-fetoprotein, carcinoembryonic antigen (CEA), β-human chorionic gonadotrophin (β-HCG), CGRP, GRP, PYY, hCGα, N Peptide K, neurokinin A, serotonin, neurotensin, motilin, substance P, histamine, catecholamines, dopa, various rarer peptide hormones, synaptotagmin and HISL-19. Newer (as of 2005) markers include N-terminally truncated variant of heat shock protein 70 (Hsp70), CDX-2, a homeobox gene product and neuroendocrine secretory protein-55. Aside from their use in diagnosis, some markers can track the progress of therapy while the patient avoids the detrimental side-effects of CT scan contrast.

On dynamic CT these tumors appear as enhancing small well-circumscribed lesions and are usually multiple. The functional state of these lesions can be assessed by a combination of radionucleide MIBG (metaiodobenzylguanidine) or an octreotide scan. MIBG has a structure similar to noradrenaline and is therefore taken up by cells of neural crest origin and APUD cells and concentrated in chromaffin granules. Tagging the compound with I^{131} allows detection of cells that preferentially concentrate MIBG. A number of carcinoids have somatostatin receptors on their cells and this forms the basis of a labeled octreotide scan which is an effective targeting agent.

The management of carcinoid disease is complex. Asymptomatic patients with small tumor volume can be observed as these tumors have an indolent course. If the patient is symptomatic, a variety of treatment options can be tried, including short- and long-acting somatostatin analogs for symptom control.

Surgery is indicated for symptom control or relieving pressure effects by debulking. Where surgery is not possible, targeted therapy with radiolabelled octreotide or MIBG can be used to treat these tumors. Alternatively the tumors can be chemoembolized via the appropriate feeding hepatic artery to allow regression of tumor growth and hypertrophy of normal liver. Local ablation with radiofrequency or a cryoprobe can also be used where appropriate. In refractory cases in the absense of demonstrable extrahepatic disease a liver transplant can be considered.

Biliary cystadenocarcinomas

Biliary cystadenocarcinoma is a rare tumor arising in a healthy liver. Prognosis is better than other malignant tumors of the liver. It frequently develops in a pre-existing benign biliary cystadeonoma and usually occurs in middle-aged women. This tumor is difficult to diagnose because of the lack of specificity of clinical, biologic and radiologic features.

The tumor is believed to arise from intrahepatic bile ducts or simple liver cyst, occasionally originating from benign cystadenoma. There is some evidence that cystadenocarcinoma is derived from a primitive hepatobiliary stem cell, since the neoplasm involves primarily the hepatic parenchyma. It is estimated that cystic neoplasm constitutes approximately 5% of liver cysts, among which the malignancy is about 5%. The overall incidence among hepatic malignant tumors is lower than 0.41%. Although rare, these cystic neoplasms are being revealed with increasing frequency due to the advances in abdominal imaging, particularly ultrasonography, CT, and MRI.

Grossly, most cystadenocarcinomas are multilocular cysts with internal septa and nodularity of the inner wall. The presence of septa without nodularity also can be seen in cystadenomas. The fluid of the cystic cavity often consists of a high-molecular-weight glycoprotein called mucin. However, hemorrhagic, bilious, clear, and mixed fluid contents have also been observed. Histologically, cystadenocarcinomas are lined by cuboid or columnar epithelium and surrounded by dense collagenous tissues. The tumor cells are well differentiated and have malignant predisposition with atypia, abnormal mitotic figure and invasion of the basement membrane.

Clinical manifestations of cystadenocarcinomas can vary widely. The majority of patients present with upper abdominal pain or discomfort. Unusual manifestations include jaundice, cholangitis, tumor rupture, intracystic hemorrhage, compression of the portal vein or vena cava, which can result in ascites formation, edema, and stone formation. The most frequent finding on physical examination is a palpable upper abdominal mass. Occasionally, a patient may have the cystadenoma found incidentally by surgical exploration.

Liver function tests are usually normal unless the biliary tree is compressed. The elevation of alkaline phosphatase and bilirubin occurs in cases of bile duct obstruction. CA19-9 may be elevated, but the CEA and fetoprotein are usually normal. Although none of these tumor markers offer specific evidence for dignosis, they should be considered in patients suspected of having a cystadenocarcinoma.

Preoperative imaging is critically important since to date there is no special marker for a definite diagnosis of these lesions. US, CT and MRI are more accurate in locating the tumor than distinguishing between benign and malignant tumor. Appearances that suggest cystadenocarcinoma include the presence of one or more of the following items: multilocular hypodense mass with echogenic internal septations and papillary projections into the cystic space, and coarse or rugged mass wall, hemorrhage or necrosis in the cyst, and mass wall with fine septal calcifications.

The only curative therapy for cystadenocarcinoma is complete resection with at least 1-cm margins, for which a major liver resection is usually required. Partial removal or enucleation inevitably fails after relapse of disease. Biopsy is necessary for confirmation of the surgical removal. Cystadenocarcinomas have a high recurrence rate even after total surgical resection. Neither chemotherapy nor radiotherapy are effective for cystadenocarcinoma.

Conclusion

Liver lesions are increasingly being diagnosed and referred to hepatobiliary MDTs for evaluation. Common benign lesions and rare liver tumors are part of the differential diagnosis for a liver lesion. To establish a diagnosis, information from a variety of sources needs to be collated and analysed to draw valid conclusions. An MDT approach ensures that the information has been collected and that the treatments offered are either evidence-based or would be considered as best practice. This is especially important as very little about the natural history of these tumors is known.

References

Belli L, De Carlis L, Beati C, Rondinara G, Sansalone V, Brambilla G. (1992) Surgical treatment of symptomatic giant hemangiomas of the liver. *Surg Gynecol Obstet* 174(6): 474–8.

Benhamou JP. (1997) [Oral contraceptives and benign tumors of the liver.] *Gastroenterol Clin Biol* 21(12): 913–15.

Boffetta P, Matisane L, Mundt KA, Dell LD. (2003) Meta-analysis of studies of occupational exposure to vinyl chloride in relation to cancer mortality. *Scand J Work Environ Health* 29(3): 220–9.

Caballes RL, Caballes RA. (1999) Multiple hepatocellular adenomas in a patient with a history of oral contraception. *Int J Gynaecol Obstet* 64(2): 177–80.

Cillo U, Ciarleglio FA, Bassanello M *et al.* (2003) Liver transplantation for the management of hepatoblastoma. *Transplant Proc* 35(8): 2983–5.

Cooper K, Hadley G, Moodley P. (1989) Mesenchymal hamartoma of the liver. A report of 5 cases. *S Afr Med J* 75(6): 295–8.

Daniel E, Kifle A. (1989) An unusual presentation of hepatoblastoma. *Ethiop Med J* 27(4): 231–4.

Davenport M, Hansen L, Heaton ND, Howard ER. (1995) Hemangioendothelioma of the liver in infants. *J Pediatr Surg* 30(1): 44–8.

Davies JQ, de la Hall PM, Kaschula RO *et al.* (2004) Hepatoblastoma—evolution of management and outcome and significance of histology of the resected tumor. A 31-year experience with 40 cases. *J Pediatr Surg* 39(9): 1321–7.

Dehner LP, Ewing SL, Sumner HW. (1975) Infantile mesenchymal hamartoma of the liver. Histologic and ultrastructural observations. *Arch Pathol* 99(7): 379–82.

Emre S, McKenna GJ. (2004) Liver tumors in children. *Pediatr Transplant* 8(6): 632–8.

Foster JH, Berman MM. (1994) The malignant transformation of liver cell adenomas. *Arch Surg* 129(7): 712–17.

Gandolfi L, Leo P, Solmi L, Vitelli E, Verros G, Colecchia A. (1991) Natural history of hepatic haemangiomas: clinical and ultrasound study. *Gut* 32(6): 677–80.

Geiser CF, Baez A, Schindler AM, Shih VE. (1970) Epithelial hepatoblastoma associated with congenital hemihypertrophy and cystathioninuria: presentation of a case. *Pediatrics* 46(1): 66–73.

Geyik S, Akhan O, Abbasoglu O *et al.* (2006) Radiofrequency ablation of unresectable hepatic tumors. *Diagn Interv Radiol* 12(4): 195–200.

Hagspiel KD, Neidl KF, Eichenberger AC, Weder W, Marincek B. (1995) Detection of liver metastases: comparison of superparamagnetic iron oxide-enhanced and unenhanced MR imaging at 1.5 T with dynamic CT, intraoperative US, and percutaneous US. *Radiology* 196(2): 471–8.

Hanajiri K, Maruyama T, Kaneko Y *et al.* (2006) Microbubble-induced increase in ablation of liver tumors by high-intensity focused ultrasound. *Hepatol Res* 36(4): 308–14.

Heinemann LA, Weimann A, Gerken G, Thiel C, Schlaud M, DoMinh T. (1998) Modern oral contraceptive use and benign liver tumors: the German Benign Liver Tumor Case-Control Study. *Eur J Contracept Reprod Health Care* 3(4): 194–200.

Horsmans Y, Laka A, Gigot JF, Geubel AP. (1996) Serum and cystic fluid CA19-9 determinations as a diagnostic help in liver cysts of uncertain nature. *Liver* 16(4): 255–7.

Ishak KG. (1995) Benign tumours of the liver. In: Berk JE, ed. *Gastroenterology*, 5th edn, pp. 2428–43. WB Saunders, Philadelphia.

Ishak KG, Rabin L. (1975) Benign tumors of the liver. *Med Clin North Am* 59(4): 995–1013.

Ishak KG, Sesterhenn IA, Goodman ZD, Rabin L, Stromeyer FW. (1984) Epithelioid hemangioendothelioma of the liver: a clinicopathologic and follow-up study of 32 cases. *Hum Pathol* 15(9): 839–52.

Ishak KG, Anthony PP, Sobin LH (2003) *Histological Typing of Tumours of the Liver*. Springer-Verlag.

Jones OM, Rees M, John TG, Bygrave S, Plant G. (2005) Biopsy of resectable colorectal liver metastases causes tumour dissemination and adversely affects survival after liver resection. *Br J Surg* 92(9): 1165–8.

Kaczynski J, Hansson G, Wallerstedt S. (1996) Incidence of primary liver cancer and aetiological aspects: a study of a defined population from a low-endemicity area. *Br J Cancer* 73(1): 128–32.

Kim HG. (2006) [Biliary cystic neoplasm: biliary cystadenoma and biliary cystadenocarcinoma.] *Korean J Gastroenterol* 47(1): 5–14.

Kim SH, Lim HK, Lee WJ, Cho JM, Jang HJ. (2000) Needle-tract implantation in hepatocellular carcinoma: frequency and CT findings after biopsy with a 19.5-gauge automated biopsy gun. *Abdom Imaging* 25(3): 246–50.

Kosugi C, Furuse J, Ishii H *et al.* (2004) Needle tract implantation of hepatocellular carcinoma and pancreatic carcinoma after ultrasound-guided percutaneous puncture: clinical and pathologic characteristics and the treatment of needle tract implantation. *World J Surg* 28(1): 29–32.

Koufos A, Hansen MF, Copeland NG, Jenkins NA, Lampkin BC, Cavenee WK. (1985) Loss of heterozygosity in three embryonal tumours suggests a common pathogenetic mechanism. *Nature* 316(6026): 330–4.

Koufos A, Grundy P, Morgan K *et al.* (1989) Familial Wiedemann–Beckwith syndrome and a second Wilms tumor locus both map to 11p15.5. *Am J Hum Genet* 44(5): 711–19.

Lauffer JM, Zimmermann A, Krahenbuhl L, Triller J, Baer HU. (1996) Epithelioid hemangioendothelioma of the liver. A rare hepatic tumor. *Cancer* 78(11): 2318–27.

Levy AD, Murakata LA, Abbott RM, Rohrmann CA Jr. (2002) From the archives of the AFIP. Benign tumors and tumorlike lesions of the gallbladder and extrahepatic bile ducts: radiologic-pathologic correlation. Armed Forces Institute of Pathology. *Radiographics* 22(2): 387–413.

Lewis, R, Rempala G. (2003) A case–cohort study of angiosarcoma of the liver and brain cancer at a polymer production plant. *J Occup Environ Med* 45(5): 538–45.

Little MH, Thomson DB, Hayward NK, Smith PJ. (1988) Loss of alleles on the short arm of chromosome 11 in a hepatoblastoma from a child with Beckwith–Wiedemann syndrome. *Hum Genet* 79(2): 186–9.

Liu YW, Chen CL, Chen YS, Wang CC, Wang SH, Lin CC. (2007) Needle tract implantation of hepatocellular carcinoma after fine needle biopsy. *Dig Dis Sci* 52(1): 228–31.

Makhlouf HR, Ishak KG, Goodman ZD. (1999) Epithelioid hemangioendothelioma of the liver: a clinicopathologic study of 137 cases. *Cancer* 85(3): 562–82.

Mamada Y, Onda M, Tajiri T *et al.* (2001) Liver cell adenoma in a 26-year-old man. *J Nippon Med Sch* 68(6): 516–19.

Mascarello JT, Krous HF. (1992) Second report of a translocation involving 19q13.4 in a mesenchymal hamartoma of the liver. *Cancer Genet Cytogenet* 58(2): 141–2.

Mehrabi A, Kashfi A, Fonouni H *et al.* (2006) Primary malignant hepatic epithelioid hemangioendothelioma: a comprehensive review of the literature with emphasis on the surgical therapy. *Cancer* 107(9): 2108–21.

Ninane J, Perilongo G, Stalens JP, Guglielmi M, Otte JB, Mancini A. (1991) Effectiveness and toxicity of cisplatin and doxorubicin (PLADO) in childhood hepatoblastoma and hepatocellular carcinoma: a SIOP pilot study. *Med Pediatr Oncol* 19(3): 199–203.

Otte JB, Pritchard J, Aronson DC *et al.* (2004) Liver transplantation for hepatoblastoma: results from the International Society of Pediatric Oncology (SIOP) study SIOPEL-1 and review of the world experience. *Pediatr Blood Cancer* 42(1): 74–83.

Park KH, Kim JS, Lee JH *et al.* (2006) [Significances of serum level and immunohistochemical stain of CA19–9 in simple hepatic cysts and intrahepatic biliary cystic neoplasms.] *Korean J Gastroenterol* 47(1): 52–8.

Pelloni A, Gertsch P. (2000) [Risks and consequences of tumor seeding after percutaneous fine needle biopsy four diagnosis of hepatocellular carcinoma.] *Schweiz Med Wochenschr* 130(23): 871–7.

Perilongo G, Shafford E, Maibach R *et al.* (2004) Risk-adapted treatment for childhood hepatoblastoma. final report of the second study of the International Society of Paediatric Oncology—SIOPEL 2. *Eur J Cancer* 40(3): 411–21.

Pollock BH, Jenson HB, Leach CT *et al.* (2003) Risk factors for pediatric human immunodeficiency virus-related malignancy. *JAMA* 289(18): 2393–9.

Powers C, Ros PR, Stoupis C, Johnson WK, Segal KH (1994) Primary liver neoplasms: MR imaging with pathologic correlation. *Radiographics* 14: 459–82.

Rabe T, Feldmann K, Grunwald K, Runnebaum B. (1994) Liver tumours in women on oral contraceptives. *Lancet* 344(8936): 1568–9.

Rainier S, Dobry CJ, Feinberg AP. (1995) Loss of imprinting in hepatoblastoma. *Cancer Res* 55(9): 1836–8.

Reyes JD, Carr B, Dvorchik I *et al.* (2000) Liver transplantation and chemotherapy for hepatoblastoma and hepatocellular cancer in childhood and adolescence. *J Pediatr* 136(6): 795–804.

Rojiani AM, Owen DA, Berry K *et al.* (1991) Hepatic hemangioblastoma. An unusual presentation in a patient with von Hippel-Lindau disease. *Am J Surg Pathol* 15(1): 81–6.

Rooks JB, Ory HW, Ishak KG *et al.* (1979) Epidemiology of hepatocellular adenoma. The role of oral contraceptive use. *JAMA* 242(7): 644–8.

Sasaki F, Matsunaga T, Iwafuchi M *et al.* (2002) Outcome of hepatoblastoma treated with the JPLT-1 (Japanese Study Group for Pediatric Liver Tumor) Protocol-1: A report from the Japanese Study Group for Pediatric Liver Tumor. *J Pediatr Surg* 37(6): 851–6.

Schnater JM, Kuijper CF, Zsiros J, Heij HA, Aronson DC. (2005) Pre-operative diagnostic biopsy and surgery in paediatric liver tumours—the Amsterdam experience. *Eur J Surg Oncol* 31(10): 1160–5.

Scrable HJ, Witte DP, Lampkin BC, Cavenee WK. (1987) Chromosomal localization of the human rhabdomyosarcoma locus by mitotic recombination mapping. *Nature* 329(6140): 645–7.

Simms LA, Reeve AE, Smith PJ. (1995) Genetic mosaicism at the insulin locus in liver associated with childhood hepatoblastoma. *Genes Chromosomes Cancer* 13(1): 72–3.

Simonato L, L'Abbe KA, Andersen A *et al.* (1991) A collaborative study of cancer incidence and mortality among vinyl chloride workers. *Scand J Work Environ Health* 17(3): 159–69.

Sotelo-Avila C, Gonzalez-Crussi F, Fowler JW. (1980) Complete and incomplete forms of Beckwith-Wiedemann syndrome: their oncogenic potential. *J Pediatr* 96(1): 47–50.

Suita S, Tajiri T, Takamatsu H *et al.* (2004) Improved survival outcome for hepatoblastoma based on an optimal chemotherapeutic regimen—a report from the study group for pediatric solid malignant tumors in the Kyushu area. *J Pediatr Surg* 39(2): 195–8.

Takamori R, Wong LL, Dang C, Wong L. (2000) Needle-tract implantation from hepatocellular cancer: is needle biopsy of the liver always necessary?. *Liver Transpl* 6(1): 67–72.

Towu E, Kiely E, Pierro A, Spitz L. (2004) Outcome and complications after resection of hepatoblastoma. *J Pediatr Surg* 39(2): 199–202.

Wanless IR, Mawdsley C, Adams R. (1985) On the pathogenesis of focal nodular hyperplasia of the liver. *Hepatology* 5(6): 1194–1200.

Weimann A, Ringe B, Klempnauer J *et al.* (1997) Benign liver tumors: differential diagnosis and indications for surgery. *World J Surg* 21(9): 983–90.

Weinberg AG, Finegold MJ. (1983) Primary hepatic tumors of childhood. *Hum Pathol* 14(6): 512–37.

Weinberg AG, Finegold MJ (1986) Primary hepatic tumours in childhood. In: Finegold MJ, ed. *Pathology of Neoplasia in Children and Adolescents - Major problems in Pathology*, 1st edn, pp. 333–72. WB Saunders, Philadelphia.

Weitz J, Klimstra DS, Cymes K *et al.* (2007) Management of primary liver sarcomas. *Cancer* 109(7): 1391–6.

Wu F. (2006) Extracorporeal high intensity focused ultrasound in the treatment of patients with solid malignancy. *Minim Invasive Ther Allied Technol* 15(1): 26–35.

Ye MQ, Suriawinata A, Ben Haim M, Parsons R, Schwartz ME. (1999) A 42-year-old woman with liver masses and long-term use of oral contraceptives. *Semin Liver Dis* 19(3): 339–44.

Yu J, Zhong S. (1999) Intraoperative ultrasound for hepatic neoplasm during surgery. *Chin Med Sci J* 14(3): 170–3.

25 Cystic neoplasms of the pancreas

Edited by Peter J. Allen

Diagnosis and imaging

John Mansour & Lawrence Schwartz

Introduction

Cystic neoplasms of the pancreas present some of the most challenging diagnostic and treatment problems confronting pancreatic clinicians today. The primary difficulty in the management of these patients arises from the fact that in many instances the specific histopathologic diagnosis cannot be determined without operative resection. Cystic lesions of the pancreas may represent benign lesions without malignant potential, premalignant lesions that may progress to malignancy, or malignant processes. Resection could be avoided in many instances if the histopathologic diagnosis could be established with laboratory assessment, imaging, aspiration or biopsy.

The most important question when formulating a treatment plan for a patient with a cystic neoplasm of the pancreas is whether that lesion has the potential for harboring or progressing into malignancy. Serous lesions tend to follow a benign course, but mucinous lesions (intraductal papillary mucinous neoplasms and mucinous cystic neoplasms) may present with or progress to malignancy. Formulating a rational treatment plan requires physicians to be familiar with the clinical, epidemiologic, histologic, radiographic, and pathologic features of all lesions that may present as pancreatic cysts.

In this section, we will describe the clinical presentation and diagnostic work-up for the most common types of primary pancreatic cystic lesions. The focus will be on patient presentation, and typical radiographic findings of these lesions. Endoscopic features, particularly those features seen with endoscopic ultrasound (EUS), are the focus of a subsequent section.

Gastrointestinal Oncology: A Critical Multidisciplinary Team Approach.
Edited by J. Jankowski, R. Sampliner, D. Kerr, and Y. Fong.

Presentation

Most authors have reported that cystic neoplasms of the pancreas comprise approximately 15% of pancreatic cystic lesions and 1% of pancreatic cancers (Becker *et al.* 1965; Cubilla 1984; Horvath & Chabot 1999). Because of an increased use of high-quality cross-sectional imaging the identification of pancreatic cysts seems to be increasing. At Massachusetts General Hospital, cystic lesions of the pancreas comprised 16% of cases in 1991 and 30% of cases in 1998. In a series of 539 patients with cystic lesions of the pancreas seen at Memorial Sloan-Kettering Cancer Center, the annual number of patients evaluated increased from 7 patients in 1995 to 117 patients in 2004. In addition, as the study period progressed, the initial size of the evaluated lesions decreased (from 4.5 cm to 3.0 cm) and the percentage of patients with incidentally identified lesions increased (from 70% to 85%) (Allen *et al.* 2003).

Patient characteristics

The distribution of cystic lesions between genders varies according to histologic type (Brugge *et al.* 2004a). If all histologic types are included, women account for 63–71% of all patients with cystic neoplasms of the pancreas (Walsh *et al.* 2005; Allen *et al.* 2006). Much of this gender difference is explained by the near-complete predisposition of mucinous cystic neoplasms (MCN) to occur in women (Table 25.1). More than 95% of MCN have been described in the female population (Warshaw *et al.* 1990; Le Borgne *et al.* 1999). Some authors have even suggested that these lesions never develop in men (Thompson *et al.* 1999). Serous cystic neoplasms (SCN) and intraductal papillary mucinous neoplasms (IPMN) are more evenly distributed between genders but tend to occur more often in women (Sarr *et al.* 2001; Sohn *et al.* 2004).

The mean age at diagnosis for pancreatic cystic lesions is approximately 56–64 years (Walsh *et al.* 2005; Allen *et al.* 2006). Patients with IPMN tend to be several years older on average (Sarr *et al.* 2003; Sohn *et al.* 2004). Some authors have noted that malignant IPMN tend to occur in slightly older patients

Table 25.1 Patient and cyst characteristics.

	Pseudocyst	Serous cystic neoplasm	Mucinous cystic neoplasm	Intraductal papillary mucinous neoplasm
Age (mean, years)	45–50	62	50–55	62–67
Gender (% male)	65–75	30	5	45
Pancreatitis history (%)	80	Uncommon	Uncommon	20
Location (% proximal)	34	50	25	70
Symptomatic (%)	>80	20–30	30–40	>50

than do benign IPMN (mean 68.2 years vs 63.2 years). A study from Johns Hopkins suggested that this difference in mean age was reflective of a 5-year time period for progression from adenoma to malignant IPMN (Sohn *et al.* 2004). This finding has also been reported for MCN of the pancreas. Malignant MCN have been reported to have a higher median age at diagnosis by approximately 15 years when compared to their benign counterparts (de Calan *et al.* 1995; Sakorafas & Sarr 2005).

Included in the differential diagnosis of any pancreatic cystic lesion is pancreatitis-associated pseudocyst. As with cystic pancreatic neoplasms, pseudocysts can present with symptoms including abdominal pain, nausea, early satiety or jaundice (Warshaw & Rutledge 1987). Although difficult to pinpoint from retrospective series, a history of pancreatitis may be reported in up to 36% of patients with cystic lesions of the pancreas (Warshaw *et al.* 1990; Talamini *et al.* 1992; Fernandez-del Castillo *et al.* 2003; Kitagawa *et al.* 2003; D'Angelica *et al.* 2004). Interestingly, among patients with a history of pancreatitis, approximately 50% will have a diagnosis other than pseudocyst.

Presenting symptoms

The presence of symptoms among patients with cystic lesions of the pancreas varies between 25 and 67% (Allen *et al.* 2003; Fernandez-del Castillo *et al.* 2003; Walsh *et al.* 2005). As the use of high-quality cross-sectional imaging has increased, the identification of asymptomatic cystic lesions has become more common (Allen *et al.* 2003). When present, the most common symptoms include abdominal pain, weight loss, back pain, or jaundice (Fernandez-del Castillo *et al.* 2003). Incidental cysts typically present among older patients and are significantly smaller than among symptomatic patients.

The presence of symptoms in any patient with a cystic lesion of the pancreas should alert the clinician to the possibility of underlying malignancy (Hashimoto *et al.* 1998; Fernandez-del Castillo *et al.* 2003). Mucinous lesions have been associated with symptoms more frequently than serous lesions (Sarr *et al.* 2001). Symptomatic patients may harbor malignancy in up to 40% of cases.

Among patients with malignant mucinous tumors, a palpable mass, obstructive jaundice, or weight loss may be observed in approximately 50% of cases (Kerlin *et al.* 1987; de Calan *et al.* 1995; Sohn *et al.* 2004). Jaundice appears to be a particularly ominous sign and may be associated with malignancy in as many as 75% of cases (Sohn *et al.* 2004). Biliary obstruction is a component of the presentation of invasive IPMN more often than with non-invasive IPMN (33% vs 7%) (Sohn *et al.* 2004).

The absence of symptoms, however, does not preclude the possibility of malignancy (Le Borgne *et al.* 1999). Some series have shown that as many as 20% of incidentally discovered lesions may be malignant when resected (Fernandez-del Castillo *et al.* 2003). In addition, premalignant entities such as MCN and IPMN may be present in as many as 45% of asymptomatic patients (Fernandez-del Castillo *et al.* 2003).

Histologic classification

A wide range of histologies can present as cystic lesions of the pancreas (Kloppel *et al.* 1996). These lesions can range from adenocarcinoma to premalignant mucinous tumors to benign serous adenomas to non-neoplastic pseudocysts. In addition to these more common types, unusual histologies can present as a pancreatic cyst. Uncommon histologies include neuroendocrine tumors, solid pseudopapillary tumors, acinar cell carcinoma, and lymphoepithelial cysts (Allen *et al.* 2006). These distinctions impact upon the treatment, follow-up, and prognosis of patients presenting with cystic lesions of the pancreas.

This section will describe the criteria used to classify cystic neoplasms, focusing on the most common histologic subtypes. These criteria are summarized in Table 25.2.

Serous cystic neoplasm

The overwhelming majority of SCN of the pancreas are benign serous cystadenomas. Approximately 30% of cystic neoplasms of the pancreas are serous cystadenomas (Fernandez-del Castillo & Warshaw 1995; Le Borgne 1998). These tumors were initially termed 'microcystic adenoma' because of their tendency to form clusters of small (<2 cm) cysts. This finding is not consistent however, as some SCN will present as a single unilocular cyst and have been termed oligocystic SCN (Santos *et al.* 2002).

Table 25.2 Cyst characteristics.

	Pseudocyst	Serous cystic neoplasm	Mucinous cystic neoplasm	Intraductal papillary mucinous neoplasm
Cyst pattern	Unilocular	Microcystic	Macrocystic	Macrocystic
Average size (cm)	6	7	5	3–4
Calcifications (%)	60–75	30	Uncommon	Uncommon
Calcifications (location)	Ductal	Central	Peripheral	Peripheral
Multifocal (%)	15–30	Uncommon	Uncommon	15–20
Nodules (%)	No	No	40–50	60
Septa	Rare	Uncommon	70–80	70–80
Duct involvement	Common	Rare	<10%	Always
Malignant (%)	No	Rare	10–20	35

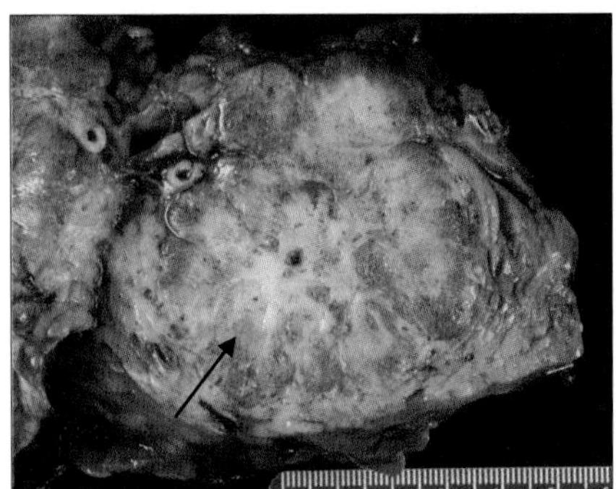
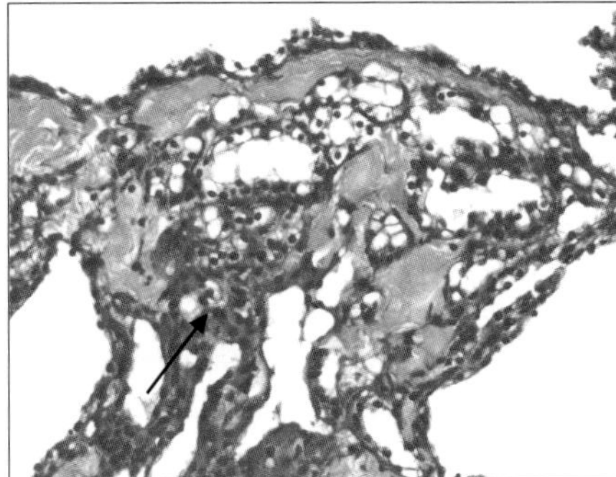

Fig. 25.1 (a) Serous cystadenoma with arrow demonstrating stellate stromal distribution seen as central scar. (b) Serous cystadenoma with stellate stroma on gross pathology.

SCN may occur anywhere in the pancreas. Lesions located in the head and uncinate are more likely to be symptomatic (Fernandez-del Castillo *et al.* 2003; Allen *et al.* 2006). Rarely, these lesions can involve the entire pancreas.

SCN can be as large as 25 cm, but most series report a mean size of 5–10 cm. (Fernandez-del Castillo & Warshaw 1995; Le Borgne *et al.* 1999; Allen *et al.* 2003, 2006). In lesions followed radiographically, the average growth rate appears to be approximately 0.5 cm/year (Allen *et al.* 2006). The development of symptoms does appear to be associated with the size of the lesion. Lesions < 5 cm in diameter rarely cause symptoms (Yeo & Sarr 1994; Allen *et al.* 2003). This finding, however, is not entirely consistent, and even large SCN may be asymptomatic (Sarr *et al.* 2003).

Histologically, these lesions appear very bland. A well-demarcated cluster of small cysts is surrounded by a thin fibrous capsule with minimal pericystic reaction. This feature can differentiate SCN from non-neoplastic pseudocysts and invasive adenocarcinoma. Cystic spaces are separated by a fibrous, vascular, frequently calcified stroma (Fig. 25.1). This finding is the histologic correlate to the nearly pathognomonic central stellate scar seen on cross-sectional imaging of serous lesions.

A layer of glycogen-rich, homogenous cells represent the epithelial lining of the cyst. This cuboidal epithelium contains clear cytoplasm and round nuclei with no dysplastic features. Stains for mucin, chromogranin, and carcinoembryonic antigen (CEA) are routinely negative in these tumors, suggesting a cellular origin other than ductal epithelium (Pyke *et al.* 1992; Tanaka *et al.* 2006). Interestingly, a gene associated with von Hippel-Lindau disease on chromosome 3p25 is deleted or mutated in the majority of serous cystadenomas (Vortmeyer *et al.* 1997; Mohr *et al.* 2000).

Case reports have been published of malignant variants of serous cystadenoma. These serous cystadenocarcinomas are exceedingly rare (George *et al.* 1989; Ohta *et al.* 1993). Serous cystic neoplasms should be considered to have extremely low malignancy.

Mucinous cystic neoplasm

Mucinous cystic neoplasms are lesions that may present as either benign or malignant entities. These lesions comprise 44–49% of primary cystic neoplasms of the pancreas (Fernandez-del Castillo & Warshaw 1995; Le Borgne 1998). Less recent literature commonly refer to these lesions by the outdated term 'macrocystic,' because the individual cystic areas are typically larger than 2 cm in diameter (Fig. 25.2) (Longnecker *et al.* 2000).

Mucinous cystic neoplasms are classically solitary lesions located in the body or tail of the pancreas (Le Borgne

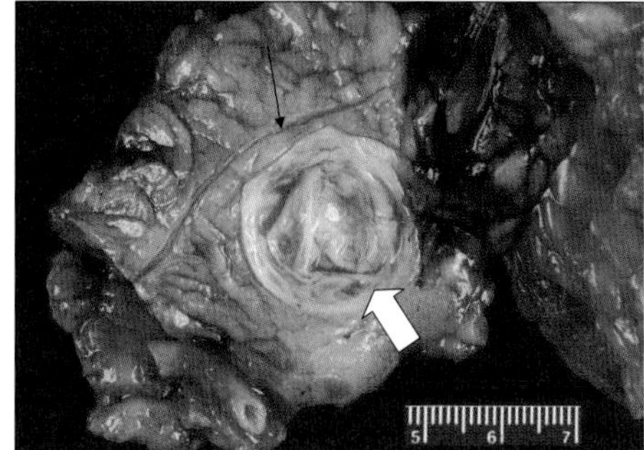
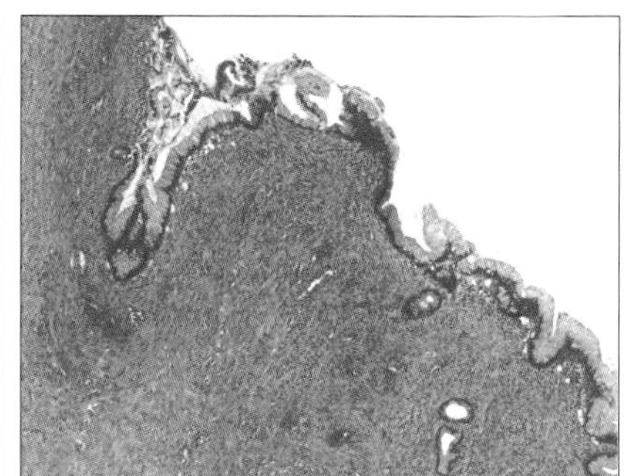

Fig. 25.2 (a) Well-circumscribed mucinous cystic neoplasm (large block arrow) distinct from normal-caliber main pancreatic duct (linear arrow). (b) H&E-stained micrograph of MCN.

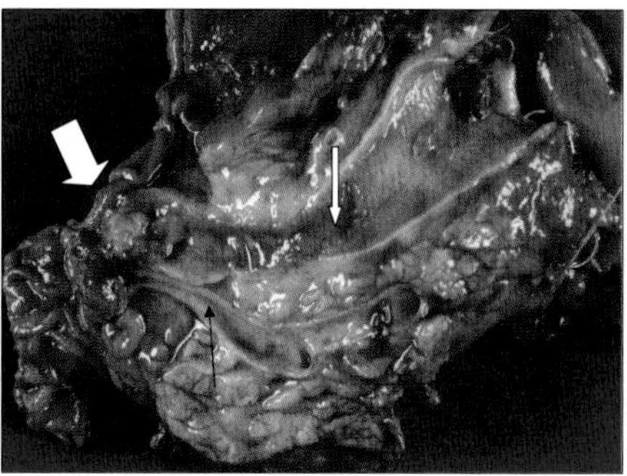
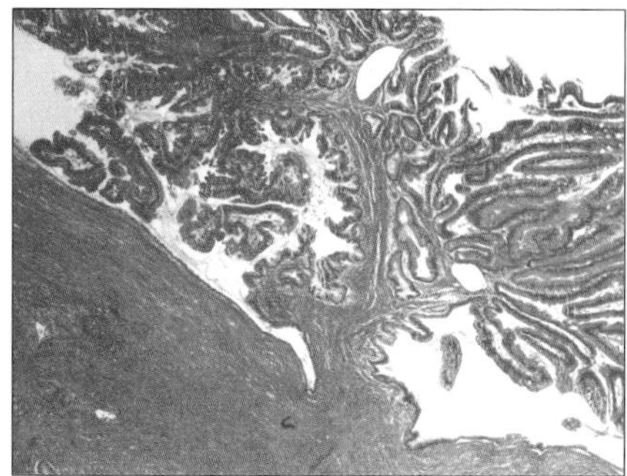

Fig. 25.3 (a) Branch duct IPMN (large block arrow) at junction of dilated branching duct (narrow block arrow) and normal caliber main pancreatic duct (linear arrow). (b) Corresponding intraductal papilloma on H&E staining.

et al. 1999; Tanaka *et al.* 2006). The mean size of MCN reported in the literature is approximately 5 cm (Sarr *et al.* 2001).

Histologically, these lesions have several defining characteristics. The *sine qua non* of the mucinous cystic neoplasm is the presence of ovarian stroma (Thompson *et al.* 1999; Zamboni *et al.* 1999; Reddy *et al.* 2004). The other class of mucinous cystic pancreas lesion, IPMN, do not contain ovarian stroma (Compagno & Oertel 1978). The stromal cells strongly resemble the cells seen in ovarian mucinous cystadenoma (Tanaka *et al.* 2006). Even in men and post-menopausal women with MCN, the stroma stains positively for estrogen, progesterone, and occasionally human chorionic gonadotrophin (hCG) (Wouters *et al.* 1998; Izumo *et al.* 2003; Reddy *et al.* 2004). Some have proposed that MCN arise from ovarian rests within the pancreas and therefore this lesion is almost exclusively seen in women (Zamboni *et al.* 1999).

The epithelial layer of MCNs is comprised of columnar, mucin-secreting cells. Often, the epithelial lining is discontinuously denuded and necrotic, likely due to pressure exerted by the mucin within the cyst (Sarr *et al.* 2001). Interruptions in the epithelial lining can lead to sampling error if a limited biopsy of the cyst wall is performed.

The absence of communication between the lesion and the pancreatic duct is one characteristic that allows distinction between this entity and IPMN. Only rarely can a connection between an MCN and the pancreatic duct be identified (Yamao *et al.* 2003).

Mucinous cystic neoplasms have a significant risk of harboring malignancy. The prevalence of invasive carcinoma in resected MCN is between 6% and 27% (Zamboni *et al.* 1999; Reddy *et al.* 2004). A broad range of dysplasia can be present within one lesion, suggesting a progression from normal columnar epithelium to dysplastic cells to frankly invasive carcinoma. Malignant cells may appear in a discontinuous pattern throughout the epithelial lining.

When MCN without frank invasion are completely resected, recurrence or distant metastasis do not occur (Wilentz *et al.* 1999; Zamboni *et al.* 1999). On the other hand, once the lesion has progressed to mucinous cystadenocarcinoma, these neoplasms have a low rate of resectability and a poor prognosis approaching that of ductal adenocarcinoma (Wilentz *et al.* 1999; Sarr *et al.* 2000).

Intraductal papillary mucinous neoplasm

Intraductal papillary mucinous neoplasms were originally described by Ohashi in the early 1980s (Ohashi *et al.* 1982). He described a triad of findings including a dilated pancreatic duct, significant intraluminal mucin production, and a bulging ampulla of Vater seen at endoscopy. IPMN are characterized by an intraductal proliferation of mucinous cells. Neoplastic mucinous cells proliferate within either the main pancreatic duct or branching side ducts to form papillae (Fig. 25.3). The papillae can then obstruct and dilate the main duct or its branches. Approximately half of resected IPMN specimens contain at least a focus of invasive carcinoma (Falconi *et al.* 2001; Doi *et al.* 2002; Kitagawa *et al.* 2003; D'Angelica *et al.* 2004).

Since their initial description, these lesions have been referred to as papillary carcinoma, mucin-producing tumors of the pancreas, ductectatic mucinous cystadenoma, and intraductal villous adenoma. A more recent classification system has been developed by the World Health Organization (WHO). This system classifies these lesions into three categories: benign adenoma, borderline atypia, and invasive malignancy (Kloppel *et al.* 1996; Longnecker *et al.* 2000).

The anatomic distribution of IPMN throughout the pancreas differs slightly from the distribution of other cystic pancreas lesions. Approximately 60–70% are located within the head/uncinate process, and 12–25% are located within the body or tail of the pancreas (Sarr *et al.* 2000; Sohn *et al.* 2004). Up to 15% of patients will have a diffuse pattern of IPMN with lesions in multiple areas of the pancreas. This finding emphasizes the current hypothesis that this histologic entity represents a process that has the ability to affect the entire ductal system within the gland.

IPMN may arise predominantly from the main pancreatic duct, the branch ducts, or both. Differentiating between those lesions predominantly within the main pancreatic duct and those within the branch ducts allows one to predict more accurately the presence of underlying carcinoma. Most investigations have demonstrated that IPMN arising from the main pancreatic duct have a significantly higher incidence of malignancy than branch-duct variants (D'Angelica *et al.* 2004; Serikawa *et al.* 2006). The risk of *in situ* malignancy approaches 95% in some series of main-duct variant IPMN. The risk of malignancy among main-duct IPMN is approximately double that of branch-duct variants (Kobari *et al.* 1999; Terris *et al.* 2000; Doi *et al.* 2002; Sohn *et al.* 2004).

Histologically, the epithelial lining of IPMN can display a wide array of dysplastic changes from benign columnar cells to invasive cancer. As with MCN, epithelial changes can be discontinuous. Copious mucin production from the epithelium is one of the hallmarks of these tumors. In contrast to MCN, IPMN stroma does not contain stroma of ovarian origin. Stroma is also devoid of calcifications as commonly found in serous neoplasms.

The subtypes of IPMN papillae have been well described and are associated with different prevalence rates of invasive malignancy. Papillae have been classified as intestinal (35% of cases), pancreatobiliary (22%), null (31%), and unclassifiable (12%) (Yonezawa *et al.* 1999; Adsay *et al.* 2000; Adsay *et al.* 2002; Nakamura *et al.* 2002).

A multi-institutional review revealed that the incidence of invasive cancer is 56–62% in the intestinal and pancreatobiliary subtypes, but only 17% among those lesions from the null subtype (Adsay *et al.* 2004). When carcinoma develops in the setting of IPMN, the two most common subtypes are colloid and tubular carcinomas. Colloid carcinoma is associated with a favorable 5-year survival compared to tubular carcinoma (Sohn *et al.* 2004).

Recently, several interesting observations have been made regarding the genetics and expression profiles of invasive and non-invasive IPMN. Loss of heterozygosity (LOH) has been observed in two well-described tumor suppressor genes, 9p21 (*p16*) and 17p13 (*p53*) among patients with IPMN. The prevalence of p16 LOH increased from 12.5% in cases of IPMN adenoma to 75% in tumors with invasive carcinoma (Wada *et al.* 2004). Loss of heterozygosity in the *p53* gene was observed only in patients with invasive carcinoma (Sakai *et al.* 2000). All specimens with invasive carcinoma demonstrated this *p53* LOH (Wada *et al.* 2004).

Mucin marker MUC2 is uniformly expressed in colloid carcinomas and intestinal-type papillae and is considered to be a marker of indolent phenotype (Adsay *et al.* 2002; Adsay *et al.* 2004; D'Angelica *et al.* 2004; Luttges *et al.* 2002; Luttges *et al.* 2004). Conversely, diffuse expression of MUC1 is associated with a significantly worse survival and is seen more commonly in the pancreaticobiliary subtype (Adsay *et al.* 2004).

Diagnostic work-up

The diagnostic workup of any cystic lesion of the pancreas must take into consideration three important principles: (i) pseudocysts related to pancreatitis are the most common pancreatic cyst; (ii) serous lesions have an extremely small risk of malignancy; (iii) mucinous lesions carry variable risk of harboring or developing into malignancy. A thoughtful, cost-effective approach to diagnosing cystic lesions of the pancreas is directed at answering three questions.

1 Is this lesion a pseudocyst related to pancreatitis?
2 Is the lesion more likely serous or mucinous?
3 If the lesion is likely a mucinous neoplasm, what is the probability that it harbors or may develop into malignancy?

Is the lesion a pseudocyst?

The most common type of pancreatic cystic lesion is a pseudocyst (Cubilla 1984; ReMine *et al.* 1987; Warshaw & Rutledge 1987; Sand *et al.* 1996; Buetow *et al.* 1998; Curry *et al.* 2000). The development of a pseudocyst is typically presaged by a history of clinical pancreatitis. Patients may complain of abdominal pain, nausea, early satiety, or weight loss weeks to months prior to the identification of the pancreatic lesion. Most patients with pancreatic pseudocyst will have a personal history of gallstones, heavy alcohol use, or abdominal trauma suggesting increased risk of pancreatitis. In addition, up to 75% of the time, a history of increased serum amylase will support the diagnosis of pancreatitis leading to pseudocyst (Shatney & Lillehei 1979; Warshaw & Rattner 1985). In a series of seven patients with mucinous cystadenoma or cystadenocarcinoma initially diagnosed as pancreatic pseudocysts, none had a history of pancreatitis, gallstones, alcohol use, or trauma.

Pseudocysts comprise the majority of all unilocular cysts. Other lesions appearing as unilocular cysts include IPMN, SCN, and lymphoepithelial cysts. Generally cysts are bland-appearing with little or no intracystic debris or hemorrhage (Sahani *et al.* 2005). If a lesion with the features described above occurs in a patient with a history of pancreatitis, the lesion is nearly always a pseudocyst (Sahani *et al.* 2005).

The presence of multiple cysts throughout the pancreas is commonly found in patients with IPMN and pseudocyst (Frey 1978; Bradley & Austin 1982). The incidence of multiple cysts is tripled in patients with acute pancreatitis compared to those with chronic pancreatitis (Nealon & Walser 2003). Communication between the pancreatic duct and the cyst suggests that the lesion is either a pseudocyst or an IPMN (Sugiyama *et al.* 1997; Tanaka 2004).

The surrounding pancreas can also give important clues as to the nature of the cystic lesion. In patients with pseudocyst, the non-cystic pancreas is often inflamed, indistinct, and adherent to the gastric wall (Hodgkinson *et al.* 1978). Contrast-enhanced imaging may demonstrate hypovascularity and displacement of vessels as opposed to the hypervascularity and invasion of vessels seen in neoplastic lesions (Uflacker *et al.* 1980; Kehagias *et al.* 2002). Linear calcifications may appear throughout the gland in patients with a history of pancreatitis predisposed to pseudocyst formation (Nealon & Walser 2003).

Pseudocysts contain no epithelium. The presence of epithelium within a cyst wall biopsy eliminates pseudocyst from the differential diagnosis. Unfortunately, lack of epithelium within the biopsy specimen may reflect the discontinuous epithelium commonly found in mucinous neoplasms.

In a series of 212 patients with pancreatic cystic lesions, 36% of patients with symptoms undergoing resection had a history of pancreatitis. Of these 48 patients, only 23 (48%) had a final diagnosis of pseudocyst. Most of the remaining patients had an IPMN discovered at final pathology (Fernandez-del Castillo *et al.* 2003).

Acute pancreatitis can be the presenting complaint in 10–15% of patients with IPMN and a further third may have a history of pancreatitis (Kitagawa *et al.* 2003; D'Angelica *et al.* 2004). Symptoms may be due to intraductal mucin secretion and functional ductal obstruction. Among patients without a history of pancreatitis or a condition predisposing to pancreatitis, the diagnosis of pseudocyst should be questioned.

Is the lesion serous or mucinous?

Because the majority of cystic neoplasms of the pancreas will represent either a serous or mucinous cyst it is important to understand the typical differences between these groups of lesions. Serous pancreatic cystic lesions are considered benign. Mucinous lesions such as MCN or IPMN can be associated with malignancy in up to 50% of patients. For this reason, categorizing a lesion as serous allows the option of non-operative management for nearly all of these lesions when asymptomatic.

In several series of patients undergoing resection, 30–50% of primary cystic pancreas lesions were serous cystadenomas (Carlson *et al.* 1998; Le Borgne 1998; Ooi *et al.* 1998; Thompson *et al.* 1999; Fernandez-del Castillo & Warshaw 2001). Recommending an operation which is associated with operative morbidity of approximately 45% and operative mortality of 2–5% for this class of benign lesions is impractical in the asymptomatic population. Conversely, up to 50% of pancreatic cystic neoplasms may be mucinous and carry a significant risk of malignancy (Zamboni *et al.* 1999; Procacci *et al.* 2001; Walsh *et al.* 2002; Allen *et al.* 2006). Routinely observing all of these lesions with a high risk of developing or harboring cancer would certainly be unwise.

History and physical exam may not provide much insight into the distinction between serous and mucinous lesions. IPMN and serous cystadenomas do not have a strong predilection for either gender. Mucinous cystic neoplasms, however, occur almost exclusively in women. In addition, MCN occur in the body or tail of the pancreas more frequently than in the head or uncinate process. Mucinous lesions are more likely to be symptomatic than serous neoplasms. However, up to 40% of serous lesions may be diagnosed based on the presence of symptoms (Sarr *et al.* 2001; Fernandez-del Castillo *et al.* 2003).

As described above, serous cystic neoplasms often have a characteristic appearance on cross-sectional imaging. These microcystic lesions are commonly comprised of small (less than 2 cm in diameter) cysts in the setting of normal-appearing pancreas with no findings of ductal obstruction. A honeycomb pattern of many small cysts is observed in up to 20% of cases of SCN (Sarr *et al.* 2003). In fewer than 10% of cases, SCN can be arranged in a macrocystic or oligocystic variant (Procacci *et al.* 1999). The macrocystic subtype of SCN may be particularly difficult to distinguish from a mucinous cystic neoplasm.

Large (>2 cm diameter) cysts commonly comprise mucinous cystic neoplasms. MCN contain debris or hemorrhage more frequently than serous lesions or pseudocysts. In addition, cysts greater than 2 cm in diameter are more likely to be mucinous than smaller lesions (Curry *et al.* 2000).

One of the classic findings of SCN on computed tomography is the presence of a central scar representing the fibrous septa between microcysts (Fig. 25.4). This finding is highly specific for serous neoplasms but is only present in 20–30% of cases (Curry *et al.* 2000; Sahani *et al.* 2005). Alternatively, calcifications located peripherally are more often associated with mucinous cystic neoplasms (Loftus *et al.* 1996; Curry *et al.* 2000). Only 29% of mucinous lesions demonstrated peripheral calcifications on CT scan imaging. These calcifications are often missed on magnetic resonance cholangiopancreatography (MRCP) (Sahani *et al.* 2006a).

MRCP may be helpful in identifying the communication between IPMN or pancreatic pseudocyst and the pancreatic duct (Irie *et al.* 2000). The cyst itself and any connections with

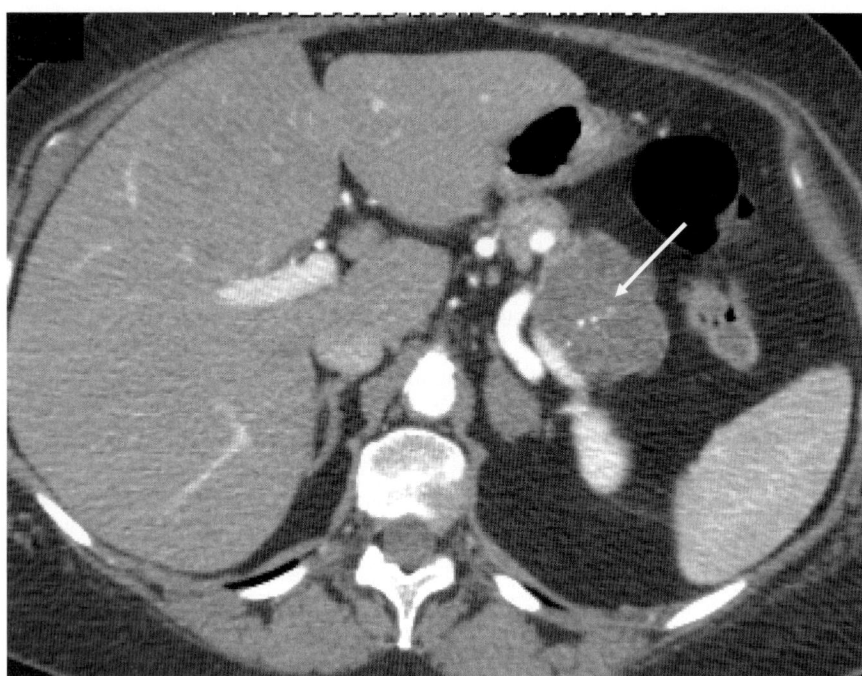

Fig. 25.4 Serous cystadenoma on CT scan. White arrow marks lesion with central calcifications and microcystic morphology.

the duct appear bright on T2-weighted images (Minami *et al.* 1989). This connection is not seen in patients with SCN or mucinous cystic neoplasms. Identifying a communication between the pancreatic duct and the cyst in a patient with no history or findings consistent with pancreatitis strongly implies the presence of an IPMN.

The accuracy of cross-sectional imaging for identifying lesions as either serous or mucinous is difficult to determine. Reports of accuracy rates for correctly identifying serous neoplasms in the range of 23–41% seem surprisingly low (Curry *et al.* 2000). This discrepancy may be an artifact of selecting only pathologically confirmed SCN with radiologic malignant features motivating resection.

Endoscopy can be helpful when trying to determine whether a lesion is a mucinous or serous cystic neoplasm. Ohashi *et al.* described a triumvirate of findings at endoscopy in his initial description of mucinous cystic neoplasms of the pancreas. He described a bulging papilla of Vater, mucin secretion from the ampulla, and a dilated pancreatic duct (Ohashi *et al.* 1982). Since that time, the diagnostic role of endoscopic retrograde cholangiopancreaticogram (ERCP) has been supplanted by MRCP in most major centers; however, enthusiasm has grown for the utility of EUS to provide additional clues as to the nature of cystic lesions of the pancreas. The role of EUS is described elsewhere in this text.

Is a mucinous lesion malignant?

Those lesions most at risk of harboring or developing malignancy are the mucinous lesions. The prevalence of invasive malignancy in resected MCN is 6–27% (Zamboni *et al.* 1999; Reddy *et al.* 2004). IPMN harbor invasive cancers in 50% of cases (Procacci *et al.* 2001; Sohn *et al.* 2004; Brugge *et al.* 2004b; Allen *et al.* 2006). Such a high incidence of malignancy necessitates surgical resection for many of these lesions not only to treat existing malignancy, but also to prevent the future development of malignancy.

Resection of suspicious lesions almost uniformly requires pancreaticoduodenectomy, distal pancreatectomy, central pancreatectomy, or total pancreatectomy. In addition, splenectomy is often added to distal pancreas resection in the setting of presumed malignancy. An operation may be modified or avoided entirely in those patients with an extremely low risk of developing or harboring malignancy. For this reason, identifying characteristics which may distinguish malignant mucinous tumors from benign mucinous neoplasms can help guide therapeutic decision-making.

Most clinicians recommend resection for lesions associated with symptoms. In a series of 75 patients with resected symptomatic mucinous neoplasms, 38 (50%) were malignant on final pathology (Fernandez-del Castillo *et al.* 2003). As mentioned earlier, it is important to remember that the absence of symptoms does not preclude the presence of malignancy. In a highly selected population of patients undergoing resection for their asymptomatic mucinous neoplasms, 17% of patients had a malignant diagnosis (Fernandez-del Castillo *et al.* 2003).

For patients with asymptomatic mucinous pancreas lesions, the risk of malignant IPMN or MCN is associated with several radiologic findings observed on cross-sectional imaging. MRCP and CT scanning have been employed with nearly equal success in identifying characteristics found to predict malignancy in these tumors. A review of 25 patients with pathologically proven IPMN undergoing MRCP and CT scan found that both modalities were equally adept at identifying malignant features of these lesions (Sahani *et al.* 2006a).

Most investigators have identified size of the mucinous neoplasm as one of the strongest predictors of the presence of malignancy within the lesion (Fig. 25.5). Lesions greater than 30 mm in diameter carry an increased risk of malignancy compared to smaller lesions.

In a series of over 500 patients evaluated for a cystic pancreatic neoplasm at Memorial Sloan-Kettering Cancer Center, no patient with a mucinous cyst smaller than 3 cm was found to have an invasive malignancy. A single patient in the group of 56 patients had *in situ* disease (Allen *et al.* 2006). Among patients with resected lesions greater than 3 cm, 49% of lesions contained either invasive or *in situ* malignancy. Several other large studies have failed to identify invasive malignancy in lesions smaller than 3 cm in diameter (Zamboni *et al.* 1999; Goh *et al.* 2006; Sahani *et al.* 2006b). Importantly, the association between cyst size and risk of malignancy does not apply to patients with ductal adenocarcinoma presenting as retention cysts adjacent to the malignancy (Allen *et al.* 2006).

Mural nodularity has also been associated with the presence of malignancy within mucinous neoplasms (Fig. 25.5). Several authors have concluded that the presence of mural nodularity can as much as double the risk of a lesion harboring malignancy (37% vs. 86%) (Yamaguchi & Tanaka 2001; Sugiyama & Atomi 2003). Multivariate analysis of malignancy-determining factors in one series of IPMN from Korea estimated a hazard ratio of 6.75 for the presence of mural nodules compared to those lesions without nodularity (Jang *et al.* 2005). Mural nodularity may be the strongest predictor of malignancy among resected IPMN for both multidetector row CT with 2D curved reformations and MRCP (Sahani *et al.* 2006a). Ductal calcifications or inspissated mucin can be mistaken for mural nodules on MR imaging (Irie *et al.* 2000).

As mentioned earlier, IPMN arising from the main pancreatic duct are more likely to be malignant than their branch-duct counterparts. Both CT and MRCP are effective at identifying involvement of branch and main ducts. Accuracy ranged from 96 to 100% in a comparative study of 25 IPMN. The employed technique for MR imaging in this series was T2-weighted MRCP without IV contrast including fat saturation as well as thin- and thick-slab series.

Branch duct IPMN typically demonstrate a non-dilated main pancreatic duct with a sectoral duct communicating with the cystic neoplasm (Koito *et al.* 1998; Yamaguchi *et al.* 1998; Procacci *et al.* 2001). The branch duct variant can be multifocal in up to 30% of cases (Fig. 25.6) (Kaneko *et al.* 1998; Kaneko *et al.* 2001). Main duct IPMN are associated with dilation of the main duct to a diameter of more than 1 cm. The involvement of the main pancreatic duct can help distinguish main-duct IPMNs from mucinous cystic neoplasms (Fig. 25.7).

A series of 208 patients with IPMN from Korea correlated radiologic features with the presence of malignancy in the

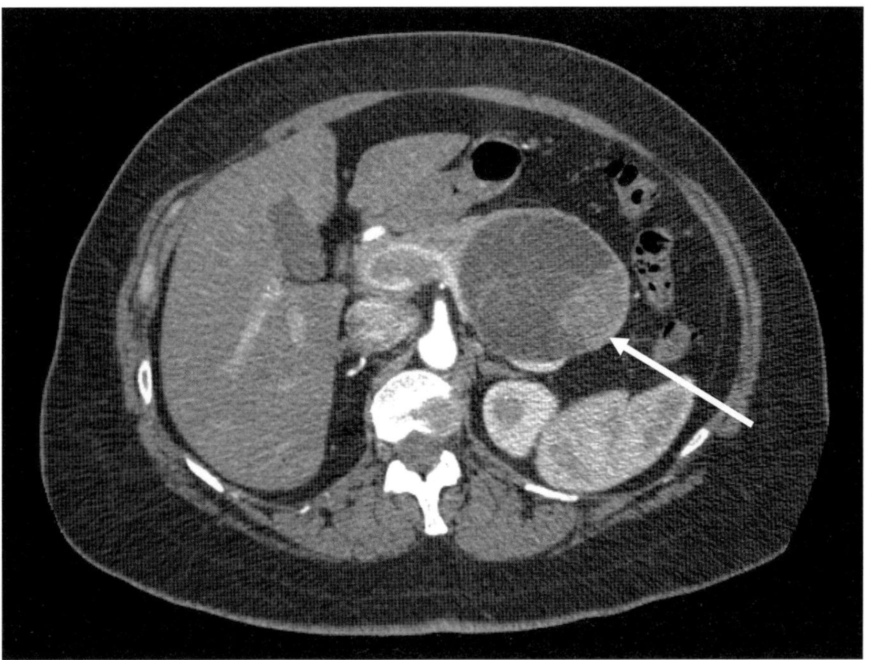

Fig. 25.5 Malignant-appearing mucinous neoplasm in tail of the pancreas. Arrow marks peripheral solid component. Fine septations visible in center of lesion.

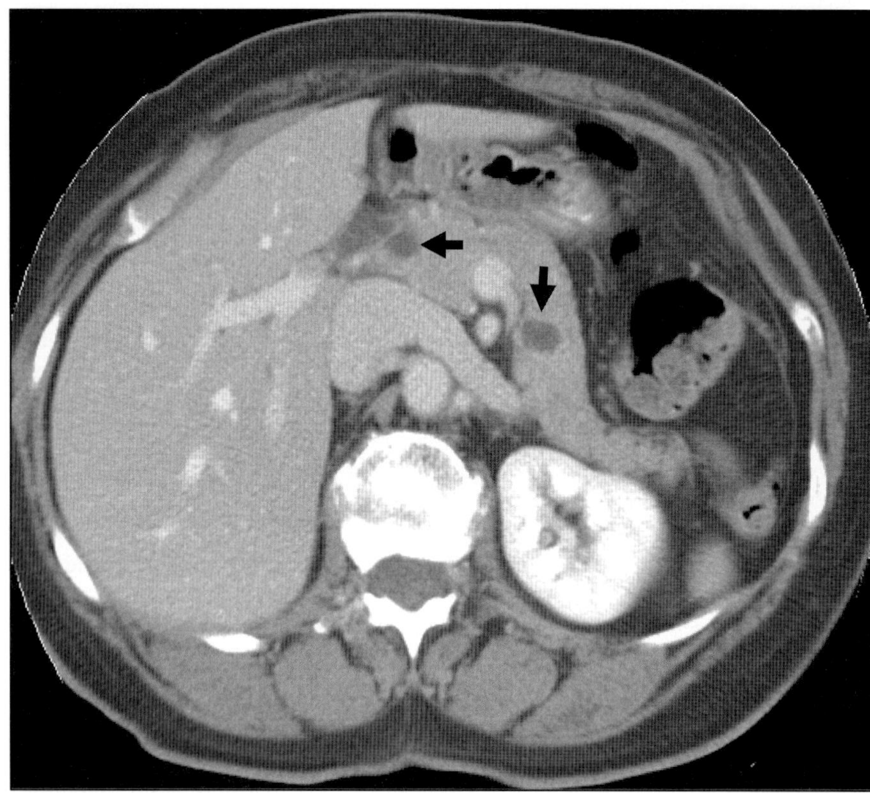

Fig. 25.6 Multifocal branch-duct benign-appearing IPMN with non-dilated main pancreatic duct. Block arrows mark lesions.

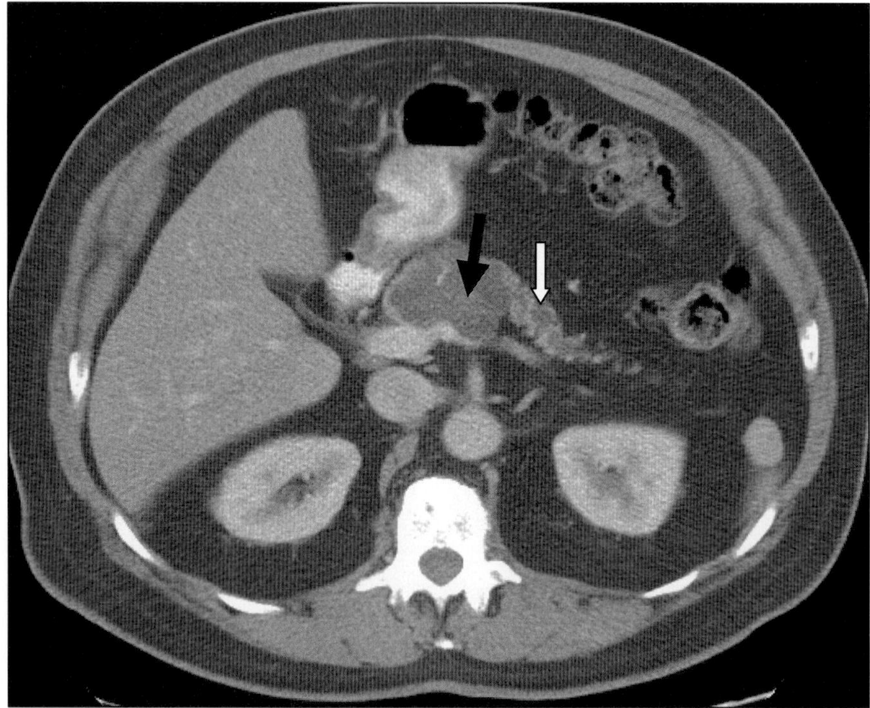

Fig. 25.7 Main duct variant IPMN. Block arrow marks lesion. Open arrow marks dilated main pancreatic duct with associated atrophic distal pancreas.

resected specimen (Jang *et al.* 2005). In addition to the presence of mural nodules and tumor size greater than 3 cm as described above, the authors identified dilation of the main pancreatic duct to greater than 12 mm as a factor predictive of the presence of malignancy. Multivariate analysis of factors predictive of malignancy calculated a hazard ratio of 6.71 for IPMN with pancreatic ducts more than 12 mm in diameter.

Jang *et al.* calculated that the following three characteristics could accurately define the risk of a lesion harboring malignancy: mural nodularity, main pancreatic duct wider than 12 mm, and tumor diameter greater than 3 cm. Among patients with none of these features, 10% were found to have a malignant lesion. For patients meeting all three criteria, the risk of malignancy was greater than 90% (Jang *et al.* 2005).

Overall, the sensitivity of CT scanning or MRCP for detecting malignancy based in part on the criteria described in the studies above is approximately 70%. Specificity and accuracy range between 87% and 92% and 76% and 80% respectively.

Ductal adenocarcinoma can also present as a pancreatic cyst. Retention cysts may herald the presence of an obstructing ductal adenocarcinoma. In a series of more than 500 patients evaluated with cystic lesions of the pancreas, 13 patients were found to have ductal adenocarcinoma. In this series, the cystic lesions within the pancreas did not appear to represent central necrosis of the tumor but rather adjacent retention cysts. The resected lesions all demonstrated retention cysts adjacent to the area of malignancy (Allen *et al.* 2006). This highlights the importance of assessing both the cyst and the adjacent parenchyma when assessing a cystic lesion of the pancreas.

Positron emission tomography (PET) imaging has been described by some authors as predictive of the presence of malignancy within these lesions (Sperti *et al.* 2001; Sperti *et al.* 2003; Sperti *et al.* 2005). Review of 68 patients from our institution with pancreatic cystic lesions evaluated with PET imaging demonstrated that only 57% of patients with malignancy were identified by PET (Mansour *et al.* 2006).

In summary, cystic pancreas lesions with associated symptoms, mural nodularity, a dilated pancreatic duct, main-duct origin, and size greater than 3 cm have a significantly increased risk of malignancy. The risk of malignancy accumulates with an increased tally of these risk factors, such that a category of lesions may carry a preoperative risk of malignancy of greater than 90%. Conversely, a subpopulation of cystic lesions can be defined preoperatively to have an associated risk of malignancy below 10%.

References

Adsay NV, Longnecker DS, Klimstra DS. (2000) Pancreatic tumors with cystic dilatation of the ducts: intraductal papillary mucinous neoplasms and intraductal oncocytic papillary neoplasms. *Semin Diagn Pathol* 17: 16–30.

Adsay NV, Conlon KC, Zee SY, Brennan MF, Klimstra DS. (2002) Intraductal papillary-mucinous neoplasms of the pancreas: an analysis of *in situ* and invasive carcinomas in 28 patients. *Cancer* 94: 62–77.

Adsay NV, Merati K, Basturk O *et al.* (2004) Pathologically and biologically distinct types of epithelium in intraductal papillary mucinous neoplasms: delineation of an 'intestinal' pathway of carcinogenesis in the pancreas. *Am J Surg Pathol* 28: 839–48.

Allen PJ, Jaques DP, D'angelica M, Bowne WB, Conlon KC, Brennan MF. (2003) Cystic lesions of the pancreas: selection criteria for operative and nonoperative management in 209 patients. *J Gastrointest Surg* 7: 970–7.

Allen PJM, Gonen M, Jaques DP *et al.* (2006) A Selective approach to the resection of cystic lesions of the pancreas: results from 539 consecutive patients. *Ann Surg* 244: 572–82.

Becker WF, Welsh RA, Pratt HS. (1965) Cystadenoma and cystadenocarcinoma of the pancreas. *Ann Surg* 161: 845–63.

Bradley EL 3rd, Austin H. (1982) Multiple pancreatic pseudocysts: the principle of internal cystocystostomy in surgical management. *Surgery* 92: 111–6.

Brugge WR, Lauwers GY, Sahani D, Fernandez-Del Castillo C, Warshaw AL. (2004a) Cystic neoplasms of the pancreas. *N Engl J Med* 351: 1218–26.

Brugge WR, Lewandrowski K, Lee-Lewandrowski E *et al.* (2004b) Diagnosis of pancreatic cystic neoplasms: a report of the cooperative pancreatic cyst study. *Gastroenterology* 126: 1330–6.

Buetow PC, Rao P, Thompson LD. (1998) From the Archives of the AFIP. Mucinous cystic neoplasms of the pancreas: radiologic-pathologic correlation. *Radiographics* 18: 433–49.

Carlson SK, Johnson CD, Brandt KR, Batts KP, Salomao DR. (1998) Pancreatic cystic neoplasms: the role and sensitivity of needle aspiration and biopsy. *Abdom Imaging* 23: 387–93.

Compagno J, Oertel JE. (1978) Mucinous cystic neoplasms of the pancreas with overt and latent malignancy (cystadenocarcinoma and cystadenoma). A clinicopathologic study of 41 cases. *Am J Clin Pathol* 69: 573–80.

Cubilla AL, Fitzgerald PJ. (1984) Tumors of the exocrine pancreas. In: *Pathology Atlas of Tumor Pathology.* Armed Forces Institute of Pathology, Washington DC.

Curry CA, Eng J, Horton KM *et al.* (2000) CT of primary cystic pancreatic neoplasms: can CT be used for patient triage and treatment? *AJR Am J Roentgenol* 175: 99–103.

D'Angelica M, Brennan MF, Suriawinata AA, Klimstra D, Conlon KC. (2004) Intraductal papillary mucinous neoplasms of the pancreas: an analysis of clinicopathologic features and outcome. *Ann Surg* 239: 400–8.

De Calan L, Levard H, Hennet H, Fingerhut A. (1995) Pancreatic cystadenoma and cystadenocarcinoma: diagnostic value of preoperative morphological investigations. *Eur J Surg* 161: 35–40.

Doi R, Fujimoto K, Wada M, Imamura M. (2002) Surgical management of intraductal papillary mucinous tumor of the pancreas. *Surgery* 132: 80–5.

Falconi M, Bassi C, Dervenis C *et al.* (2001) Cystic tumours of the pancreas: a review. *Chir Ital* 53: 595–608.

Fernandez-Del Castillo C, Warshaw AL. (1995) Cystic tumors of the pancreas. *Surg Clin North Am* 75: 1001–16.

Fernandez-Del Castillo C, Warshaw AL. (2001) Cystic neoplasms of the pancreas. *Pancreatology* 1: 641–7.

Fernandez-Del Castillo C, Targarona J, Thayer SP, Rattner DW, Brugge WR, Warshaw AL. (2003) Incidental pancreatic cysts: clinicopathologic characteristics and comparison with symptomatic patients. *Arch Surg* 138: 427–3; discussion 433–4.

Frey CF. (1978) Pancreatic pseudocyst–operative strategy. *Ann Surg* 188: 652–62.

George DH, Murphy F, Michalski R, Ulmer BG. (1989) Serous cystadenocarcinoma of the pancreas: a new entity? *Am J Surg Pathol* 13: 61–6.

Goh BK, Tan YM, Chung YF *et al.* (2006) A review of mucinous cystic neoplasms of the pancreas defined by ovarian-type stroma: clinicopathological features of 344 patients. *World J Surg* 30: 2236–45

Hashimoto L, Walsh RM, Vogt D, Henderson JM, Mayes J, Hermann R. (1998) Presentation and management of cystic neoplasms of the pancreas. *J Gastrointest Surg* 2: 504–8.

Hodgkinson DJ, Remine WH, Weiland LH. (1978) Pancreatic cystadenoma. A clinicopathologic study of 45 cases. *Arch Surg* 113: 512–9.

Horvath KD, Chabot JA. (1999) An aggressive resectional approach to cystic neoplasms of the pancreas. *Am J Surg* 178: 269–74.

Irie H, Honda H, Aibe H *et al.* (2000) MR cholangiopancreatographic differentiation of benign and malignant intraductal mucin-producing tumors of the pancreas. *AJR Am J Roentgenol* 174: 1403–8.

Izumo A, Yamaguchi K, Eguchi T *et al.* (2003) Mucinous cystic tumor of the pancreas: immunohistochemical assessment of 'ovarian-type stroma'. *Oncol Rep* 10: 515–25.

Jang JY, Kim SW, Ahn YJ *et al.* (2005) Multicenter analysis of clinicopathologic features of intraductal papillary mucinous tumor of the pancreas: is it possible to predict the malignancy before surgery? *Ann Surg Oncol* 12: 124–32.

Kaneko T, Nakao A, Nomoto S *et al.* (1998) Intraoperative pancreatoscopy with the ultrathin pancreatoscope for mucin-producing tumors of the pancreas. *Arch Surg* 133: 263–7.

Kaneko T, Nakao A, Inoue S *et al.* (2001) Intraoperative ultrasonography by high-resolution annular array transducer for intraductal papillary mucinous tumors of the pancreas. *Surgery* 129: 55–65.

Kehagias D, Smyrniotis V, Kalovidouris A *et al.* (2002) Cystic tumors of the pancreas: preoperative imaging, diagnosis, and treatment. *Int Surg* 87: 171–4.

Kerlin DL, Frey CF, Bodai BI, Twomey PL, Ruebner B. (1987) Cystic neoplasms of the pancreas. *Surg Gynecol Obstet* 165: 475–8.

Kitagawa Y, Unger TA, Taylor S, Kozarek RA, Traverso LW. (2003) Mucus is a predictor of better prognosis and survival in patients with intraductal papillary mucinous tumor of the pancreas. *J Gastrointest Surg* 7: 12–8; discussion 18–9.

Kloppel G, Solcia E, Longnecker DS. (1996) Histological typing of tumours of the exocrine pancreas. In: *World Health Organization International Classification of Tumors,* 2nd edn. Springer, Berlin.

Kobari M, Egawa S, Shibuya K *et al.* (1999) Intraductal papillary mucinous tumors of the pancreas comprise 2 clinical subtypes: differences in clinical characteristics and surgical management. *Arch Surg* 134: 1131–6.

Koito K, Namieno T, Ichimura T *et al.* (1998) Mucin-producing pancreatic tumors: comparison of MR cholangiopancreatography with endoscopic retrograde cholangiopancreatography. *Radiology* 208: 231–7.

Le Borgne J. (1998) Cystic tumours of the pancreas. *Br J Surg* 85: 577–9.

Le Borgne J, De Calan L, Partensky C. (1999) Cystadenomas and cystadenocarcinomas of the pancreas: a multiinstitutional retrospective study of 398 cases. French Surgical Association. *Ann Surg* 230: 152–61.

Loftus EV Jr, Olivares-Pakzad BA, Batts KP *et al.* (1996) Intraductal papillary-mucinous tumors of the pancreas: clinicopathologic features, outcome, and nomenclature. Members of the Pancreas Clinic, and Pancreatic Surgeons of Mayo Clinic. *Gastroenterology* 110: 1909–18.

Longnecker DS, Adler G, Hruban RH, Kloppel G. (2000) Intraductal papillary-mucinous neoplasms of the pancreas. In: Hamilton SR, Aaltonen LA, eds. *World Health Organization Classification of Tumors. Pathology and Genetics of Tumors of the Digestive System.* IARC Press, Lyon.

Luttges J, Feyerabend B, Buchelt T, Pacena M, Kloppel G. (2002) The mucin profile of noninvasive and invasive mucinous cystic neoplasms of the pancreas. *Am J Surg Pathol* 26: 466–71.

Luttges J, Hahn S, Kloppel G. (2004) Where and when does pancreatic carcinoma start? *Med Klin (Munich)* 99: 191–5.

Mansour JC, Schwartz L, Pandit-Taskar N *et al.* (2006) The utility of F-18 fluorodeoxyglucose whole body PET imaging for determining malignancy in cystic lesions of the pancreas. *J Gastrointest Surg* 10: 1354–60.

Minami M, Itai Y, Ohtomo K, Yoshida H, Yoshikawa K, Iio M. (1989) Cystic neoplasms of the pancreas: comparison of MR imaging with CT. *Radiology* 171: 53–6.

Mohr VH, Vortmeyer AO, Zhuang Z *et al.* (2000) Histopathology and molecular genetics of multiple cysts and microcystic (serous) adenomas of the pancreas in von Hippel-Lindau patients. *Am J Pathol* 157: 1615–21.

Nakamura A, Horinouchi M, Goto M *et al.* (2002) New classification of pancreatic intraductal papillary-mucinous tumour by mucin expression: its relationship with potential for malignancy. *J Pathol* 197: 201–10.

Nealon WH, Walser E. (2003) Duct drainage alone is sufficient in the operative management of pancreatic pseudocyst in patients with chronic pancreatitis. *Ann Surg* 237: 614–20; discussion 620–2.

Ohashi K, Murakami K, Murayama M. (1982) Four cases of 'mucin-producing' cancer of the pancreas on specific findings of papilla of Vater. *Proc Dig Endosc* 20: 348–51.

Ohta T, Nagakawa T, Itoh H, Fonseca L, Miyazaki I, Terada T. (1993) A case of serous cystadenoma of the pancreas with focal malignant changes. *Int J Pancreatol* 14: 283–9.

Ooi LL, Ho GH, Chew SP, Low CH, Soo KC. (1998) Cystic tumours of the pancreas: a diagnostic dilemma. *Aust N Z J Surg* 68: 844–6.

Procacci C, Biasiutti C, Carbognin G *et al.* (1999) Characterization of cystic tumors of the pancreas: CT accuracy. *J Comput Assist Tomogr* 23: 906–12.

Procacci C, Carbognin G, Accordini S *et al.* (2001) CT features of malignant mucinous cystic tumors of the pancreas. *Eur Radiol* 11: 1626–30.

Pyke CM, Van Heerden JA, Colby TV, Sarr MG, Weaver AL. (1992) The spectrum of serous cystadenoma of the pancreas. Clinical, pathologic, and surgical aspects. *Ann Surg* 215: 132–9.

Reddy RP, Smyrk TC, Zapiach M *et al.* (2004) Pancreatic mucinous cystic neoplasm defined by ovarian stroma: demographics, clinical features, and prevalence of cancer. *Clin Gastroenterol Hepatol* 2: 1026–31.

Remine SG, Frey D, Rossi RL, Munson JL, Braasch JW. (1987) Cystic neoplasms of the pancreas. *Arch Surg* 122: 443–6.

Sahani DV, Kadavigere R, Saokar A, Fernandez-Del Castillo C, Brugge WR, Hahn PF. (2005) Cystic pancreatic lesions: a simple imaging-based classification system for guiding management. *Radiographics* 25: 1471–84.

Sahani DV, Kadavigere R, Blake M, Fernandez-Del Castillo C, Lauwers GY, Hahn PF. (2006a) Intraductal papillary mucinous neoplasm of pancreas: multi-detector row CT with 2D curved reformations–correlation with MRCP. *Radiology* 238: 560–9.

Sahani DV, Saokar A, Hahn PF, Brugge WR, Fernandez-Del Castillo C. (2006b) Pancreatic cysts 3 cm or smaller: how aggressive should treatment be? *Radiology* 238: 912–9.

Sakai Y, Yanagisawa A, Shimada M *et al.* (2000) K-ras gene mutations and loss of heterozygosity at the p53 gene locus relative to histological characteristics of mucin-producing tumors of the pancreas. *Hum Pathol* 31: 795–803.

Sakorafas GH, Sarr MG. (2005) Cystic neoplasms of the pancreas; what a clinician should know. *Cancer Treat Rev* 31: 507–35.

Sand JA, Hyoty MK, Mattila J, Dagorn JC, Nordback IH. (1996) Clinical assessment compared with cyst fluid analysis in the differential diagnosis of cystic lesions in the pancreas. *Surgery* 119: 275–80.

Santos LD, Chow C, Henderson CJ *et al.* (2002) Serous oligocystic adenoma of the pancreas: a clinicopathological and immunohistochemical study of three cases with ultrastructural findings. *Pathology* 34: 148–56.

Sarr MG, Carpenter HA, Prabhakar LP *et al.* (2000) Clinical and pathologic correlation of 84 mucinous cystic neoplasms of the pancreas: can one reliably differentiate benign from malignant (or premalignant) neoplasms? *Ann Surg* 231: 205–12.

Sarr MG, Kendrick ML, Nagorney DM, Thompson GB, Farley DR, Farnell MB. (2001) Cystic neoplasms of the pancreas: benign to malignant epithelial neoplasms. *Surg Clin North Am* 81: 497–509.

Sarr MG, Murr M, Smyrk TC *et al.* (2003) Primary cystic neoplasms of the pancreas. Neoplastic disorders of emerging importance-current state-of-the-art and unanswered questions. *J Gastrointest Surg* 7: 417–28.

Serikawa MM, Sasaki TT, Fujimoto YY, Kuwahara KK, Chayama KK. (2006) Management of intraductal papillary-mucinous neoplasm of the pancreas: treatment strategy based on morphologic classification. *J Clin Gastroenterol* 40: 856–62.

Shatney CH, Lillehei RC. (1979) Surgical treatment of pancreatic pseudocysts. Analysis of 119 cases. *Ann Surg* 189: 386–94.

Sohn TA, Yeo CJ, Cameron JL *et al.* (2004) Intraductal papillary mucinous neoplasms of the pancreas: an updated experience. *Ann Surg* 239: 788–97; discussion 797–9.

Sperti C, Pasquali C, Chierichetti F, Liessi G, Ferlin G, Pedrazzoli S. (2001) Value of 18-fluorodeoxyglucose positron emission tomography in the management of patients with cystic tumors of the pancreas. *Ann Surg* 234: 675–80.

Sperti C, Pasquali C, Chierichetti F, Ferronato A, Decet G, Pedrazzoli S. (2003) 18-Fluorodeoxyglucose positron emission tomography in predicting survival of patients with pancreatic carcinoma. *J Gastrointest Surg* 7: 953–9; discussion 959–60.

Sperti C, Pasquali C, Decet G, Chierichetti F, Liessi G, Pedrazzoli S. (2005) F-18-fluorodeoxyglucose positron emission tomography in differentiating malignant from benign pancreatic cysts: a prospective study. *J Gastrointest Surg* 9: 22–8; discussion 28–9.

Sugiyama M, Atomi Y. (2003) Recent topics in mucinous cystic tumor and intraductal papillary mucinous tumor of the pancreas. *J Hepatobiliary Pancreat Surg* 10: 123–4.

Sugiyama M, Atomi Y, Kuroda A. (1997) Two types of mucin-producing cystic tumors of the pancreas: diagnosis and treatment. *Surgery* 122: 617–25.

Talamini MA, Pitt HA, Hruban RH, Boitnott JK, Coleman J, Cameron JL. (1992) Spectrum of cystic tumors of the pancreas. *Am J Surg* 163: 117–23; discussion 123–4.

Tanaka M. (2004) Intraductal papillary mucinous neoplasm of the pancreas: diagnosis and treatment. *Pancreas* 28: 282–8.

Tanaka M, Chari S, Adsay V *et al.* (2006) International consensus guidelines for management of intraductal papillary mucinous neoplasms and mucinous cystic neoplasms of the pancreas. *Pancreatology* 6: 17–32.

Terris B, Ponsot P, Paye F *et al.* (2000) Intraductal papillary mucinous tumors of the pancreas confined to secondary ducts show less aggressive pathologic features as compared with those involving the main pancreatic duct. *Am J Surg Pathol* 24: 1372–7.

Thompson LD, Becker RC, Przygodzki RM, Adair CF, Heffess CS. (1999) Mucinous cystic neoplasm (mucinous cystadenocarcinoma of low-grade malignant potential) of the pancreas: a clinicopathologic study of 130 cases. *Am J Surg Pathol* 23: 1–16.

Uflacker R, Amaral NM, Lima S, Aakhus T, Pereira E, Kuroda K. (1980) Angiography in cystadenoma and cystadenocarcinoma of the pancreas. *Acta Radiol Diagn (Stockh)* 21: 189–95.

Vortmeyer AO, Lubensky IA, Fogt F, Linehan WM, Khettry U, Zhuang Z. (1997) Allelic deletion and mutation of the von Hippel-Lindau (VHL) tumor suppressor gene in pancreatic microcystic adenomas. *Am J Pathol* 151: 951–6.

Wada K, Takada T, Yasuda H *et al.* (2004) Does 'clonal progression' relate to the development of intraductal papillary mucinous tumors of the pancreas? *J Gastrointest Surg* 8: 289–96.

Walsh RM, Henderson JM, Vogt DP *et al.* (2002) Prospective preoperative determination of mucinous pancreatic cystic neoplasms. *Surgery* 132: 628–33; discussion 633–4.

Walsh RM, Vogt DP, Henderson JM *et al.* (2005) Natural history of indeterminate pancreatic cysts. *Surgery* 138: 665–70; discussion 670–1.

Warshaw AL, Rattner DW. (1985) Timing of surgical drainage for pancreatic pseudocyst. Clinical and chemical criteria. *Ann Surg* 202: 720–4.

Warshaw AL, Rutledge PL. (1987) Cystic tumors mistaken for pancreatic pseudocysts. *Ann Surg* 205: 393–8.

Warshaw AL, Compton CC, Lewandrowski K, Cardenosa G, Mueller PR. (1990) Cystic tumors of the pancreas. New clinical, radiologic, and pathologic observations in 67 patients. *Ann Surg* 212: 432–43; discussion 444–5.

Wilentz RE, Albores-Saavedra J, Zahurak M *et al.* (1999) Pathologic examination accurately predicts prognosis in mucinous cystic neoplasms of the pancreas. *Am J Surg Pathol* 23: 1320–7.

Wouters K, Ectors N, Van Steenbergen W *et al.* (1998) A pancreatic mucinous cystadenoma in a man with mesenchymal stroma, expressing oestrogen and progesterone receptors. *Virchows Arch* 432: 187–9.

Yamaguchi K, Tanaka M. (2001) Radiologic imagings of cystic neoplasms of the pancreas. *Pancreatology* 1: 633–6.

Yamaguchi K, Chijiwa K, Shimizu S, Yokohata K, Morisaki T, Tanaka M. (1998) Comparison of endoscopic retrograde and magnetic resonance cholangiopancreatography in the surgical diagnosis of pancreatic diseases. *Am J Surg* 175: 203–8.

Yamao K, Nakamura T, Suzuki T *et al.* (2003) Endoscopic diagnosis and staging of mucinous cystic neoplasms and intraductal papillary-mucinous tumors. *J Hepatobiliary Pancreat Surg* 10: 142–6.

Yeo CJ, Sarr MG. (1994) Cystic and pseudocystic diseases of the pancreas. *Curr Probl Surg* 31: 165–243.

Yonezawa S, Horinouchi M, Osako M *et al.* (1999) Gene expression of gastric type mucin (MUC5AC) in pancreatic tumors: its relationship with the biological behavior of the tumor. *Pathol Int* 49: 45–54.

Zamboni G, Scarpa A, Bogina G *et al.* (1999) Mucinous cystic tumors of the pancreas: clinicopathological features, prognosis, and relationship to other mucinous cystic tumors. *Am J Surg Pathol* 23: 410–22.

Treatment recommendations

John Mansour & Peter J. Allen

Introduction

The management of cystic neoplasms of the pancreas is controversial. This controversy arises from the incidental presentation of many of these lesions, the uncertainty in preoperative diagnosis for most cysts, the unclear risk reduction benefits of removing potentially premalignant neoplasms, and the operative morbidity commonly associated with pancreatic resection. The central question in this debate is: which cystic neoplasms should be resected and which can be safely observed?

Because of the unknown natural history of many premalignant cystic neoplasms, and the diagnostic uncertainty, some authors have recommended resection of all pancreatic cysts (Ooi *et al.* 1998; Siech *et al.* 1998; Horvath & Chabot 1999). These authors argue that because of the inability to differentiate between benign and malignant, and because the potential adverse consequences of not resecting a potentially malignant cyst are significant, all patients with pancreatic cysts should undergo resection. This approach can provide a guarantee to patients that no premalignant or malignant lesions will be observed; however it exposes patients with benign lesions to the risks of operation without defined benefit.

Several recent reports, including a report from our institution, have recommended a selective approach to resection (Allen *et al.* 2003; Spinelli *et al.* 2004; Walsh *et al.* 2005). This selective approach argues that with improved radiographic imaging techniques, and an improved understanding of the various histologic entities, a group of patients can be identified with an extremely low risk of malignancy. Within this group of patients the risk of malignancy within the given lesion approximates the risk of mortality from resection, and therefore the reports argue that within this group of patients routine resection should not be recommended. Studies reporting this selective approach to resection have typically recommended non-operative management for patients with small, incidentally discovered cysts of the pancreas (Allen *et al.* 2003; Spinelli *et al.* 2004; Walsh *et al.* 2005). This approach avoids the risks of operation in patients with benign lesions, but with current limitations in non-resectional diagnosis, it cannot guarantee that a malignancy is not mistakenly being observed.

In some instances the histopathology of a given cyst can be determined with a high level of certainty without resection. In these instances treatment recommendations can be made based on what is known of the natural history of the specific histologic entity. In other circumstances—typically patients with small cysts—the exact histopathology of the lesion cannot be determined without resection. In these instances treatment recommendations must be based on the radiographic characteristics, and the inferred histopathology, once the diagnostic work-up is complete. Several reports have noted that over 85% of neoplastic lesions will represent serous cystadenomas, intraductal papillary mucinous neoplasms, or mucinous cystic neoplasms (Le Borgne *et al.* 1999; Allen *et al.* 2006). The following discussion will focus on these three most commonly identified cystic neoplasms of the pancreas.

Treatment recommendations for specific histopathologic entities

Serous cystadenoma

Serous cystadenoma is generally considered a benign lesion. Fewer than 15 cases of metastatic serous cystadenoma have been reported in the world literature (Abe *et al.* 1998). Resection for serous cystadenoma should generally be reserved for symptomatic patients, young patients in whom significant growth has been observed, or patients who have very large lesions that are marginally resectable at presentation. In the asymptomatic patient the risk of mortality from resection certainly exceeds the risk of malignancy. Data from our institution as well as others confirms the non-metastatic nature of serous cystadenomas (Le Borgne *et al.*1999; Tseng *et al.* 2005). These lesions however can become symptomatic, and resection remains indicated in the presence of symptoms.

Because the size at which a serous lesion will become symptomatic is unknown, and because the growth rate of serous cystadenomas has not been defined, the appropriate management of the young patient with an asymptomatic small serous lesion is controversial. In a report from Massachusetts General Hospital a growth rate of 0.6 cm/year was reported for patients with serous cystadenomas of the pancreas (Tseng *et al.* 2005). In this report, serial radiography was obtained for a group of 24 patients who had a median radiographic follow-up of 23 months. This study reported a difference in the growth rate of tumors < 4 cm at presentation (0.48 cm/year) compared to those ≥ 4 cm (1.98 cm/year) (Tseng *et al.* 2005). Because of this observed increased rate of growth in larger lesions, this study recommended resection for asymptomatic patients with serous cystadenomas > 4 cm. We previously reported a similar overall growth rate of approximately 0.5 cm/year, but have not found an association between the size of the lesion and the rate of growth (Allen *et al.* 2006). We feel that asymptomatic patients with lesions characteristic of serous cystadenoma can be safely followed with the possible exception of those patients who have large lesions that are marginally resectable at presentation.

Intraductal papillary mucinous neoplasm

Many surgeons recommend resection for all patients with IPMN of the pancreas. These recommendations should generally be considered because of the reported high rate of malignancy within these lesions as well as the ability of non-invasive IPMN to progress to invasive malignancy. When cross-sectional imaging and endoscopic studies are characteristic of main duct IPMN, and/or when there are concerning radiographic features such as a solid component, septations, or size > 3 cm our standard approach is to perform resection (Allen *et al.* 2006). Lesions in the head of the pancreas are resected by pancreaticoduodenectomy, and lesions in the tail of the pancreas undergo distal pancreatectomy with or without splenectomy.

The goal of resection for patients who present with IPMN is to achieve complete resection with a negative margin. Because many consider IPMN to represent a defect within the entire ductal system of the pancreas there is concern that removal of just part of the pancreas is inadequate (Lai & Lau 2005; Sarr *et al.* 2003). For patients with invasive IPMN the clinical significance of gland recurrence does not appear to be great, as the timing and site of recurrence (early and distant) is more similar to that of conventional pancreatic adenocarcinoma. Patients who undergo resection of non-invasive IPMN, however, may develop recurrent disease in the pancreatic remnant. These patients must be followed carefully after initial resection for the development of gland recurrence. We recently reviewed a group of 79 patients who underwent resection for non-invasive IPMN and identified gland recurrence in 8% of patients after a median follow-up of 36 months (White *et al.* 2006). The majority of patients have not developed local recurrence, and therefore at this time we feel the morbidity of total pancreatectomy is not justified at the time of initial resection. We do emphasize however the need to follow these patients over the long term with cross-sectional imaging for evidence of gland recurrence.

The more difficult clinical scenario is the management of the patient who presents with a small branch duct IPMN, particularly when it arises in the head of the pancreas of an elderly patient. We are currently evaluating over 100 patients per year with incidentally discovered small cysts of the pancreas. Many of these patients have cysts that are between 3 mm and 2 cm in diameter, have no concerning radiographic features, and have been found to have an elevated CEA level on EUS/FNA cyst fluid analysis. These patients are presumed to have small branch duct IPMN (or possibly MCN in female patients), and as noted above, the current ability to determine present or future malignancy in these lesions is extremely limited. A recent review of our institutional experience with these lesions identified the size of the lesion to be associated with the presence of malignancy as well as with the decision to recommend operative or non-operative management (Allen *et al.* 2006). We have not identified invasive malignancy in any mucinous lesion less than 3 cm in diameter (Fig. 25.8). Multiple other studies have also failed to identify invasive disease in small (<3 cm) mucinous cysts of the pancreas (Compagno & Oertel 1978; Zamboni *et al.* 1999; Sahani *et al.* 2006). Current consensus guidelines suggest that branch duct IPMNs < 3 cm in size may be managed with careful observation in selected patients (Tanaka *et al.* 2006).

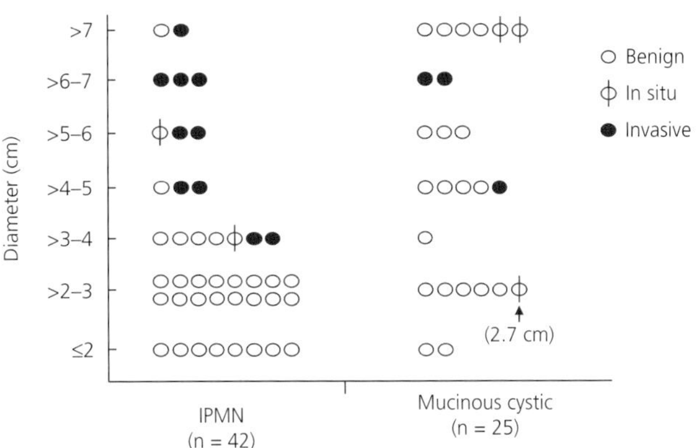

Fig. 25.8 The presence of benign, *in situ*, and invasive disease in patients who underwent resection for a mucinous cystic tumor of the pancreas.

Because of the low risk of malignancy in small mucinous cysts of the pancreas, and because of the risks associated with pancreatectomy, our current approach to resection of the small mucinous cyst is selective. Resection is generally performed when symptoms are present (which are typically not present), when there are concerning radiographic features (solid component, increasing size), or in the younger patient with anxiety over non-operative management. The majority of these patients at our institution (isolated, <3 cm cyst, without solid component) however will undergo non-operative management. Non-operative management typically consists of high-quality cross-sectional imaging every 6 months for 2 years, and then annually thereafter. Upper endoscopy with EUS and cyst aspiration is generally reserved for patients where additional information regarding the nature of the lesion is needed to determine whether or not resection should be performed. During radiographic follow-up, resection is typically recommended when there is any significant change within the lesion on imaging. These changes may consist of cyst growth, the development of a solid component, or other features of concern for malignancy (main pancreatic ductal dilatation or bile duct dilatation).

Mucinous cystic neoplasm (cystadenoma and cystadenocarcinoma)

Because of the inability to distinguish between branch-duct IPMN and MCN of the pancreas, we recommend a similar approach to MCN as that of branch-duct IPMN. Differences in the biology of MCN that should be considered are that they are much more common in the tail of the pancreas, and after complete resection of benign MCN there does not appear to be an increased risk of recurrence within the pancreatic remnant. Because of their location, MCN of the pancreas may be amenable to both splenic preservation as well as laparoscopic resection. Laparoscopic resection has been shown to be feasible and safe (Root *et al.* 2005; D'Angelica *et al.* 2006).

Treatment recommendations in the setting of a radiographically indeterminate lesion

For many patients a non-operative histologic diagnosis cannot be made, and in this setting treatment recommendations must be based primarily on radiographic characteristics and information gained from endoscopic ultrasound with or without cyst aspiration. The majority of patients with these indeterminate lesions will have small (<2 cm) asymptomatic cysts. Characteristics that have been reported to be associated with malignancy in this group of patients have included the presence of symptoms, cyst diameter, the presence of a solid component, and the presence of septations (Walsh *et al.* 2005; Allen *et al.* 2006; Sahani *et al.* 2006).

We recently reported on our institutional experience with cystic lesions of the pancreas between 1995 and 2005 (Allen *et al.* 2006). The majority of patients in this series (369/539, 68%) were managed non-operatively. Patients who were initially managed non-operatively were more likely to have asymptomatic, small (mean diameter 2.4 cm) cysts that were without a solid component. After a median follow-up of 2 years, the average change in diameter of these lesions was 0.2 cm, and 29 patients (29/369, 8%) developed changes that resulted in resection (Table 25.3). The majority of patients within this group had radiographically indeterminate lesions. No patient with a malignant mucinous tumor was followed radiographically however, adenocarcinoma was identified in eight of the 369 patients (2%) who did not undergo immediate resection. None of these eight patients presented with a large adenocarcinoma with cystic degeneration, however in five cases the cysts appeared to represent retention cysts that developed adjacent to a radiographically occult malignancy. The risk of malignancy in patients followed radiographically in this study (2%) was lower than the reported mortality rate of pancreatectomy (Birkmeyer *et al.* 1999a; Birkmeyer *et al.* 1999b). Decision tree analysis from this group of 539 patients is presented in Fig. 25.9.

Because of these findings our current approach for the patient with an incidentally discovered cyst of the pancreas that is 2.5 cm in diameter is to initially obtain high-quality pancreatic imaging. This is most often performed with a triphasic multidetector CT with 2-mm cuts through the pancreas. MRCP may also be performed. This imaging is then reviewed at a multidisciplinary conference attended by both surgeons and radiologists who are dedicated to the treatment of pancreatic disease. Attention must be paid to both the cyst characteristics, as well as to the characteristics of the adjacent pancreatic parenchyma. The presence of a solid component or mural nodularity within the cyst, or any evidence of a mass adjacent to the cyst, is viewed as suspicious and will most often result in additional testing (endoscopy/EUS) or resection. We emphasize the importance of evaluating the adjacent pancreatic parenchyma because the only cases of malignancy that underwent delayed resection in the series discussed above were patients with small retention cysts that were adjacent to a radiographically occult adenocarcinoma. Patients with incidentally discovered cysts < 2.5–3.0 cm

Table 25.3 Histopathology of patients undergoing initial operative management (n = 170), and delayed operative management (n = 29).

Initial operative management (n = 170)				
Benign (n = 138; 82%)		**Malignant (n = 32; 18%)**		
Histopathology	*n*	*Histopathology*		*n*
Serous cystadenoma	72 (52%)	IPMN	*in situ*	2 (6%)
IPMN benign/borderline	25 (18%)		invasive	10 (31%)
Mucinous cystic benign/borderline	16 (12%)	Mucinous cystic	*in situ*	3 (9%)
Pseudocyst	9 (6%)		invasive	3 (9%)
Retention cyst	8 (6%)	Neuroendocrine		6 (19%)
Other	8 (6%)	Adenocarcinoma		4 (13%)
		Solid pseudopapillary		4 (13%)
Delayed operative management (n = 29)				
Benign (n = 18; 62%)		**Malignant (n = 11; 38%)**		
Histopathology	*n*	*Histopathology*		*n*
Serous cystadenoma	4	IPMN	*in situ*	0
IPMN benign/borderline	5		invasive	0
Mucinous cystic benign/borderline	3	Mucinous cystic	*in situ*	0
Pseudocyst	2		invasive	0
Retention cyst	3	Neuroendocrine		3
Other	1	Adenocarcinoma		8
		Solid pseudopapillary		0

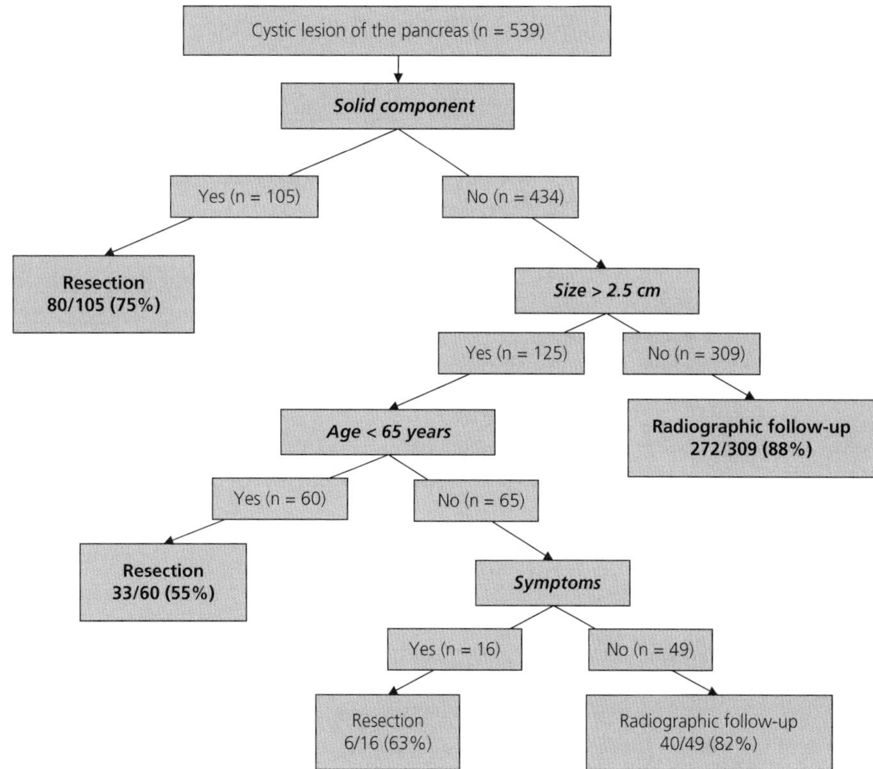

Fig. 25.9 Decision tree analysis for the selection of initial operative management in the 539 patients evaluated for a pancreatic cyst.

in size, without solid component, are most often followed radiographically. Radiographic imaging is typically performed every 6 months for 2 years, and then annually thereafter.

Conclusion

The number of patients being identified with asymptomatic small cysts of the pancreas is increasing. The majority of cystic neoplasms will represent serous cystadenomas, IPMN, or MCN. Serous cystadenomas should be considered benign, and in the absence of symptoms, can be safely followed radiographically. The majority of patients who present with mucinous cysts should undergo resection as many of these will have *in situ* or invasive carcinoma. The presence of a solid component appears to be associated with malignancy in patients with mucinous cysts and cyst size appears to be associated with malignancy in patients with MCN and branch-duct IPMN. Branch-duct IPMN (<3 cm) without a solid component or other features of concern for malignancy may be followed radiographically. When radiographic follow-up is recommended, we typically obtain high-quality cross-sectional imaging every 6 months for 2 years and then annually thereafter. Upper endoscopy with EUS and cyst aspiration should be performed in any patient where additional information might be helpful.

In the setting of a radiographically indeterminate cyst (histologic diagnosis not possible) many institutions are now reporting a selective approach to resection. Routine resection of all pancreatic cysts is currently impractical, and given the large numbers of patients being identified with <2-cm lesions routine resection would result in a mortality rate that approximate the rate of malignancy. Most studies advocating a selective approach have reported the characteristics of a solid component, cyst size, and symptoms to be associated with treatment recommendations. We feel that radiographic follow-up is warranted in any patient where the presumed risk of malignancy is less than the risk of mortality from resection (no solid component, <3 cm, asymptomatic). The majority of patients with incidentally discovered cysts, <3 cm in diameter, and without a solid component can be safely followed radiographically. In the young patient with a small mucinous tumor the additional factors to be considered are the likelihood of progression to malignancy, and patient anxiety about radiographic follow-up.

Efforts should be made to improve the ability to distinguish histopathologic subtypes without resection. The current challenges are to improve the sensitivity and specificity for the identification of mucinous subtype, to better characterize the progression of IPMN and mucinous cystic tumors, and to develop better methods for identifying the presence of *in situ* or invasive disease in these patients. Continued improvements in cross-sectional imaging and endoscopic techniques, as well as further investigation into markers in the serum and cyst fluid, should allow better identification of mucinous subtypes.

References

Abe H, Kubota K, Mori M *et al.* (1998) Serous cystadenoma of the pancreas with invasive growth: benign or malignant? *Am J Gastroenterol* 93: 1963–6.

Allen PJ, Jaques DP, D'Angelica M *et al.* (2003) Cystic lesions of the pancreas: selection criteria for operative and nonoperative management in 209 patients. *J Gastrointest Surg* 7: 970–7.

Allen PJ, D'Angelica M, Gonen M *et al.* (2006) A selective approach to the resection of cystic lesions of the pancreas: results from 539 consecutive patients. *Ann Surg* 244: 572–82.

Birkmeyer JD, Finlayson SR, Tosteson AN *et al.* (1999a) Effect of hospital volume on in-hospital mortality with pancreaticoduodenectomy. *Surgery* 125: 250–6.

Birkmeyer JD, Warshaw AL, Finlayson SR *et al.* (1999b) Relationship between hospital volume and late survival after pancreaticoduodenectomy. *Surgery* 126: 178–83.

Compagno J, Oertel JE. (1978) Mucinous cystic neoplasms of the pancreas with overt and latent malignancy (cystadenocarcinoma and cystadenoma). A clinicopathologic study of 41 cases. *Am J Clin Pathol* 69: 573–80.

D'Angelica M, Are C, Jarnagin W *et al.* (2006) Initial experience with hand-assisted laparoscopic distal pancreatectomy. *Surg Endosc* 20: 142–8.

Horvath KD, Chabot JA. (1999) An aggressive resectional approach to cystic neoplasms of the pancreas. *Am J Surg* 178: 269–74.

Lai EC, Lau WY. (2005) Intraductal papillary mucinous neoplasms of the pancreas. *Surgeon* 3: 317–24.

Le Borgne J, De Calan L, Partensky C. (1999) Cystadenomas and cystadenocarcinomas of the pancreas: a multiinstitutional retrospective study of 398 cases. French Surgical Association. *Ann Surg* 230: 152–61.

Ooi LL, Ho GH, Chew SP *et al.* (1998) Cystic tumours of the pancreas: a diagnostic dilemma. *Aust N Z J Surg* 68: 844–6.

Root J, Nguyen N, Jones B *et al.* (2005) Laparoscopic distal pancreatic resection. *Am Surg* 71: 744–9.

Sahani DV, Saokar A, Hahn PF *et al.* (2006) Pancreatic cysts 3 cm or smaller: how aggressive should treatment be? *Radiology* 238: 912–19.

Sarr MG, Murr M, Smyrk TC *et al.* (2003) Primary cystic neoplasms of the pancreas. Neoplastic disorders of emerging importance-current state-of-the-art and unanswered questions. *J Gastrointest Surg* 7: 417–28.

Siech M, Tripp K, Schmidt-Rohlfing B *et al.* (1998) Cystic tumours of the pancreas: diagnostic accuracy, pathologic observations and surgical consequences. *Langenbecks Arch Surg* 383: 56–61.

Spinelli KS, Fromwiller TE, Daniel RA *et al.* (2004) Cystic pancreatic neoplasms: observe or operate. *Ann Surg* 239: 651–7.

Tanaka M, Chari S, Adsay V *et al.* (2006) International consensus guidelines for management of intraductal papillary mucinous neoplasms and mucinous cystic neoplasms of the pancreas. *Pancreatology* 6: 17–32.

Tseng JF, Warshaw AL, Sahani DV *et al.* (2005) Serous cystadenoma of the pancreas: tumor growth rates and recommendations for treatment. *Ann Surg* 242: 413–19.

Walsh RM, Vogt DP, Henderson JM *et al.* (2005) Natural history of indeterminate pancreatic cysts. *Surgery* 138: 665–70.

White R, D'Angelica M, Tang L *et al.* (1999) *The fate of the remnant pancreas following resection of non-invasive intraductal papillary mucinous neoplasm.* Abstract. Presented at Southern Surgical Association December 5, 2006, Palm Beach, Florida.

Zamboni G, Scarpa A, Bogina G *et al.* (1999) Mucinous cystic tumors of the pancreas: clinicopathological features, prognosis, and relationship to other mucinous cystic tumors. *Am J Surg Pathol* 23: 410–22.

Endoscopic assessment and treatment

Mark Greaves & Mark Schattner

Introduction

In the United States, the incidence of pancreatic cancer has been relatively stable since the 1970s at a rate of 37,170 new cases per year (Jemal *et al.* 2007). Because of the late presentation of this disease, only 20% of patients are resectable and survival remains extremely poor with 33,370 deaths per year. Traditional risk factors have included chronic pancreatitis, smoking, diabetes, and hereditary cancer syndromes. In 1982, the first intraductal mucinous papillary neoplasm (IPMN) was described (Ohashi *et al.* 1982). Since then, it has been recognized that a proportion of pancreatic cysts represent a small, but definable population of premalignant pancreatic lesions.

Cystic lesions of the pancreas can be classified clinically as neoplastic, inflammatory, or congenital. These lesions are increasingly being detected as incidental findings on imaging studies (Gorin *et al.* 1997), and are becoming a more frequent indication for resection at major referral centers (Balcom *et al.* 2001). The biggest challenge in managing pancreatic cystic lesions lies in making the correct diagnosis, since deciding whether the lesion represents a premalignant lesion or not will determine whether pancreatic surgery is necessary. Highlighting the difficulty in diagnosing these lesions, it has been noted that up to 40% of cystic neoplasms were originally misdiagnosed as pseudocysts (Warshaw *et al.* 1990).

The American Society of Gastrointestinal Endoscopy (ASGE) guidelines for cystic lesions of the pancreas state that these lesions, regardless of size or symptoms, require a diagnostic evaluation since they may represent a malignant or premalignant process (Jacobson *et al.* 2005). Traditionally, this evaluation has included various imaging modalities (primarily CT and MRI) and surgery. Endoscopic retrograde cholangiopancreaticogram (ERCP) has had a limited role in the work-up of pancreatic cysts (primarily in patients with IPMN tumors) and has not been found to be reliable when trying to differentiate between benign and malignant lesions (Gazelle *et al.* 1993). The role of endoscopic ultrasound (EUS) in the evaluation of pancreatic cysts was described in 1998 (Maguchi *et al.* 1998). The importance of EUS in managing these lesions increased with the advent of EUS-guided fine needle aspiration (EUS-FNA). More recently, researchers have focused on ways to eradicate these cysts via endoscopic methods, such as cyst ablation techniques and cyst gastrostomies. This section will review the various cystic lesions of the pancreas and present the current roles for both EUS and EUS-FNA in the diagnosis and treatment of these lesions.

Endoscopic ultrasonography

Technique

Endoscopic ultrasonography involves the introduction of an endoscope-mounted ultrasonic transducer directly into the gastrointestinal lumen, bringing the instrument into close proximity to the pancreas, which lies posterior to the stomach and adjacent to the duodenum. This eliminates the artifacts usually created by intraluminal air and food that are seen with traditional transabdominal ultrasonography and CT imaging. Although it does require conscious sedation, EUS is performed with the same ease and comfort as routine upper gastrointestinal endoscopy, with minimal risk, and is well tolerated by most patients.

The 5-, 7.5-, 12-, and 20-MHz probes allow assessment of the tissue planes of the gastrointestinal tract, including the mucosa, submucosa, muscularis propria, and serosa. The lower frequencies permit the evaluation of nearby extramural organs, including regional lymph nodes and adjacent organs such as the liver, spleen, and pancreas.

With the transducer in the duodenum, the uncinate process, ampulla of Vater, head of the pancreas, pancreatic duct, and the bile duct are all readily seen. Moving the transducer into the stomach allows for visualization of the pancreatic neck, body and tail, the celiac trunk, the splenic and hepatic blood vessels, and regional lymph nodes. Normal pancreatic parenchyma usually has a homogenous echogenic appearance, whereas tumors and cysts appear as hypoechoic or anechoic lesions. Specific EUS characteristics associated with the various cystic lesions will be discussed in more detail later.

EUS-FNA technique

The development of linear-array echoendoscopes, which scan the area orthogonally in line with the scope, and in line with the biopsy channel, has allowed for the development of fine needle aspiration (FNA). EUS-FNA has several theoretical advantages: it has a high sensitivity for detecting small lesions (due to the close proximity of the imaging device, i.e. the echoendoscope); the biopsy is generally performed through a segment of duodenal wall that will be removed as part of a resection should the patient require surgery (thus reducing the risk of needle tract seeding); and direct ultrasound guidance provides confirmation of correct placement and avoidance of other structures (such as intervening bowel, blood vessels, and neighboring organs).

Diagnostic EUS should be performed immediately before any EUS-FNA procedure. This allows for proper characterization of the lesion in question before an attempt at biopsy. The linear-array echoendoscope is then positioned as close as possible to the target lesion, typically less than 3 cm away. Doppler ultrasonography is used to ensure there is no significant vascular structure crossing the needle path, and then a fine needle aspiration is performed under real-time ultrasonography with a 25-, 22-, or 19-gauge needle. Once the needle has entered the lesion of interest, the stylet is removed and negative pressure is applied with a 10 mL syringe. Ideally, a cytopathologist or cytotechnician should be present to confirm the adequacy of the specimen. If this is not possible, multiple passes (up to seven) should be performed to try to ensure specimen adequacy (LeBlanc *et al.* 2004). Of note, antibiotic prophylaxis has been recommended for all patients undergoing aspiration of pancreatic cysts (Jacobson *et al.* 2005). Antibiotic prophylaxis is not necessary when attempting aspiration of pancreatic solid lesions, unless otherwise indicated by endocarditis prophylaxis guidelines.

EUS-guided aspiration of pancreatic cysts carries a low-risk of complications. A review of 603 procedures demonstrated a complication rate of 2.2%; including pancreatitis, abdominal pain, bleeding, and infection (Lee *et al.* 2005). In that review, no patient or cyst characteristics were predictive of adverse events.

EUS characteristics of pancreatic cysts

Pancreatic cysts are generally characterized by their size (macrocystic versus microcystic), the presence/absence of septations or solid components, and whether or not there is communication between the cyst and the pancreatic or biliary ducts. Mucinous neoplasms (MCN) often appear as hypoechoic complex cysts, whereas serous cysts often display a honeycomb pattern. IPMN lesions classically demonstrate a dilated, tortuous main pancreatic duct, mural nodules, and pancreatic atrophy. The EUS/EUS-FNA characteristics of the different pancreatic cysts are compared in Table 25.4.

Mucinous cystic neoplasms

Mucinous cystic neoplasms, previously referred to as 'macrocystic tumors', form a group of tumors composed of mucin-producing columnar epithelial cells overlying a fibrous stroma. These lesions can run a spectrum from mucinous cystadenoma to mucinous cystadenocarcinoma. Many of these lesions can have elements of both benign and malignant tissue within the same tumor (Sarr *et al.* 2000). Therefore, all mucinous lesions should be considered premalignant or malignant and be considered for excision. They typically occur in middle-aged women, and are usually located in the body/tail of the pancreas. Symptoms can include abdominal pain, presence of abdominal mass or jaundice, or the patient can be asymptomatic. The lesion is usually composed of one or more macrocystic spaces lined by mucus-secreting cells (Fig. 25.10). However, the cellular lining of the cyst is frequently denuded, making diagnosis by biopsy/aspiration difficult.

Table 25.4 Endoscopic ultrasound-guided fine needle aspiration characteristics of pancreatic cysts.

Cyst	EUS morphology	Communication with pancreatic duct	Fluid amylase	Fluid CEA	Fluid cytology
Mucinous neoplasm	Macrocystic; thick septations	Occasionally	Variable	High	(+) mucin stain
IPMN	Dilated, tortuous pancreatic duct	Yes	Variable	High	(+) mucin stain
Serous cystadenoma	Microcystic; central calcification	Rarely	Variable	Low	Thin, clear, small cuboidal cells; (+) glycogen stain
Pseudopapillary neoplasm	Solid and cystic components	Occasionally			Branching papillary fragments; (+) vimentin stain
Pseudocyst	Thick-walled; debris	Frequently	Very high	Low	Inflammatory cells, no epithelial cells
Retention cyst	Thin walled; no septations	Occasionally	Variable	Low	Normal cell

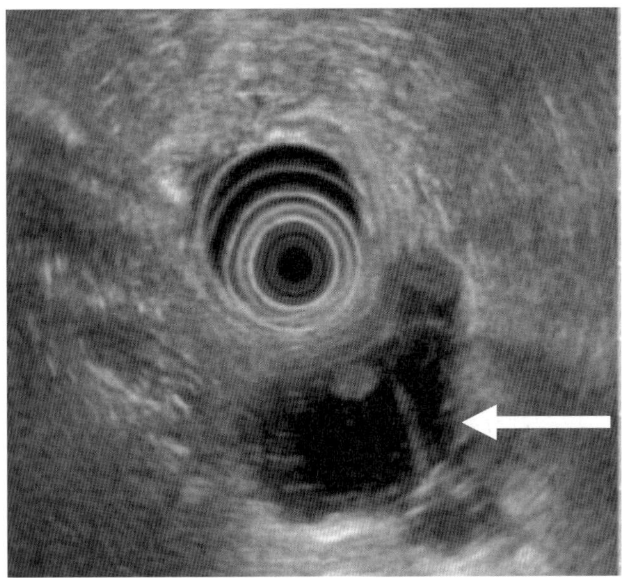

Fig. 25.10 Endoscopic ultrasound image of a mucinous cystadenoma demonstrating a thick-walled macrocyst with septations (arrow).

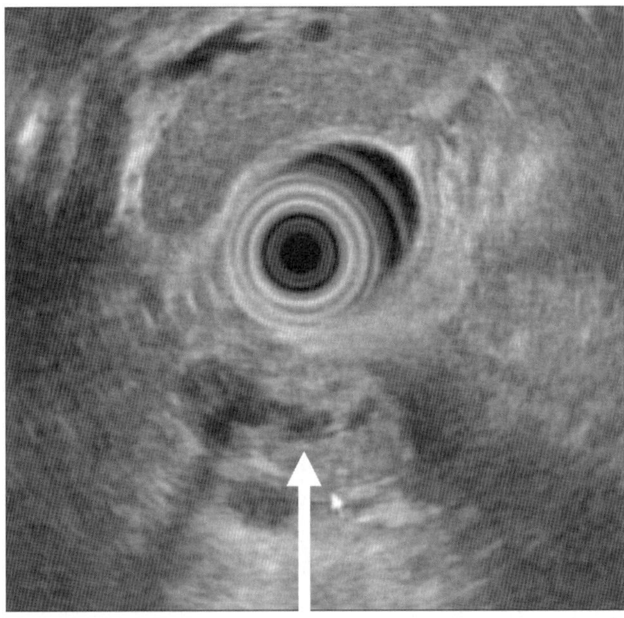

Fig. 25.11 Endoscopic ultrasound image of an intraductal papillary mucinous neoplasm demonstrating ectasia of the main pancreatic duct (arrow).

Intraductal papillary mucinous neoplasm (IPMN)

IPMN (formerly known as intraductal papillary mucinous tumor, IPMT) lesions are composed of mucinous cells lining the pancreatic ducts. They can involve the main duct of Wirsung (less common), the branch ducts, or both. The mucinous material distends the duct causing ductal ectasia and creating a multiloculated 'mass' (Fig. 25.11). More common in men, they are usually located in the head of the pancreas, although they can be present more diffusely throughout the pancreas. Patients with IPMN can present with recurrent attacks of pancreatitis due to intermittent duct obstruction due to mucous plugs. These lesions have a risk of transformation to malignancy, with more than one-third of them being associated with invasive adenocarcinoma (Bernard *et al.* 2002). As with mucinous cystadenomas, these lesions should be considered for resection when diagnosed due to the risk of developing into invasive cancer.

Serous cystadenoma

Serous cystadenoma, formerly known as 'microcystic neoplasm, is the second most common cystic tumor of the pancreas. These lesions are generally considered benign, despite some reports of serous cystadenocarcinomas (George *et al.* 1989). It occurs most frequently in middle-aged women, and has an equal distribution throughout the pancreas. It is typically composed of a myriad of small cysts, lined by glycogen-rich cells (Fig. 25.12). A classic finding is a calcified central stellate star, although it is only present in 13–18% of lesions (Johnson *et al.* 1988). Similar to mucinous cystadenomas, these lesions can also have denuded lining, again making the diagnosis difficult. Serous cystadenomas can grow quite large, causing symptoms as a result of local organ displacement. Since the risk of progression to malignancy is low, these cysts can be followed if they are small, asymptomatic, or non-enlarging. The optimal interval for surveillance imaging in such patients is currently unknown. It should be noted that a macrocystic variant of serous cystadenomas has been defined (Lewandrowski *et al.* 1992). While also considered benign, these lesions share considerable morphologic overlap with mucinous cystadenomas, making distinction between the two sometimes difficult. O'Toole *et al.* have advocated using EUS, combined with cyst fluid analysis, to aid in distinguishing between the two lesions (O'Toole *et al.* 2004).

Papillary cystic neoplasm

Also referred to as solid and pseudopapillary neoplasm, this lesion is the least common of the cystic neoplasms of the pancreas. Although it can be locally invasive, distant metastases are rare. It usually occurs in young women, most commonly in the body/tail of the pancreas (Fig. 25.13). Due to the risk of local invasion, treatment is resection, when possible.

Pseudocysts

Pseudocysts are the most common cystic lesion of the pancreas and develop in the setting of pancreatic inflammation and necrosis. Most patients will have had a history of symptoms that suggest clinical pancreatitis (abdominal pain, jaundice, hyperamylasemia). The cysts can be single or multiple, small or large, and can be located within or outside of the pancreas. Extrapancreatic location, in particular, helps favor a diagnosis of pseudocyst over cystic neoplasm. Most communicate with the pancreatic ducts, and therefore contain a high concentration of digestive enzymes such as amylase. Ductal communication also tends to favor a diagnosis of pseudocyst, although a significant portion of mucinous cystic neoplasms can communicate with the duct. By definition, pseudocysts lack a true epithelial lining. Instead the lining consists of fibrous and granulation tissue and the walls are formed by adjacent structures such as the stomach, transverse mesocolon, omentum, and pancreas. Symptoms can arise due to local organ displacement. Management of these pseudocysts depends largely on the size of the lesion, the presence or absence of symptoms, and chronicity. Lesions can be followed expectantly if they are smaller in size and asymptomatic (Vitas *et al.* 1992). All other pseudocysts should be drained, either surgically, percutaneously, or via endoscopic cyst gastrostomy.

Retention cysts

Also known as simple or true cysts, these lesions are small, developmental, fluid-filled spaces lined by normal duct and

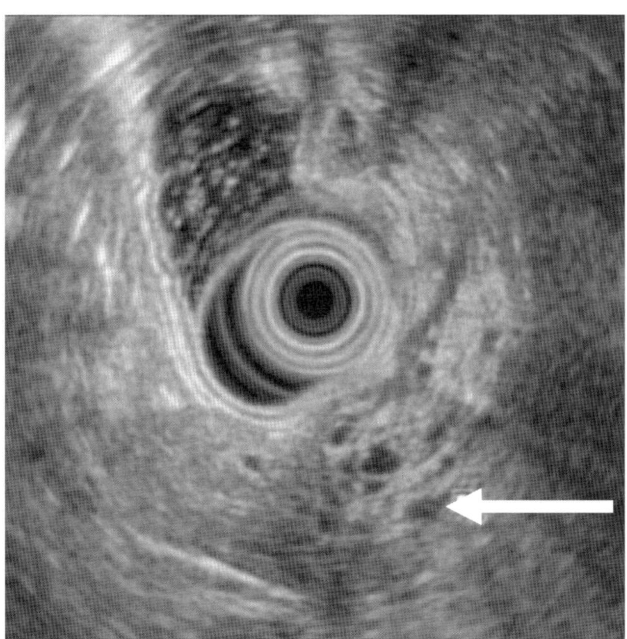

Fig. 25.12 Endoscopic ultrasound image of a serous cystadenoma demonstrating multiple microcystic spaces (arrow).

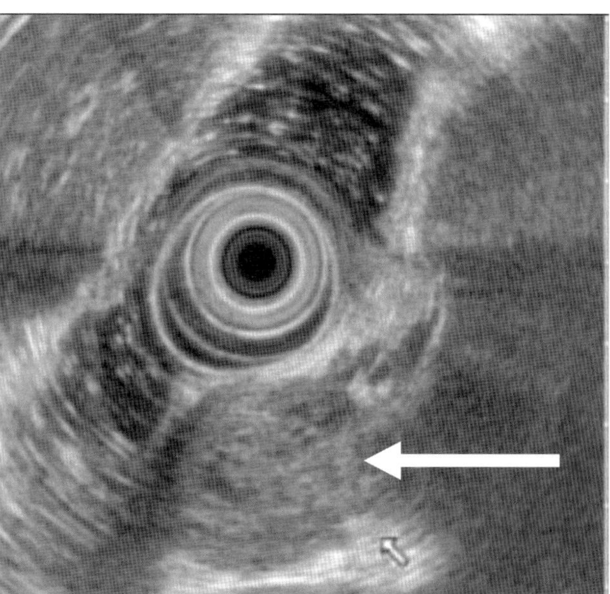

Fig. 25.13 Endoscopic ultrasound image of a papillary cystic neoplasm demonstrating both solid and cystic components within the same mass (arrow).

centroacinar cells. They are usually incidental findings of no clinical significance. Their only clinical significance occurs when they are confused with cystic neoplasms, leading to an unnecessary work-up, since further evaluation or treatment is usually not indicated.

Evaluating the role of EUS and EUS-FNA in the work-up of pancreatic cysts

As already stated, EUS offers two methods for diagnosing cystic lesions of the pancreas: morphologic imaging and guidance for fine needle aspiration. In one of the initial studies that looked at EUS imaging to diagnose pancreatic cystic lesions, Koito *et al.* demonstrated an accuracy for differentiating benign and malignant tumors of 96% and 92%, respectively, by two observers (Koito *et al.* 1997). Comparing the EUS morphologic findings to the surgical findings in thirty-four patients, a later study showed that EUS alone had 91% sensitivity, 60% specificity, and 82% accuracy in identifying malignant and premalignant lesions (Sedlack *et al.* 2002). In yet another study, parenchymal changes within the cysts (more common in pseudocysts) and mural nodules (more common in cystic tumors) were found to be independent predictors in differentiating pseudocysts and cystic tumors (Song *et al.* 2003). The mural nodules (more common in mucinous lesions) also helped in differentiating serous cystadenomas from mucinous lesions.

Other trials looking at the utility of EUS morphology have been less promising. EUS did not reliably differentiate between benign and malignant cystic lesions in one study that looked at 98 patients with pancreatic cysts, who had non-diagnostic cross-sectional imaging prior to the EUS procedure (Ahmad *et al.* 2001). This study also reported poor interobserver agreement among experienced endosonographers when it came to differentiating neoplastic versus non-neoplastic cysts (Ahmad *et al.* 2003).

When evaluating the literature on EUS-FNA, it is important to remember that its usefulness is a reflection of the usefulness of the various tests that the cyst fluid is submitted for. As such, the ability of FNA to contribute to the diagnosis of pancreatic cystic lesions should continue to improve as the field of cyst fluid analysis evolves. That being said, most of the trials to date that have looked at EUS-FNA have submitted the cyst fluid for cytology (most common) and sometimes tumor markers as well.

In one such trial, EUS alone correctly identified the cystic lesion in 73% of the cases, whereas the addition of FNA yielded a correct diagnosis in 97% of cases (Frossard *et al.* 2003). In this study, the cyst fluid was submitted for cytology and various tumor markers. Brandwein *et al.* found that EUS-FNA had only 50% sensitivity for detecting malignancy in cystic lesions, but had 100% accuracy (Brandwein *et al.* 2001).

Finally, recent work has looked at using a tru-cut needle when performing EUS-guided biopsies of pancreatic cysts (Levy *et al.* 2005). A tru-cut biopsy yields a core biopsy sample, which may improve diagnostic accuracy. Comparison studies with traditional FNA have not been carried out as of yet.

Comparing EUS to other imaging modalities

In 2002, a retrospective review of 149 tissue samples showed that EUS-guided biopsies were as accurate as CT/US-guided sampling (Mallery *et al.* 2002). A more recent study compared the results of EUS-FNA, ultrasound-FNA, and CT-FNA in 1050 pancreatic FNA procedures (Volmar *et al.* 2005). The study showed that for lesions < 3 cm, the EUS method had a higher accuracy than ultrasound or CT. No difference was seen for larger lesions. Of note, the number of FNA passes did not affect outcome.

Pancreatic cyst fluid analysis

Cytology

Cytologic examination remains the most common test for which pancreatic cyst fluid is submitted. However, many neoplastic lesions have a denuded epithelial lining, which can lead to a false-negative result. Furthermore, the sampling of a heterogeneous cyst may miss small foci of malignancy (Hernandez *et al.* 2002). Several studies have confirmed these limitations, with the sensitivity of cytology of a pancreatic cyst aspirate being reported at 20–50% (Lewandrowski *et al.* 1995; Brandwein *et al.* 2001; Sedlack *et al.* 2002). As a result, a negative aspiration cannot rule out a malignant lesion.

Cyst fluid tumor markers

Given the poor results seen when using cytology alone, several investigators have turned to tumor markers in an attempt to improve the accuracy in differentiating among the various cystic lesions. One of the larger studies in this area prospectively gathered the results of EUS imaging, cytology, and several cyst fluid tumor markers (CEA, CA19-9, CA15-3, CA125, and CA72-4) in 341 patients (Brugge *et al.* 2004). The accuracy of CEA (85%) in predicting which lesions were mucinous (premalignant) versus non-mucinous (benign) was higher than EUS morphology (51%) and cytology (59%). Furthermore, no combination of tests yielded a greater accuracy than CEA alone. Of note, it was determined that the optimal cut-off value for CEA in this study was 192 ng/mL. Several other trials have also found that CEA has a high sensitivity and specificity for diagnosing mucinous lesions (Sperti *et al.* 1996; Hammel *et al.* 1997; Frossard *et al.* 2003). It is worth mentioning though, that an important limitation of cyst fluid CEA analysis is that it requires at least 1 mL of cyst fluid to be aspirated. This can be difficult if the cyst cavities are small or the cyst fluid is too viscous to aspirate through the needle. Khlaid *et al.* demonstrated that, even in expert hands, 25% of EUS-FNA aspirations do not produce sufficient fluid for CEA measurement (Khalid *et al.* 2005).

In the study by Brugge *et al.* that demonstrated the utility of CEA levels, CA72-4 (with a cut-off value > 7) provided the next greatest level of accuracy out of all of the tumor markers at 72% (Brugge *et al.* 2004). CA72-4 was shown to have a high specificity for detecting mucinous lesions (98% and 94%, respectively) in two additional studies (Sperti *et al.* 1997; Hammel *et al.* 1998). The sensitivities varied widely though in these studies.

Finally, in a study comparing EUS-FNA results to surgical findings, CA19-9 levels were evaluated (Frossard *et al.* 2003). A CA19-9 level greater than 50,000 U/mL had only 15% sensitivity and an 81% specificity in distinguishing mucinous cysts from other cysts. However, it had 86% sensitivity and 85% specificity to distinguish cystadenocarcinoma from other cystic lesions.

Mutation analysis

Recent research in the field of cyst-fluid analysis has focused on analysing the DNA of the cellular material obtained from a FNA specimen to attempt to identify mutations that might help differentiate benign versus malignant lesions. Broad-panel microsatellite loss and k-ras point mutations have been linked to IPMN (Schoedel *et al.* 2006) and malignant lesions (Khalid *et al.* 2006). Other markers, such as p53, are being investigated. One advantage of these tests is that results can be obtained with very small fluid sample sizes. As more mutations are discovered, these techniques could represent a major advance for the field of cyst fluid analysis.

Novel endoscopic therapeutics

Cyst ablation

Based on success in treating cystic lesions in other parts of the body, researchers have attempted to ablate pancreatic cysts via ethanol lavage. A recent trial demonstrated complete resolution of pancreatic cysts in 35% of patients, with an additional 20% showing histologic evidence of epithelial ablation in the surgically-resected specimen (Gan *et al.* 2005). Long-term data on safety, efficacy, and malignancy prevention are lacking. Because of this, ethanol ablation remains at this time a purely experimental therapy.

Cystogastrostomies

The role for using EUS in the drainage of pseudocysts has been established by several studies (Norton *et al.* 2001; Antillon *et al.* 2006; Kahaleh *et al.* 2006). In a prospective series, EUS-guided drainage of pancreatic pseudocysts and abscesses was performed in 35 patients (Kruger *et al.* 2006). Initial stent placement was successful in 94% of patients. Overall, there was an 88% resolution rate in the lesions, although many required multiple endoscopic interventions to achieve complete resolution. Complications included ineffective drainage, stent occlusion, and cyst infection.

A case report recently illustrated the potential role for EUS-guided cystogastrostomy in palliating symptoms associated with malignant pancreatic cysts (Silva *et al.* 2006). In the report, a patient with unresectable pancreatic cystadenocarcinoma causing gastric outlet obstruction underwent a EUS-guided cystogastrostomy with subsequent dramatic improvement in symptoms. The long-term safety of such procedures (including risks of seeding, etc) is currently not known.

Summary

More than 20 years after their discovery, pancreatic cysts remain a diagnostic challenge for clinicians. The most common lesions (mucinous cystic neoplasms, IPMN, serous cystadenomas, and pseudocysts) often have overlapping radiologic and clinical features that make a precise diagnosis difficult. The evaluation of pancreatic cysts should therefore focus on attempting to differentiate between benign and malignant/premalignant cystic lesions.

As outlined in this chapter, EUS has been shown to be useful in the evaluation of pancreatic cysts. The role of EUS and EUS-FNA in the work-up of these lesions continues to increase as experience grows. As the field of cyst-fluid analysis is refined further, the accuracy of FNA will continue to improve. EUS-guided therapeutic interventions, while still in their infancy, offer an exciting new pathway in the treatment of pancreatic cystic lesions.

When cross-sectional imaging fails to reveal a clear diagnosis, consideration should be given to EUS-FNA. At the time of the procedure, a cytotechnician or a cytopathologist should be present in the room to help confirm specimen adequacy. Diagnostic tests that may be helpful include cytology (with special staining to attempt to detect mucin), CEA level, molecular studies, and amylase if the lesion is felt to communicate with the pancreatic duct.

It is important to note that surgery remains the gold standard for both diagnosis and treatment. Currently, most pancreatic surgeons reserve FNA for low- to moderate-risk lesions, poor surgical candidates, or to help gain more evidence to attempt to convince reluctant patients with suspicious lesions to undergo surgery. It is also important to remember that, due to the limitations, a negative EUS-FNA result should not dissuade from a surgical intervention if the lesion was otherwise felt to be suspicious.

References

Ahmad N, Kochman M, Lewis J *et al.* (2001) Can EUS alone differentiate between malignant and benign cystic lesions of the pancreas? *Am J Gastroenterol* 96: 3295.

Ahmad N, Kochman M, Brensinger C *et al.* (2003) Interobserver agreement among endosonographers for the diagnosis of neoplastic verus non-neoplastic pancreatic cystic lesions. *Gastrointest Endosc* 58: 59.

Antillon MR, Shah RJ, Stiegmann G *et al.* (2006) Single-step EUS-guided transmural drainage of simple and complicated pancreatic pseudocysts. *Gastrointest Endosc* 63: 797.

Balcom JH, Rattner DW, Warshaw AL *et al.* (2001) Ten-year experience with 733 pancreatic resections: changing indications, older patients, and decreasing length of hospitalization. *Arch Surg* 136: 391.

Bernard P, Scoazec J-Y, Joubert M *et al.* (2002) Intraductal papillary-mucinous tumors of the pancreas: predictive criteria of malignancy according to pathological examination of 53 cases. *Arch Surg* 137: 1274.

Brandwein S, Farrell J, Centeno B *et al.* (2001) Detection and tumor staging of malignancy in cystic, intraductal, and solid tumors of the pancreas by EUS. *Gastrointest Endosc* 53: 722.

Brugge WR, Lewandrowski K, Lee-Lewandrowski E *et al.* (2004) Diagnosis of pancreatic cystic neoplasms: a report of the cooperative pancreatic cyst study. *Gastroenterol* 126: 1330.

Frossard JL, Amouyal P, Amouyal G *et al.* (2003) Performance of endosonography-guided fine needle aspiration and biopsy in the diagnosis of pancreatic cystic lesions. *Am J Gastroenterol* 98: 1516.

Gan SI, Thompson CC, Lauwers GY *et al.* (2005) Ethanol lavage of pancreatic cystic lesions: initial pilot study. *Gastrointest Endosc* 61: 746.

Gazelle GS, Mueller PR, Raafat N *et al.* (1993) Cystic neoplasms of the pancreas: evaluation with endoscopic retrograde pancreatography. *Radiology* 188: 633.

George DH, Murphy F, Michalski R *et al.* (1989) Serous cystadenocarcinoma of the pancreas: a new entity? *Am J Surg Pathol* 13: 61.

Gorin AD, Sackier JM. (1997) Incidental detection of cystic neoplasms of the pancreas. *Maryland Med J* 46: 79.

Hammel PR, Forgue-Lafitte ME, Levy P *et al.* (1997) Detection of gastric mucins (M1 antigens) in cyst fluid for the diagnosis of cystic lesions of the pancreas. *Int J Cancer* 74: 286.

Hammel P, Voitot H, Vilgrain V *et al.* (1998) Diagnostic value of CA 72-4 and carcinoembryonic antigen determination in the fluid of pancreatic cystic lesions. *Eur J Gastroenterol Hepatol* 10: 345.

Hernandez LV, Mishra G, Forsmark C *et al.* (2002) Role of endoscopic ultrasound (EUS) and EUS-guided fine needle aspiration in the diagnosis and treatment of cystic lesions of the pancreas. *Pancreas* 25: 222.

Jacobson BC, Baron TH, Adler DG *et al.* (2005) ASGE guideline: the role of endoscopy in the diagnosis and the management of cystic lesions and inflammatory fluid collections of the pancreas. *Gastrointest Endosc* 61: 363.

Jemal A, Siegel R, Ward E *et al.* (2007) Cancer statistics, 2007. *Cancer J Clin* 57: 43.

Johnson CD, Stephens DH, Charboneau JW *et al.* (1988) Cystic pancreatic tumors: CT and sonographic assessment. *Am J Roentgenol* 151: 1133.

Kahaleh M, Shami VM, Conaway MR *et al.* (2006) Endoscopic ultrasound drainage of pancreatic pseudocyst: a prospective comparison with conventional endoscopic drainage. *Endoscopy* 38: 355.

Khalid A, McGrath KM, Zahid M *et al.* (2005) The role of pancreatic cyst fluid molecular analysis in predicting cyst pathology. *Clin Gastroenterol Hepatol* 3: 967.

Khalid A, Nodit L, Zahid M *et al.* (2006) Endoscopic ultrasound fine needle aspirate DNA analysis to differentiate malignant and benign pancreatic masses. *Am J Gastroenterol* 101: 1.

Koito K, Namieno T, Nagakawa T *et al.* (1997) Solitary cystic tumor of the pancreas: EUS-pathologic correlation. *Gastrointest Endosc* 45: 268.

Kruger M, Schneider AS, Manns MP *et al.* (2006) Endoscopic management of pancreatic pseudocysts or abscesses after EUS-guided 1-step procedure for initial access. *Gastrointest Endosc* 63: 409.

LeBlanc JK, Ciaccia D, Al-Assi MT *et al.* (2004) Optimal number of EUS-guided fine needle passes needed to obtain a correct diagnosis. *Gastrointest Endosc* 59: 475.

Lee LS, Saltzman JR, Bounds BC *et al.* (2005) EUS-guided fine needle aspiration of pancreatic cysts: a retrospective analysis of complications and their predictors. *Clin Gastroenterol Hepatol* 3: 231.

Levy MJ, Smyrk TC, Reddy RP *et al.* (2005) Endoscopic ultrasound-guided trucut biopsy of the cyst wall for diagnosing cystic pancreatic tumors. *Clin Gastroenterol Hepatol* 3: 974.

Lewandrowski K, Warshaw A, Compton C. (1992) Macrocystic serous cystadenoma of the pancreas: a morphologic variant differing from microcystic adenoma. *Hum Pathol* 23: 871.

Lewandrowski K, Lee J, Southern J *et al.* (1995) Cyst fluid analysis in the differential diagnosis of pancreatic cysts: a new approach to the preoperative assessment of pancreatic cystic lesions. *Am J Roentgenol* 164: 815.

Maguchi H, Osanai M, Yanagawa N *et al.* (1998) Endoscopic ultrasonography diagnosis of pancreatic cystic disease. *Endoscopy* 30: A108.

Mallery J, Centeno B, Hahn P *et al.* (2002) Pancreatic tissue sampling guided by EUS, CT/US, and surgery: A comparison of sensitivity and specificity. *Gastrointest Endosc* 56: 218.

Norton ID, Clain JE, Wiersema MJ *et al.* (2001) Utility of endoscopic ultrasonography in endoscopic drainage of pancreatic pseudocysts in selected patients. *Mayo Clin Proc* 76: 794.

Ohashi KM, Maruyama MY. (1982) Four cases of mucin producing cancer of the pancreas on specific findings of the papilla of vater. *Prog Dig Endosc* 20: 348.

O'Toole D, Palazzo L, Hammel P *et al.* (2004) Macrocystic pancreatic cystadenoma: the role of EUS and cyst fluid analysis in distinguishing mucinous and serous lesions. *Gastrointest Endosc* 59: 823.

Sarr MG, Carpenter HA, Prabhakar LP *et al.* (2000) Clinical and pathologic correlation of 84 mucinous cystic neoplasms of the pancreas: can one reliably differentiate benign from malignant (or premalignant) neoplasms? *Ann Surg* 231: 205.

Schoedel K, Finkelstein S, Ohori N. (2006) K-Ras and microsatellite marker analysis of fine-needle aspirates from intraductal papillary mucinous neoplasms of the pancreas. *Diagn Cytopathol* 34: 605.

Sedlack R, Affi A, Vazquez-Sequeiros E *et al.* (2002) Utility of EUS in the evaluation of cystic pancreatic lesions. *Gastrointest Endosc* 56: 543.

Silva RG, Silverman WB, Gerke H. (2006) Palliative endoscopic ultrasound-guided drainage of a malignant pancreatic cyst causing gastric outlet obstruction. *Pancreatology* 6: 472.

Song MH, Lee SK, Kim MH *et al.* (2003) EUS in the evaluation of pancreatic cystic lesions. *Gastrointest Endosc* 57: 891.

Sperti C, Pasquali C, Guolo P *et al.* (1996) Serum tumor markers and cyst fluid analysis are useful for the diagnosis of pancreatic cystic tumors. *Cancer* 78: 237.

Sperti C, Pasquali C, Pedrazzoli S *et al.* (1997) Expression of mucin-like carcinoma-associated antigen in the cyst fluid differentiates mucinous from nonmucinous pancreatic cysts. *Am J Gastroenterol* 92: 672.

Vitas GJ, Sarr MG. (1992) Selected management of pancreatic pseudocysts: operative versus expectant management. *Surgery* 111: 123.

Volmar KE, Vollmer RT, Jowell PS. (2005) Pancreatic FNA in 1000 cases: a comparison of imaging modalities. *Gastrointest Endosc* 61: 854.

Warshaw AL, Compton CC, Lewandrowski K *et al.* (1990) Cystic tumors of the pancreas. New clinical, radiologic, and pathologic observation in 67 patients. *Ann Surg* 212: 432.

INDEX

Note: page numbers in *italics* refer to figures, those in **bold** refer to tables

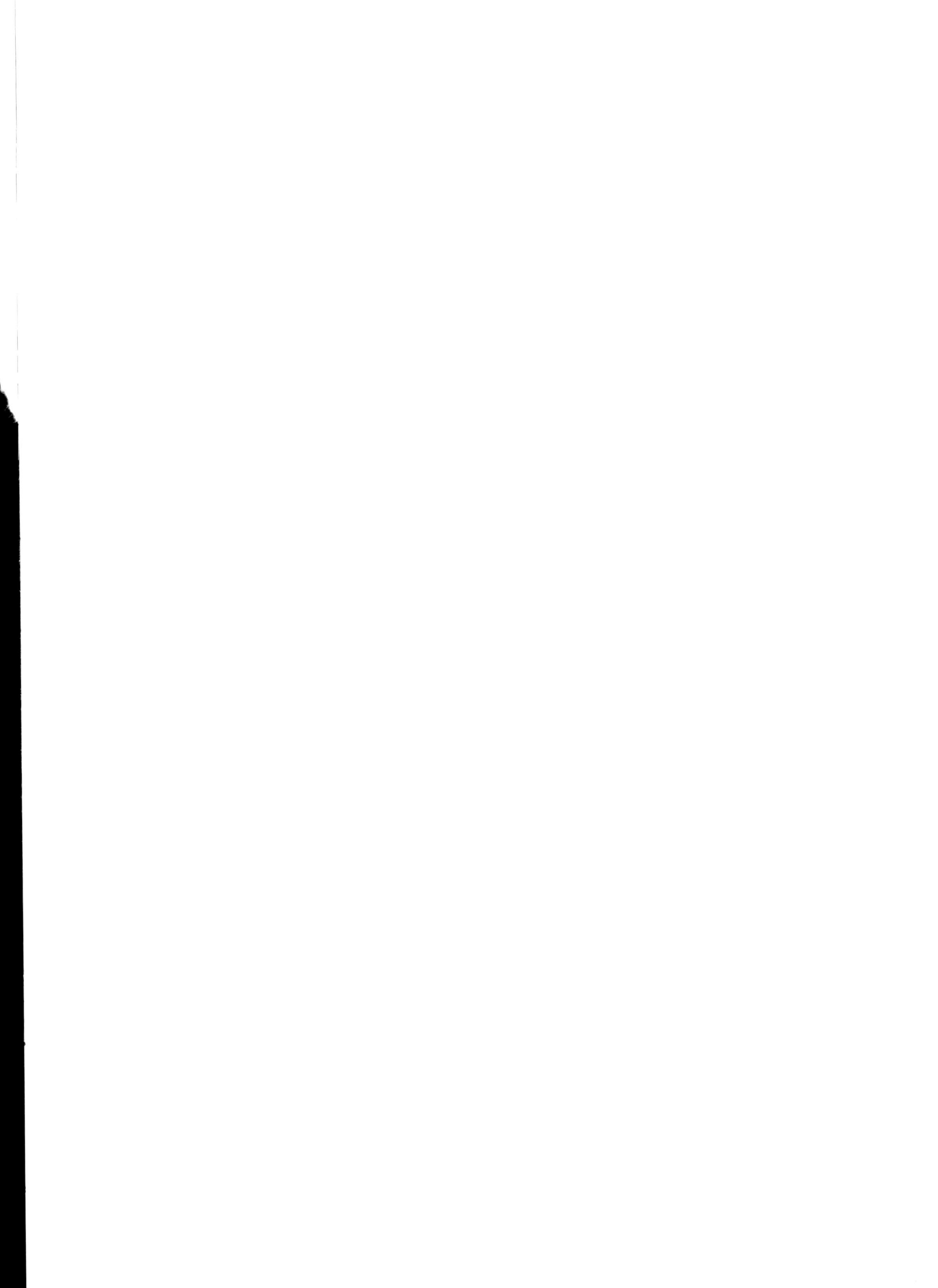